CLINICAL HANDBOOK
OF PSYCHOLOGICAL DISORDERS

CLINICAL HANDBOOK OF PSYCHOLOGICAL DISORDERS

A Step-by-Step Treatment Manual

FIFTH EDITION

Edited by

David H. Barlow

THE GUILFORD PRESS
New York   London

© 2014 The Guilford Press
A Division of Guilford Publications, Inc.
370 Seventh Avenue, Suite 1200, New York, NY 10001
www.guilford.com

Printed in the United States of America

This book is printed on acid-free paper.

Last digit is print number: 9   8   7   6   5   4

The authors have checked with sources believed to be reliable in their efforts to
provide information that is complete and generally in accord with the standards
of practice that are accepted at the time of publication. However, in view of the
possibility of human error or changes in behavioral, mental health, or medical
sciences, neither the authors, nor the editor and publisher, nor any other party who
has been involved in the preparation or publication of this work warrants that the
information contained herein is in every respect accurate or complete, and they are
not responsible for any errors or omissions or the results obtained from the use of such
information. Readers are encouraged to confirm the information contained in this
book with other sources.

Library of Congress Cataloging-in-Publication Data

Clinical handbook of psychological disorders : a step-by-step treatment manual /
edited by David H. Barlow.—Fifth edition.
    pages cm
  Includes bibliographical references and index.
  ISBN 978-1-4625-1326-0 (hardcover)
    1. Behavior therapy—Handbooks, manuals, etc.   2. Medical protocols—
Handbooks, manuals, etc.   I. Barlow, David H., editor of compilation.
  RC489.B4C584 2014
    616.89′142—dc23

                                                                    2013027134

To Beverly
For love, loyalty, and dedication

About the Editor

David H. Barlow, PhD, ABPP, is Professor of Psychology and Psychiatry and Founder and Director Emeritus of the Center for Anxiety and Related Disorders at Boston University. He has published over 500 articles and book chapters and over 60 books and clinical manuals—some translated into more than 20 languages, including Arabic, Chinese, Hindi, and Russian—primarily in the areas of emotional disorders and clinical research methodology. Dr. Barlow's books include *Handbook of Assessment and Treatment Planning for Psychological Disorders, Second Edition*, and *Anxiety and Its Disorders, Second Edition*. He has been the recipient of numerous awards, including, most recently, the Career/Lifetime Achievement Award from the Association for Behavioral and Cognitive Therapies. He is past president of the Society of Clinical Psychology and the Association for Behavioral and Cognitive Therapies and past editor of the journals *Clinical Psychology: Science and Practice* and *Behavior Therapy*. Dr. Barlow's research has been continually funded by the National Institutes of Health for over 40 years.

Contributors

David H. Barlow, PhD, Center for Anxiety and Related Disorders and Department of Psychology, Boston University, Boston, Massachusetts

Aaron T. Beck, MD, Department of Psychiatry, Perelman School of Medicine at the University of Pennsylvania, Philadelphia, Pennsylvania; Beck Institute for Cognitive Behavior Therapy, Bala Cynwyd, Pennsylvania

Larry E. Beutler, PhD, ABPP, Department of Clinical Psychology, Palo Alto University, Palo Alto, California

Kathryn L. Bleiberg, PhD, Department of Psychiatry, Weill Cornell Medical College, Cornell University, New York, New York

Andrew Christensen, PhD, Department of Psychology, University of California, Los Angeles, California

Zafra Cooper, DPhil, Department of Psychiatry, University of Oxford, Oxford, United Kingdom

Michelle G. Craske, PhD, Department of Psychology, University of California, Los Angeles, California

Sona Dimidjian, PhD, Department of Psychology and Neuroscience, University of Colorado, Boulder, Colorado

Brian D. Doss, PhD, Department of Psychology, University of Miami, Coral Gables, Florida

Kristen K. Ellard, PhD, Department of Psychiatry, Massachusetts General Hospital, Boston, Massachusetts

Christopher G. Fairburn, DM, Department of Psychiatry, University of Oxford, Oxford, United Kingdom

Christopher P. Fairholme, PhD, Center for Anxiety and Related Disorders, Boston University, Boston, Massachusetts

Todd J. Farchione, PhD, Center for Anxiety and Related Disorders and Department of Psychology, Boston University, Boston, Massachusetts

Edna B. Foa, PhD, Department of Psychiatry and Center for the Treatment and Study of Anxiety, University of Pennsylvania, Philadelphia, Pennsylvania

Martin E. Franklin, PhD, Department of Psychiatry, Perelman School of Medicine at the University of Pennsylvania, Philadelphia, Pennsylvania

Allison G. Harvey, PhD, Department of Psychology, University of California, Berkeley, California

Sarah H. Heil, PhD, Vermont Center on Behavior and Health, Departments of Psychiatry and Psychology, University of Vermont, Burlington, Vermont

Richard G. Heimberg, PhD, Adult Anxiety Clinic and Department of Psychology, Temple University, Philadelphia, Pennsylvania

Ruth Herman-Dunn, PhD, private practice and Department of Psychology, University of Washington, Seattle, Washington

Stephen T. Higgins, PhD, Vermont Center on Behavior and Health, Departments of Psychiatry and Psychology, University of Vermont, Burlington, Vermont

Samuel Hubley, MA, Department of Psychology and Neuroscience, University of Colorado, Boulder, Colorado

Neil S. Jacobson, PhD (deceased), Department of Psychology, University of Washington, Seattle, Washington

Katherine A. Kaplan, PhD, Department of Psychiatry and Behavioral Sciences, Stanford University School of Medicine, Stanford, California

Marsha M. Linehan, PhD, Department of Psychology, University of Washington, Seattle, Washington

Leanne Magee, PhD, Division of Plastic and Reconstructive Surgery, Department of Child and Adolescent Psychiatry and Behavioral Sciences, The Children's Hospital of Philadelphia, Philadelphia, Pennsylvania

John C. Markowitz, MD, Department of Psychiatry, Columbia University College of Physicians and Sugeons; Department of Psychiatry, New York State Psychiatric Institute; Department of Psychiatry, Weill Medical College, Cornell University, New York, New York

Christopher R. Martell, PhD, Martell Behavioral Activation Research Consulting, and Department of Psychology, University of Wisconsin, Milwaukee, Wisconsin

Barbara S. McCrady, PhD, Center on Alcoholism, Substance Abuse, and Addictions, and Department of Psychology, University of New Mexico, Albuquerque, New Mexico

David J. Miklowitz, PhD, Department of Psychiatry, Semel Institute for Neuroscience and Human Behavior, David Geffen School of Medicine, Los Angeles, California

Candice M. Monson, PhD, Department of Psychology, Ryerson University, Toronto, Ontario, Canada

Andrada D. Neacsiu, PhD, Department of Psychiatry and Behavioral Sciences, Duke University Medical Center, Durham, North Carolina

John C. Norcross, PhD, ABPP, private practice and Department of Psychology, University of Scranton, Scranton, Pennsylvania

Susan M. Orsillo, PhD, Department of Psychology, Suffolk University, Boston, Massachusetts

Laura A. Payne, PhD, Department of Pediatrics, David Geffen School of Medicine, University of California, Los Angeles, California

Patricia A. Resick, PhD, Department of Psychiatry and Behavioral Sciences, Duke University School of Medicine, Durham, North Carolina

Shireen L. Rizvi, PhD, Graduate School of Applied and Professional Psychology, Rutgers, The State University of New Jersey, Piscataway, New Jersey

Lizabeth Roemer, PhD, Department of Psychology, University of Massachusetts, Boston, Massachusetts

Jayne L. Rygh, PhD, private practice, New York, New York

Stacey C. Sigmon, PhD, Vermont Center on Behavior and Health, Departments of Psychiatry and Psychology, University of Vermont, Burlington, Vermont

Nicholas Tarrier, PhD, Institute of Psychiatry, King's College London, London, United Kingdom

Rumina Taylor, DClinPsy, Institute of Psychiatry, King's College London, and South London and Maudsley NHS Foundation Trust, London, United Kingdom

Arthur D. Weinberger, PhD (retired), Cognitive Therapy Center of New York, New York, New York

Jennifer G. Wheeler, PhD, private practice, Seattle, Washington

Jeffrey E. Young, PhD, Department of Psychiatry, Columbia University, and Schema Therapy Institute of New York, New York, New York

Preface

Evidence-based practice (EBP) is one of those ideas that comes along occasionally and takes the world by storm. Although some of the tenets of EBP have been around for decades (as has this handbook), it is only in the past 15 years that EBP has been formally identified as a systematic method of delivering clinical care (Institute of Medicine, 2001; Sackett, Strauss, Richardson, Rosenberg, & Haynes, 2000).

Since that time, the "tipping point" (Gladwell, 2000) for EBP has clearly occurred, and health care policymakers and governments, as well as professional societies around the world, have collectively decided that the delivery of health care, including behavioral health care, should be based on evidence (APA Task Force on Evidence-Based Practice, 2006). Fulfilling this mandate comprises the goals of EBP, and has also been the goal of this book since the first edition was published in 1985.

The fifth edition of this book continues to represent a distinct departure from any number of similar books reviewing advances in the treatment of psychological disorders from the perspective of EBP. Over the past two decades, we have developed a technology of behavior change that necessarily differs from disorder to disorder.

This technology comprises a variety of techniques or procedures with more or less proven effectiveness for a given disorder (and increasingly for classes of disorders). Naturally, we have more evidence of the effectiveness of these treatments for some disorders than for others. It also has become more apparent since the earlier editions that considerable clinical skill is required to apply this technology most effectively. Therefore, this book, in its fifth edition, is *not* another review of therapeutic procedures for a given problem with recommendations for further research. Rather, it is a detailed description of actual treatment protocols in which experienced clinicians implement the technology of behavior change in the context of the most frequently encountered disorders.

In this edition, the originators of some of the best-known treatment protocols have revised and updated the descriptions of their interventions to reflect the latest developments in an increasingly powerful array of psychological therapies. Among these revisions to existing chapters, several deserve comment. Monson, Resick, and Rizvi (Chapter 2) have updated their chapter on posttraumatic stress disorder, describing the tragic case of a soldier fresh from the battlefields of Iraq. Their successful treatment of this individual suffering from the unspeakable (and intolerable) trauma of war is one consequence of today's headline news stories that seldom makes it into print. Drug abuse continues as a scourge that ruins individual lives, the functioning of families, and the very fabric of society. Higgins, Sigmon, and Heil (Chapter 14) present the latest iterations of their approach, which is applicable to all serious drugs of abuse. Chapters on schizophrenia and other psychotic disorders, borderline personality disorder, bipolar disorder, and a number of anxiety disorders, along with depression, written in almost all cases by the originators of these leading protocols, have been updated considerably to reflect the latest evidence for the most effective approaches to these common but debilitating problems.

In addition, three original treatment protocols make their appearance for the first time in this edition. Brief psychological treatments for insomnia represent one of the success stories in EBP, with marked superiority to popular sleep medications, yet many clinicians who frequently confront severe sleep problems and disorders among their patients are unaware of these strategies. Because of the success of these treatment approaches, the American Academy of Sleep Medicine recommends these protocols as a first-line treatment for people with all forms of insomnia, including those currently using hypnotic drugs. The protocol described by Kaplan and Harvey (Chapter 16) represents an advanced and successful approach to this problem.

Roemer and Orsillo (Chapter 5) describe a new acceptance-based treatment for generalized anxiety disorder that reflects in a clever and creative way many of the principles espoused by the so-called "third-wave" approach to psychological disorders. Initial results from this protocol are impressive.

Norcross and Beutler (Chapter 15), experienced and well-known therapists, present their "treatment matching" strategic approach in the context of a young woman suffering from polysubstance abuse and depression. While standard cognitive-behavioral and systems approaches are recognizable in this treatment description, in an explicit manner the authors highlight transdiagnostic but empirically supported therapist and relationship factors that clearly deserve description in this book.

Finally, there is growing consensus that the future of EBP will be to distill principles of effective change that cut across diagnostic conditions, making them more generally applicable. Two of these "unified" or "transdiagnostic" protocols appear in this fifth edition. In Chapter 6 (Payne, Ellard, Farchione, Fairholme, and Barlow), we present our own unified transdiagnostic approach to emotional disorders, and Fairburn and Cooper (Chapter 17) describe a transdiagnostic approach to eating disorders that they originated with their colleagues.

In all chapters, the nuts and bolts of clinical application are emphasized.

As with the previous editions, this book was motivated by countless clinical psychology graduate students, psychiatric residents, and other mental health professionals, either in training or in practice, asking, "But how do I do it?" Realizing that there is no single source in which to find step-by-step treatment protocols for use as a guide to practice, this book attempts to fill the void. To accomplish this purpose, a number of specific topics are common to most chapters. Each chapter begins with a brief review of our knowledge of the specific disorder (or class of disorders), followed by a description of the particular model or mini-theory that guides the technology utilized with the disorder in question. This model, or mini-theory, typically answers the question: What particular facets of the disorder should be assessed and treated? While clinical application always dilutes theoretical models, clinicians will recognize cognitive-behavioral and systems approaches, with some psychodynamic contributions, as the predominant theoretical context.

This model is followed by a description of the typical setting in which the treatment is carried out. The setting varies from disorder to disorder, ranging from the more usual office setting to the home environment of the patient. Authors provide similar detailed descriptions of the social context of treatment (e.g., the importance of the involvement of family or friends) as well as therapist and client variables that are important within the context of the particular problem. For example, therapist variables that may be important in implementing techniques for treatment of agoraphobia or couple distress are described. In addition, authors discuss the implications for treatment of client variables, such as dependency and unassertiveness in individuals with panic disorder with agoraphobia.

A detailed description of the actual step-by-step process of assessment and treatment follows, liberally sprinkled in many chapters with transcripts of therapy sessions. Important components of this process are the specifics of the rationale given to the patient before treatment, as well as typical problems that arise during the implementation of the technology. Where data exist, authors provide information on clinical predictors of success or failure.

In accomplishing the rather ambitious goals just described, I was very fortunate in this edition of the book, as in previous editions, to have leading clinicians and researchers document in some detail how they actually treat their patients. Once again, these authorities reported that the number of details they had to include in order to convey how they actually applied their treatment programs went far beyond their expectations. My hope is that practicing clinicians and clinical students everywhere will benefit from acquaintance with these details.

In closing, I would like to express my deep appreciation to Amantia Ametaj, my research and administrative assistant during the editing of this book. She worked with me and the authors every step of the way. I am sure this information will come in handy as she is now pursuing her own doctorate in clinical psychology.

DAVID H. BARLOW, PhD

REFERENCES

APA Task Force on Evidence-Based Practice. (2006). Evidence-based practice in psychology. *American Psychologist, 61*, 271–285.

Gladwell, M. (2000). *The tipping point: How little things can make a big difference.* Boston: Little, Brown.

Institute of Medicine. (2001). *Crossing the quality chasm: A new health system for the 21st century.* Washington, DC: National Academies Press.

Sackett, D. L., Strauss, S. E., Richardson, W. S., Rosenberg, W., & Haynes, R. B. (2000). *Evidence-based medicine: How to practice and teach EBM* (2nd ed.). London: Churchill Livingstone.

Contents

CHAPTER 1

Panic Disorder and Agoraphobia

MICHELLE G. CRASKE
DAVID H. BARLOW

> The treatment protocol described in this chapter represents one of the success stories in the development of evidence-based psychological treatments. Results from numerous studies indicate that this approach provides substantial advantages over placebo medication or alternative psychosocial approaches containing "common" factors, such as positive expectancies and helpful therapeutic alliances. In addition, this treatment forms an important part of every clinical practice guideline in either public health or other sources from countries around the world, describing effective treatments for panic disorder and agoraphobia. Results from numerous studies evaluating this treatment protocol, both individually and in combination with leading pharmacological approaches, suggest that this appvroach is equally effective as the best pharmacological approaches in the short term and more durable over the long term. But this treatment protocol has not stood still. For example, we have learned a great deal in recent years about neurobiological mechanisms of action in fear reduction, and the best psychological methods for effecting these changes and newly developed acceptance-based procedures have proven efficacious. In this chapter we present the latest version of this protocol, incorporating these changes and additions in the context of changes to diagnostic criteria in DSM-5, all as illustrated in a comprehensive account of the treatment of "Julie."—D. H. B.

Advances continue in the development of biopsychosocial models and cognitive-behavioral treatments for panic disorder and agoraphobia. The conceptualization of panic disorder as an acquired fear of certain bodily sensations, and agoraphobia as a behavioral response to the anticipation of related bodily sensations or their crescendo into a full-blown panic attack, continues to be supported by experimental, clinical, and longitudinal research. Furthermore, the efficacy of cognitive-behavioral treatments that target fear of bodily sensations and associated agoraphobic situations is well established. In addition to presenting an up-to-date review of treatment outcome data, this chapter covers recent theoretical and empirical developments in reference to etiological factors, the role of comorbid diagnoses in treatment, ways of optimizing learning during exposure therapy, and the effect of medication on cognitive-behavioral treatments. The chapter concludes with a detailed, session-by-session outline of cognitive-behavioral treatment for panic disorder and agoraphobia. This protocol has been developed in our clinics; the full protocol is detailed in available treatment manuals (Barlow & Craske, 2006; Craske & Barlow, 2006).

NATURE OF PANIC AND AGORAPHOBIA

Panic Attacks

"Panic attacks" are discrete episodes of intense fear or discomfort, accompanied by physical and cognitive symptoms, as listed in the DSM-5 panic attack checklist (American Psychiatric Association, 2013). Panic attacks are discrete by virtue of their sudden or abrupt onset and brief duration, as opposed to gradually building anxious arousal. Panic attacks in panic disorder often have an unexpected quality, meaning that from the patient's perspective, they appear to happen without an obvious trigger or at unexpected times. Indeed, the diagnosis of panic disorder is defined by recurrent "unexpected" panic attacks, followed by at least 1 month of persistent concern about their recurrence and their consequences, or by a significant change in behavior consequent to the attacks (American Psychiatric Association, 2013).

As with all basic emotions (Izard, 1992), panic attacks are associated with strong action tendencies: Most often, these are urges to escape, and less often, urges to fight. These fight and flight tendencies usually involve elevated autonomic nervous system arousal needed to support such fight–flight reactivity. Furthermore, perceptions of imminent threat or danger, such as death, loss of control, or social ridicule, often accompany such fight–flight reactivity. However, the features of urgency to escape, autonomic arousal, and perception of threat are not present in every self-reported occurrence of panic. For example, despite evidence for elevated heart rate or other indices of sympathetic nervous system activation during panic attacks on average (e.g., Wilkinson et al., 1998), Margraf, Taylor, Ehlers, Roth, and Agras (1987) found that 40% of self-reported panic attacks were not associated with accelerated heart rate. Moreover, in general, patients with panic disorder are more likely than nonanxious controls to report arrhythmic heart rate in the absence of actual arrhythmias (Barsky, Cleary, Sarnie, & Ruskin, 1994). Heightened anxiety about signs of autonomic arousal may lead patients to perceive cardiac events when none exist (Barlow, Brown, & Craske, 1994; Craske & Tsao, 1999). We believe that self-reported panic in the absence of heart rate acceleration or other indices of autonomic activation reflects anticipatory anxiety rather than true panic (Barlow et al., 1994), especially because more severe panic attacks are more consistently associated with accelerated heart rate (Margraf et al., 1987). Sometimes

individuals report intense abrupt fear in the absence of perceptions of threat or danger. This has been termed "noncognitive" panic (Rachman, Lopatka, & Levitt, 1988; see Kircanski, Craske, Epstein, & Wittchen, 2009). Finally, the urgency to escape is sometimes weakened by situational demands for continued approach and endurance, such as performance expectations or job demands, thus creating discordance between behavioral responses on the one hand, and verbal or physiological fear responses on the other.

A subset of individuals with panic disorder experience nocturnal panic attacks. "Nocturnal panic" refers to waking from sleep in a state of panic with symptoms that are very similar to panic attacks during wakeful states (Craske & Barlow, 1989; Uhde, 1994). Nocturnal panic does *not* refer to waking from sleep and panicking after a lapse of waking time, or nighttime arousals induced by nightmares or environmental stimuli (e.g., unexpected noises). Instead, nocturnal panic is an abrupt waking from sleep in a state of panic, without an obvious trigger. Nocturnal panic attacks reportedly most often occur between 1 and 3 hours after sleep onset, and only occasionally more than once per night (Craske & Barlow, 1989). Surveys of select clinical groups suggest that nocturnal panic is relatively common among individuals with panic disorder: 44–71% report having experienced nocturnal panic at least once, and 30–45% report repeated nocturnal panics (Craske & Barlow, 1989; Krystal, Woods, Hill, & Charney, 1991; Mellman & Uhde, 1989; Roy-Byrne, Mellman, & Uhde, 1988; Uhde, 1994). Individuals who suffer frequent nocturnal panic often become fearful of sleep and attempt to delay sleep onset. Avoidance of sleep may result in chronic sleep deprivation, which in turn precipitates more nocturnal panics (Uhde, 1994).

"Nonclinical" panic attacks occur occasionally in approximately 3–5% of people in the general population who do not otherwise meet criteria for panic disorder (Norton, Cox, & Malan, 1992). Also, panic attacks occur across a variety of anxiety and mood disorders (Barlow et al., 1985), as well as substance use, personality disorders and psychoses (Craske et al., 2010) and are not limited to panic disorder. Indeed, the ubiquity of panic attacks has been emphasized in DSM-5 (American Psychiatric Association, 2013) where panic attacks are designated as a potential specifier for any DSM disorder. As stated earlier, the defining feature of panic disorder is not the presence of panic attacks per se, but involves additional anxiety about the recurrence of panic or its consequences, or a significant behavioral change because of the panic attacks. It is the additional anxiety about panic combined with catastrophic cognitions in the face of panic that differentiate between the person with panic disorder and the occasional nonclinical panicker (e.g., Telch, Lucas, & Nelson, 1989) or the person with other anxiety disorders who also happens to panic. The following scenario exemplifies the latter point.

PATIENT: Sometimes I lay awake at night thinking about a million different things. I think about what is going to happen to my daughter if I get sick. Who will look after her, or what would happen if my husband died and we didn't have enough money to give my daughter a good education? Then I think about where we would live and how we would cope. Sometimes I can work myself up so much that my heart starts to race, my hands get sweaty, and I feel dizzy and scared. So I have to stop myself from thinking about all those things. I usually get out of bed and turn on the TV—anything to get my mind off the worries.

THERAPIST: Do you worry about the feelings of a racing heart, sweating, and dizziness happening again?

PATIENT: No. They're unpleasant, but they are the least of my concerns. I am more worried about my daughter and our future.

This scenario illustrates the experience of panic that is *not* the central focus of the person's anxiety. More likely, this woman has generalized anxiety disorder, and her uncontrollable worry leads her to panic on occasion. The next example is someone with social anxiety disorder, who becomes very concerned about panicking in social situations, because the possibility of a panic attack increases her concerns about being judged negatively by others.

PATIENT: I am terrified of having a panic attack in meetings at work. I dread the thought of others noticing how anxious I am. They must be able to see my hands shaking, the sweat on my forehead, and worst of all, my face turning red.

THERAPIST: What worries you most about others noticing your physical symptoms?

PATIENT: That they will think that I am weird or strange.

THERAPIST: Would you be anxious in the meetings if the panic attacks were gone?

PATIENT: I would still be worried about doing or saying the wrong thing. It is not just the panic attacks that worry me.

THERAPIST: Are you worried about panic attacks in any other situations?

PATIENT: Formal social events and sometimes when I meet someone for the first time.

In this case, even though the patient experiences panic attacks, the real concern is about being judged negatively by others consequent to panic attacks, and the panic attacks do not occur in situations other than social ones. Hence, this presentation is most aptly described as social anxiety.

Agoraphobia

"Agoraphobia" refers to avoidance or endurance with dread of situations from which escape might be difficult or help is unavailable in the event of a panic-like symptoms (including but not limited to panic attacks) or other incapacitating symptoms, such as loss of bowel control or vomiting, disorientation (especially in children), or sense of falling (especially in older adults) (American Psychiatric Association, 2013). Typical agoraphobic situations include shopping malls, waiting in line, movie theaters, traveling by car or bus, crowded restaurants, and being alone. "Mild" agoraphobia is exemplified by the person who hesitates about driving long distances alone but manages to drive to and from work, prefers to sit on the aisle at movie theaters but still goes to movies, and avoids crowded places. "Moderate" agoraphobia is exemplified by the person whose driving is limited to a 10-mile radius from home and only if accompanied, who shops at off-peak times and avoids large supermarkets, and who avoids flying or traveling by train. "Severe" agoraphobia refers to very limited mobility, sometimes even to the point of becoming housebound.

Relationship between Panic and Agoraphobia

The relationship between panic and agoraphobia is complex. On the one hand, not all persons who panic develop agoraphobia, and the extent of agoraphobia that emerges is highly variable (Craske & Barlow, 1988). Various factors have been investigated as potential predictors of agoraphobia. Although agoraphobia tends to increase as history of panic lengthens, a significant proportion of individuals panic for many years without developing agoraphobic limitations. Nor is agoraphobia related to age of onset or frequency of panic (Cox, Endler, & Swinson, 1995; Craske & Barlow, 1988; Kikuchi et al., 2005; Rapee & Murrell, 1988). Some studies report more intense physical symptoms during panic attacks when there is more agoraphobia (e.g., de Jong & Bouman, 1995; Goisman et al., 1994; Noyes, Clancy, Garvey, & Anderson, 1987; Telch, Brouillard, Telch, Agras, & Taylor, 1989). Others fail to find such differences (e.g., Cox et al., 1995; Craske, Miller, Rotunda, & Barlow, 1990). On the one hand, fears of dying, going crazy, or losing control do not relate to level of agoraphobia (Cox et al., 1995; Craske, Rapee, & Barlow, 1988). On the other hand, concerns about social consequences of panicking may be stronger when there is more agoraphobia (Amering et al., 1997; de Jong & Bouman, 1995; Rapee & Murrell, 1988; Telch, Brouilard, et al., 1989). In addition, Kikuchi and colleagues (2005) found that individuals who develop agoraphobia within 6 months of the onset of panic disorder have a higher prevalence of generalized anxiety disorder but not major depression. However, whether social evaluation concerns or comorbidity are precursors or are secondary to agoraphobia remains to be determined. Occupational status also predicts agoraphobia, accounting for 18% of the variance in one study (de Jong & Bouman, 1995). Perhaps the strongest predictor of agoraphobia is sex; the ratio of males to females shifts dramatically in the direction of female predominance as level of agoraphobia worsens (e.g., Thyer, Himle, Curtis, Cameron, & Nesse, 1985).

On the other hand, not everyone with agoraphobia has a history of panic attacks or even panic-like symptoms, although a history of panic is much more common in treatment-seeking samples of individuals with agoraphobia than in epidemiological samples (Wittchen, Gloster, Beesdo-Baum, Fava, & Craske, 2010). Nonetheless, the prevalence of agoraphobia without a history of panic disorder, panic attacks, or panic-like symptoms was reported to be at least as high as the combined rates of panic disorder with and without agoraphobia across all epidemiological studies (Wittchen et al., 2010). Approximately 50% of individuals from community samples who endorse agoraphobia do not endorse panic attacks. Furthermore, agoraphobia without panic-like features appears to be as impairing as panic disorder without agoraphobia, although the combination is usually associated with even more impairment. In addition, some differences exist between

them in terms of incidence, comorbidity, and response to treatment (Wittchen et al., 2010). For these reasons, panic disorder and agoraphobia are now recognized as two distinct, albeit highly comorbid, disorders in DSM-5 (American Psychiatric Association, 2013).

PRESENTING FEATURES

From the latest epidemiological study, the National Comorbidity Survey Replication (NCS-R; Kessler, Berglund, Demler, Jin, & Walters, 2005; Kessler, Chiu, Demler, & Walters, 2005) 12-month prevalence estimates for panic disorder are approximately 2% in adults and adolescents. Lower estimates have been reported for some Asian, African and Latin American countries, ranging from 0.1 to 0.8% (Lewis-Fernandez et al., 2010). The 12-month rates for agoraphobia are approximately 1.7%, and the lifetime morbid risk is 3.7% (Kessler et al., 2012).

The modal age of onset for panic disorder is late teenage years and early adulthood (Kessler, Berglund, et al., 2005). In fact, although panic disorder is rare below the age of 14, a substantial proportion of adolescents report panic attacks (e.g., Hayward et al., 1992), and panic disorder in children and adolescents tends to be chronic and comorbid with other anxiety, mood, and disruptive disorders (Biederman, Faraone, Marrs, & Moore, 1997). Treatment is usually sought much later, around age 34 (e.g., Noyes et al., 1986). Similarly, agoraphobia may occur in childhood but the incidence peaks in late adolescence and early adulthood (Beesdo, Knappe, & Pine, 2007; Bittner et al., 2007); the mean age of onset is 17 years (Kessler et al., 2012), and older in the absence of history of panic disorder or panic attacks. Rates of panic disorder decline in older adults, possibly diminishing to subclinical levels (Wolitzky-Taylor, Castriotti, Lenze, Stanley, & Craske, 2010). Similarly, 12-month prevalence rates for agoraphobia reduce to 0.4% in individuals over the age of 65 years (Kessler et al., 2006). The overall ratio of females to males is approximately 2:1 (Kessler et al., 2006) and, as mentioned already, the ratio shifts dramatically in the direction of female predominance as level of agoraphobia worsens (e.g., Thyer et al., 1985).

Rarely do the diagnoses of panic disorder or agoraphobia occur in isolation. Commonly co-occurring Axis I conditions include specific phobias, social phobia, dysthymia, generalized anxiety disorder, major depressive disorder, and substance abuse (e.g., Brown,

Campbell, Lehman, Grishman, & Mancill, 2001; Goisman, Goldenberg, Vasile, & Keller, 1995; Kessler, Chiu, et al., 2005). Also, 25–60% of persons with panic disorder also meet criteria for a personality disorder, mostly avoidant and dependent personality disorders (e.g., Chambless & Renneberg, 1988). However, the nature of the relationship with personality disorders remains unclear. For example, comorbidity rates are highly dependent on the method used to establish Axis II diagnosis, as well as the co-occurrence of depressed mood (Alneas & Torgersen, 1990; Chambless & Renneberg, 1988). Moreover, the fact that abnormal personality traits improve and some "personality disorders" even remit after successful treatment of panic disorder (Black, Monahan, Wesner, Gabel, & Bowers, 1996; Mavissakalian & Hamman, 1987; Noyes, Reich, Suelzer, & Christiansen, 1991) raises questions about the validity of Axis II diagnoses. The issue of comorbidity with personality disorders and its effect on treatment for panic disorder and agoraphobia is described in more detail in a later section.

Finally, panic disorder and agoraphobia tend to be chronic conditions, with severe financial and interpersonal costs (Wittchen et al., 2010). Only a minority of untreated individuals remit without subsequent relapse within a few years if not treated (Emmelkamp & Wittchen, 2009; Katschnig & Amering, 1998; Roy-Byrne & Cowley, 1995). Also, individuals with panic disorder overutilize medical resources compared to the general public and individuals with other "psychiatric" disorders (e.g., Katon et al., 1990; Roy-Byrne et al., 1999).

HISTORY OF PSYCHOLOGICAL TREATMENT FOR PANIC DISORDER AND AGORAPHOBIA

It was not until the publication of DSM-III (American Psychiatric Association, 1980) that panic disorder with or without agoraphobia was recognized as a distinct anxiety problem. Until that time, panic attacks were viewed primarily as a form of free-floating anxiety. Consequently, psychological treatment approaches were relatively nonspecific. They included relaxation and cognitive restructuring for stressful life events in general (e.g., Barlow, O'Brien, & Last, 1984). Many presumed that pharmacotherapy was necessary for the control of panic. In contrast, the treatment of agoraphobia was quite specific from the 1970s onward, with primarily exposure-based approaches to target fear and

avoidance of specific situations. However, relatively little consideration was given to panic attacks in either the conceptualization or treatment of agoraphobia. The development of specific panic control treatments in the middle to late 1980s shifted interest away from agoraphobia. Interest in agoraphobia was subsequently renewed, specifically in terms of whether panic control treatments are sufficient for the management of agoraphobia, and whether their combination with treatments that directly target agoraphobia is superior overall. We address these questions in more detail after describing the conceptualization that underlies cognitive-behavioral approaches to the treatment of panic and agoraphobia.

CONCEPTUALIZATION OF ETIOLOGICAL AND MAINTAINING FACTORS FOR PANIC DISORDER AND AGORAPHOBIA

Several independent lines of research (Barlow, 1988; Clark, 1986; Ehlers & Margraf, 1989) converged in the 1980s on the same basic conceptualization of panic disorder as an acquired fear of bodily sensations, particularly sensations associated with autonomic arousal. Psychological and biological predispositions are believed to enhance the vulnerability to acquire such fear. These interacting vulnerabilities have been organized into an etiological conception of anxiety disorders in general, referred to as "triple vulnerability theory" (Barlow, 1988, 2002; Suárez, Bennett, Goldstein, & Barlow, 2008). First, genetic contributions to the development of anxiety and negative affect constitute a generalized (heritable) biological vulnerability. Second, evidence supports a generalized psychological vulnerability to experience anxiety and related negative affective states, characterized by a diminished sense of control arising from early developmental experiences. Although the unfortunate co-occurrence of generalized biological and psychological vulnerabilities may be sufficient to produce anxiety and related states, particularly generalized anxiety disorder and depression, a third vulnerability seems necessary to account for the development of at least some specific anxiety disorders, including panic disorder; that is, early learning experiences in some instances seem to focus anxiety on particular areas of concern. In panic disorder, the experience of certain somatic sensations becomes associated with a heightened sense of threat and danger. This specific psychological vulnerability, when coordinated with the generalized biological and psychological vulnerabilities mentioned earlier, seems to contribute to the development of panic disorder. Fear conditioning, avoidant responding, and information-processing biases are believed to perpetuate such fear. It is the perpetuating factors that are targeted in the cognitive-behavioral treatment approach. What follows is a very brief review of some contributory factors with practical relevance for panic disorder.

Vulnerability Factors

Genetics and Temperament

The temperament most associated with anxiety disorders, including panic disorder, is neuroticism (Eysenck, 1967; Gray, 1982), or proneness to experience negative emotions in response to stressors. A closely linked construct, "negative affectivity," is the tendency to experience a variety of negative emotions across a variety of situations, even in the absence of objective stressors (Watson & Clark, 1984). Structural analyses confirm that negative affect is a higher-order factor that distinguishes individuals with each anxiety disorder (and depression) from controls with no mental disorder: Lower-order factors discriminate among anxiety disorders, with "fear of fear" being the factor that discriminates panic disorder from other anxiety disorders (Brown, Chorpita, & Barlow, 1998; Prenoveau et al., 2010; Zinbarg & Barlow, 1996). The anxiety disorders load differentially on negative affectivity, with more pervasive anxiety disorders, such as generalized anxiety disorder, loading more heavily, panic disorder loading at an intermediate level, and social anxiety disorder loading the least (Brown et al., 1998).[1] However, these findings derive from cross-sectional datasets.

Longitudinal prospective evidence for the role of neuroticism in predicting the onset of panic disorder is relatively limited. Specifically, neuroticism predicted the onset of panic attacks in adolescents (Hayward, Killen, Kraemer, & Taylor, 2000; Schmidt, Lerew, & Jackson, 1997, 1999), and "emotional reactivity" at age 3 was a significant variable in the classification of panic disorder in 18- to 21-year-old males (Craske, Poulton, Tsao, & Plotkin, 2001). Ongoing studies, such as the Northwestern/UCLA Youth Emotion Project, are comprehensively evaluating the role of neuroticism in the prediction of subsequent panic disorder.

Numerous multivariate genetic analyses of human twin samples consistently attribute approximately 30–50% of variance in neuroticism to additive genetic factors (Eley, 2001; Lake, Eaves, Maes, Heath, & Martin, 2000). In addition, anxiety and depression appear to be variable expressions of the heritable tendency toward neuroticism (Kendler, Heath, Martin, & Eaves, 1987). Symptoms of panic (i.e., breathlessness, heart pounding) may be additionally explained by a unique source of genetic variance that is differentiated from symptoms of depression and anxiety (Kendler et al., 1987) and neuroticism (Martin, Jardine, Andrews, & Heath, 1988).

Analyses of specific genetic markers remain preliminary and inconsistent. For example, panic disorder has been linked to a locus on chromosome 13 (Hamilton et al., 2003; Schumacher et al., 2005) and chromosome 9 (Thorgeirsson et al., 2003), but the exact genes remain unknown. Findings regarding markers for the cholecystokinin-B receptor gene have been inconsistent (cf. Hamilton et al., 2001; van Megen, Westenberg, Den Boer, & Kahn, 1996). Also, association and linkage studies implicate the adenosine receptor gene in panic disorder (Deckert et al., 1998; Hamilton et al., 2004). An allele of the neuropeptide S receptor gene on chromosome 7 was linked in a male-specific manner to panic disorder and not to schizophrenia or attention deficit disorder (Okamura et al., 2011), whereas the same gene was linked in a female-specific manner to panic disorder compared to healthy controls (Domschke et al., 2011). Thus, at this stage, the results are rather piecemeal and sometimes inconsistent, and there is no evidence at this point for a specific link between genetic markers and temperament, on the one hand, and panic disorder on the other. Rather, neurobiological factors seem to comprise a nonspecific biological vulnerability.

Anxiety Sensitivity

As described earlier, neuroticism is viewed as a higher-order factor characteristic of all anxiety disorders, with "fear of fear" being more unique to panic disorder. The construct "fear of fear" overlaps with the construct "anxiety sensitivity," or the belief that anxiety and its associated symptoms may cause deleterious physical, social, and psychological consequences that extend beyond any immediate physical discomfort during an episode of anxiety or panic (Reiss, 1980). Anxiety sensitivity is elevated across most anxiety disorders, but it is particularly elevated in panic disorder (e.g., Taylor, Koch, & McNally, 1992; Zinbarg & Barlow, 1996), especially the Physical Concerns subscale of the Anxiety Sensitivity Index (Zinbarg & Barlow, 1996; Zinbarg,

Barlow, & Brown, 1997). Therefore, beliefs that physical symptoms of anxiety are harmful seem to be particularly relevant to panic disorder and may comprise a specific psychological vulnerability.

Anxiety sensitivity is presumed to confer a risk factor for panic disorder because it primes fear reactivity to bodily sensations. In support, anxiety sensitivity predicts subjective distress and reported symptomatology in response to procedures that induce strong physical sensations, such as CO_2 inhalation (Forsyth, Palav, & Duff, 1999), balloon inflation (Messenger & Shean, 1998), and hyperventilation (Sturges, Goetsch, Ridley, & Whittal, 1998) in nonclinical samples, even after researchers control for the effects of trait anxiety (Rapee & Medoro, 1994). In addition, several longitudinal studies indicate that high scores on the Anxiety Sensitivity Index predict the onset of panic attacks over 1- to 4-year intervals in adolescents (Hayward et al., 2000), college students (Maller & Reiss, 1992), and community samples with specific phobias or no anxiety disorders (Ehlers, 1995). The predictive relationship remains after researchers control for prior depression (Hayward et al., 2000). In addition, Anxiety Sensitivity Index scores predicted spontaneous panic attacks and worry about panic (and anxiety more generally), during an acute military stressor (i.e., 5 weeks of basic training), even after researchers control for history of panic attacks and trait anxiety (Schmidt et al., 1997, 1999). Finally, panic attacks themselves elevate anxiety sensitivity over a 5-week period in adults (Schmidt et al., 1999), and over a 1-year period in adolescents, albeit to a lesser extent (Weems, Hayward, Killen, & Taylor, 2002).

However, Bouton, Mineka, and Barlow (2001) have noted that the relationship between anxiety sensitivity and panic attacks in these studies is relatively small, not exclusive to panic, and weaker than the relationship between panic and neuroticism. Furthermore, these studies have evaluated panic attacks and worry about panic but not the prediction of diagnosed panic disorder. Thus, the causal significance of anxiety sensitivity for panic disorder remains to be fully understood.

History of Medical Illness and Abuse

Other studies highlight the role of medical illnesses as contributing to a specific psychological vulnerability for panic disorder. For example, using the Dunedin Multidisciplinary Study database, we found that experience with personal respiratory disturbance (and parental poor health) as a youth predicted panic disorder

at age 18 or 21 (Craske et al., 2001). This finding is consistent with reports of more respiratory disturbance in the history of patients with panic disorder compared to other patients with anxiety disorders (Verburg, Griez, Meijer, & Pols, 1995). Furthermore, first-degree relatives of patients with panic disorder had a significantly higher prevalence of chronic obstructive respiratory disease, and asthma in particular, than first-degree relatives of patients with other anxiety disorders (van Beek, Schruers, & Friez, 2005).

Childhood experiences of sexual and physical abuse may also prime panic disorder. Retrospective reports of such childhood abuse were associated with panic disorder onset at ages 16–21 years in a longitudinal analysis of New Zealanders from birth to age 21 (Goodwin, Fergusson, & Horwood, 2005). This finding is consistent with multiple cross-sectional studies in both clinical and community samples (e.g., Bandelow et al., 2002; Kendler et al., 2000; Kessler, Davis, & Kendler, 1997; Moisan & Engels, 1995; Stein et al., 1996). The association with childhood abuse is stronger for panic disorder than for other anxiety disorders, such as social phobia (Safren, Gershuny, Marzol, Otto, & Pollack, 2002; Stein et al., 1996) and obsessive–compulsive disorder (Stein et al., 1996). In addition, some studies report an association between panic disorder and exposure to violence between other family members, generally interparental violence (e.g., Bandelow et al., 2002; Moisan & Engels, 1995), whereas another study did not (Goodwin et al., 2005). Retrospective reporting of childhood abuse and familial violence in all of these studies, however, limits the findings.

Interoceptive Awareness

Patients with panic disorder, as well as nonclinical panickers, appear to have heightened awareness of, or ability to detect, bodily sensations of arousal (e.g., Ehlers & Breuer, 1992, 1996; Ehlers, Breuer, Dohn, & Feigenbaum, 1995; Zoellner & Craske, 1999). Discrepant findings (e.g., Antony et al., 1995; Rapee, 1994) exist but have been attributed to methodological artifact (Ehlers & Breuer, 1996). Ability to perceive heartbeat, in particular, appears to be a relatively stable individual-difference variable given that it does not differ between untreated and treated patients with panic disorder (Ehlers & Breuer, 1992), or from before to after successful treatment (Antony, Meadows, Brown, & Barlow, 1994; Ehlers et al., 1995). Thus, interoceptive accuracy may be a predisposing trait for panic disorder that increases the probability of perceiving sensations that in turn may trigger a panic attack. Whether interoceptive awareness is learned, and represents another specific psychological vulnerability, or is more dispositional remains to be determined.

Separate from interoception is the issue of propensity for intense autonomic activation. As noted earlier, some evidence points to a unique genetic influence on the reported experience of breathlessness, heart pounding, and a sense of terror (Kendler et al., 1987). Conceivably, cardiovascular reactivity presents a unique physiological predisposition for panic disorder. In support of this, cardiac symptoms and shortness of breath predict later development of panic attacks and panic disorder (Keyl & Eaton, 1990). Unfortunately, these data derive from *report* of symptoms, which is not a good index of actual autonomic state (Pennebaker & Roberts, 1992) and may instead reflect interoception.

Initial Panic Attacks

From an evolutionary standpoint, fear is a natural and adaptive response to threatening stimuli. However, the fear experienced during the first unexpected panic attack is often unjustified due to the lack of an identifiable trigger or antecedent; hence, it represents a "false alarm" (Barlow, 1988, 2002). The large majority of initial panic attacks are recalled as occurring outside of the home, while driving, walking, at work, or at school (Craske et al., 1990), generally in public (Lelliott, Marks, McNamee, & Tobena, 1989), and on a bus, plane, subway, or in social-evaluative situations (Shulman, Cox, Swinson, Kuch, & Reichman, 1994). Barlow (1988) and Craske and Rowe (1997b) believe situations that set the scene for initial panic attacks are ones in which bodily sensations are perceived as posing the most threat because of impairment of functioning (e.g., driving), entrapment (e.g., air travel, elevators), negative social evaluation (e.g., job, formal social events), or distance from safety (e.g., unfamiliar locales). Entrapment concerns may be particularly salient for the subsequent development of agoraphobia (Faravelli, Pallanti, Biondi, Paterniti, & Scarpato, 1992).

Maintenance Factors

Acute "fear of fear" (or, more accurately, anxiety focused on somatic sensations) that develops after initial panic attacks in *vulnerable individuals* refers to anxiety about certain bodily sensations associated with panic attacks (e.g., racing heart, dizziness, paresthe-

sias) (Barlow, 1988; Goldstein & Chambless, 1978), and is attributed to two factors. The first is interoceptive conditioning, or conditional fear of internal cues, such as elevated heart rate, because of their association with intense fear, pain, or distress (Razran, 1961). Specifically, interoceptive conditioning refers to low-level somatic sensations of arousal or anxiety becoming conditional stimuli, so that early somatic components of the anxiety response come to elicit significant bursts of anxiety or panic (Bouton et al., 2001). An extensive body of experimental literature attests to the robustness of interoceptive conditioning (e.g., Dworkin & Dworkin, 1999), particularly with regard to early interoceptive drug-onset cues becoming conditional stimuli for larger drug effects (e.g., Sokolowska, Siegel, & Kim, 2002). In addition, interoceptive conditional responses are not dependent on conscious awareness of triggering cues (Razran, 1961); thus, they have been observed in patients under anesthesia (e.g., Block, Ghoneim, Fowles, Kumar, & Pathak, 1987). Within this model, then, slight changes in relevant bodily functions that are not consciously recognized may elicit conditional anxiety or fear and panic due to previous pairings with panic (Barlow, 1988; Bouton et al., 2001); the result would be an unexpected panic attack. Further support for a conditioning model comes from evidence that individuals with panic disorder, as well as other anxiety disorders, show elevated fear conditioning and weakened fear extinction in laboratory paradigms (Lissek et al., 2005), suggesting that they are more prone to developing fear through negative associations, and once acquired, their fear is less likely to diminish with time. This pattern seems to be compounded for individuals with panic disorder who additionally show impaired safety learning (Lissek et al., 2009) and greater fear generalization (Lissek et al., 2010) in laboratory paradigms. In other words, once fear of specific bodily sensations is acquired, individuals with panic disorder may have difficulty perceiving other sensations as being harmless and may be more likely to generalize their fear to various bodily states.

The second factor, offered by Clark (1986) to explain acute fear of panic-related body sensations, is catastrophic misappraisals of bodily sensations (misinterpretation of sensations as signs of imminent death, loss of control, etc.). We have taken issue with the purely cognitive model of panic disorder by stating that it cannot account for panic attacks devoid of conscious cognitive appraisal without turning to constructs such as "automatic appraisals," which prove to be untestable

(Bouton et al., 2001). Catastrophic misappraisals may accompany panic attacks because they are a natural part of the constellation of responses that go with panic, or because they have been encouraged and reinforced much like sick role behaviors during childhood. In addition, such thoughts may become conditioned stimuli that trigger anxiety and panic, as demonstrated via panic induction through presentation of pairs of words involving sensations and catastrophic outcomes (Clark et al., 1988). In this case, catastrophic cognitions may well be sufficient to elicit conditioned panic attacks, but not necessary.

Whether cognitively or noncognitively based, excessive anxiety over panic-related bodily sensations in panic disorder is well supported. Persons with panic disorder endorse strong beliefs that bodily sensations associated with panic attacks cause physical or mental harm (e.g., Chambless, Caputo, Bright, & Gallagher, 1984; McNally & Lorenz, 1987). They are more likely to interpret bodily sensations in a catastrophic fashion (Clark et al., 1988) and to allocate more attentional resources to words that represent physical threat, such as "disease" and "fatality" (e.g., Ehlers, Margraf, Davies, & Roth, 1988; Hope, Rapee, Heimberg, & Dombeck, 1990); catastrophe words, such as "death" and "insane" (e.g., Maidenberg, Chen, Craske, Bohn, & Bystritsky, 1996; McNally, Riemann, Louro, Lukach, & Kim, 1992); and heartbeat stimuli (Kroeze & van den Hout, 2000; however, attentional bias is not always found; e.g., DeCort, Hermans, Spruyt, Griez, & Schruers, 2008). Also, individuals with panic disorder show enhanced brain potentials in response to panic-related words (Pauli, Amrhein, Muhlberger, Dengler, & Wiedemann, 2005). In addition, they are more likely to become anxious in procedures that elicit bodily sensations similar to the ones experienced during panic attacks, including benign cardiovascular, respiratory, and audiovestibular exercises (Antony, Ledley, Liss, & Swinson, 2006; Jacob, Furman, Clark, & Durrant, 1992), as well as more invasive procedures, such as CO_2 inhalations, compared to patients with other anxiety disorders (e.g., Perna, Bertani, Arancio, Ronchi, & Bellodi, 1995; Rapee, 1986; Rapee, Brown, Antony, & Barlow, 1992) or healthy controls (e.g., Gorman et al., 1994). The findings are not fully consistent, however, because patients with panic disorder did not differ from patients with social phobia in response to an epinephrine challenge (Veltman, van Zijderveld, Tilders, & van Dyck, 1996). Nonetheless, individuals with panic disorder also fear signals that ostensibly reflect heightened arousal and false physiological feedback (Craske & Freed, 1995; Craske, Lang, et al., 2002; Ehlers, Margraf, Roth, Taylor, & Birnbaumer, 1988).

Distress over bodily sensations is likely to generate ongoing distress for a number of reasons. First, in the immediate sense, autonomic arousal generated by fear in turn intensifies the feared sensations, thus creating a reciprocating cycle of fear and sensations that is sustained until autonomic arousal abates or the individual perceives safety. Second, because bodily sensations that trigger panic attacks are not always immediately obvious, they may generate the perception of unexpected or "out of the blue" panic attacks (Barlow, 1988) that causes even further distress (Craske, Glover, & DeCola, 1995). Third, the perceived uncontrollability, or inability to escape or terminate bodily sensations, again, is likely to generate heightened anxiety (e.g., Maier, Laudenslager, & Ryan, 1985; Mineka, Cook, & Miller, 1984). Unpredictability and uncontrollability, then, are seen as enhancing general levels of anxiety about "When is it going to happen again?" and "What do I do when it happens?", thereby contributing to high levels of chronic anxious apprehension (Barlow, 1988, 2002). In turn, anxious apprehension increases the likelihood of panic by directly increasing the availability of sensations that have become conditioned cues for panic and/or attentional vigilance for these bodily cues. Thus, a maintaining cycle of panic and anxious apprehension develops. Also, subtle avoidance behaviors are believed to maintain negative beliefs about feared bodily sensations (Clark & Ehlers, 1993). Examples include holding onto objects or persons for fear of fainting, sitting and remaining still for fear of a heart attack, and moving slowly or searching for an escape route because one fears acting foolish (Salkovskis, Clark, & Gelder, 1996). Such avoidance includes "experiential avoidance," or being unwilling to remain in contact with particular private experiences, in this case bodily sensations and catastrophic cognitions. Experiential avoidance is believed to contribute to overall distress and dysfunction in general (Hayes et al., 1996), and appears to correlate with panic-related worries and disability in individuals with panic disorder (Kampfe et al., 2012). Further support for the role of experiential avoidance comes from evidence for instructions to accept symptoms of panic to result in less fear and avoidance in patients with panic disorder (Campbell-Sills, Barlow, Brown, & Hofmann, 2006; Eifert & Heffner, 2003), including CO_2 inhalation challenges (Levitt, Brown, Orsillo, & Barlow, 2004). Finally, anxiety may develop over specific contexts in which the occurrence of panic would be particularly troubling (i.e., situations associated with impairment, entrapment, negative social evaluation, and distance from safety). These anxieties may contribute to agoraphobia, which in turn maintains distress by preventing disconfirmation of catastrophic misappraisals and extinction of conditioned responding. Clearly, this model targets panic disorder and agoraphobia, and is not as relevant to agoraphobia in the absence of panic attacks or panic-like symptoms.

TREATMENT VARIABLES

Setting

There are several different settings for conducting cognitive-behavioral therapy for panic disorder and agoraphobia. The first, the outpatient clinic–office setting, is suited to psychoeducation, cognitive restructuring, assignment, and feedback regarding homework assignments and role-play rehearsals. In addition, certain exposures can be conducted in the office setting, such as interoceptive exposure to feared bodily sensations we describe later. Outpatient settings have extended from mental health settings to primary care suites (e.g., Craske, Roy-Byrne, et al., 2002; Craske et al., 2011; Roy-Byrne, Craske, et al., 2005; Roy-Byrne et al., 2010; Sharp, Power, Simpson, Swanson, & Anstee, 1997). This extension is particularly important because of the higher prevalence of panic disorder in primary care settings (e.g., Shear & Schulberg, 1995; Tiemens, Ormel, & Simon, 1996). However, whether a mental health or a primary care office is being used, the built-in safety signals of such an office may limit the generalizability of learning that takes place in that setting. For example, learning to be less afraid in the presence of the therapist, or in an office located near a medical center, may not necessarily generalize to conditions in which the therapist is not present, or when the perceived safety of a medical center is not close by. For this reason, homework assignments to practice cognitive-behavioral skills in a variety of different settings are particularly important.

In the second setting, the natural environment, cognitive restructuring and other anxiety management skills are put into practice as the patient faces feared situations. The latter is called *in vivo* exposure and can be conducted with the aid of the therapist or alone. Therapist-directed exposure is particularly use-

ful for patients who lack a social network to support *in vivo* exposure assignments, and more valuable than self-directed exposure for patients with more severe agoraphobia (Holden, O'Brien, Barlow, Stetson, & Infantino, 1983). Therapist-directed exposure is essential to "guided mastery exposure," in which the therapist gives corrective feedback about the way the patient faces feared situations to minimize unnecessary defensive behaviors. For example, patients are taught to drive in a relaxed position and to walk across a bridge without holding the rail. On the one hand, guided mastery exposure has been shown to be more effective than "stimulus exposure" when patients attempt simply to endure the situation alone until fear subsides, without the benefit of ongoing therapist feedback (Williams & Zane, 1989). On the other hand, self-directed exposure is very valuable also, especially to the degree that it encourages independence and generalization of the skills learned in treatment to conditions in which the therapist is not present. Thus, the most beneficial approach in the natural environment is to proceed from therapist-directed to self-directed exposure.

In telephone-guided treatment, an interesting variation that combines the office and the natural environment, therapists direct patients with agoraphobia by phone to conduct *in vivo* exposure to feared situations (NcNamee, O'Sullivan, Lelliot, & Marks, 1989; Swinson, Fergus, Cox, & Wickwire, 1995) or provide instruction in panic control skills (Cote, Gauthier, Laberge, Cormier, & Plamondon, 1994). In addition, one small study showed that cognitive-behavioral therapy was as effective when delivered by videoconference as in person (Bouchard et al., 2004).

Self-directed treatments, with minimal direct therapist contact, take place in the natural environment and are beneficial for highly motivated and educated patients (e.g., Ghosh & Marks, 1987; Gould & Clum, 1995; Gould, Clum, & Shapiro, 1993; Lidren et al., 1994; Schneider, Mataix-Cols, Marks, & Bachofen, 2005). On the other hand, self-directed treatments are less effective for more severely affected patients (Holden, O'Brien, Barlow, Stetson, & Infantino, 1983); for those with more comorbidity (Hecker, Losee, Roberson-Nay, & Maki, 2004), less motivation, and less education; or for patients who are referred as opposed to recruited through advertisement (Hecker, Losee, Fritzler, & Fink, 1996). Self-directed treatments have expanded beyond workbooks and manuals to computerized and Internet versions (e.g., Carlbring, Ekselius, & Andersson, 2003; Richards, Klein, & Austin, 2006; Richards, Klein, & Carlbring, 2003). In general, these treatments yield very positive results with strong effect sizes (Andrews, Cuijpers, Craske, McEvoy, & Titov, 2010), and at least two studies indicate that they are as effective as therapist-led cognitive-behavioral therapy for panic disorder (Carlbring et al., 2005; Kiropoulos et al., 2008). However, attrition rates may be higher with self-directed computer/Internet programs in the absence of any therapist contact (e.g., Carlbring et al., 2003).

The third setting, the inpatient facility, is most appropriate when conducting very intensive cognitive-behavioral therapy (e.g., daily therapist contact) or treating severely disabled persons who can no longer function at home. In addition, certain medical or drug complications may warrant inpatient treatment. The greatest drawback to the inpatient setting is poor generalization to the home environment. Transition sessions and follow-up booster sessions in an outpatient clinic–office or in the patient's own home facilitate generalization.

Format

Cognitive-behavioral therapy for panic disorder and agoraphobia may be conducted in individual or group formats. Several clinical outcome studies have used group treatments (e.g., Bohni, Spindler, Arendt, Hougaaard, & Rosenberg, 2009; Craske, DeCola, Sachs, & Pontillo, 2003; Craske et al., 2007; Evans, Holt, & Oei, 1991; Feigenbaum, 1988; Hoffart, 1995; Telch et al., 1993). The fact that their outcomes are generally consistent with the summary statistics obtained from individually formatted treatment suggests that group treatment is as effective as individual therapy. In direct comparisons, albeit few in number, a slight advantage is shown for individual formats. Specifically, Neron, Lacroix, and Chaput (1995) compared 12–14 weekly sessions of individual or group cognitive-behavioral therapy ($N = 20$), although the group condition received two additional 1-hour individual sessions. The two conditions were equally effective for measures of panic and agoraphobia at posttreatment and 6-month follow-up. However, the individual format was more successful in terms of generalized anxiety and depressive symptoms by the follow-up point. In addition, individual treatments resulted in more clinically significant outcomes than group formats in primary care (Sharp, Power, & Swanson, 2004). Furthermore, 95% of individuals assigned to the waiting-list condition in the latter study

stated a clear preference for individual treatment when given the choice at the end of the waiting list.

Most studies of cognitive-behavioral therapy for panic and agoraphobia involve 10–20 weekly treatment sessions. Several studies show that briefer treatments may be effective as well. Evans and colleagues (1991) compared a 2-day group cognitive-behavioral treatment to a waiting-list condition, although without random assignment. The 2-day program comprised lectures (3 hours); teaching skills, such as breathing, relaxation, and cognitive challenge (3 hours); *in vivo* exposure (9 hours); and group discussion plus a 2-hour support group for significant others. Eighty-five percent of treated patients were reported to be either symptom-free or symptomatically improved, and these results were maintained 1 year later. In contrast, the waiting-list group did not demonstrate significant changes. A pilot study similarly indicated effectiveness with intensive cognitive-behavioral therapy over 2 days (Deacon & Abramowitz, 2006). Other studies have evaluated the effectiveness of cognitive-behavioral therapy when delivered over fewer sessions. In a randomized study, patients with panic disorder with agoraphobia who awaited pharmacotherapy treatment were assigned to four weekly sessions of either cognitive-behavioral therapy or supportive nondirective therapy (Craske, Maidenberg, & Bystritsky, 1995). Cognitive-behavioral therapy was more effective than supportive therapy, particularly with less severely affected patients, although the results were not as positive as those typically seen with more sessions. Also, we found that up to six sessions (average of three sessions) of cognitive-behavioral therapy combined with medication recommendations yielded significantly greater improvements on an array of measures, including quality of life, compared to treatment as usual for individuals with panic disorder in primary care settings (Roy-Byrne, Craske, et al., 2005). Notably, however, the treatment effects substantially increased as the number of cognitive-behavioral therapy sessions (up to six) and follow-up booster phone call sessions (up to six) increased (Craske et al., 2006). In our subsequent primary care study, an average of seven sessions of cognitive-behavioral therapy and/or medication recommendations was superior to usual care, and in this case, usual care often involved several active treatment elements (Craske et al., 2011). Finally, in a direct comparison, results were equally effective whether cognitive-behavioral therapy was delivered across the standard 12 sessions or across approximately six sessions (Clark et al., 1999).

Interpersonal Context

Interpersonal context variables have been researched in terms of the development, maintenance, and treatment of agoraphobia. The reason for this research interest is apparent from the following vignettes:

> "My husband really doesn't understand. He thinks it's all in my head. He gets angry at me for not being able to cope. He says I'm weak and irresponsible. He resents having to drive me around, and doing things for the kids that I used to do. We argue a lot because he comes home tired and frustrated from work only to be frustrated more by the problems I'm having. But I can't do anything without him. I'm so afraid that I'll collapse into a helpless wreck without him, or that I'll be alone for the rest of my life. As cruel as he can be, I feel safe around him because he always has everything under control. He always knows what to do."

This vignette illustrates dependency on the significant other for a sense of safety despite a nonsympathetic response that may only serve to increase background stress for the patient. The second vignette illustrates inadvertent reinforcement of fear and avoidance through attention from the significant other:

> "My boyfriend really tries hard to help me. He's always cautious of my feelings and doesn't push me to do things that I can't do. He phones me from work to check on me. He stays with me and holds my hand when I feel really scared. He never hesitates to leave work to help me if I'm having a bad time. Only last week we visited some of his friends, and we had to leave. I feel guilty because we don't do the things we used to enjoy doing together. We don't go to the movies anymore. We used to love going to ball games, but now it's too much for me. I am so thankful for him. I don't know what I would do without him."

Perhaps some forms of agoraphobia represent a conflict between desire for autonomy and dependency in interpersonal relationships (Fry, 1962; Goldstein & Chambless, 1978). In other words, the "preagoraphobic" is trapped in a domineering relationship without the skills needed to activate change. However, the concept of a distinct marital system that predisposes toward agoraphobia lacks empirical evidence. That is not to say that marital or interpersonal systems are un-

important to agoraphobia. For example, interpersonal discord/dissatisfaction may represent one of several possible stressors that precipitate panic attacks. Also, interpersonal relations may be negatively impacted by the development of agoraphobia (Buglass, Clarke, Henderson, & Presley, 1977) and in turn contribute to its maintenance. Not unlike one of the earlier vignettes, consider the woman who has developed agoraphobia and now relies on her husband to do the shopping and other errands. These new demands upon the husband lead to resentment and marital discord. The marital distress adds to background stress, making progress and recovery even more difficult for the patient.

Aside from whether interpersonal dysregulation contributes to the onset or maintenance of panic disorder or agoraphobia, some studies suggest that poor marital relations adversely impact exposure-based treatments (Bland & Hallam, 1981; Dewey & Hunsley, 1989; Milton & Hafner, 1979). However, other studies show no relationship between marital distress and outcome from cognitive-behavioral therapy (Arrindell & Emmelkamp, 1987; Emmelkamp, 1980; Himadi, Cerny, Barlow, Cohen, & O'Brien, 1986). Another line of research suggests that involving significant others in every aspect of treatment may override potential negative impacts of poor marital relations on phobic improvement (Barlow et al., 1984; Cerny, Barlow, Craske, & Himadi, 1987). Furthermore, involvement of significant others resulted in better long-term outcomes from cognitive-behavioral therapy for agoraphobia (Cerny et al., 1987). Similarly, communications training with significant others, compared to relaxation training, after 4 weeks of *in vivo* exposure therapy, resulted in significantly greater reductions on measures of agoraphobia by posttreatment (Arnow, Taylor, Agras, & Telch, 1985), an effect that was maintained over an 8-month follow-up. Together, these studies suggest the value of including significant others in the treatment for agoraphobia. On the other hand, treatment focused specifically on interpersonal relationships, via interpersonal therapy, was not as effective as cognitive-behavioral therapy for panic disorder and agoraphobia (Vos, Huibers, Diels, & Arntz, 2012).

Yet another question is the degree to which treatment for panic disorder and agoraphobia influences marital/interpersonal relations. Some have noted that successful treatment can have deleterious effects (Hafner, 1984; Hand & Lamontagne, 1976). Others note that it has no effect or a positive effect on marital functioning (Barlow, O'Brien, & Last, 1984; Himadi et al., 1986) and interpersonal functioning in general (Hoffart, 1997). We (Barlow et al., 1983) suggested that when negative effects do occur, it may be because exposure therapy is conducted intensively, without the significant other's involvement, which causes major role changes that the significant other perceives as being beyond his or her control. This again speaks to the value of involving significant others in the treatment process.

Therapist Variables

Only a few studies have evaluated therapist variables in relation to cognitive-behavioral treatments for anxiety disorders, let alone panic disorder or agoraphobia. Williams and Chambless (1990) found that patients with agoraphobia who rated their therapists as caring/involved, and as modeling self-confidence, achieved better outcomes on behavioral approach tests. However, an important confound in this study was that patient ratings of therapist qualities may have depended on patient responses to treatment. Keijsers, Schaap, Hoogduin, and Lammers (1995) reviewed findings on therapist relationship factors and behavioral outcome. They concluded that empathy, warmth, positive regard, and genuineness assessed early in treatment predict positive outcome; patients who view their therapists as understanding and respectful improve the most; and patient perceptions of therapist expertness, self-confidence, and directiveness relate positively to outcome, although not consistently. In their own study of junior therapists who provided cognitive-behavioral treatment for panic disorder with or without agoraphobia, Keijsers and colleagues found that more empathic statements and questioning occurred in Session 1 than in later sessions. In Session 3, therapists became more active and offered more instructions and explanations. In Session 10, therapists employed more interpretations and confrontations than previously. Most importantly, directive statements and explanations in Session 1 predicted poorer outcome. Empathic listening in Session 1 related to better behavioral outcome, whereas empathic listening in Session 3 related to poorer behavioral outcome. Thus, they demonstrated the advantages of different interactional styles at different points in therapy.

Most clinicians assume that therapist training and experience improve the chances of successful outcome. Some believe this to be the case particularly with respect to the cognitive aspects of cognitive-behavioral therapy (e.g., Michelson et al., 1990), and some indirect evidence for this supposition exists. Specifically,

cognitive-behavioral therapy conducted by "novice" therapists in a medical setting (Welkowitz et al., 1991) was somewhat less effective in comparison to the same therapy conducted by inexperienced but highly trained therapists in a psychological setting (Barlow, Craske, Czerny, & Klosko, 1989), or by experienced and highly trained therapists in a community mental health setting (Wade, Treat, & Stuart, 1998). Huppert and colleagues (2001), who directly evaluated the role of therapist experience, found that, in general, therapist experience positively related to outcome, seemingly because these therapists were more flexible in administering the treatment and better able to adapt it to the individual being treated. Obviously, there is a need for more evaluation of the role of therapist experience and training in cognitive-behavioral therapy.

In our primary care work, we developed a computer guide to assist novice clinicians in implementing a cognitive-behavioral program for panic disorder (plus other anxiety disorders and depression) (Craske et al, 2009), called Calm Tools for Living. The clinician and patient sit side by side as both view the program on-screen. Throughout, the program prompts clinicians to engage in specific tasks, such as helping patients to establish a fear hierarchy, demonstrating breathing skills, practicing cognitive skills, conducting interoceptive exposure, or designing *in vivo* exposure assignments. The program also provides learning tools for patients, such as didactic information, interactive exercises, video vignettes, and quizzes. The goal of the computerized program is to enhance the integrity of cognitive-behavioral therapy in the hands of novice and relatively untrained clinicians.

Patient Variables

There has been interest in the effect of comorbidity upon the outcomes of cognitive-behavioral therapy for panic disorder and agoraphobia. Brown, Antony, and Barlow (1995) found that comorbidity with other anxiety disorders did not predict response to cognitive-behavioral therapy overall, although social phobia was unexpectedly associated with superior outcome for panic disorder and agoraphobia. In contrast, Tsao, Lewin, and Craske (1998) found a trend for comorbidity that comprised mostly other anxiety disorders to be associated with slightly lower rates of overall success. In a subsequent study, however, we replicated the finding by Brown and colleagues of no relationship between baseline comorbidity comprising mostly other anxiety disorders, and either immediate or 6-month outcome for panic disorder and agoraphobia (Tsao, Mystkowski, Zucker, & Craske, 2002).

Research on how comorbid depression affects the course and outcome of panic disorder treatment has yielded mixed results. Studies focused on cognitive-behavioral therapy for all anxiety disorders and treatment participation have found that comorbidity with depression is associated with increased rates of refusal to enter treatment (Issakidis & Andrews, 2004); however, once patients have entered treatment, the comorbidity has no effect on rates of attrition (Allen et al., 2010; Brown et al., 1995). Preliminary research investigating the effects of comorbidity on engagement with treatment has revealed that comorbid depression has no effect on compliance with cognitive-behavioral therapy homework (McLean, Woody, Taylor, & Koch, 1998) or compliance with cognitive-behavioral treatment as a whole (Murphy, Michelson, Marchione, Marchione, & Testa, 1998), though it does increase levels of distress associated with treatment (Murphy et al., 1998). Interestingly, comorbid depression has no effect on the response to cognitive-behavioral therapy for panic disorder at posttreatment or follow-up and in both referred and primary care settings (Allen et al., 2010; McLean et al., 1998; Roy-Byrne, Craske, et al., 2005). It seems contradictory that comorbid depression would have significant impact on the severity and persistence of panic disorder (Baldwin, 1998) but would not affect the outcomes of panic disorder treatment. This may be a product of limitations to the current treatment literature. For example, studies have recruited patients for the treatment of panic disorder and have often excluded patients who are very extremely depressed or suicidal. Thus, the majority of patients are mildly to moderately depressed. Many of these studies also exclude patients with bipolar disorder, and therefore exclude an entire group of individuals who experience major depressive episodes. However, it may also be that the effects of cognitive-behavioral therapy for panic disorder are sufficiently potent to impact depressive symptoms either directly or indirectly.

A relatively high co-occurrence exists between panic disorder and agoraphobia, and avoidant, dependent, and histrionic personality disorders (e.g., Reich et al., 1994). Questions of diagnostic reliability and validity aside, comorbid personality disorders are sometimes associated with poorer response than usual to cognitive-behavioral therapy for panic disorder or agoraphobia (e.g., Hoffart & Hedley, 1997; Marchand, Goyer, Dupuis, & Main-guy, 1998). However, closer examination reveals that although individuals with comorbid personality disorders have greater severity of panic or agoraphobia pre- and post–cognitive-behavioral therapy, the rate of decrease in panic or agoraphobia symptoms usually is not affected by the comorbid personality disorder. Thus, Dreessen, Arntz, Luttels, and Sallaerts (1994) and van den Hout, Brouwers, and Oomen (2006) found that comorbid personality disorders did not affect response to cognitive-behavioral therapy for panic or agoraphobia. Moreover, Hofmann and colleagues (1988) found that scores on questionnaire subscales reflecting Axis II personality disorders did not predict panic disorder treatment response to either cognitive-behavioral therapy or to medication. In fact, some personality traits may associate positively with outcome, as was reported by Rathus, Sanderson, Miller, and Wetzler (1995) with respect to compulsive personality features.

Substance-related disorders also commonly co-occur with panic disorder and agoraphobia, but very few treatment studies have addressed this important comorbidity. In a series of single cases (N = 3), Lehman, Brown, and Barlow (1998) demonstrated successful control of panic attacks in individuals who were abusing alcohol. Also, the addition of anxiety treatment to a relapse prevention program for abstinent individuals with a primary diagnosis of alcohol dependence and a comorbid diagnosis of panic disorder or social phobia decreased anxiety symptoms relative to a relapse prevention program alone (Schade et al., 2005). However, adding the anxiety treatment did not affect rates of alcohol relapse in that study.

Another source of comorbidity is medical conditions, such as cardiac arrhythmias or asthma, that may slow improvement rates given the additional complications involved in discriminating between anxiety and disease symptomatology, increases in actual medical risk, and the stress of physical diseases. We found that medically ill patients with panic disorder, although more severely affected than their nonmedically ill counterparts at baseline, responded just as favorably to cognitive-behavioral therapy with psychotropic medication recommendations (Roy-Byrne, Stein, et al., 2005). Also, cognitive-behavioral therapy for panic disorder has been shown to alleviate self-reported physical health symptoms (Schmidt et al., 2003). Similarly, we found that cognitive-behavioral therapy and/or psychotropic medication recommendations for anxiety disorders (including panic disorder) significantly improve physical health functioning (Niles et al., 2013).

Other patient variables include socioeconomic status and general living conditions. We evaluated perceived barriers to receiving mental health treatment in our primary care study of panic disorder (Craske, Golinelli, et al., 2005). Commonly reported barriers included inability to find out where to go for help (43%), worry about cost (40%), lack of coverage by one's health plan (35%), and inability to get an appointment soon enough (35%). Also, in our multicenter trial, attrition from cognitive-behavioral and/or medication treatment for panic disorder with minimal agoraphobia was predicted by lower education, which in turn was dependent on lower income (Grilo et al., 1998). Similarly, levels of education and motivation were associated with dropout rates in another sample, although the effects were small (Keijsers, Kampman, & Hoogduin, 2001). Low education–income may reflect less discretionary time to engage in activities such as weekly treatment. Consider a woman who is the mother of two, a full-time clerk, whose husband is on disability due to a back injury, or the full-time student who works an extra 25 hours a week to pay his way through school. Under these conditions, treatment assignments of daily *in vivo* exposure exercises are much less likely to be completed. Frustration with lack of treatment progress is likely to result. Therapeutic success requires either a change in lifestyle that allows the cognitive-behavioral treatment to become a priority or termination of therapy until a later time, when life circumstances are less demanding. In fact, these kinds of life circumstance issues may explain the trend for African Americans to show less treatment benefit, in terms of mobility, anxiety, and panic attacks, than European Americans (Friedman & Paradis, 1991; Williams & Chambless, 1994). Although, in contrast to these two studies, Friedman, Paradis, and Hatch (1994) found equivalent outcomes across the two racial groups, and the results from another study yielded outcomes from a female African American sample that were judged to be comparable to those of European Americans (Carter, Sbrocco, Gore, Marin, & Lewis, 2003). The influence of ethnic and cultural differences on treatment outcome and delivery clearly needs more evaluation.

Finally, patients' understanding of the nature of their problem may be important to the success of cognitive-behavioral treatments. Given the somatic nature of panic disorder, many patients seek medical help first. Beyond that, however, differences in the way the problem is conceptualized could lead to the perception that pharmacological or analytical treatment approaches are more credible than cognitive-behavioral treatment approaches. For example, individuals who strongly believe their condition is due to "a neurochemical imbalance" may be more likely to seek medication and to refute psychological treatments. Similarly, individuals who attribute their condition to "something about my past—it must be unconscious influences" may resist cognitive-behavioral interpretations. Also, Grilo and colleagues (1998) found that patients with panic disorder or agoraphobia who attributed their disorder to specific stressors in their lives were more likely to drop out of cognitive-behavioral or medication treatment, perhaps because they saw the offered treatment as irrelevant.

Concurrent Pharmacological Treatment

Many more patients receive medications than cognitive-behavioral therapy for panic disorder and agoraphobia, partly because primary care physicians are usually the first line of treatment. Thus, one-half or more of patients with panic disorder who attend psychology research clinics already are taking anxiolytic medications. The obvious questions, therefore, are the extent to which cognitive-behavioral therapy and medications have a synergistic effect, and how medications impact cognitive-behavioral therapy.

Results from large clinical trials, including our own multisite trial (Barlow, Gorman, Shear, & Woods, 2000), suggest no advantage during or immediately after treatment of combining cognitive-behavioral and pharmacological approaches. Specifically, both individual cognitive-behavioral and drug treatment, and a combination treatment were immediately effective following treatment. Furthermore, following medication discontinuation, the combination of medication and cognitive-behavioral therapy fared worse than cognitive-behavioral therapy alone, suggesting the possibility that state- (or context-) dependent learning in the presence of medication may have attenuated the new learning that occurs during cognitive-behavioral therapy. In contrast, in the primary care setting, we found that the addition of even just one component of cognitive-behavioral therapy to medications for panic disorder resulted in statistically and clinically significant improvements at posttreatment and 12 months later (Craske, Golinelli, et al., 2005).

More recently, our multisite collaborative team has been investigating long-term strategies in the treatment of panic disorder. We examined sequential combination strategies to determine whether this approach is more advantageous than simultaneously combining treatments. In the initial phase, 256 patients with panic disorder and all levels of agoraphobia completed 3 months of initial treatment with cognitive-behavioral therapy (Aaronson et al., 2008; White et al., 2010). Patients were then triaged into two clinical trials. Responders were randomized to 9 months of monthly booster sessions ($N = 79$) or no booster sessions ($N = 78$), then followed for an additional 12 months without treatment (White et al., 2013). Booster sessions produced significantly lower relapse rates (5.2%) and reduced work and social impairment compared to the assessment-only condition without booster sessions (18.4%) at 21-month follow-up. Multivariate Cox proportional hazards models showed that residual symptoms of agoraphobia at the end of acute-phase treatment were independently predictive of time to relapse during 21-month follow-up (hazard rate = 1.15, $p < .01$). Thus, booster sessions aimed at reinforcing acute treatment gains to prevent relapse and offset disorder recurrence improved long-term outcome for panic disorder with and without agoraphobia. Fifty-eight of the original patients did not reach an optimal level of functioning (high end-state functioning) and entered a trial in which they received either continued cognitive-behavioral therapy for 3 months or paroxetine for 3 months. Patients doing well with one treatment or the other continued with the respective treatment for an additional 9 months (Payne et al., 2012). Results indicated significantly lower panic disorder symptoms for individuals in the paroxetine condition compared to those in continued cognitive-behavioral therapy at 3 months. However, group differences had disappeared 9 months later. Results were maintained when excluding individuals with comorbid major depression. These data suggest a more rapid treatment response when switching to paroxetine after not responding optimally to cognitive-behavioral therapy; however, both treatments ultimately achieved similar outcomes.

In another study with similar results, patients who did not respond to cognitive-behavioral therapy also benefited more from the addition of a serotonergic drug (paroxetine) to continued cognitive-behavioral therapy than from the addition of a drug placebo, with substantially different effect sizes (Kampman, Keijsers, Hoogduin, & Hendriks, 2002). Conversely, individuals who are resistant to pharmacotherapy may respond positively to cognitive-behavioral therapy, although these findings were part of an open trial without randomization (Heldt et al., 2006).

Findings from the combination of fast-acting anxiolytics, specifically, the high-potency benzodiazepines, and behavioral treatments for agoraphobia are contradictory (e.g., Marks et al., 1993; Wardle et al., 1994). Nevertheless, several studies have reliably demonstrated the detrimental effects of chronic use of high-potency benzodiazepines on short-term and long-term outcome in cognitive-behavioral treatments for panic or agoraphobia (e.g., Otto, Pollack, & Sabatino, 1996; van Balkom, de Beurs, Koele, Lange, & van Dyck, 1996; Wardle et al., 1994). Specifically, there is evidence for more attrition, poorer outcome, and more relapse with chronic use of high-potency benzodiazepines. In addition, use of benzodiazepines as needed was associated with poorer outcome than regular use or no use in one small naturalistic study (Westra, Stewart, & Conrad, 2002).

Finally, the cost-effectiveness of cognitive-behavioral and medication treatments alone rather than in combination requires further evaluation; currently, cognitive-behavioral therapy is considered to be more cost-effective (e.g., disability costs, work days missed, health care use) than pharmacotherapy (Heuzenroeder et al., 2004).

Understanding the ways in which psychotropic medications influence cognitive-behavioral therapy may prove useful for developing methods that optimize the combination of these two approaches to treatment. First, medications, particularly fast-acting, potent medications that cause a *noticeable* shift in state and are used on an as-needed basis (e.g., benzodiazepines, beta-blockers), may contribute to relapse because therapeutic success is attributed to them rather than to cognitive-behavioral therapy. Patients' resultant lack of perceived self-control may increase relapse potential when medication is withdrawn or contribute to maintenance of a medication regimen under the assumption that it is necessary to functioning. In support, attribution of therapeutic gains to alprazolam, and lack of confidence in coping without alprazolam, even when given in conjunction with behavioral therapy, predicted relapse (Basoglu, Marks, Kilic, Brewin, & Swinson, 1994). Second, medications may assume the role of safety signals, or objects to which persons erroneously attribute their safety from painful, aversive outcomes. Safety signals may contribute to maintenance of fear and avoidance in the long term (Hermans, Craske, Mineka, & Lovibond, 2006) and may interfere with corrections of misappraisals of bodily symptoms (see below for further discussion of this issue). Third, medications may reduce the motivation to engage in practices of cognitive-behavioral skills, yet completion of between-session assignments is a positive predictor of outcome from cognitive-behavioral therapy (e.g., Glenn et al., in press). Finally, learning that takes place under the influence of medications may not necessarily generalize to the time when medications are removed, thus contributing to relapse (Bouton & Swartzentruber, 1991). Some of these points are illustrated in the following vignettes:

"I had been through a program of cognitive-behavioral therapy, but it was really the Paxil that helped. Because I was feeling so much better, I considered tapering off the medication. At first I was very concerned about the idea. I had heard horror stories about what people go through when withdrawing. However, I thought it would be OK as long as I tapered slowly. So, I gradually weaned myself off. It really wasn't that bad. Well, I had been completely off the medication for about a month when the problem started all over again. I remember sitting in a restaurant, feeling really good because I was thinking about how much of a problem restaurants used to be for me before, and how easy it seemed now. Then, whammo. I became very dizzy and I immediately thought, 'Oh no, here it comes.' I had a really bad panic attack. All I could think of was why didn't I stay on the medication?"

"I started to lower my dose of Xanax. I was OK for the first couple of days. . . . I felt really good. Then, when I woke up on Friday morning, I felt strange. My head felt really tight and I worried about having the same old feelings all over again. The last thing I want to do is to go through that again. So I took my usual dose of Xanax and, within a few minutes, I felt pretty good again. I need the medication. I can't manage without it right now."

In what ways might such negative effects of medications be offset? One possibility is that continuation of exposure after medication is withdrawn may offset relapse because it enhances attributions of personal mastery and reduces the safety signal function of medications. In addition, opportunities to practice exposure and cognitive and behavioral strategies without the aid of medication overcome state dependency and enhance generalization of therapeutic gains once treatment is over.

CASE STUDY

Julie, a 33-year-old European American mother of two, lives with Larry, her husband of 8 years. For the past 3 years she has been chronically anxious and panic stricken. She describes her panic attacks as unbearable and increasing in frequency. The first time she felt panicky was just over 3 years ago, when she was rushing to be by her grandmother's side in the last moments before she died. Julie was driving alone on the freeway. She remembers feeling as if everything were moving in slow motion, as if the cars were standing still, and things around her seemed unreal. She recalled feeling short of breath and detached. However, it was so important to reach her destination that she did not dwell on how she felt until later. After the day was over, she reflected on how lucky she was not to have had an accident. A few weeks later, she experienced the same feeling again when driving on the freeway. This time it occurred without the pressure of getting to her dying grandmother. It scared Julie because she was unable to explain the feelings. She pulled to the side of the road and called her husband, who came to meet her. She followed him home, feeling anxious the entire way.

Now, Julie has these feelings in many situations. She describes her panic attacks as feelings of unreality, detachment, shortness of breath, a racing heart, and a general fear of the unknown. It is the unreality that scares her the most. Consequently, Julie is sensitive to anything that produces "unreal" types of feelings, such as the semiconsciousness that occurs just before falling asleep, the period when daylight changes to night, bright lights, concentrating on the same thing for long periods of time, alcohol or drugs, and being anxious in general. Even though she has a prescription for Klonopin (a high-potency benzodiazepine), she rarely, if ever, uses it because of her general fear of being under the influence of a drug, or of feeling an altered state of consciousness. She wants to be as alert as possible at all times, but she keeps the Klonopin with her in the event that she has no other way of managing her panic. She does not leave home without the Klonopin. Julie is very sensitive to her body in general; she becomes scared of anything that feels a little different than usual. Even coffee, which she used to enjoy, is distressing to her now because of its agitating and racy effects. She was never a big exerciser, but to think of exerting herself now is also scary. Julie reports that she is constantly waiting for the next panic attack to occur. She avoids freeways, driving on familiar surface streets only. She limits herself to a 10-mile radius from home. She avoids crowds and large groups as well, partly because of the feeling of too much stimulation and partly because she is afraid to panic in front of others. In general, she prefers to be with her husband or her mother. However, she can do most things as long as she is within her "safety" region.

Julie describes how she differs from the way she used to be: how weak and scared she is now. The only other incident that is similar to her current panic attacks occurred in her early 20s, when she had a negative reaction to smoking marijuana. Julie became very scared of the feeling of losing control and feared that she would never return to reality. She has not taken drugs since then. Otherwise, there is no history of serious medical conditions or any previous psychological treatment. Julie had some separation anxiety and was shy as a young child and throughout her teens. However, her social anxiety improved throughout her 20s to the point that until the onset of her panic attacks, she was mostly very comfortable around people. Since the onset of her panic attacks, Julie has become concerned that others will notice that she appears anxious. However, her social anxiety is limited to panic attacks and does not reflect a broader social phobia.

In general, Julie's appetite is good, but her sleep is restless. At least once a week she wakes abruptly in the middle of the night, feeling short of breath and scared, and she has great difficulty going to sleep when her husband travels. In addition to worrying about her panic attacks, Julie worries about her husband and her children, although these latter worries are secondary to her worry about panicking and not excessive. She has some difficulty concentrating but is generally able to function at home and at work because of the familiarity of her environment and the safety she feels in the presence of her husband. Julie works part time as the manager of a business that she and her husband own. She sometimes becomes depressed about her panic and the limitations on how far she can travel. Occasionally she feels hopeless about the future, doubting whether she will ever be able to escape the anxiety. Although the feelings of hopelessness and the teariness never last than more than a few days, Julie has generally had a low-grade depressed mood since her life became restricted by the panic attacks.

Julie's mother and her uncle both had panic attacks when they were younger. Julie is now worried that her oldest child is showing signs of being overly anxious because he is hesitant about trying new things or spending time away from home.

ASSESSMENT

A functional behavioral analysis depends on several different modes of assessment, which we describe next.

Interviews

An in-depth interview is the first step in establishing diagnostic features and the profile of symptomatic and behavioral responses. Several semistructured and fully structured interviews exist. The Anxiety Disorders Interview Schedule for DSM-IV (ADIS-IV; Di Nardo, Brown, & Barlow, 1994) and for DSM-5 (ADIS-5; Brown & Barlow, in press) primarily assesses anxiety disorders, as well as mood and somatoform disorders. Psychotic and drug conditions are screened by this instrument also. The ADIS facilitates gathering the necessary information to make a differential diagnosis among anxiety disorders and offers a means to distinguish between clinical and subclinical presentations of a disorder. Data on the frequency, intensity, and duration of panic attacks, as well as details on avoidance behavior, are embedded within the ADIS; this information is necessary for tailoring treatment to each individual's presentation. The value of structured interviews is their contribution to a differential diagnosis and interrater reliability. Interrater agreement ranges from satisfactory to excellent for the various anxiety disorders using the ADIS-IV (Brown, Di Nardo, Lehman, & Campbell, 2001). Similar analysis for the ADIS-5 are under way.

Similarly, the Schizophrenia and Affective Disorders Schedule—Lifetime Version (modified for the study of anxiety) produces reliable diagnoses for most of the anxiety disorders (generalized anxiety disorder and simple phobia are the exceptions) (Manuzza, Fyer, Liebowitz, & Klein, 1990), as does the Structured Clinical Interview for DSM (SCID), which covers all of the mental disorders (First, Spitzer, Gibbon, & Williams, 1994), and will be updated for DSM-5 diagnostic criteria.

Differential diagnosis is sometimes difficult because, as described earlier, panic is a ubiquitous phenomenon (Barlow, 1988) that occurs across a wide variety of emotional disorders. It is not uncommon for persons with specific phobias, social phobia, generalized anxiety disorder, obsessive–compulsive disorder, and posttraumatic stress disorder to report panic attacks. For Julie, there was a differential diagnostic question regarding social anxiety disorder, and panic disorder and agoraphobia. Shown in Figure 1.1 are the ADIS-IV questions that address this differentiation (Julie's answers are in italics).

Parts of ADIS-IV Panic Disorder Section

Do you currently have times when you feel a sudden rush of intense fear or discomfort? *Yes.*

In what kinds of situations do you have those feelings? *Driving, especially on freeways . . . alone at home . . . at parties or in crowds of people.*

Did you ever have those feelings come "from out of the blue," for no apparent reason, or in situations where you did not expect them to occur? *Yes.*

How long does it usually take for the rush of fear/discomfort to reach its peak level? *It varies, sometimes a couple of seconds and at other times it seems to build more slowly.*

How long does the fear/discomfort usually last at its peak level? *Depends on where I am at the time. If it happens when I'm alone, sometimes it is over within a few minutes or even seconds. If I'm in a crowd, then it seems to last until I leave*

In the last month, how much have you been worried about, or how fearful have you been about having another panic attack?

0	1	2	3	4	5	6	7	8
No worry no fear		Rarely worried/mild fear		Occasionally worried/moderate fear		Frequently worried/ severe fear		Constantly worried/ extreme fear

Parts of ADIS-IV Social Phobia Section

In social situations, where you might be observed or evaluated by others, or when meeting new people, do you feel fearful, anxious, or nervous? *Yes.*

Are you overly concerned that you might do and/or say something that might embarrass or humiliate yourself in front of others, or that others may think badly of you? *Yes.*

What are you concerned will happen in these situations? *That others will notice that I am anxious. My face turns white and my eyes look strange when I panic. I am worried that I'll flip out in front of them, and they won't know what to do.*

Are you anxious about these situations because you are afraid that you will have an unexpected panic attack? *Yes (either a panic or that I'll feel unreal).*

Other than when you are exposed to these situations, have you experienced an unexpected rush of fear/anxiety? *Yes.*

FIGURE 1.1. Julie's responses to ADIS-IV questions.

As demonstrated in Figure 1.1, Julie experiences panic attacks in social situations and is concerned about being negatively evaluated by others if her anxiety becomes visibly apparent. However, despite her history of shyness, Julie's current social discomfort is based primarily on the possibility of panicking. Because of this, and because she meets the other criteria for panic disorder (i.e., unexpected /nonsocial panic attacks and pervasive apprehension about future panic attacks), the social distress is best subsumed under the domain of panic disorder and agoraphobia. If Julie reported that she experiences panic attacks in social situations only, or that she worries about panic attacks in social situations only, then a diagnosis of social anxiety disorder would be more probable. A report of unexpected panic attacks, as well as self-consciousness about things that she might do or say in social situations regardless of the occurrence of panic, would be consistent with a dual diagnosis of panic disorder–agoraphobia and social anxiety disorder. In general, an individual with panic disorder may continue to feel anxious even when playing a passive role in a social setting, whereas a patient with social phobia is more likely to feel relaxed when he or she is not the center of attention and does not anticipate being evaluated or judged (Dattilio & Salas-Auvert, 2000).

The same types of diagnostic questioning are useful for distinguishing between panic disorder–agoraphobia and claustrophobia. Other differential diagnostic issues can arise with respect to somatoform disorders, real medical conditions, and avoidant or dependent personality disorders.

Following completion of a diagnostic assessment, a dimensional assessment specifically designed for panic disorder, such as the Panic Disorder Severity Scale (PDSS; Shear et al., 1997), may be helpful. This clinician-completed scale rates seven areas of responding using a 0- to 4-point severity rating scale: panic attack frequency; distress; anticipatory anxiety; agoraphobic and interoceptive-related fears; avoidant behavior; and work and social impairment. A cutoff score of 8 on the PDSS identifies patients with panic disorder with high sensitivity and acceptable specificity (Shear et al., 2001).

Medical Evaluation

A medical evaluation is generally recommended because several medical conditions should be ruled out before assigning the diagnosis of panic disorder. These include thyroid conditions, caffeine or amphetamine intoxication, drug withdrawal, or pheochromocytoma (a rare adrenal gland tumor). Furthermore, certain medical conditions can exacerbate panic disorder, although panic disorder is likely to continue even when the symptoms are under medical control. Mitral valve prolapse, asthma, allergies, and hypoglycemia fall into this latter category. According to the model described earlier, these medical conditions exacerbate panic disorder to the extent that they elicit the feared physical sensations. For example, mitral valve prolapse sometimes produces the sensation of a heart flutter, asthma produces shortness of breath, and hypoglycemia produces dizziness and weakness, all of which overlap

with symptoms of panic and may therefore become conditional cues for panic.

Self-Monitoring

Self-monitoring is a very important part of assessment and treatment for panic disorder and agoraphobia. Retrospective recall of past episodes of panic and anxiety, especially when made under anxious conditions, may inflate estimates of panic frequency and intensity (Margraf et al., 1987; Rapee, Craske, & Barlow, 1990). Moreover, such inflation may contribute to apprehension about future panic. In contrast, ongoing self-monitoring generally yields more accurate, less inflated estimates (for a comprehensive review of self-monitoring for panic and anxiety, see Craske & Tsao, 1999). Also, ongoing self-monitoring is believed to contribute to an objective self-awareness. Objective self-monitoring replaces negative, affect-laden self-statements such as "I feel horrible. This is the worst it has ever been—my whole body is out of control" with "My anxiety level is 6. My symptoms include tremulousness, dizziness, unreal feelings, and shortness of breath—and this episode lasted 10 minutes." Objective self-awareness usually reduces negative affect. Finally, self-monitoring provides feedback for judging progress and useful material for in-session discussions.

Panic attacks are recorded in the Panic Attack Record, a version of which is shown in Figure 1.2. This record, which is to be completed as soon as possible after a panic attack occurs, is therefore carried on-person (wallet size). Daily levels of anxiety, depression, and worry about panic are monitored with the Daily Mood Record shown in Figure 1.3. This record is completed at the end of each day. Finally, activities may be recorded by logging daily excursions in a diary, or by checking off activities completed from an agoraphobia checklist.

A common problem with self-monitoring is noncompliance. Sometimes noncompliance is due to misunderstanding or lack of perceived credibility in self-monitoring. Most often, however, noncompliance is due to anticipation of more anxiety as a result of monitoring. This is particularly true for individuals whose preferred style of coping is to distract themselves as much as possible because thoughts of panic might otherwise become overwhelming: "Why should I make myself worse by asking myself how bad I feel?" In Julie's case, the self-monitoring task was particularly difficult because explicit reminders of her anxiety elicited strong

Date _2/16/06_   Time began _5:20 P.M._

Triggers _Home alone and shortness of breath_

Expected _x_   Unexpected _____

Maximum Fear   0——1——2——3——4——5——6——7——8——9——10
                None   Mild   Moderate   Strong   Extreme

Check all symptoms present to at least a mild degree:

Chest pain or discomfort	_____	Sweating	_x_____
Heart racing/palpitations/pounding	_x_____	Nausea/upset stomach	_____
Short of breath	_x_____	Dizzy/unsteady/lightheaded/faint	_____
Shaking/trembling	_x_____	Chills/hot flushes	_____
Numbness/tingling	_____	Feelings of unreality	_x_____
Feelings of choking	_____	Fear of dying	_____
Fear of losing control/going crazy	_x_____		

Thoughts: _I am going crazy, I will lose control_

Behaviors: _Called my mother_

FIGURE 1.2. Julie's Panic Attack Record.

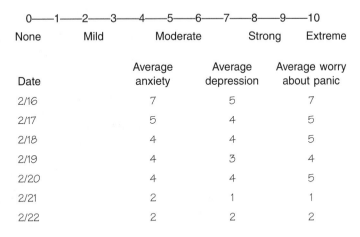

0——1——2——3——4——5——6——7——8——9——10
None   Mild   Moderate   Strong   Extreme

Date	Average anxiety	Average depression	Average worry about panic
2/16	7	5	7
2/17	5	4	5
2/18	4	4	5
2/19	4	3	4
2/20	4	4	5
2/21	2	1	1
2/22	2	2	2

FIGURE 1.3. Julie's Daily Mood Record.

concerns about losing touch with reality. Prompting, reassurance that anxiety would subside with perseverance at self-monitoring, and emphasis on objective versus subjective self-monitoring were helpful for Julie. In addition, therapist attention to the self-monitored information and corrective feedback about the method of self-monitoring at the start of each treatment session reinforced Julie's self-monitoring.

Standardized Inventories

Several standardized self-report inventories provide useful information for treatment planning and are sensitive markers of therapeutic change. The Anxiety Sensitivity Index (Reiss, Peterson, Gursky, & McNally, 1986) and the multidimensional Anxiety Sensitivity Index–3 (Taylor et al., 2007) have received wide acceptance as a trait measure of threatening beliefs about bodily sensations. Both display good psychometric properties and tend to discriminate panic disorder and agoraphobia from other anxiety disorders (e.g., Taylor et al., 1992; Telch, Sherman, & Lucas, 1989), especially the Physical Concerns subscale (Zinbarg et al., 1997). More specific information about which particular bodily sensations are feared most and what specific misappraisals occur most often may be obtained from the Body Sensations Questionnaire and the Agoraphobia Cognitions Questionnaire, respectively (Chambless, Caputo, Bright, & Gallagher, 1984). Both scales have strong to excellent psychometric properties and are sensitive to change following treatment (see Keller & Craske, 2008). The Mobility Inventory (Chambless, Caputo, Gracely, Jasin, & Williams, 1985) lists agoraphobic situations, which are rated in terms of degree of avoidance when alone and when accompanied. This instrument is very useful for establishing *in vivo* exposure hierarchies and, again, is well supported psychometrically.

In addition, we have developed two standardized self-report inventories that are useful for panic disorder and agoraphobia. The first, the Albany Panic and Phobia Questionnaire (Rapee, Craske, & Barlow, 1995), assesses fear and avoidance of activities that produce feared bodily sensations (e.g., exercise, caffeine), as well as more typical agoraphobia and social situations. Factor analyses confirmed three distinct factors labeled Agoraphobia, Social Phobia, and Interoceptive Fears. The questionnaire has adequate psychometric properties and is useful in profiling agoraphobic versus interoceptive avoidance. The second, the Anxiety Control Questionnaire, assesses perceived lack of control over anxiety-related events and occurrences, such as internal emotional reactions or externally threatening cues (Rapee, Craske, Brown, & Barlow, 1996). This scale is designed to assess locus of control, but in a more specific and targeted manner relevant to anxiety and anxiety disorders compared to more general locus-of-control scales. A revised 15-item version yields three factors—Emotion Control, Threat Control, and Stress Control—with a higher-order dimension of perceived control (Brown, White, Forsyth, & Barlow, 2004). Changes in this scale from pre to posttreatment predicted reductions in comorbidity at follow-up in one study (Craske et al., 2007). A more detailed review of each questionnaire listed herein and the complete assessment for panic disorder and agoraphobia is provided by Keller and Craske (2008).

Behavioral Tests

The behavioral test is a useful measure of degree of avoidance of specific interoceptive cues and external situations. Behavioral approach tests can be standardized or individually tailored. The standardized behavioral test for agoraphobic avoidance usually involves walking or driving a particular route, such as a 1-mile loop around the clinic setting. Standardized behavioral tests for anxiety about physical sensations involve exercises that induce panic-like symptoms, such as spinning in a circle, running in place, hyperventilating, and breathing through a straw (Barlow & Craske, 2006). Anxiety levels are rated at regular intervals throughout the behavioral tests, and actual distance or length of time is measured. The disadvantage of standardized behavioral tests is that the specific task may not be relevant to all patients (e.g., a 1-mile walk or running in place may be only mildly anxiety provoking to some but highly distressing to others); hence, the value of individually tailored tasks. In the case of agoraphobia, this usually entails attempts at three to five individualized situations that the patient has identified as ranging from *Somewhat difficult* to *Extremely difficult*, such as driving two exits on freeway, waiting in a bank line, or shopping in a local supermarket for 15 minutes. For anxiety about physical sensations, individually tailored behavioral tests entail exercises designed specifically to induce the sensations feared most by a given patient (e.g., nose plugs to induce sensations of difficulty breathing). As with standardized tests, ongoing levels of anxiety and degree of approach behavior are measured in relation to individually tailored behavioral tests.

Individually tailored behavioral tests are more informative for clinical practice, although they confound between-subject comparisons for research purposes. Behavioral tests are an important supplement to self-report of agoraphobic avoidance because patients tend to underestimate what they can actually achieve (Craske et al., 1988). In addition, behavioral tests often reveal important information for treatment planning of which the individual is not yet fully aware. For example, the tendency to remain close to supports, such as railings or walls, may not be apparent until one observes the patient walking through a shopping mall. In Julie's case, the importance of change from daylight to night was not apparent until she was asked to drive on a section of road as a behavioral test. Her response was that it was too late in the day to drive because dusk made her feel as if things were unreal. Similarly, it was not until Julie completed a behavioral test that we recognized the importance of air-conditioning when she was driving. Julie believed that the cool air blowing on her face helped her to remain "in touch with reality." Finally, we noticed that her physical posture while driving was a factor that contributed to anxiety: Julie's shoulders were hunched, and she leaned toward the steering wheel and held it very tightly. All of these were targeted in the treatment: Driving at dusk was included in her hierarchy; air-conditioning was regarded as a safety signal from which she should be weaned; and driving in a more relaxed position was part of mastery exposure.

Psychophysiology

Ongoing physiological measures are not very practical tools for clinicians, but they can provide important information. In particular, the discrepancy described earlier between reports of symptoms and actual physiological arousal (i.e., report of heart rate acceleration in absence of actual heart rate acceleration) may serve as a therapeutic demonstration of the role of attention and cognition in symptom production. Similarly, actual recordings provide data to disconfirm misappraisals such as "My heart feels like it's going so fast that it will explode" or "I'm sure my blood pressure is so high that I could have a stroke at any minute." Finally, resting levels of physiological functioning, which are sometimes dysregulated in anxious individuals, may be sensitive measures of treatment outcome (e.g., Craske, Lang, et al., 2005).

Functional Analysis

The various methods of assessment provide the material for a full functional analysis for Julie. Specifically, the topography of her panic attack is as follows: The most common symptoms include a feeling of unreality, shortness of breath, and racing heart; average frequency of panic attacks is three per week; each panic attack on average lasts from a few seconds to 5 minutes, if Julie is not in a crowd, where the panicky feelings last until she exits the crowd; in terms of apprehension, Julie worries about panic 75% of the day; and most of her panic attacks are expected, but she has some unexpected ones as well. Julie has both situational and internal antecedents to her panic attacks. The situational antecedents include driving on freeways; crowds of people; being alone, especially at night; restaurants; dusk; reading and concentrating for long periods of time; and aerobic activity. The internal antecedents include heart rate fluctuations, lightheaded feelings, hunger feelings, weakness due to lack of food, thoughts of the "big one" happening, thoughts of not being able to cope with this for much longer, and anger. Her misappraisals about panic attack symptoms include beliefs that she will never return to normality, that she will go crazy or lose control, and that others will think she is weird. Her behavioral reactions to panic attacks include escape behaviors such as pulling off to the side of the road, leaving restaurants and other crowded places, calling her husband or mother, and checking for her Klonopin. Her behavioral reactions to the anticipation of panic attacks include avoidance of driving long distances alone, driving on unfamiliar roads and freeways or at dusk, crowded areas, exercise, quiet time with nothing to do, and doing one thing for a long period of time. In addition, she tries not to think about anxiety or feelings of unreality. Her safety signals and safety-seeking behaviors include having her Klonopin on hand at all times, always knowing the location of her husband, and having the air-conditioning on. The consequences of her panic disorder with agoraphobia affect her family: Julie's husband is concerned and supportive, but her mother thinks she should pull herself together because "it's all in her head." In addition, Julie works but has cut back the number of hours, and she travels and socializes much less. Her general mood includes some difficulty concentrating and sleeping, restlessness, headaches, and muscular pains and aches. In addition, she is occasionally tearful, sad, and hopeless, and generally feels down.

COMPONENTS OF COGNITIVE-BEHAVIORAL THERAPY

The components of the cognitive-behavioral treatment described in this section are integrated into a session-by-session treatment program in the next section.

Education

The treatment begins with education about the nature of panic disorder, the causes of panic and anxiety, and the ways panic and anxiety are perpetuated by feedback loops among physical, cognitive, and behavioral response systems. In addition, specific descriptions of the psychophysiology of the fight–flight response are provided, as well as an explanation of the adaptive value of the various physiological changes that occur during panic and anxiety. The purpose of this education is to correct the common myths and misconceptions about panic symptoms (i.e., beliefs about going crazy, dying, or losing control) that contribute to panic and anxiety. The survival value of alarm reactions (i.e., panic attacks) is emphasized throughout.

Education also distinguishes between the state of anxiety and the emotion of fear/panic, both conceptually and in terms of its three response modes (subjective, physiological, and behavioral). This distinction is central to the model of panic disorder and to the remainder of the treatment. Anxiety is viewed as a state of preparation for future threat, whereas panic is the fight–flight emotion elicited by imminent threat. Panic/fear is characterized by perceptions of imminent threat, sudden autonomic discharge, and fight–flight behavior. In contrast, anxiety is characterized by perceptions of future threat and chronic tension, cautiousness, avoidance, and disruption of performance.

Self-Monitoring

Self-monitoring is essential to the personal scientist model of cognitive-behavioral therapy. Self-monitoring is introduced as a way to enhance objective self-awareness and increase accuracy in self-observation. As noted earlier, patients are asked to keep at least two types of records. The first, the Panic Attack Record, is completed as soon after each panic attack as possible; this record provides a description of cues, maximal distress, symptoms, thoughts, and behaviors. The second, the Daily Mood Record, is completed at the end of each day to record overall or average levels of anxiety, de-pression, and whatever else is considered important to record. Additionally, patients may keep a daily record of activities or situations completed or avoided.

Breathing Retraining and Capnometry-Assisted Respiratory Training

Breathing retraining is a central component early on in the development of panic control treatments because many panic patients describe symptoms of hyperventilation as being very similar to their panic attack symptoms. It is noteworthy, however, that a hyperventilation symptom report does not always accurately represent hyperventilation physiology: Only 50% or fewer patients show actual reductions in end-tidal CO_2 values during panic attacks (Hibbert & Pilsbury, 1989; Holt & Andrews, 1989; Hornsveld, Garssen, Fiedelij Dop, & van Spiegel, 1990).

In early conceptualizations, panic attacks were related to stress-induced respiratory changes that provoke fear either because they are perceived as threatening or they augment fear already elicited by other phobic stimuli (Clark, Salkovskis, & Chalkley, 1985). Several studies illustrated a positive effect of breathing retraining, involving slow abdominal breathing exercises (e.g., Kraft & Hoogduin, 1984). The value of breathing retraining was subsequently questioned. For example, several studies suggested that the addition of breathing retraining alone did not improve on *in vivo* exposure (e.g., de Beurs, van Balkom, Lange, Koele, & van Dyck, 1995). We found breathing retraining to be slightly less effective than interoceptive exposure when each was added to cognitive restructuring and *in vivo* exposure (Craske, Rowe, Lewin, & Noriega-Dimitri, 1997), and in another study, the inclusion of breathing retraining resulted in poorer outcomes than cognitive-behavioral therapy without breathing retraining, although the findings were not robust (Schmidt et al., 2000). From their review of efficacy and mechanisms of action, Garssen, de Ruiter, and van Dyck (1992) concluded that breathing retraining probably effects change not through breathing per se but through distraction and/or a sense of control. Thus, breathing retraining is no longer considered a central component of cognitive-behavioral therapy for panic disorder. Furthermore, to the extent that it might become misused as a means for avoiding physical symptoms, it may even be countertherapeutic. That being said, there may be occasions when breathing retraining is a useful tool, such as for the individual showing obvious signs of irregular breathing (e.g., rapid, shallow breathing, frequent deep breaths), as long as breathing retraining does not become a method of avoidance or safety seeking.

In contrast to traditional breathing retraining, capnometry-assisted respiratory training (CART) targets respiratory dysregulation, in particular hypocapnia (Meuret, Rosenfield, Seidel, Bhaskara, & Hofmann, 2010; Meuret, Wilhelm, Ritz, & Roth, 2008). CART is a brief, 4-week training that uses immediate feedback of end-tidal partial pressure CO_2 (pCO_2) to teach patients how to raise their subnormal levels of pCO_2 (hyperventilation) and thereby gain control over dysfunctional respiratory patterns and associated panic symptoms (e.g., shortness of breath, dizziness). The device, a portable capnometer, offers breath-by-breath feedback of expired CO_2 and rate of breathing (both measured via a nasal canula). Due to the novelty of CART, randomized controlled trials are limited but promising. In a first randomized-controlled study, Meuret and colleagues (2008) tested the efficacy of 4 weeks of CART ($N = 20$) compared to a delayed wait-list control group (WL, $N = 17$). CART, but not WL, led to sustained increases in pCO2 levels and reduced panic severity and frequency. Reductions in panic symptom severity (PDSS; Shear et al., 1997) were comparable to standard cognitive-behavioral therapy, and improvements were maintained at 12-month follow-up. In a second study, patients with panic disorder were randomly assigned to receive either 4 weeks of CART ($N = 21$) or cognitive therapy ($N = 20$). An initial 4 weeks of skills training was followed by three sessions of *in vivo* exposure and a fourth session at a 2-months follow-up. Respective skills acquisition trainings led to significant and comparable reductions in panic symptom severity and panic-related cognitions, irrespective of modality. However, only CART, not cognitive therapy, led to a correction of hypocapnic levels of pCO_2 (Meuret et al., 2010; Seidel, Rosenfield, Bhaskara, Hofmann, & Meuret, 2009). However, an evaluation of the degree to which CART augments exposure therapy (relative to exposure therapy alone) awaits testing.

Applied Relaxation

A form of relaxation known as applied relaxation has shown good results as a treatment for panic attacks. Two studies by Öst (Öst & Westling, 1995; Öst, Westling, & Hellström, 1993) indicate that applied relaxation is as effective as *in vivo* exposure and cognitive therapy. In contrast, Barlow and colleagues (1989) found that applied progressive muscle relaxation (PMR) is relatively ineffective for panic attacks, although we excluded all forms of interoceptive exposure from the hierarchy of tasks to which PMR was applied, which was not necessarily the case in the studies by Öst. Clark and colleagues (1994) found cognitive therapy to be superior to applied PMR when conducted with equal amounts of *in vivo* exposure, whereas Beck, Stanley, Baldwin, Deagle, and Averill (1994) found very few differences between cognitive therapy and PMR when each was administered without exposure procedures.

Cognitive Restructuring

Cognitive restructuring is a skills set in which patients learn to recognize cognitive errors and generate alternative, noncatastrophic explanations for the sensations that are feared during panic attacks. Cognitive therapy begins with a treatment rationale and discussion of the role of thoughts in generating emotions. Next, thoughts are recognized as hypotheses rather than as fact, and are therefore open to being questioned and challenged. Detailed self-monitoring of emotions and associated cognitions is instituted to identify specific beliefs, appraisals, and assumptions. Once identified, relevant cognitions are categorized into types of typical errors that occur during heightened emotion, such as overestimations of risk of negative events or catastrophization of meaning of events. The process of categorization, or labeling of thoughts, is consistent with a personal scientist model and facilitates an objective perspective by which the validity of the thoughts can be evaluated. Thus, in labeling the type of cognitive distortion, the patient is encouraged to use an empirical approach to examine the validity of his or her thoughts by considering all of the available evidence. Therapists use Socratic questioning to help patients make guided discoveries and question their anxious thoughts. Next, more evidence-based alternative hypotheses are generated. In addition to surface-level appraisals (e.g., "That person is frowning at me because I look foolish"), core-level beliefs or schemas (e.g., "I am not strong enough to withstand further distress" or "I am unlikable") are questioned in the same way. Importantly, cognitive restructuring is not intended as a direct means of minimizing fear, anxiety, or unpleasant symptoms. Instead, cognitive restructuring is intended to correct distorted thinking; eventually fear and anxiety are expected to subside, but their diminution is not the first goal of cognitive therapy.

Cognitive therapy is often intermingled with behavioral techniques (e.g., "behavioral experiments," "hypothesis testing," "instructions" involving exposure) that complicate direct testing of the efficacy of cognitive therapy in its "pure" form (e.g., Hoffart, Sexton, Hedley, & Martinsen, 2008; Hofmann et al., 2007; Öst et al., 1993; Teachman, Marker, & Smith-Janik, 2008). Nonetheless, there is some evidence that training in cognitive procedures in full isolation from exposure and behavioral procedures is efficacious in reducing aspects of panic (Beck et al., 1994; Meuret et al., 2010; Salkovskis, Clark, & Hackmann, 1991; van den Hout, Arntz, & Hoekstra, 1994). Similarly, in a study by Bouchard and colleagues (1996), cognitive restructuring was as effective as exposure therapy in reducing panic symptoms. However, the effects of cognitive therapy alone on agoraphobia are unclear. One study found that cognitive therapy was less effective than exposure therapy for agoraphobia (Williams & Falbo, 1996). Another study (Hoffart, 1995) found that cognitive therapy was as effective as guided mastery exposure delivered intensively over 6 weeks for individuals with moderate to severe agoraphobia, although some elements of exposure (e.g., hyperventilation tests to elicit sensations) were included in the cognitive therapy condition.

A few studies have evaluated the effects of cognitive therapy combined with exposure in comparison to exposure alone or in combination with other coping skills. Most often, cognitive therapy combined with exposure does not yield an additional benefit over *in vivo* exposure alone (Öst, Thulin, & Ramnero, 2004; van den Hout et al., 1994; see Murphy et al., 1998, for an exception).

Exposure

Exposure is a critical phase of treatment and, once begun, is a major focus of treatment sessions as well as between-treatment session homework, since limited exposure practice is of small benefit and may even be detrimental. The exposure is designed to disconfirm misappraisals and extinguish conditional emotional responses to external situations and contexts, through *in vivo* exposure, as well as to bodily sensations, through interoceptive exposure. Growing evidence suggests that exposure represents the most powerful component of cognitive-behavioral therapy for panic disorder and agoraphobia, including meta-analyses that fail to show any additional benefit of either cognitive restructuring or somatic coping skills beyond exposure therapy alone

(Norton & Price, 2007). A large trial reported a dose–response relationship between exposure and improvement in agoraphobia (Gloster et al., 2011).

In Vivo *Exposure*

In vivo exposure refers to repeated and systematic, real-life exposure, in this case, to agoraphobic situations. A long history of research has established the efficacy of *in vivo* exposure for agoraphobia.

Most often, *in vivo* exposure is conducted in a graduated manner, proceeding from the least to the most anxiety-provoking situations on an avoidance hierarchy. However, there is some evidence to suggest that intensive or ungraduated exposure may be effective. In a study by Feigenbaum (1988), treatment sessions were conducted in a massed format over the course of 6–10 consecutive days. One group received ungraded exposure ($N = 25$), beginning with the most feared items from avoidance hierarchies. Another group received graded exposure ($N = 23$), beginning with the least feared hierarchy items. Approximately one-third of this severely agoraphobic sample was housebound at initial assessment. At posttreatment and 8 months later, the conditions proved to be equally effective (although, intriguingly, the graded group reported the treatment to be more distressing). However, ungraded exposure was clearly superior at the 5-year follow-up assessment: 76% of the intensive group versus 35% of the graded group reported themselves to be completely free of symptoms. When 104 subjects were added to the intensive exposure format, the same results were obtained. Of 129 subjects, 78% were reportedly completely symptom-free 5 years later. This dramatic set of results suggests that an intensive approach, which is likely to produce higher levels of arousal than a graduated approach, can be very beneficial (at least when conducted in a massed format). Unfortunately, the validity of the outcome measures in this study is somewhat questionable, and replication by independent investigators has yet to be reported.

The amount of time devoted to *in vivo* exposure is very dependent on the patient's agoraphobia profile. Obviously, more time is needed for patients with more severe agoraphobia.

Interoceptive Exposure

In interoceptive exposure, the goal is deliberately to induce feared physical sensations a sufficient number of times, and long enough each time, so that misappraisals about the sensations are disconfirmed and conditional anxiety responses are extinguished. A standard list of exercises, such as hyperventilating and spinning, is used to establish a hierarchy of interoceptive exposures. With a graduated approach, exposure begins with the less distressing physical exercises and continues with the more distressing exercises. It is essential that the patient endure the sensations beyond the point at which they are first noticed, for at least 30 seconds to 1 minute, because early termination of the task may eliminate the opportunity to learn that the sensations are not harmful and that the anxiety can be tolerated. The exercise is followed by a discussion of what the patient learned about the physical sensations. These interoceptive exercises are practiced daily outside of the therapy session to consolidate the process of learning. Interoceptive exposure extends to naturalistic activities that induce somatic sensations (e.g., caffeine consumption, exercise).

A series of studies reported on the effects of interoceptive exposure independent of other therapeutic strategies. Early on, Bonn, Harrison, and Rees (1971) and Haslam (1974) observed successful reduction in reactivity with repeated infusions of sodium lactate (a drug that produces panic-type bodily sensations). However, panic was not monitored in these investigations. Griez and van den Hout (1986) compared six sessions of graduated CO_2 inhalations to a treatment regimen of propranolol (a beta-blocker chosen because it suppresses symptoms induced by CO_2 inhalations), both conducted over the course of 2 weeks. CO_2 inhalation treatment resulted in a mean reduction from 12 to four panic attacks, which was superior to the results from propranolol. In addition, inhalation treatment resulted in significantly greater reductions in reported fear of sensations. A 6-month follow-up assessment suggested maintenance of treatment gains, although panic frequency was not reported. Beck and Shipherd (1997) similarly found a positive effect from repeated CO_2 inhalations, although it had little effect on agoraphobia (Beck, Shipherd, & Zebb, 1997). Broocks and colleagues (1998) tested the effects of exercise (with once-weekly supportive contact from a therapist) in comparison to clomipramine or drug placebo over 10 weeks. The exercise group was trained to run 4 miles, three times per week. Despite high attrition from exercise (31%), exercise was more effective than the drug placebo condition. However, clomipramine was superior to exercise.

In the first comparison to other cognitive and behavioral treatments, Barlow and colleagues (1989) compared applied PMR, interoceptive exposure plus breathing retraining and cognitive restructuring, their combination with applied PMR, and a waiting-list control, in a sample with panic disorder with limited agoraphobia. The two conditions involving interoceptive exposure, breathing retraining and cognitive restructuring, were significantly superior to applied PMR and wait-list conditions. The results were maintained 24 months following treatment completion for the group receiving interoceptive exposure, breathing retraining, and cognitive restructuring without PMR, whereas the combined group tended to deteriorate over follow-up (Craske, Brown, & Barlow, 1991). As already mentioned, we compared interoceptive exposure, cognitive therapy, and *in vivo* exposure to breathing retraining, cognitive therapy, and *in vivo* exposure for individuals with varying levels of agoraphobia. The condition that included interoceptive exposure was slightly superior to breathing retraining at posttreatment and 6 months later (Craske et al., 1997). Similarly, Ito, Noshirvani, Basoglu, and Marks (1996) found a trend for those who added interoceptive exposure to their self-directed *in vivo* exposure and breathing retraining to be more likely to achieve at least a 50% improvement in phobic fear and avoidance. However, the combination of breathing education, breathing retraining, and repeated interoceptive exposure to hyperventilation did not increase the effectiveness of *in vivo* exposure for agoraphobia (de Beurs, Lang, van Dyck, & Koele, 1995).

Interoceptive exposure is now a standard component of cognitive-behavioral therapy for panic disorder (e.g., Barlow et al., 2000; Craske, Lang, Aikins, & Mystkowski, 2005), although different groups give different emphases to interoceptive exposure, with some emphasizing it as a means for extinguishing fear responses (Barlow & Craske, 2006) and others, as a vehicle for disconfirming misappraisals (Clark, 1996).

Optimizing Learning during Exposure

Our understanding of the mechanisms of exposure therapy has evolved over time. One of the most influential theories is emotional processing theory, which emphasized habituation of fear responding within an exposure trial as a necessary precursor to habituation across treatment sessions, that in turn leads to long-term corrective learning (Foa & Kozak, 1986; Foa & McNally, 1996). Most recently, we have emphasized optimizing inhibitory learning and its retrieval in ways that are not necessarily dependent on reductions in fear throughout trials of exposure (Craske et al., 2008); we discuss this approach below.

Emotional processing theory emphasizes mechanisms of habituation as precursors to cognitive correction. Specifically, emotional processing theory purports that the effects of exposure therapy derive from activation of a "fear structure" and integration of information that is incompatible with it, resulting in the development of a non-fear structure that replaces or competes with the original one. Incompatible information derives first from within-session habituation, or reduction in fear responding with prolonged exposure to the fear stimulus. Within-session habituation is seen as a prerequisite for the second piece of incompatible information, which derives from between-session habituation over repeated occasions of exposure. Between-session habituation is purported to form the basis for long-term learning and to be mediated by changes in "meaning," or lowered probability of harm (i.e., risk) and lessened negativity (i.e., valence) of the stimulus. Emotional processing theory guides clinicians to focus on the initial elevation of fear followed by within- and between-session reductions in fear as signs of treatment success. Although enticing in its face validity, support for the theory has been inconsistent at best (Craske et al., 2008; Craske, Liao, Brown, & Vervliet, 2012). Rather, the evidence suggests that the amount by which fear habituates from the beginning to the end of an exposure practice is not a good predictor of overall outcomes, and that evidence for between-session habituation is mixed (Craske et al., 2008, 2012).

A return to the science of fear learning and extinction may help to explain the effects of exposure therapy and thereby optimize its implementation. It is now thought that inhibitory learning is central to extinction (Bouton, 1993). Inhibitory pathways are also recognized in the neurobiology of fear extinction (see Sotres-Bayon, Cain, & LeDoux, 2006). Within a Pavlovian conditioning approach, inhibitory learning means that the original conditioned stimulus–unconditioned stimulus (CS-US) association learned during fear conditioning is not erased during extinction, but rather is left intact as a new, secondary learning about the CS-US develops (Bouton, 1993). The degree to which inhibitory associations shape fear responding at retest (the index of strength and stability of new "learning") is independent of fear levels expressed throughout extinction and instead is dependent on factors such as context and time.

Based on the inhibitory retrieval model of extinction, outcomes may be enhanced by strategies that do not rely on fear reduction within a trial of exposure (Craske et al., 2008, 2012). Indeed, fear reduction may become a safety behavior for persons with panic disorder (since fear reduction eradicates the very thing that is feared), such that a more appropriate goal may be to maintain high levels of fear and anxiety in order to disconfirm the expectancy of negative consequences. One translational possibility is "deepened extinction" (Rescorla, 2006), in which multiple fear conditional stimuli are first extinguished separately before being combined during extinction, and in animal studies, decrease spontaneous recovery and reinstatement of fear. Indeed, this is what is essentially done when interoceptive exposure is conducted in feared agoraphobic situations (Barlow & Craske, 1994) and recent experimental data supports the beneficial effects of deepened extinction in human conditioning studies (Culver, Vervliet, & Craske, in press).

In addition, the effects of exposure therapy may be enhanced by the prevention or removal of "safety signals" or "safety behaviors." Common safety signals and behaviors for clients with panic disorder are the presence of another person, therapists, medications, or food or drink. In the experimental literature, safety signals alleviate distress in the short term, but when they are no longer present, the fear returns (Lovibond, Davis, & O'Flaherty, 2000), an effect that may derive in part from interference with the development of inhibitory associations. In phobic samples, the availability and use of safety signals and behaviors has been shown to be detrimental to exposure therapy (Sloan & Telch, 2002), whereas instructions to refrain from using safety behaviors improved outcomes (Salkovskis, 1991). Similarly, the use of safety signals was associated with poorer outcomes for panic (Helbig-Lang & Petermann, 2010). However, recent data have presented contradictory findings (Rachman, Shafran, Radomsky, & Zysk, 2011).

Further options include stimulus variability throughout exposure, since variability has been shown to enhance the storage capacity of newly learned information. Two studies with clinical analogues have demonstrated positive benefits in terms of spontaneous recovery (Lang & Craske, 2000; Rowe & Craske, 1998), while a third showed trends only (Kircanski et al., 2011). In the treatment for panic disorder with agoraphobia, this implies conducting exposure for varying durations, at varying levels of intensity, rather than continuing exposure in one situation until fear declines before moving to the next situation. Notably, such variability typically elicits higher levels of anxiety during exposure, but without detrimental effects and sometimes with beneficial effects in the long term.

Based on evidence for fear extinction to be weakened by antagonists of the glutamate receptors in the amygdala, Walker and Davis (2002) tested and demonstrated that drug agonists of the same receptors, and in particular, D-cycloserine, enhance extinction in animal studies. In a meta-analysis of the efficacy of D-cycloserine for anxiety disorders, Norberg, Krystal, and Tolin (2008) reported effect sizes of $d = 0.60$ at posttreatment and 0.47 at follow-up in clinical anxiety samples. D-Cycloserine in combination with interoceptive exposure for panic clients has resulted in a greater reduction in symptom severity, and a greater likelihood of achieving a change in clinical status at posttreatment and 1-month follow-up compared to exposure plus placebo (Otto et al., 2010). Notably, D-cycloserine has been shown to have positive effects without influencing the level of fear during exposure per se.

A number of options for enhancing retrieval of the extinction memory have been tested. One option during extinction training is to include retrieval cues to be used in other contexts once extinction is over. This has been shown to be effective in animal studies and human conditioning studies (see Craske et al., 2012, for a review). In clinical analogue samples, the effects of a retrieval cue upon context renewal were very weak in one study (Culver et al., 2012), although instructions to reinstate what was learned mentally during exposure had more robust effects in reducing context renewal in another study (Mystkowski, Craske, Echiverri, & Labus, 2006). In the treatment of panic disorder, this approach simply suggests that clients carry with them cues (e.g., wristband) to remind them what they learned during exposure therapy (as long as the cues do not become safety signals), or are prompted to remind themselves of what they learned in exposure therapy each time they experience previously feared sensations or situations.

Another option is to provide multiple contexts in which extinction takes place. This approach has been shown to offset context renewal in rodent samples, and in a clinical analogue study of exposure therapy (Vansteenwegen et al., 2007) although the results are not always consistent (Neumann, Lipp & Cory, 2007). In the treatment of panic disorder and agoraphobia, this would mean asking clients to conduct their interoceptive and *in vivo* exposures in multiple different contexts,

such as when alone, in unfamiliar places, or at varying times of day or varying days of the week.

A recent (re-)discovery is that retrieving already stored memories induces a process of reconsolidation (Nader, Schafe, & Le Doux, 2000), since the memory is written into long-term memory again, requiring de novo neurochemical processes. Thus, it may be possible to change memories during the reconsolidation time frame upon retrieval. Propranolol, a beta-blocker, has been shown to block the reconsolidation of memories, and Debiec and Le Doux (2004) found that infusions of propranaolol blocked the reconsolidation of a previously formed CS-US memory, and led to erasure of the fear response and resistance to reinstatement effects. This suggests that propranolol upon retrieval may be a useful clinical tool, and indeed, two fear conditioning studies in healthy humans (Kindt, Soeter, & Vervliet, 2009; Soeter & Kindt, 2010) have replicated the effects. However, the effects have not been tested in the context of exposure therapy for panic disorder.

Role of Acceptance during Exposure

Cognitive and somatic coping skills are central to cognitive-behavioral therapy and are taught to facilitate and improve exposure therapy. Newer approaches that explore acceptance and cognitive defusion (e.g., acceptance and commitment therapy; Hayes, Strosahl, & Wilson, 1999) have been gaining interest, especially given evidence that experiential avoidance is a correlate of anxious psychopathology and acceptance increases willingness to experience and lessens emotional distress over induced anxiety symptoms in individuals with panic disorder (e.g., Campbell-Sills et al., 2006; Eifert & Heffner, 2003), including CO_2 inhalation challenges (Levitt et al., 2004). Interestingly, the acceptance approach is entirely consistent with our formulation of interoceptive exposure, in which patients are encouraged to experience the feared physical sensations without any attempt to lessen them or to think differently about them in the moment of exposure. We recently extended this model of acceptance during interoceptive exposure to acceptance during *in vivo* exposure in an open trial of 11 patients with panic disorder (Meuret, Twohig, Rosenfield, Hayes, & Craske, 2012). In general, the exposures were an opportunity for patients to behave *with* their panic-related thoughts, feelings, and bodily sensations; in other words, patients were encouraged to realize that they can drive for and reach life goals, even in the presence of unpleasant inner experiences. To that end, it was explicitly stated that the level of anxiety or fear was not the determining factor. Rather, it was explained that "willingness can do surprising things to one's inner experiences. If one is willing to experience anxiety it may or may not show up. Thus, we are not going to judge the success of these exposures on how high the anxiety gets, but instead in how open you are to what might show up." To plan effectively for interoceptive (i.e., eliciting panic sensations such as a racing heart or shortness of breath) and *in vivo* exposures (i.e., seeking places and situations that one previously avoided because of the fear of panic sensations), a hierarchy of least to most anxiety-provoking items was created. Movement up the hierarchy was not based on reductions in anxiety at the preceding step but high willingness to experience panic-related inner experiences. During the exposures, patients were encouraged to maintain an open, nonjudgmental stance toward whatever thoughts, feelings, and bodily sensations arose in a given moment, experiencing them for what they were, and moving toward them while anxious. Treatment was associated with clinically significant improvements in panic symptom severity, willingness to allow inner experiences to occur, and reductions in avoidant behavior. In another study of a mixed anxiety disorder sample, we found very few differences in outcome between acceptance and commitment therapy (Hayes et al., 1999) and cognitive-behavioral therapy, although the treatments were matched on amount of time spent on exposure therapy, albeit framed differently within for each condition (Arch et al., 2012). Thus, the data to date suggest that both a cognitive therapy coping approach and an acceptance-based exposure approach are effective.

OVERALL EFFICACY OF COGNITIVE-BEHAVIORAL THERAPY

An extensive body of research has evaluated the efficacy of cognitive-behavioral therapy for panic disorder and agoraphobia. Cognitive-behavioral therapy, involving most or all of the components just listed, yields panic-free rates in the range of 70–80% and high end-state rates (i.e., within normative ranges of functioning) in the range of 50–70% for panic disorder with minimal agoraphobia (e.g., Barlow et al., 1989; Clark et al., 1994). Although agoraphobic avoidance is sometimes associated with less positive response (e.g., Dow et al., 2007), the overall within-group effect size for change in panic disorder and agoraphobia from pre- to post-

treatment is very large (e.g., effect size = 1.53; Norton & Price, 2007). Moreover, the between-group effect size is substantial in comparison to wait-list conditions (e.g., effect size = 0.64; Haby, Donnelly, Corry, & Vos, 2006). However, more research is needed comparing cognitive-behavioral therapy to alternative active treatment conditions.

The effectiveness extends to clients who experience nocturnal panic attacks (Craske, Lang, et al., 2005). Furthermore, cognitive-behavioral therapy results in improvements in rates of comorbid anxiety and mood disorders (e.g., Craske et al., 2007; Tsao, Mystkowksi, Zucker, & Craske, 2005), although one study suggested that the benefits for comorbid conditions may lessen over time, when assessed 2 years later (Brown et al., 1995). Finally, applications of cognitive-behavioral therapy lower relapse rates upon discontinuation of high-potency benzodiazepines (e.g., Spiegel, Bruce, Gregg, & Nuzzarello, 1994). The effects of cognitive-behavioral therapy are sustained over time, as meta-analyses show little change (i.e., maintenance of treatment effects) from posttreatment to follow-up (effect size = 0.12; Norton & Price, 2007). From their review of meta-analyses for cognitive behavioral therapy across all disorders, Butler, Chapman, Forman, and Beck (2006) concluded that evidence for maintenance of treatment gains was particularly strong for panic disorder, where the rate of relapse was almost half the rate of relapse following pharmacotherapy. Continuing improvement after acute treatment is facilitated by involvement of significant others in every aspect of treatment for agoraphobia (e.g., Cerny et al., 1987). Also, booster sessions enhance long-term outcomes (Craske et al., 2006).

Efficacy data from research settings are now being complemented by effectiveness data from real-world, primary care settings. In a randomized controlled trial in primary care settings with novice therapists, cognitive-behavioral therapy combined with expert recommendations for medication regimens was more effective than treatment as usual (Roy-Byrne, Craske, et al., 2005). The effects appeared primarily to be due to cognitive-behavioral therapy rather than mediation (Craske, Golinelli, et al., 2005). In the more recent CALM study (Craske et al., 2011), the effectiveness of cognitive-behavioral therapy for panic disorder in primary care settings was demonstrated in the hands of nonexperienced therapists with the aid of a computerized guide, combined with expert recommendations for medication, relative to treatment as usual.

Even though cognitive-behavioral therapy for panic disorder and agoraphobia is efficacious and effective, there is room for improvement. One study estimated that 30% of clients continue to function poorly at follow-up and only 48% reached high end-state status (Brown & Barlow, 1995). In a landmark study (Barlow et al., 2000), only 32% of clients with panic disorder assigned to cognitive-behavioral therapy alone demonstrated strong treatment response 12 months after acute treatment. Finally, of those who do start treatment, the mean dropout rate is 19%, with a range of 0–54% (Haby et al., 2006).

TREATMENT DESCRIPTION: PROTOCOL

What follows is a description of a 12-session cognitive-behavioral therapy for panic disorder and agoraphobia tailored to Julie's presentation. Of course, the degree to which the various components of treatment are emphasized vary by the functional assessment conducted for each patient.

Overview

The basic aim of the treatment protocol is to influence directly the catastrophic misappraisals and avoidance of bodily sensations and agoraphobic situations. This is done first through the provision of accurate information as to the nature of the fight–flight response. By provision of such information, patients are taught that they experience sensations that are normal and harmless. Second, treatment aims to teach a set of skills for developing evidence-based appraisals regarding bodily sensations and agoraphobic situations. At the same time, specific information concerning the effects of hyperventilation and its role in panic attacks is provided, with practice of breathing retraining if deemed appropriate. Then, the crux of the treatment involves repeated exposure to feared internal cues and agoraphobic situations.

Session 1

The goals of Session 1 are to describe fear and anxiety; to help patients understand the cyclical influences among behavioral, physiological, and cognitive responses; to understand that panic attack symptoms are not harmful; and to begin self-monitoring, if it was not already begun with the initial assessment. Therapy begins with identifying anxiety patterns and the situa-

tions in which anxiety and panic attacks are likely to occur. Many patients have difficulty identifying specific antecedents, reporting that panic can occur at almost any time. Therapists help patients to identify internal triggers, specifically, negative verbal cognitions, catastrophic imagery, and physical sensations. The following interchange took place for Julie:

THERAPIST: In what situations are you most likely to panic?

JULIE: Crowded restaurants and when I'm driving on the freeway. But sometimes I am driving along, feeling OK, when all of a sudden it hits. And other times I can be sitting at home feeling quite relaxed and it just hits. That's when I really get scared because I can't explain it.

THERAPIST: So, when you are driving on the freeway, what is the very first thing you notice that tells you you're about to panic?

JULIE: Well, the other cars on the road look as if they are moving really slowly . . . it's as if I am in a dream.

THERAPIST: And what is the first thing you notice when you're at home?

JULIE: An unreal feeling, like I'm floating.

THERAPIST: So, what does that tell you? What is the common factor that started these two panic attacks?

JULIE: The feeling as if things are unreal? Wow, I always thought the physical feelings were the panic attack, but maybe they start the panic attack.

Next, the three-response system model for describing and understanding anxiety and panic is introduced. This model contributes to an objective self-awareness—to becoming a personal scientist—and provides the groundwork for an alternative conceptual framework for explaining panic and anxiety that replaces the patient's own misassumptions. Patients are asked to describe cognitive, physiological, and behavioral aspects to their responding: to identify the things that they *feel, think,* and *do* when they are anxious and panicky. As described earlier, differences between the response profiles of anxiety and panic are highlighted. After grasping the notion of three responses that are partially independent, interactions among the response systems are described. The patient is asked to describe the three-response system components in a recent panic attack and to identify ways in which they interacted to produce heightened distress. For example,

THERAPIST: How would you describe the three parts to the panic attack you had at home last week?

JULIE: Well, physically, my head felt really light, and my hands were clammy. I thought that I would either pass out or that I would somehow dissolve into nothingness. My behavior was to lie down and phone my husband.

THERAPIST: Ok that's a great description of your thoughts, physical feelings, and behaviors. Now let's look at the sequence of events. What was the very first thing you noticed?

JULIE: When I stood up, my head started to feel really weird, as if it was spinning inside.

THERAPIST: What was your very next reaction to that feeling?

JULIE: I held onto the chair. I thought something was wrong. I thought it could get worse and that I'd collapse.

THERAPIST: So it began with a physical sensation, and then you had some very specific thoughts about those sensations. What happened next?

JULIE: I felt very anxious.

THERAPIST: And what happened next?

JULIE: Well, the dizziness seemed to be getting worse and worse. I became really concerned that it was different from any other experience I had ever had. I was convinced that this was "it."

THERAPIST: So, as you became more anxious, the physical feelings and the thoughts that something bad was going to happen intensified. What did you do next?

JULIE: I called my husband and lay on the bed until he came home. It was horrible.

THERAPIST: Can you see how one thing fed off another, creating a cycle? That it began with a sensation, then some anxious thoughts, then feeling anxious, then more sensations and more thoughts, and more fear, and so on?

Next, the reasons why panic attacks first began are addressed briefly. Patients are informed that it is not necessary to understand the reasons why they began to panic to benefit from the treatment because factors involved in onset are not necessarily the same as the factors involved in the maintenance of a problem. Nev-

ertheless, the initial panic attack is described as a manifestation of anxiety/stress. The stressors surrounding the time of the first panic attack are explored with the patient, particularly in terms of how stressors may have increased levels of physical arousal and primed certain danger-laden cognitive schemas.

Also, the therapist briefly describes the physiology underlying anxiety and panic, and the myths about what the physical sensations might mean. The main concepts covered in this educational phase are (1) the survival value or protective function of anxiety and panic; (2) the physiological basis to the various sensations experienced during panic and anxiety, and the survival function of the underlying physiology; and (3) the role of specific learned and cognitively mediated fears of certain bodily sensations. The model of panic we described earlier in this chapter is explained. In particular, the concepts of misappraisals and interoceptive conditioning are explained as accounting for panic attacks that seem to occur from out of the blue—that are triggered by very subtle internal cues or physical sensations that may occur at any time. Not only does this information reduce anxiety by decreasing uncertainty about panic attacks but it also enhances the credibility of the subsequent treatment procedures. This information is detailed in a handout given to the patient to read over the next week (for the handout, see Barlow & Craske, 2006).

This information was very important for Julie because the inability to explain her panic attacks was a major source of distress. Here are some of the questions she asked in her attempt to understand more fully:

JULIE: So, if I understand you correctly, you're saying that my panic attacks are the same as the fear I experienced the time we found a burglar in our house. It doesn't feel the same at all.

THERAPIST: Yes, those two emotional states—an unexpected panic attack and fear when confronted with a burglar—are essentially the same. However, in the case of the burglar, where were you focusing your attention—on the burglar or on the way you were feeling?

JULIE: The burglar, of course, although I did notice my heart was going a mile a minute.

THERAPIST: And when you have a panic attack, where are you focusing your attention—on the people around you or on the way you are feeling?

JULIE: Well, mostly on the way I'm feeling, although it depends on where I am at the time.

THERAPIST: Being most concerned about what's going on inside can lead to a very different type of experience than being concerned about the burglar, even though basically the same physiological response is occurring. For example, remember our description of the way fear of sensations can intensify the sensations.

JULIE: I get that. But what about the feelings of unreality? How can they be protective or how can feeling unreal help me deal with a dangerous situation?

THERAPIST: OK, remember that it's the physiological events that are protective—not the sensations. The sensations are just the end result of those events. Now, feelings of unreality can be caused by changes in your blood flow to your brain (although not dangerously so), or from overbreathing, or from concentrating too intensely on what's going on inside you. So the unreality sensation may not be protective, but the changes in blood flow and overbreathing are.

JULIE: I understand how I can create a panic attack by being afraid of my physical feelings, like my heart racing or feeling unreal. But sometimes it happens so quickly that I don't have time to think.

THERAPIST: Yes, these reactions can occur very quickly, at times automatically. But remember, we are tuned to react instantaneously to things that we believe to be dangerous. Imagine yourself walking through a dark alley, and you have reason to believe that somewhere in the darkness lurks a killer. Under those conditions, you would be extremely attentive to any sign, any sound, or any sight of another person. If you were walking through the same alley and were sure there were no killers, you might not hear or detect the same signals you picked up on in the first case. Now let's translate this to panic; the killer in the dark alley is the panic attack, and the signs, sounds, and smells are the physical sensations you think signal the possibility of a panic attack. Given the acute degree of sensitivity to physical symptoms that signal a panic attack, it is likely that you are noticing normal "noises" in your body that you would otherwise not notice, and on occasion, immediately become fearful because of those "noises." In other words, the sensations are often noticeable because you attend to them.

Next, the method of self-monitoring was described and demonstrated with in-session practice of completing a Panic Attack Record. Julie was concerned that self-monitoring would only elevate her distress, by reminding of the very thing she was afraid of (panic and unreality). The therapist clarified the difference between objective and subjective self-monitoring, and explained that distress would subside as Julie persevered with self-monitoring.

The homework for this session was to self-monitor panic attacks, daily anxiety, and mood, and to read the handout. In fact, we encourage patients to reread the handout several times, and to actively engage in the material by circling or marking the most personally relevant sections or areas in need of clarification, because effort enhances long-term retention of the material learned. Of course, for some patients, reading the material draws their attention to things they fear (just as with self-monitoring). In this case, therapists can discuss the role of avoidance, and how, with repeated readings, distress levels will most likely subside.

At the end of the session, Julie suddenly became highly anxious. She felt unable to tolerate either the treatment procedures or her anticipation of them. She became very agitated in the office and reported feelings of unreality. She opened the office door to find her husband, who was waiting outside. The therapist helped Julie understand how the cycle of panic had emerged just at that moment: (1) The trigger was the treatment description—having to face eventually feared sensations and situations; (2) this was anxiety producing because Julie believed that she could not cope with the treatment demands, that the treatment would cause her so much anxiety that she would "flip out" and lose touch with reality permanently, or that she would never improve because she could not tolerate the treatment; (3) the current anxiety in the office elicited sensations of unreality and a racing heart; (4) Julie began to worry that she might panic and lose touch with reality permanently within the next few minutes; (5) the more anxious Julie felt, and the stronger her attempts to escape and find safety, the stronger the physical sensations became; and (6) she felt some relief upon finding her husband because his presence reassured her that she would be safe. Julie was reassured that treatment would progress at a pace with which she was comfortable, but at the same time she was helped to understand that her acute distress about the feeling of unreality would be the precise target of this type of treatment, therefore attesting to the relevance of this treatment for her. She was also calmed by preliminary cognitive restructuring of the probability of permanently losing touch with reality. After a lengthy discussion, Julie became more receptive to treatment. A team approach to treatment planning and progress was agreed upon, so that Julie did not feel that she would be forced to do things she did not think she could do.

Session 2

The goals of this session are to begin the development of a hierarchy of agoraphobic situations and coping skills of breathing retraining and cognitive restructuring. The individualized hierarchy comprises situations that range from mild to moderate anxiety, all the way up to extreme anxiety. These situations become the basis of graduated *in vivo* exposure. Although *in vivo* exposure exercises are not scheduled to take place until Session 4, the hierarchy is introduced now, so that cognitive restructuring skills can be practiced in relation to each situation on the hierarchy before *in vivo* exposure begins. Moreover, the hierarchy will be refined as a result of the cognitive restructuring practice because the latter highlights specific features of agoraphobic situations that are most anxiety provoking.

Julie was asked to develop a hierarchy over the following week. She expressed some doubt that she would ever be able to accomplish any, let alone all, of the items on her hierarchy. The therapist helped Julie by asking her to think of any situation in her lifetime that used to be difficult but became easier with practice. Julie remembered how anxious she used to be when she first started working with customers at her husband's office—and how that discomfort subsided over time. This was used to help Julie realize that the same might happen with the situations listed on her hierarchy. Julie's final hierarchy comprised the following situations: driving home from work alone; sitting in a crowded movie theater; spending 2 hours alone at home during the day; being alone at home as day turned to night; driving on surface streets to her brother's house (10 miles) alone; driving two exits on Freeway 444, with her husband following in the car behind; driving two exits on Freeway 444, alone; driving four exits on Freeway 444; and driving on the freeway to her brother's house alone. Then, Julie was to repeat all of these tasks without taking Klonopin, and without knowing the location of her husband.

Breathing retraining also is begun in this session. Patients are asked to hyperventilate voluntarily by standing and breathing fast and deep, as if blowing up a balloon, for 1½ minutes. With prompting and encouragement from the therapist, patients can often complete the full 1½ minutes, after which time they are asked to sit, close their eyes, and breathe very slowly, pausing at the end of each breath, until the symptoms have abated. The experience is then discussed in terms of the degree to which it produced symptoms similar to those that occur naturally during anxiety or panic. Approximately 50–60% of patients report that the symptoms of hyperventilation are very similar to their panic attack symptoms. Often, however, similarity of the symptoms is confused with similarity of the anxiety. Because the exercise is conducted in a safe environment and the symptoms have an obvious cause, most patients rate the experience as less anxiety provoking than if the same symptoms had occurred naturally. This distinction is important to make because it demonstrates the significance of perceived safety for the degree of anxiety experienced. Julie rated the hyperventilation exercise as very anxiety provoking (8 on a 0- to 10-point scale), and rated the symptoms as being quite similar to her panic symptoms (6 on a 0- to 10-point scale). She terminated the task after approximately 40 seconds, in anticipation of experiencing a full-blown panic attack. The therapist and Julie discussed this experience in terms of the three response systems, and the role of misappraisals and interoceptive conditioning described during the previous session.

Then, Julie was briefly educated about the physiological basis to hyperventilation (see Barlow & Craske, 2006). As before, the goal of the didactic presentation was to allay misinterpretations of the dangers of overbreathing, and to provide a factual information base on which to draw when actively challenging misinterpretations. The educational content is tailored to the patient's own educational level and covered only to the degree that it is relevant to the patient.

In the next step, the therapist teaches breathing retraining, which begins by teaching patients to rely more on the diaphragm (abdomen) than on chest muscles. In addition, patients are instructed to concentrate on their breathing by counting on their inhalations and thinking the word "relax" on exhalations. (Slow breathing is introduced in Session 3.) Therapists model the suggested breathing patterns, then provide corrective feedback to patients while they practice in the office setting.

(Note that CART uses a different method of breathing retraining that is based on raising levels of CO_2 in the blood through biofeedback.)

Initial reactions to the breathing exercise may be negative for patients who are afraid of respiratory sensations because the exercise directs their attention to breathing. It also can be difficult for patients who are chronic overbreathers, and patients for whom any interruption of habitual breathing patterns initially increases respiratory symptomatology. In both cases, continued practice is advisable, with reassurance that sensations such as shortness of breath are not harmful. The goal is to use breathing skills training to encourage continued approach toward anxiety and anxiety-producing situations. On occasion, patients mistakenly view breathing retraining as a way of relieving themselves of terrifying symptoms, thus falling into the trap of fearing dire consequences should they not succeed in correcting their breathing. This is what happened for Julie:

JULIE: So, all I have to do is to slow down my breathing, then everything will be OK?

THERAPIST: Certainly, slowing down your breathing will help to decrease the physical symptoms that you feel, but I am not sure what you mean when you ask whether everything will be OK.

JULIE: That proper breathing will prevent me from losing touch with reality—that I won't disappear.

THERAPIST: Breathing retraining will help you to regulate your breathing, which may lessen your physical symptoms, including the sense of unreality. Your question, though, is the reason for our next treatment skill of changing your thinking, so you can learn that the sense of unreality is not a sign of actual loss of touch with reality and disappearance.

The homework is to practice diaphragmatic breathing for at least 10 minutes, two times a day in relaxing environments.

Therapists introduce in this session cognitive restructuring, by explaining that everyone has errors in thinking when anxious, thus helping the patient to expect his or her thinking to be distorted. Patients are informed that these distortions have an adaptive function: Chances of survival are greater if we perceive danger as probable and worthy of attention rather than minimize it. Therefore, anxiety leads us to judge threatening events as being more likely and more threatening

than they really are. However, the cognitive distortions are unnecessary because there is no real threat in the case of panic disorder.

Then, patients are taught to treat their thoughts as hypotheses or guesses rather than as facts. The notions of automatic thinking and discrete predictions are also explained, to emphasize the need to become an astute observer of one's own habitual self-statements in each situation. This leads to a "downward arrow technique" to identify specific predictions made at any given moment, as shown with Julie.

THERAPIST: What is it that scared you about feeling detached in the movie theater last night?

JULIE: It is just such a horrible feeling.

THERAPIST: What makes it so horrible?

JULIE: I can't tolerate it.

THERAPIST: What makes you think you cannot tolerate it? What is the feeling of detachment going to do to you that makes you think it is horrible and intolerable?

JULIE: It might become so intense that it overwhelms me.

THERAPIST: And if it overwhelms you, what would happen?

JULIE: I could become so distressed that I lose touch with reality.

THERAPIST: What would it mean if you lost touch with reality?

JULIE: That I would be in a different mind state forever—I would never come back to reality. That I would be so crazy that I would have to be carted out of the movie theater to a mental hospital and locked away forever.

Overly general self-statements, such as "I feel terrible—something bad could happen," are insufficient, nontherapeutic, and may serve to intensify anxiety by virtue of their global and nondirective nature. Instead, detail in thought content, such as "I am afraid that if I get too anxious while driving, then I'll lose control of the wheel and drive off the side of the road and die," permits subsequent cognitive restructuring.

Analysis of anxious thought content yields two broad factors that are labeled as "risk" and "valence." These two main types of cognitive errors are described to patients. Risk translates to overestimation, or jumping to conclusions by viewing negative events as being probable events, when in fact they are unlikely to occur. The patient is asked to identify overestimations from the anxiety and panic incidents over the past couple of weeks: "Can you think of events that you felt sure were going to happen when you panicked, only to find out in the end that they did not happen at all?" Usually, patients can identify such events easily, but with protestations. For example,

JULIE: Well, several times I thought that I really was going to lose it this time . . . that I would flip out and never return to reality. It never actually happened, *but* it could still happen.

THERAPIST: Why do you think "it" could still happen?

JULIE: Part of me feels like I've always managed to escape it just in time, by either removing myself from the situation or by having my husband help me, or by holding on long enough for the feeling to pass. But what if I can't hold on the next time?

THERAPIST: Knowing what we know about our thoughts when we are anxious, can you classify any of the ideas you just expressed, of "just holding on" or "just escaping in time," as overestimations?

JULIE: I suppose you're saying that I can hold on or I can always escape in time.

THERAPIST: More that you feel the need to hold on and the need to escape because you are overestimating the likelihood of flipping out and never returning to reality.

JULIE: But it really feels like I will.

THERAPIST: The confusion between what you think will happen and what actually happens is the very problem that we are addressing in this session.

The reasons why overestimations persist despite repeated disconfirmation are explored. Typically, patients misattribute the absence of danger to external safety signals or safety behaviors (e.g., "I only made it because I managed to find help in time," "If I had not taken Xanax last week when I panicked in the store, I'm sure I would have passed out," or "I wouldn't have made it if I hadn't pulled off the road in time"), or to "luck," instead of realizing the inaccuracy of the original prediction. Similarly, patients may assume that the only reason they are still alive, sane, and safe is because the "big one" has not happened. In this case, patients err by

assuming that intensity of panic attacks increases the risk of catastrophic outcomes.

The method for countering overestimation errors is to question the evidence for probability judgments. The general format is to treat thoughts as hypotheses or guesses rather than as facts, and to examine the evidence and generate alternative, more realistic predictions. This is best done by the therapist using a Socratic style, so that patients learn the skill of examining the content of their statements and arrive at alternative statements or predictions after they have considered all of the evidence. Questioning of the logic (e.g., "How does a racing heart lead to heart attack?"), or the bases from which judgments are made (e.g., misinformation from others, unusual sensations) is useful in this regard. Continuing with the previous example from Julie, the questioning took the following course:

THERAPIST: One of the specific thoughts you have identified is that you will flip out and never return to reality. What specifically leads you to think that that is likely to happen?

JULIE: Well, I guess it really feels like that.

THERAPIST: Describe the feelings?

JULIE: Well, I feel spacey and unreal, like things around me are different and that I'm not connected.

THERAPIST: And why do you think those feelings mean that you have actually lost touch with reality?

JULIE: I don't know—it feels as if I have.

THERAPIST: So, let's examine that assumption. What is your behavior like when you feel unreal? For example, do you respond if someone asks you a question during those episodes?

JULIE: Well, I respond to you even though I feel that way sometimes in here.

THERAPIST: OK, and can you walk or write or drive when you feel that way?

JULIE: Yes, but it feels different.

THERAPIST: But you do perform those functions despite feeling detached. So, what does that tell you?

JULIE: Well, maybe I haven't lost complete touch with reality. But what if I do?

THERAPIST: How many times have you felt detached?

JULIE: Hundreds and hundreds of times.

THERAPIST: And how many times have you lost touch with reality permanently?

JULIE: Never. But what if the feelings don't go away? Maybe I'll lose it then?

THERAPIST: So what else tells you that this is a possibility?

JULIE: Well, what about my second cousin? He lost it when he was about 25, and now he's just a mess. He can hardly function at all, and he is constantly in and out of psychiatric hospitals. They have him on a bunch of heavy-duty drugs. I'll never forget the time I saw him totally out of it. He was talking to himself in jibberish.

THERAPIST: So, do you make a connection between him and yourself?

JULIE: Yes.

THERAPIST: What are the similarities between the two of you?

JULIE: There are none really. It's just that he *is* what I think I will become.

THERAPIST: Did he ever feel the way you feel now?

JULIE: I don't know.

THERAPIST: And if another one of your cousins had severe back problems, would you be concerned that you would end up with severe back problems?

JULIE: No.

THERAPIST: Why not?

JULIE: Because it never crosses my mind. It is not something that I worry about.

THERAPIST: So, it sounds like you think you will end up like your cousin because you are afraid of ending up like him.

JULIE: I suppose so.

THERAPIST: So, let's look at all of the evidence and consider some alternatives. You have felt unreal hundreds of times, and you've never lost touch with reality because you've continued to function in the midst of those feelings, and they have never lasted. You are afraid of becoming like your cousin, but there are no data to show that you and he have the same problem. In fact, the data suggest otherwise because you function and he does not. So what is the realistic probability that you will lose touch with reality permanently? Use a scale of 0 to 100, where 0 = *No chance at all* and 100 = *Definitely will happen.*

JULIE: Well, maybe it is lower than I thought. Maybe 20%.

THERAPIST: So that would mean that you have actually lost touch with reality in a permanent way once every five times you have felt unreal.

JULIE: When it's put like that, I guess not. Maybe it's a very small possibility.

THERAPIST: Yes, so what is an alternative explanation?

JULIE: Perhaps the feelings of unreality are caused by feeling anxious or overbreathing, and having those feelings does not mean that I am actually losing touch with reality, and that I am not like my cousin at all.

For homework, in addition to continuation of self-monitoring and practice of diaphragmatic breathing, Julie was asked to identify her anxious thoughts in relation to every item on her agoraphobia hierarchy, and to use the in-session steps of examining the evidence and generating alternative evidence based interpretations for errors of overestimating the risk. She was to do the same for every panic attack that occurred over the next week.

Session 3

The goals of this session are to develop breathing retraining and to continue active cognitive restructuring. The therapist reviews the patient's week of diaphragmatic breathing practice. Julie was disappointed with her attempts to practice.

JULIE: I just didn't seem to be able to do it the right way. Sometimes I would start off OK and then the more I tried, the more it felt like I was running out of air, and I'd have to take a big gulp between breaths. At other times, I felt dizzy and the unreal feelings would start, at which point I would stop and do "busy work" to keep my mind occupied.

THERAPIST: It sounds like quite a few things were going on. First of all, remember that this is a skill, just like learning to ride a bike, and you cannot expect it to be easy from the get-go. Second, it sounds like you experienced some uncomfortable physical symptoms that worried you. You said it felt like you were running out of air. Based on what we talked about last week, what do you think might have caused that feeling?

JULIE: Well, maybe I wasn't getting enough air into my

lungs because it's really hard for me to use my diaphragm muscle. I felt like I was suffocating myself.

THERAPIST: Possibly it's just a matter of learning to use the diaphragm muscle, but were you really suffocating or was it an interpretation that you might be suffocating?

JULIE: I don't know. I've had the feeling of suffocating before, especially when I'm trapped in a crowded room.

THERAPIST: So, how do you know you were suffocating?

JULIE: I don't know. It just felt that way.

THERAPIST: So, let's put the evidence together. You've had the feelings before and never suffocated. As we discussed last time, anxiety can sometimes create a sensation of shortness of breath even though you are getting plenty of air. Can you think of an alternative explanation?

JULIE: Well, maybe I wasn't suffocating. Maybe it just felt like that.

Julie's complaints represent typical concerns that should be addressed. The next step is to slow the rate of breathing until the patient can comfortably span a full inhalation and exhalation cycle of 6 seconds. Again, the therapist models slowed breathing, then provides corrective feedback on practice in the session. The patient is instructed to continue to practice slow breathing in "safe" or relaxing environments, and is discouraged from applying slow breathing when anxious or panicking, until fully skilled in its application.

Also, cognitive restructuring is continued by addressing the second cognitive error, which involves viewing an event as "dangerous," "insufferable," or "catastrophic." Typical examples of catastrophic errors are "If I faint, people will think that I'm weak, and that would be unbearable" or "Panic attacks are the worst thing I can imagine," and "The whole evening is ruined if I start to feel anxious." "Decatastrophizing" means to face the worst, to realize that the occurrences are not as "catastrophic" as stated, and to think about actual ways to cope with negative events rather than how "bad" they are. A key principle underlying decatastrophizing is that events can be endured even though they are uncomfortable. Recognition of the time-limited nature of discomfort contributes to the development of a sense of being able to cope. The critical distinction here is that although patients might prefer that these events not

occur, they can tolerate the discomfort, if necessary. Thus, for the person who states that negative judgments from others are unbearable, it is important to discuss what he or she would do to cope should someone else make a direct negative judgment. Similarly, for the person who states that the physical symptoms of panic are intolerably embarrassing, the following type of questioning is helpful:

JULIE: I am really worried that I might lose control and do something crazy, like yell and scream.

THERAPIST: Let's face the worst and find out what is so bad about it. What would be so horrible about yelling and screaming?

JULIE: I could never live it down.

THERAPIST: Well, let's think it through. What are the various things you could do in the situation? You have just yelled and screamed—now what?

JULIE: Well, I guess the yelling and screaming would eventually stop.

THERAPIST: That's right—at the very least you would eventually exhaust yourself. What else?

JULIE: Well, maybe I would explain to the people around me that I was having a really bad day but that I would be OK. In other words, reassure them.

THERAPIST: Good. What else?

JULIE: Maybe I would just get away—find someplace to calm down and reassure myself that the worst is over.

THERAPIST: Good.

JULIE: But what if the police came and took me away, locked me up in a mental ward?

THERAPIST: Again, let's face the worst. What if the police did come when you were yelling and screaming, and what if the police did take you away? As scary as that may sound to you, let's consider what actually would happen.

JULIE: I have this image of myself not being able to tell them what is really going on—that I am so out of it I don't have the ability to let them know I am just anxious.

THERAPIST: If you were so distraught that you could not clearly communicate, how long would that last?

JULIE: You're right. I would eventually exhaust myself and then I could speak more clearly. But what if they didn't believe me?

THERAPIST: What if they did not believe you at first? How long would it take before they would realize that you were not crazy?

JULIE: I guess that after a while they would see that I was OK, and maybe I could call a friend or my doctor to explain what was going on.

The homework for this session, in addition to continued self-monitoring, is to practice slow and diaphragmatic breathing in relaxing environments, and to identify errors of catastrophizing in relation to each item on the agoraphobia hierarchy, followed by practice of decatastrophizing and generation of ways to cope. In addition, Julie was to use the skill of decatastrophizing for panic attacks that occurred over the following week.

Session 4

The main goal of this session is to use breathing retraining skills as a coping tool, to review cognitive restructuring skills, and to begin *in vivo* exposure to the first item on the agoraphobia hierarchy.

Now that patients have practiced slow and diaphragmatic breathing sufficiently in relaxing environments, they are ready to use these methods in distracting environments and in anxious situations. Patients are encouraged to use breathing skills as a coping technique as they face fear, anxiety, and anxiety-provoking situations. Some patients use breathing skills as a safety signal or a safety behavior; in other words, they believe that they will be at risk for some mental, physical, or social calamity if they do not breathe correctly. This issue came up with Julie:

JULIE: When I panicked during the week, I tried to use the breathing. It didn't work. It made me feel worse.

THERAPIST: It sounds as if you might have attempted to use the breathing exercise as a desperate attempt to control the feelings you were experiencing.

JULIE: Yes, that's right.

THERAPIST: What did you think would have happened if you had not been able to control the feelings?

JULIE: I was really worried that I might not be able to handle the feelings.

THERAPIST: And if you weren't able to handle the feelings, what would happen?

JULIE: It just feels like I will lose it, permanently.

THERAPIST: So this is one of those thoughts that we were talking about last time. What does your evidence tell you about the likelihood of losing touch with reality permanently?

JULIE: So you mean even if I don't control my breathing, then I will be OK?

THERAPIST: Well, you had not lost touch with reality permanently before you learned the breathing exercise, so what does that tell you?

JULIE: OK, I get it.

THERAPIST: The breathing exercise is best thought of as a tool to help you face whatever is provoking anxiety. So, as you face situations and your anxiety increases, use the breathing exercise to help you to face rather than run away from anxiety.

Patients who consistently use the breathing skills as a safety behavior might be discouraged from using the breathing skills because they learn that what they are most worried about either does not happen or it can be managed without using the breathing skills.

In terms of the cognitive restructuring, therapists give corrective feedback to patients on the methods of questioning the evidence to generate realistic probabilities, facing the worst, and generating ways to cope with each item on the agoraphobia hierarchy and any panic attacks that occurred over the past week. Particular "corrective" feedback is given when patients lack specificity in their cognitive restructuring (e.g., patients who record that they are most worried about panicking should be encouraged to detail what it is about panicking that worries them) or rely on blanket reassurance (e.g., patients who record that "Everything will be OK" as their evidence and/or ways of coping should be encouraged to list the evidence and/or generate actual coping steps).

Next, attention is given to how to practice the first item on the agoraphobia hierarchy. If appropriate, reasons why previous attempts at *in vivo* exposure may have failed are reviewed. Typical reasons for patients' past failures at *in vivo* exposure include attempts that are too haphazard and/or brief, or spaced too far apart, and attempts conducted without a sense of mastery, or while maintaining beliefs that catastrophe is very possible. Julie had tried to face agoraphobic situations in the past, but each time she had escaped, feeling overwhelmed by panic and terrified of losing touch with reality permanently. The therapist helped Julie realize how to approach the agoraphobic situations differently to benefit from the exposure. Julie's typical safety signals were the presence of her husband, or at least knowing his whereabouts, and Klonopin (which she carried but rarely used). The therapist discussed the importance of eventual weaning from those safety signals.

As mentioned earlier, the goal of exposure therapy is not immediate reduction in fear and anxiety; rather, the goal is for the patient to learn something new as a result of exposure. Clarification of what patients are most worried about as they face their feared situations and the conditions that best help them to learn that what worries them most never or rarely happens, and/or that they can cope with the situation and tolerate anxiety, is essential for effective exposure. If a patient is most worried that fear and anxiety will remain elevated for the duration of the practice, then corrective learning involves toleration of sustained anxiety. For Julie, the first situation on her hierarchy was to drive home from work, alone. She stated that what most worried her in that situation was that she would panic and lose touch with reality, and as a result, lose control of the car and die in an accident. She also stated that to drive at dusk was the condition under which she was most convinced of these eventualities. Thus, the task that the therapist considered most effective in teaching Julie that she would not lose touch with reality, or that she could cope with the sensations of unreality and panic, was to drive home from work at dusk.

Delineate the exposure task as concretely as possible, so that patients clearly understand exactly what the practice entails (e.g., "Walk around inside of mall for 10 minutes by myself"). Importantly, the practice should not be ended because of anxiety (e.g., "Continue driving on the freeway until I feel anxious") because the exposure practice would then reinforce avoidance of anxiety.

Julie was reminded to use her coping skills should she panic as she practiced the task; that is, in moments of fear, patients are encouraged to use their breathing and thinking skills to complete the assigned task; the coping skills are not intended as means to reduce fear and anxiety, but to tolerate it. Acceptance and nonjudgmental observation of physical sensations and thoughts can be another strategy to use in the midst of exposure therapy.

Patients are encouraged to maintain a regular schedule of repeated *in vivo* exposure practices at least three times per week, and to conduct these practices regardless of internal (e.g., having a "bad day," feeling ill) or external (e.g., inclement weather, busy schedules) factors that may prompt postponement of practices. Julie expressed some concerns about being able to practice at least three times over the following week:

JULIE: I don't know if I can practice three times because more days than not I feel pretty worn down; maybe I can practice on just Monday and Tuesday because they are the days I typically feel better.

THERAPIST: What is it you are worried about happening if you practice on a day when you already feel worn down?

JULIE: I feel more fragile on those days.

THERAPIST: And if you feel more fragile, what might happen?

JULIE: I just don't think I could do it. It would be too hard. I might really freak out and lose touch with reality for ever.

THERAPIST: OK, so let's think about that thought. What does your experience tell you? How many times have you permanently lost touch with reality, including days when you were worn down?

JULIE: Well, never.

THERAPIST: So, what does that tell you?

JULIE: OK, but it still feels difficult to drive on those days.

THERAPIST: How about you start with Monday or Tuesday, but quickly move to the other days of the week when you are feeling worn down, so that you get a really good opportunity to learn whether you permanently lose touch with reality or not?

Julie's homework for this session involves continued self-monitoring, continued use of cognitive restructuring and breathing retraining in the event of elevated anxiety or panic, and practicing the first item on the agoraphobia hierarchy at least three times, with at least one of those times being without her husband Larry.

Session 5

The goals of this session are to review the practice of *in vivo* exposure, to design another exposure task to be practiced over the next week, and to begin interoceptive exposure. Note that *in vivo* and interoceptive exposure can be done simultaneously or sequentially. For Julie, *in vivo* exposure was begun in Session 4, whereas interoceptive exposure was begun in this session, but they could easily have been done in the opposite order.

It is essential to review the week's practice of *in vivo* exposure. An objective evaluation of performance is considered necessary to offset subjective and damaging self-evaluations. As demonstrated in experimental literature on learning and conditioning, appraisals of aversive events after they have occurred can influence anxiety about future encounters with the same types of aversive events. Any practice that is terminated prematurely is to be reviewed carefully for contributing factors that can then be incorporated into subsequent trials of *in vivo* exposure. Recognition of the precipitant to escape is very important because the urge to escape is usually based on the prediction that continued endurance would result in some kind of danger. For example, patients may predict that the sensations will become intense and lead to an out-of-control reaction. This prediction can be discussed in terms of jumping to conclusions and blowing things out of proportion. At the same time, escape itself need not be viewed catastrophically (i.e., as embarrassing, or as a sign of failure). In addition, therapists reinforce the use of breathing and cognitive skills (or acceptance skills) to help patients remain in the situation until the specified duration or task has been completed, despite uncomfortable sensations.

Again, it is important for patients to recognize that the goal is repeatedly to face situations despite anxiety, not to achieve a total absence of anxiety. Toleration of fear rather than immediate fear reduction is the goal for each exposure practice; this approach leads to an eventual fear reduction over time. Anxiety that does not decline over repeated days of *in vivo* exposure may result from too much emphasis on immediate fear and anxiety reduction; that is, trying too hard or wishing too much for anxiety to decline typically maintains anxiety.

Julie had success with her first *in vivo* exposure practice; she managed to drive home from work at dusk, alone, four different times. She noted that the first time was easier than she had expected; the second was harder, and the one time she pulled off to the side of the road. The therapist helped Julie identify the thoughts and sensations that led her to "escape" from the situation: the sensations of unreality and fears of losing touch with reality. Julie had waited for a few minutes, then continued driving home—an action that was highly reinforced by the therapist. The third and fourth times were easier.

Julie's husband, Larry, attended Session 5, so that he could learn how to help Julie overcome her panic and agoraphobia. He was supportive and eager to help in any way possible, expressing frustration at having had no idea how to help in the past.

There are general principles for involvement of significant others in treatment. First, a treatment conceptualization is provided to the significant other to reduce his or her frustration and/or negative attributions about the patient's emotional functioning (e.g., "Oh, she's just making it up. There's nothing really wrong with her" or "He has been like this since before we were married, and he'll never change"). The way in which the agoraphobic problem has disrupted daily routines and distribution of home responsibilities is explored and discussed also. Examples might include social activities, leisure activities, and household chores. The therapist explains that family activities may be structured around the agoraphobic fear and avoidance to help the patient function without intense anxiety. At the same time, reassignment of the patient's tasks to the significant other may actually reinforce the agoraphobic pattern of behavior. Consequently, the importance of complying with *in vivo* exposure homework instructions, even though the patient may experience some distress initially, is emphasized.

The significant other is encouraged to become an active participant by providing his or her perception of the patient's behavior and fearfulness, and the impact on the home environment. Sometimes the significant other provides information of which the patient is not fully aware, or did not report, particularly in relation to how the patient's behavior affects his or her own daily functioning. Larry, for example, described how he felt restricted at home in the evenings; whereas, before, he occasionally played basketball with his friends at the local gym, he now stays at home because he feels guilty if he leaves Julie alone.

The next step is to describe the role of the significant other regarding *in vivo* exposure tasks. The significant other is viewed as a coach, and the couple is encouraged to approach the tasks as a problem-solving team. This includes deciding exactly where and when to practice *in vivo* exposure. In preparation for practices, the patient identifies his or her misappraisals about the task and generates cognitive alternatives. The significant other is encouraged to help the patient question his or her own "anxious" thoughts. Role plays of this type of questioning of the patient by the significant other may be conducted in the session, so that the therapist can provide corrective feedback to each partner. Throughout *in vivo* exposure, the significant other reminds the patient to apply coping skills, whether it be cognitive challenges, breathing skills, or acceptance skills. Because the significant other is usually a safety signal, tasks are less anxiety provoking. However, the patient must be weaned from the safety signal eventually. Therefore, initial attempts at facing agoraphobic situations are conducted with the significant other, and later trials are conducted alone. Weaning from the significant other may be graduated, as in the case of Julie (1) driving first with Larry in the car, (2) with him in a car behind, (3) meeting him at a destination point, and (4) driving alone.

Very important to the success of this collaboration is style of communication. On the one hand, the significant other is discouraged from magnifying the experience of panic and encouraged to help the patient apply coping statements when anxious. On the other hand, the significant other is encouraged to be patient given the fact that progress for the patient may be erratic. The patient and the significant other are instructed to use a 0- to 10-point rating scale to communicate with each other about the patient's current level of anxiety or distress, as a way of diminishing the awkwardness associated with discussion of anxiety, especially in public situations. The patient is warned about the potential motivation to avoid discussing his or her feelings with the significant other, due to embarrassment or an attempt to avoid the anxiety for fear that such discussion and concentration on anxiety may intensify his or her distress level. Avoidance of feelings is discouraged because distraction is viewed as less beneficial in the long term than objectively facing whatever is distressing and learning that predicted catastrophes do not occur. The patient is reassured that the initial discomfort and embarrassment will most likely diminish as the partners become more familiar with discussing anxiety levels and their management. Furthermore, the patient's concerns about the significant other being insensitive or too pushy are addressed. For example, a significant other may presume to know the patient's level of anxiety and anxious thoughts without confirmation from the patient, or the significant other may become angry at the patient for avoiding or escaping from situations, or being fearful. All of these issues are described as relatively common and understandable patterns of communication that are nevertheless in need of correction. In-session role playing of more adaptive communication styles during episodes of heightened anxiety is a useful learning technique. On occasion, more specific communications training may be beneficial, especially if the partners frequently argue in their attempts to generate items or methods for conducting *in vivo* exposure.

The next *in vivo* exposure task for Julie was to sit in a crowded movie theater, gradually moving away from the aisle, toward the middle of the row, because that was the condition in which she was most concerned that she would lose control and draw attention to herself. Julie and Larry rehearsed their approach to the *in vivo* exposure task in session, while the therapist provided corrective feedback using the principles of communication and coping described earlier. They were instructed to practice this task at least three times over the next week. On at least one occasion, Julie was to practice the task alone.

Next, interoceptive exposure was introduced. As with *in vivo* exposure, through repeated exposures to feared sensations, patients learn that they are not harmed by the sensations, and they achieve increased confidence in their ability to tolerate symptoms of anxiety. The procedure begins with assessment of the patient's response to a series of standardized exercises. The therapist models each exercise first. Then, after the patient has completed the exercise, the therapist records the sensations, anxiety level (0 to 10), sensation intensity (0 to 10), and similarity to naturally occurring panic sensations (0 to 10). The exercises include shaking the head from side to side for 30 seconds; placing the head between the legs for 30 seconds and lifting the head to an upright position quickly; running in place or using steps for 1 minute; holding one's breath for as long as possible; complete body muscle tension for 1 minute or holding a push-up position for as long as possible; spinning in a swivel chair for 1 minute; hyperventilating for 1 minute; breathing through a narrow straw (with closed nasal passages) or breathing as slowly as possible for 2 minutes; and staring at a spot on the wall or at one's mirror image for 90 seconds. If none of these exercises produce sensations at least moderately similar to those that occur naturally, other, individually tailored exercises are generated. For example, tightness around the chest may be induced by a deep breath before hyperventilating; heat may be induced by wearing heavy clothing in a heated room; choking sensations may be induced by a tongue depressor, a high-collared sweater, or a necktie; and startle may be induced by an abrupt, loud noise in the midst of relaxation. For Julie, the sensations produces by hyperventilating, spinning, and staring at a spot on the wall were most anxiety provoking.

Patients who report little or no fear because they feel safe in the presence of the therapist are asked to attempt each exercise alone, either at home or with the therapist out of the office. At the same time, discussing the influence of perceived safety as a moderating factor in the amount of fear experienced reinforces the value of cognitive restructuring. For a minority of patients, the known cause and course of the sensations override the fear response; that is, because the sensations are predictably related to a clear cause (the interoceptive exercise), and because the sensations can be relatively easily controlled by simply terminating the interoceptive exercise, fear is minimal. Under these conditions, discussion can productively center on the misassumptions that render naturally occurring sensations more frightening than the ones produced by the interoceptive exercises. Typically, these misassumptions are that naturally occurring sensations are unpredictable; that unpredictable sensations are more harmful; and that if naturally occurring sensations are not controlled, then they pose a potential threat. The majority of patients fear at least several of the interoceptive exercises despite knowing the cause of the sensations and their controllability.

Interoceptive exercises rated as producing at least somewhat similar sensations to naturally occurring panic (at least 3 on the 0- to 10-point scale) are selected for repeated exposure. A graduated approach is used for interoceptive exposure, beginning with the lowest item on the hierarchy established in Session 4. For each trial of exposure, the patient is asked to begin the induction, to indicate when the sensations are first experienced (e.g., by raising a hand), and to continue the induction for at least 30 seconds longer to permit corrective learning. After terminating the induction, anxiety is rated, and the patient is given time to apply cognitive and breathing coping skills. Finally, the therapist reviews the induction experience and the application of management strategies with the patient. During this review, the therapist emphasizes the importance of experiencing the sensations fully during the induction, of concentrating objectively on the sensations versus distracting from them, and the importance of identifying specific cognitions and challenging them by considering all of the evidence. In addition, the therapist asks key questions to help the patient realize his or her safety (e.g., "What would have happened if you had continued spinning for another 60 seconds?"), and to generalize to naturally occurring experiences (e.g., "How is this different from when you feel dizzy at work?"). In other

words, cognitive restructuring extends the cognitive reprocessing already taking place implicitly as a result of repeated interoceptive exposure.

Specific, previously unrecognized cognitions sometimes become apparent during repeated exposure. For example, when Julie began to conduct repeated exposures to hyperventilation and spinning, she became more aware of her implicit assumption that sensations of spaciness or lightheadedness would lead her to lose control of her limbs. This related to her concern about causing an accident when driving. During repeated hyperventilation exercises, and with prompting of "what ifs" from the therapist, Julie discovered her fear of not being able to move her arms or legs. The therapist then behaviorally challenged this assumption by having Julie overbreathe for longer periods of time, followed immediately by walking, picking up objects, and so on.

Homework practice is very important because safety signals present in the clinic setting or that derive from the therapist per se may, again, prevent generalizability to the natural setting. Patients are instructed to practice the interoceptive items conducted in session on a daily basis, three times each day. Julie was to practice hyperventilation over the following week. She expressed some concern at doing the exercises alone, so the therapist helped Julie to use her cognitive restructuring skills in relation to being alone. In addition, more graduation of homework was suggested, so that Julie would practice hyperventilating when her husband was at home the first couple of days, then when he was not at home the rest of the time.

Sessions 6 and 7

The primary goal of these sessions is to review the past week of *in vivo* exposure practices, design new exposures, review between-session practices of interoceptive exposure, conduct repeated interoceptive exposure in session, and assign those as homework for the next week.

The *in vivo* exposure is reviewed, as in the previous session. In this case, Julie and Larry had done well with the movie theater practice. Julie even practiced going to the movies on her own. On that occasion she reported higher anxiety than when she was with Larry for fear of having to get up and leave the theater and worries about bothering others in the audience. The therapist helped Julie to identify what worry led her to think about leaving in the first place; in other words, what did she think might happen if she could not leave? When

Julie indicated that she had thoughts of losing control and causing a scene, she was then prompted to apply her cognitive restructuring skills of evidence-based analyses and decatastrophizing. She was ready to move to the next items on her hierarchy: to spend 2 hours alone at home during the day and to stay alone at home as day turned to night. As with every *in vivo* exposure task, Julie identified what she most feared happening in those situations, and the best practice conditions under which to learn that either those eventualities would not happen and/or she could cope with the worst.

The past week of interoceptive exposure practice is reviewed in session with a mind toward avoidance: either overt failure to practice or covert avoidance by minimizing the intensity or duration of the sensations induced, or by limiting practice to the presence of a safety signal (e.g., a significant other) or times when background anxiety is minimal. Reasons for avoidance may include continued misinterpretation of the dangers of bodily sensations (i.e., "I don't want to hyperventilate because I'm afraid that I won't be able to stop overbreathing and no one will be there to help me") or the belief that anxiety will not reduce with repetition of the task.

For the first week, Julie practiced interoceptive exposure exercises about half of the days between sessions. The therapist used a "downward arrow" method to explore Julie's reasons for not practicing every day.

JULIE: I tried hyperventilating on my own. However, I wasn't very successful because I felt too scared and I stopped it as soon as I noticed the strange feelings.

THERAPIST: What did you think would happen if the sensations became more intense?

JULIE: I thought the feelings would get worse and worse and worse, and just overwhelm me. I didn't want to have that feeling of panic again.

THERAPIST: If you did become overwhelmed, then what would happen to you?

JULIE: Then I'd feel really terrible.

THERAPIST: And if you felt really terrible?

JULIE: Well, nothing. I'd just feel terrible.

THERAPIST: The word "terrible" carries a lot of meaning. Let's see if we can pin down your anxious thoughts that make the feelings so terrible.

JULIE: I just can't tolerate the feeling.

THERAPIST: What tells you that you cannot tolerate it? How do you know you can't tolerate it?

And the discussion continued, so that Julie realized what was most important for her to learn by the repeated hyperventilation: She could tolerate the sensations and anxiety. However, after the subsequent week of repeated practice, Julie remained cautious for fear that the exercises would cause her to revert to her state of several weeks earlier; that is, she was concerned that the inductions would leave her in a persistent symptomatic state. Furthermore, she was particularly reluctant to practice interoceptive exposure at the end of the day, when she was more likely to feel unreal, or on a day when an important social event was scheduled. Again, these avoidance patterns were related to fears that the symptoms would become too intense or result in some type of mental or social catastrophe. These types of avoidance patterns are addressed in the following vignette:

THERAPIST: When did you practice deliberately spinning and hyperventilating?

JULIE: Usually in the mornings. One day I left it until the end of the day, and that turned out to be a bad idea. I felt terrible.

THERAPIST: Let's think about that a bit more. What made it terrible when you practiced at the end of the day?

JULIE: Well, I was already feeling pretty unreal—I usually do around that time of the day. So I was much more anxious about the symptoms.

THERAPIST: Being more anxious implies that you thought the symptoms were more harmful. Is that what happened on the day that you practiced interoceptive exposure when you were already feeling unreal?

JULIE: Yes, I felt that because I was already feeling unreal, I was on the edge, and that I might push myself over the edge if I tried to increase the feelings of unreality.

THERAPIST: What do you mean by "push myself over the edge"?

JULIE: That I would make the feelings so intense that I really would lose it—go crazy.

THERAPIST: So there is one of those hypotheses: to feel more intense unreality means to be closer to going crazy. Let's examine the evidence. Is it necessarily the case that more intense unreality means you are closer to craziness?

In sessions, the therapist continued practice of interoceptive exposure with the next item on Julie's hierarchy, which was to stare at a spot on the wall and to spin around.

The homework from this session is to continue self-monitoring, *in vivo* exposure to an item from the agoraphobia hierarchy at least three times, and daily practice of interoceptive exposure.

Sessions 8 and 9

The primary goals of these sessions are to continue *in vivo* exposure, as described in the prior sessions, and to extend interoceptive exposure to natural activities. Julie had practiced staying at home for 2 hours alone during the day and as daylight turned to dusk, with good results. In particular, despite experiencing a couple of panic attacks during these *in vivo* exposure practices, she continued with the assigned practice. This was critical for Julie because it allowed her to learn that she could survive the feeling of panic; it was the first time she had remained in a situation despite panicking.

In reviewing the week's practice of interoceptive exposure, it became apparent that Julie was separating the practices from real-life experiences of bodily sensations in a way that would limit generalization. This was addressed as follows:

JULIE: After spinning and hyperventilating several times, I really do feel much less anxious. I was terrified at the start, but now I am only mildly anxious, if at all. But this is different than what happens to me when I'm on the freeway or at home.

THERAPIST: How is it different?

JULIE: I don't know when the feelings of dizziness and unreality are going to hit.

THERAPIST: From our previous discussions, let's think of potential reasons why you might feel dizzy or unreal at a particular time?

JULIE: I know. I have to keep remembering that it could be my breathing, or just feeling anxious, or tired, or a bunch of different things.

THERAPIST: OK. And why is it so important to know when those feelings will occur?

JULIE: Because I don't want them to be there at all.

THERAPIST: And why not . . . what are you afraid of?

JULIE: I guess it's the same old thing . . . that I'll lose it somehow?

THERAPIST: So let's go back to the cognitive restructuring that you have been doing. What specifically are you afraid of? How likely is it to happen? What are the alternatives?

JULIE: I understand.

THERAPIST: So, now you see that whether the sensations of dizziness or unreality are produced by anxiety, overbreathing, diet, or the exercises we do here, they're all the same—they are just uncomfortable physical sensations. The only reason they perturb you more when you are driving or at home is because of the meaning you still give to them in those situations.

"Naturalistic" interoceptive exposure refers to exposure to daily tasks or activities that have been avoided or endured with dread because of the associated sensations. Typical examples include aerobic exercise or vigorous physical activity, running up flights of stairs, eating foods that create a sensation of fullness or are associated with sensations of choking, saunas or steamy showers, driving with the windows rolled up and the heater on, caffeine consumption, and so on. (Of course, these exercises may be modified in the event of actual medical complications, such as asthma or high blood pressure.) From a list of typically feared activities and generation of items specific to the individual's own experience, a hierarchy is established. Each item is ranked in terms of anxiety ratings (0–10). Julie's hierarchy was as follows: looking out through venetian blinds (anxiety = 3); watching *One Flew over the Cuckoo's Nest* (anxiety = 4); playing tennis (anxiety = 4); scanning labels on a supermarket shelf (anxiety = 5); concentrating on needlework for an hour (anxiety = 6); driving with windows closed and heater on (anxiety = 7); a nightclub with strobe lights (anxiety = 8); and rides at Disneyland (anxiety = 10).

Like the symptom exercises, the activity exercises are designed to be systematically graduated and repetitive. Patients may apply the breathing and cognitive skills while the activity is ongoing. This is in contrast to the symptom induction exercises, in which coping skills are used only after completion of the symptom exercise, because the activities often are considerably longer than the symptom induction exercises. Nevertheless, patients are encouraged to focus on the sensations and experience them fully throughout the activity, and not use the coping skills to prevent or remove the sensations.

Patients are instructed to identify maladaptive cognitions and rehearse cognitive restructuring before beginning each activity. In-session rehearsal of the cognitive preparation allows therapists to provide corrective feedback. Julie did this with her therapist for her first two naturalistic activities, which were to look at venetian blinds and to watch *One Flew over the Cuckoo's Nest*. Julie realized that she was most worried about sensations of unreality and fears of going crazy, although, as a result of her various exposure exercises up to this point, she quickly was able to recognize that such sensations were harmless and that she could tolerate them, and that such fears were unrealistic based on the evidence.

As with all exposures, it is important to identify and remove (gradually, if necessary) safety signals or protective behaviors, such as portable phones, lucky charms, walking slowly, standing slowly, and staying in close proximity to medical facilities. These safety signals and behaviors reinforce catastrophic misappraisals about bodily sensations. Julie's safety behaviors were identified as checking the time on the clock (as a reassurance that she was in touch with reality) and pinching herself (again, to feel reality). She was asked to practice the two naturalistic interoceptive exposures at least three times each before the next treatment session, without the safety behaviors.

Sessions 10 and 11

The primary goals of these sessions are to review the *in vivo* and naturalistic exposure exercises over the past week, and to combine exposure to feared and avoided agoraphobic situations with deliberate induction of feared sensations into those situations. As with earlier interoceptive exposure homework assignments, it is important to evaluate and correct tendencies to avoid naturalistic interoceptive exposure tasks, mainly by considering the underlying misassumptions that lead to avoidance. Remember also that a form of avoidance is to rely on safety signals or safety behaviors, so careful questioning of the way in which the naturalistic exposure was conducted, and under what conditions, may help to identify inadvertent reliance on these unnecessary precautions. Julie reported that she was successful in looking at the venetian blinds, even though she experienced sensations of unreality. She had more difficulty watching *One Flew over the Cuckoo's Nest* because it tapped directly into her worst fears of losing touch with reality permanently; she tried but terminated the film

early. The second time, she watched it with Larry, who prompted Julie to remember her cognitive and breathing skills, and she was able to watch the entire film. She watched the film one more time on her own. Two new naturalistic exposure items were selected for the coming week, with special attention to weaning or removing safety signals and safety behaviors, and rehearsal of cognitive restructuring in session. For Julie, these were playing tennis (something she had avoided for years) and scanning items on supermarket shelves.

The notion of deliberately inducing feared bodily symptoms within the context of feared agoraphobic situations derives from the evidence that compound relationships between external and internal cues can be the most potent anxiogenic agent (i.e., deepened extinction, as reviewed in earlier sections); that is, neither just the situation nor just the bodily sensation triggers distress. It is the combination of the bodily sensation and the situation that is most distressing. Thus, effective exposure targets both types of cues. Otherwise, patients run the risk of later return of fear. For example, repeated practice walking through a shopping mall without feeling dizzy does not adequately prepare patients for occasions on which they feel dizzy walking through a shopping mall, and without such preparation, patients may be likely to panic and escape should they feel dizzy in this or similar situations in the future. Wearing heavy clothing in a restaurant helps patients to learn to be less afraid of not only the restaurant but also of feeling hot in a restaurant. Other examples include drinking coffee before any of the agoraphobic tasks, turning off the air-conditioning or turning on the heater while driving, breathing very slowly in a crowded area, and so on.

Patients choose an item from their hierarchy of agoraphobia situations, either one already completed or a new item, and also choose which symptom to induce and ways of inducing that symptom in that situation. Julie's task was to drink coffee as she went to a movie. She expressed the following concerns:

JULIE: Do you really think I am ready to drink coffee and go to the movie?

THERAPIST: What worries you about the combination of coffee and the movie theater?

JULIE: Well, I've practiced in the movie theaters a lot, so that feels pretty good, but the coffee is going to make me feel very anxious.

THERAPIST: And if you feel very anxious in the movie theater, then what?

JULIE: Then, I don't know what. Maybe I will get those old feelings again, like I have to get out.

THERAPIST: Based on everything you have learned, how can you manage those feelings?

JULIE: Well, I guess my number one rule is never to leave a situation because I am feeling anxious. I will stick it out, no matter what.

THERAPIST: That sounds great. It means you are accepting the anxiety and taking the opportunity to learn that you can tolerate it. What else?

JULIE: I can ask myself what is the worst that can happen. I know I am not going to die or go crazy. I will probably feel my heart rate going pretty fast because of the coffee.

THERAPIST: And if your heart rate goes fast, what does that mean?

JULIE: I guess it just means that my heart rate will go fast.

THERAPIST: This will be a really good way for you to learn that you can tolerate the anxiety and the symptoms of a racing heart.

The homework for this session is to continue self-monitoring, to practice *in vivo* exposure combined with interoceptive exposure, and to continue naturalistic interoceptive exposure.

Session 12

The last treatment session reviews the principles and skills learned and provides the patient with a template of coping techniques for potentially high-risk situations in the future. Julie finished the program after 12 sessions, by which time she had not panicked in 8 weeks, rarely experienced dizziness or feelings of unreality, and was driving further distances. There were some situations still in need of exposure practices (e.g., driving very long distances away from home and on the freeway at dusk). However, Julie and Larry agreed to continue *in vivo* exposure practices over the next few months to consolidate her learning and to continue her improvement.

CONCLUSION

As noted earlier in this chapter, cognitive-behavioral treatments for panic disorder and agoraphobia are highly effective and represent one of the success stories of psychotherapy. Between 80 and 100% of patients undergoing these treatments will be panic free at the end of treatment and maintain these gains for up to 2 years. These results reflect substantially more durability than medication treatments. Furthermore, between 50 and 80% of these patients reach a point of "high end state," which means their symptoms and functioning are within normative realms, and many of the remainder have only residual symptomatology. Nevertheless, major difficulties remain.

First, these treatments are not foolproof. As many as 50% of patients retain substantial symptomatology despite improvement from baseline, and this is particularly likely for those with more severe agoraphobia. Further research must determine how treatments can be improved or better individualized to alleviate continued suffering. For example, one of us (D. H. B.) saw a patient several years ago who had completed an initial course of treatment but required continued periodic visits for over 4 years. This patient was essentially improved for approximately 9 months but found himself relapsing during a particularly stressful time at work. A few booster sessions restored his functioning, but he was back in the office 6 months later with reemerging symptomatology. This pattern essentially continued for 4 years and was characterized by symptom-free periods followed by (seemingly) stress-related relapses. Furthermore, the reemerging panic disorder would sometimes last from 3 to 6 months before disappearing again, perhaps with the help of a booster session.

Although this case was somewhat unusual in our experience, there was no easy explanation for this pattern of relapses and remissions. The patient, who has a graduate degree, understood and accepted the treatment model and fully implemented the treatment program. There was also no question that he fully comprehended the nature of anxiety and panic, and the intricacies of the therapeutic strategies. While in the office, he could recite chapter and verse on the nature of these emotional states, as well as the detailed process of his own reaction while in these states. Nevertheless, away from the office, the patient found himself repeatedly hoping that he would not "go over the brink" during a panic attack, despite verbalizing very clearly the irrationality of this concept while in the office. In addition, he continued to attempt to reduce minor physiological symptoms associated with anxiety and panic, despite a full rational understanding of the nature of these symptoms (including the fact that they are the same symptoms he experienced during a state of excitement, which he enjoyed). His limited tolerance of these physical sensations was also puzzling in view of his tremendous capacity to endure pain.

Any number of factors might account for what seemed to be "overvalued ideation" or very strongly held irrational ideas during periods of anxiety, including the fact that the patient has several relatives who have repeatedly been hospitalized for emotional disorders (seemingly mood disorders or schizoaffective disorder). Nevertheless, the fact remains that we do not know why this patient did not respond as quickly as most people. Eventually he made a full recovery, received several promotions at work, and considered treatment to be the turning point in his life. But it took 5 years.

Other patients, as noted earlier, seem uninterested in engaging in treatment, preferring to conceptualize their problems as chemical imbalances. Still others have difficulty grasping some of the cognitive strategies, and further attempts are necessary to make these treatments more "user-friendly."

It also may seem that this structured, protocol-driven treatment is applied in a very standard fashion across individuals. Nothing could be further from the truth. The clinical art involved in this, and in all treatments described in this book, requires a careful adaptation of these treatment strategies to the individual case. Many of Julie's symptoms revolved around feelings of unreality (derealization and depersonalization). Emphasizing rational explanations for the production of such feelings, as well as adapting cognitive and exposure exercises to maximize these sensations, is an important part of this treatment program. Although standard interoceptive provocation exercises seemed sufficient to produce relevant symptomatology in Julie's case, we have had to develop new procedures to deal with people with more idiosyncratic symptoms and fears, particularly those involving feelings of unreality or dissociation. Other innovations in both cognitive and behavioral procedures will be required by individual therapists as they apply these procedures.

Although these new treatments seem highly successful when applied by trained therapists, treatment is not readily available to individuals with these disorders. In fact, these treatments, although brief and structured, are far more difficult to deliver than, for example, pharmacological treatments (which are also often misapplied). Furthermore, few people are currently skilled in the application of these treatments. What seems to be needed for these and other successful psychosocial treatments is a new method of disseminating them, so that they reach the maximum number of patients. Modification of these treatment protocols into more user-friendly formats, as well as brief periods of training for qualified therapists to a point of certification, would be important steps in successfully delivering these treatments. This may be difficult to accomplish.

NOTE

1. Specific phobias were not assessed, but by being most circumscribed, they would be hypothesized to load the least on negative affectivity.

REFERENCES

Aaronson, C. J., Shear, M. K., Goetz, R. R., Allen, L. B., Barlow, D. H., White, K. S., et al. (2008). Predictors and time course of response among panic disorder patients treated with cognitive-behavioral therapy. *Journal of Clinical Psychiatry, 69,* 418–424.

Allen, L. B., White, K. S., Barlow, D. H., Shear, M. K., Gorman, J. M., & Woods, S. W. (2010). Cognitive-behavior therapy (CBT) for panic disorder: Relationship of anxiety and depression comorbidity with treatment outcome. *Journal of Psychopathology and Behavioral Assessment, 32,* 185–192.

Alneas, R., & Torgersen, S. (1990). DSM-III personality disorders among patients with major depression, anxiety disorders, and mixed conditions. *Journal of Nervous and Mental Disease, 178,* 693–698.

American Psychiatric Association. (1980). *Diagnostic and statistical manual of mental disorders* (3rd ed.). Washington, DC: Author.

American Psychiatric Association. (2013). *Diagnostic and statistical manual of mental disorders* (5th ed.). Arlington, VA: Author.

Amering, M., Katschnig, H., Berger, P., Windhaber, J., Baischer, W., & Dantendorfer, K. (1997). Embarrassment about the first panic attack predicts agoraphobia in disorder patients. *Behaviour Research and Therapy, 35,* 517–521.

Andrews, G., Cuijpers, P., Craske, M. G., McEvoy, P., & Titov, N. (2010). Computer therapy for the anxiety and depressive disorders is effective, acceptable and practical health care: A meta-analysis. *PLoS ONE, 5,* e13196.

Antony, M. M., Brown, T. A., Craske, M. G., Barlow, D. H., Mitchell, W. B., & Meadows, E. A. (1995). Accuracy of heartbeat perception in panic disorder, social phobia, and nonanxious subjects. *Journal of Anxiety Disorders, 9,* 355–371.

Antony, M. M., Ledley, D. R., Liss, A., & Swinson, R. P. (2006). Responses to symptom induction exercises in panic disorder. *Behaviour Research and Therapy, 44,* 85–98.

Antony, M. M., Meadows, E. A., Brown, T. A., & Barlow, D. H. (1994). Cardiac awareness before and after cognitive-behavioral treatment for panic disorder. *Journal of Anxiety Disorders, 8,* 341–350.

Arch, J. J., Eifert, G. H., Davies, C., Plumb, J. C., Rose, R. D., & Craske, M. G. (2012). Randomized trial of cognitive behavioral therapy versus acceptance and commitment therapy for the treatment of mixed anxiety disorders. *Journal of Consulting and Clinical Psychology, 80,* 750–765.

Arnow, B. A., Taylor, C. B., Agras, W. S., & Telch, M. J. (1985). Enhancing agoraphobia treatment outcome by changing couple communication patterns. *Behavior Therapy, 16,* 452–467.

Arrindell, W., & Emmelkamp, P. (1987). Psychological states and traits in female agoraphobics: A controlled study. *Journal of Psychopathology and Behavioral Assessment, 9,* 237–253.

Baldwin, D. S. (1998). Depression and panic: Comorbidity. *European Psychiatry, 13,* 65s–70s.

Bandelow, B., Spath, C., Tichaner, G. A., Brooks, A., Hajak, G., & Ruther, E. (2002). Early traumatic life events, parental attitudes, family history, and birth risk factors in patients with panic disorder. *Comprehensive Psychiatry, 43,* 269–278.

Barlow, D. H. (1988). *Anxiety and its disorders: The nature and treatment of anxiety and panic.* New York: Guilford Press.

Barlow, D. H. (2002). *Anxiety and its disorders: The nature and treatment of anxiety and panic* (2nd ed.). New York: Guilford Press.

Barlow, D. H., Brown, T. A., & Craske, M. G. (1994). Definitions of panic attacks and panic disorder in the DSM-IV: Implications for research. *Journal of Abnormal Psychology, 103,* 553–564.

Barlow, D. H., Cohen, A., Waddell, M., Vermilyea, J., Klosko, J., Blanchard, E., et al. (1984). Panic and generalized anxiety disorders: Nature and treatment. *Behavior Therapy, 15,* 431–449.

Barlow, D. H., & Craske, M. G. (1994). *Mastery of your anxiety and panic* (2nd ed.) San Antonio, TX: Harcourt Brace.

Barlow, D. H., & Craske, M. G. (2006). *Mastery of your anxiety and panic: Patient workbook* (4th ed.). New York: Oxford University Press.

Barlow, D. H., Craske, M. G., Cerny, J. A., & Klosko, J. S. (1989). Behavioral treatment of panic disorder. *Behavior Therapy, 20,* 261–282.

Barlow, D. H., Gorman, J. M., Shear, M. K., & Woods, S. W. (2000). Cognitive-behavioral therapy, imipramine, or their combination for panic disorder: A randomized controlled trial. *Journal of the American Medical Association, 283*(19), 2529–2536.

Barlow, D. H., O'Brien, G. T., & Last, C. G. (1984). Couples treatment of agoraphobia. *Behavior Therapy, 15*(1), 41–58.

Barlow, D. H., O'Brien, G. T., Last, C. G., & Holden, A. E. (1983). Couples treatment of agoraphobia. In K. D. Craig & R. J. McMahon (Eds.), *Advances in clinical behavior therapy* (pp. 99–127). New York: Brunner/Mazel.

Barlow, D. H., Vermilyea, J., Blanchard, E., Vermilyea, B., Di Nardo, P., & Cerny, J. (1985). Phenomenon of panic. *Journal of Abnormal Psychology, 94,* 320–328.

Barsky, A. J., Cleary, P. D., Sarnie, M. K., & Ruskin, J. N. (1994). Panic disorder, palpitations, and the awareness of cardiac activity. *Journal of Nervous and Mental Disease, 182,* 63–71.

Basoglu, M., Marks, I. M., Kilic, C., Brewin, C. R., & Swinson, R. P. (1994). Alprazolam and exposure for panic disorder with agoraphobia: Attribution of improvement to medication predicts subsequent relapse. *British Journal of Psychiatry, 164,* 652–659.

Beck, J. G., & Shipherd, J. C. (1997). Repeated exposure to interoceptive cues: Does habituation of fear occur in panic disorder patients?: A preliminary report. *Behaviour Research and Therapy, 35,* 551–557.

Beck, J. G., Shipherd, J. C., & Zebb, B. J. (1997). How does interoceptive exposure for panic disorder work?: An uncontrolled case study. *Journal of Anxiety Disorders, 11,* 541–556.

Beck, J. G., Stanley, M. A., Baldwin, L. E., Deagle, E. A., & Averill, P. M. (1994). Comparison of cognitive therapy and relaxation training for panic disorder. *Journal of Consulting and Clinical Psychology, 62,* 818–826.

Beesdo, K., Knappe, S., & Pine, D. S. (2007). Anxiety and anxiety disorders in children and adolescents: developmental issues and implications for DSM-V. *Psychiatric Clinics of North America, 32,* 483–524.

Biederman, J., Faraone, S. V., Marrs, A., & Moore, P. (1997). Panic disorder and agoraphobia in consecutively referred children and adolescents. *Journal of the American Academy of Child and Adolescent Psychiatry, 36*(12), 214–223.

Bittner, A., Egger, H. L., Erkanli, A., Costello, J., Foley, D. L., & Angold, A. (2007). What do childhood anxiety disorders predict? *Journal of Child Psychology and Psychiatry, 48,* 1174–1183.

Black, D. W., Monahan, P., Wesner, R., Gabel, J., & Bowers, W. (1996). The effect of fluvoxamine, cognitive therapy, and placebo on abnormal personality traits in 44 patients with panic disorder. *Journal of Personality Disorders, 10,* 185–194.

Bland, K., & Hallam, R. (1981). Relationship between response to graded exposure and marital satisfaction in agoraphobics. *Behaviour Research and Therapy, 19,* 335–338.

Block, R. I., Ghoneim, M. M., Fowles, D. C., Kumar, V., & Pathak, D. (1987). Effects of a subanesthetic concentration of nitrous oxide on establishment, elicitation and semantic and phonemic generalization of classically conditioned skin conductance responses. *Pharmacological and Biochemical Behavior, 28*, 7–14.

Bohni, M. K., Spindler, H., Arendt, M., Hougaard, E., & Rosenberg, N. K. (2009). A randomized study of massed three-week cognitive behavioural therapy schedule for panic disorder. *Acta Psychiatrica Scandinavica, 120*(3), 187–195.

Bonn, J. A., Harrison, J., & Rees, W. (1971). Lactate-induced anxiety: Therapeutic application. *British Journal of Psychiatry, 119*, 468–470.

Bouchard, S., Gauthier, J., Laberge, B., French, D., Pelletier, M., & Godbout, D. (1996). Exposure versus cognitive restructuring in the treatment of panic disorder with agoraphobia. *Behaviour Research and Therapy, 34*, 213–224.

Bouchard, S., Paquin, B., Payeur, R., Allard, M., Rivard, V., Gournier, T., et al. (2004). Delivering cognitive-behavior therapy for panic disorder with agoraphobia in videoconference [Special issue: Telemedicine in Canada]. *Telemedicine Journal and E-Health, 10*(1), 13–24.

Bouton, M. E. (1993). Context, time and memory retrieval in the interference paradigms of Pavlovian learning. *Psychological Bulletin, 114*, 90–99.

Bouton, M. E., Mineka, S., & Barlow, D. H. (2001). A modern learning-theory perspective on the etiology of panic disorder. *Psychological Review, 108*(1), 4–32.

Bouton, M. E., & Swartzentruber, D. (1991). Sources of relapse after extinction in Pavlovian conditioning and instrumental conditioning. *Behavioral Neuroscience, 104*, 44–55.

Broocks, A., Bandelow, B., Pekrun, G., George, A., Meyer, T., Bartmann, U., et al. (1998). Comparison of aerobic exercise, clomipramine, and placebo in the treatment of panic disorder. *American Journal of Psychiatry, 155*, 603–609.

Brown, T. A., Antony, M. M., & Barlow, D. H. (1995). Diagnostic comorbidity in panic disorder: Effect on treatment outcome and course of comorbid diagnoses following treatment. *Journal of Consulting and Clinical Psychology, 63*, 408–418.

Brown, T. A., & Barlow, D. H. (1995). Long-term outcome in cognitive-behavioral treatment of panic disorder: Clinical predictors and alternative strategies for assessment. *Journal of Consulting and Clinical Psychology, 63*, 754–765.

Brown, T. A., & Barlow, D. H. (in press). *Anxiety Disorders Interview Schedule–5*. New York: Oxford University Press.

Brown, T. A., Campbell, L. A., Lehman, C. L., Grisham, J. R., & Mancill, R. B. (2001). Current and lifetime comorbidity of the DSM-IV anxiety and mood disorders in a large clinical sample. *Journal of Abnormal Psychology, 110*(4), 585–599.

Brown, T. A., Chorpita, B. F., & Barlow, D. H. (1998). Structural relationships among dimensions of the DSM-IV anxiety and mood disorders and dimensions of negative affect, positive affect, and autonomic arousal. *Journal of Abnormal Psychology, 107*(2), 179–192.

Brown, T. A., Di Nardo, P. A., Lehman, C. L., & Campbell, L. A. (2001). Reliability of DSM-IV anxiety and mood disorders: Implications for the classification of emotional disorders. *Journal of Abnormal Psychology, 110*(1), 49–58.

Brown, T. A., White, K. S., Forsyth, J. P., & Barlow, D. H. (2004). The structure of perceived emotional control: Psychometric properties of a revised Anxiety Control Questionnaire. *Behavior Therapy, 35*(1), 75–99.

Buglass, P., Clarke, J., Henderson, A., & Presley, A. (1977). A study of agoraphobic housewives. *Psychological Medicine, 7*, 73–86.

Butler, A. C., Chapman, J. E., Forman, E. M., & Beck, A. T. (2006). The empirical status of cognitive-behavioral therapy: A review of meta-analyses. *Clinical Psychology Review, 26*, 17–31.

Campbell-Sills, L., Barlow, D. H., Brown, T. A., & Hofmann, S. G. (2006). Acceptability and suppression of negative emotion in anxiety and mood disorders. *Emotion, 6*(4), 587–595.

Carlbring, P., Ekselius, L., & Andersson, G. (2003). Treatment of panic disorder via the Internet: A randomized trial of CBT vs. applied relaxation. *Journal of Behavior Therapy and Experimental Psychiatry, 34*, 129–140.

Carlbring, P., Nilsson-Ihrfelt, E., Waara, J., Kollenstam, C., Buhrman, M, Klado, V., et al. (2005). Treatment of panic disorder: live therapy vs. self-help via the internet. *Behaviour Research and Therapy, 43*, 1321–1333.

Carter, M. M., Sbrocco, T., Gore, K. L., Marin, N. W., & Lewis, E. L. (2003). Cognitive-behavioral group therapy versus a wait-list control in the treatment of African American women with panic disorder. *Cognitive Therapy and Research, 27*(5), 505–518.

Cerny, J. A., Barlow, D. H., Craske, M. G., & Himadi, W. G. (1987). Couples treatment of agoraphobia: A two-year follow-up. *Behavior Therapy, 18*, 401–415.

Chambless, D. L. (1990). Spacing of exposure sessions in treatment of agoraphobia and simple phobia. *Behavior Therapy, 21*, 217–229.

Chambless, D. L., Caputo, G., Bright, P., & Gallagher, R. (1984). Assessment of fear in agoraphobics: The Body Sensations Questionnaire and the Agoraphobic Cognitions Questionnaire. *Journal of Consulting and Clinical Psychology, 52*, 1090–1097.

Chambless, D. L., Caputo, G., Gracely, S., Jasin, E., & Williams, C. (1985). The Mobility Inventory for Agoraphobia. *Behaviour Research and Therapy, 23*, 35–44.

Chambless, D. L., & Renneberg, B. (1988, September). *Personality disorders of agoraphobics*. Paper presented at World Congress of Behavior Therapy, Edinburgh, Scotland.

Clark, D. M. (1996). Panic disorder: From theory to therapy. In P. M. Salkovskis (Ed.), *From frontiers of cognitive therapy: The state of art and beyond* (pp. 318–344). New York: Guilford Press.

Clark, D. M. (1986). A cognitive approach to panic. *Behaviour Research and Therapy, 24*, 461–470.

Clark, D. M., & Ehlers, A. (1993). An overview of the cognitive theory and treatment of panic disorder. *Applied and Preventive Psychology, 2*, 131–139.

Clark, D. M., Salkovskis, P., & Chalkley, A. (1985). Respiratory control as a treatment for panic attacks. *Journal of Behavior Therapy and Experimental Psychiatry, 16*, 23–30.

Clark, D. M., Salkovskis, P., Gelder, M., Koehler, C., Martin, M., Anastasiades, P., et al. (1988). Tests of a cognitive theory of panic. In I. Hand & H. Wittchen (Eds.), *Panic and phobias II* (pp. 71–90). Berlin: Springer-Verlag.

Clark, D. M., Salkovskis, P. M., Hackmann, A., Middleton, H., Anastasiades, P., & Gelder, M. (1994). A comparison of cognitive therapy, applied relaxation and imipramine in the treatment of panic disorder. *British Journal of Psychiatry, 164*, 759–769.

Clark, D. M., Salkovskis, P. M., Hackmann, A., Wells, A., Ludgate, J., & Gelder, M. (1999). Brief cognitive therapy for panic disorder: A randomized controlled trial. *Journal of Consulting and Clinical Psychology, 67*, 583–589.

Cote, G., Gauthier, J. G., Laberge, B., Cormier, H. J., & Plamondon, J. (1994). Reduced therapist contact in the cognitive behavioral treatment of panic disorder. *Behavior Therapy, 25*, 123–145.

Cox, B. J., Endler, N. S., & Swinson, R. P. (1995). An examination of levels of agoraphobic severity in panic disorder. *Behaviour Research and Therapy, 33*, 57–62.

Craske, M. G., & Barlow, D. H. (1988). A review of the relationship between panic and avoidance. *Clinical Psychology Review, 8*, 667–685.

Craske, M. G., & Barlow, D. H. (1989). Nocturnal panic. *Journal of Nervous and Mental Disease, 177*(3), 160–167.

Craske, M. G., & Barlow, D. H. (2006). *Mastery of your anxiety and panic: Therapist guide* (3rd ed.). New York: Oxford University Press.

Craske, M. G., Brown, T. A., & Barlow, D. H. (1991). Behavioral treatment of panic disorder: A two-year follow-up. *Behavior Therapy, 22*, 289–304.

Craske, M. G., DeCola, J. P., Sachs, A. D., & Pontillo, D. C. (2003). Panic control treatment of agoraphobia. *Journal of Anxiety Disorders, 17*(3), 321–333.

Craske, M. G., Farchione, T., Allen, L., Barrios, V., Stoyanova, M., & Rose, D. (2007). Cognitive behavioral therapy for panic disorder and comorbidity: More of the same or less of more. *Behaviour Research and Therapy, 45*(6), 1095–1109.

Craske, M. G., & Freed, S. (1995). Expectations about arousal and nocturnal panic. *Journal of Abnormal Psychology, 104*, 567–575.

Craske, M. G., Glover, D., & DeCola, J. (1995). Predicted versus unpredicted panic attacks: Acute versus general distress. *Journal of Abnormal Psychology, 104*, 214–223.

Craske, M. G., Golinelli, D., Stein, M. B., Roy-Byrne, P., Bystritsky, A., & Sherbourne, C. (2005). Does the addition of cognitive behavioral therapy improve panic disorder treatment outcome relative to medication alone in the primary-care setting? *Psychological Medicine, 35*(11), 1645–1654.

Craske, M. G., Kircanski, K., Epstein, A., Wittchen, H.-U., Pine, D.S., Lewis-Fernandez, R., et al. (2010). Panic disorder: A review of DSM-IV panic disorder and proposals for DSM-V. *Depression and Anxiety, 27*, 93–112.

Craske, M. G., Kircanski, K., Zelikowsky, M., Mystkowski, J., Chowdhury, N., & Baker, A. (2008). Optimizing inhibitory learning during exposure therapy. *Behaviour Research and Therapy, 46*, 5–27.

Craske, M. G., Lang, A. J., Aikins, D., & Mystkowski, J. L. (2005). Cognitive behavioral therapy for nocturnal panic. *Behavior Therapy, 36*, 43–54.

Craske, M. G., Lang, A. J., Rowe, M., DeCola, J. P., Simmons, J., Mann, C., et al. (2002). Presleep attributions about arousal during sleep: Nocturnal panic. *Journal of Abnormal Psychology, 111*, 53–62.

Craske, M. G., Liao, B., Brown, L., & Vervliet, B. (2012). Role of inhibition in exposure therapy. *Journal of Experimental Psychopathology, 3*(3), 322–345.

Craske, M. G., Maidenberg, E., & Bystritsky, A. (1995). Brief cognitive-behavioral versus non directive therapy for panic disorder. *Journal of Behavior Therapy and Experimental Psychiatry, 26*, 113–120.

Craske, M. G., Miller, P. P., Rotunda, R., & Barlow, D. H. (1990). A descriptive report of features of initial unexpected panic attacks in minimal and extensive avoiders. *Behaviour Research and Therapy, 28*, 395–400.

Craske, M. G., Poulton, R., Tsao, J. C. I., & Plotkin, D. (2001). Paths to panic–agoraphobia: An exploratory analysis from age 3 to 21 in an unselected birth cohort. *American Journal of Child and Adolescent Psychiatry, 40*, 556–563.

Craske, M. G., Rapee, R. M., & Barlow, D. H. (1988). The significance of panic–expectancy for individual patterns of avoidance. *Behavior Therapy, 19*, 577–592.

Craske, M. G., Rose, R. D., Lang, A., Welch, S., Campbell-Sills, L., Sullivan, G., et al. (2009). Computer-assisted delivery of cognitive-behavioral therapy for anxiety disorders in primary care settings. *Depression and Anxiety, 26*, 235–242.

Craske, M. G., & Rowe, M. K. (1997a). A comparison of behavioral and cognitive treatments of phobias. In G. C. L. Davey (Ed.), *Phobias—a handbook of theory, research and treatment* (pp. 247–280). West Sussex, UK: Wiley.

Craske, M. G., & Rowe, M. K. (1997b). Nocturnal panic. *Clinical Psychology: Science and Practice, 4*, 153–174.

Craske, M. G., Rowe, M., Lewin, M., & Noriega-Dimitri, R. (1997). Interoceptive exposure versus breathing retraining within cognitive-behavioural therapy for panic disorder with agoraphobia. *British Journal of Clinical Psychology, 36*, 85–99.

Craske, M. G., Roy-Byrne, P., Stein, M. B., Donald-Sherbourne, C., Bystritsky, A., Katon, W., et al. (2002). Treating panic disorder in primary care: A collaborative care intervention. *General Hospital Psychiatry, 24*(3), 148–155.

Craske, M. G., Roy-Byrne, P., Stein, M. B., Sullivan, G., Hazlett-Stevens, H., Bystritsky, A., et al. (2006). CBT intensity and outcome for panic disorder in a primary care setting. *Behavior Therapy, 37*, 112–119.

Craske, M. G., Stein, M. B., Sullivan, G., Sherbourne, C., Bystritsky, A., Rose, D., et al. (2011). Disorder specific impact of CALM treatment for anxiety disorders in primary care. *Archives of General Psychiatry, 68*, 378–388.

Craske, M. G., & Tsao, J. C. I. (1999). Self-monitoring with panic and anxiety disorders. *Psychological Assessment, 11*, 466–479.

Culver, N., Stoyanova, M. S., & Craske, M. G. (2012). Emotional variability and sustained arousal during exposure. *Journal of Behavior Therapy and Experimental Psychiatry, 43*, 787–793.

Culver, N., Vervliet, B., & Craske, M. G. (in press). Compound extinction: Using the Rescorla–Wagner model to maximize the effects of exposure therapy for anxiety disorders. *Clinical Psychological Science.*

Dattilio, F. M., & Salas-Auvert, J. A. (2000). *Panic disorder: Assessment and treatment through a wide-angle lens.* Phoenix, AZ: Zeig, Tucker.

Deacon, B., & Abramowitz, J. (2006). A pilot study of two-day cognitive-behavioral therapy for panic disorder. *Behaviour Research and Therapy, 44*, 807–817.

de Beurs, E., Lange, A., van Dyck, R., & Koele, P. (1995). Respiratory training prior to exposure *in vivo* in the treatment of panic disorder with agoraphobia: Efficacy and predictors of outcome. *Australian and New Zealand Journal of Psychiatry, 29*, 104–113.

de Beurs, E., van Balkom, A. J., Lange, A., Koele, P., & van Dyck, R. (1995). Treatment of panic disorder with agoraphobia: Comparison of fluvoxamine, placebo, and psychological panic management combined with exposure and of exposure *in vivo* alone. *American Journal of Psychiatry, 152*, 683–691.

Debiec, J., & Le Doux, J. E. (2004). Disruption of reconsolidation but not consolidation of auditory fear conditioning by noradrenergic blockade in the amygdala. *Neuroscience, 129*(2), 267–272.

Deckert, J., Nothen, M. M., Franke, P., Delmo, C., Fritze, J., Knapp, M., et al. (1998). Systematic mutation screening and association study of the A1 and A2a adenosine receptor genes in panic disorder suggest a contribution of the A2a gene to the development of disease. *Molecular Psychiatry, 3*, 81–85.

De Cort, K., Hermans, D., Spruyt, A., Griez, E., & Schruers, K. (2008). A specific attentional bias in panic disorder? *Depression and Anxiety, 25*(11), 951–955.

de Jong, M. G., & Bouman, T. K. (1995). Panic disorder: A baseline period: Predictability of agoraphobic avoidance behavior. *Journal of Anxiety Disorders, 9*, 185–199.

Dewey, D., & Hunsley, J. (1990). The effects of marital adjustment and spouse involvement on the behavioral treatment of agoraphobia: A meta-analytic review. *Anxiety Research, 2*(2), 69–83.

Di Nardo, P., Brown, T. A., & Barlow, D. H. (1994). *Anxiety Disorders Interview Schedule—Fourth Edition (ADIS-IV).* New York: Oxford University Press.

Domschke, K., Agineszka, G., Winter, B., Hermann, M. J., Warrings B., Muhlberger, A., et al. (2011). ADORA2A gene variation, caffeine, and emotional processing: A multi-level interaction on startle reflex. *Neuropsychopharmacology, 37*, 759–769.

Dow, M., Kenardy, J., Johnston, D., Newman, M., Taylor, C., & Thomson, A. (2007). Prognostic indices with brief and standard CBT for panic disorder: I. Predictors of outcome. *Psychological Medicine, 27*, 1493–1502.

Dreessen, L., Arntz, A., Luttels, C., & Sallaerts, S. (1994). Personality disorders do not influence the results of cognitive behavior therapies for anxiety disorders. *Comprehensive Psychiatry, 35*(4), 265–274.

Dworkin, B. R., & Dworkin, S. (1999). Heterotopic and homotopic classical conditioning of the baroreflex. *Integrative Physiological and Behavioral Science, 34*(3), 158–176.

Ehlers, A. (1995). A 1–year prospective study of panic attacks: Clinical course and factors associated with maintenance. *Journal of Abnormal Psychology, 104*, 164–172.

Ehlers, A., & Breuer, P. (1992). Increased cardiac awareness in panic disorder. *Journal of Abnormal Psychology, 101*, 371–382.

Ehlers, A., & Breuer, P. (1996). How good are patients with panic disorder at perceiving their heartbeats? *Biological Psychology, 42*, 165–182.

Ehlers, A., Breuer, P., Dohn, D., & Fiegenbaum, W. (1995). Heartbeat perception and panic disorder: Possible explanations for discrepant findings. *Behaviour Research and Therapy, 33*, 69–76.

Ehlers, A., & Margraf, J. (1989). The psychophysiological model of panic attacks. In P. M. G. Emmelkamp (Ed.), *Anxiety disorders: Annual series of European research in behavior therapy* (Vol. 4, pp. 1–29). Amsterdam: Swets.

Ehlers, A., Margraf, J., Davies, S., & Roth, W. T. (1988). Selective processing of threat cues in subjects with panic attacks. *Cognition and Emotion, 2*, 201–219.

Ehlers, A., Margraf, J., Roth, W. T., Taylor, C. B., & Birnbaumer, N. (1988). Anxiety induced by false heart rate feedback in patients with panic disorder. *Behaviour Research and Therapy, 26*(1), 1–11.

Eifert, G. H., & Heffner, M. (2003). The effects of acceptance versus control contexts on avoidance of panic-related symptoms. *Journal of Behavior Therapy and Experimental Psychiatry, 34*(3–4), 293–312.

Eley, T. C. (2001). Contributions of behavioral genetics research: Quantifying genetic, shared environmental and nonshared environmental influences. In M. W. Vasey & M. R. Dadds (Eds.), *The developmental psychopathology of anxiety* (pp. 45–59). New York: Oxford University Press.

Emmelkamp, P. (1980). Agoraphobic's interpersonal problems. *Archives of General Psychiatry, 37*, 1303–1306.

Emmelkamp, P. M., & Wittchen, H.-U. (2009). Specific phobias. In G. Andrews (Ed.), *Stress-induced and fear circuitry disorders: Advancing the research agenda for DSM-V* (pp. 77–104). Arlington, VA: American Psychiatric Association.

Evans, L., Holt, C., & Oei, T. P. S. (1991). Long term follow-up of agoraphobics treated by brief intensive group cognitive behaviour therapy. *Australian and New Zealand Journal of Psychiatry, 25*, 343–349.

Eysenck, H. J. (1967). *The biological basis of personality.* Springfield, IL: Thomas.

Faravelli, C., Pallanti, S., Biondi, F., Paterniti, S., & Scarpato, M. A. (1992). Onset of panic disorder. *American Journal of Psychiatry, 149*, 827–828.

Feigenbaum, W. (1988). Long-term efficacy of ungraded versus graded massed exposure in agoraphobics. In I. Hand & H. Wittchen (Eds.), *Panic and phobias: Treatments and variables affecting course and outcome* (pp. 83–88). Berlin: Springer-Verlag.

First, M. B., Spitzer, R. L., Gibbon, M., & Williams, J. B. W. (1994). *Structured Clinical Interview for Axis I DSM-IV Disorders.* New York: Biometric Research Department, New York State Psychiatric Institute.

Foa, E. B., & Kozak, M. J. (1986). Emotional processing of fear: exposure to corrective information. *Psychological Bulletin, 99*, 20–35.

Foa, E. B., & McNally, R. J. (1996). Mechanisms of change in exposure therapy. In R. M. Rapee (Ed.), *Current controversies in the anxiety disorders* (pp. 329–343). New York: Guilford Press.

Forsyth, J. P., Palav, A., & Duff, K. (1999). The absence of relation between anxiety sensitivity and fear conditioning using 20% versus 13% CO_2-enriched air as unconditioned stimuli. *Behaviour Research and Therapy, 37*(2), 143–153.

Friedman, S., & Paradis, C. (1991). African-American patients with panic disorder and agoraphobia. *Journal of Anxiety Disorders, 5*, 35–41.

Friedman, S., Paradis, C. M., & Hatch, M. (1994). Characteristics of African-American and white patients with panic disorder and agoraphobia. *Hospital and Community Psychiatry, 45*, 798–803.

Fry, W. (1962). The marital context of an anxiety syndrome. *Family Process, 1*, 245–252.

Garssen, B., de Ruiter, C., & van Dyck, R. (1992). Breathing retraining: A rational placebo? *Clinical Psychology Review, 12*, 141–153.

Ghosh, A., & Marks, I. M. (1987). Self-treatment of agoraphobia by exposure. *Behavior Therapy, 18*, 3–16.

Glenn, D., Golinelli, D., Rose, R., Roy-Byrne, P., Stein, M.,

Sullivan, G., et al. (in press). Who gets the most out of cognitive behavioral therapy for anxiety disorders: The role of treatment dose and patient engagement. *Journal of Consulting and Clinical Psychology.*

Gloster, A. T., Wittchen, H.-U., Einsle, F., Lang, T., Helbig-Lang, S., Fydrich, T., et al. (2011). Psychological treatment for panic disorder with agoraphobia: A randomized controlled trial to examine the role of therapist-guided exposure in situ in CBT. *Journal of Consulting and Clinical Psychology, 79*, 406–420.

Goisman, R. M., Goldenberg, I., Vasile, R. G., & Keller, M. B. (1995). Comorbidity of anxiety disorders in a multicenter anxiety study. *Comprehensive Psychiatry, 36*, 303–311.

Goisman, R. M., Warshaw, M. G., Peterson, L. G., Rogers, M. P., Cuneo, P., Hunt, M. F., et al. (1994). Panic, agoraphobia, and panic disorder with agoraphobia: Data from a multicenter anxiety disorders study. *Journal of Nervous and Mental Disease, 182*, 72–79.

Goldstein, A. J., & Chambless, D. L. (1978). A reanalysis of agoraphobia. *Behavior Therapy, 9*, 47–59.

Goodwin, R. D., Fergusson, D. M., & Horwood, L. J. (2005). Childhood abuse and familial violence and the risk of panic attacks and panic disorder in young adulthood. *Psychological Medicine, 35*, 881–890.

Gorman, J. M., Papp, L. A., Coplan, J. D., Martinez, J. M., Lennon, S., Goetz, R. R., et al. (1994). Anxiogenic effects of CO_2 and hyperventilation in patients with panic disorder. *American Journal of Psychiatry, 151*(4), 547–553.

Gould, R. A., & Clum, G. A. (1995). Self-help plus minimal therapist contact in the treatment of panic disorder: A replication and extension. *Behavior Therapy, 26*, 533–546.

Gould, R. A., Clum, G. A., & Shapiro, D. (1993). The use of bibliotherapy in the treatment of panic: A preliminary investigation. *Behavior Therapy, 24*, 241–252.

Gray, J. A. (1982). *The neuropsychology of anxiety: An enquiry into the functions of the septo-hippocampal system.* New York: Oxford University Press.

Griez, E., & van den Hout, M. A. (1986). CO_2 inhalation in the treatment of panic attacks. *Behaviour Research and Therapy, 24*, 145–150.

Grilo, C. M., Money, R., Barlow, D. H., Goddard, A. W., Gorman, J. M., Hofmann, S. G., et al. (1998). Pretreatment patient factors predicting attrition from a multicenter randomized controlled treatment study for panic disorder. *Comprehensive Psychiatry, 39*, 323–332.

Haby, M., Donnelly, M., Corry, J., & Vos, T. (2006). Cognitive behavioural therapy for depression, panic disorder and generalized anxiety disorder: A meta-regression of factors that may predict outcome. *Australian and New Zealand Journal of Psychiatry, 40*, 9–19.

Hafner, R. J. (1984). Predicting the effects on husbands of behavior therapy for agoraphobia. *Behaviour Research and Therapy, 22*, 217–226.

Hamilton, S. P., Fyer, A. J., Durner, M., Heiman, G. A., Baisre de Leon, A., Hodge, S. E., et al. (2003). Further genetic evidence for a panic disorder syndrome mapping to chromosome 13q. *Proceedings of National Academy of Science USA, 100,* 2550–2555.

Hamilton, S. P., Slager, S. L., De Leon, A. B., Heiman, G. A., Klein, D. F., Hodge, S. E., et al. (2004). Evidence for genetic linkage between a polymorphism in the adenosine 2A receptor and panic disorder. *Neuropsychopharmacology, 29,* 558–565.

Hamilton, S. P., Slager, S. L., Helleby, L., Heiman, G. A., Klein, D. F., Hodge, S. E., et al. (2001). No association or linkage between polymorphisms in the genes encoding cholecystokinin and the cholecystokinin B receptor and panic disorder. *Molecular Psychiatry, 6,* 59–65.

Hand, I., & Lamontagne, Y. (1976). The exacerbation of interpersonal problems after rapid phobia removal. *Psychotherapy: Theory, Research and Practice, 13,* 405–411.

Haslam, M. T. (1974). The relationship between the effect of lactate infusion on anxiety states and their amelioration by carbon dioxide inhalation. *British Journal of Psychiatry, 125,* 88–90.

Hayes, S. C., Strosahl, K. D., & Wilson, K. G. (1999). *Acceptance and commitment therapy: An experiential approach to behavior change.* New York: Guilford Press.

Hayes, S. C., Wilson, K. G., Gifford, E. V., & Follette, V. M. (1996). Experiential avoidance and behavioral disorders: A functional dimensional approach to diagnosis and treatment. *Journal of Consulting and Clinical Psychology, 64*(6), 1152–1168.

Hayward, C., Killen, J. D., Hammer, L. D., Litt, I. F., Wilson, D. M., Simmonds, B., et al. (1992). Pubertal stage and panic attack history in sixth- and seventh-grade girls. *American Journal of Psychiatry, 149,* 1239–1243.

Hayward, C., Killen, J. D., Kraemer, H. C., & Taylor, C. B. (2000). Predictors of panic attacks in adolescents. *Journal of the American Academy of Child and Adolescent Psychiatry, 39*(2), 1–8.

Hecker, J. E., Losee, M. C., Fritzler, B. K., & Fink, C. M. (1996). Self-directed versus therapist-directed cognitive behavioral treatment for panic disorder. *Journal of Anxiety Disorders, 10,* 253–265.

Hecker, J. E., Losee, M. C., Roberson-Nay, R., & Maki, K. (2004). Mastery of your anxiety and panic and brief therapist contact in the treatment of panic disorder. *Journal of Anxiety Disorders, 18*(2), 111–126.

Helbig-Lang, S., & Petermann, F. (2010). Tolerate or eliminate?: A systematic review on the effects of safety behavior across anxiety disorders. *Clinical Psychology: Science and Practice, 17*(3), 218–233.

Heldt, E., Manfro, G. G., Kipper, L., Blaya, C., Isolan, L., & Otto, M. W. (2006). One-year follow-up of pharmacotherapy-resistant patients with panic disorder treated with cognitive-behavior therapy: Outcome and predictors of remission. *Behaviour Research and Therapy, 44*(5), 657–665.

Hermans, D., Craske, M. G., Mineka, S., & Lovibond, P. F. (2006). Extinction in human fear conditioning. *Biological Psychiatry, 60,* 361–368.

Heuzenroeder, L., Donnelly, M., Haby, M. M., Mihalopoulos, C., Rossell, R., Carter, R., et al. (2004). Cost-effectiveness of psychological and pharmacological interventions for generalized anxiety disorder and panic disorder. *Australian and New Zealand Journal of Psychiatry, 38*(8), 602–612.

Hibbert, G., & Pilsbury, D. (1989). Hyperventilation: Is it a cause of panic attacks? *British Journal of Psychiatry, 155,* 805–809.

Himadi, W., Cerny, J., Barlow, D., Cohen, S., & O'Brien, G. (1986). The relationship of marital adjustment to agoraphobia treatment outcome. *Behaviour Research and Therapy, 24,* 107–115.

Hoffart, A. (1995). A comparison of cognitive and guided mastery therapy of agoraphobia. *Behaviour Research and Therapy, 33,* 423–434.

Hoffart, A. (1997). Interpersonal problems among patients suffering from panic disorder with agoraphobia before and after treatment. *British Journal of Medical Psychology, 70*(2), 149–157.

Hoffart, A., & Hedley, L. M. (1997). Personality traits among panic disorder with agoraphobia patients before and after symptom-focused treatment. *Journal of Anxiety Disorders, 11,* 77–87.

Hoffart, A., Sexton, H., Hedley, L., & Martinsen, E. W. (2008). Mechanisms of change in cognitive therapy for panic disorder with agoraphobia. *Journal of Behavior Therapy and Experimental Psychiatry, 39*(3), 262–275.

Hofmann, S. G., Shear, M. K., Barlow, D. H., Gorman, J. M., Hershberger, D., Patterson, M., et al. (1988). Effects of panic disorder treatments on personality disorder characteristics. *Depression and Anxiety, 8*(1), 14–20.

Hofmann, S. G., Suvak, M. K., Barlow, D. H., Shear, M. K., Meuret, A. E., et al. (2007). Preliminary evidence for cognitive mediation during cognitive-behavioral therapy of panic disorder. *Journal of Consulting and Clinical Psychology, 75*(3), 374–379.

Holden, A. E. O., O'Brien, G. T., Barlow, D. H., Stetson, D., & Infantino, A. (1983). Self-help manual for agoraphobia: A preliminary report of effectiveness. *Behavior Therapy, 14,* 545–556.

Holt, P., & Andrews, G. (1989). Hyperventilation and anxiety in panic disorder, agoraphobia, and generalized anxiety disorder. *Behaviour Research and Therapy, 27,* 453–460.

Hope, D. A., Rapee, R. M., Heimberg, R. G., & Dombeck, M. J. (1990). Representations of the self in social phobia: Vulnerability to social threat. *Cognitive Therapy and Research, 14,* 177–189.

Hornsveld, H., Garssen, B., Fiedeldij Dop, M., & van Spiegel, P. (1990). Symptom reporting during voluntary hyperventilation and mental load: Implications for diagnosing hyperventilation syndrome. *Journal of Psychosomatic Research, 34,* 687–697.

Huppert, J. D., Bufka, L. F., Barlow, D. H., Gorman, J. M., Shear, M. K., & Woods, S. W. (2001). Therapist, therapist variables, and cognitive-behavioral therapy outcome in a multicenter trial for panic disorder. *Journal of Consulting and Clinical Psychology, 69*(5), 747–755.

Issakidis, C., & Andrews, G. (2004). Pretreatment attrition and dropout in an outpatient clinic for anxiety disorders. *Acta Psychiatrica Scandinavica, 109*(6), 426–433.

Ito, L. M., Noshirvani, H., Basoglu, M., & Marks, I. M. (1996). Does exposure to internal cues enhance exposure to external exposure to external cues in agoraphobia with panic. *Psychotherapy and Psychosomatics, 65,* 24–28.

Izard, C. E. (1992). Basic emotions, relations among emotions, and emotion cognition relations. *Psychological Review, 99,* 561–565.

Jacob, R. G., Furman, J. M., Clark, D. B., & Durrant, J. D. (1992). Vestibular symptoms, panic, and phobia: Overlap and possible relationships. *Annals of Clinical Psychiatry, 4*(3), 163–174.

Kampfe, C. K., Gloster, A. T., Wittchen, H.-U., Helbig-Lang, S., Lang, T., & Gerlach, A. L. (2012). Experiential avoidance and anxiety sensitivity in patients with panic disorder and agoraphobia: Do both constructs measure the same? *International Journal of Clinical and Health Psychology, 12,* 5–22.

Kampman, M., Keijsers, G. P. J., Hoogduin, C. A. L., & Hendriks, G.-J. (2002). A randomized, double-blind, placebo-controlled study of the effects of adjunctive paroxetine in panic disorder patients unsuccessfully treated with cognitive-behavioral therapy alone. *Journal of Clinical Psychiatry, 63*(9), 772–777.

Katon, W., Von Korff, M., Lin, E., Lipscomb, P., Russo, J., Wagner, E., et al. (1990). Distressed high utilizers of medical care: DSM-III-R diagnoses and treatment needs. *General Hospital Psychiatry, 12*(6), 355–362.

Katschnig, H., & Amering, M. (1998). The long-term course of panic disorder and its predictors. *Journal of Clinical Psychopharmacology, 18*(6, Suppl. 2), 6S–11S.

Keijsers, G. P., Kampman, M., & Hoogduin, C. A. (2001). Dropout prediction in cognitive behavior therapy for panic disorder. *Behavior Therapy, 32*(4), 739–749.

Keijsers, G. P., Schaap, C. P., Hoogduin, C. A., & Lammers, M. W. (1995). Patient–therapist interaction in the behavioral treatment of panic disorder with agoraphobia. *Behavior Modification, 19,* 491–517.

Keller, M. L., & Craske, M. G. (2008). Panic disorder and agoraphobia. In J. Hunsley & E. J. Mash (Eds.), *A guide to assessments that work* (pp. 229–253). New York: Oxford University Press.

Kendler, K. S., Bulik, C. M., Silberg, J., Hettema, J. M., Myers, J., & Prescott, C. A. (2000). Childhood sexual abuse and adult psychiatric and substance use disorders in women: An epidemiological and co-twin analysis. *Archives of General Psychiatry, 57,* 953–959.

Kendler, K. S., Heath, A. C., Martin, N. G., & Eaves, L. J. (1987). Symptoms of anxiety and symptoms of depression: Same genes, different environments? *Archives of General Psychiatry, 44,* 451–457.

Kessler, R. C., Berglund, P., Demler, O., Jin, R., & Walters, E. E. (2005). Lifetime prevalence and age-of-onset distributions of DSM-IV disorders in the National Comorbidity Survey Replication. *Archives of General Psychiatry, 62,* 593–602.

Kessler, R. C., Chiu, W. T., Demler, O., & Walters, E. E. (2005). Lifetime prevalence and age-of-onset distributions of DSM-IV disorders in the National Comorbidity Survey Replication. *Archives of General Psychiatry, 62*(6), 593–602.

Kessler, R. C., Chiu, W. T., Jin, R., Ruscio, A. M., Shear, K., & Walters, E. E. (2006). The epidemiology of panic attacks, panic disorder, and agoraphobia in the National Comorbidity Survey Replication. *Archives of General Psychiatry, 63,* 415–424.

Kessler, R. C., Davis, C. G., & Kendler, K. S. (1997). Childhood adversity and adult psychiatric disorder in the U.S. National Comorbidity Survey. *Psychological Medicine, 27,* 1101–1119.

Kessler, R. C., McGonagle, K. A., Zhao, S., Nelson, C. B., Hughes, M., Eshleman, S., et al. (1994). Lifetime and 12 month prevalence of DSM-III-R psychiatric disorders in the United States: Results from the National Comorbidity Study. *Archives of General Psychiatry, 51,* 8–19.

Kessler, R. C., Petukhova, M., Sampson, N. A., Zaslavsky, A. M., & Wittchen, H.-U. (2012). Twelve-month and life time prevalence and lifetime morbid risk of anxiety and mood disorders in the United States. *International Journal of Methods in Psychiatric Research, 21*(3), 169–184.

Keyl, P. M., & Eaton, W. W. (1990). Risk factors for the onset of panic disorder and other panic attacks in a prospective, population-based study. *American Journal of Epidemiology, 131,* 301–311.

Kikuchi, M., Komuro, R., Hiroshi, O., Kidani, T., Hanaoka, A., & Koshino, Y. (2005). Panic disorder with and without agoraphobia: Comorbidity within a half-year of the onset of panic disorder. *Psychiatry and Clinical Neurosciences, 58,* 639–643.

Kindt, M., Soeter, M., & Vervliet, B. (2009). Beyond extinction: Erasing human fear responses and preventing the return of fear. *Nature Neuroscience, 12,* 256–258.

Kircanski, K., Craske, M. G., Epstein, A. M., & Wittchen, H.-U. (2009). Subtypes of panic attacks: A critical review of the empirical literature. *Depression and Anxiety, 26,* 878–887.

Kircanski, K., Mortazavi, A., Castriotta, N., Baker, A., Mystkowski, J., Yi, R., et al. (2011). Challenges to the traditional exposure paradigm: variability in exposure therapy for contamination fears. *Journal of Behavior Therapy and Experimental Psychiatry, 43,* 745–751.

Kiropoulos, L. A., Klein, B., Austin, D. W., Gilson, K., Pier, C., Mitchell J., et al. (2008). Is internet-based CBT for panic disorder and agoraphobia as effective as face-to-face CBT? *Journal of Anxiety Disorders, 22,* 1273–1284.

Kraft, A. R., & Hoogduin, C. A. (1984). The hyperventilation syndrome: A pilot study of the effectiveness of treatment. *British Journal of Psychiatry, 145,* 538–542.

Kroeze, S., & van den Hout, M. A. (2000). Selective attention for cardiac information in panic patients. *Behaviour Research and Therapy, 38,* 63–72.

Krystal, J. H., Woods, S. W., Hill, C. L., & Charney, D. S. (1991). Characteristics of panic attack subtypes: Assessment of spontaneous panic, situational panic, sleep panic, and limited symptom attacks. *Comprehensive Psychiatry, 32*(6), 474–480.

Lake, R. I., Eaves, L. J., Maes, H. H., Heath, A. C., & Martin, N. G. (2000). Further evidence against the environmental transmission of individual differences in neuroticism from a collaborative study of 45,850 twins and relatives of two continents. *Behavior Genetics, 30*(3), 223–233.

Lang, A. J., & Craske, M. G. (2000). Manipulations of exposure based therapy to reduce return of fear: a replication. *Behaviour Research and Therapy, 38,* 1–12.

Lehman, C. L., Brown, T. A., & Barlow, D. H. (1998). Effects of cognitive-behavioral treatment for panic disorder with agoraphobia on concurrent alcohol abuse. *Behavior Therapy, 29,* 423–433.

Lelliott, P., Marks, I., McNamee, G., & Tobena, A. (1989). Onset of panic disorder with agoraphobia: Toward an integrated model. *Archives of General Psychiatry, 46,* 1000–1004.

Levitt, J. T., Brown, T. A., Orsillo, S. M., & Barlow, D. H. (2004). The effects of acceptance versus suppression of emotion on subjective and psychophysiological response to carbon dioxide challenge in patients with panic disorder. *Behavior Therapy, 35,* 747–766.

Lewis-Fernandez, R., Hinton, D. E., Laria, A. J., Patterson, E. H., Hofmann, S. G., Craske, M. et al. (2010). Culture and the anxiety disorders: recommendations for DSM-V. *Depression and Anxiety, 27,* 212–229.

Lidren, D. M., Watkins, P., Gould, R. A., Clum, G. A., Asterino, M., & Tulloch, H. L. (1994). A comparison of bibliotherapy and group therapy in the treatment of panic disorder. *Journal of Consulting and Clinical Psychology, 62,* 865–869.

Lovibond, P. F., Davis, N. R., & O'Flaherty, A. S. (2000). Protection from extinction in human fear conditioning. *Behaviour Research and Therapy, 38,* 967–983.

Lissek, S., Powers, A. S., McClure, E. B., Phelps, E. A., Wolderhawariat, G., et al. (2005). Classical fear conditioning in the anxiety disorders: A meta-analysis. *Behaviour Research and Therapy, 43,* 1391–1424.

Lissek, S., Rabin, S. J., Heller, R. E., Lukenbaugh, D., Geraci,

M., Pine, D. S., et al. (2010). Overgeneralization of conditioned fear as a pathogenic marker of panic disorder. *American Journal of Psychiatry, 167*(1), 47–55.

Lissek, S., Rabin, S. J., McDowell, D. J., Divir, S., Bradford, D. E., Geraci, M., et al. (2009). Impaired discriminative fear-conditioning resulting from elevated fear responding to learned safety cues among individuals with panic disorder. *Behaviour Research and Therapy, 47*(2), 111–118.

Maidenberg, E., Chen, E., Craske, M., Bohn, P., & Bystritsky, A. (1996). Specificity of attentional bias in panic disorder and social phobia. *Journal of Anxiety Disorders, 10,* 529–541.

Maier, S. F., Laudenslager, M. L., & Ryan, S. M. (1985). Stressor controllability, immune function and endogenous opiates. In F. R. Brush & J. B. Overmeier (Eds.), *Affect, conditioning and cognition: Essays on the determinants of behavior* (pp. 183–201). Hillsdale, NJ: Erlbaum.

Maller, R. G., & Reiss, S. (1992). Anxiety sensitivity in 1984 and panic attacks in 1987. *Journal of Anxiety Disorders, 6*(3), 241–247.

Mannuzza, S., Fyer, A. J., Liebowitz, M. R., & Klein, D. F. (1990). Delineating the boundaries of social phobia: Its relationship to panic disorder and agoraphobia. *Journal of Anxiety Disorders, 4*(1), 41–59.

Marchand, A., Goyer, L. R., Dupuis, G., & Mainguy, N. (1998). Personality disorders and the outcome of cognitive-behavioural treatment of panic disorder with agoraphobia. *Canadian Journal of Behavioural Science, 30*(1), 14–23.

Margraf, J., Taylor, C. B., Ehlers, A., Roth, W. T., & Agras, W. S. (1987). Panic attacks in the natural environment. *Journal of Nervous and Mental Disease, 175,* 558–565.

Marks, I. M., Swinson, R. P., Basoglu, M., Kuck, K., Noshirvani, H., O'Sullivan, G., et al. (1993). Alprazolam and exposure alone and combined in panic disorder with agoraphobia: A controlled study in London and Toronto. *British Journal of Psychiatry, 162,* 776–787.

Martin, N. G., Jardine, R., Andrews, G., & Heath, A. C. (1988). Anxiety disorders and neuroticism: Are there genetic factors specific to panic? *Acta Psychiatrica Scandinavica, 77,* 698–706.

Mavissakalian, M., & Hamman, M. (1987). DSM-III personality disorder in agoraphobia: II. Changes with treatment. *Comprehensive Psychiatry, 28,* 356–361.

McLean, P. D., Woody, S., Taylor, S., & Koch, W. J. (1998). Comorbid panic disorder and major depression: Implications for cognitive-behavioral therapy. *Journal of Consulting and Clinical Psychology, 66,* 240–247.

McNally, R. J., & Lorenz, M. (1987). Anxiety sensitivity in agoraphobics. *Journal of Behavior Therapy and Experimental Psychiatry, 18*(1), 3–11.

McNally, R. J., Riemann, B. C., Louro, C. E., Lukach, B. M., & Kim, E. (1992). Cognitive processing of emotional information in panic disorder. *Behaviour Research and Therapy, 30,* 143–149.

McNamee, G., O'Sullivan, G., Lelliott, P., & Marks, I. M. (1989). Telephone-guided treatment for housebound agoraphobics with panic disorder: Exposure vs. relaxation. *Behavior Therapy, 20,* 491–497.

Mellman, T. A., & Uhde, T. W. (1989). Sleep panic attacks: New clinical findings and theoretical implications. *American Journal of Psychiatry, 146,* 1204–1207.

Messenger, C., & Shean, G. (1998). The effects of anxiety sensitivity and history of panic on reactions to stressors in a non-clinical sample. *Journal of Behavior Therapy, 29,* 279–288.

Meuret, A. E., Rosenfield, D., Seidel, A., Bhaskara, L., & Hofmann, S. G. (2010). Respiratory and cognitive mediators of treatment change in panic disorder: Evidence for intervention specificity. *Journal of Consulting and Clinical Psychology, 78,* 691–704.

Meuret, A. E., Twohig, M. P., Rosenfield, D., Hayes, S. C., & Craske, M. G. (2012). Brief acceptance and commitment therapy and exposure for panic disorder: A pilot study. *Cognitive and Behavioral Practice, 19*(4), 606–618.

Meuret, A. E., Wilhelm, F. H., Ritz, T., & Roth, W. T. (2008). Feedback of end-tidal pCO2 as a therapeutic approach for panic disorder. *Journal of Psychiatric Research, 42*(7), 560–568.

Michelson, L., Mavissakalian, M., Marchione, K., Ulrich, R., Marchione, N., & Testa, S. (1990). Psychophysiological outcome of cognitive, behavioral, and psychophysiologically based treatments of agoraphobia. *Behaviour Research and Therapy, 28,* 127–139.

Milton, F., & Hafner, J. (1979). The outcome of behavior therapy for agoraphobia in relation to marital adjustment. *Archives of General Psychiatry, 36,* 807–811.

Mineka, S., Cook, M., & Miller, S. (1984). Fear conditioned with escapable and inescapable shock: The effects of a feedback stimulus. *Journal of Experimental Psychology: Animal Behavior Processes, 10,* 307–323.

Moisan, D., & Engels, M. L. (1995). Childhood trauma and personality disorder in 43 women with panic disorder. *Psychological Reports, 76,* 1133–1134.

Murphy, M. T., Michelson, L. K., Marchione, K., Marchione, N., & Testa, S. (1998). The role of self-directed *in vivo* exposure in combination with cognitive therapy, relaxation training, or therapist-assisted exposure in the treatment of panic disorder with agoraphobia. *Behaviour Research and Therapy, 12,* 117–138.

Mystkowski, J. L., Craske, M. G., Echiverri, A. M., & Labus, J. S. (2006). Mental reinstatement of context and return of fear in spider-fearful participants. *Behavior Therapy, 37*(1), 49–60.

Nader, K., Schafe, G. E., & Le Doux, J. E. (2000). Fear memories require protein synthesis in the amygdala for reconsolidation after retrieval. *Nature, 406,* 722–726.

Neron, S., Lacroix, D., & Chaput, Y. (1995). Group vs individual cognitive behaviour therapy in panic disorder: An open clinical trial with a six month follow-up. *Canadian Journal of Behavioural Science, 27,* 379–392.

Neumann, D. L., Lipp, O. V., & Cory, S. E. (2007). Conducting extinction in multiple contexts does not necessarily attenuate the renewal of shock expectancy in a fear-conditioning procedure with humans. *Behaviour Research and Therapy, 45,* 385–394.

Niles, A. N., Sherbourne, C., Roy-Byrne, P., Stein, M., Sullivan, G., Bystritsky, A., et al. (2013). Anxiety treatment improves physical functioning with oblique scoring of the SF-12 Short Form Health Survey. *General Hospital Psychiatry, 35*(3), 291–296.

Norberg, M. M., Krystal, J. H., & Tolin, D. F. (2008). A meta-analysis of D-cycloserine and the facilitation of fear extinction and exposure therapy. *Biological Psychiatry, 63,* 1118–1126.

Norton, G. R., Cox, B. J., & Malan, J. (1992). Nonclinical panickers: A critical review. *Clinical Psychology Review, 12,* 121–139.

Norton, P., & Price, E. (2007). A meta-analytic review of adult cognitive-behavioral treatment outcome across the anxiety disorders. *Journal of Nervous and Mental Disease, 195,* 521–531.

Noyes, R., Clancy, J., Garvey, M. J., & Anderson, D. J. (1987). Is agoraphobia a variant of panic disorder or a separate illness? *Journal of Anxiety Disorders, 1,* 3–13.

Noyes, R., Crowe, R. R., Harris, E. L., Hamra, B. J., McChesney, C.M., & Chaudhry, D. R. (1986). Relationship between panic disorder and agoraphobia: A family study. *Archives of General Psychiatry, 43,* 227–232.

Noyes, R., Reich, J., Suelzer, M., & Christiansen, J. (1991). Personality traits associated with panic disorder: Change associated with treatment. *Comprehensive Psychiatry, 32,* 282–294.

Okamura, N., Garau, C., Duangdao, D. M., Clark, S. D., Jungling, K., Hans-Christian, P., et al. (2011). Neuropeptide S enhances memory during the consolidation phase and interacts with noradrenergic systems in the brain. *Neuropsychopharmacology, 36*(4), 744–752.

Öst, L.-G. (1988). Applied relaxation vs. progressive relaxation in the treatment of panic disorder. *Behaviour Research and Therapy, 26,* 13–22.

Öst, L.-G., Thulin, U., & Ramnero, J. (2004). Cognitive behavior therapy vs exposure *in vivo* in the treatment of panic disorder with agoraphobia. *Behaviour Research and Therapy, 42*(1), 1105–1127.

Öst, L. G., & Westling, B. E. (1995). Applied relaxation vs cognitive behavior therapy in the treatment of panic disorder. *Behaviour Research and Therapy, 33,* 145–158.

Öst, L. G., Westling, B. E., & Hellström, K. (1993). Applied relaxation, exposure *in vivo*, and cognitive methods in the treatment of panic disorder with agoraphobia. *Behaviour Research and Therapy, 31,* 383–394.

Otto, M. W., Pollack, M. H., & Sabatino, S. A. (1996). Maintenance of remission following cognitive behavior therapy for panic disorder: Possible deleterious effects of concurrent medication treatment. *Behavior Therapy, 27,* 473–482.

Otto, M. W., Tolin, D. F., Simon, N. M., Pearlson, G. D., Basden, S., Meunier, S. A., et al. (2010). Efficacy of D-cycloserine for enhancing response to cognitive-behavior therapy for panic disorder. *Biological Psychiatry, 67*(4), 365–370.

Pauli, P., Amrhein, C., Muhlberger, A., Dengler, W., & Wiedemann, G. (2005). Electrocortical evidence for an early abnormal processing of panic-related words in panic disorder patients. *International Journal of Psychophysiology, 57,* 33–41.

Payne, L. A., White, K. S., Gallagher, M. W., Woods, S. W., Shear, M. K., Gorman, J. M., et al. (2012). *Second-stage treatments for relative non-responders to cognitive-behavioral therapy (CBT) for panic disorder with and without agoraphobia.* Manuscript submitted for publication.

Pennebaker, J. W., & Roberts, T. (1992). Toward a his and hers theory of emotion: Gender differences in visceral perception. *Journal of Social and Clinical Psychology, 11*(30), 199–212.

Perna, G., Bertani, A., Arancio, C., Ronchi, P., & Bellodi, L. (1995). Laboratory response of patients with panic and obsessive–compulsive disorders to 35% CO_2 challenges. *American Journal of Psychiatry, 152,* 85–89.

Prenoveau, J. M., Zinbarg, R. E., Craske, M. G., Mineka, S., Griffith, J. W., & Epstein, A. (2010). Testing a hierarchical model of anxiety and depression in adolescents: A trilevel model. *Journal of Anxiety Disorders, 24,* 334–344.

Rachman, S., Lopatka, C., & Levitt, K. (1988). Experimental analyses of panic: II. Panic patients. *Behaviour Research and Therapy, 26,* 33–40.

Rachman, S., Shafran, R., Radomsky, A. S., & Zysk, E. (2011). Reducing contamination by exposure plus safety behaviour. *Journal of Behavior Therapy and Experimental Psychiatry, 42,* 397–404.

Rapee, R. (1986). Differential response to hyperventilation in panic disorder and generalized anxiety disorder. *Journal of Abnormal Psychology, 95,* 24–28.

Rapee, R. M. (1994). Detection of somatic sensations in panic disorder. *Behaviour Research and Therapy, 32,* 825–831.

Rapee, R. M., Brown, T. A., Antony, M. M., & Barlow, D. H. (1992). Response to hyperventilation and inhalation of 5.5% carbon dioxide-enriched air across the DSM-III-R anxiety disorders. *Journal of Abnormal Psychology, 101,* 538–552.

Rapee, R. M., Craske, M. G., & Barlow, D. H. (1990). Subject described features of panic attacks using a new self-monitoring form. *Journal of Anxiety Disorders, 4,* 171–181.

Rapee, R. M., Craske, M. G., & Barlow, D. H. (1995). Assessment instrument for panic disorder that includes fear of sensation-producing activities: The Albany Panic and Phobia Questionnaire. *Anxiety, 1,* 114–122.

Rapee, R. M., Craske, M. G., Brown, T. A., & Barlow, D. H. (1996). Measurement of perceived control over anxiety-related events. *Behavior Therapy, 27*(2), 279–293.

Rapee, R. M., & Medoro, L. (1994). Fear of physical sensations and trait anxiety as mediators of the response to hyperventilation in nonclinical subjects. *Journal of Abnormal Psychology, 103*(4), 693–699.

Rapee, R. M., & Murrell, E. (1988). Predictors of agoraphobic avoidance. *Journal of Anxiety Disorders, 2,* 203–217.

Rathus, J. H., Sanderson, W. C., Miller, A. L., & Wetzler, S. (1995). Impact of personality functioning on cognitive behavioral treatment of panic disorder: A preliminary report. *Journal of Personality Disorders, 9,* 160–168.

Razran, G. (1961). The observable unconscious and the inferable conscious in current soviet psychophysiology: Interoceptive conditioning, semantic conditioning, and the orienting reflex. *Psychological Review, 68,* 81–147.

Reich, J., Perry, J. C., Shera, D., Dyck, I., Vasile, R., Goisman, R. M., et al. (1994). Comparison of personality disorders in different anxiety disorder diagnoses: Panic, agoraphobia, generalized anxiety, and social phobia. *Annals of Clinical Psychiatry, 6*(2), 125–134.

Reiss, S. (1980). Pavlovian conditioning and human fear: An expectancy model. *Behavior Therapy, 11,* 380–396.

Reiss, S., Peterson, R., Gursky, D., & McNally, R. (1986). Anxiety sensitivity, anxiety frequency, and the prediction of fearfulness. *Behaviour Research and Therapy, 24,* 1–8.

Rescorla, R. A. (2006). Deepened extinction from compound stimulus presentation. *Journal of Experimental Psychology: Animal Behavior Processes, 32,* 135–144.

Richards, J., Klein, B., & Carlbring, P. (2003). Internet-based treatment for panic disorder. *Cognitive Behaviour Therapy, 32,* 125–135.

Richards, J. C., Klein, B., & Austin, D. W. (2006). Internet cognitive behavioural therapy for panic disorder: Does the inclusion of stress management information improve end-state functioning? *Clinical Psychologist, 10*(1), 2–15.

Rowe, M. K., & Craske, M. G. (1998). Effects of an expanding-spaced vs massed exposure schedule on fear reduction and return of fear. *Behaviour Research and Therapy, 36,* 701–717.

Roy-Byrne, P. P., & Cowley, D. S. (1995). Course and outcome in panic disorder: A review of recent follow-up studies. *Anxiety, 1,* 151–160.

Roy-Byrne, P., Craske, M. G., Stein, M. B., Sullivan, G., Bystritsky, A., Katon, W., et al. (2005). A randomized effectiveness trial of cognitive-behavioral therapy and medication for primary care panic disorder. *Archives of General Psychiatry, 62,* 290–298.

Roy-Byrne, P., Craske, M. G., Sullivan, G., Rose, R. D., Edlund, M. J., Lang, A. J., et al. (2010). Delivery of evidence-based treatment for multiple anxiety disorders in primary care. *Journal of American Medicine, 303*(19), 1921–1928.

Roy-Byrne, P., Stein, M. B., Russo, J., Craske, M. G., Katon, W., Sullivan, G., et al. (2005). Medical illness and response to treatment in primary care panic disorder. *General Hospital Psychiatry, 27*(4), 237–243.

Roy-Byrne, P. P., Mellman, T. A., & Uhde, T. W. (1988). Biologic findings in panic disorder: Neuroendocrine and sleep-related abnormalities [Special issue: Perspectives on Panic-Related Disorders]. *Journal of Anxiety Disorders, 2*, 17–29.

Roy-Byrne, P. P., Stein, M. B., Russo, J., Mercier, E., Thomas, R., McQuaid, J., et al. (1999). Panic disorder in the primary care setting: Comorbidity, disability, service utilization, and treatment. *Journal of Clinical Psychiatry, 60*(7), 492–499.

Safren, S. A., Gershuny, B. S., Marzol, P., Otto, M. W., & Pollack, M. H. (2002). History of childhood abuse in panic disorder, social phobia, and generalized anxiety disorder. *Journal of Nervous and Mental Disease, 190*(7), 453–456.

Salkovskis, P., Clark, D., & Hackmann, A. (1991). Treatment of panic attacks using cognitive therapy without exposure or breathing retraining. *Behaviour Research and Therapy, 29*, 161–166.

Salkovskis, P. M. (1991). The importance of behaviour in the maintenance of anxiety and panic: A cognitive account [Special issue: The changing Face of Behavioural Psychotherapy]. *Behavioural Psychotherapy, 19*(1), 6–19.

Salkovskis, P. M., Clark, D. M., & Gelder, M. G. (1996). Cognition–behaviour links in the persistence of panic. *Behaviour Research and Therapy, 34*, 453–458.

Schade, A., Marquenie, L. A., van Balkom, A. J., Koeter, M. W., de Beurs, E., van den Brink, W., et al. (2005). The effectiveness of anxiety treatment on alcohol-dependent patients with a comorbid phobic disorder: A randomized controlled trial. *Alcoholism: Clinical and Experimental Research, 29*(5), 794–800.

Schmidt, N. B., Lerew, D. R., & Jackson, R. J. (1997). The role of anxiety sensitivity in the pathogenesis of panic: Prospective evaluation of spontaneous panic attacks during acute stress. *Journal of Abnormal Psychology, 106*, 355–364.

Schmidt, N. B., Lerew, D. R., & Jackson, R. J. (1999). Prospective evaluation of anxiety sensitivity in the pathogenesis of panic: Replication and extension. *Journal of Abnormal Psychology, 108*, 532–537.

Schmidt, N. B., McCreary, B. T., Trakowski, J. J., Santiago, H. T., Woolaway-Bickel, K., & Ialong, N. (2003). Effects of cognitive behavioral treatment on physical health status in patients with panic disorder. *Behavior Therapy, 34*(1), 49–63.

Schmidt, N. B., Woolaway-Bickel, K., Trakowski, J., Santiago, H., Storey, J., Koselka, M., et al. (2000). Dismantling cognitive-behavioral treatment for panic disorder: Questioning the utility of breathing retraining. *Journal of Consulting and Clinical Psychology, 68*(3), 417–424.

Schneider, A. J., Mataix-Cols, D., Marks, I. M., & Bachofen, M. (2005). Internet-guided self-help with or without exposure therapy for phobic and panic disorders. *Psychotherapy and Psychosomatics, 74*(3), 154–164.

Schumacher, J., Jamra, R. A., Becker, T., Klopp, N., Franke, P., Jacob, C., et al. (2005). Investigation of the DAOA/G30 locus in panic disorder. *Molecular Psychiatry, 10*, 428–429.

Seidel, A., Rosenfield, D., Bhaskara, L., Hofmann, S. G., & Meuret, A. E. (2009). *Pathways of biobehavioral change in exposure therapy of panic disorder.* Paper presented at the 43rd Annual Convention of the Association of Advancement for Behavioral and Cognitive Therapies, New York.

Sharp, D. M., Power, K. G., Simpson, R. J., Swanson, V., & Anstee, J. A. (1997). Global measures of outcome in a controlled comparison of pharmacological and psychological treatment of panic disorder and agoraphobia in primary care. *British Journal of General Practice, 47*, 150–155.

Sharp, D. M., Power, K. G., & Swanson, V. (2004). A comparison of the efficacy and acceptability of group versus individual cognitive behaviour therapy in the treatment of panic disorder and agoraphobia in primary care. *Clinical Psychology and Psychotherapy, 11*(2), 73–82.

Shear, M. K., Brown, T. A., Barlow, D. H., Money, R., Sholomskas, D. E, Woods, S. W., et al. (1997). Multicenter collaborative Panic Disorder Severity Scale. *American Journal of Psychiatry, 154*, 1571–1575.

Shear, M. K., Rucci, P., Williams, J., Frank, E., Grochocinski, V., Vander-Bilt, J., et al. (2001). Reliability and validity of the Panic Disorder Severity Scale: Replication and extension. *Journal of Psychiatric Research, 35*(5), 293–296.

Shear, M. K., & Schulberg, H. C. (1995). Anxiety disorders in primary care. *Bulletin of the Menninger Clinic, 59*(2, Suppl. A), A73–A85.

Shulman, I. D., Cox, B. J., Swinson, R. P., Kuch, K., & Reichman, J. T. (1994). Precipitating events, locations and reactions associated with initial unexpected panic attacks. *Behaviour Research and Therapy, 32*, 17–20.

Sloan, T., & Telch, M. J. (2002). The effects of safety-seeking behavior and guided threat reappraisal on fear reduction during exposure: An experimental investigation. *Behaviour Research and Therapy, 40*(3), 235–251.

Soeter, M., & Kindt, M. (2010). Dissociating response systems: Erasing fear from memory. *Neurobiology of Learning and Memory, 94*(1), 30–41.

Sokolowska, M., Siegel, S., & Kim, J. A. (2002). Intraadministration associations: Conditional hyperalgesia elicited by morphine onset cues. *Journal of Experimental Psychology: Animal Behavior Processes, 28*(3), 309–320.

Sotres-Bayon, F., Cain, C. K., & LeDoux, J. E. (2006). Brain mechanisms of fear extinction: historical perspectives on the contribution of prefrontal cortex. *Biological Psychiatry, 60*, 329–336.

Spiegel, D. A., Bruce, T. J., Gregg, S. F., & Nuzzarello, A. (1994). Does cognitive behavior therapy assist slow-taper alprazolam discontinuation in panic disorder? *American Journal of Psychiatry, 151*(6), 876–881.

Stein, M. B., Walker, J. R., Anderson, G., Hazen, A. L., Ross, C. A., Eldridge, G., et al. (1996). Childhood physical and sexual abuse in patients with anxiety disorders and a community sample. *American Journal of Psychiatry, 153,* 275–277.

Sturges, L. V., Goetsch, V. L., Ridley, J., & Whittal, M. (1998). Anxiety sensitivity and response to hyperventilation challenge: Physiologic arousal, interoceptive acuity, and subjective distress. *Journal of Anxiety Disorders, 12*(2), 103–115.

Suárez, L., Bennett, S., Goldstein, C., & Barlow, D. H. (2008). Understanding anxiety disorders from a "triple vulnerabilities" framework. In M. M. Anthony & M. B. Stein (Eds.), *Oxford handbook of anxiety and related disorders* (pp. 153–172). New York: Oxford University Press.

Swinson, R. P., Fergus, K. D., Cox, B. J., & Wickwire, K. (1995). Efficacy of telephone-administered behavioral therapy for panic disorder with agoraphobia. *Behaviour Research and Therapy, 33,* 465–469.

Taylor, S., Koch, W. J., & McNally, R. J. (1992). How does anxiety sensitivity vary across the anxiety disorders? *Journal of Anxiety Disorders, 6,* 249–259.

Taylor, S., Zvolensky, M. J., Cox, B .J., Deacon, B., Heimberg, R. G., Ledley, D. R., et al. (2007). Robust dimensions of anxiety sensitivity: development and initial validation of the Anxiety Sensitivity Index–3. *Psychological Assessment, 19*(2), 176–188.

Teachman, B. A., Marker, C. D., & Smith-Janik, S. B. (2008). Automatic associations and panic disorder: Trajectories of change over the course of treatment. *Journal of Consulting and Clinical Psychology, 76*(6), 988–1002.

Telch, M. J., Brouillard, M., Telch, C. F., Agras, W. S., & Taylor, C. B. (1989). Role of cognitive appraisal in panic-related avoidance. *Behaviour Research and Therapy, 27,* 373–383.

Telch, M. J., Lucas, J. A., & Nelson, P. (1989). Nonclinical panic in college students: An investigation of prevalence and symptomatology. *Journal of Abnormal Psychology, 98,* 300–306.

Telch, M. J., Lucas, J. A., Schmidt, N. B., Hanna, H. H., LaNae, Jaimez, T., et al. (1993). Group cognitive-behavioral treatment of panic disorder. *Behaviour Research and Therapy, 31,* 279–287.

Telch, M. J., Sherman, M., & Lucas, J. (1989). Anxiety sensitivity: Unitary personality trait or domain specific appraisals? *Journal of Anxiety Disorders, 3,* 25–32.

Thorgeirsson, T. E., Oskarsson, H., Desnica, N., Kostic, J. P., Stefansson, J. G., Kolbeinsson, H., et al. (2003). Anxiety with panic disorder linked to chromosome 9q in Iceland. *American Journal of Human Genetics, 72,* 1221–1230.

Thyer, B. A., Himle, J., Curtis, G. C., Cameron, O. G., & Nesse, R. M. (1985). A comparison of panic disorder and agoraphobia with panic attacks. *Comprehensive Psychiatry, 26,* 208–214.

Tiemens, B. G., Ormel, J., & Simon, G. E. (1996). Occurrence, recognition, and outcome of psychological disorders in primary care. *American Journal of Psychiatry, 153,* 636–644.

Tsao, J. C. I., Lewin, M. R., & Craske, M. G. (1998). The effects of cognitive-behavior therapy for panic disorder on comorbid conditions. *Journal of Anxiety Disorders, 12,* 357–371.

Tsao, J. C. I., Mystkowski, J. L., Zucker, B. G., & Craske, M. G. (2002). Effects of cognitive-behavioral therapy for panic disorder on comorbid conditions: Replication and extension. *Behavior Therapy, 33,* 493–509.

Tsao, J. C. I., Mystkowski, J. L., Zucker, B. G., & Craske, M. G. (2005). Impact of cognitive-behavioral therapy for panic disorder on comorbidity: A controlled investigation. *Behaviour Research and Therapy, 43,* 959–970.

Uhde, T. W. (1994). The anxiety disorders: Phenomenology and treatment of core symptoms and associated sleep disturbance. In M. Kryger, T. Roth, & W. Dement (Eds.), *Principles and practice of sleep medicine* (pp. 871–898). Philadelphia: Saunders.

van Balkom, A. J., de Beurs, E., Koele, P., Lange, A., & van Dyck, R. (1996). Long-term benzodiazepine use is associated with smaller treatment gain in panic disorder with agoraphobia. *Journal of Nervous and Mental Disease, 184,* 133–135.

van Beek, N., Schruers, K. R., & Friez, E. J. (2005). Prevalence of respiratory disorders in first-degree relatives of panic disorder patients. *Journal of Affective Disorders, 87,* 337–340.

van den Hout, M., Arntz, A., & Hoekstra, R. (1994). Exposure reduced agoraphobia but not panic, and cognitive therapy reduced panic but not agoraphobia. *Behaviour Research and Therapy, 32,* 447–451.

van den Hout, M., Brouwers, C., & Oomen, J. (2006). Clinically diagnosed Axis II co-morbidity and the short term outcome of CBT for Axis I disorders. *Clinical Psychology and Psychotherapy, 13*(1), 56–63.

van Megen, H. J., Westenberg, H. G., Den Boer, J. A., & Kahn, R. S. (1996). The panic-inducing properties of the cholecystokinin tetrapeptide CCK4 in patients with panic disorder. *European Neuropsychopharmacology, 6,* 187–194.

Vansteenwegen, D., Vervliet, B., Iberico, C., Baeyens, F., van den Bergh, O., & Hermans, D. (2007). The repeated confrontation with videotapes of spiders in multiple contexts attenuates renewal of fear in spider-anxious students. *Behavior Research and Therapy, 45*(6), 1169–1179.

Veltman, D. J., van Zijderveld, G., Tilders, F. J., & van Dyck, R. (1996). Epinephrine and fear of bodily sensations in panic disorder and social phobia. *Journal of Psychopharmacology, 10*(4), 259–265.

Verburg, K., Griez, E., Meijer, J., & Pols, H. (1995). Respiratory disorders as a possible predisposing factor for panic disorder. *Journal of Affective Disorders, 33*, 129–134.

Vos, S. P., Huibers, M. J., Diels, L., & Arntz, A. (2012). A randomized clinical trial of cognitive behavioral therapy and interpersonal psychotherapy for panic disorder with agoraphobia. *Psychological Medicine, 42*(12), 2661–2672.

Wade, W. A., Treat, T. A., & Stuart, G. L. (1998). Transporting an empirically supported treatment for panic disorder to a service clinic setting: A benchmarking strategy. *Journal of Consulting and Clinical Psychology, 66*, 231–239.

Walker, D. L., & Davis, M. (2002). The role of amygdala glutamate receptors in fear learning, fear-potentiated startle, and extinction. *Pharmacology, 71*, 379–392.

Wardle, J., Hayward, P., Higgitt, A., Stabl, M., Blizard, R., & Gray, J. (1994). Effects of concurrent diazepam treatment on the outcome of exposure therapy in agoraphobia. *Behaviour Research and Therapy, 32*, 203–215.

Watson, D., & Clark, L. A. (1984). Negative affectivity: The disposition to experience aversive emotional states. *Psychological Bulletin, 96*(3), 465–490.

Weems, C. F., Hayward, C., Killen, J., & Taylor, C. B. (2002). A longitudinal investigation of anxiety sensitivity in adolescence. *Journal of Abnormal Psychology, 111*(3), 471–477.

Welkowitz, L., Papp, L., Cloitre, M., Liebowitz, M., Martin, L., & Gorman, J. (1991). Cognitive-behavior therapy for panic disorder delivered by psychopharmacologically oriented clinicians. *Journal of Nervous and Mental Disease, 179*, 473–477.

Westra, H. A., Stewart, S. H., & Conrad, B. E. (2002). Naturalistic manner of benzodiazepine use and cognitive behavioral therapy outcome in panic disorder and agoraphobia. *Journal of Anxiety Disorders, 16*(3), 223–246.

White, K. S., Allen, L. B., Barlow, D. H., Gorman, J. M., Shear, M. K., & Woods, S. W. (2010). Attrition in a multicenter clinical trial of panic disorder. *Journal of Nervous and Mental Diseases, 198*, 665–671.

White, K. S., Payne, L. A., Gorman, J. M., Shear, M. K., Woods, S. W., Saska, J. R., et al. (2013). Does maintenance CBT contribute to long-term treatment response of panic disorder with or without agoraphobia?: A randomized controlled clinical trial. *Journal of Consulting and Clinical Psychology, 81*, 47–57.

Wilkinson, D. J., Thompson, J. M., Lambert, G. W., Jennings, G. L., Schwarz, R. G., Jefferys, D., et al. (1998). Sympathetic activity in patients with panic disorder at rest, under laboratory mental stress, and during panic attacks. *Archives of General Psychiatry, 55*(6), 511–520.

Williams, K. E., & Chambless, D. (1990). The relationship between therapist characteristics and outcome of *in vivo* exposure treatment for agoraphobia. *Behavior Therapy, 21*, 111–116.

Williams, K. E., & Chambless, D. L. (1994). The results of exposure-based treatment in agoraphobia. In S. Friedman (Ed.), *Anxiety disorders in African Americans* (pp. 149–165). New York: Springer.

Williams, S. L., & Falbo, J. (1996). Cognitive and performance-based treatments for panic attacks in people with varying degrees of agoraphobic disability. *Behaviour Research and Therapy, 34*, 253–264.

Williams, S. L., & Zane, G. (1989). Guided mastery and stimulus exposure treatments for severe performance anxiety in agoraphobics. *Behaviour Research and Therapy, 27*, 237–245.

Wittchen, H.-U., Gloster, A. T., Beesdo-Baum, K., Fava, G. A., & Craske, M. G. (2010). Agoraphobia: A review of the diagnostic classificatory position and criteria. *Depression and Anxiety, 27*, 113–133.

Wolitzky-Taylor, K., Castriotta, N., Lenze, E., Stanley, M. A., & Craske, M. G. (2010). Anxiety disorders in older adults: A comprehensive review. *Depression and Anxiety, 27*, 190–211.

Zinbarg, R. E., & Barlow, D. H. (1996). Structure of anxiety and the anxiety disorders: A hierarchical model. *Journal of Abnormal Psychology, 105*(2), 184–193.

Zinbarg, R. E., Barlow, D. H., & Brown, T. A. (1997). Hierarchical structure and general factor saturation of the Anxiety Sensitivity Index: Evidence and implication. *Psychological Assessment, 9*, 277–284.

Zoellner, L. A., & Craske, M. G. (1999). Interoceptive accuracy and panic. *Behaviour Research and Therapy, 37*, 1141–1158.

CHAPTER 2

Posttraumatic Stress Disorder

CANDICE M. MONSON
PATRICIA A. RESICK
SHIREEN L. RIZVI

Severe, unexpected trauma may occur in less than a minute but have lifelong consequences. The tragedy that is posttraumatic stress disorder (PTSD) is brought into stark relief when the origins of the trauma occur in the context of people's inhumanity to others. In this chapter, the case of "Tom" illustrates the psychopathology associated with PTSD in all its nuances and provides a very personal account of its impact. In one of any number of events summarized dryly every day in the middle pages of the newspaper, Tom, in the fog of war in Iraq, shoots and kills a pregnant woman and her young child in the presence of her husband and father. The impact of this event devastates him. The sensitive and skilled therapeutic intervention described in this chapter is a model for new therapists, and belies the notion that, in these severe cases, manualized therapy can be rote and automated. In addition, the next generation of treatment for PTSD, termed "cognitive processing therapy" by the authors, is sufficiently detailed to allow knowledgeable practitioners to incorporate this treatment program into their practice. This comprehensive treatment program takes advantage of the latest developments in our knowledge of the psychopathology of trauma impact by incorporating treatment strategies specifically tailored to overcome trauma-related psychopathology, and does so in the context of the significant changes to diagnostic criteria in DSM-5.—D. H. B.

DIAGNOSIS

Unlike most other psychological disorders, posttraumatic stress disorder (PTSD) requires the occurrence of a specific type of event from which the person affected does not recover. First, to qualify for a diagnosis of PTSD according to the fifth edition of the *Diagnostic and Statistical Manual of Mental Disorders* (DSM-5; American Psychiatric Association, 2013), the individual must have experienced, witnessed, or otherwise been confronted with an event or events that involved actual or threatened death, serious injury, or sexual violence. Exposure to traumatic events may take

the form of experiencing an event directly, witnessing the event happen to someone else, learning of violent or accidental trauma that happened to a close friend or family member, or being repeatedly or extremely exposed to aversive elements of a traumatic event (e.g., a rescue worker collecting body parts). Symptom criteria fall into four broad categories: reexperiencing (criterion B), avoidance (criterion C), negative alterations in cognition and mood (criterion D; e.g., memory difficulties, feeling detached, persistent negative beliefs) and hyperarousal (criterion E). According to criterion B, the reexperiencing symptoms must be experienced in one of the following ways: Memories of the trauma may intrude into consciousness repetitively, without warning, seemingly "out of the blue," without triggers or reminders to elicit them. The person with PTSD may experience intensely vivid reenactment experiences, or flashbacks. Intrusive memories may also occur during the sleeping state in the form of thematically related nightmares. Additionally, when faced with cues associated with the traumatic event, whether actual or symbolic, the individual may exhibit intense psychological reactions (e.g., terror, disgust, depression) and/or physiological responses (e.g., increased heart rate, perspiration, rapid breathing).

These reexperiencing symptoms are generally distressing and intrusive because the individual has no control over when or how they occur, and they elicit strong negative emotions associated with the initial trauma (Janoff-Bulman, 1992; Resick & Schnicke, 1992). Fear stimuli (cues) are sometimes obvious, such as the combat veteran who ducks in fear when a car backfires and sounds like gunfire. But sometimes the relationship between the trauma and the cue is not immediately clear. For example, one survivor of rape was fearful of taking showers, even though the rape had occurred away from her home. However, as she began to process the rape in treatment, she realized that every time she took a shower, she felt very vulnerable because she was alone, naked, had no escape routes, and had diminished vision and hearing—all stimuli that reminded her of the rape.

Avoidance symptoms (criterion C) reflect the individual's attempt to gain physical and psychological distance from the trauma. Some have suggested that avoidance symptoms are a response to reexperiencing symptoms (Buckley, Blanchard, & Hickling, 1998; Creamer, Burgess, & Pattison, 1992; Taylor, Kuch, Koch, Crockett, & Passey, 1998). As traumatic memories intrude into consciousness, so do the painful negative emotions associated with the trauma. Thus, the individual may avoid thoughts and feelings about the trauma, may avoid situations and events reminiscent of the trauma, or may actually forget significant aspects of the trauma (criterion D1). Avoidance of the trauma memory leads to a temporary decrease in painful emotions but, paradoxically, increases avoidance behavior. Trauma survivors frequently report highly constricted lifestyles after the traumatic experience due to the need to avoid reminders of the traumatic memory and associated emotions. At least three types of avoidance behavior are required before a diagnosis can be made.

Similarly, detachment or numbing symptoms (part of criterion D) are attempts to cut off the aversive feelings associated with intrusive memories (Astin, Layne, Camilleri, & Foy, 1994; Resick & Schnicke, 1992). This detachment may then generalize to all emotions, both positive and negative. Trauma survivors commonly state that they no longer have any strong feelings, or that they feel numb a great deal of the time. This sort of pervasive detachment may interfere profoundly with the individual's ability to relate to others, enjoy daily life, remain productive, and plan for the future. It is also important to note that not all trauma survivors experience emotional numbing. On the contrary, some find themselves experiencing continuous, intense negative emotions such as anger or shame. Trauma survivors may experience persistent cognitive symptoms, also classified under criterion D. These include negative beliefs about about themselves, others, or life in general (e.g., "I'll never be able to have a normal relationship," "Nowhere is 100% safe"). They may have distorted perceptions, often involving self-blame, about why the trauma occurred or its consequences.

The trauma survivor may also experience symptoms of hyperarousal (criterion E). This suggests that the individual is in a constant state of "fight or flight," which is similar to how the individual's body responded during the actual traumatic event. In this state of alert, the individual is primed to react to new threats of danger, even in relatively safe situations. During a crisis, this is adaptive because it facilitates survival. However, as a steady state, hyperarousal interferes with daily functioning and leads to exhaustion. In this state, the individual spends a great deal of energy scanning the environment for danger cues (hypervigilance). The individual is likely to experience sleep disturbance, decreased concentration, irritability, and overreactivity to stimuli (exaggerated startle response). There is evidence to suggest that this constant state of tension has deleterious effects on overall physical health (e.g., Kulka et al., 1990). At least two criterion E behaviors must be present for a diagnosis of PTSD.

The previously described symptom criteria must be met concurrently for at least 1 month to warrant a diagnosis of PTSD, and the symptoms must be perceived as distressing or cause functional impairment. A substantial proportion of trauma survivors exhibit symptoms consistent with a PTSD diagnosis immediately after the traumatic event. However, these rates drop almost in half within 3 months posttrauma, then tend to stabilize. For example, rape trauma survivors assessed at 2 weeks, 1 month, 3 months, 6 months, and 9 months posttrauma exhibited PTSD diagnostic rates of 94, 65,

47, 42, and 42%, respectively (Rothbaum & Foa, 1992). Thus, after 3 months, PTSD rates did not decrease substantially. Another study that assessed survivors of rape trauma at approximately 2 weeks and at 3 months postassault found very similar rates of PTSD (Gutner, Rizvi, Monson, & Resick, 2006). At the first assessment, 81% of the rape survivors met symptom criteria for PTSD (minus the time criterion), and at 3 months postrape, 53% continued to meet criteria. Other, more heterogeneous events (greater variability in the severity of the event), such as combat, disasters, or physical assaults, are associated with lower rates of PTSD than rape (Kessler, Sonnega, Bromet, Hughes, & Nelson, 1995). Delayed onset of PTSD is rare and may reflect earlier subthreshold symptoms (perhaps due to dissociation, amnesia, or extensive avoidance) or a change in the meaning of the event at a later time (e.g., the perpetrator kills a later victim, thereby changing the meaning of the event for the survivor).

The introduction of DSM-5 in 2013 brought about changes in diagnostic criteria that impact research and treatment of PTSD. Whereas PTSD was classified as an anxiety disorder in previous DSM editions, it is currently listed among trauma- and stressor-related disorders. This change makes sense given that PTSD does not group cleanly with the anxiety disorders based on factor analyses (e.g., Cox, Clara, & Enns, 2002; Miller, Greif, & Smith, 2003; Miller, Kaloupek, Dillon, & Keane, 2004; Miller & Resick, 2007) and may include a range of emotions such as anger, sadness, guilt, or horror (see DSM-5 criterion D). DSM-5 also tightened the stressor criterion, and criterion D (negative alterations in cognitions and mood) is new to DSM-5.

The intrusion criterion clearly does not include ruminating about the event but it does include at least one of the following: spontaneous or cued distressing memories of the traumatic event; recurrent distressing dreams in which the content or emotions are related to the event; dissociative reactions in which the individual feels or acts as if the traumatic event(s) are happening again; psychological distress when confronted with internal or external cues that symbolize or resemble the traumatic event; or marked physiological reactions to reminders of the traumatic event(s).

The avoidance criterion includes two items: avoidance of internal reminders or avoidance of external reminders of the traumatic event. Only one of the two is required for diagnosis.

The third symptom criterion includes some clarified items and some items newly introduced in DSM-5. The individual must experience at least two of the following types of symptoms: inability to remember an important aspect of the traumatic event(s); persistent and exaggerated negative cognitions about one's self, others, or the world; distorted blame of self or others about the cause or consequences of the event(s); global negative emotional states (e.g., fear, horror, anger, guilt, shame); markedly diminished interest or participation in significant activities; feeling of detachment or estrangement from others; or persistent inability to experience positive emotions (e.g., inability to have loving feelings, psychic numbing).

Compared to DSM-IV, in DSM-5 the fourth symptom criterion is expanded beyond physiological arousal to dysfunctional and impulsive behaviors, and includes irritable or aggressive behavior; reckless or self-destructive behavior; hypervigilance; exaggerated startle response; problems with concentration; and sleep disturbance.

Unlike DSM-IV, DSM-5 stipulates that symptoms cannot be due to the direct physiological effects of a substance or a general medical condition (e.g., traumatic brain injury, coma).

New to DSM-5 is a dissociative subtype of PTSD, which has been added due to a convergence of literature from epidemiological studies (e.g., Wolf et al., 2012), psychophysiological studies (e.g., Griffin, Resick & Mechanic, 1997); neuroimaging studies (e.g., Lanius et al., 2010), and treatment studies (Cloitre, Petkova, Wang, & Lu Lassell, 2012; Resick, Williams, Suvak, Monson, & Gradus, 2012) that have found a small group (15%) of people with severe PTSD who are also highly dissociative. These individuals appear to respond differently to treatment than those with severe PTSD without dissociative features.

In addition, DSM-5 offers separate classification for PTSD in young children, as well as PTSD in which symptom onset is not for at least 6 months after the trauma.

PREVALENCE

Epidemiological studies document high rates of trauma exposure and PTSD in the population (Kessler et al., 1995; Kilpatrick, Saunders, Veronen, Best, & Von, 1987; Kulka et al., 1990). In a national (U.S.) random probability sample of 4,008 women, Resnick, Kilpatrick, Dansky, Saunders, and Best (1993) found a high rate of trauma experiences (69%). When they extrapolated their results to the U.S. population based on census statistics for 1989, they estimated that 66 million women in the United States had experienced at least one major traumatic event. Of those who had experienced a criterion A stressor, Resnick and colleagues found the following lifetime PTSD rates: completed rape, 32%; other sexual assault, 31%; physical assault, 39%; homicide of family or friend, 22%; any crime victimization, 26%; and noncrime trauma (e.g., natural and manmade disasters, accidents, injuries), 9%.

In the first large national civilian prevalence study of the psychological effects of trauma, Kessler and colleagues (1995) surveyed a representative U.S. national sample of 5,877 persons (2,812 men and 3,065 women). This study assessed 12 categories of traumatic stressors and found that a majority of people had experienced at least one major traumatic event. They found that whereas 20.4% of women and 8.2% of men were likely to develop PTSD following exposure to trauma, the rates for specific traumas were often much higher. For example, rape was identified as the trauma most likely to lead to PTSD among men, as well as women, and 65% of men and 46% of women who identified rape as their most distressing trauma were diagnosed with PTSD. Among men who identified other traumas as most distressing, the probability of having PTSD was 39% for those with combat exposure, 24% for those who suffered childhood neglect, and 22% of those who experienced childhood physical abuse. Among women, aside from rape, PTSD was associated with physical abuse in childhood (49%), threat with a weapon (33%), sexual molestation (27%), and physical attack (21%). As with Resnick and colleagues' (1993) study, accidents and natural disasters were much less likely to precipitate PTSD among men and women. On the other hand, Norris (1992) pointed out that although motor vehicle accidents (MVAs) occur less frequently than some traumas (e.g., tragic death or robbery) and are less traumatic than some events (sexual and physical assault), when both frequency and impact are considered together, MVAs may be the single most significant event. The lifetime frequency of MVAs is 23%, and the PTSD rate is 12%, which results in a rate of 28 seriously distressed people for every 1,000 adults in the United States, just from one type of event.

More recently, Kessler and his colleagues (Kessler, Berglund, et al., 2005; Kessler, Chiu, Demler, Merikangas, & Walters, 2005) reported on another large National Comorbidity Survey with over 9,200 respondents. The overall prevalence of PTSD was 6.8% in this

study; this compares to the 7.8% population prevalence reported in the 1995 study.

The largest study of combat veterans to date, the National Vietnam Veterans Readjustment Study (NVVRS; Kulka et al., 1990), was mandated by the U.S. Congress in 1983 to assess PTSD and other psychological problems following the Vietnam War. During the years of the war, over 8 million people served in the U.S. military. Of those, 3.1 million served in Vietnam (theater veterans) and the remainder served in other areas abroad or in the United States (era veterans). Women comprised 7,200 of those serving in Vietnam, and over 255,000 of those serving elsewhere during the Vietnam era. The NVVRS conducted in-depth interviews and assessments with three groups: 1,632 Vietnam theater veterans, 716 Vietnam era veterans, and 668 nonveterans/civilian counterparts, for a total of 3,016 participants.

The results of the NVVRS indicated that the majority of Vietnam theater veterans made a successful readjustment to civilian life and did not suffer from PTSD or other problems. However, the researchers also found that 31% of men and 27% of women veterans had a full diagnosis of PTSD at some time during their lives. Furthermore, 15% of men and 9% of women veterans had PTSD at the time of the study, over a decade after the end of the war. These rates translated to 479,000 Vietnam veterans with current PTSD. In addition, 11% of men and 8% of women veterans were found to have significant symptoms and distress but did not meet the full criteria for PTSD. This translated to an additional 350,000 men and women in the United States alone who were still suffering in the aftermath of the Vietnam War.

Data from the NVVRS were reevaluated using very strict criteria that only included those incidents that could be verified through historical records. Dohrenwend and colleagues (2006) found very little falsification of events and a strong relationship between the amount of trauma exposure and rates of PTSD (i.e., dose–response relationship). They did, however, find lower rates of PTSD after controlling for people who developed PTSD before or after their deployment to Vietnam and eliminating those people with unverifiable events. Using these stricter criteria, they found that 18.7% of the veterans met the criteria for war-related PTSD at some point, and 9.1% still had PTSD when assessed 11 to 12 years later. These rates should be considered minimum likelihood rates given that people can be traumatized by events that may not be verifiable (e.g., rape, accidents) in historical accounts of war. Currently under way is a study of the participants of the NVVRS, called the National Vietnam Veterans Longitudinal Study (NVVLS), which will inform us about the long-term effects of PTSD.

More recent conflicts in Iraq and Afghanistan saw the first attempts to assess PTSD *during* a war (Hoge et al., 2004; Hoge, Auchterlonie, & Milliken, 2006). Hoge and his colleagues (2004) studied 2,530 Army soldiers and Marines before and 3,671 after deployment to Iraq or Afghanistan. They found that mental health problems were significantly greater among those who returned from deployment than among those not yet deployed, and that mental health problems were greater in those who deployed to Iraq compared with Afghanistan. Prior to deployment, 9% of the service personnel exceeded the cutoff used for likely PTSD, whereas 11.5% of those deployed to Afghanistan and 18–20% of those deployed to Iraq exceeded the cutoff. There was a linear relationship between the number of firefights reported and the severity of PTSD. Being wounded or otherwise physically injured was also associated with greater PTSD symptomatology.

Because the military began screening all military personnel for PTSD following deployment, a population-based study of 303,905 Army soldiers and Marines who deployed to Afghanistan, Iraq, or other locations could be conducted for a 1-year period (May 2003 to April 2004; Hoge et al., 2006). As with the previous report, service men and women were more likely to report mental health problems after serving in Iraq (19.1%) than after serving in Afghanistan (11.3%) or other locations (8.5%). In this study 32,500 women were also assessed, comprising 10.7% of the total sample. There was an overall sex difference in mental health concerns, with 23.6% of women compared with 18.6% of men reporting a mental health concern. However, this sex comparison did not take into account preexisting traumas or PTSD, exposure to combat traumas or sexual assault, or other variables that might explain these differences. Also, the PTSD screen was a four-item questionnaire in which two "yes" answers indicated possible PTSD. On this screen, 9.8% of those who had served in Iraq met criteria for possible PTSD, and there was again an association between the amount of combat exposure and PTSD.

Recently, Vogt and colleagues (2011) reported on the effects of combat on women, which is a change from prior wars, as well as predictors of PTSD with a national random survey of veterans of Iraq and Afghanistan who had returned from deployment within the previous year. The researchers attempted to contact 2,000 veterans, oversampling female veterans to have equal numbers of men and women. The sample comprised 579 veterans who completed the survey. Significantly more men (49%) than women (43%) reported warfare exposure. Women also reported significantly lower levels of relationship concerns. However, men and women did not differ with regard to perceived threat, childhood family functioning, prior stressors, postdeployment stressors, postdeployment social support, or PTSD symptom severity. This study did not examine military sexual trauma, which has been found to be higher among women, perhaps explaining the equal rates of PTSD for men and women in this sample (Street, Gradus, Vogt, Giasson, & Resick, 2013).

THEORETICAL MODELS OF PTSD

As researchers and clinicians began to study and treat survivors of rape trauma and Vietnam veterans in the 1970s, they began to draw upon learning theory as an explanation for the symptoms they were observing. Mowrer's two-factor theory (1947) of classical and operant conditioning was first proposed to account for posttrauma symptoms (Becker, Skinner, Abel, Axelrod, & Cichon, 1984; Holmes & St. Lawrence, 1983; Keane, Zimering, & Caddell, 1985; Kilpatrick, Veronen, & Best, 1985; Kilpatrick, Veronen, & Resick, 1982). Classical conditioning was used to explain the high levels of distress and fear observed in trauma victims in reaction to trauma-related stimuli. Operant conditioning explained the onset of PTSD avoidance symptoms and maintenance of fear over time, despite the fact that the unconditioned stimulus, the traumatic stressor, does not recur. Because the trauma memory and other cues (conditioned stimuli) elicit fear and anxiety (conditioned emotional responses), people avoid (or escape from) these cues, and the result is a reduction in fear and anxiety. In this manner, avoidance of the conditioned stimuli is negatively reinforced, which prevents deterioration of the link between the trauma cues and anxiety that would normally be expected without repetition of the trauma itself.

Although learning theory accounts for much of the onset and maintenance of the fear and avoidance in PTSD, it does not fully explain "intrusion symptoms" (i.e., repetitive memories of the trauma that intrude into survivors' thoughts in both conscious and unconscious, states such as nightmares). Based on Lang's (1977) information-processing theory of anxiety development, Foa, Steketee, and Rothbaum (1989) suggested that PTSD emerges due to the development of a fear network in memory that elicits escape and avoidance behavior. Mental fear structures include stimuli, response, and meaning elements. Anything associated with the trauma may elicit the fear structure or schema and subsequent avoidance behavior. The fear network in people with PTSD is thought to be stable and to generalize broadly, so that it is easily accessed. Chemtob, Roitblat, Hamada, Carlson, and Twentyman (1988) proposed that these structures are always at least weakly activated in individuals with PTSD and guide their interpretation of events as potentially dangerous. When the fear network is activated by reminders of the trauma, the information in the network enters consciousness (intrusive symptoms). Attempts to avoid this activation result in the avoidance symptoms of PTSD. According to information-processing theory, repetitive exposure to the traumatic memory in a safe environment results in habituation of fear and subsequent changes in the fear structure. As emotion decreases, clients with PTSD begin to modify their meaning elements spontaneously, and consequently change their self-statements and reduce their generalization.

Cognitive theories are also concerned with information processing, but they focus on the effect of trauma on the survivor's belief system and the adjustments that are necessary to reconcile a traumatic event with prior beliefs and expectations. The first and most influential cognitive theorist, Horowitz (1986), moved from a more psychodynamic view to a cognitive processing theory. Horowitz proposed that processing is driven by a "completion tendency," the psychological need for new, incompatible information to be integrated with existing beliefs. The completion tendency keeps the trauma information in active memory until the processing is complete and the event is resolved. Horowitz also theorized that there is a basic conflict between the person's need to resolve and reconcile the event into his or her history, and the desire to avoid emotional pain. When images of the event (flashbacks, nightmares, intrusive recollections), thoughts about the meanings of the trauma, and emotions associated with the trauma become overwhelming, psychological defense mechanisms take over, and the person exhibits numbing or avoidance. Horowitz suggested that a person with PTSD oscillates between phases of intrusion and avoidance, and that if successfully processed, the oscillations become less frequent

and less intense. According to this theory, chronic PTSD occurs because the trauma remains in active memory without becoming fully integrated; therefore, it is still able to stimulate intrusive and avoidant reactions.

Several other social-cognitive researchers and theorists who have focused more on the content of the cognitions in PTSD propose that basic assumptions about the world and oneself are "shattered." Constructivist theories are based on the idea that people actively create their own internal representations of the world (and themselves). New experiences are assigned meaning based on a person's model of the world (Janoff-Bulman, 1985, 1992; Mahoney & Lyddon, 1988; McCann & Pearlman, 1990). The task for recovery is to reconstruct fundamental beliefs and establish equilibrium. Janoff-Bulman (1985) suggested that this process is accomplished by reinterpreting the event to reduce the distance between the prior beliefs and the new beliefs. Other theorists have proposed that if one's preexisting beliefs are particularly positive or particularly negative, then more severe PTSD symptoms result (McCann & Pearlman, 1990; Resick & Schnicke, 1992; Resick, Monson, & Chard, 2007). Foa, Steketee, and Rothbaum (1989) focused particularly on beliefs regarding the predictability and controllability of the trauma, whereas McCann and Pearlman (1990) proposed that several areas of cognition might be either disrupted or seemingly confirmed, that is, beliefs regarding safety, trust, control/power, esteem, and intimacy. The Resick and colleauges (2007) model focuses particularly on the "just world" myth and the human desire (and illusion) that we can predict and control our lives.

In a cognitive model, affective expression is needed, not for habituation, but for the trauma memory to be processed fully. It is assumed that the natural affect, once accessed, dissipates rather quickly, and that the work of accommodating the memory with beliefs can begin. Once faulty beliefs regarding the event (self-blame, guilt) and overgeneralized beliefs about oneself and the world (e.g., safety, trust, control, esteem, intimacy) are challenged, then the secondary emotions also decrease, along with the intrusive reminders. The fact that both stress inoculation training without trauma exposure exercises (Foa, Rothbaum, Riggs, & Murdock, 1991; Foa et al., 1999) and cognitive therapy without written or oral accounts of the traumatic experience (e.g., Ehlers et al., 2003; Resick et al., 2008; Tarrier et al., 1999) are effective treatments for PTSD undermines the assumption that habituation is the sole mechanism of change.

Ehlers and Clark (2000) proposed a cognitive model of PTSD that focuses on perceived threat and memory. Although the event occurred in the past, Ehlers and Clark propose that people with PTSD are unable to see the event as time-limited and assume that it has larger implications for the future. Individuals with PTSD appraise the event such that they believe themselves to be currently at risk. There are several ways in which this misappraisal happens. One is to overgeneralize based on the event and assume that normal activities are more dangerous than they objectively are. Individuals may overestimate the probability that the event will recur. After the trauma happens, they may misconstrue the meaning of their PTSD symptoms such that they perceive themselves to be in greater danger (false alarms are assumed to be true alarms) or interpret their symptoms to mean that they cannot cope with events in the future.

Ehlers and Clark's (2000) cognitive theory also considers the apparent memory disturbance that occurs, such that persons with PTSD may have trouble intentionally accessing their memory of the event but have involuntary intrusions of parts of the event. They propose that because memory encoded at the time of the trauma is poorly elaborated and integrated with other memories with regard to details, context of time, sequence, and so forth, this might explain why people with PTSD have poor autobiographical memory, yet may be triggered to have memory fragments that have a here-and-now quality (no time context) or lack appropriate posttrauma appraisals (e.g., "I did not die"). Like the emotional processing models, Ehlers and Clark also propose that strong associative learning is paired with fear responses and may generalize. In response to perceptions of threat, people with PTSD adopt various maladaptive coping strategies, depending on their appraisals. For example, people who believe they will go crazy if they think about the traumatic event try to avoid thoughts about the trauma and keep their minds occupied as much as possible. Someone who believes that he or she must figure out why the traumatic event occurred to keep it from happening again will ruminate about how it could have been prevented. Those who think they were being punished for their actions may become immobilized and be unable to make decisions. These maladaptive strategies, most often avoidance behaviors, may (1) increase symptoms, (2) prevent change in negative appraisals, or (3) prevent change in the trauma memory.

In an attempt to reconcile the theories of PTSD, Brewin, Dalgleish, and Joseph (1996) proposed a dual-representation theory that incorporates both information-processing and social-cognitive theories, and introduces research and theory from cognitive science with regard to memory. They have suggested that the concept of a single emotional memory is too narrow to describe the full range of memory that has been evident in research and clinical observations. Based on prior research, they proposed that sensory input is subject to both conscious and nonconscious processing. The memories that are conscious and can be deliberately retrieved, termed "verbally accessible memories" (VAMs), contain some sensory information, information about emotional and physical reactions, and the personal meaning of the event. Although VAMs might be reasonably detailed, they may also be very selective because attention is narrowed under conditions of stress, and short-term memory capacity may be decreased.

The other type of memories are theorized to be nonconsious and are termed "situationally accessed memories" (SAMs). This type of information, which is probably much more extensive than autobiographical memories of the event, cannot be accessed deliberately and is not as easily altered or edited as the more explicitly accessed VAMs. SAMs comprise sensory (e.g., auditory, visual, tactile), physiological, and motoric information that may be accessed automatically when a person is exposed to a stimulus situation similar in some fashion to the trauma, or when that person consciously thinks about the trauma. SAMs are then experienced as intrusive sensory images or flashbacks accompanied by physiological arousal.

Dual-representation theory posits two types of emotional reactions: One type is conditioned during the event (e.g., fear, anger), recorded in the SAMs, and activated along with reexperienced sensory and physiological information. The other type, secondary emotions, result from the consequences and implications (meaning) of the trauma. These secondary emotions may include not only fear and anger but also guilt, shame, and sadness.

Brewin and colleagues (1996) proposed that emotional processing of the trauma has two elements. One element of the processing is the activation of SAMS (as suggested by information-processing theories), the purpose of which is to aid in cognitive readjustment by supplying detailed sensory and physiological information concerning the trauma. The activation of SAMs may eventually diminish in frequency when they are blocked by the creation of new SAMs, or when they are altered by the incorporation of new information. When the SAMs are brought into consciousness, they can be altered by being paired with different bodily states (e.g., relaxation or habituation) or different conscious thoughts. Eventually, if the SAMs are replaced or altered sufficiently, there is a reduction in negative emotions and a subsequent reduction in attentional bias and accessibility of the memory.

The second element (as proposed by the social-cognitive theorists) is the conscious attempt to search for meaning, to ascribe cause or blame, and to resolve conflicts between the event and prior expectations and beliefs. The goal of this process is to reduce the negative emotions and to restore a sense of relative safety and control in one's environment. To obtain this second goal, the traumatized person may have to edit his or her autobiographical memory (VAMs) to reconcile conflicts between the event and the person's belief system. The traumatized person may either alter the memory of the event in some way to reestablish the preexisting belief system or alter preexisting beliefs and expectations to accommodate this new information.

Brewin and colleagues (1996) suggest that for cases in which the emotions are primary and driven by SAMs, exposure therapy may be all that is needed. However, when secondary emotions such as self-blame, guilt, or shame are present, cognitive therapy may be needed. Although both exposure and cognitive therapies have been found to be effective in treating PTSD, no research thus far has matched types of therapy to client profiles.

Another multirepresentational cognitive model called SPAARS (Dalgleish, 2004) was originally proposed to explain everyday emotional experience and was then applied to PTSD. This model also endeavors to encompass previous theories. The model proposes four types or levels of mental representation systems: schematic, propositional, analogue, and associative representational systems. The schematic level represents abstract generic information, or schemas. Propositional-level information is verbally accessible meanings, similar to VAMs, whereas information at the analogue level is stored as "images" across all types of sensory systems, similar to SAMs. Associative representations are similar to the fear structures hypothesized in emotional processing theory as representing

the connections between other types of representations. In the SPAARS model, emotions are generated through two routes. One, similar to the Ehlers and Clark (2000) cognitive model, is through appraisals at the schematic level, in which events are compared against important goals. A person appraises an event to be threatening if it blocks an important goal, then experiences fear. Because traumatic events are threats to survival, they are appraised as threatening and elicit fear. The second route to emotion is through associative learning, which is automatic and similar to the fear activation described by Foa and her colleagues (1989).

Within the SPAARS model, a traumatic event triggers intense appraisal-driven fear, helplessness, or horror, as well as a range of other emotions. Information about the traumatic event is encoded in the schematic, propositional, and analogue levels simultaneously. Because the memory of the traumatic event represents an ongoing threat to goals, the person is left with low-level fear activation, cognitive bias to attend to threat appraisals, and intrusive sensory images and appraisals. The trauma memory exists across different levels of mental representation but is unincorporated into the person's larger mental representations; the memory may be elicited as flashbacks or nightmares. Such strong memory and emotional intrusions result in efforts to cope through avoidance.

ASSESSMENT

Any comprehensive assessment of PTSD must capture whether or not a life event meets the seriousness and subjective response requirements of a traumatic stressor (criterion A), as well as the presence and severity of the DSM-IV-TR 20 associated symptoms (criteria B–E). Although interview-based measures are considered the "gold standard" for assessing PTSD, a number of self-report measures have been developed in recent years to provide a quicker, less resource-heavy method for assessing PTSD. New DSM-5 criteria continue to be psychometrically validated, and assessment and research are adapting accordingly.

Assessment of Traumatic Events

The first essential step in the assessment of PTSD is to identify traumas in the patient's history. Often this is difficult to achieve because many trauma survivors, especially rape and child sexual abuse trauma survivors, do not spontaneously disclose their trauma history. This is consistent with general patterns of avoidance of trauma-related reminders and may reflect shame, embarrassment, and self-blame regarding the incidents. Even when seeking treatment for mental health problems, trauma survivors often fail to recognize that their psychological difficulties may be associated with their trauma history. Kilpatrick (1983) suggested several other reasons survivors might not be forthcoming with this information, including fear of a negative reaction to disclosure, especially if previous disclosure has resulted in disbelief or blame. Additionally, many trauma survivors do not recognize or label their experience as "trauma," "rape," or "abuse," especially if the assailant was an acquaintance or a relative, or if the trauma was experienced by many people, as in combat. Finally, in the absence of a strong alliance with the therapist, many people choose not to disclose such deeply personal information. It is therefore important for the clinician to forge a positive alliance as early as possible and be forthcoming about the purpose of the questioning, any limits of confidentiality, and how the obtained information may be used (i.e., diagnosis, treatment planning, research purposes).

In terms of questions regarding the presence of traumatic experiences, a behavioral, descriptive prompt such as "Has anyone ever made you have unwanted sexual contact by physical force or threat of force?" is more detailed and is preferable to asking, "Have you ever been raped?" In the latter case, someone who is married (or dating) and has been sexually assaulted may say "no," because "rape" might not be a term that he/she associates with forced sex by one's partner. The same problem may exist with child abuse. A client may indicate that he was not abused as a child but readily admit, when asked, that a parent whipped him with a belt until he had welts. In general, it is recommended that clinicians always begin with broad questions about experiences, then move to more specific, behaviorally anchored questions.

Some structured interviews have been developed with the primary purpose of assessing traumas in more detail. The Potential Stressful Events Interview (Kilpatrick, Resnick, & Freedy, 1991) has behaviorally anchored questions that are particularly good for assessing interpersonal victimization, as well as a range of other traumatic stressors. The DSM-IV version of the Clinician-Administered PTSD Scale (CAPS; Blake et al., 1995; reviewed in more detail later, and used

in the majority of extant PTSD research), includes a self-report screening scale (Life Events Checklist), followed by interviewer prompts to establish whether a trauma meets criterion A. Validation of the most recent CAPS (Weathers, Blake, et al., 2013), reflecting current DSM-5 criteria, is ongoing.

Many clinicians may choose to circumvent some of these extensive questions by using self-report measures, such as checklists, to acquire some initial information. Although clinicians should not rely on them exclusively, a number of checklists can be used as a springboard for further inquiry. In addition to the Life Events Checklist, the Traumatic Stress Schedule (Norris, 1990), the Trauma History Questionnaire (THQ; Green, 1996), the Traumatic Life Events Questionnaire (TLEQ; Kubany, Haynes, et al., 2000), and the Traumatic Events Scale (Vrana & Lauterbach, 1994) all assess a number of different types of trauma, including accidents, natural disaster, sexual assault, and threats of, or actual, physical harm. The Posttraumatic Stress Diagnostic Scale (PDS; Foa, 1995) has two sections prior to assessment of symptoms. The first section assesses 13 potentially traumatic events, whereas the second has questions to determine whether an event meets the definition of criterion A. With regard to combat in particular, the Combat Exposure Scale (Keane, Fairbank, Caddell, & Zimering, 1989) has been used widely to assess the degree of combat exposure.

Structured Diagnostic Interviews

The CAPS, developed by Blake and colleagues (1995), has become a "gold-standard" assessment of PTSD and is now the most widely used diagnostic interview (Weathers, Keane, & Davidson, 2001; Weathers, Ruscio, & Keane, 1999). The CAPS has several attractive features. In addition to a detailed assessment of individual trauma experiences, it assesses both severity and frequency of symptoms, using specific criteria. Furthermore, the CAPS includes questions on associated features of PTSD, including dissociation, survivor guilt, and social and occupational impairment. Additionally, it gives clear guidelines for assessing changes in behavior following exposure to trauma. The CAPS has a large body of research demonstrating its reliability and validity across a wide variety of trauma populations. One disadvantage is its length of administration, which, on average, takes about 1 hour, and the need for administration by a mental health clinician. The length of administration may be decreased slightly by assessing only the 17 core DSM-IV symptoms. As mentioned, the CAPS has been revised to be consistent with DSM-5 criteria (Weathers, Blake, et al., 2013) and is currently undergoing testing.

The Structured Clinical Interview for DSM-IV (SCID; First, Spitzer, Williams, & Gibbon, 1995), one of the most widely used diagnostic scales, includes assessment of PTSD symptomatology and was developed for use by experienced clinicians. Although it assesses all of the symptoms of PTSD and can provide information about whether an individual meets criteria for the diagnosis, it is important to note that the interview does not assess for frequency or severity of individual symptoms. Furthermore, by using the SCID, one can only determine a count of the number of positive symptoms, thereby limiting its utility in research or clinical settings in which a continuous measure of severity may be desirable. Resnick, Kilpatrick, and Lipovsky (1991) recommended certain modifications of the SCID for use with rape victims, including more sensitive screening questions for history of rape and other major traumatic events. The SCID is being modified to reflect current DSM-5 criteria for PTSD.

Another highly structured interview, the Diagnostic Interview Schedule (DIS; Robins, Helzer, Croughan, & Ratcliff, 1981), has the advantage of requiring less training and experience to administer than the CAPS and the SCID. Like the SCID, the DIS results in diagnosis but does not have continuous severity scores. One potential problem is that the PTSD section assesses exposure to civilian trauma, including sexual assault, but uses the term "rape" without any further specification. Thus, the modifications suggested by Resnick and colleagues (1991) relative to rape may be appropriate for this instrument, as well as when assessing interpersonal traumas. Kessler and colleagues (1995) also have modified the DIS for better diagnosis of PTSD in large studies with lay interviewers.

The PTSD Symptom Scale—Interview (PSS-I; Foa, Riggs, Dancu, & Rothbaum, 1993) has a particular advantage in its ease of administration and brevity. The PSS-I originally comprised 17 items and prompts matching the 17-symptom PTSD criteria in DSM-IV, and an updated version reflecting DSM-5 criteria is undergoing validation. The PSS-I can result in continuous scores to reflect frequency of symptoms or to determine PTSD diagnosis. Another advantage is its companion self-report measure (PSS-SR), to which scores on the interview can be compared. Thus, after conducting an initial interview, one could administer the PSS-SR on a more regular basis (e.g., biweekly) to monitor symptom change, without having to readminister the interview frequently. A disadvantage of the interview is that symptoms are assessed only over a current, 2-week period instead of 1 month, so it is possible that some diagnoses may be incorrect per DSM-5. The time frame should be modified for careful diagnosis.

Self-Report Instruments

There are now a number of self-report scales of PTSD that have good psychometric properties. Among them are the PSS-SR (Falsetti, Resnick, Resick, & Kilpatrick, 1993; Foa et al., 1993), the Purdue PTSD Scale—Revised (Lauterbach & Vrana, 1996), the PTSD Checklist (PCL; Weathers, Litz, Herman, Huska, & Keane, 1993), the Distressing Event Questionnaire (DEQ; Kubany, Leisen, Kaplan, & Kelly, 2000), the Mississippi Scale for Combat-Related PTSD (Mississippi Scale; Keane, Caddell, & Taylor, 1988), and the PDS (Foa, 1995). Most of these scales were developed with specific populations, such as rape trauma survivors (e.g., PSS) or combat veterans (e.g., Mississippi Scale, PCL), and research on their validity with other populations in some cases is minimal. Thus, it is important for clinicians to think about their target population before adopting a measure. Moreover, as with any self-report measure, there are limitations to relying exclusively on questionnaires for diagnosis or symptom severity. Used in conjunction with structured interviews, however, they can be useful for screening purposes or for demonstrating changes over time as a result of a particular intervention. There is also evidence that self-report and clinician interview of PTSD symptoms are correlated over the course of treatment (Monson et al., 2008).

The Impact of Event Scale—Revised (IES-R; Weiss & Marmar, 1997) and the Mississippi Scale (Keane et al., 1988, 1989) are two of the oldest self-report measures. The IES-R is useful for measuring trauma impact and maps onto DSM-IV criteria, including symptoms of avoidance, intrusion and arousal (Weiss & Marmar, 1997). The original 35-item Mississippi Scale assessed both diagnostic criteria and associated features of PTSD in combat veterans; a newer version has been created for use with civilians (Lauterbach, Vrana, King, & King, 1997). The PDS (Foa, 1995), a 49-item scale designed to assess all five PTSD criteria, has strong psychometrics. Griffin, Uhlmansiek, Resick, and Mechanic (2004) found a strong correlation between the PDS and the CAPS.

Two measures of PTSD have been empirically derived from other scales. The Keane PTSD Scale (PK) of the Minnesota Multiphasic Personality Inventory (MMPI) and MMPI-2 has been used successfully to discriminate between Vietnam combat veterans with and without PTSD (Keane, Malloy, & Fairbank, 1984; Weathers & Keane, 1999). The Symptom Checklist 90—Revised (SCL-90-R; Derogatis, 1983) has also been examined by Saunders, Arata, and Kilpatrick (1990) and by Weathers and colleagues (1999), who developed PTSD subscales derived from different sets of items for female crime victims and combat veterans, respectively.

The PCL is widely used in Department of Veterans Affairs (VA) and military settings with a Military Version (PCL-M) that refers specifically to military-related traumas. The Civilian Version of the scale (PCL-C) assesses civilian traumas, and the Specific Version (PCL-S) allows the assessor to identify the specific trauma of reference. Like the PDS, the PCL reflects DSM-IV symptoms of PTSD and like the CAPS, the PCL has now been revised to reflect the DSM-5 and is undergoing testing (Weathers, Litz, et al., 2013).

In response to a need to screen large numbers of people for PTSD after combat or disasters, or in medical settings when time is limited, a brief PTSD screen has been developed for use in primary care settings or for large-group administrations, such as those with military personnel following deployment (Prins et al., 2004). The Primary Care PTSD Screen (PC-PTSD) was developed for such a purpose and is now being used routinely in the United States with anyone returning from military deployment or receiving any kind of treatment in the VA medical system (Hoge et al., 2006). This scale has four yes–no items that represent the four major symptom clusters found in most PTSD factor-analytic studies that separate effortful avoidance from numbing. These four items were found to be highly associated with PTSD as measured by the CAPS. In fact, the PC-PTSD outperformed the PCL with regard to sensitivity and specificity, as well as efficiency. A cutoff of 3 was recommended as an optimally efficient score for both men and women, and a cutoff of 2 was recommended for maximum sensitivity.

Finally, it should be noted that only one trauma-related scale, the Trauma Symptom Inventory (TSI; Briere, 1995), includes scales to assess response bias. For forensic purposes, in which response bias may be of particular concern, the assessor may wish to include the TSI or administer the MMPI-2, which contains both the PK scale and Validity subscales. In addition to clinical scales, the TSI also includes subscales assessing tendencies to overendorse unusual or bizarre symptoms, to respond in an inconsistent or random manner, and to deny symptoms that others commonly endorse. In addition to PTSD-related subscales, such as Intrusive Experiences, Defensive Avoidance, and Anxious Arousal, it also includes subscales that measure frequently observed problems: Depression, Anger, Dissociation, Tension-Reduction Behaviors, and Disruptions in Self-Perception and Sexual Functioning.

Psychophysiological Assessment

The ideal assessment includes measurement in multiple response channels, including physiological responses. This is especially true in PTSD assessment because physiological reactivity to trauma cues is one of the criteria of the disorder. However, a psychophysiological test might not be feasible in clinical settings because the required technology and expertise are not always available. Despite this limitation, it is important to be aware of the research in this area and to be alert to obvious physiological symptoms in patients when talking about their trauma experiences (e.g., signs of agitation, sweating, flushing). Research has demonstrated consistent group differences in physiological reactivity between individuals with and without PTSD when exposed to trauma-related stimuli, such as through the use of individualized trauma scripts (for a systematic review of this body of research, see Orr, Metzger, Miller, & Kaloupek, 2004). Vietnam veterans with PTSD have consistently been found to be more reactive to combat imagery than combat veterans without PTSD, even when the comparison samples had other anxiety disorders or other psychological problems (Keane et al., 1998; Pitman, Orr, Forgue, & Altman, 1990; Pitman, Orr, Forgue, de Jong, & Claiborn, 1987). Similar results have been found in people with PTSD as a result of MVAs and child sexual abuse (Blanchard, Hickling, Buckley, & Taylor, 1996; Orr et al., 1998).

The largest investigation of physiological reactivity was a multisite study of over 1,300 veterans (Keane et al., 1998). Using four psychophysiological measures, Keane and colleagues (1998) were able to classify correctly two-thirds of those who had PTSD. This indicates that whereas psychophysiological reactivity can help to distinguish between many members of PTSD and non-PTSD groups, it should not be used as a sole measure of diagnostic assessment. In fact, a number of factors may affect physiological reactivity, and these must be taken into account when assessing the validity of psychophysiological findings. For example, the presence of psychotropic drugs (i.e., benzodiazepines, beta-adrenergic blockers) can affect an individual's response. In addition to people who do not respond physiologically, some people appear to have an alternative response to arousal. Griffin and colleagues (1997) studied psychophysiological reactivity in recent rape trauma survivors using a methodology that differed in two significant ways from prior studies. First, rather than listening to generated scripts, participants were asked to talk for 5 minutes on both a neutral recall topic and their rapes. These neutral and trauma phases were interspersed with baseline conditions. Second, instead of looking at the PTSD group as a whole, the researchers examined physiological reactivity by degree of "peritraumatic dissociation" (PD), which refers to the extent to which someone dissociated during the traumatic event. Griffin and colleagues found that a small group of women with high PD responded in a very different manner than other women with PTSD. Whereas skin conductance and heart rate of women with low PD scores increased as expected while they were talking about the rape, those with high PD scores showed a decrease in the physiological measures. When the participants' subjective distress during each of the phases was examined, the high-PD group reported the same level of distress as the low-PD group. Therefore, despite experiencing distress, the physiological responses of the high-PD group were suppressed. Griffin and colleagues speculated that there may be a dissociative subtype of individuals with PTSD who physiologically respond quite differently than those with the more phobic type of PTSD. The addition of neuroimaging has demonstrated that instead of a strong amygdala response, individuals who are highly dissociative appear to have an overmodulated response and strong activation of the frontal lobes (Lanius et al., 2010). Research such as this supports the dissociative subtype found in DSM-5.

In general, there are two major aims in assessment in clinical practice: diagnosis and treatment planning. Whether the primary purpose of assessment is diagnosis or treatment planning, a multidimensional, multiaxial approach is desirable. Because a cross-sectional view taken at a single point in time may fail to capture the full range and pattern of symptoms, a longitudinal approach to assessment has been advocated by Denny, Robinowitz, and Penk (1987), and Sutker, Uddo-Crane, and Allain (1991). Certainly for the purposes of treat-

ment, ongoing assessment of symptom patterns and treatment effectiveness is essential. Even when measuring PTSD cross-sectionally, it has been suggested that multiple measures and methods be used, depending on the purpose of the assessment (Keane, Brief, Pratt, & Miller, 2007; Weathers & Keane, 1999).

Some final notes regarding assessment are in order. First, given the empirical evidence linking PTSD with increased risk of suicide, suicide risk should always be carefully assessed and monitored. The National Women's Study (Kilpatrick, Edmunds, & Seymour, 1992) found that 13% of rape survivors had made a suicide attempt compared with 1% of nonvictims. Additionally, 33% of rape survivors, compared with 8% of nonvictims, stated that they had seriously considered suicide at some point. Furthermore, the presence of comorbid PTSD has been associated with a greater number of suicide attempts among individuals with major depressive disorder (Oquendo et al., 2003). These data highlight the need for careful monitoring of suicidal ideation and self-harm behavior among individuals being assessed or treated for PTSD.

Second, a growing body of research suggests that individuals with PTSD are at increased risk of perpetrating physical aggression against others. McFall, Fontana, Raskind, and Rosenheck (1999) found that male Vietnam veteran inpatients with PTSD were more likely than inpatients without PTSD or a community sample of Vietnam veterans to perpetrate acts of violence toward objects or others. Results from the NVVRS indicated that 33% of Vietnam veterans with PTSD had assaulted their partner within the previous year (Jordan et al., 1992). Risk of violence is not limited to Vietnam veterans. There is evidence of increased risk of violence in other traumatized populations, including women (e.g., Miller et al., 2004). Given also that outbursts of anger are one of the DSM-5 symptoms of PTSD, it is important that history of aggressive acts (under criterion E), as well as current impulses toward aggression (e.g., angry mood in criterion D), be carefully assessed and addressed.

TREATMENT

Types of Therapy for PTSD

There have been four predominant forms of therapy for PTSD: coping, skills-focused treatments; exposure-based treatments; cognitive therapy; combination treatments; and eye movement desensitization and reprocessing (EMDR; which may be a combination treatment). Before reviewing the research on treatment outcome for PTSD, we describe some of the treatment protocols.

Stress Inoculation Training

The earliest comprehensive approach described specifically for use with rape survivors was stress inoculation training (SIT; Kilpatrick & Amick, 1985; Kilpatrick et al., 1982). Based on Meichenbaum's (1985) approach to anxiety, its aim is to give clients a sense of mastery over their fears by teaching a variety of coping skills. The approach is tailored to the individual problems and needs of each client, so it is flexible and can be used in individual or group settings. SIT is approached in phases. The first phase, preparation for treatment, includes an educational element to provide an explanatory or conceptual framework from which the client can understand the nature and origin of his/her fear and anxiety, and make sense of the trauma and its aftermath. In SIT, a social learning theory explanation is used. Along with this, fear and anxiety reactions are explained as occurring along three channels (Lang, 1968): (1) the physical or autonomic channel; (2) the behavioral or motoric channel; and (3) the cognitive channel. Specific examples are given for each, and the patient identifies his/her own reactions within each channel. Interrelationships among the three channels are explained and discussed. The second phase of SIT is the training of coping skills directed at each of these channels of response. It includes, in sequence, a definition of the coping skill, a rationale, an explanation of the mechanism by which the skill works, a demonstration of the skill, application by the client of the skill to a problem area unrelated to the target behaviors, a review of how well the skill worked, and, finally, application and practice of the skill with one of the target fears. Skills taught most often for coping with fear in the physical channel are muscle relaxation and breathing control.

For the behavioral channel, covert modeling and role playing are the coping skills usually taught. The client is taught to visualize a fear- or anxiety-provoking situation and to imagine him/herself confronting it successfully. For the cognitive channel, the client is taught guided self-dialogue. The client is taught to focus on his/her internal dialogue and trained to label negative, irrational, and maladaptive self-statements. He/she is then taught to substitute more adaptive self-verbalizations.

Self-dialogue is taught in four categories: preparation, confrontation and management, coping with feelings of being overwhelmed, and reinforcement. For each of these categories, a series of questions and/or statements is generated that encourages the client to assess the actual probability that the negative event will occur, to manage the overwhelming fear and avoidance behavior, to control self-criticism and self-devaluation, to engage in the feared behavior, and finally to reinforce him/herself for making the attempt and following the steps.

Exposure Techniques

Beginning in the early 1980s, forms of exposure therapy were investigated as a treatment for PTSD. Although systematic desensitization (SD) has been demonstrated to be effective for treating PTSD in a number of case study reports and controlled studies, it was not widely adopted as a preferred treatment (Bowen & Lambert, 1986; Brom, Kleber, & Defares, 1989; Frank et al., 1988; Frank & Stewart, 1983, 1984; Schindler, 1980; Shalev, Orr, & Pitman, 1992). Because people with PTSD may fear and avoid a wide range of trauma-related stimuli, SD may require a number of hierarchies that can be quite inefficient.

Extended exposure to feared cues or to the trauma memory itself is a more efficient treatment and has been employed more widely. Known variously as direct therapeutic exposure (DTE), flooding, or prolonged exposure, these exposure techniques require clients to confront feared situations *in vivo*, to imagine themselves in a fear-producing situation, or to recall their particular trauma for extended periods of time. Rothbaum, Hodges, Ready, Graap, and Alarcon (2001) experimented with the use of virtual reality for treating veterans. The veteran with PTSD can take a virtual helicopter trip in Vietnam, complete with gunfire, or drive a vehicle in Middle Eastern streets, as well as experience other stimuli that may evoke memories of traumatic events.

Foa and colleagues (1991; Rothbaum & Foa, 1992) were the first to focus extensively on the specific trauma memory rather than fear-producing stimuli. Prolonged exposure (PE) is conducted individually in 9–12 weekly or biweekly 90-minute sessions. The first two sessions are for information gathering, treatment planning, and explanation of the treatment rationale. Clients are also taught breathing retraining. A hierarchical list of major stimuli that are feared and avoided is created. Clients are instructed to confront feared cues for at least

45 minutes a day, starting with a moderately anxiety-provoking stimulus on the hierarchy. Beginning with Session 3, the trauma scene is relived in imagination, and the client is asked to describe it aloud in the present tense. The level of detail is left to the client for the first two exposures, but thereafter he/she is encouraged to include more and more detail about external cues and internal cues, such as thoughts, physiological responses, and feared consequences. Descriptions are repeated several times each session (for 60 minutes) and audio-recorded. Clients are assigned as homework listening to the recording and engaging in *in vivo* tasks. Care is taken in sessions to ensure that the client's anxiety decreases before the session is terminated, aided by the therapist, if necessary (Foa & Rothbaum, 1998).

Marks, Lovell, Noshirvani, Livanou, and Thrasher (1998) have conducted exposure therapy somewhat differently. Their version of the therapy includes five sessions of imaginal exposure, then five sessions of live exposure. During the imaginal exposure, clients are asked to relive aloud in the first person, present tense, the details of their experience, then to imagine and describe critical aspects of the event (rewind and hold). Clients listen to their therapy recordings daily between sessions. During the live exposure portion of therapy, clients (most often therapist-accompanied) progress through a hierarchy of feared, avoided, and disabling trauma-related stimuli. They are asked to practice the live exposure for an hour a day between sessions.

Cognitive Interventions

Cognitive therapy for PTSD has generally taken two forms. One form is more present-focused and typically uses daily diaries or monitoring forms to elicit current thoughts that the client has recorded during the week. These homework sheets form the basis of the cognitive interventions that occur during treatment through the use of teaching and Socratic questioning. Clients are taught to identify and to dispute their unrealistic or exaggerated thoughts about themselves, the world, and their futures with more probabilistic reasoning and evidence-based argument. Examples of researchers who have used this model of cognitive restructuring are Blanchard and colleagues (2003) and Foa and colleagues (2005).

The other form of cognitive therapy is trauma-focused and constructivist, focusing on the particular meanings that the traumatic event(s) has for the client and how those interpretations of the event contradict or seemingly confirm previously held beliefs about self and others. These distorted assumptions about the event (e.g., "I should have been able to stop the event, so it is my fault that it happened") may maintain a belief in a just world or a sense of controllability, but at the cost of reduced self-esteem, shame, or guilt. The focus of treatment is on how clients may have distorted the event itself to maintain prior beliefs about justice or the role of others (assimilation), or conversely, how they may have changed their beliefs about themselves and the world too much (overaccommodation) in an attempt to regain a sense of control or safety in the present or the future ("I cannot trust other people at all any more"). Treatment includes Socratic questioning and using cognitive worksheets to teach clients to challenge their thinking about their traumatic events and the implications they have constructed. Examples of trauma-focused cognitive therapy are studies by Resick and colleagues (2002, 2008) and Tarrier and colleagues (1999).

Cognitive processing therapy (CPT) initially was developed specifically to treat the specific symptoms of PTSD in sexual assault survivors (Resick & Schnicke, 1992, 1993), but it has since been updated and applied to other populations (Resick et al., 2007). CPT, which can be delivered in either individual or group formats, is a 12-session, structured therapy program that is predominantly a cognitive therapy. After an introduction to PTSD symptoms and the therapy, clients are asked to write an Impact Statement, which is a description of how their most distressing traumatic event has affected them. Clients are asked to focus on any self-blame they experience regarding the trauma and the effects of the event on their beliefs about self and others. This statement is used to understand how they may have distorted the cause of the event or overgeneralized its meaning, such that their functioning has been compromised. For example, if someone thinks that he/she should have been able to stop the event, then the individual might feel guilt afterward. If a client has decided that the event means no one is to be trusted, then he/she will behave as though this is true.

Before examining the trauma in depth, the client is taught to label emotions and recognize the connection among events, thoughts, and feelings, then is asked to write a detailed account of the index traumatic event and read it to him/herself every day. In sessions he/she reads it to the therapist and is encouraged to feel whatever emotions emerge and to complete worksheets on identified stuck points about the trauma. The therapist begins to challenge problematic thinking about the traumatic event with Socratic dialogue. After writing and reading the account for a second time, the therapist focuses on teaching the client the skill of challenging thoughts and assumptions with Socratic questions for him/herself through a series of worksheets. The client is first taught to question a single thought, then look for patterns of problematic thinking, and, finally, to generate alternative, more balanced thoughts about the event itself, then overgeneralized assumptions about self and world. In the last five sessions, clients are provided modules to assist them in thinking about specific themes that are commonly disrupted following traumatic events: safety, trust, power and control, esteem, and intimacy. In an alternative version that is receiving increased research attention, the written account is omitted. This is discussed below in the research section.

Combination Treatments/Additive Studies

Some studies that we review below refer to the protocols as cognitive-behavioral therapy (CBT; e.g., Blanchard et al., 2003). These therapy packages are typically combinations of various forms of exposure (imaginal, *in vivo*) and cognitive therapy, but they may also include relaxation or other coping skills. Some of these protocols were developed as a combination treatment at the outset or reflect additive studies in which a new component is added to an existing treatment to determine whether the extra component adds value to the existing therapy. An important distinction between these two types of protocols is that the combination treatments were designed to be a specific length to accommodate the components of the treatment. In other words, the therapy package was designed to achieve the optimal goals of the exposure or cognitive components. Additive studies must accommodate to the original protocol length; therefore, they may not be designed with the optimal amount of therapy needed to achieve the goals of the components. In additive studies, the amount of exposure, stress management, or cognitive therapy in combination is shortened to maintain the length of the original protocol being compared.

STAIR/MPE

Cloitre, Koenen, Cohen, and Han (2002) proposed that survivors of child sexual abuse trauma have problems of affect regulation and interpersonal effectiveness, in addition to their PTSD, that compromise their ability to profit from trauma-focused interventions. Thus, they developed a protocol called STAIR (i.e., skills training in affective and interpersonal regulation) that includes treatment for these problems prior to implementing a modification of prolonged exposure (MPE). This combination treatment first trains patients in emotion management and interpersonal skills for 8 weeks, followed by a second phase of treatment with imaginal exposure. The imaginal exposure phase also includes postexposure emotional management and cognitive therapy.

Eye Movement Desensitization and Reprocessing

Eye movement desensitization and reprocessing (EMDR) is a controversial therapy that evolved not from theory or application of effective techniques for other disorders, but from a personal observation. As originally developed by Shapiro (1989, 1995), EMDR was based on a chance observation that troubling thoughts were resolved when her eyes followed the waving of leaves during a walk in the park. Shapiro developed EMDR on the basis of this observation and argues that lateral eye movements facilitate cognitive processing of the trauma. Subsequently, EMDR has been conceptualized as a cognitive-behavioral treatment aimed at facilitating information processing of traumatic events and cognitive interventions for negative, trauma-related cognitions. In the early presentations, EMDR was touted as a one-session cure for a range of disorders. However, more recent studies are typically of trauma-related symptoms, with a course more similar to the other trauma therapies. EMDR is now described as an eight-phase treatment that includes history taking, client preparation, target assessment, desensitization, installation, body scan, closure, and reevaluation of treatment effects. EMDR includes exposure and cognitive components, as well as the lateral eye movements.

In the basic EMDR protocol, clients are asked to identify and focus on a traumatic image or memory (target assessment phase). Next, the therapist elicits negative cognitions or belief statements about the memory. Clients are asked to assign a rating to the memory and negative cognitions on an 11-point scale of distress and to identify the physical location of the anxiety. The therapist helps clients generate positive cognitions that would be preferable to associate with the memory. These are rated on a 7-point scale of how much the clients believe the statement. Once the therapist has instructed a client in the basic EMDR procedure, he/she is asked to do four things simultaneously (desensitization phase): (1) visualize the memory; (2) rehearse the negative cognitions; (3) concentrate on the physical sensations of the anxiety; and (4) visually track the therapist's index finger. While the client does this, the therapist rapidly moves his/her index finger back and forth from right to left, 30–35 centimeters from the client's face, with two back-and-forth movements per second (there are now light bars available to do this). These are repeated 24 times. Then the client is asked to blank out the memory and take a deep breath. Subsequently, she or he brings back the memory and cognitions and rates the level of distress. Sets of eye movements (saccades) are repeated until the distress rating equals 0 or 1. At this point, the client is asked how she or he feels about the positive cognition and gives a rating for it (installation phase).

Evidence for Treatment Efficacy

CBT and EMDR have been established as efficacious treatments in multiple meta-analyses (e.g., Bradley, Greene, Russ, Dutra, & Westen, 2005; Powers, Halpern, Ferenschak, Gillihan, & Foa, 2010; van Etten & Taylor, 1998). They have also been recommended as first-line treatments in multiple treatment guidelines for PTSD (e.g., Foa, Keane, Friedman, & Cohen, 2008; National Institute of Clinical Excellence, 2005; U.S. Departments of Veterans Affairs and Defense, 2010).

Randomized controlled trials have consistently shown CBT to be superior to waiting-list and treatment-as-usual conditions (e.g., Chard, 2005; Foa et al., 1999; Monson et al., 2006; Resick et al., 2002), and generally better than therapies designed to control for the essential and nonspecific elements of efficacious psychotherapy (e.g., Blanchard et al., 2003; Neuner, Schauer, Klaschik, Karunakara, & Elbert, 2004; Schnurr et al., 2007). Head-to-head trials have shown few differences between different CBT packages at posttreatment (e.g., Bryant, Moulds, Guthrie, Dang, & Nixon, 2003; Foa et al., 1999; Resick et al., 2002; Tarrier et al., 1999), and there have been equivocal results regarding differential efficacy at longer-term follow-up (i.e., ≥ 5 years posttreatment; Resick et al., 2012; Tarrier & Sommerfield, 2004). The addition or removal of different elements of CBT protocols have not generally affected the efficacy of these packages (e.g., Foa et al., 1999; Resick et al., 2008).

Randomized controlled trials show EMDR to be superior to waiting-list conditions (e.g., Rothbaum,

Astin, & Marsteller, 2005). However, several studies have shown CBT to be more efficacious than EMDR (e.g., Devilly & Spence, 1999; Taylor et al., 2003), others have reported no difference (e.g., Ironson, Freund, Strauss, & Williams, 2002; Power et al., 2002; Rothbaum et al., 2005), and still others report EMDR to be superior to CBT for at least intrusive symptoms (Lee, Gavriel, Drummond, Richards, & Greenwald, 2002). Although Shapiro maintains that lateral eye movements are an essential therapeutic component of EMDR, dismantling studies examining this have yielded mixed results (e.g., Pitman, Orr, Altman, Longpre, Poire, & Macklin, 1996; Renfrey & Spates, 1994; Wilson, Silver, Covi, & Foster, 1996).

In summary, different forms of CBT focused on skills development or trauma processing through cognitive or behavioral methods have been found to be efficacious in the treatment of PTSD and to have long-term, sustained effects. Studies have documented the efficacy of EMDR, although the evidence supporting lateral eye movements as an active treatment ingredient are equivocal.

Therapist, Client, and Setting Variables

Gender and Ethnicity

According to the National Comorbidity Survey Replication study (Kessler, Berglund, et al., 2005) lifetime prevalence rates of PTSD are nearly three times higher in women (9.7%) than in with men (3.6%). Tolin and Foa's (2006) meta-analysis of sex differences in the risk for exposure to potentially traumatic events and PTSD indicated that women are more likely than men to meet criteria for PTSD but less likely to have experienced potentially traumatic events. Women are more likely than men to experience sexual assault and child sexual abuse but less likely to experience accidents and nonsexual assaults; to witness death and injury; and to experience disaster, fire, and war-related trauma. Within specific types of traumatic events, women still exhibited greater PTSD, suggesting that risk of exposure to particular types of trauma only partially explains the differential PTSD risk in men and women.

Because sexual assault is predominantly perpetrated by men, and is a highly personal and intimate crime, survivors of sexual assault often distrust men. Consequently, the issue of therapist sex can be relevant. Frequently, clients prefer or insist on a female therapist. The effectiveness of male therapists has not been studied specifically, but they may be quite effective, if well trained (Resick, Jordan, Girelli, Hutter, & Marhoeder-Dvorak, 1988). Issues for male therapists, discussed by Silverman (1977) and Koss and Harvey (1991), include the tendency for men to view rape more as a sexual crime than as a crime of violence (Burt, 1980), therefore focusing too much on sexual aspects of the experience and its aftermath.

In treating survivors of sexual assault, regardless of therapist sex, it is essential that the therapist be knowledgeable about rape and PTSD. This includes the literature on reactions to rape, rape myths, and attitudes about rape. Therapists bring their culturally learned perceptions with them, as do clients, and these can interfere with their effectiveness if they adhere to any of the common misperceptions about rape (e.g., rape is primarily about sex, most rapists are strangers, it is not rape unless the woman actively resists). Sexual assault survivors are extremely sensitive to insinuations that they might have been to blame, for example, and many drop out of treatment if they sense that the therapist might harbor victim-blaming attributions.

Similarly, combat veterans are often hesitant to start treatment with novice therapists who may not know particular war details or relevant history. It is important for therapists to acknowledge their level of familiarity and work with clients to understand more fully their trauma experiences and the context surrounding them.

The role of ethnicity in CBT for PTSD has received little attention in outcome research. This limitation, unfortunately, is not restricted to PTSD treatment research; the minority-focused supplement of the Surgeon General's report on mental health (U.S. Department of Health and Human Services, 2001) made clear that there is a paucity of empirical research on treatment for depression and anxiety in minorities. The few studies of prevalence rates among ethnic groups have shown mixed results that, in part, may reflect differential rates of trauma exposure (Breslau, Davis, & Andreski, 1995; Norris, 1992).

Two program evaluation studies compared African American and European American male veterans with PTSD. Rosenheck, Fontana, and Cottrol (1995) found less improvement among African American veterans on some measures. However, Rosenheck and Fontana's (1996) study did not support this finding. Only a few studies to date have examined the efficacy of CBT with African American women with PTSD. Zoellner, Feeny, Fitzgibbons, and Foa (1999) compared African American and European American women who were survi-

vors of either sexual or nonsexual assault. Treatment comprised PE, SIT, or a combination of the two. There were no ethnic group differences in treatment efficacy. These results were achieved in spite of an inability to match clients and therapists on ethnicity. Lester, Resick, Young-Xu, and Artz (2010) combined the datasets from both Resick and colleagues (2002, 2008) studies to examine the dropout and outcomes of treatment among 94 African American and 214 European American female victims of interpersonal trauma. The dropout rate was significantly greater for African-American patients (45% vs. 73% completed all sessions). However, despite that, in the intention-to-treat analyses in which everyone was randomized, there were no differences between the racial groups in treatment outcome. The differences appeared to be due to the fact that African American patients who dropped out of therapy benefited more from treatment than the European American patients who dropped out. Although these results are encouraging, continued attention to racial, ethnic, and cultural issues in treatment is important (see McNair & Neville, 1996).

Vicarious Traumatization

Working with trauma victims can have negative effects on therapists that have been labeled "secondary" or "vicarious" traumatization by some. McCann and Pearlman (1990) discuss this impact as disruption of the therapist's own cognitive schemas about self and the world. Hearing clients' traumatic experiences may be shocking and lead to lasting alterations in assumptions and expectations, which in turn affect therapists' feelings, behaviors, and relationships. Working with trauma victims may challenge therapists' assumptions about personal invulnerability and safety, as well as beliefs that the world is a meaningful, orderly place filled with trustworthy people. According to McCann and Pearlman's model, an individual therapist's reaction depends on the degree of discrepancy between the survivor's trauma and the therapist's cognitive schemas. For example, if the therapist's own complex experiences have led to the development of safety assumptions (schemas) as central to his/her well-being, working with trauma survivors may be distressing due to a heightened sense of vulnerability. In addition, the therapist's memory system may be altered to incorporate traumatic imagery that can become intrusive.

To counteract the negative effects of working with traumatized individuals, therapists should be prepared to recognize and acknowledge these effects and take steps to deal with them. McCann and Pearlman (1990) recommend the use of one's professional network as a source of support and to prevent isolation. Talking to other professionals who work with trauma survivors is especially useful because they can help the therapist to recognize these effects and normalize these reactions. Other coping strategies suggested by McCann and Pearlman include balancing one's caseload with trauma and nontrauma cases, engaging in other professional and personal activities, recognizing one's own limitations, working for social change, and focusing on the positive personal impact of work with trauma survivors and ways it can enrich one's life.

"Resistance"

Clients with PTSD can be difficult to engage and treat due to their ambivalence about therapy. They may want help, but they fear confronting their memories and have difficulty trusting others, including therapists. They may also have strong feelings of shame about the traumatic event that interfere with their willingness to disclose information that they feel may lead to rejection by others. Of course, it is important to remember that avoidance behaviors, including avoiding thoughts about the trauma, are part of the criteria for PTSD. Therefore, it is to be expected that avoidance will also occur in the context of treatment. No-shows are common, and both subtle and obvious avoidance behaviors are seen throughout the beginning stages of therapy. If possible, therapists should consider treatment as starting on the telephone prior to the first session. The no-show rate is likely to decrease if the therapist expresses understanding of the client's hesitance to come in and encourages attendance. Early in therapy, the therapist should describe avoidance as a symptom of PTSD and an ineffective, though understandable, means of coping. Labeling this as "resistance" likely only increases judgmentalness toward the client and hinders therapist effectiveness. This and other challenges in working with rape trauma survivors are discussed by Koss and Harvey (1991) and Kilpatrick and Veronen (1983). Shay and Munroe (1999) discuss the challenges of working with combat veterans with complex PTSD.

Multiply Traumatized Victims

The treatment approaches presented here have been shown to produce significant improvement in civilian trauma victims within a brief time. The studies presented typically did not exclude anyone for his/her trauma history, and most had extensive trauma histories, even when there was an identified trauma that was the primary inclusion criterion (rape, combat). Moreover, in a secondary analysis of Resick and colleagues' (2002) trial, Resick and colleagues (2003) showed that the 42% of patients with childhood sexual abuse (CSA) experiences in addition to their adult index trauma had significant improvements in their PTSD and did not differ from those without a CSA history. In recent years, there has been a surge in evidence of treatment success in individuals with more chronic or repeated trauma histories, such as domestic violence (Kubany et al., 2004), combat (Monson et al., 2006), and long-standing CSA (Chard, 2005; Cloitre, Stovall-McClough, Miranda, & Chemtob, 2004). This research points to the utility of evidence-based treatment for complex cases and debunks the myth that CBT only works for "simple" cases of a single trauma. That said, therapists should be aware of attending to special issues in working with these cases. For example, some research suggests that PTSD in sexual assault trauma survivors may play a role in repeat traumatization (e.g., Kilpatrick et al., 1987), although this relationship appears to be complex (Wilson, Calhoun, & Bernat, 1999). Survivors of CSA may present additional challenges (Cloitre, 1998) because their traumatization may have interfered with processes of normal development. Given that the abuse often involves a relative or trusted adult, it represents a serious betrayal by someone on whom the child depended for basic safety and protection. They may need more help with skills development as well, especially interpersonal and emotion regulation skills. In some cases, sexual dysfunctions must be addressed. This can be added to an individual treatment program or the client may be referred to a sex therapy specialist, but only after the treatment for other trauma-related problems is complete. Veterans may present with issues specific to committing acts of violence or killing others, distrust of the government and authority figures, ethnic/racial stereotyping, and protracted grief reactions (Monson, Price, & Ranslow, 2005).

Group Treatment

The decision whether to use a group or an individual format for treatment is usually made on the basis of clinical judgment and practicality. There is scant research comparing the two formats. Some interventions that have been used with trauma victims are adaptable for use in either format. Recent research has shown that standardized group treatments may be successful for combat veterans and CSA trauma survivors (Chard, 2005; Creamer, Morris, Biddle, & Elliott, 1999). Recently Morland, Hynes, Macintosh, Resick, and Chard (2011) produced pilot data for an ongoing study in which group CPT was conducted through telehealth with a group on one of the Hawaiian islands while the therapist was on another island. Although the main randomized trial has not been completed yet, the findings appear promising that there will be equivalence between telehealth and in-person groups.

Group treatment has several advantages that make it popular with both trauma survivors and professionals. Koss and Harvey (1991) discussed a number of these. Group treatment reduces the sense of isolation felt by most survivors, who withdraw from interactions and believe that others cannot understand their feelings. It provides social support that is unambiguous and non-blaming. It helps to validate and to normalize feelings and reactions to the trauma. Group treatment confirms the reality of the traumatic experience and allows sharing of coping strategies. It counteracts self-blame and promotes self-esteem. Because it is more egalitarian than individual therapy, group treatment can promote empowerment and decrease dependency. It provides a safe environment for developing attachment and intimacy with others, and an opportunity for sharing grief and loss. Finally, group treatment can help trauma survivors assign meaning to the event, promoting cognitive processing.

Group approaches have drawbacks as well, and care should be taken to screen clients to assess their readiness for joining a group. McCann and Pearlman (1990) suggest that clients with severe PTSD should be in individual therapy simultaneously with group treatment because groups may elicit strong affect and memories that can overwhelm an unprepared client. For similar reasons, Resick and Markaway (1991) warn against having group members share their rape experiences during the first few sessions. Although important for recovery, the sharing of "war stories" should be done later in the group process or in individual sessions, to avoid frightening other group members or sensitizing them to other vulnerable situations. Poor candidates for group treatment, as suggested by Koss and Harvey (1991) and McCann and Pearlman, are suicidal clients; those with heavy substance abuse problems; self-mutilating or substance-abusing clients with a borderline personality disorder diagnosis; clients with very unstable, disorganized lives; and clients who have never before spoken about the trauma or whose memory of it is incomplete.

CASE STUDY

"Tom" is a 23-year-old, single, white male who presented for treatment approximately 1 year after a traumatic event that occurred during his military service in Iraq. Tom received CPT while on active duty in the Army.

Background

Tom was born the third of four children to his parents. He described his father as an alcoholic who was frequently absent from the home due to work travel prior to his parents' divorce. Tom indicated that his father was always emotionally distant from the family, especially after the divorce. Tom had close relationships with his mother and siblings. He denied having any significant mental health or physical health problems in his childhood. However, he described two significant traumatic events in his adolescence. Specifically, he described witnessing his best friend commit suicide by gunshot to the head. Tom indicated that this event severely affected him, as well as his entire community. He went on to report that he still felt responsible for not preventing his friend's suicide. The second traumatic event was the death of Tom's brother in an automobile accident when Tom was 17 years old. Tom did not receive any mental health treatment during his childhood or after these events, though he indicated that he began using alcohol and illicit substances after these traumatic events in his youth. He admitted to using cannabis nearly daily during high school, as well as daily use of alcohol, drinking as much as a 24-pack of beer per day until he passed out. Tom reported that he decreased his alcohol consumption and ceased using cannabis after his enlistment.

Tom served in the Infantry. He went to Basic Training, then attended an advanced training school prior to being deployed directly to Iraq. While in Iraq, Tom witnessed and experienced a number of traumatic incidents. He spoke about fellow soldiers who were killed and injured in service, as well as convoys that he witnessed being hit by improvised explosive devices (IEDs). However, the traumatic event that he identified as most distressing and anxiety-provoking was shooting a pregnant woman and child.

Tom described this event as follows: Suicide bombers had detonated several bombs in the area where Tom served, and a control point had been set up to contain the area. During the last few days of his deployment, Tom was on patrol at this control point. It was dark outside. A car began approaching the checkpoint, and officers on the ground signaled for the car to stop. The car did not stop in spite of these warnings. It continued to approach the control point, entering the area where the next level of Infantrymen were guarding the entrance. Per protocol, Tom fired a warning shot to stop the approaching car, but the car continued toward the control point. About 25 yards from the control point gate, Tom and at least one other soldier fired upon the car several times.

After a brief period of disorientation, a crying man with clothes soaked with blood emerged from the car with his hands in the air. The man quickly fell to his knees, with his hands and head resting on the road. Tom could hear the man sobbing. According to Tom, the sobs were guttural and full of despair. Tom looked over to find in the pedestrian seat a dead woman who was apparently pregnant. A small child in the backseat was also dead. Tom never confirmed this, but he and his fellow soldiers believed that the man crying on the road was the husband of the woman and the father of the child and fetus.

Tom was immediately distressed by the event, and a Combat Stress Control unit in the field eventually had him sent back to a Forward Operating Base because of his increasing reexperiencing and hypervigilance symptoms. Tom was eventually brought to a major Army hospital and received individual CPT within this setting.

Tom was administered the CAPS at pretreatment; his score was in the severe range, and he met diagnostic criteria for PTSD. He also completed the Beck Depression Inventory–II (BDI-II) and the State–Trait Anxiety Inventory (STAI). His depression and anxiety symptoms at pretreatment were in the severe range. Tom was provided feedback about his assessment results in a session focused on an overview of his psychological assessment results and on obtaining his informed consent for a course of CPT. After providing feedback about his assessment, the therapist gave Tom an overview of CPT, with an emphasis on its trauma-focused nature, expectation of out-of-session practice adherence, and

the client's active role in getting well. Tom signed a "CPT Treatment Contract" detailing this information and was provided a copy of the contract for his records. The CPT protocol began in the next session.

Session 1

Tom arrived 15 minutes prior to his first scheduled appointment of CPT. He sat down in the chair the therapist gestured that he sit in, but he was immediately restless and repositioned frequently. Tom quickly asked to move to a different chair in the room, so that his back was not facing the exterior door and his gaze could monitor both the door and the window. He asked the therapist how long his session would take and whether he would have to "feel anything." The therapist responded that this session would last 50–60 minutes, and that, compared with other future sessions, she would be doing most of the talking. She added that, as discussed during the treatment contracting session, the focus would be on Tom's feelings in reaction to the traumatic event but that the current session would focus less on this. The therapist also explained that she would have the treatment manual in her lap, and would refer to it throughout to make sure that she delivered the psychotherapy as it was prescribed. She encouraged Tom to ask any questions he might have as the session unfolded.

The therapist explained that at the beginning of each session they would develop an agenda for the session. The purposes of the first therapy session were to (1) describe the symptoms of PTSD; (2) give Tom a framework for understanding why these symptoms had not remitted; (3) present an overview of treatment to help Tom understand why practice outside of session and therapy attendance were important to elicit cooperation and to explain the progressive nature of the therapy; (4) build rapport between Tom and the therapist; and (5) give the client an opportunity to talk briefly about his most distressing traumatic event or other issues.

The therapist then proceeded to give didactic information about the symptoms of PTSD. She asked Tom to provide examples of the various clusters of PTSD symptoms that he was experiencing, emphasizing how reexperiencing symptoms are related to hyperarousal symptoms, and how hyperarousal symptoms elicit a desire to avoid or become numb. The paradoxical effect of avoidance and numbing in maintaining, or even increasing, PTSD symptoms was also discussed. Tom indicated that this was the first time someone had explained the symptoms of PTSD in this way, putting them "in motion" by describing how they interact with one another.

The therapist transitioned to a description of trauma aftereffects within an information-processing framework. She described in lay terms how traumas may be schema-discrepant events; traumatic events often do not fit with prior beliefs about oneself, others, or the world. To incorporate this event into one's memory, the person may alter his/her perception of the event (assimilate the event into an existing belief system). Examples of assimilation include looking back on the event and believing that some other course of action should have been taken ("undoing" the event) or blaming oneself because it occurred. The therapist went on to explain that Tom could have also attempted to change his prior belief system radically to overaccommodate the event to his prior beliefs. "Overaccommodation" was described as changing beliefs too much as a result of the traumatic event (e.g., "I can't trust myself about anything"). She explained that several areas of beliefs are often affected by trauma, including safety, trust, power/control, esteem, and intimacy. She further explained that these beliefs could be about the self and/or others. The therapist also pointed out that if Tom had negative beliefs prior to the traumatic event relative to any of these topics, the event could serve to strengthen these preexisting negative beliefs.

At this point, Tom described his childhood and adolescent experiences, and how they had contributed to his premilitary trauma beliefs. The therapist noted that Tom tended to blame himself and to internalize the bad things that had happened in his family and the suicide of his friend. She also noted his comment, "I wonder if my father drank to cope with me and my siblings." In Tom's case, it seemed likely that the traumatic experience served more to confirm his preexisting beliefs that he had caused or contributed to bad things happening around and to him.

Tom then spent some time describing how drastically things had changed after his military traumas. Prior to his military experiences and, specifically, the shooting of the woman and child, Tom described himself as "proud of being a soldier" and "pulling his life together." He indicated that the military structure had been very good for him in developing self-discipline and improving his self-esteem. He indicated that he felt good about "the mission to end terrorism" and was proud to serve his country. He felt camaraderie with his fellow soldiers and considered a career in the military.

He denied any authority problems and in fact believed that his commanding officers had been role models of the type of leader he wished to be. Prior to his deployment to Iraq, Tom met and married his wife, and they appeared to have a stable, intimate relationship. After his return from Iraq, Tom indicated that he did not trust anyone, especially anyone associated with the U.S. government. Tom expressed his disillusionment with the war effort and distrust of the individuals who commanded his unit. He also articulated distrust of himself: "I always make bad decisions when the chips are down." He stated that he felt completely unsafe in his environment. In his immediate postdeployment period, Tom had occasionally believed snipers on the base grounds had placed him in their crosshairs to kill him. He indicated that he minimally tolerated being close to his wife, including sexual contact between the two of them.

The therapist introduced the notion of "stuck points," or ways of making sense of the trauma or of thinking about himself, others, and the world, as getting in the way of Tom's recovery from the traumatic events. The therapist noted that a large number of individuals are exposed to trauma. In fact, military personnel are among the most trauma-exposed individuals. However, most people recover from their trauma exposure. Thus, a primary goal of the therapy was to figure out what had prevented Tom from recovering (i.e., how his thinking had got him "stuck," leading to the maintenance of his PTSD symptoms).

The therapist then asked Tom to provide a 5-minute account of his index traumatic event. Tom immediately responded, "There were so many bad things over there. How could I pick one?" The therapist asked, "Which of those events do you have the most thoughts or images about? Which of those events do you dislike thinking about the most?" The therapist indicated that Tom did not need to provide a fine-grained description of the event, but rather a brief overview of what happened. Tom provided a quick account of the shooting of the woman and child. The therapist praised Tom for sharing about the event with her and asked about his feelings as a result of sharing the information. Tom said that he felt anxious and wanted the session to be over. The therapist used this as an opportunity to describe the differences between "natural" and "manufactured" emotions.

The therapist first described "natural" emotions as those feelings that are commensurate reactions to experiences that have occurred. For example, if we perceive that someone has wronged us, it is natural to feel anger. If we encounter a threatening situation, it is natural to feel fear. Natural emotions have a self-limited and diminishing course. If we allow ourselves to feel these natural emotions, they will naturally dissipate. The therapist used the analogy of the energy contained in a bottle of carbonated soda to illustrate this concept. If the top of the bottle is removed, the pressure initially comes out with some force, but that force subsides and eventually has no energy forthcoming. On the other hand, there are "manufactured" emotions, or emotions that a person has a role in making. Our thoughts contribute to the nature and course of these emotions. The more that we "fuel" these emotions with our self-statements, the more we can increase the "pressure" of these emotions. For example, if a person tells himself over and over that he is a stupid person and reminds himself of more and more situations in which he perceived that he made mistakes, then he is likely to have more and more anger toward himself. The therapist reiterated that the goals of the therapy were (1) to allow Tom to feel the natural emotions he has "stuffed," which keep him from recovering from his trauma; and (2) to figure out how Tom was manufacturing emotions that were unhelpful to him.

The therapist summarized for Tom the three major goals of the therapy: (1) to remember and to accept what happened to him by not avoiding those memories and associated emotions; (2) to allow himself to feel his natural emotions and let them run their course, so the memory could be put away without such strong feelings still attached; and (3) to balance beliefs that had been disrupted or reinforced, so that Tom did not manufacture unhelpful emotions.

The therapist made a strong pitch for the importance of out-of-session practice adherence before assigning Tom the first practice assignment. The therapist told Tom that there appeared to be no better predictor of response to the treatment than how much effort a patient puts into it. She pointed out that of the 168 hours in a week, Tom would be spending 1–2 hours of that week in psychotherapy sessions (*Note.* We have found it helpful to do twice-weekly sessions, at least in the initial portion of the therapy, to facilitate rapport building, to overcome avoidance, and to capitalize on early gains in the therapy.) If Tom only spent the time during psychotherapy sessions focused on these issues, he would be spending less than 1% of his week focused on his recovery. To get better, he would be using daily worksheets and other writing assignments to promote

needed skills in his daily life and to decrease his avoidance. The therapist also pointed out that at the beginning of each session they would review the practice assignments that Tom had completed. The therapist asked Tom if this made sense, and he responded, "Sure. It makes sense that you get out of it what you put into it."

Tom's first assignment was to write an Impact Statement about the meaning of the event to determine how he had made sense of the traumatic event, and to help him begin to determine what assimilation, accommodation, and overaccommodation had occurred since the event. Stuck points that get in the way of recovery are identified with this first assignment. Tom was instructed to start writing the assignment later that day to address directly any avoidance about completing the assignment. He was specifically reminded that this was *not* a trauma account (that would come later) and that this assignment was specifically designed to get at the meaning of the event in his life, and how it had impacted his belief systems.

The specific assignment was as follows:

> Please write at least one page on what it means to you that you that this traumatic experience happened. Please consider the effects that the event has had on your beliefs about yourself, your beliefs about others, and your beliefs about the world. Also consider the following topics while writing your answer: safety, trust, power/competence, esteem, and intimacy. Bring this with you to the next session.

Session 2

The purposes of the second session are (1) to discuss the meaning of the event and (2) to help Tom begin to recognize thoughts, label emotions, and see the connection between what he says to himself and how he feels. Tom arrived with obvious anger and appeared defensive throughout most of the session. He stated that he had been feeling quite angry all week, and that he was "disgusted" with society and particularly politicians, who were "all self-interested or pandering to those with money." He expressed a great deal of anger over the reports of alleged torture at Abu Ghraib prison, which was a major news item during his therapy. The therapist was interested in the thinking behind Tom's anger about the events at Abu Ghraib. However, she first reviewed Tom's practice assignment, writing the first Impact Statement, to reinforce the completion of this work and to maintain the session structure she had outlined in the first session.

The therapist asked Tom to read his Impact Statement aloud. Clients in individual CPT are always asked to read their practice assignments aloud. Should the therapist read them, the client could dissociate or otherwise avoid his/her own reactions to their material. Tom had written:

The reason that this traumatic event happened is because I was friggin' stupid and made a bad decision. I killed an innocent family, without thinking. I murdered a man's wife and child. I can't believe that I did it. I took that man's wife and child, and oh, yeah, his unborn child, too. I feel like I don't deserve to live, let alone have a wife and child on the way. Why should I be happy when that man was riddled with despair, and that innocent woman, child, and unborn child died? Now, I feel like I'm totally unsafe. I don't feel safe even here on the hospital grounds, let alone in the city or back home with my family. I feel like someone is watching me and is going to snipe at me and my family because the terrorists had information about the situation and passed it on. I also don't feel that people are safe around me. I might go off and hurt someone, and God forbid it be my own family. With my wife pregnant, I am really concerned that I might hurt her. I don't trust anyone around me, and especially the government. I don't even trust the military treating me. I also don't trust myself. If I made a bad decision at that time, who is to say that I won't make a bad decision again? About power and control, I feel completely out of control of myself, and like the military and my commanding officer have complete control over me. My self-esteem is in the toilet. Why wouldn't it be given the crappy things that I have done? I don't think there are many positive things that I've done with my life, and when the chips are down, I always fail and let others down. I'm not sure what other-esteem is, but I do like my wife. In fact, I don't think she deserves to have to deal with me, and I think they would be better without me around. I don't want to be close to my wife, or anyone else for that matter. It makes me want to crawl out of my skin when my wife touches me. I feel like I'll never get over this. It wasn't supposed to be like this.

The therapist asked Tom what it was like to write and then read the Impact Statement aloud. Tom responded that it had been very difficult, and that he had avoided the assignment until the evening before his psychotherapy session. The therapist immediately reinforced Tom for his hard work in completing the assignment. She also used the opportunity to gently address the role of avoidance in maintaining PTSD symptoms. She asked specific Socratic questions aimed at elucidating the distress associated with anticipatory anxiety, and wondered aloud with Tom about what it would have been like to have completed the assignment earlier in the week. She also asked Socratic questions aimed at highlighting the fact that Tom felt better, not worse, after completing the assignment.

Tom's first Impact Statement and the information he shared in the first session made evident the stuck points that would have to be challenged. In CPT, areas of assimilation are prioritized as the first targets of treatment. Assimilation is targeted first because changes in the interpretation of the event itself are integrally related to the other, more generalized beliefs involved in overaccommodation. In Tom's case, he was assimilating the event by blaming himself. He used the term "murderer" to describe his role in the event, disregarding important contextual factors that surrounded the event. These beliefs would be the first priority for challenging. Tom's overaccommodation is evident in his general distrust of society and authority figures, and his belief that he will make bad decisions in difficult situations. His overaccommodation is also evident in his sense of threat in his environment (e.g., snipers), difficulty being emotionally and physically intimate with his wife, and low esteem for others and himself.

The therapist returned to Tom's anger about Abu Ghraib to get a better sense of possible stuck points, and also to experiment with Tom's level of cognitive rigidity or openness to cognitive challenging. The following exchange ensued between Tom and the therapist:

THERAPIST: Earlier you mentioned that you were feeling angry about the reports from Abu Ghraib. Can you tell me what makes you angry?

TOM: I can't believe that they would do that to those prisoners.

THERAPIST: What specifically upsets you about Abu Ghraib?

TOM: Haven't you heard the reports? I can't believe that they would humiliate and hurt them like that. Once again, the U.S. military's use of force is unacceptable.

THERAPIST: Do you think your use of force as a member of the U.S. military was unacceptable?

TOM: Yes. I murdered innocent civilians. I am no different than those military people at Abu Ghraib. In fact, I'm worse because I murdered them.

THERAPIST: "Murder." That's a strong word.

TOM: Yeah?

THERAPIST: From what you've told me, it seems like you killed some people who may or may not have been "innocent." Your shooting occurred in a very specific place and time, and under certain circumstances.

TOM: Yes, they died at my hands.

THERAPIST: Yes, they died, and it seems, at least in part, because of your shooting. Does that make you a murderer?

TOM: Innocent people died and I pulled the trigger. I murdered them. That's worse than what happened at Abu Ghraib.

THERAPIST: (*quietly*) Really, you think it is worse?

TOM: Yes. In one case, people died, and in another they didn't. Both are bad, and both were caused by soldiers, but I killed people and they didn't.

THERAPIST: The outcomes are different—that is true. I'm curious if you think *how* it happened matters?

TOM: Huh?

THERAPIST: Does it matter what the soldiers' intentions were in those situations, regardless of the outcome?

TOM: No. The bottom line is killing versus no killing.

THERAPIST: (*realizing that there was minimal flexibility at this point*) I agree that there is no changing the fact that the woman and child died, and that your shooting had something to do with that. However, I think we might slightly disagree on the use of the term "murder." It is clear that their deaths have been a very difficult thing for you to accept, and that you are trying to make sense of that. The sense that you appear to have made of their deaths is that you are a "murderer." I think this is a good example of one of those stuck points that seem to have prevented you from recovering from this traumatic event. We'll definitely be spending more time together on understanding your role in their deaths.

In addition to testing Tom's cognitive flexibility, the therapist also wanted to plant the seeds of a different interpretation of the event. She was careful not to push too far and retreated when it was clear that Tom was not amenable to an alternative interpretation at this point in the therapy. He was already defensive and somewhat angry, and she did not want to exacerbate his defensiveness or possibly contribute to dropout from the therapy.

From there, the therapist described how important it was to be able to label emotions and to begin to identify what Tom was saying to himself. The therapist and Tom discussed how different interpretations of events can lead to very different emotional reactions. They generated several examples of how changes in thoughts result in different feelings. The therapist also reminded Tom that some interpretations and reactions follow naturally from situations and do not need to be altered. For example, Tom indicated that he was saddened by the death of the family; the therapist did not challenge that statement. She encouraged Tom to feel his sadness and to let it run its course. He recognized that he had lost something, and it was perfectly natural to feel sad as a result. At this point Tom responded, "I don't like to feel sad. In fact, I don't like to feel at all. I'm afraid I'll go crazy." The therapist gently challenged this belief. "Have you ever allowed yourself to feel sad?" Tom responded that he worked very hard to avoid any and all feelings. The therapist encouraged Tom, "Well, given that you don't have much experience with feeling your feelings, we don't *know* that you're going to go crazy if you feel your feelings, right?" She also asked him whether he had noticed anyone in his life who had felt sad and had not gone crazy. He laughed. The therapist added, "Not feeling your feelings hasn't been working for you so far. This is your opportunity to experiment with feeling these very natural feelings about the traumatic event to see whether it can help you recover now from what has happened."

Tom was given a number of A-B-C Sheets as practice assignments to begin to identify what he was telling himself and his resulting emotions. In the first column, under A, "Something happens," Tom was instructed to write down an event. Under the middle column, B, "I tell myself something," he was asked to record his thoughts about the event. Under column C, "I feel and/ or do something," Tom was asked to write down his behavioral and emotional responses to the event. The therapist pointed out that if Tom says something to himself a lot, it becomes automatic. After a while, he does not need to think the thought consciously, he can go straight to the feeling. It is important to stop and recognize automatic thoughts to decide whether they either make sense or should be challenged and changed.

Session 3

Tom handed the therapist his practice assignments as soon as he arrived. The therapist went over the individual A-B-C Sheets Tom had completed and emphasized that he had done a good job in identifying his feelings and recognizing his thoughts. Some of this work is shown in Figure 2.1.

The purpose of reviewing this work at this point in the therapy is to identify thoughts and feelings, not to heavily challenge the content of those thoughts. The therapist did a minor correction of Tom's identification of the thought "I feel like I'm a bad person" (bolded in Figure 2.1) as a feeling. She commented that feelings are almost always one word and what you feel in your "gut," and that adding the stem "I feel . . . " does not necessarily make it a feeling. The therapist noticed the pattern of thoughts that Tom tended to record (i.e., internalizing and self-blaming), as well as the characteristic emotions he reported.

The therapist noted the themes of assimilation that again emerged (i.e., self-blame) and chose to focus on mildly challenging these related thoughts. She specifically chose to focus on Tom's thoughts and feelings related to his wife's pregnancy, which ultimately seemed to be related to his assimilation of the traumatic event.

THERAPIST: You don't think you deserve to have a family? Can you say more about that?

TOM: Why should I get to have a family when I took someone else's away?

THERAPIST: OK, so it sounds like this relates to the first thought that you wrote down on the A-B-C Sheet about being a murderer. When you say to yourself, "I took someone else's family away," how do you feel?

TOM: I feel bad.

THERAPIST: Let's see if we can be a bit more precise. What brand of bad do you feel? Remember how we talked about the primary colors of emotion? Which of those might you feel?

TOM: I feel so angry at myself for doing what I did.

THERAPIST: OK. Let's write that down—anger at self. So, I'm curious, Tom, do the other people you've told about this situation, or who were there at the time, think what you did was wrong?

TOM: No, but they weren't the ones who did it, and they don't care about the Iraqi people like I do.

ACTIVATING EVENT A "Something happens"	BELIEF B "I tell myself something"	CONSEQUENCE C "I feel something"
I killed an innocent family.	"I am a murderer."	**I feel like I'm a bad person.** Avoid talking about it.
My wife is pregnant.	"I don't deserve to have a family."	Guilty
Abu Ghraib	"The government sucks."	Angry
Going to therapy	"I'm weak. I shouldn't have PTSD. PTSD is only for the weak."	Angry

Are my thoughts in B *realistic*?

Yes.

What can you tell yourself on such occasions in the future?

?

FIGURE 2.1. A-B-C Sheet.

THERAPIST: Hmm . . . that makes me think about something, Tom. In the combat zone in which you were involved in Iraq, how easy was it to determine who you were fighting?

TOM: Not always particularly easy. There were lots of insurgents who looked like everyday people.

THERAPIST: Like civilians? *Innocent* civilians? (*pause*)

TOM: I see where you are going. I feel like it is still wrong because they died.

THERAPIST: I believe you when you say that it *feels* that way. However, feeling a certain way doesn't necessarily mean that it is based on the facts or the truth. We're going to work together on seeing whether that feeling of guilt or wrongdoing makes sense when we look at the situation very carefully in our work together.

Because the goal is for Tom to challenge and dismantle his own beliefs, the therapist probed and planted seeds for alternative interpretations of the traumatic event but did not pursue the matter too far. Although Tom did move some from his extreme stance within the session, the therapist was not expecting any dramatic changes. She focused mostly on helping Tom get the connections among thoughts, feelings, and behaviors, and developing a collaborative relationship in which cognitive interventions could be successfully delivered.

The therapist praised Tom for his ability to recognize and label thoughts and feelings, and said that she wanted Tom to attend to both during the next assignment, which was writing about the index traumatic event. Tom was asked to write as his practice assignment a detailed account of the event, and to include as many sensory details as possible. He was asked to include his thoughts and feelings during the event. He was instructed to start as soon as possible on the assignment, preferably that day, and to pick a time and place where he would have privacy and could allow himself to experience his natural emotions. Wherever he had to stop writing his account of the event, he was asked to draw a line. (The place where the client stops is often the location of a stuck point in the event, where the client gave up fighting, where something particularly heinous occurred, etc.) Tom was also instructed to read the account to himself every day until his next session. The therapist predicted that Tom would want to avoid writing the account and procrastinate until as late as possible. She asked Tom why it would be important for him to do the assignment and do it as soon as possible.

This was a technique to determine how much Tom was able to recount the rationale for the therapy, and to strengthen his resolve to overcome avoidance. Tom responded that he needed to stop avoiding, or he would remain scared of his memory. The therapist added that the assignment was to help Tom get his full memory back, to feel his emotions about it, and for therapist and client to begin to look for stuck points. She also reassured Tom that although doing so could be difficult for a relatively brief period of time, it would not continue to be so intense, and he would soon be over the hardest part of the therapy.

Session 4

During the settling-in portion of the session, Tom indicated that he had written the account of the event the evening before, although he had thought about and dreaded it every day prior to that. He admitted that he had been avoidant due to his anxiety. The therapist asked Tom to read his account aloud to her. Before starting, Tom asked why it was important to read it in the session. The therapist reminded Tom of what they had talked about the previous session, and added that the act of reading aloud would help him to access the whole memory and his feelings about it. Tom read what he wrote quickly, like a police report, and without much feeling:

There were several of us who were assigned to guard a checkpoint south of Baghdad. We were there because insurgents were beginning to take over the particular area, and we were there to contain the area. I was placed on top of the checkpoint. It was dusk. It had been a fairly routine day, with people coming through the checkpoint like they were going through a toll booth. Off in the distance I noticed a small, dark car that was going faster than most cars. I could tell it was going faster because there was more sand smoke kicking up behind it. Men out in front of the checkpoint were motioning for the car to slow down, but it didn't seem to be slowing down. Someone shot into the air to warn them, but they kept on coming. I could see two heads in the car coming toward us. We had been told to shoot at any vehicle that came within 25 yards of the gate to protect those around the gate, and the area beyond the gate. The car kept coming. I shot a bunch of rounds at the car.

At least one other person shot, too. There was so much chaos after that. I remember feeling my gun in my hand as I stood there. After a few moments, I also remember my legs carrying me down to the car. I don't really remember how I got there, but I did. Several men had surrounded the car, and a man got out of it. The man was crying. No, sobbing. He was speaking fast while he cried. He turned toward the car, resisting the men who attempted to remove him from the scene. I turned to see what the man was looking at and saw them for the first time. I saw the woman first.

There was blood everywhere, and her face had been shot. Then I saw the little girl in the backseat slumped over, holding a doll. There was blood all over her, too. I saw the gunshots through the car. I looked back at the woman, but avoided looking at her face. I saw a bump under her dress. She was pregnant.

I don't remember much else after that. I know I went back to camp and basically fell apart. They took me off duty for a couple of days, but eventually they sent me back to the Forward Operating Base because I was such a mess.

After reading the account, Tom quickly placed it in his binder of materials and closed the binder as if to indicate that he was ready to move onto something else. The therapist asked Tom what he was feeling, and he indicated that he was feeling "nothing." The therapist followed up, saying, "Nothing at all?" Tom reluctantly admitted that he was feeling anxious. The therapist then asked him to read the account again, but this time to slow down his reading rate, and allow himself to experience the emotions he had felt at the time of the event.

After reading the account for the second time, the therapist sought to flush out details of the event that Tom had "glossed over" and to focus on what appeared to be the most difficult aspects of the situation.

THERAPIST: What part of what you just read to me is the most difficult?

TOM: It is all difficult. The whole thing is horrible.

THERAPIST: What is the worst of it, though?

TOM: I guess the worst of it is seeing that small girl in the backseat of the car.

THERAPIST: What did she look like when you saw her?

(Tom describes his memory of the girl when he arrived at the car.)

THERAPIST: What are you feeling right now?

TOM: I feel sick to my stomach. I feel like I did at the time—that I want to throw up. I am also disgusted and sad. I killed an innocent child. There are so many things I could have done differently not to have taken her life.

(The therapist is aware of the assimilation process in Tom's use of hindsight bias. She stores that information away for future reference because she wants to make sure that Tom is feeling strongly as many of his natural emotions as possible about the traumatic event.)

THERAPIST: Continue to feel those feelings. Don't run away from them. Anything else that you're feeling?

TOM: I feel mad at myself and guilty.

THERAPIST: Were you feeling mad at yourself and guilty at the time?

TOM: No. I was horrified.

THERAPIST: OK, let's stay with that feeling.

TOM: *(Pauses.)* I don't want to feel this anymore.

THERAPIST: I know you don't want to feel this anymore. You're doing a great job of not avoiding your feelings here. In order to not feel like this for a long time, you need to feel these absolutely natural feelings. Let them run their course. They'll decrease if you stay with them.

After a period in which Tom experienced his feelings related to the situation and allowed them to dissipate, a discussion ensued regarding how hurtful it was to Tom to hear other people's reaction to the war. He expressed specific frustration with the presidential administration and its policy on the war. The therapist gently redirected Tom's more philosophical discussion of international policy to the effects of the trauma on him. Tom then told a story of how he had shared his traumatic experience with a high school friend. He felt that this person had a negative reaction to him as a result of sharing the story. Tom felt judged and unsupported by this friend. Since this experience with his friend, Tom had refrained from telling others about his combat experience. Using Socratic questioning, the therapist asked Tom if there might be any reason, outside of his actions, that someone might have a negative reaction to hearing about the shooting. Through this exchange, Tom was able to recognize that when others hear about traumatic events, they also are trying to make sense of these experiences in light of their existing belief systems. In other words, others around him might fall prey to the "just world" belief that bad things only happen to bad people. They also might not take into account the entire context in which Tom shot the passengers in the car. This recognition resulted in Tom feeling less angry at his friend for this perceived judgment. He was also somewhat willing to admit that his interpretation of his friend's reaction might have been skewed by his own judgment of himself. In fact, later in the therapy, when Tom was able to ask his friend directly about the perceived reaction, the friend indicated that it had been hard for him to hear, but that he had not been judging Tom at all. In actuality, he was thinking about the terrible predicament Tom had endured at the time.

The therapist asked Tom what stuck points he had identified in writing and reading his account. The following dialogue then occurred:

TOM: I'm not sure what the stuck points are, but from what you've been asking me, I guess you question whether or not I murdered this family.

THERAPIST: That's true. I think it is worthwhile for us to discuss the differences between blame and responsibility. Let's start with responsibility. From your account, it sounds like you were *responsible* for shooting the family. It sounds like other people may have been responsible, too, given that you were not the only person who shot at them.

(The therapist stores this fact in her mind to challenge Tom later about the appropriateness of his actions. This also provides a good opportunity to reinforce Tom for performing well in a stressful situation.)

The bottom line is that responsibility is about your behavior causing a certain outcome. *Blame* has to do with your intentionality to cause harm. It has to do with your motivations at the time. In this case, did you go into the situation with the motivation and intention to kill a family?

TOM: No, but the outcome was that they were murdered.

THERAPIST: Some *died*. From what you've shared, if we put ourselves back into the situation at the time, it was not at all your intention for them to die. They were coming down the road too fast, not responding to the very clear efforts to warn them to stop. Your own and others' intentions were to get them to stop at the checkpoint. Your intention at the time did not seem to be to kill them. In fact, wasn't your intention quite the opposite?

TOM: Yes. (*Begins to cry.*)

THERAPIST: (*Pauses until Tom's crying subsides somewhat.*) It doesn't seem that your intention was to *kill* them at all. Thus, the word "blame" is not appropriate. Murder or considering yourself a murderer does not seem accurate in this situation. The reason I've questioned the term "murder" or "murderer" all

along was because it doesn't seem like your intention was to have to shoot them.

TOM: But why do I feel like I am to blame?

THERAPIST: That's a good question. What's your best guess about why that is?

TOM: (*Still crying*) If someone dies, someone should take responsibility.

THERAPIST: Do you think it is possible to take responsibility without being to blame? What would be a better word for a situation that is your responsibility, but that you didn't intend to happen? If a person shot someone but didn't intend to do that, what would we call that?

TOM: An accident, I guess.

THERAPIST: That's right. In fact, what would you call shooting a person when you are trying to protect something or someone?

TOM: Self-defense.

THERAPIST: Yes, very good. Weren't you responsible for guarding the checkpoint?

TOM: Yeah.

THERAPIST: So, if you were responsible for guarding that checkpoint, and they continued through, wouldn't that have put the area at risk?

TOM: Yes, but it was a family—not insurgents.

THERAPIST: How did you know that at the time?

TOM: There was woman and child in the car.

THERAPIST: But, did you know that at the time?

TOM: No.

THERAPIST: So only in hindsight do you know that it was a family that *might* have had no bad intention. We actually don't know the family's intention, do we? They didn't heed the several warnings, right?

TOM: Yes. (*Pauses.*) I hadn't thought that they would be looking to do something bad with a woman and child in the car.

THERAPIST: We don't know, and won't ever know, bottom line. However, what we do know is what *you* knew at the time. What you knew at the time is that they did not heed the warnings, that you were responsible for securing the checkpoint, and that you took action when you needed to take action to protect the post. Thinking about those facts of what happened and what you knew at the time, how do you feel?

TOM: Hmm . . . I guess I'd feel less guilty.

THERAPIST: You'd feel less guilty, or you feel less guilty?

TOM: When I think through it, I do feel less guilty.

THERAPIST: There may be points when you start feeling guiltier again. It will be important for you to hold onto the facts of what happened versus going to your automatic interpretation that you've had for awhile now. Is there any part of it that makes you proud?

TOM: Proud?

THERAPIST: Yes. It seems like you did exactly what you were supposed to do in a stressful situation. Didn't you show courage under fire?

TOM: It's hard for me to consider my killing them as courageous.

THERAPIST: Sure. You haven't been thinking about it in this way for a long time, but it is something to consider.

The therapist's Socratic dialogue was designed to help Tom consider the entire context in which he was operating. She also began to plant the seed that Tom not only did nothing wrong but he also did what he was supposed to do to protect the checkpoint. Whenever possible, pointing out acts of heroism or courage can be powerful interventions with trauma survivors.

Prior to ending the session, the therapist checked Tom's emotional state to make sure he was calmer than he had been during the session. She also inquired about his reaction to the therapy session. He commented that it had been very difficult, but that he felt better than he expected in going into the "nitty-gritty" of what happened. He also noted that there were things he had not considered about the event that were "food for thought." The therapist praised Tom for doing a great job on the writing assignment and reinforced the importance of not quitting now. She commented that he had completed one of the hardest steps of the therapy, which would help him recover.

The therapist took the first account of the trauma and gave Tom his next practice assignment: to write the entire account again. The therapist asked Tom to add any details he might have left out of the first account and to provide even more sensory details. She also asked him to record any thoughts and feelings he was having in the here-and-now in parentheses, along with his thoughts and feelings at the time of the event.

Session 5

Tom arrived at Session 5 looking brighter and making more eye contact with the therapist. He indicated that he had written the account again, right after the previous session. He commented that the writing was hard, but not as hard as the first time. The therapist used this as an opportunity to reinforce how natural emotions resolve *naturally* as they are allowed expression. Tom noted that he had talked with his wife more this week, avoiding her less. Their increased communication allowed Tom's wife to express her concerns about Tom's well-being. She shared that he seemed disinterested in her and in their unborn child. Tom had previously told his wife about the incident, but he had not shared the specific detail that the woman in the vehicle was pregnant. Tom perceived his wife as having a very good reaction to his disclosure about the pregnant woman. He noted that she asked him questions, and that her comments indicated that she did not blame him for his actions. For example, she asked, "How could you have known at the time that it was a family?" She also reportedly said, "It's hard to know with terrorism if they were actually just a family traveling." Tom laughed when he reported that their conversation sounded like his last psychotherapy session.

The therapist asked Tom to read his second account out loud, with as many emotions as possible. Tom had written more about the event, and the therapist noted that he had included more information about what he and the other guards had done to warn the passengers in the car to slow down for the checkpoint. Tom read the second account more slowly and was not as tense as he had been the first time he read aloud. Tom's second account included much more detail and focused more on the vehicle and its occupants after he had fired upon them.

THERAPIST: I notice that you wrote more about the car and the family. What are you feeling about that right now?

TOM: I feel sad.

THERAPIST: Do you feel as sad as you felt the first time you wrote about it?

TOM: I think I may feel sadder about it now.

THERAPIST: Hmm . . . Why do you think that might be?

TOM: I think it's like what I wrote in the parenthesis about what I'm thinking now. Now, instead of feeling so much guilt that I shot them, I think it's sad that they didn't heed the warnings.

THERAPIST: You mentioned that you're feeling less guilt now. Why is that?

TOM: I'm beginning to realize that I was not the only one there that was trying to stop them. Several of us were trying to get them to stop. There is still some guilt that *I* was the one who shot them.

THERAPIST: If one of the other guards had shot them, would you blame him or her for the shooting? Would you expect him or her to feel guilty for their behavior?

TOM: (*Laughs.*) I started thinking about that this week. It made me wonder if it was really me who even shot them. As I was writing and thinking about it more, I realized that there is a possibility that another of the guards may have been shooting at the same time.

THERAPIST: What would it mean if he or she was shooting at the same time?

TOM: If he was shooting at the same time, it means that he thought that shooting at them might be the right thing to do in that situation.

THERAPIST: *Might* have been the right thing to do?

TOM: (*smiling*) Yeah, I still have questions that we might have been able to do something else.

THERAPIST: It seems like you're still trying to "undo" what happened. I'm curious, what else could you have done?

TOM: Not have shot at them.

THERAPIST: Then what would have happened?

TOM: They might have stopped. (*Pauses.*) Or I guess they could have gone through the checkpoint and hurt other people past the checkpoint. I guess they could have also been equipped with a car bomb that could have hurt many other people. That seems hard to believe, though, because of the woman and child in the car.

THERAPIST: It is impossible for us to know their intentions, as we discussed before. The bottom line is that you've tended to assume that doing something different, or doing nothing, would have led to a better outcome.

TOM: That is true. I still feel sad.

THERAPIST: Sure you do—that's natural. I take it as a good sign that you feel sad. Sadness seems like a very natural and appropriate reaction to what happened— much more consistent with what happened than the guilt and self-blame that you've been experiencing.

Tom and the therapist discussed how the goal of the therapy was not to forget what had happened, but to have the memory without all of the anxiety, guilt, and other negative emotions attached to it. Tom indicated that he was becoming less afraid and more able to tolerate his feelings, even when they were intense. Tom acknowledged that reading his account, talking about his trauma, and coming to psychotherapy sessions were becoming easier and that his negative feelings were beginning to diminish.

After discussing Tom's reactions to his memories, with a focus on how he had attempted to assimilate the memory into his existing beliefs, the therapist began to discuss areas of overaccommodation. One area of overaccommodation was Tom's beliefs about the U.S. military. He had entered the service with a very positive view of the military. Tom had a family history of military service and believed in service to country and the "rightfulness" of the military.

Subsequent to his traumatic event and military service in Iraq, he developed a negative view of the military that had extended to the Federal government in general. The therapist used this content to introduce the first series of tools to help challenge Tom's stuck points. She also emphasized how he would gradually be taking over as his own therapist, capable of challenging his own patterns of thinking that kept him "stuck."

THERAPIST: It seems that you have some very strong beliefs about the military and the U.S. government since your service. I'd like to use those beliefs to introduce some new material that will be helpful to you in starting to challenge stuck points on your own. You've done an outstanding job of considering the way that you think and feel about things. You've been very open to considering alternative interpretations of things. Starting in this session, I'm going to help you to become your own therapist and to attack your own stuck points directly.

TOM: OK.

THERAPIST: Today we will cover the first set of skills. We're going to be building your skills over the next few sessions. The first tool is a sheet called the Challenging Questions Sheet. Our first step is to identify a single belief you have that may be a stuck point.

As I mentioned before, I'd like us to use your beliefs about the Federal government now. So, if you were to boil down what you believe about the Federal government or the military, what is it?

TOM: I don't know. I'm not sure. I guess I'd say that the U.S. military is extremely corrupt.

THERAPIST: Good. That is very clear and to the point. So let's go over these questions and answer them as they relate to this belief. The first question you ask yourself is, "What's the evidence for and against this idea?"

TOM: The evidence for this is Abu Ghraib. Can you believe that they would do that? I would have also put my own shooting under the "for" list, but I'm beginning to question that.

THERAPIST: What other evidence is there of corruption?

TOM: Oh, and these defense contractors . . . what a scam! That leads me to the current administration and its vested interests in going to war to make money on defense contracting. And, oh, of course, to make money on the oil coming out of these countries!

THERAPIST: OK. Sounds like you have some "for" evidence. What about the "against" evidence?

TOM: Well, some of my fellow soldiers were very good. They were very committed in their service and to the mission. I also had mostly good leaders, although some of them were real pigs. Some were really power-hungry a—holes, frankly.

THERAPIST: So, it sounds like you have some pros and cons that support your belief that the U.S. military is completely corrupt. In the process of changing, it is not uncommon to have thoughts on both sides. That is great news! It means that you are considering different alternatives, and are not "stuck" on one way of seeing things. Let's take the next one. . . .

The therapist spent the balance of the session going over the list of questions to make sure that Tom understood them. Although most of the questions focused on the issue of corruption in the military, other issues were also brought in to illustrate the meaning of the questions. For example, the therapist introduced the probability questions with the example from Tom's life in which he believed that he was going to be shot by an insurgent sniper while back home. These questions are best illustrated with regard to issues of safety. The

therapist pointed out that perhaps not all of the questions applied to the belief on which Tom was working. The question "Are you thinking in all-or-none terms?" seemed to resonate with Tom the most because it applied to his belief about the military. He commented that he was applying a few examples of what seemed to be corruption to the entire military. Tom also indicated that his description of the military as "extremely" corrupt was consistent with the question "Are you using words or phrases that are extreme or exaggerated?" Indicative of his grasp of the worksheet, Tom also noticed that the question "Are you taking selected examples out of context?" applied to his prior view of his behavior as a murder in the traumatic event.

For his practice assignment prior to Session 6, Tom agreed to complete one Challenging Questions Sheet each day. He and the therapist brainstormed about potential stuck points prior to the end of the session to facilitate practice assignment completion. These stuck points included "I don't deserve to have a family," "I murdered an innocent family," and "I am weak because I have PTSD."

Session 6

Tom completed Challenging Questions Sheets about all of the stuck points he and the therapist had generated. The therapist reviewed these worksheets to determine whether Tom had used the questions as designed. She asked Tom which of the worksheets he had found *least* helpful. He responded that he had had the most difficulty completing the sheet about deserving to have a family. The therapist then reviewed this sheet in detail with Tom (see Figure 2.2).

THERAPIST: So, I notice that in your answer about the evidence for and against this idea about deserving a family, you included as evidence that you took some other man's family. I'm glad to see that you didn't include the word "murder"—that's progress. But, how is that evidence for *you* not deserving a family?

TOM: It is evidence because I feel like I took someone else's; therefore, I don't deserve one for myself. It seems fair.

THERAPIST: Remind me to make sure and look what you put for item 9 about confusing feelings and facts. For now, though, help me understand the math of why you don't deserve your family, and your happiness about your family, because of what happened?

Challenging Questions Sheet

Below is a list of questions to be used in helping you challenge your maladaptive or problematic beliefs. Not all questions will be appropriate for the belief you choose to challenge. Answer as many questions as you can for the belief you have chosen to challenge below.

Belief: _I don't deserve to have a family._

1. What is the evidence for and against this idea?
   FOR: *I took some other man's family.*

   AGAINST: *I didn't want to have to shoot anyone. An "eye for an eye" does not apply here.*

2. Is your belief a habit or based on facts?
   It is a habit for me to think this way. The facts are that I didn't do something wrong to deserve to be punished in this way.

3. Are your interpretations of the situation too far removed from reality to be accurate?
   My interpretation of the original situation has been fairly unrealistic, which is where I get this belief.

4. Are you thinking in all-or-none terms?
   N/A

5. Are you using words or phrases that are extreme or exaggerated? (i.e., always, forever, never, need, should, must, can't, and every time)
   I guess maybe "deserve" could be an extreme word.

6. Are you taking the situation out of context and only focusing on one aspect of the event?
   Yes, like #3, I tend to forget what all was going on at the time of my shooting.

7. Is the source of information reliable?
   No, I'm not very reliable these days.

8. Are you confusing a low probability with a high probability?
   N/A

9. Are your judgments based on feelings rather than facts?
   I'm feeling guilty like I did something wrong when the truth is that I did what I was supposed to do.

10. Are you focused on irrelevant factors?
    Maybe my deserving a family has nothing to do with someone else losing theirs?

FIGURE 2.2. Challenging Questions Sheet.

TOM: I don't know—it just seems fair.

THERAPIST: Fair? That implies that you did something bad that requires you to be punished.

TOM: As I've been thinking about it more, I don't think I did something wrong when I really look at it, but it still *feels* like I did something wrong and that I shouldn't have something good like a wife and child in my life.

THERAPIST: Maybe we should look at your response to item 9 now. What did you put in response to the question "Are your judgments based on feelings rather than facts?"

TOM: I wrote, "I'm feeling guilty, like I did something wrong when the truth is that I did what I was supposed to do." I try to remember what we talked about, and what my wife also has said to me about them not responding to the warnings and my shooting them, which may have prevented something else that was bad. I still feel bad—not as bad as I did—but I still feel like I did something wrong.

(The therapist uses this as an opportunity to talk about the need for practicing new alternative thoughts in order to elicit emotional change.)

THERAPIST: You are well on your way, Tom, to getting unstuck and recovering. Your head is starting to get it, and your feelings need to catch up. You've been thinking about what happened and what you did in a certain way for awhile now. You blamed yourself over and over and over again, telling yourself that you did something wrong. You gave yourself a steady diet of that type of thinking, which resulted in you feeling guilty about what happened. It is like a well-worn rut of thinking in your brain that automatically leads you down the path of feeling guilty. What you need to do now is start a new road of more realistic and truthful thinking about the situation that will eventually be a well-worn path. What is the more realistic view of your role in this event?

TOM: *(tearfully)* I had to shoot at the car, and people died.

THERAPIST: That's right. And, let's pretend for a second that you really do believe that thought. If so, what would you feel?

TOM: I'd feel so much lighter. I wouldn't feel guilty. I'd continue to feel sad about this horrible situation, but I wouldn't blame myself.

THERAPIST: Let's take it the next step. If you didn't blame yourself and feel guilty, then would you believe that you deserve to be happy with your wife and the baby that will soon be here?

TOM: Sure.

THERAPIST: So, Tom, your work is to practice, practice, practice this new and more accurate way of looking at what happened and your role in it. With practice, your feelings will start matching the truth about what happened and the fact that you are not to blame.

TOM: It is kind of like training to use a weapon. They made us do certain things with our guns over and over again, until it was automatic. It was very automatic after a while.

THERAPIST: That's right. There are other questions on this sheet that might be helpful in convincing you of the truth about this in your practice. What did you put for the question "Is your belief a habit or based on a fact?"

This dialogue illustrates a common occurrence at this stage in the therapy. Tom was starting to experience cognitive change, but his emotional change was lagging. The therapist reinforced the need to practice the new ways of thinking to feel different. It is also important to highlight clients' gains in changing their thinking, even if their feelings have not changed or are ambivalent. A change in thinking is framed as more than halfway to a change in feeling. In effect, changed thinking involves competing thoughts or learning, and with more repetitions of the new thought, the associated feelings follow and eventually win out.

In the latter portion of this session the therapist introduced the Patterns of Problematic Thinking Sheet and provided an explanation of how this list was different from the Challenging Questions Sheet (see Figure 2.3). More specifically, she indicated that the Patterns of Problematic Thinking Sheet pertains to more general patterns of thinking versus challenging individual thoughts that Tom might have. The Patterns of Problematic Thinking Sheet lists seven types of faulty thinking patterns (e.g., oversimplifying, overgeneralizing, emotional reasoning).

Tom and the therapist went through the list and generated examples for each of the patterns. For example, for "Disregarding important aspects of a situation," the therapist pointed out something that Tom had brought up several times during therapy. Initially Tom had not included the important information that he and the other guards had attempted to stop the car before shooting at it. She also pointed out that emotional reasoning was similar to confusing a feeling with a fact, which had been a primary focus of the session.

When they got to the item "Overgeneralizing from a single incident," Tom said that he had noticed he was beginning to change his thoughts about the government and its leaders. He commented that it had been very powerful for him to consider that, in a number of instances, his fellow soldiers had operated with integrity and were committed to the mission, and to the safety and protection of others. Tom said spontaneously, "I guess that is also kind of like drawing conclusions when evidence is lacking or even contradictory." He said that he had started stereotyping after the traumatic event—applying negative attributes and opinions to everyone in the military and the government too broadly. Tom and the therapist discussed how the goal of the therapy was to have a balanced and realistic view of things versus the overly ideal version he had pretrauma or the overly pessimistic version he had posttrauma. In other words, the goal was to find shades of gray and balance in his thinking about the government, the military, and their leadership. Tom added an example of this thinking: "There are at least some people in government who want to do good for others."

Tom was given the practice assignment to read over the list in the Patterns of Problematic Thinking Sheet and to note examples of times he used each of the problematic thinking patterns.

Session 7

Tom began the session by stating that he was feeling better, and that his wife had also noted a difference in him and was feeling less concerned about the therapy making him worse rather than better. The therapist had given Tom the PCL and the BDI-II to complete while he was waiting for his appointment. She quickly scored these assessment measures and gave Tom feedback

Patterns of Problematic Thinking

Listed below are several types of patterns of problematic thinking that people use in different life situations. These patterns often become automatic, habitual thoughts that cause us to engage in self-defeating behavior. Considering your own stuck points, find examples for each of these patterns. Write in the stuck point under the appropriate pattern and describe how it fits that pattern. Think about how that pattern affects you.

1. **Jumping to conclusions** when the evidence is lacking or even contradictory.
   I tend to jump to the conclusion that I have done something wrong when bad things happen. I assume things are my fault.

2. **Exaggerating or minimizing** a situation (blowing things way out of proportion or shrinking their importance inappropriately).
   I minimize the things that I have done well in the military.

3. **Disregarding important aspects** of a situation.
   In the past I have tended to neglect the important aspect that several of us tried to stop the car from going through the checkpoint.

4. **Oversimplifying** things as good–bad or right–wrong.
   I can sometimes think of all Iraqis as all bad.

5. **Overgeneralizing** from a single incident (a negative event is seen as a never-ending pattern).
   I have assumed that because of my traumatic event, I could not be safe with my baby to be born.

6. **Mind reading** (you assume people are thinking negatively of you when there is no definite evidence for this).
   I assume that everyone thinks I am a terrible person, a murderer, because of what I did.

7. **Emotional reasoning** (you have a feeling and assume there must be a reason).
   This one is easy—I feel guilty, and therefore I must be.

FIGURE 2.3. Patterns of Problematic Thinking Sheet.

about his scores at the beginning of this session. His PCL score had decreased from 68 to 39, which was a clear and clinically meaningful change in his PTSD symptomatology. She noticed that his avoidance and reexperiencing symptoms had decreased the most; his hyperarousal symptoms had also decreased, but less so. His score on the BDI-II had decreased from 28 to 14, clearly indicating a reduction in his depressive symptoms.

The therapist asked whether Tom had completed his practice assignment, the Patterns of Problematic Thinking Sheet. He indicated that he had not, but that he had thought about it over the week. He also laughed and said that he had noticed the thinking patterns in his wife and others. The therapist asked Tom to complete some of the sheet in session. At this point in therapy, the therapist was sitting back more as Tom took on the role of challenging his own cognitions. The therapist provided both minimal clarification and additional examples that she had noticed in working with Tom.

In this session, the therapist introduced the Challenging Beliefs Worksheet. She was careful to point out that the worksheet integrated all of the previous work Tom had done and added a few new elements. The following dialogue illustrates the introduction of this sheet (see Figure 2.4).

THERAPIST: I want to show you the final worksheet that we're going to be using for the rest of the therapy.

TOM: OK. Wow—that looks complicated!

THERAPIST: Actually, you've done pretty much everything on this worksheet already. This worksheet brings together into one place everything that we've been working on.

TOM: I'll take your word for it, Doc.

THERAPIST: Remember the A-B-C Sheets from way back when?

TOM: Yes.

THERAPIST: (*pointing to first three columns on the Challenging Beliefs Worksheet*) This is A, B, and C. You have in column A the situation, or "Activating Event" that you had on the A-B-C Sheet. In column B you have "Automatic Thoughts," which is the "Belief" portion of the A-B-C Sheet. Last, column C, "Emotions," is the "Consequence" portion of the A-B-C Sheet.

TOM: OK. So far, so good.

THERAPIST: Column D is where you identify the "Challenging Questions" from that sheet that apply to the thought or stuck point that you're working on. In column E, you identify the type of "Patterns of Problematic Thinking" that apply to the thought or stuck point that you're working on. Make sense?

TOM: Yes.

THERAPIST: So, only column F, "Alternative Thought," is new. Here you identify alternative thoughts that you could have about the situation. In other words, we're looking for alternative statements that you can tell yourself or different interpretations of the event. In columns G and H, you get to see how your belief in your original thoughts may change and how the new thoughts affect your feelings.

TOM: OK.

THERAPIST: So, let's pick a stuck point and start using this Challenging Beliefs Worksheet. We're going to be talking about safety as one of the first topics of the next few sessions. Can you think of a stuck point that relates to your ability to keep yourself safe or to how safe others are around you?

TOM: Well, I still wonder if there are people out in the world who want to hurt me, even if I now realize that no sniper is going to take me out.

THERAPIST: So, let's pick a specific event—the more specific, the better.

TOM: I was in the grocery store, and I had my uniform on. There was this guy who seemed to have a chip on his shoulder about it—like he hated me or something.

THERAPIST: So, write down the event in Column A. (*Pauses.*) What was your thought? You've already mentioned one of them.

TOM: This guy has a chip on his shoulder about me because I'm in the military.

THERAPIST: Good. How strongly do you believe that thought?

TOM: 100%.

THERAPIST: OK, let's write that next to the thought. We are now rating how much you believe in your thoughts because you're going to see at the end how much your thought has changed. What feeling or feelings are associated with that thought?

TOM: Definitely anger.

A. Situation	B. Thoughts	D. Challenging Thoughts	E. Problematic Patterns	F. Alternative Thought
Describe the event, thought, or belief leading to the unpleasant emotion(s).	Write thought(s) related to Column A. Rate belief in each thought below from 0–100%. (How much do you believe this thought?)	Use **Challenging Questions** to examine your automatic thoughts from Column B. Is the thought balanced and factual or extreme?	Use the **Problematic Thinking Patterns** sheet to decide if this is one of your problematic patterns of thinking.	What else can I say instead of Column B? How else can I interpret the event instead of Column B? Rate belief in alternative thought(s) from 0–100%.
	"This guy has a chip on his shoulder because I am in the military." (100%)	Evidence? **Habit or Fact?** *Habit to think everyone dislikes me because I was in Iraq.*	Jumping to conclusions	*"I don't know if he has a chip on his shoulder."* (60%)
		Interpretations not accurate?	Exaggerating or minimizing	*"If he does have a chip on his shoulder, I don't know what it is about – maybe it isn't even about me, let alone having served in Iraq."* (80%)
		All or none?	Disregarding important aspects	
		Extreme or exaggerated?	Oversimplifying	
At store in uniform		Out of context?	Overgeneralizing	
	C. Emotion(s)	**Source unreliable?** *Me*		**G. Rerate Old Thoughts**
	Specify sad, angry, etc., and rate how strongly you feel each emotion from 0–100%.	Low versus high probability?	**Mind reading** *I am assuming that he is thinking the worst of me.*	Rerate how much you now believe the thought in Column B from 0–100%. 35%
		Based on feelings or facts?	Emotional reasoning	**H. Emotion(s)**
	Anger (80%) *Fear (30%)*	Irrelevant factors?		Now what do you feel? 0–100% *Anger (20%)* *Fear (15%)*

FIGURE 2.4. Challenging Beliefs Worksheet completed in session.

THERAPIST: Makes sense, given your thought. How much anger from 0 to 100%, with 100% being as much anger as you could possibly imagine having?

TOM: Hmm . . . I'd say 80%.

THERAPIST: Any other feelings? You can have more than one.

TOM: I guess when I stop and think about it, there is some fear there, too.

THERAPIST: That makes sense, too. How much fear from 0 to 100%?

TOM: Oh, maybe 30%. It's not the strongest feeling, but it's there, because I'm wondering if he is going to say something or do something.

THERAPIST: Nice job. Let's move onto the next column that relates to the Challenging Questions Sheet you've already done. Take a look at this list. What questions might apply here?

TOM: I guess I might be confusing a habit with a fact. It seems like it is a habit for me to assume that everyone dislikes me because I was in Iraq. I really don't know if that is why he seemed to have a chip on his shoulder. I guess I also don't know for sure if he had a chip on his shoulder. He didn't say anything to me. (*Pauses.*) I guess that is also an example of the source of information being unreliable, and that source is me! (*Laughs.*)

THERAPIST: While you were talking, I was thinking that the same things applied. So you'd write those in this column. You can also pick out other challenging questions that might apply, but usually two or three will do the trick. In the next column, we're going to refer to the Patterns of Problematic Thinking Sheet. What might fit here?

TOM: I guess one jumps out—mind reading.

THERAPIST: How so?

TOM: I'm assuming that he is thinking the worst about me and about my having served my country in this war. I'm good at that.

THERAPIST: Write that down. You can add others later if something seems to apply. The next column is very important. This is where you start coaching yourself to come up with alternative thoughts or perceptions about the situation. Based on having asked yourself these questions and noticing the problematic thinking patterns, what other ways might you think about this situation?

TOM: I guess one thing I could say to myself is, "I don't know if he has chip on his shoulder." I could also say, "If he does have a chip on his shoulder, I don't know what it is about—maybe it isn't even about me, let alone about my having served in Iraq."

THERAPIST: Wow! You're doing great at this. Let's get those written down. Let's also add how much you believe those two new thoughts. Below those alternative thoughts is the column that asks you to reconsider how much you believe your original thoughts over here in column B. How much do you believe them after walking through this process? Before you said 100%.

TOM: Oh, I'd say now it is only about 35%.

THERAPIST: That is a big change. You went from 100% certainty to 35% certainty that he had a chip on his shoulder because you fought in the war.

TOM: I'm a little surprised by that myself.

THERAPIST: Let's take it the final step. How about your feelings now? Let's rerate those here.

TOM: My anger is way down—I'd say only about 20%. The anxiety is still there because I really wouldn't want to have to protect myself, and he might have had a chip on his shoulder at me. It is down a little, though, because I realize I'm not 100% certain he was out to get me. I'd say maybe 15% on fear.

THERAPIST: Do you have questions about what we just did here?

TOM: Not at the moment. I'll get back to you.

THERAPIST: I'm going to ask that you do one of these sheets on a stuck point per day until I see you again. I'm also going to give you some example sheets other patients have done that might be helpful to you.

TOM: OK. Should be interesting. . . .

The therapist reminded Tom that he might find he is not using problematic thinking, and in that case, no change in feelings would be expected. She also cautioned Tom that he should not expect his beliefs and feelings always to change completely in the process of doing the sheet. The old thought would need to be completely dismantled and the new thought would need to become more habitual for him to see a more permanent change. The therapist suggested that Tom read the sheets he completed over to himself a number of times to facilitate the process.

The Safety module was then introduced. Safety is the first of five modules (two- to three-page handouts) that also include Trust, Power/Control, Esteem, and Intimacy. The therapist oriented Tom to the format of the module, which included discussion about how beliefs about the self and others in this area can be disrupted or seemingly confirmed after a traumatic event, depending on one's history prior to the traumatic event. The modules describe how these problematic beliefs are manifested emotionally and behaviorally (e.g., not leaving one's home because of the belief that the world is unsafe). It also provides alternative self-statements that are more balanced and realistic in each area.

Tom had felt safe with others before the traumatic event occurred, and this sense of safety about others had been disrupted, as evidenced by his sense that others around him were out to get him. Pretrauma, Tom had also felt as though he was not a danger to others. Posttrauma, he believed that he could not be safe with others, which specifically manifested in his concerns about being around his pregnant wife. The therapist suggested that Tom complete at least one worksheet on his stuck points about others being safe, as well as his being a possible danger to others. The therapist also reminded Tom that he needed to finish the Patterns of Problematic Thinking Sheet assignment from last session.

Session 8

Tom arrived at the session having completed the Patterns of Problematic Thinking Sheet, as well as two Challenging Beliefs Worksheets. The therapist spent a little time looking at his answers to the Patterns of Problematic Thinking Sheet because she did not want to send the message inadvertently that completing the assignments was unimportant. She asked Tom to read the patterns that he had completed at home, as opposed to those in their previous session.

Tom completed two Challenging Beliefs Worksheets related to the topic of safety, as the therapist had instructed. He did one each on self and other safety beliefs. He did not seem to understand that he could use the Challenging Beliefs Worksheets on everyday events that were distressing or even positive for him. Thus, the therapist emphasized how Tom might use this process more generally in his day-to-day life, and highlighted how more practice would lead to more results. She noted that using the process on less emotionally distressing topics could actually be very helpful in getting the process down. It is always easier to learn something when one is not dealing with the most challenging circumstances. She used a military analogy with Tom about learning to load and shoot a gun—best learned in a nonconflict situation, so that it is a more rote behavior when under fire.

The therapist skimmed the two sheets Tom had completed and noticed that he had struggled most coming up with alternative statements about his own sense of dangerousness related to his wife's impending delivery of their child. The following dialogue ensued (see Figure 2.5):

THERAPIST: I notice that you might have had the most trouble coming up with alternative thoughts about how safe you can be with your wife and your child who is about to be born.

TOM: Yeah, I don't really like to talk about it. It freaks my wife out. I'm uncomfortable being around my wife, which makes her feel bad, but I'm just afraid I'm going to hurt her or the child.

THERAPIST: Let's take your first thought because it is kind of general. How is it that you think you're going to hurt them? Are we talking physically or mentally?

TOM: Oh, physically is what I mean. I don't know how exactly, but somehow, some way, I guess.

THERAPIST: That makes it a bit more concrete. How do you physically think you're going to hurt them? Do you think you'll shoot them, given your trauma history?

TOM: No. Absolutely not. There are no firearms in my house, and I don't go hunting or have friends or family who hunt—nothing that would make guns a part of our life.

THERAPIST: So, what have you considered in your mind?

TOM: I guess I'm worried that, out of nowhere, I'll get physically violent.

THERAPIST: OK, now we're cooking. Let's write that down. "Out of nowhere I'll get physically violent." I noticed that in column C you didn't mention anything about probabilities. Safety issues are almost always about gauging probabilities. The world is not a completely safe place, and every day we all make calculated risks about our safety based on the probability of bad things happening to us or to someone

A. Situation	B. Thoughts	C. Emotion(s)	D. Challenging Thoughts	E. Problematic Patterns	F. Alternative Thought
Describe the event, thought, or belief leading to the unpleasant emotion(s).	Write thought(s) related to Column A. Rate belief in each thought below from 0–100%. (How much do you believe this thought?)	Specify sad, angry, etc., and rate how strongly you feel each emotion from 0–100%.	Use **Challenging Questions** to examine your automatic thoughts from Column B. Is the thought balanced and factual or extreme?	Use the **Problematic Thinking Patterns** sheet to decide if this is one of your problematic patterns of thinking.	What else can I say instead of Column B? How else can I interpret the event instead of Column B? Rate belief in alternative thought(s) from 0–100%.
Being around my wife and child	*"Out of nowhere, I'll get physically violent."* (80%)		Evidence?	Jumping to conclusions	
			Habit or fact?		
			Interpretations not accurate?	**Exaggerating or minimizing** *I'm exaggerating the likelihood that I'd be violent.*	*"It is unlikely that I'll hurt my family, and even more unlikely that it will be sudden and unexpected."* (95%)
			All or none?	Disregarding important aspects	
			Extreme or exaggerated?	Oversimplifying	
		C. Emotion(s)	Out of context?		**G. Rerate Old Thoughts**
		Fear (85%)	Source unreliable?	**Overgeneralizing** *I'm assuming because I shot once in a certain situation, I'll be violent in general.*	Rerate how much you now believe the thought in Column B from 0–100%.
			Low versus high probability? *Given my history, it is actually a low probability not high.*		*10%*
			Based on feelings or facts?	Mind reading	**H. Emotion(s)**
					Now what do you feel? 0–100%
			Irrelevant factors?	Emotional reasoning	*Fear (< 10%)*

FIGURE 2.5. Challenging Beliefs Worksheet regarding safety.

else. How do you think the probability questions might apply?

TOM: Are you getting at the idea that I'm confusing a low probability with a high probability?

THERAPIST: Precisely. How do you think that applies here?

TOM: I'm convinced that "somehow, some way" I'm going to hurt my family, so I believe that it is a high probability that it will happen and not a low probability. I think you think that the probability I will do that is low. But, I'm still concerned about it.

THERAPIST: Let's talk about the actual probability. How often have you hurt your family physically?

TOM: Never. Are you kidding?

THERAPIST: I thought as much, but you made it sound like it was very likely to happen. I guess that's part of the problem, right?

TOM: You're right.

THERAPIST: How often have you been physically violent against anyone?

TOM: I haven't, besides the shooting. And it surely hasn't been unexpected. Now that we're talking through it, it feels a little silly.

THERAPIST: So, it sounds like figuring out the actual probability of this is right where we needed to go. Given what we've talked about, what is an alternative statement you can tell yourself and how much do you believe it?

TOM: It is unlikely that I'll hurt my family, and even more unlikely that it will be sudden and unexpected given that it has never happened.

THERAPIST: Let's keep going to see how that might change how you feel. You wrote that you had 85% fear. What is that rating now?

TOM: Less than 10%. There is some fear now that I know I am capable of hurting a family, but like we've talked about before—and what I have to remember—is that it occurred in a certain situation and not in my everyday life now as a civilian in my family.

This exchange between Tom and the therapist illustrates the hallmark role of probability in assessments and beliefs about safety. It is important to realize that there are some objectively unsafe situations or behaviors, and these should not be minimized or challenged. If there are unreasonable safety precautions or beliefs,

the actual probability of harm should be carefully evaluated, keeping in mind that 100% safety is rarely, if ever, guaranteed.

The therapist transitioned the session to introduce the Trust module. Tom noted that he had pretty good trust of himself and others prior to his best friend committing suicide when they were in high school. Tom said that after the experience, he sometimes did not trust his judgments about other people, and that he felt responsible for not anticipating his friend's suicide. The military traumatic event served to confirm his belief that he could not trust his judgments about others' intentions. Tom's concerns about his ability to be safe with his wife and unborn child also dovetailed with the issue of trust. The therapist and Tom went over the information in the Trust module handout, and Tom seemed to resonate with all of the potential effects. He reported that he had really been trying to open up with his wife and not avoid her. He noted that they were communicating more, which made both of them more relaxed and comfortable in the final days of her pregnancy.

The therapist closed the session by assigning daily Challenging Beliefs Worksheets, asking Tom to do at least one on the topic of trust. She reminded him that, like other areas, the goal is to develop balanced alternative thoughts. In the case of trust, she noted that stuck points about trust often revolve around making all-or-none judgments, either trusting or not. The goal is to consider trust as multidimensional, with different types of issues resulting in different levels of trust in different situations.

Session 9

Tom arrived at this session having completed a number of Challenging Beliefs Worksheets. Several of them were about trust, including his level of trust of the government and trust of himself in being a father. He had also used the worksheets on non-trust-related topics related to his daily life. He commented that the worksheets had been helpful in working out his thinking before he behaved impulsively or felt miserable.

The therapist praised Tom for completing the worksheets so well, and asked him whether he felt he could use assistance with any of the worksheets. Tom quickly responded that he wanted to focus on the sheet about fatherhood because he was experiencing so much anxiety about his child's impending birth. In turning their attention to this worksheet, the therapist immediately noticed that Tom had probably struggled with this worksheet because he had listed so many different types of thoughts that were fueling his anxiety about becoming a father. She used this as an opportunity to fine-tune Tom's use of the worksheets. The therapist's choice in thoughts to challenge first also illustrates the prioritization of treatment targets in the therapy. She chose to go after the more directly trauma-related thoughts that contained remnants of assimilation. Tom's thoughts about deserving to be happy about starting a family, given the death of the woman, fetus, and child, suggested that he had not fully accepted the traumatic event and the circumstances surrounding it. Thus, she addressed this thought first (see Figure 2.6).

THERAPIST: Wow, you've got lots of thoughts going on in your head about becoming a father, don't you? I'm going to suggest that we use a different worksheet for each of the clusters of thoughts you're having on this topic. I think that will make your use of the Challenging Beliefs Worksheet better. It seems that some thoughts are directly related to your traumatic experience, others are specifically related to your wife's labor and delivery, and still others are related more generally to being a parent. Let's focus on those that are directly related to your trauma. You wrote that one of your feelings was guilt (85%), and I'm assuming that it is related to your thought that it isn't right that you're happy with a soon-to-be-born baby given what happened.

TOM: That's right. If I'm really honest, I still feel guilty that the Iraqi woman was pregnant and getting ready to have a child, and the shooting deprived her of the ability to have that child and be happy, and I'm getting ready to have that happiness.

THERAPIST: We've talked about this before, but we've been more focused on the man involved in the situation.

TOM: Yeah, I think the closer my wife gets to delivery, the more I think about the Iraqi woman. I've been imagining that she wasn't part of a potential plot for terrorist activity and was more an innocent participant. Then, I go back and forth, thinking that she might have actually been involved and didn't care that she was pregnant. Or maybe it was just an accident, and they truly didn't understand that they needed to stop. Uggghhhh, it is exhausting.

THERAPIST: And we'll never know. If your friend were saying all of this to you, what would be your response to him?

TOM: I'd be telling him to quit beating himself up and feeling guilty.

THERAPIST: Easier said than done. Anything else? Maybe it would help to look at the Challenging Questions and Patterns of Problematic Thinking Sheets. I'm wondering if you are focusing on irrelevant factors—item 10 on the Challenging Questions Sheet.

TOM: Hmm . . . what is irrelevant in this case?

THERAPIST: How relevant are *her* intentions to deserving to be happy yourself about having a child?

TOM: (*Pauses.*) I'm going to have to think about that for a second.

THERAPIST: Aren't *your* intentions in that situation what is relevant? Were your intentions at that time to deprive her of the right to bear her child and live happily ever after?

TOM: No, not at all.

THERAPIST: So, why the guilt? What did you do wrong that you should be punished about?

TOM: Oh, wow. I hadn't thought of that. Her intentions are irrelevant. It only makes me crazy to try to get in her head. I guess that would be mind-reading, now wouldn't it?

THERAPIST: Very good—a different spin on mind-reading. So what is the alternative, more balanced and realistic thought?

TOM: My intentions are what matter. I didn't intend for her to lose her own or her baby's life.

THERAPIST: Go on . . . do you have a right to experience happiness?

TOM: I guess I do. It just feels weird.

THERAPIST: Sure—it feels different. It is different than what you've been thinking about it for awhile. I'm curious—what would you feel if you said to yourself, "I did not intentionally do anything to deprive someone else of family happiness. I deserve to be happy in becoming a father."

TOM: I'd feel less guilty for sure, and even happy.

THERAPIST: Let's get this all written down. Now you have the job of holding on to these new insights and practicing them. Read over this worksheet every day until you see me again. I'd also like you to take these other thoughts on your original Challenging Beliefs Worksheet about this topic and put them on separate worksheets and work through them. Can you commit to doing that?

A. Situation	B. Thoughts		C. Emotion(s)	D. Challenging Thoughts	E. Problematic Patterns	F. Alternative Thought
Describe the event, thought, or belief leading to the unpleasant emotion(s).	Write thought(s) related to Column A. Rate belief in each thought below from 0–100%. (How much do you believe this thought?)		Specify sad, angry, etc., and rate how strongly you feel each emotion from 0–100%.	Use **Challenging Questions** to examine your automatic thoughts from Column B. Is the thought balanced and factual or extreme?	Use the **Problematic Thinking Patterns** sheet to decide if this is one of your problematic patterns of thinking.	What else can I say instead of Column B? How else can I interpret the event instead of Column B? Rate belief in alternative thought(s) from 0–100%.
Killing a pregnant Iraqi woman and her son.	*"It isn't right that I'm happy with a baby on the way, given what happened."* *(80%)* *"She might not have been part of a terrorist plot, but just a passenger."* *(50%)*		*Guilt (85%)*	Evidence? Habit or fact? Interpretations not accurate? All or none? Extreme or exaggerated? Out of context? Source unreliable? Low versus high probability? Based on feelings or facts? **Irrelevant factors?** ***Her intentions are not relevant. Mine are.***	Jumping to conclusions Exaggerating or minimizing Disregarding important aspects Oversimplifying Overgeneralizing **Mind reading** *I'm trying to figure out what was in her head.* Emotional reasoning	*"My intentions are what matter. I didn't intend to do anything to deprive someone else of family happiness."* *(85%)*
					G. Rerate Old Thoughts	
				Rerate how much you now believe the thought in Column B from 0–100%.		
				15% *(2nd doesn't matter)*		
				H. Emotion(s)		
				Now what do you feel? 0–100%		
				Guilt (5%) *Happy (10%)*		

FIGURE 2.6. Challenging Beliefs Worksheet regarding trauma.

103

TOM: Yes, I already feel lighter.

THERAPIST: This is an exciting time—you've got to continue to work on this, so that you can have the enjoyment you deserve!

At this point, the therapist introduced the Power/Control module. Tom admitted that prior to the traumatic event, he was someone who liked to be in control. He did not like unpredictability, and he noticed that this tendency had gotten especially bad after his friend's suicide. The military lifestyle seemed to be congruent with this tendency. Tom indicated that he had not had authority issues prior to the traumatic event, but he had noticed himself questioning authority much more since his military trauma. As with previous sessions, Tom was given the practice assignment to complete Challenging Beliefs Worksheets every day prior to the next session, and at least one was assigned on power/control.

Session 10

Tom began the session by saying that his wife had gone to her obstetrician the previous day, and that her labor would be induced in 1 week if she did not naturally go into labor before then. Tom indicated that the last session had been very good in helping him to become happier about his child's impending birth, and that he had read the Challenging Questions Worksheet about deserving to be happy several times since the last session. He believed it more and more. He stated that he was still having some anxiety about becoming a father, and about everything going OK with his wife's labor and delivery. The therapist normalized some of Tom's anxiety, stressing how it was very natural for a first-time father, and Tom was able to recognize the typicality of this anxiety in others he had witnessed becoming parents.

Tom stated that since reading the Power/Control module after the last session, he had started to realize that not everyone in authority over him had wielded his/her authority malevolently. This was very important in light of Tom's preexisting history of desiring to exert control; he had directly confronted his illusion of control. The therapist and Tom went over this worksheet.

Tom went on to describe how his belief that he could and *should* have control over everything had resulted in low self-esteem. In general, when things did not go as he desired, Tom felt as though he was a failure for not controlling the outcome. This belief structure led

him to think that he should have been able to control his friend and stop him from committing suicide. It also led him to believe that he should have been able to create a positive outcome in the military traumatic event. This discussion served as a natural segue to the next topic—esteem. Tom admitted that he had become someone who thrived too much on accomplishment. This had affected his self-esteem and was especially relevant to his belief that he had not accomplished his goal in the military because he had to be taken from the field after the traumatic event at the checkpoint.

After reviewing the Esteem module, the therapist asked Tom to complete Challenging Beliefs Worksheets on his remaining stuck points, as well as any stuck points relating to esteem. He was also given two other assignments: to practice giving and receiving compliments every day, and to do one nice thing for himself every day that was not contingent on "achieving" something. These assignments were to help him with his self- and other-esteem.

Session 11

Tom completed a worksheet on self-esteem related to his belief that he had not achieved his goal within the military. The therapist and Tom went over this worksheet, and both noted that he had made significant progress by using the worksheet to change the way he thought and felt about himself. He asserted that he was beginning to see that people are much more than their professional accomplishments. They also have other activities and relationships with their families, friends, and themselves.

The therapist inquired about the assignment of giving and receiving compliments. Tom replied that it had gone well, even though it felt a bit awkward and forced. He was even able to notice that when he gave compliments and was more positive toward other people, he seemed to get more positive responses back from them. The therapist noticed that several of the compliments were to his wife, and she pointed out that Tom seemed more connected to his wife. He said that he was actually beginning to feel glimmers of excitement about the birth of their child. He reported that he was still feeling some anxiety about becoming a father, and about how the labor and delivery would go, but that the anxiety was less and more manageable. When the therapist asked about Tom *receiving* compliments, he reported more difficulties. She asked what Tom typically did when he received compliments, and it became clear that he often deflected or minimized them. Correspondingly, Tom also said that he had only done one nice thing for himself since the last session, and that it had felt uncomfortable. This pattern seemed to fit with Tom's overall schema of being unworthy and undeserving. The following dialogue ensued between the therapist and Tom:

THERAPIST: It seems like you have a hard time letting someone be nice to you and being nice to yourself.

TOM: Yes.

THERAPIST: Why do you think that is?

TOM: I don't know. (*Pauses.*) I don't like it. It feels like *they* shouldn't be nice to me, and *I* shouldn't be nice to me.

THERAPIST: Hmm . . . I wonder if there is anything "off" about that thinking? What do you think?

TOM: As I hear myself say it, it sounds a little weird. It sounds like I don't deserve to have nice things for me. Kind of like not deserving to have a family . . .

THERAPIST: This seems like a larger tendency in your life—one of those problematic thinking patterns. What pattern do you hear in your thinking? Look at the worksheet if you want to.

TOM: Maybe emotional reasoning. I feel like I don't deserve it; therefore, I must not deserve it. That seems like the best one. Maybe I'm also drawing a conclusion when the evidence is lacking.

THERAPIST: I agree. Given how much you seem to follow this pattern of thinking, I'm betting it has been around for awhile—maybe even before the shooting occurred in Iraq.

TOM: It has. I think it had to do with my dad, his alcoholism, and not being close to me. As a kid, I always thought I had done something wrong, or that I was so bad that he didn't want to be around me.

THERAPIST: Now, with adult eyes, what do you think about your dad not being close to you?

TOM: I figure that he drank for a reason, and that it might have been me and my other brothers and sisters.

THERAPIST: Why do you assume that he drank because of you kids?

TOM: I don't know. I figure it was stressful having four kids.

THERAPIST: It probably was at times, but as you hear yourself talk about this, what is amiss in how you've made sense of his drinking and being close to you?

TOM: I've known other people who had four kids and didn't have drinking problems. There were a lot of big families where I grew up. Plus, I know that he and my mom had money problems when we were young, and that they fought a lot.

THERAPIST: So, again, why then do you assume it was *you* who caused his drinking and alienation?

TOM: When we talk about it, I guess I see that it might not have been me alone.

THERAPIST: Or not even you *at all*. Everybody has a choice about how they handle their stress, and it seems that he was distant from everyone, not just you.

TOM: True. It still *feels* that way.

THERAPIST: There seems to be a well-worn path in your brain that when something goes wrong, you blame yourself. The next step is that you deserve to be punished, or at least you don't deserve anything good. I don't think this tendency is going to change overnight. You're going to need to work hard at talking to yourself more rationally to change how you feel. For that new path to get worn, you're going to have to walk down it a number of times. Pretty soon, the path will be more worn and automatic. It will take some effort, but you can change the way you automatically feel. I'd like you to do a Challenging Beliefs Worksheet about what we've just talked about. Once we get a good one about it, you can read and refer to it as part of forging that new path. Can you do that?

TOM: Yes. I think it would be good.

This exchange regarding Tom's dad dovetailed nicely with the final module, Intimacy. The therapist noted that people tend to think of intimacy as it relates to romantic relationships, and especially in terms of sexual intimacy. She stressed that there are all kinds of intimacy with different people. In essence, intimacy relates to how close and open we feel with other people. She went on to discuss the notion of self-intimacy, or how well we take care of, support, and soothe ourselves. In other words, it reflects how good a relationship we have with ourselves. Tom admitted that he struggled with being close to other people, which had most obviously manifested in the work he had done relative to his wife and unborn child. As noted earlier, Tom also struggled with doing nice things and taking good care of himself. Both of these areas seemed to be affected by Tom's underlying schema that he was undeserving and unworthy.

The therapist assigned daily Challenging Beliefs Worksheets and requested that he do worksheets on being nice to himself and being close to his wife. In addition, she asked Tom to write a final Impact Statement, specifically about his understanding of the trauma now, after all the work he had done. The therapist asked him to write about his current thoughts/beliefs in the areas of safety, trust, power/control, esteem, and intimacy.

Session 12

The day after Session 11, Tom left a message indicating that his wife had delivered a healthy baby girl. He indicated in his voice mail message that he felt happy and relieved. He went on about how beautiful the baby was, how well his wife had done in labor and delivery, and how he had enjoyed holding his daughter in his arms the first time. The 12th session was delayed an extra week because of the baby's arrival.

Tom's wife and new daughter accompanied him to the final session. The therapist spent some time admiring Tom's new baby and congratulating his wife before starting the final session. Tom seemed genuinely proud and happy about his daughter, and noted that becoming a father had been more natural than he had anticipated. He commented that he had been worried that he would not want to hold the infant for fear of hurting her or because he would do something wrong. Instead, he found it almost "instinctual" to hold her, and that soothing her had come more naturally than he expected. Tom seemed surprised about how natural his role as a father had come.

The therapist inquired about how the assignments had gone. Tom said that he had not done as much as he had hoped given the baby's arrival, but that he had done worksheets about his father and about being close to his wife. The therapist looked over these worksheets, which Tom had done very well. She asked Tom about how helpful they had been, and he reported that they had been very helpful. He added that he was still struggling about his father, but that he was beginning to think that it was not all about him, which had made him feel better about himself and less guilty in general. He mentioned that he was considering writing a letter to his father about his daughter's arrival, and that he was thinking about asking his father about why he drank

and distanced himself from his family. The therapist reinforced Tom for considering this and for not blindly making assumptions about his role in his father's drinking. However, she also attempted to inoculate Tom to the possibility that his father could blame him or his siblings for his alcoholism (given that she did not know his father or his history), and that this did not necessarily mean that it was true. She reminded him that he needed to consider the source of information, and that any good detective would get multiple reports. Tom seemed to like the idea of getting more information from others, mentioning that he and his siblings had never really talked about his belief that they were to blame for their father's alcoholism.

Tom also shared that he better understood the idea of having intimacy, without sex, in his relationship with his wife. He said that since the birth of their child, he felt closer to his wife and had generally been more open and present to her. The therapist asked him about doing nice things for himself, and Tom laughed and said that he was more open to that but was finding less time to do it with a new baby.

The therapist then asked Tom to read the final Impact Statement about the meaning of the event for him after the work that he had done. He wrote:

> There is no doubt that this traumatic event has deeply impacted me. My thoughts about myself, others, and the world were changed. When I started therapy, I believed that I was a murderer. I blamed myself completely. Now, I believe that I shot a family, but I did not murder them. I realize that I and others around me had to do what we did at the time, and that we chose to shoot because we had to. I will never know what that man, or maybe even the family, was trying to do by going through that checkpoint, but I know now that I had no choice but to shoot to stop them. Regarding safety, I used to think that there were people out to get me, but now I realize that the probability of that is slim. I still feel a little anxious about me, my wife, and now my daughter, getting hurt, but not by a sniper. That seems unlikely. Now I worry about the stuff that everyone worries about—like crazy drivers, illness, or some accident. About safety, I used to worry that I was going to go "off" and hurt my family. I don't believe that I will do that because I've never done that before and basically this trauma messed with my head about how likely I would be to hurt someone unless I had to. I'm trusting myself more in terms of the decisions I make, and I have some more faith and trust in my government now that I realize I really needed to shoot in that situation. I think I may always struggle with wanting to have

power and control over things, but I'm working on not having control over everything. The fact is, I don't have control, even though I like to think that I do. My self-esteem is improving. I have to remember that not every bad thing that happens is my fault, and that I deserve to be happy even if I don't fully believe it yet. One of the biggest things that seems to be changing is that I'm enjoying being close to my wife and my new daughter. I used to avoid my wife because I thought I didn't deserve to be happy and that I might hurt her. Slowly I'm realizing that it is not very likely that I'll hurt my wife or my new daughter, or at least hurt them intentionally. My wife seems much happier now. I want to hold on to this time in my life and provide a good life for my daughter and wife. I'm happy to know that my daughter is not going to know someone who thought that snipers were out to get him, and who was anxious, avoiding everything and everyone. It sounds silly, but I'm kind of glad that I went through this because I think I'm going to be better dad and person because of it.

Tom was a bit teary as he finished reading. The therapist asked Tom whether he remembered what he wrote the first time. Tom said no, so the therapist read to him his first Impact Statement. She pointed out that Tom had come a long way, and he agreed. The therapist and Tom reviewed the whole therapy process, what they had covered, and the "stuck points" that Tom had challenged. Tom said that he was going to continue using the worksheets because they had been so helpful in making him slow down to think about things instead of just reacting. They did some lapse planning, and the therapist asked Tom what he could do if he sensed that he was struggling with PTSD or depressive symptoms, or second-guessing his new ways of thinking. He mentioned that he was going to share the materials with his wife because she was very good at helping him to "get his head on straight." He also included on his list a review of the materials he had completed during the course of therapy. The therapy session ended with a discussion of Tom's goal to write his father a letter and to increase his contact with his siblings. He was planning to use these contacts to discover more about the reasons his father was alcoholic and had seemed to abandon the family. Tom also shared his goals about the type of father and husband he hoped to be, and what his professional future held as he left the military. The therapist congratulated Tom on his willingness to do the hard work to recover from what happened to him and wished him the best with his family and future. Tom expressed his appreciation for the therapy.

REFERENCES

American Psychiatric Association. (1994). *Diagnostic and statistical manual of mental disorders* (4th ed.). Washington, DC: Author.

American Psychiatric Association. (2013). *Diagnostic and statistical manual of mental disorders* (5th ed.). Arlington, VA: Author.

Astin, M. C., Layne, C. M., Camilleri, A. J., & Foy, D. W. (1994). Posttraumatic stress disorder in victimization-related traumata. In I. J. Briere (Ed.), *Assessing and treating victims of violence: New directions for mental health services* (pp. 39–51). San Francisco: Jossey-Bass.

Becker, J. V., Skinner, L. J., Abel, G. G., Axelrod, R., & Cichon, J. (1984). Sexual problems of sexual assault survivors. *Women and Health, 9,* 5–20.

Beckham, J. C., Feldman, M. E., & Kirby, A. C. (1998). Atrocities exposure in Vietnam combat veterans with chronic posttraumatic stress disorder: Relationship to combat exposure, symptom severity, guilt, and interpersonal violence. *Journal of Traumatic Stress, 11,* 777–785.

Blake, D. D., Weathers, F. W., Nagy, L. M., Kaloupek, D. G., Gusman, F. D., Charney, D. S., et al. (1995). The development of a Clinician-Administered PTSD Scale. *Journal of Traumatic Stress, 8,* 75–90.

Blanchard, E. B., Hickling, E. J., Buckley, T. C., & Taylor, A. E. (1996). Psychophysiology of posttraumatic stress disorder related to motor vehicle accidents: Replication and extension. *Journal of Consulting and Clinical Psychology, 64,* 742–751.

Blanchard, E. B., Hickling, E. J., Devinei, T., Veazey, C. H., Galovski, T. E., & Mundy, E. (2003). A controlled evaluation of cognitive behavioral therapy for posttraumatic stress in motor vehicle accident survivors. *Behaviour Research and Therapy, 41,* 79–96.

Bowen, G. R., & Lambert, J. A. (1986). Systematic desensitization therapy with post-traumatic stress disorder cases. In C. R. Figley (Ed.), *Trauma and its wake: Vol. II. Traumatic stress theory, research, and intervention* (pp. 280–291). New York: Brunner/Mazel.

Bradley, R., Greene, J., Russ, E., Dutra, L., & Westen, D. (2005). A multidimensional meta-analysis of psychotherapy for PTSD. *American Journal of Psychiatry, 162,* 214–227.

Breslau, N., Davis, G. C., & Andreski, P. (1995). Risk factors for PTSD-related traumatic events: A prospective analysis. *American Journal of Psychiatry, 152,* 529–535.

Brewin, C. R., Dalgleish, T., & Joseph, S. (1996). A dual representation theory of posttraumatic stress disorder. *Psychological Review, 103,* 670–686.

Briere, J. (1995). *The Trauma Symptom Inventory (TSI): Professional manual.* Odessa, FL: Psychological Assessment Resources.

Brom, D., Kleber, R. J., & Defares, P. B. (1989). Brief psychotherapy for PTSD. *Journal of Consulting and Clinical Psychology, 57,* 607–612.

Bryant, R. A., Moulds, M. L., Guthrie, R. M., Dang, S. T., & Nixon, R. D. V. (2003). Imaginal exposure alone and imaginal exposure with cognitive restructuring in treatment of posttraumatic stress disorder. *Journal of Consulting and Clinical Psychology, 71,* 706–712.

Buckley, T. C., Blanchard, E. B., & Hickling, E. J. (1998). A confirmatory factor analysis of posttraumatic stress symptoms. *Behaviour Research and Therapy, 36,* 1091–1099.

Burt, M. R. (1980). Cultural myths and supports for rape. *Journal of Personality and Social Psychology, 38,* 217–230.

Chard, K. M. (2005). An evaluation of cognitive processing therapy for the treatment of posttraumatic stress disorder related to childhood sexual abuse. *Journal of Consulting and Clinical Psychology, 73,* 965–971.

Chemtob, C., Roitblat, H. L., Hamada, R. S., Carlson, J. G., & Twentyman, C. T. (1988). A cognitive action theory of post-traumatic stress disorder. *Journal of Anxiety Disorders, 2,* 253–275.

Cloitre, M. (1998). Sexual revictimization: Risk factors and prevention. In V. M. Follette, J. I. Ruzek, & F. R. Abueg (Eds.), *Cognitive-behavioral therapies for trauma* (pp. 278–304). New York: Guilford Press.

Cloitre, M., Koenen, K. C., Cohen, L. R., & Han, H. (2002). Skills training in affective and interpersonal regulation followed by exposure: A phase-based treatment for PTSD related to childhood abuse. *Journal of Consulting and Clinical Psychology, 70,* 1067–1074.

Cloitre, M., Petkova, E., Wang, J., & Lu Lassell, F. (2012). An examination of the influence of a sequential treatment on the course and impact of dissociation among women with PTSD related to childhood abuse. *Depression and Anxiety, 29,* 707–717.

Cloitre, M., Stovall-McClough, K. C., Miranda, R., & Chemtob, C. M. (2004). Therapeutic alliance, negative mood regulation, and treatment outcome in child abuse-related posttraumatic stress disorder. *Journal of Consulting and Clinical Psychology, 72,* 411–416.

Cox, B. J., Clara, I. P., & Enns, M. W. (2002). Posttraumatic stress disorder and the structure of common mental disorders. *Depression and Anxiety, 15,* 168–171.

Creamer, M., Burgess, P., & Pattison, P. (1992). Reactions to trauma: A cognitive processing model. *Journal of Abnormal Psychology, 101,* 452–459.

Creamer, M., Morris, P., Biddle, D., & Elliott, P. (1999). Treatment outcome in Australian veterans with combat-related posttraumatic stress disorder: A cause for cautious optimism? *Journal of Traumatic Stress, 12,* 545–558.

Dalgleish, T. (2004). Cognitive approaches to posttraumatic stress disorder: The evolution of multirepresentational theorizing. *Psychological Bulletin, 130,* 228–260.

Denny, N., Robinowitz, R., & Penk, W. (1987). Conduct-

ing applied research on Vietnam combat-related posttraumatic stress disorder. *Journal of Clinical Psychology, 43,* 56–66.

Derogatis, L. R. (1983). *SCL-90-R: Administration, scoring and procedures manual–II.* Towson, MD: Clinical Psychometric Research.

Devilly, G. J., & Spence, S. H. (1999). The relative efficacy and treatment distress of EMDR and a cognitive-behavior trauma treatment protocol in the amelioration of posttraumatic stress disorder. *Journal of Anxiety Disorders, 13,* 131–157.

Dohrenwend, B. P., Turner, J. B., Turse, N. A., Adams, B. G., Koenen, K. C., & Marshall, R. (2006). The psychological risks of Vietnam for U.S. veterans: A revisit with new data and methods. *Science, 313,* 979–982.

Ehlers, A., & Clark, D. M. (2000). A cognitive model of posttraumatic stress disorder. *Behaviour Research and Therapy, 38,* 319–345.

Ehlers, A., Clark, D. M., Hackmann, A., McManus, F., Fennell, M., Herbert, C., et al. (2003). A randomized controlled trial of cognitive therapy, a self-help booklet, and repeated assessments as early interventions for posttraumatic stress disorder. *Archives of General Psychiatry, 60,* 1024-1032.

Ehlers, A., Hackmann, A., Steil, R., Clohessy, S., Wenninger, K., & Winter, H. (2002). The nature of intrusive memories after trauma: The warning signal hypothesis. *Behaviour Research and Therapy, 40,* 995–1002.

Falsetti, S. A., Resnick, H. S., Resick, P. A., & Kilpatrick, D. G. (1993). The Modified PTSD Symptom Scale: A brief self-report measure of posttraumatic stress disorder. *Behavior Therapist, 16,* 161–162.

First, M. B., Spitzer, R. L., Williams, J. B. W., & Gibbon, M. (1995). *Structured Clinical Interview for DSM-IV—Patient Edition (SCID-P).* Washington, DC: American Psychiatric Press.

Foa, E. B. (1995). *Posttraumatic Stress Diagnostic Scale (manual).* Minneapolis, MN: National Computer Systems.

Foa, E. B., Dancu, C. V., Hembree, E. A., Jaycox, L. H., Meadows, E. A., & Street, G. P. (1999). A comparison of exposure therapy, stress inoculation training, and their combination for reducing posttraumatic stress disorder in female assault victims. *Journal of Consulting and Clinical Psychology, 67,* 194–200.

Foa, E. B., Hembree, E. A., Cahill, S. E., Rauch, S. A. M., Riggs, D. S., Feeny, N. C., et al. (2005). Randomized trial of prolonged exposure for posttraumatic stress disorder with and without cognitive restructuring: Outcome at academic and community clinics. *Journal of Consulting and Clinical Psychology, 73,* 953–964.

Foa, E. B., Keane, T. M., Friedman, M. J., & Cohen, J. A. (Eds.). (2008). *Effective treatments for PTSD: Practice guidelines from the International Society for Traumatic Stress Studies* (2nd ed.). New York: Guilford Press.

Foa, E. B., Riggs, D. S., Dancu, C. V., & Rothbaum, B. O.

(1993). Reliability and validity of a brief instrument for assessing post-traumatic stress disorder. *Journal of Traumatic Stress, 6*, 459–473.

Foa, E. B., & Rothbaum, B. O. (1998). *Treating the trauma of rape: Cognitive-behavioral therapy for PTSD*. New York: Guilford Press.

Foa, E. B., Rothbaum, B., Riggs, D., & Murdock, T. (1991). Treatment of posttraumatic stress disorder in rape victims: A comparison between cognitive-behavioral procedures and counseling. *Journal of Consulting and Clinical Psychology, 59*, 715–723.

Foa, E. B., Steketee, G., & Rothbaum, B. O. (1989). Behavioral/cognitive conceptualizations of post-traumatic stress disorder. *Behavior Therapy, 20*, 155–176.

Frank, E., Anderson, B., Stewart, B. D., Dancu, C., Hughes, C., & West, D. (1988). Efficacy of cognitive behavior therapy and systematic desensitization in the treatment of rape trauma. *Behavior Therapy, 19*, 403–420.

Frank, E., & Stewart, B. D. (1983). Treating depression in victims of rape. *Clinical Psychologist, 36*, 95–98.

Frank, E., & Stewart, B. D. (1984). Depressive symptoms in rape victims: A revisit. *Journal of Affective Disorders, 1*, 269–277.

Green, B. L. (1996). Trauma History Questionnaire. In B. H. Stamm (Ed.), *Measurement of stress, trauma, and adaptation* (pp. 366–369). Lutherville, MD: Sidran.

Griffin, M. G., Resick, P. A., & Mechanic, M. B. (1997). Objective assessment of peritraumatic dissociation: Psychophysiological indicators. *American Journal of Psychiatry, 154*, 1081–1088.

Griffin, M. G., Uhlmansiek, M. H., Resick, P. A., & Mechanic, M. B. (2004). Comparison of the Posttraumatic Stress Disorder Scale versus the Clinician-Administered Posttraumatic Stress Disorder Scale in domestic violence survivors. *Journal of Traumatic Stress, 17*, 497–504.

Gutner, C., Rizvi, S. L., Monson, C. M., & Resick, P. A. (2006). Changes in coping strategies, relationship to the perpetrator, and posttraumatic stress disorder in female crime victims. *Journal of Traumatic Stress, 19*, 813–823.

Hoge, C. W., Auchterlonie, J. L., & Milliken, C. S. (2006). Mental health problems, use of mental health services, and attrition from military service after returning from deployment to Iraq or Afghanistan. *Journal of the American Medical Association, 295*, 1023–1032.

Hoge, C. W., Castro, C. A., Messer, S. C., McGurk, D., Cotting, D. I., & Koffman, R. L. (2004). Combat duty in Iraq and Afghanistan, mental health problems, and barriers to care. *New England Journal of Medicine, 351*, 13–22.

Holmes, M. R., & St. Lawrence, J. S. (1983). Treatment of rape-induced trauma: Proposed behavioral conceptualization and review of the literature. *Clinical Psychology Review, 3*, 417–433.

Horowitz, M. J. (1986). *Stress response syndromes* (2nd ed.). New York: Aronson.

Ironson, G., Freund, B., Strauss, J. L., & Williams, J. (2002). Comparison of two treatments for traumatic stress: A community-based study of EMDR and prolonged exposure. *Journal of Clinical Psychology, 58*, 113–128.

Janoff-Bulman, R. (1985). The aftermath of victimization: Rebuilding shattered assumptions. In C. R. Figley (Ed.), *Trauma and its wake: Vol. I. The study and treatment of posttraumatic stress disorder* (pp. 15–35). New York: Brunner/Mazel.

Janoff-Bulman, R. (1992). *Shattered assumptions: Towards a new psychology of trauma*. New York: Free Press.

Jordan, B. K., Marmar, C. R., Fairbank, J. A., Schlenger, W. E., Kulka, R. A., Hough, R. L., et al. (1992). Problems in families of male Vietnam veterans with posttraumatic stress disorder. *Journal of Consulting and Clinical Psychology, 60*, 916–926.

Keane, T. M., Brief, D. J., Pratt, E. M., & Miller, M. W. (2007). Assessment and its comorbidities in adults. In M. J. Friedman, T. M. Keane, & P. A. Resick (Eds.), *Handbook of PTSD: Science and practice* (pp. 279–305). New York: Guilford Press.

Keane, T. M., Caddell, J. M., & Taylor, K. L. (1988). Mississippi Scale for Combat-Related Posttraumatic Stress Disorder: Three studies in reliability and validity. *Journal of Consulting and Clinical Psychology, 56*, 85–90.

Keane, T. M., Fairbank, J. A., Caddell, J. M., & Zimering, R. T. (1989). Implosive (flooding) therapy reduces symptoms of PTSD in Vietnam combat veterans. *Behavior Therapy, 20*, 245–260.

Keane, T. M., Kolb, L. C., Kaloupek, D. G., Orr, S. P., Blanchard, E. B., Thomas, R. G., et al. (1998). Utility of psychophysiology measurement in the diagnosis of posttraumatic stress disorder: Results from a Department of Veteran's Affairs cooperative study. *Journal of Consulting and Clinical Psychology, 66*, 914–923.

Keane, T. M., Malloy, P. F., & Fairbank, J. A. (1984). Empirical development of an MMPI subscale for the assessment of combat-related posttraumatic stress disorder. *Journal of Consulting and Clinical Psychology, 52*, 888–891.

Keane, T. M., Zimering, R. T., & Caddell, J. M. (1985). A behavioral formulation of posttraumatic stress disorder. *Behavior Therapist, 8*, 9–12.

Kessler, R. C., Berglund, P., Demler, O., Jin, R., Merikangas, K. R., & Walters, E. E. (2005). Lifetime prevalence and age-of-onset distributions of DSM-IV disorders in the National Comorbidity Survey Replication. *Archives of General Psychiatry, 62*, 593–602.

Kessler, R. C., Chiu, W. T., Demler, O., Merikangas, K. R., & Walters, E. E. (2005). Prevalence, severity, and comorbidity of 12-month DSM-IV disorders in the National Comorbidity Survey Replication. *Archives of General Psychiatry, 62*, 617–627.

Kessler, R. C., Sonnega, A., Bromet, E., Hughes, M., & Nelson, C. B. (1995). Posttraumatic stress disorder in the National Comorbidity Survey. *Archives of General Psychiatry, 52*, 1048–1060.

Kilpatrick, D. G. (1983). Rape victims: Detection, assessment and treatment. *Clinical Psychologist, 36*, 92–95.

Kilpatrick, D. G., & Amick, A. E. (1985). Rape trauma. In M. Hersen & C. Last (Eds.), *Behavior therapy casebook* (pp. 86–103). New York: Springer.

Kilpatrick, D. G., Edmunds, C. N., & Seymour, A. K. (1992). *Rape in America: A report to the nation.* Arlington, VA: National Victim Center.

Kilpatrick, D. G., Resnick, H. S., & Freedy, J. R. (1991). *The Potential Stressful Events Interview.* Unpublished instrument, National Crime Victims Research and Treatment Center, Medical University of South Carolina, Charleston.

Kilpatrick, D. G., Saunders, B. E., Veronen, L. J., Best, C. L., & Von, J. M. (1987). Criminal victimization: Lifetime prevalence, reporting to police, and psychological impact. *Crime and Delinquency, 33*, 479–489.

Kilpatrick, D. G., & Veronen, L. J. (1983). Treatment for rape-related problems: Crisis intervention is not enough. In L. H. Cohen, W. L. Claiborn, & G. A. Specter (Eds.), *Crisis intervention* (pp. 165–185). New York: Human Sciences Press.

Kilpatrick, D. G., Veronen, L. J., & Best, C. L. (1985). Factors predicting psychological distress among rape victims. In C. R. Figley (Ed.), *Trauma and its wake: Vol. I. The study and treatment of posttraumatic stress disorder* (pp. 114–141). New York: Brunner/Mazel.

Kilpatrick, D. G., Veronen, L. J., & Resick, P. A. (1982). Psychological sequelae to rape: Assessment and treatment strategies. In D. M. Doleys, R. L. Meredith, & A. R. Ciminero (Eds.), *Behavioral medicine: Assessment and treatment strategies* (pp. 473–497). New York: Plenum Press.

Koss, M. P., & Harvey, M. R. (1991). *The rape victim: Clinical and community interventions* (2nd ed.). Thousand Oaks, CA: Sage.

Kubany, E. S., Haynes, S. N., Leisen, M. B., Owens, J. A., Kaplan, A. S., Watson, S. B., et al. (2000). Development and preliminary validation of a brief broad-spectrum measure of trauma exposure: The Traumatic Life Events Questionnaire. *Psychological Assessment, 12*, 210–224.

Kubany, E. S., Hill, E. E., Owens, J. A., Iannce-Spencer, C., McCaig, M. A., & Tremayne, K. J. (2004). Cognitive trauma therapy for battered women with PTSD (CTT-BW). *Journal of Consulting and Clinical Psychology, 72*, 3–18.

Kubany, E. S., Leisen, M. B., Kaplan, A. S., & Kelly, M. P. (2000). Validation of a brief measure of posttraumatic stress disorder: The Distressing Event Questionnaire (DEQ). *Psychological Assessment, 12*, 197–209.

Kulka, R. A., Schlenger, W. E., Fairbank, J. A., Hough, R. L., Jordan, B. K., Marmar, C. R., et al. (1990). *Trauma and the Vietnam war generation: Report of findings from the National Vietnam Veterans Readjustment Study.* New York: Brunner/Mazel.

Lang, P. J. (1968). Fear reduction and fear behavior: Problems in treating a construct. In J. M. Schlien (Ed.), *Research in psychotherapy* (pp. 90–102). Washington, DC: American Psychological Association.

Lang, P. J. (1977). Imagery in therapy: An information processing analysis of fear. *Behavior Therapy, 8*, 862–886.

Lanius, R. A., Vermetten, E., Loewenstein, R. J., Brand, B., Schmahl, C., Bremner, J. D., et al. (2010). Emotion modulation in PTSD: Clinical and neurobiological evidence for a dissociative subtype. *American Journal of Psychiatry, 167*(6), 640–647.

Lauterbach, D., & Vrana, S. R. (1996). Three studies on the reliability and validity of a self-report measure of posttraumatic stress disorder. *Assessment, 3*, 17–25.

Lauterbach, D., Vrana, S., King, D. W., & King, L. A. (1997). Psychometric properties of the civilian version of the Mississippi PTSD scale. *Journal of Traumatic Stress, 10*, 499–513.

Lee, C., Gavriel, H., Drummond, P., Richards, J., & Greenwald, R. (2002). Treatment of PTSD: Stress inoculation training with prolonged exposure compared to EMDR. *Journal of Clinical Psychology, 58*, 1071–1089.

Lester, K. M., Resick, P. A., Young-Xu, Y., & Artz, C. E. (2010). Impact of ethnicity on early treatment termination and outcomes in PTSD treatment. *Journal of Consulting and Clinical Psychology, 4*, 480-489.

Mahoney, M. J., & Lyddon, W. J. (1988). Recent developments in cognitive approaches to counseling and psychotherapy. *Counseling Psychologist, 16*, 190–234.

Marks, I., Lovell, K., Noshirvani, H., Livanou, M., & Thrasher, S. (1998). Treatment of posttraumatic stress disorder by exposure and/or cognitive restructuring: A controlled study. *Archives of General Psychiatry, 55*, 317–325.

McCann, I. L., & Pearlman, L. A. (1990). Vicarious traumatization: A framework for understanding the psychological effects of working with victims. *Journal of Traumatic Stress, 3*, 131–149.

McFall, M., Fontana, A., Raskind, M., & Rosenheck, R. (1999). Analysis of violent behavior in Vietnam combat veteran psychiatric inpatients with posttraumatic stress disorder. *Journal of Traumatic Stress, 12*, 501–517.

McNair, L. D., & Neville, H. A. (1996). African American women survivors of sexual assault: The intersection of race and class. In M. Hill & E. D. Rothblum (Eds.), *Classism and feminist therapy: Counting costs* (pp. 107–118). New York: Haworth.

Meichenbaum, D. H. (1985). *Stress inoculation training.* Elmsford, NY: Pergamon.

Miller, M. W., Greif, J. L., & Smith, A. A. (2003). Multidimensional Personality Questionnaire profiles of veterans with traumatic combat exposure: Externalizing and internalizing subtypes. *Psychological Assessment, 15*, 205–215.

Miller, M. W., Kaloupek, D. G., Dillon, A. L., & Keane, T. M. (2004). Externalizing and internalizing subtypes of combat-related PTSD: A replication and extension using the PSY-5 scales. *Journal of Abnormal Psychology, 113*, 636–645.

Miller, M. W., & Resick, P. A. (2007). Internalizing and externalizing subtypes in female sexual assault survivors: Implications for the understanding of complex PTSD. *Behavior Therapy, 38*, 58–71.

Monson, C. M., Gradus, J. L., Young-Xu, Y., Schnurr, P. P., Price, J. A., Schumm, J. A. (2008). Change in posttraumatic stress disorder symptoms: Do clinicians and patients agree? *Psychological Assessment, 20*, 131–138.

Monson, C. M., Price, J. L., & Ranslow, E. (2005, October). Treating combat PTSD through cognitive processing therapy. *Federal Practitioner, 22*(10), 75–83.

Monson, C. M., Schnurr, P. P., Resick, P. A., Friedman, M. J., Young-Xu, Y., & Stevens, S. P. (2006). Cognitive processing therapy for veterans with military-related posttraumatic stress disorder. *Journal of Consulting and Clinical Psychology, 74*, 898–907.

Morland, L. A., Hynes, A. K., Mackintosh, M., Resick, P. A., & Chard, K. M. (2011). Group cognitive processing therapy delivered to veterans via telehealth: A pilot cohort. *Journal of Traumatic Stress, 24*, 465–469.

Mowrer, O. H. (1947). On the dual nature of learning—a reinterpretation of "conditioning" and "problem-solving." *Harvard Educational Review, 14*, 102–148.

National Institute of Clinical Excellence. (2005). *Posttraumatic stress disorder (PTSD): The treatment of PTSD in adults and children.* London: Author.

Neuner, F., Schauer, M., Klaschik, C., Karunakara, U., & Elbert, T. (2004). A comparison of narrative exposure therapy, supportive counseling, and psychoeducation for treating posttraumatic stress disorder in an African refugee settlement. *Journal of Consulting and Clinical Psychology, 72*, 579–587.

Norris, F. H. (1990). Screening for traumatic stress: A scale for use in the general population. *Journal of Applied Social Psychology, 20*, 1704–1718.

Norris, F. H. (1992). Epidemiology of trauma: Frequency and impact of different potentially traumatic events on different demographic groups. *Journal of Consulting and Clinical Psychology, 60*, 409–418.

Oquendo, M. A., Friend, J. M., Halberstam, B., Brodsky, B. S., Burke, A. K., Grunebaum, M. F., et al. (2003). Association of comorbid posttraumatic stress disorder and major depression with greater risk for suicidal behavior. *American Journal of Psychiatry, 160*, 580–582.

Orr, S. P., Lasko, N. B., Metzger, L. J., Berry, N. J., Ahern, C. E., & Pitman, R. K. (1998). Psychophysiologic assessment of women with posttraumatic stress disorder resulting from childhood sexual abuse. *Journal of Consulting and Clinical Psychology, 66*, 906–913.

Orr, S. P., Metzger, L. J., Miller, M. W., & Kaloupek, D. G. (2004). Psychophysiological assessment of PTSD. In J. P. Wilson & T. M. Keane (Eds.), *Assessing psychological trauma and PTSD* (2nd ed., pp. 289–343). New York: Guilford Press.

Pitman, R. K., Orr, S. P., Altman, B., Longpre, R. E., Poire, R. E., & Macklin, M. L. (1996). Emotional processing during eye movement desensitization and reprocessing therapy of Vietnam veterans with chronic posttraumatic stress disorder. *Comprehensive Psychiatry, 37*, 419–429.

Pitman, R. K., Orr, S. P., Forgue, D. F., & Altman, B. (1990). Psychophysiologic responses to combat imagery of Vietnam veterans with posttraumatic stress disorder versus other anxiety disorders. *Journal of Abnormal Psychology, 99*, 49–54.

Pitman, R. K., Orr, S. P., Forgue, D. F., de Jong, J., & Claiborn, J. M. (1987). Psychophysiologic assessment of posttraumatic stress disorder imagery in Vietnam combat veterans. *Archives of General Psychiatry, 44*, 970–975.

Power, K., McGoldrick, T., Brown, K., Buchanan, R., Sharp, D., & Swanson, V. (2002). A controlled comparison of eye movement desensitization and reprocessing versus exposure plus cognitive restructuring versus wait list in the treatment of posttraumatic stress disorder. *Clinical Psychology and Psychotherapy, 9*, 299–318.

Powers, M. B., Halpern, J. M., Ferenschak, M. P., Gillihan, S. J., & Foa, E. B. (2010). A meta-analytic review of prolonged exposure for posttraumatic stress disorder. *Clinical Psychology Review, 30*, 635–641.

Prins, A., Ouimette, P., Kimerling, R., Camerond, R. P., Hugelshofer, D. S., Shaw-Hegwer, J., et al. (2004). The Primary Care PTSD Screen (PC-PTSD): Development and operating characteristics. *Primary Care Psychiatry, 9*, 9–14.

Renfrey, G., & Spates, C. R. (1994). Eye movement desensitization: A partial dismantling study. *Journal of Behavior Therapy and Experimental Psychiatry, 25*, 231–239.

Resick, P. A., Galovski, T. E., Uhlmansiek, M. O., Scher, C. D., Clum, G., & Young-Xu, Y. (2008). A randomized clinical trial to dismantle components of cognitive processing therapy for posttraumatic stress disorder in female victims of interpersonal violence. *Journal of Consulting and Clinical Psychology, 76*, 243–258.

Resick, P. A., Jordan, C. G., Girelli, S. A., Hutter, C. K., & Marhoeder-Dvorak, S. (1988). A comparative outcome study of behavioral group therapy for sexual assault victims. *Behavior Therapy, 19*, 385–401.

Resick, P. A., & Markaway, B. E. (1991). Clinical treatment of adult female victims of sexual assault. In C. R. Hollin & K. Howells (Eds.), *Clinical approaches to sex offenders and their victims* (pp. 261–284). London: Wiley.

Resick, P. A., Monson, C. M., & Chard, K. M. (2007). *Cognitive processing therapy: Veteran/military version.* Washington, DC: Department of Veterans Affairs.

Resick, P. A., Nishith, P., & Griffin, M. G. (2003). How well does cognitive-behavioral therapy treat symptoms of complex PTSD?: An examination of child sexual abuse survivors within a clinical trial. *CNS Spectrums, 8*, 340–355.

Resick, P. A., Nishith, P., Weaver, T. L., Astin, M. C., & Feuer, C. A. (2002). A comparison of cognitive processing therapy, prolonged exposure and a waiting condition for the treatment of posttraumatic stress disorder in female rape victims. *Journal of Consulting and Clinical Psychology, 70,* 867–879.

Resick, P. A., & Schnicke, M. K. (1992). Cognitive processing therapy for sexual assault victims. *Journal of Consulting and Clinical Psychology, 60,* 748–756.

Resick, P. A., & Schnicke, M. K. (1993). *Cognitive processing therapy for rape victims: A treatment manual.* Newbury Park, CA: Sage.

Resick, P. A., Williams, L. F., Suvak, M. K., Monson, C. M., & Gradus, J. L. (2012). Long-term outcomes of cognitive-behavioral treatments for posttraumatic stress disorder among female rape survivors. *Journal of Consulting and Clinical Psychology, 80,* 201–210.

Resnick, H. S., Kilpatrick, D. G., Dansky, B. S., Saunders, B. E., & Best, C. L. (1993). Prevalence of civilian trauma and posttraumatic stress disorder in a representative national sample of women. *Journal of Consulting and Clinical Psychology, 61,* 984–991.

Resnick, H. S., Kilpatrick, D. G., & Lipovsky, J. A. (1991). Assessment of rape-related posttraumatic stress disorder: Stressor and symptom dimensions. *Psychological Assessment, 3,* 561–572.

Robins, L. N., Helzer, J. E., Croughan, J., & Ratcliff, K. S. (1981). National Institute of Mental Health Diagnostic Interview Schedule: Its history, characteristics, and validity. *Archives of General Psychiatry, 38,* 381–389.

Rosenheck, R., & Fontana, A. (1996). PTSD and community-based treatment: A commentary on "PTSD diagnosis and treatment for mental health clinicians." *Community Mental Health Journal, 32,* 191–193.

Rosenheck, R., Fontana, A., & Cottrol, C. (1995). Effect of clinician–veteran racial pairing in the treatment of posttraumatic stress disorder. *American Journal of Psychiatry, 152,* 555–563.

Rothbaum, B. O., Astin, M. C., & Marsteller, F. (2005). Prolonged exposure versus eye movement desensitization and reprocessing (EMDR) for PTSD rape victims. *Journal of Traumatic Stress, 18,* 607–616.

Rothbaum, B. O., & Foa, E. B. (1992). Exposure therapy for rape victims with post-traumatic stress disorder. *Behavior Therapist, 15,* 219–222.

Rothbaum, B. O., Hodges, L. F., Ready, D., Graap, K., & Alarcon, R. (2001). Virtual reality exposure therapy for Vietnam veterans with PTSD. *Journal of Clinical Psychiatry, 62,* 617–622.

Saunders, B. E., Arata, C. M., & Kilpatrick, D. G. (1990). Development of a crime-related posttraumatic stress disorder scale for women within the Symptom Checklist—90—Revised. *Journal of Traumatic Stress, 3,* 439–448.

Schindler, F. E. (1980). Treatment by systematic desensitization of a recurring nightmare of a real life trauma. *Journal of Behavior Therapy and Experimental Psychiatry, 11,* 53–54.

Schnurr, P. P., Friedman, M. J., Engel, C. C., Foa, E. B., Shea, T., Chow, B. K., et al. (2007). Cognitive-behavioral therapy for posttraumatic stress disorder in women: A randomized controlled trial. *Journal of the American Medical Association, 297,* 820–830.

Shalev, A. Y., Orr, S. P., & Pitman, R. K. (1992). Psychophysiologic response during script-driven imagery as an outcome measure in posttraumatic stress disorder. *Journal of Clinical Psychiatry, 53,* 324–326.

Shapiro, F. (1989). Eye movement desensitization: A new treatment for post-traumatic stress disorder. *Journal of Behavior Therapy and Experimental Psychiatry, 20,* 211–217.

Shapiro, F. (1995). *Eye movement desensitization and reprocessing: Basic principles, protocols, and procedures.* New York: Guilford Press.

Shay, J., & Munroe, J. (1999). Group and milieu therapy for veterans with complex posttraumatic stress disorder. In P. A. Saigh & J. D. Bremner (Eds.), *Posttraumatic stress disorder: A comprehensive text* (pp. 391–413). Needham Heights, MA: Allyn & Bacon.

Silverman, D. (1977). First do no more harm: Female rape victims and the male counselor. *American Journal of Orthopsychiatry, 47,* 91–96.

Street, A. E., Gradus, J. L., Vogt, D. S., Giasson, H. L., & Resick, P. A. (2013). Gender differences among veterans deployed in support of the wars in Afghanistan and Iraq. *Journal of General Internal Medicine, 28*(Suppl. 2), 556–562.

Sutker, P. B., Uddo-Crane, M., & Allain, A. N. (1991). Clinical and research assessment of posttraumatic stress disorder: A conceptual overview. *Psychological Assessment, 3,* 520–530.

Tarrier, N., Pilgrim, H., Sommerfield, C., Faragher, B., Reynolds, M., Graham, E., et al. (1999). A randomized trial of cognitive therapy and imaginal exposure in the treatment of chronic posttraumatic stress disorder. *Journal of Consulting and Clinical Psychology, 67,* 13–18.

Tarrier, N., & Sommerfield, C. (2004). Treatment of chronic PTSD by cognitive therapy and exposure: 5-year follow-up. *Behavior Therapy, 35,* 231–246.

Taylor, S., Kuch, K., Koch, W. J., Crockett, D. J., & Passey, G. (1998). The structure of posttraumatic stress symptoms. *Journal of Abnormal Psychology, 107,* 154–160.

Taylor, S., Thordarson, D. S., Maxfield, L., Fedoroff, I. C., Lovell, K., & Orgodniczuk, J. (2003). Comparative efficacy, speed, and adverse effects of three PTSD treatments: Exposure therapy, EMDR, and relaxation training. *Journal of Consulting and Clinical Psychology, 71,* 330–338.

Tolin, D. F., & Foa, E. B. (2006). Sex differences in trauma and posttraumatic stress disorder: A quantitative review of 25 years of research. *Psychological Bulletin, 132,* 959–992.

U.S. Department of Health and Human Services. (2001). *Mental health: A report of the Surgeon General.* Washington, DC: Author.

U.S. Departments of Veterans Affairs and Defense. (2010). *VA/DoD clinical practice guideline for the management of PTSD*. Washington, DC: Author.

van Etten, M. L., & Taylor, S. (1998). Comparative efficacy of treatments for post-traumatic stress disorder: A meta-analysis. *Clinical Psychology and Psychotherapy, 5*, 126–144.

Vogt, D., Smith, B., Elwy, R., Martin, J., Schultz, M., Drainoni, M.-L., et al.(2011). Predeployment, deployment, and postdeployment risk factors for posttraumatic stress symptomatology in female and male OEF/OIF veterans. *Journal of Abnormal Psychology, 120*, 819–831.

Vrana, S., & Lauterbach, D. (1994). Prevalence of traumatic events and post-traumatic psychological symptoms in a nonclinical sample of college students. *Journal of Traumatic Stress, 7*, 289–302.

Weathers, F. W., Blake, D. D., Schnurr, P. P., Kaloupek, D. G., Marx, B. P., & Keane, T. M. (2013). *Clinician-Administered PTSD Scale for DSM-5*. Washington, DC: U.S. Veterans Affairs National Center for Posttraumatic Stress Disorder.

Weathers, F., Litz, B. T., Herman, D. S., Huska, J. A., & Keane, T. M. (1993, October). *The PTSD Checklist (PCL): Reliability, validity, and diagnostic utility*. Presentation at the International Society for Traumatic Stress Studies, San Antonio, TX.

Weathers, F. W., & Keane, T. M. (1999). Psychological assessment of traumatized adults. In P. A. Saigh & J. D. Bremner (Eds.), *Posttraumatic stress disorder: A comprehensive text* (pp. 219–247). Boston: Allyn & Bacon.

Weathers, F. W., Keane, T. M., & Davidson, J. R. (2001). Clinician-Administered PTSD Scale: A review of the first ten years of research. *Depression and Anxiety, 13*, 132–156.

Weathers, F. W., Litz, B., Keane, K. M., Palmieri, P. A., Marx, B., & Schnurr, P. P. (2013). *PTSD Checklist–5*. Washington, DC: U.S. Veterans Affairs National Center for Posttraumatic Stress Disorder.

Weathers, F. W., Ruscio, A. M., & Keane, T. M. (1999). Psychometric properties of nine scoring rules for the Clinician-Administered Posttraumatic Stress Disorder Scale. *Psychological Assessment, 11*, 124–133.

Weiss, D. S., & Marmar, C. R. (1997). The Impact of Event Scale—Revised. In J. P. Wilson & T. M. Keane (Eds.), *Assessing psychological trauma and PTSD* (pp. 399–411). New York: Guilford Press.

Wilson, A. E., Calhoun, K. S., & Bernat, J. A. (1999). Risk recognition and trauma-related symptoms among sexually revictimized women. *Journal of Consulting and Clinical Psychology, 67*, 705–710.

Wilson, D., Silver, S. M., Covi, W., & Foster, S. (1996). Eye movement desensitization and reprocessing: Effectiveness and automatic correlates. *Journal of Behavior Therapy and Experimental Psychiatry, 27*, 219–229.

Wolf, E. J., Lunney, C. A., Miller, M. W., Resick, P. A., Friedman, M. J., & Schnurr, P. P. (2012). The dissociative subtype of PTSD: A replication and extension. *Depression and Anxiety, 29*, 679–688.

Zoellner, L. A., Feeny, N. C., Fitzgibbons, L. A., & Foa, E. B. (1999). Response of African American and Caucasian women to cognitive behavioral therapy for PTSD. *Behavior Therapy, 30*, 581–595.

CHAPTER 3

Social Anxiety Disorder

RICHARD G. HEIMBERG
LEANNE MAGEE

Many people are very shy and somewhat inhibited. For this reason, the suffering associated with social anxiety disorder is often minimized as a common trait in the population that does not require a heavy artillery of formalized treatment interventions (either drugs or psychological treatments). Nothing could be further from the truth. For members of a very large segment of the population with debilitating social anxiety (over 12% and increasing), at some point in their lives, the seemingly simple process of interacting with people or forming relationships provokes overwhelming terror and is often avoided. The effects on career and quality of life can be devastating. This chapter examines the latest iteration of an established psychological treatment for social anxiety disorder. As is increasingly true of our new generation of psychological interventions, cognitive-behavioral therapy has proven to be significantly better than equally credible but less focused psychological interventions, and its effect is increasingly powerful over time. As such, this treatment is among the best of the new generation of psychological treatments characterized by power and specificity. The case of Josie, with a report of her progress at a 5-year follow-up that is new to this edition, also illustrates the maturity and clinical sophistication of this remarkable approach to social anxiety.—D. H. B.

The National Comorbidity Survey Replication Study (NCS-R), which assessed over 9,000 noninstitutionalized individuals throughout the United States, found that 12.1% of people have social anxiety disorder at some point during their lives (Kessler et al., 2005). In this survey, social anxiety disorder (also known as social phobia; Liebowitz, Heimberg, Fresco, Travers, & Stein, 2000) was the fourth most common psychiatric disorder, with only major depressive disorder, alcohol abuse, and specific phobia being more prevalent. More conservative lifetime prevalence estimates suggest that clinically significant social anxiety affects a compelling but more modest 4% of the population (Narrow, Rae, Robins, & Regier, 2002).

When social anxiety disorder was first included as a diagnostic category in the third edition of the *Diagnostic and Statistical Manual of Mental Disorders* (DSM-III; American Psychiatric Association, 1980), it was thought to result in only minimal disruption in role functioning. Research has since revealed that social anxiety disorder can be quite incapacitating. The vast majority of individuals with social anxiety disorder report that their work, academic, and social functioning have been seriously impaired by their fears (Acarturk, de Graaf, van Straten, ten Have, & Cuijpers, 2008; Aderka et al., 2012; Katzelnick et al., 2001; Schneier et al., 1994). Compared to their nonanxious peers, individuals with social anxiety disorder report fewer friends and dating partners (Rodebaugh, 2009; Wenzel, 2002), and they are less likely to marry, even in comparison to persons with other anxiety disorders. In one study, despite a mean age in the early 30s, 50% of individuals with social anxiety disorder had never married, compared to 36% of individuals with panic disorder and agoraphobia, and 18% of those with generalized anxiety disorder (Sanderson, Di Nardo, Rapee, & Barlow, 1990). In another study, individuals with social anxiety disorder were more likely than their nonanxious counterparts to work at a job below their level of educational attainment and to believe that their supervisors did not think that they fit into the work environment (Bruch, Fallon, & Heimberg, 2003). Symptoms of social anxiety are also associated with a low level of life satisfaction, even after taking into account the level of disability engendered by these symptoms (Hambrick, Turk, Heimberg, Schneier, & Liebowitz, 2003).

Social anxiety disorder most commonly begins during early childhood or adolescence (Schneier, Johnson, Hornig, Liebowitz, & Weissman, 1992) and typically follows an unremitting course in clinical samples (Bruce et al., 2005). Nevertheless, most individuals with social anxiety disorder do not seek treatment unless they develop an additional disorder (Schneier et al., 1992). In contrast, rates of remission have been higher in epidemiological than in clinical samples (Blanco et al., 2011; Vriends, Becker, Meyer, Williams, et al., 2007).

Approximately 70–80% of individuals with social anxiety disorder meet criteria for additional diagnoses, and, in most cases, social anxiety disorder predates the onset of the comorbid condition (W. J. Magee, Eaton, Wittchen, McGonagle, & Kessler, 1996; Schneier et al., 1992). In community samples, the most common additional diagnoses include specific phobia, agoraphobia, major depression, and alcohol use disorders (W. J. Magee et al., 1996; Schneier et al., 1992). Compared to individuals with uncomplicated social anxiety disorder, persons with social anxiety disorder and comorbid disorders have higher rates of suicide attempts, are more likely to report significant role impairment, and more often use medication to control their symptoms (W. J. Magee et al., 1996; Schneier et al., 1992).

Comorbidity is also associated with more severe impairment before and after cognitive-behavioral therapy (CBT), although individuals with and without comorbid conditions make similar gains (Erwin, Heimberg, Juster, & Mindlin, 2002). Comorbid mood disorders appear to be more strongly associated with impairment than do comorbid anxiety disorders (Erwin et al., 2002).

SUBTYPES OF SOCIAL ANXIETY DISORDER AND AVOIDANT PERSONALITY DISORDER

Individuals with social anxiety are a heterogeneous group in terms of the pervasiveness and severity of their fears. Many individuals have a range of social fears, including social interaction fears (e.g., dating, joining an ongoing conversation, being assertive), performance fears (e.g., public speaking, playing a musical instrument in front of others), and observation fears (e.g., working in front of others, walking down the street). In previous editions of the DSM, this was labeled as a *generalized* subtype of social anxiety disorder, a term absent in DSM-5. Instead, DSM-5 includes a *performance-only* subtype, reflecting individuals for whom the fear is restricted to speaking or performing in public (American Psychiatric Association, 2013).

Relative to the DSM-5 performance-only subtype, having social anxiety in many situations has been associated with earlier age of onset, decreased educational attainment, higher rates of unemployment, and a greater likelihood of being unmarried (Heimberg, Hope, Dodge, & Becker, 1990; Mannuzza et al., 1995). This group also experiences more depression, anxiety, avoidance, fear of negative evaluation, and functional impairment (e.g., Brown, Heimberg, & Juster, 1995; Herbert, Hope, & Bellack, 1992; Turner, Beidel, & Townsley, 1992). Nevertheless, after CBT, clients who fear many social situations improve as much as those who only fear performance situations (Brown et al., 1995; Hope, Herbert, & White, 1995; Turner, Beidel, Wolff, Spaulding, & Jacob, 1996). However, because clients with multiple social fears begin treatment with greater impairment, they remain more impaired after receiving the same number of treatment sessions. Therefore, these individuals may require a longer course of treatment to achieve outcomes similar to those of clients with the performance-only subtype. However, it has not been clearly established that the DSM-5 subtyping scheme provides more information than a simple count of the number of feared social situations (Vriends, Becker, Meyer, Michael, & Margraf, 2007).

With the exception of the performance-only subtype, social anxiety disorder has many features in common with avoidant personality disorder (APD). In the current diagnostic system, APD is characterized by a long-standing pattern "of social inhibition, feelings of inadequacy, and hypersensitivity to negative evaluation" (American Psychiatric Association, 2013, p. 672). Given the similarity between the descriptions of the two disorders, it is not surprising that many individuals who meet criteria for social anxiety disorder also meet criteria for APD. In both clinical and community samples (Cox, Pagura, Stein, & Sareen, 2009; Huppert, Strunk, Ledley, Davidson, & Foa, 2008; Marques et al., 2012), individuals who met criteria for both social anxiety disorder and APD were more depressed and demonstrated greater functional impairment and reduced quality of life. However, in one study, these differences were no longer evident when severity of social anxiety was controlled (Chambless, Fydrich, & Rodebaugh, 2008). The most parsimonious description of the relationship between social anxiety disorder and APD may be that they are not different disorders and that individuals meeting criteria for both disorders are simply the most severely impaired persons with social anxiety disorder (Chambless et al., 2008; Heimberg, Holt, Schneier, Spitzer, & Liebowitz, 1993). With regard to treatment outcome, some studies have found that clients with and without comorbid APD make similar gains (Brown et al., 1995; Hofmann, Newman, Becker, Taylor, & Roth, 1995; Hope, Herbert, et al., 1995), although others have found that comorbid APD is associated with poorer treatment response (Chambless, Tran, & Glass, 1997; Feske, Perry, Chambless, Renneberg, & Goldstein, 1996), despite greater improvement early in the treatment process in one study (Huppert et al., 2008). As with individuals meeting criteria for social anxiety disorder, clients with APD may require prolonged treatment to achieve an optimal outcome.

OVERVIEW OF THE TREATMENT OUTCOME LITERATURE

Researchers have investigated the efficacy of a broad range of treatments for social anxiety disorder, including social skills training, cognitive therapy, relaxation training, exposure, interpersonal psychotherapy, dynamically oriented supportive psychotherapy, and various pharmacotherapies. This review examines only studies that have tested the efficacy of combined exposure and cognitive treatment. The combination of exposure and cognitive restructuring has been the most frequently studied form of psychosocial intervention for social anxiety disorder and represents the focus of the intervention described in this chapter (broader reviews of the treatment outcome literature are provided by Pontoski, Heimberg, Turk, & Coles, 2010, and Wong, Gordon, & Heimberg, 2012).

Researchers have often sought to demonstrate that the efficacy of exposure is improved by the addition of cognitive restructuring. The results of these efforts have been mixed. A meta-analysis conducted by Powers, Sigmarsson, and Emmelkamp (2008) revealed no greater benefit from the addition of cognitive restructuring to exposure. However, a more recent meta-analysis by Ougrin (2011) demonstrated a significant difference in favor of this combination, assessed either immediately after treatment or at follow-up assessments. This difference was evident in the treatment of social anxiety disorder, but not in the treatment of other anxiety disorders.

Heimberg, Dodge, and colleagues (1990) conducted the first controlled trial of his group treatment for social anxiety disorder, which comprised integrated exposure, cognitive restructuring, and homework assignments (i.e., cognitive-behavioral group therapy [CBGT]). This treatment was compared to an attention control treatment that comprised education about social anxiety disorder and nondirective supportive group therapy. CBGT participants reported less anxiety during an individualized behavioral test and were more likely than control participants to be rated as improved by a clinical assessor. A 5-year follow-up of a subset of participants from the original sample indicated that individuals who had received CBGT were more likely than comparable attention control participants to maintain their gains (Heimberg, Salzman, Holt, & Blendell, 1993).

In a component analysis of CBGT, Hope, Heimberg, and Bruch (1995) reported that CBGT and exposure alone were both more effective than a waiting-list control. At posttest, there was some evidence that the exposure-alone condition was more effective than CBGT, but these differences disappeared at 6-month follow-up.

In a two-site study, 133 clients were randomly assigned to receive CBGT, the monoamine oxidase inhibitor phenelzine, pill placebo, or the attention control psychotherapy developed by Heimberg, Dodge, and colleagues (1990; Heimberg et al., 1998). At posttest, independent assessors classified 21 of 28 CBGT completers (75%; 58% of the intent-to-treat [ITT] sample) and 20 of 26 phenelzine completers (77%; 65% of the ITT sample) as treatment responders. The response rates for phenelzine and CBGT clients were significantly better than those for clients receiving pill placebo or the attention control psychotherapy. In the second phase of this study, clients who responded to CBGT or phenelzine were continued through an additional 6 months of maintenance treatment and a 6-month follow-up period (Liebowitz et al., 1999). At study's end, 50% of previously responding clients who received phenelzine relapsed, compared to only 17% of clients who received CBGT.

Another study examined the efficacy of CBGT alone, versus phenelzine, and in combination with phenelzine (Blanco et al., 2010). Response rates at posttest suggested that combined treatment was superior to placebo, but that CBGT and phenelzine alone did not differ from each other, from combined treatment, or from placebo. However, additional examination suggested that phenelzine was often superior to CBGT in these short-term analyses, not inconsistent with the findings of Heimberg and colleagues (1998).

Two studies compared CBGT to mindfulness and acceptance-based treatments. Koszyski, Benger, Shilk, and Bradwejn (2007) compared CBGT to mindfulness-based stress reduction (MBSR; Kabat-Zinn, 1990). In this study, MBSR comprised eight 2.5-hour group sessions and one full-day meditation retreat. Both treatments produced improvements in mood, functioning, and quality of life; however, CBGT was associated with significantly greater reductions in self- and clinician-rated social anxiety, as well as higher rates of response and remission. Piet, Hougaard, Hecksher, and Rosenberg (2010) compared CBGT to mindfulness-based cognitive therapy (MBCT; Segal, Williams, & Teasdale, 2002) in socially anxious young adults ages 18–25. Using a crossover design, participants were randomly assigned to eight 2-hour group sessions of MBCT and twelve 2-hour sessions of CBGT. MBCT produced moderate effects ($d = 0.78$), which were lower but not significantly different from those produced by CBGT ($d = 1.15$), and participants continued to improve during the 6-month follow-up period.

A waiting-list controlled study of the individually administered version of this treatment was recently completed (Ledley et al., 2009). The individual cognitive-behavioral treatment consistently outperformed the waiting list on both self-report and clinician-administered measures of social anxiety. Effect sizes were large, and little dropout occurred. These positive findings were essentially replicated by Goldin and colleagues (2012) in an independent sample.

Controlled trials of Clark's cognitive therapy (CT) for social anxiety disorder have also yielded large effect sizes and appear promising. CT includes exposure and cognitive restructuring, with emphasis on identifying and eliminating safety behaviors. In CT, the therapist and patient create a personalized conceptualization of the factors serving to maintain the patient's social anxiety (e.g., patient's idiosyncratic thoughts, images, safety behaviors, and attentional strategies). Throughout therapy, the patient's negatively distorted self-representations are modified using video feedback, in which predicted performance is compared to actual performance. Additionally, the therapist encourages direction of attention away from aversive internal experiences (i.e., symptoms of anxiety), toward the task at hand. CT has demonstrated efficacy for individuals with social anxiety disorder (Clark et al., 2003; 2006), as well as superiority to interpersonal therapy (Stangier, Schramm, Heidenreich, Berger, & Clark, 2011). Gains made during CT were maintained when assessed after 5 years (Mörtberg, Clark, & Bejerot, 2011).

In summary, it appears that a combined package of exposure and cognitive restructuring is an effective intervention for social anxiety disorder. Whether it is more effective than exposure alone is more difficult to determine given the limited number of studies and mixed results. However, more important to practitioners is the mounting evidence that three out of four clients with social anxiety disorder are likely to realize clinically significant change after a reasonably intensive trial of combined exposure and cognitive restructuring.

AN INTEGRATED COGNITIVE-BEHAVIORAL MODEL OF SOCIAL ANXIETY DISORDER

Rapee and Heimberg's (1997) development of an integrated cognitive-behavioral model that describes how individuals with social anxiety disorder process information when confronted with a situation that holds the potential for negative evaluation has been recently updated by Heimberg, Brozovich, and Rapee (2010). The process begins when the socially anxious individual is in the presence of an audience. The term "audience" captures the sense that socially anxious individuals have of being "on stage" in the presence of others, whether the situation is a speech, social interaction, or another situation in which the person may be observed by others. Socially anxious persons perceive this audience as inherently critical (e.g., Leary, Kowalski, & Campbell, 1988) and as having standards that they are unlikely to meet (e.g., Wallace & Alden, 1991).

In the presence of an audience, socially anxious individuals construct a mental representation of how they appear to other people. This mental representation of the self comprises negative and distorted images in which the self is viewed from an observer perspective (Hackmann, Surawy, & Clark, 1998). These images have been found to be related to memories of early adverse social events, such as being bullied (Hackmann, Clark, & McManus, 2000). For example, one client described being mercilessly teased by her peers as a young adolescent for being tall and skinny. Although at the time of treatment she was an attractive adult, she still described her appearance as "gangly," "awkward," and "ugly." Research has also shown that socially anxious individuals rate their own social behavior more harshly than do objective observers (Rapee & Lim, 1992; Stopa & Clark, 1993) and overestimate the visibility of their anxiety relative to ratings by objective observers (Bruch, Gorsky, Collins, & Berger, 1989; Norton & Hope, 2001). Undoubtedly, these beliefs negatively impact their image of how they are coming across to others. The image of the self is further influenced by internal cues (e.g., somatic sensations of perspiration may produce images of sweat dripping down one's face) and external cues such as others' reactions (e.g., someone glancing at one's clothing and frowning might lead to images of appearing disheveled).

Beliefs that they are unacceptable to other people, that other people are inherently critical, and that the evaluation of others is extremely important motivate individuals with social anxiety disorder to be hypervigilant for early indications of disapproval from others (e.g., frowns, yawns) and aspects of their own behavior or appearance that might elicit negative evaluation from others (e.g., making an inane comment, not being dressed appropriately, visibly shaking). The division of attentional resources among external social threats, the (distorted) mental representation of the self as seen by others, and the demands of the current social task *may* result in actual performance deficits, which may then elicit actual negative social feedback. In effect, socially anxious persons operate within the equivalent of a multiple-task paradigm, which increases the probability of disrupted social performance (MacLeod & Mathews, 1991). Therefore, complex social tasks are more likely than less complex tasks to result in poorer performance, due to limited processing resources.

Persons with social anxiety disorder also attempt to predict the standards that the audience holds for them in the situation. Characteristics of the audience (e.g., importance, attractiveness) and features of the situation (e.g., whether it is formal or informal) influence the projected standards of the audience. Individuals with social anxiety disorder then attempt to judge the extent to which their current mental representation of their appearance and behavior matches the predicted standards of the audience. Of course, given the negative bias present in their mental self-representation, they are likely to conclude that they are falling short of the audience's expectations, and painful outcomes such as loss of social status and rejection are likely follow. Negative predictions result in cognitive, behavioral, and physiological symptoms of anxiety that eventually feed back into the negatively biased mental representation of the self as seen by others and perpetuate the cycle of anxiety.

A significant recent change to the model addresses what is thought to be the core fear in social anxiety disorder, typically characterized as a fear of negative evaluation. However, recent research suggests that socially anxious individuals fear *any* evaluation, whether it is negative or positive (e.g., Weeks, Heimberg, Rodebaugh, & Norton, 2008). Fear of positive evaluation (FPE) may arise when successful social performance activates the belief that others will expect continued success in future social interactions, but the person doubts his/her ability to meet these increased expectations. However, the construct of FPE is derived from an evolutionary model of social anxiety disorder, which posits that socially anxious individuals work to maintain their (low) social status by not drawing attention to themselves (Gilbert, 2001). In this way, they neither risk losing status nor have to engage in conflict with more powerful others to defend any elevated social status they may have achieved. The update to the Rapee–Heimberg model reflects this line of thinking, and the model now posits that socially anxious persons fear and attend to cues of evaluation, regardless of valence. The model as updated by Heimberg and colleagues (2010) is presented in Figure 3.1. See the chapter in that book for a fuller explication of revisions to the original model.

TREATMENT RATIONALE FROM A COGNITIVE-BEHAVIORAL PERSPECTIVE

The heart of our approach to treatment is the integration of exposure and cognitive restructuring (Heimberg & Becker, 2002; Hope, Heimberg, & Turk, 2010a, 2010b). Exposure is beneficial for several reasons that are communicated to the client. One of the most important aspects of exposure is the opportunity to test dysfunctional beliefs (e.g., "I will get too anxious to finish

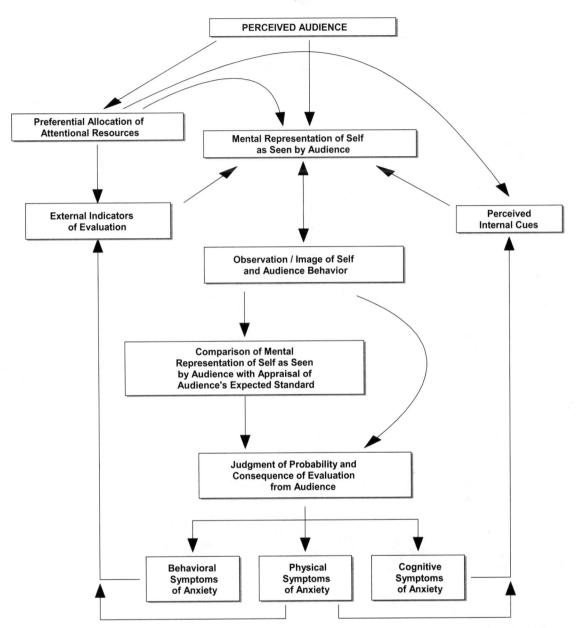

FIGURE 3.1. An updated cognitive-behavioral model of social anxiety disorder. From Heimberg, Brozovich, and Rapee (2010, Figure 15.2, p. 416). Copyright 2010 by Elsevier Limited. Reprinted by permission.

the speech") and to generate more realistic ways of understanding the self and others (e.g., "I can continue the speech even if I am anxious"). Exposure also allows clients to experience the natural anxiety reduction that comes with staying in a feared situation for a prolonged period of time on several occasions (i.e., habituation). Last, exposure allows clients to practice long-avoided behavioral skills (e.g., asking someone for a date, being assertive) and to engage in behaviors consistent with their personal goals (e.g., engaging in small talk with new people that may lead to friendships in the future).

Cognitive restructuring is also important for several reasons communicated to clients. Clients learn to treat their anxiety-provoking thoughts and beliefs as hypotheses and to explore whether there are more helpful or realistic ways of viewing the situation, the self, and others. As clients come to view social situations as less threatening, they are often more willing to confront those situations in exposures. Furthermore, addressing dysfunctional cognitions often frees up attentional resources that can be used to increase focus on the social task at hand and potentially improve performance. Additionally, cognitive restructuring may help clients to take credit for successes and cope with disappointments after exposures. The use of cognitive skills to diffuse postevent processing may be especially important given that rumination following one anxiety-provoking event is associated with greater initial anxiety prior to confronting another anxiety-provoking event (for a review, see Brozovich & Heimberg, 2008). Last, as clients' cognitive assessments of the danger inherent in social situations become more realistic, their physiological symptoms of anxiety often diminish as well.

In-session exposures, with cognitive restructuring occurring before, during, and after each exposure, are particularly crucial. With the gentle encouragement and emotional support of the therapist, clients are often willing to engage in behaviors in session that they have avoided outside of session for many years. Successful in-session exposures can provide clients with the confidence and motivation to try out these behaviors in the real world. In-session exposures may also be more easily graduated than *in vivo* exposures. For example, a client who is terrified of formal public speaking might do an initial in-session exposure that comprises reading an article aloud from a magazine while sitting down. The next exposure might involve standing up while reading the article aloud, then taking questions from a small audience. In-session exposures also provide the therapist with the opportunity to teach clients about the principles of effective exposure, such as staying in a feared social situation for a prolonged period of time without avoiding, even if anxiety escalates. In-session exposures also allow the therapist to see firsthand any subtle avoidance behaviors (i.e., safety behaviors) that the client may employ to manage anxiety. For example, a client who fears that other people might reject him if they got to know him personally may assail a conversation partner with questions and not reveal any personal information. A client who is afraid of the reaction of others to her speech might never look up from her notes, so that she never has to see any bored or critical faces (and, of course, also never has a chance to see any interested or approving faces). As noted by Clark and Wells (1995), such safety behaviors are essentially attempts to avoid feared outcomes, but they may have the unintended effect of making individuals appear socially awkward and increase the likelihood of negative reactions from others. Furthermore, clients do not learn that they might have managed the social situation as well, if not better, without engaging in safety behaviors. In-session exposures provide the therapist with the opportunity to point out these behaviors and to set goals for the next exposure that involve fully confronting the feared situation (e.g., looking at the audience during the speech, revealing personal information during a conversation). In-session exposures also provide the opportunity for clients to receive direct feedback on their social performance in a way that is often not possible in real life. For example, a client who believes that she trembles so much during public speaking that others pity her can ask her exposure audience how noticeable the trembling was and what they thought of her (rarely will an audience reply that an anxious person was pitied). Last, in-session exposures provide the opportunity for the therapist to assist clients in applying cognitive restructuring skills to an actual anxiety-provoking situation. Once in-session exposures begin, homework involves confronting similar situations outside of session. As with in-session exposures, clients are asked to engage in cognitive restructuring activities before, during, and after each *in vivo* exposure.

TREATMENT-RELATED VARIABLES

Group versus Individual Treatment

Treatment of social anxiety disorder has often been conducted in a group format (e.g., Blanco et al., 2010;

Heimberg, Dodge, et al., 1990; Heimberg et al., 1998), which has been conceptualized as having a number of advantages over the individual format. It provides opportunities for vicarious learning, support from others with similar problems, the availability of multiple role-play partners, informal exposure stemming from group participation, and a range of people to provide evidence to counter distorted thinking (Heimberg & Becker, 2002; Sank & Shaffer, 1984). Nevertheless, the group format has a number of potential disadvantages as well. Treatment cannot begin until a group of approximately six clients has been assembled, which means that the first few individuals joining the group may have to wait for an extended period before starting treatment. Some of these individuals lose motivation and drop out before the group begins. Group treatment also provides less flexibility in making up missed sessions. Although group treatment provides opportunities for vicarious learning, this benefit may be offset by the reduced time available for the idiosyncratic needs of each client. Clinically, some clients appear to get discouraged and lose motivation when they see other group members progressing at a more rapid pace than themselves. Additionally, even when efforts are made to screen potential group members, a group may include a client who is domineering, aggressive, or otherwise difficult to manage, and may have a negative impact on the group. Last, some individuals never fully habituate to the group setting, and their anxiety may interfere with their ability to process information during sessions.

Little available data speak to the issue of whether individual or group therapy provides better outcomes. In their meta-analysis, Powers and colleagues (2008) reported that group and individual cognitive-behavioral interventions for social anxiety disorder produced similar effect sizes, but another meta-analysis based on a small sample of studies (Aderka, 2009) suggested a modest advantage for individual treatment. Group and individual formats have rarely been compared within the same study. Scholing and Emmelkamp (1993) examined various combinations of exposure and cognitive restructuring delivered in group or individual formats and found no clear advantage for either treatment modality. Similarly, Wlazlo, Schroeder-Hartwig, Hand, Kaiser, and Münchau (1990) found no differences in outcome between group and individual exposure treatment. One study did find that an individual version of CBT for social anxiety disorder was superior to the group version, and that both formats were superior to a waiting list (Stangier, Heidenreich, Peitz, Lauterbach,

& Clark, 2003). However, the data do not suggest a clear advantage for either modality in the treatment of social anxiety disorder.

Heimberg and Becker (2002) provide a description of CBGT for social anxiety disorder. This chapter provides a description of the individual version of this treatment, which has been the focus of our attention in recent years (see also Hope et al., 2010a; 2010b).

Appropriate Clients

In treatment studies to date, social anxiety disorder has been the primary diagnosis of the participants. As previously discussed, social anxiety disorder is often comorbid with other disorders (W. J. Magee et al., 1996; Schneier et al., 1992). In such cases, the clinician and client need to reach a joint decision that social anxiety will be the focus of treatment for a specified period of time (e.g., 16 weeks). Clinically, it is important to clarify this issue prior to beginning treatment because some clients may express a desire to switch the focus of treatment to another problem area when it is time to begin exposures. In general, our policy is to remind the client of the original treatment contract and goals, and to encourage him/her to "avoid avoidance." In some cases, the best clinical decision is to change the focus of treatment due to changes in the client's life circumstances or symptoms. Nevertheless, we are especially wary of altering the treatment plan when the client's desire to change the focus of treatment coincides with the initiation of exposures. Therapists without a strong background in CBT or exposure therapy may be at risk for changing the focus of treatment too readily, partially due to their own discomfort with conducting in-session exposures. Sometimes a compromise can be reached in which exposures remain in the treatment plan but some session time is set aside to deal with other issues.

Appropriate Therapists

The ideal therapist has a strong background in the theoretical underpinnings of CBT for anxiety disorders, experience conducting exposures, good basic therapy skills, and experience with social anxiety in particular. Little is known about the effectiveness of manualized treatments when implemented by clinicians without extensive training in the manual's theoretical underpinnings and procedures (Chambless & Ollendick, 2001), although data are accumulating to suggest that the treatments described here or similar ones retain their efficacy when implemented in community settings (Gaston, Abbott, Rapee, & Neary, 2006; Lincoln et al., 2003; McEvoy, 2007; McEvoy, Nathan, Rapee, & Campbell, 2012). Our clinical experience suggests that with good supervision, this treatment can be successfully implemented by novice therapists seeing their very first clients (in fact, the client presented later was treated by L. Magee, who at the time was a novice therapist) and experienced therapists with a theoretical orientation other than a cognitive-behavioral one. Experienced clinicians with a good cognitive-behavioral background are likely to do quite well working independently with this manualized treatment. Moreover, our client workbook (Hope et al., 2010a) and therapist guide (Hope et al., 2010b) were designed with the intention of being sufficiently detailed to allow therapists with a wide variety of backgrounds to provide this treatment, although supervision and/or consultation with an experienced cognitive-behavioral therapist on the first few cases and the more complex cases would be beneficial.

Medication and CBT for Social Anxiety Disorder

Many clients are already taking psychotropic medications when they present for therapy. Some take medication to control their social anxiety, whereas others take medication for comorbid conditions. We do not require clients to discontinue medications prior to starting CBT (unless dictated by a specific research protocol). However, we do ask clients to stabilize their dosage before starting treatment and to refrain from changing their dosage or trying any new medications during treatment. Clinically, we want clients to attribute positive changes in their symptoms to the work they are doing in therapy rather than to changes in their medication regimen. Individuals who take medication on an as-needed basis are asked to refrain from doing so before sessions or exposure homework assignments. The same request is made of individuals who use nonprescription drugs, alcohol, or other substances to control their anxiety.

PRETREATMENT ASSESSMENT AND PREPARATION FOR TREATMENT

Assessment should play an integral part in diagnosis, case conceptualization, treatment planning, and termination decisions. Although administering all of the measures presented here is not practical in most clinical settings, we highly recommend administering a subset of the self-report and clinician-rated instruments described below, and a behavioral assessment, if at all possible (for a more thorough review of assessment of social anxiety disorder, see Heimberg & Turk, 2002).

Clinical Interview

The Anxiety Disorders Interview Schedule for DSM-IV (ADIS-IV; Brown, Di Nardo, & Barlow, 1994), the ADIS-IV—Lifetime Version (ADIS-IV-L; Di Nardo, Brown, & Barlow, 1994), as well as the ADIS for DSM-5 (ADIS-5-L; Brown, Di Nardo, & Barlow, 2013), provide a thorough diagnostic assessment of the anxiety disorders and include modules for mood disorders, substance use disorders, and disorders that overlap with anxiety disorders in clinical presentation (e.g., hypochondriasis, somatization disorder). There are screening questions for other major disorders (e.g., psychosis). A 0- to 8-point clinician's severity rating (CSR) designates the degree of distress and interference associated with each diagnosis. A CSR of 4 or higher suggests that the client meets diagnostic criteria. When multiple disorders receive a CSR of 4 or higher, the disorder receiving the highest CSR is designated as the principal diagnosis and the other disorders are designated as additional. In a major reliability study of the ADIS-IV-L, 362 individuals seeking treatment at an anxiety specialty clinic received two independent administrations of the ADIS-IV (Brown, Di Nardo, Lehman, & Campbell, 2001). Social anxiety disorder evidenced good reliability as a principal diagnosis (kappa = .77), as a clinical (principal or additional) diagnosis (kappa = .77), and as a past (lifetime) diagnosis (kappa = .72). The CSR for social anxiety disorder ($r = .80$) also evidenced good interrater reliability.

We routinely administer the ADIS during the first client visit. Semistructured interviews such as the ADIS assist with differential diagnosis and in providing systematic assessment for a broad range of comorbid conditions that may affect the course of treatment. Nevertheless, diagnostic interviews may be costly and time-consuming. Regardless of whether a semistructured or unstructured clinical interview is conducted, devoting time to a thorough and accurate diagnostic evaluation is crucial to appropriate treatment planning. Clients whose symptoms are better accounted for by another diagnosis may experience, among other things, little improvement with treatment targeting social anxiety, unnecessarily prolonged suffering as they go without the appropriate treatment, increased hopelessness, and financial hardship.

Self-Report Instruments

Self-report instruments are an important complement to the diagnostic interview. Clients may experience feelings of shame and embarrassment during a clinical interview and give descriptions of their problems that do not fully reflect the severity or pervasiveness of their social fear or avoidance. Furthermore, normative data on questionnaires allow the clinician to evaluate the severity of a client's symptoms relative to meaningful reference points. Importantly, pretreatment scores provide a baseline against which treatment progress can be assessed.

Measures of Social Anxiety

A number of questionnaires are available to assess social anxiety and avoidance. The Social Interaction Anxiety Scale (SIAS) and Social Phobia Scale (SPS) are commonly used companion measures designed specifically for the assessment of social anxiety disorder (Mattick & Clarke, 1998). The SIAS assesses fear of interacting in dyads and groups, and the SPS assesses fear of being observed by others (e.g., eating in front of others). In most published studies, the SIAS and SPS contain 20 items each. For each instrument, respondents rate how characteristic each statement is of them on a 5-point Likert-type scale (0, *Not at all*; 4, *Extremely*). Multiple studies suggest that the SIAS and SPS are reliable and valid measures, and sensitive to the effects of CBT (e.g., Brown et al., 1997; Cox, Ross, Swinson, & Direnfeld, 1998; Heimberg, Mueller, Holt, Hope, & Liebowitz, 1992; Ries et al., 1998). However, recent research suggests that the 17 straightforwardly worded items of the SIAS are more sensitive to the construct of social anxiety than the three reverse-scored items, which seem more related to the construct of extraversion (Rodebaugh, Woods, & Heimberg, 2007). A number of studies now support the use of the 17-item scale (e.g., Rodebaugh et al., 2011). Recently, even shorter forms of both instruments have been developed (Fergus, Valentiner, McGrath, Gier-Lonsway, & Kim, 2012; Kupper & Denollet, 2012; Peters, Sunderland, Andrews, Rapee, & Mattick, 2012), as has a brief instrument derived from a factor analysis of the pooled item set (Social Interaction Phobia Scale; Carleton et

al., 2009). However, it is premature at this time to suggest that it is time to set the originals aside in favor of recent variants.

Another commonly used instrument developed to assess social anxiety disorder, the Social Phobia and Anxiety Inventory (SPAI; Turner, Beidel, Dancu, & Stanley, 1989), comprises a Social Phobia subscale, an Agoraphobia subscale, and a derived Difference (or Total) score (i.e., Social Phobia–Agoraphobia subscales). The SPAI contains 45 items, 21 of which require multiple responses. For example, for the item that begins "I attempt to avoid social situations where there are .. .," the client separately rates how frequently he/she avoids situations involving strangers, authority figures, the opposite sex, and people in general. The client gives a total of 109 responses, making the administration and scoring of the SPAI relatively time-consuming. Despite the disadvantages imposed by the length of the scale, the quantity and specificity of information that it elicits can be quite helpful in case formulation and treatment planning.

The Social Phobia subscale assesses somatic, cognitive, and behavioral responses to a variety of interaction, performance, and observation situations. The Agoraphobia subscale assesses anxiety in situations commonly feared by individuals with panic disorder with agoraphobia (e.g., waiting in line). Respondents rate how frequently they feel anxious in each situation using a 7-point Likert-type scale (1, *Never*; 7, *Always*). The Difference score is intended to provide an index of social anxiety and avoidance distinct from the sometimes similar concerns of clients with agoraphobia. However, the very high correlation between the Difference score and the score of the Social Phobia subscale ($r = .91$) (Ries et al., 1998) suggests that there may be little benefit to this strategy. Multiple studies suggest that the SPAI is a reliable and valid instrument (e.g., Beidel, Turner, Stanley, & Dancu, 1989; Herbert, Bellack, & Hope, 1991; Turner et al., 1989), and sensitive to treatment-related change (e.g., Cox et al., 1998; Ries et al., 1998; Taylor, Woody, McLean, & Koch, 1997).

Another scale that may prove to be quite useful is the 17-item Social Phobia Inventory, also known as the SPIN (Antony, Coons, McCabe, Ashbaugh, & Swinson, 2006; Connor et al., 2000), which has demonstrated good reliability, significant correlations with related measures, and the ability to discriminate between clients with social anxiety disorder and those with other anxiety disorders. A three-item version of the SPIN, the Mini-SPIN, has also shown substantial utility as a screening device for social anxiety disorder in both general health care (Connor, Kobak, Churchill, Katzelnick, & Davidson, 2001) and anxiety specialty clinic (Weeks, Spokas, & Heimberg, 2007) settings.

Although developed and validated with college students prior to the inclusion of social anxiety disorder in the DSM, the original Fear of Negative Evaluation scale (FNE; Watson & Friend, 1969) and the brief version of the scale (BFNE; Leary, 1983) continue to be widely used because they target a core construct of the disorder. The FNE comprises 30 items and employs a true–false format. In treatment studies, changes on the FNE have been found to predict end-state functioning (e.g., Mattick & Peters, 1988). The FNE appears to be sensitive to the effects of treatment, although changes are typically small in magnitude (Heimberg, 1994). The BFNE contains 12 items, uses a 5-point Likert-type format (1, *Not at all characteristic of me*; 5, *Extremely characteristic of me*), and correlates highly with the original scale ($r = .96$) (Leary, 1983). In a recent study by Rodebaugh and colleagues (2004) that utilized a large sample of undergraduates, the BFNE was more sensitive than the FNE to differing degrees of fear of negative evaluation. A study by Weeks and colleagues (2005) that utilized a large sample of clients with social anxiety disorder found that the BFNE had high internal consistency, correlated with measures of social anxiety, showed good discriminant validity, and was sensitive to the effects of CBT. Both of these studies suggest quite compellingly that, similar to the SIAS, the reverse-scored items of the BFNE may detract from its validity, and we now score only the straightforwardly worded items. Others have taken a similar approach by rewording the reverse-scored items to be consistent with the straightforwardly worded items (e.g., Collins, Westra, Dozois, & Stewart, 2005).

The Social Anxiety Session Change Index (SASCI; Hayes, Miller, Hope, Heimberg, & Juster, 2008) was developed for the assessment of session-by-session change in the treatment of social anxiety disorder. Clients use a 7-point Likert-type scale to indicate how much they have changed since the beginning of therapy on four dimensions: anxiety, avoidance, concern about humiliation and embarrassment, and interference. A total score of 16 indicates no change since the beginning of treatment. Scores of 4–15 indicate improvement, whereas scores of 17–28 indicate deterioration. The internal consistency of the SASCI across sessions ranged from .84 to .94 across sessions ($M = .89$) in the study by Hayes and colleagues (2008). Change on the

SASCI was related to change in fear of negative evaluation and to clinician-rated improvement, but not to ratings of anxiety sensitivity or depression. The use of the SASCI and the BFNE as session-by-session measures is demonstrated in the case study reported later in this chapter.

Other Self-Report Measures

In addition to measures targeting social anxiety, we administer questionnaires assessing other constructs relevant to case conceptualization and treatment outcome. We routinely administer the Beck Depression Inventory–II (BDI-II; A. T. Beck, Steer, & Brown, 1996), which assesses symptoms of depression, including the affective, cognitive, behavioral, somatic, and motivational components, as well as suicidal wishes. We also use the Liebowitz Self-Rated Disability Scale (Schneier et al., 1994), which assesses impairment across 11 domains (e.g., school, work, alcohol abuse), and the Quality of Life Inventory (Frisch, 1994), which assesses the client's overall sense of well-being and satisfaction with life.

Feedback and Treatment Contract Interview

At the session following the intake session, the interviewer reviews assessment data with the client, explains diagnoses, answers questions, and offers treatment recommendations. For clients with comorbid diagnoses, the benefits of initially making social anxiety the primary focus of treatment for 12–16 weekly sessions is discussed, as noted earlier. Last, clients are assured that the severity of their social anxiety symptoms and any comorbid conditions will be reassessed following this initial course of treatment and, if necessary, additional treatment recommendations will be made at that time. Additional assessments may be conducted at this visit, or clients may be scheduled for one additional session to conduct further assessments before treatment formally begins. The additional assessments may include clinician-administered measures of social anxiety and behavior tests.

Clinician-Administered Measures of Social Anxiety

The two most commonly used clinician-administered measures of social anxiety are the Liebowitz Social Anxiety Scale (LSAS; Liebowitz, 1987) and the Brief

Social Phobia Scale (BSPS; Davidson et al., 1991, 1997). We routinely utilize the LSAS, so we describe it here. This measure is completed at the second clinic visit largely to avoid making the initial intake session unduly lengthy. The LSAS separately evaluates Fear and Avoidance of 11 interaction (e.g., talking to people in authority) and 13 performance (e.g., working while being observed) situations using 4-point Likert-type scales.

Summing the Fear and Avoidance ratings for all 24 items yields an index of overall severity. The LSAS has been shown to have good reliability and convergent/discriminant validity (e.g., Cox et al., 1998; Heimberg et al., 1999). It discriminates well between clients with social anxiety disorder and those with generalized anxiety disorder (Heimberg & Holaway, 2007). It has also demonstrated sensitivity to cognitive-behavioral and pharmacological treatment of social anxiety disorder (e.g., Blanco et al., 2010; Heimberg et al., 1998). When the LSAS is accompanied by detailed instructions, it appears that it also has good reliability and validity as a self-report instrument (Fresco et al., 2001; Rytwinski et al., 2009).

Behavioral Assessment

Behavior tests, or role plays of social situations relevant to the client, can be a very useful addition to the self-report and clinician-administered measures described here. Although these tests may be quite anxiety-provoking for the client, the information obtained during a behavior test is unique and important in several ways. Individuals with social anxiety disorder are likely to describe their social behavior as inadequate (e.g., Rapee & Lim, 1992; Stopa & Clark, 1993) and their anxiety as highly visible to others (e.g., Norton & Hope, 2001). However, behavior tests often demonstrate that these reports are largely inaccurate and are essentially examples of distorted beliefs. Furthermore, level of anxiety and quality of performance exhibited by a client during behavior tests may be used to calibrate the difficulty of exposures and increase the likelihood that the therapist creates a first exposure that provides both a challenge and a successful experience for the client.

During behavior tests, the clinician may ask for anxiety ratings before, at several points during, and after the role play. Other assessments, such as asking clients to rate the quality of their performance or list the thoughts they had during the role play, are easily incorporated. Affordable ambulatory physiological assessment de-vices, such as pulse monitors, are available and add a useful dimension. The clinician can choose to test the limits of a client's ability to perform when anxious by asking him/her to remain in the situation for a certain period of time (typically 4–5 minutes). On the other hand, the clinician may give the client explicit permission to stop (e.g., Ries et al., 1998) when the anxiety is excessive, and latency to escape the situation becomes a measure of avoidance.

Behavior tests may either be standardized or individualized. Standardized role plays allow for the observation of differences across patients for a particular task. Commonly used tasks include a conversation with a same-sex stranger, a conversation with an opposite-sex stranger, a conversation with two or more people, and a speech to a small audience. In contrast, the advantage of individualized behavior tests is that they may be designed more precisely to target idiosyncratic fears. For example, a client with a fear of displaying a hand tremor when eating in front of others may experience little anxiety during a one-on-one conversation. However, if that client is asked to engage in a one-on-one conversation while eating a bowl of soup, his or her anxiety is more likely to be activated.

INDIVIDUAL CBT FOR SOCIAL ANXIETY DISORDER

Principles and Logistics

For our studies on individual treatment of social anxiety disorder, we have established guidelines to which our therapists must adhere (Hope et al., 2010b). One issue facing manualized treatments is that it is unclear to what extent one may take liberties with how the treatment is carried out and still expect outcomes similar to those obtained during efficacy studies. Therefore, although we recognize that this treatment may be applied more flexibly in clinical settings, we present these guidelines to help therapists understand the treatment as it has been most thoroughly studied.

The treatment comprises 16 weekly 1-hour sessions within a period of 16–20 weeks. Although completing 16 sessions within 16 weeks might be ideal, up to 20 weeks are allowed to take into consideration sessions missed due to illness, vacations, holidays, and so forth. Taking longer than 20 weeks to complete 16 sessions may compromise the momentum of therapy. The two to three pretreatment sessions described earlier, as well as posttreatment assessment and feedback sessions, are not counted as part of the 16-session treatment phase.

Our individual treatment requires that the client use a workbook (Hope et al., 2010a) as he/she works with the therapist during each session and for homework assignments. This workbook comprises 13 chapters, but the treatment program does not follow a one-chapter-per-session format. Rather, treatment is divided into five segments, described below, and the therapist has flexibility in terms of the pace and, to some extent, the content of these segments. We ask clients to read assigned chapters before coming to the session.

Clients are asked to bring their workbook to every session. Therapists typically bring their own copy of the workbook and/or a copy of the therapist guide to session as well. The therapist also makes sure that there is something to write on that therapist and client can look at together during the session. In our clinic, a newsprint easel or a dry-erase board mounted to the wall is typically used (for ease, we refer to the use of an easel hereafter). However, at times, we have also just pulled two chairs side by side, so that both therapist and client can write on and view the same piece of paper on a clipboard. Importantly, every session introduces key concepts that are written down (e.g., a therapist may draw a continuum of anxiety in Session 1; client automatic thoughts and rational responses are always recorded). Writing things down during session helps clients better to track and process the information being covered and is a required component of the treatment.

The therapeutic relationship is actively fostered throughout treatment. As Kendall, Chu, Gifford, Hayes, and Nauta (1998) have pointed out, some critics assume that the therapeutic relationship is not considered relevant when a manual is utilized (see also Kendall, Gosch, Furr, & Sood, 2008). To the contrary, our therapist adherence manual (Hope, Van Dyke, Heimberg, Turk, & Fresco, 2002) includes explicit ratings of the therapeutic relationship within each segment of treatment. Therapists are rated on how well they engage in active listening, respond to verbal and nonverbal cues, facilitate the client's investment in treatment, and communicate support of and investment in the client. Additionally, therapists are expected to help clients to experience and deepen affect as appropriate to the situation at hand. For example, a therapist would be expected to help a client both to be open to the experience of anxiety during exposures and to process and grieve losses that are a consequence of many years of social avoidance. In other situations, the therapist would be

expected to help the client use uncomfortable feelings as cues for additional cognitive coping practice. For example, the therapist would help a client who experiences a deep sense of shame after making a small social mistake (e.g., spilling a drink, calling someone by the wrong name) to engage in cognitive restructuring to change the meaning of the event eliciting such emotions. Therapists are actively supervised on these aspects of treatment, and not attending to the therapeutic relationship or appropriately responding to what is going on in session is considered a serious failure to follow protocol.

Recent data suggest that the therapeutic relationship is indeed related to successful outcomes in our protocol (Hayes, Hope, Van Dyke, & Heimberg, 2007). Clients' ratings of the therapeutic alliance were positively related to their perceptions of session helpfulness. Interestingly, the relationship between the therapeutic alliance and anxiety reduction during in-session exposures was curvilinear; that is, when ratings of the alliance were higher or lower, clients showed less anxiety reduction than when the ratings of the alliance were moderate. The effect for low ratings of the alliance may not require explanation, but we have conjectured that if the client feels too comfortable with the therapist, then this may possibly interfere with anxiety evocation during exposures and thereby, emotional processing. Maintaining the "right" therapeutic alliance is important in CBT for social anxiety disorder (Hayes et al., 2007).

Therapists are also expected to engage in efficient time management. Our therapist adherence manual rates therapists' ability to cover required topics flexibly, without rushing or boring the client by belaboring various points (Hope et al., 2002). Two types of problems that tend to crop up with regard to time management may in turn negatively impact the therapeutic relationship. Some therapists fall into the trap of turning each session into a psychoeducational lecture, and this tendency may be aggravated if the therapist is working with a client who is very quiet in the early sessions. The primary recommendation in this situation is to ask open-ended questions that prompt the client to relate his/her personal experiences to the material. The client's verbalizations in response to these questions are then reinforced through the use of active listening skills, which elicit more client verbalizations. The other trap into which some therapists fall is allowing the client to dominate the session with long, detailed stories about experiences with social anxiety. In some cases, the therapist may have inadvertently taught the client to lead the session in this way, by indiscriminately using active listening skills and nonverbal cues, even when the client is discussing tangential or repetitive material. In other cases, clients may be accustomed to dominating sessions through prior experiences with traditional talk therapy, or they may even intentionally attempt to dominate the session to avoid difficult material, particularly in-session exposures. In this situation, gentle verbal redirection is required. In some cases, a straightforward discussion of time management issues and negotiation of session time may be beneficial.

Last, we want to emphasize our belief that manualized treatments such as this one do not represent an inflexible set of procedures applied indiscriminately to all clients. Rather, we expect therapists to develop an individualized conceptualization of each client's particular presenting problem, which is continually refined over the course of treatment and incorporates the unique characteristics of the client (e.g., cultural group, sex, educational background). Treatment procedures are then tailored to address the unique aspects of each case.

Segment 1: Psychoeducation

Segment 1 covers the material in Chapters 1–4 of the client workbook (Hope et al., 2010a). Establishing a good working relationship is a critical goal for this segment of therapy. If the therapist was not also the initial interviewer, three to four sessions are typically needed for the psychoeducation segment to allow adequate attention to building rapport. If a good working alliance has been established during the course of the initial assessment and if the client is especially bright and motivated, it may be possible to cover two chapters per session, finishing this portion of treatment in as little as 2 weeks. Therapists should not assign more than two chapters per week at any point in therapy because clients are unlikely to process the material fully and make the most of the associated exercises and self-monitoring homework.

One or two chapters are assigned as homework at the end of each session. Each chapter includes a variety of forms that the client attempts to complete as well. At the beginning of the next session, the therapist asks the client for reactions to and questions about the readings, and therapist and client review corresponding forms completed by the client. If the client has not made an attempt to complete a form, it is completed at the beginning of the session during homework review.

Therapists are required to review certain topics from each chapter in the client workbook in session; other topics are optional depending on the needs of the individual client. For Chapter 1, the therapist must review two topics: (1) normal versus problematic social anxiety, and (2) the investment that treatment will require. The discussion of normal and problematic social anxiety conveys to the client that social anxiety exists along a continuum, with some people rarely experiencing any social anxiety, other people frequently experiencing intense social anxiety, and most people falling somewhere between these extremes. People who fall in the middle of the continuum experience social anxiety in some situations, such as a first date or a job interview, but the anxiety is typically manageable and decreases as the person remains in the situation. Factors such as intensity and duration of anxiety before and during social situations, the number of situations eliciting anxiety, and the degree of life impairment differentiate between normal social anxiety and problematic social anxiety for which a diagnosis may be assigned. By asking what types of situations elicit social anxiety for many people and what purpose social anxiety might serve, the therapist can engage the client in illustrating the notion that social anxiety has an adaptive value (e.g., caring about what other people think might cause anxiety, but it also helps people to treat each other more kindly). A therapist typically uses this opportunity to discuss what the client should expect in terms of treatment outcome. First, the therapist points out that social anxiety is part of the human condition; thus, it is impossible to remove it completely, even if this were a desirable goal. Total freedom from social anxiety is not a reasonable expectation for treatment. However, it is reasonable to expect to move down the continuum from problematic levels of social anxiety to a level of social anxiety that is more typical of most people. Not all clients are willing to accept that social anxiety exists on a continuum or that it can have an adaptive value this early in treatment. This first session is merely an introduction to these concepts, and arguing with a client about these issues is likely to be unproductive. Rather, the therapist empathizes with the client's current worldview (e.g., "You feel you are either calm or extremely anxious, and that no middle ground is possible for you") but does not agree with it.

The discussion of the required investment in treatment involves instilling hope in the client that he/she will be able to make significant changes and conveying the time, effort, and emotional energy that treatment activities require. Research has shown that positive expectancies are associated with more favorable outcomes in CBT for social anxiety (Chambless et al., 1997; Safren, Heimberg, & Juster, 1997). The therapist shares with the client that in studies of individuals who completed CBT, approximately 75–80% were rated by independent clinical interviewers as having experienced meaningful reductions in their social anxiety (e.g., Heimberg et al., 1998). The therapist also emphasizes that attending sessions regularly, doing homework, being willing to experience anxiety during exposures, and being open to new ways of looking at the world, other people, and oneself are factors that substantially influence whether someone becomes a treatment responder, and that these factors are largely under the client's control. During this time, clients are encouraged to speak about their fears regarding treatment and their goals for a better life after treatment. Included is a motivational exercise in which the client is asked to generate pros and cons for working on his/her social anxiety and a similar list for not doing so as a means to increase commitment to the treatment process.

Next, the therapist reviews with the client the three components of anxiety presented in Chapter 2 of the client workbook (Hope et al., 2010a). Each of the three components of anxiety is described: (1) The physiological component comprises bodily reactions, such as a pounding heart; (2) the cognitive component comprises what a person thinks, such as "I look foolish"; and (3) the behavioral component comprises what a person does when he/she is anxious, such as avoiding eye contact. When presenting the behavioral component, the therapist emphasizes how escape and avoidance behaviors may reduce anxiety in the short term but lead to missed opportunities, a less satisfying life, and other negative feelings, such as guilt and shame, in the long term.

The therapist then helps the client to practice identifying each of these components with a hypothetical example. Over the years, we have found that initially using a hypothetical example is much more conducive to learning than starting with an example from the client's own experience. Issues such as fear of negative evaluation, defensiveness, anxiety, and lack of objectivity can result in a client having difficulty identifying the three components from a personal experience this early in treatment (e.g., "I wasn't thinking anything"). The default option for the therapist is simply to review the hypothetical examples from the workbook that illustrate the three components, but we generally recommend using a different hypothetical example in session

to give the client more practice. Alternatively, we use the example from the group treatment version (Heimberg & Becker, 2002), in which the client is asked to imagine a person waiting in the lobby to interview for a job that is extremely attractive in terms of responsibilities, pay, and hours. The client is told that the person is feeling anxious about the interview and then is asked what that person might be experiencing as he/she anxiously waits to be called in to the office. Using the easel, the therapist writes the client's responses under the appropriate heading (e.g., "feeling nauseous" is written under "Physiological Component"). After classifying the client's spontaneous responses, the therapist then asks questions to elicit several examples of each of the three components (e.g., "Might the person have any thoughts relating to her sweaty palms? What might she say to herself about that?"). The therapist makes an effort to draw out how each of the three components interacts with the others, resulting in an escalating spiral of anxiety (e.g., sweaty palms might lead to the thought "The interviewer will think I am anxious," which might lead to a behavior of wiping sweaty hands on one's suit). The therapist concludes that treatment involves learning ways to disrupt this spiral of anxiety. Assuming that the client does reasonably well with this exercise, the therapist then helps the client to repeat the exercise with a recent, personal experience of social anxiety. At this point in therapy, the therapist makes no effort to help the client to challenge anxiety-provoking cognitions, only to identify the three components of anxiety and to understand how they interact with each other. In addition to readings from the workbook, the client is given the homework assignment of identifying all three components of anxiety experienced in a social situation during the week.

Referring to the material covered in Chapter 3 of the client workbook, the therapist teaches the client how to use the Subjective Units of Discomfort Scale (SUDS; Wolpe & Lazarus, 1966) and construct a fear and avoidance hierarchy. The assignment from the previous week is repeated here and again over the next few sessions to solidify learning in this important domain, and weekly assessment of progress using the SASCI is initiated.

Next, the therapist describes for the client factors that are thought to be related to the development of problematic social anxiety, which are presented in Chapter 4 of the workbook. The therapist tells the client that research suggests that genetics plays a role in the etiology of social anxiety disorder. The therapist emphasizes that what is inherited is probably a tendency to be a sensitive and emotionally reactive individual rather than a gene that inevitably results in social anxiety (Barlow, 2002). This inherited sensitivity might not be at all problematic, and it may even be a good thing. For example, the person might be especially empathic toward others and have a greater capacity to experience joy, as well as anxiety. However, if a biologically sensitive individual is exposed to important social experiences during development and learns that others are threatening and hurtful, then the biological vulnerability may contribute to the development of problematic social anxiety. The therapist might inquire whether other family members seem to have problems with social anxiety or other types of anxiety, suggesting a genetic predisposition. The therapist then presents experiences within the family as another potential factor contributing to social anxiety. For example, a socially anxious mother might teach a child that the opinions of others are extremely important and that negative evaluation is to be avoided at all cost. Alternatively, a verbally abusive father might provide experiences that teach the child that other people are dangerous, and that avoidance is a good strategy for self-protection. Again, the therapist asks the client whether this information fits with his/her personal experiences. Last, the therapist describes how experiences outside of the family can similarly teach a person that others are a source of threat. For example, teasing by peers seems to be related to later social anxiety (Roth, Coles, & Heimberg, 2002). This discussion is facilitated by a homework assignment completed in advance of the session, in which the client answers a series of questions relevant to his/her own personal experiences of social anxiety and how they map onto these three major sources of input, and completes a pie chart indicating his/her belief in the relative importance of each. Throughout the discussion, the therapist emphasizes the idea that because social anxiety is largely learned through experience, it can be changed through experience.

This discussion of the etiology of social anxiety leads into a discussion of dysfunctional thoughts. Therapists might ask clients what lessons they learned about themselves and other people through a negative early-life social experience, such as being teased (e.g., "I learned that I don't fit in"). In this way, therapists educate clients about the origins of many of their automatic thoughts, which is important given that many clients view their tendency to have negative cognitions as a sign of inherent personal flaws rather than a logical consequence of their experiences. They then ask clients to think about how these dysfunctional ways of thinking color the kinds of thoughts and reactions they now have when confronting social situations (e.g., thoughts of not fitting in at parties, expecting to be made fun of by coworkers). At this point in therapy, clients are asked simply to consider the possibility that changing some of these automatic thinking biases might change the experience of anxiety. Therapists then set forth the rationale for primary interventions of cognitive restructuring, exposures, and homework.

Segment 2: Training in Cognitive Restructuring

Training in cognitive restructuring typically requires two to three sessions. The material is presented in Chapters 5 and 6 of the client workbook (Hope et al., 2010a). After three sessions, a small minority of clients may still be struggling to master the cognitive concepts due to factors such as low educational attainment and/or poor abstract thinking skills. Our experience suggests that rather than forcing the issue with such clients, it is better simply to move on to the next segment of treatment after three sessions. In this circumstance, Heimberg and Becker (2002) recommend that, for the remainder of therapy, the cognitive portion of treatment be deemphasized in favor of relying more heavily on repeated exposure. Additionally, such clients may be able to generate realistic self-statements (e.g., "I have done this before") or self-instructions (e.g., "Start by introducing myself") informally, with help from the therapist, for use in anxiety-provoking situations rather than relying on more formal cognitive restructuring.

As in the previous segment, each session begins with a homework review and ends with homework assignment. Homework assignments include readings from the client workbook, associated forms, and self-monitoring exercises. Some clients begin to attempt *in vivo* exposures spontaneously at this point in treatment, without being specifically assigned to do so. If these exposures go well, then they may be beneficial to the client. However, therapists should not actively encourage exposures as homework until completion of training in cognitive restructuring and one in-session exposure. At this point in treatment, clients still have few adaptive strategies for managing anxiety or coping with social situations that have disappointing outcomes. They are also likely to escape a situation at the first sign of trouble. Therefore, the possibility of a less than positive exposure experience at this phase of treatment could lead to resistance to attempting future exposures.

In this segment of treatment, clients are explicitly introduced to the basic tenet of the cognitive-behavioral model, which proposes that emotional reactions occur as a result of *interpretations* of situations, not situations themselves. "Automatic thoughts" are defined as negative, distorted, or irrational thoughts about oneself, the world, or the future that lead to or increase the experience of problematic anxiety. These concepts are first demonstrated with a hypothetical example rather than an emotionally charged example from the client's own life. The client workbook describes the very different thoughts of two young men after meeting a woman. Negative thoughts lead one man to give up any attempts to get to know the woman better and to experience several more unpleasant thoughts and emotions. The more neutral and realistic thoughts of the other man facilitate his continued efforts at making conversation. Additional examples are provided for therapist and client to examine whether the client appears to need further instruction on the concept of automatic thoughts. Clients are then asked to examine their own thoughts, first related to a hypothetical social situation, then as recorded on previously completed homework forms.

"Thinking errors" are defined as common categories into which automatic thoughts may fall. Clients often find that they are particularly prone to engage in certain types of distorted thinking (e.g., mind reading, fortune-telling, disqualifying the positive), and identifying these habitual thinking errors can assist in challenging automatic thoughts (e.g., "There I go, mind reading again. I have no reason to assume that they are thinking the worst"). Clients are introduced to an adaptation of the list of thinking errors outlined by Judith Beck (1995) in the first edition of her book *Cognitive Therapy: Basics and Beyond*. Ideally, the client has reviewed this list in the course of doing the readings for homework, and therapist and client can briefly discuss which thinking errors the client personally found most relevant. If the client has not done the homework, each thinking error is briefly reviewed by therapist and client in session. The therapist and client can practice identifying both the thinking errors in workbook examples and the client's automatic thoughts recorded as part of previous homework assignments, and further examine automatic thoughts the client might have about upcoming situations. For homework, clients monitor their automatic thoughts, their belief in the automatic thoughts (on a 0- to 100-point scale), the thinking errors they

contain, and the emotions they cause in one or two naturally occurring situations during the week.

The next steps in cognitive restructuring are to challenge the automatic thoughts and develop rational responses to them. The process of challenging automatic thoughts is begun with the assistance of disputing questions, originally adapted from the work of Sank and Shaffer (1984). These generic questions can be brought to bear on automatic thoughts (e.g., "Do I know for certain that _____?"; "What evidence do I have that _____?; What evidence do I have that the opposite is true?"; "What is the worst that could happen? How bad is that? How can I cope with that?"; "What does _____ mean? Does _____ really mean that I am a(n) _____?"). Before having the client apply these questions to his/her own thoughts, however, the therapist and client review a hypothetical example from the client workbook. Thereafter, the therapist addresses the client's automatic thoughts examined in the earlier discussion of thinking errors. Together client and therapist question the automatic thoughts using the disputing questions to arrive at alternative, more realistic ways of viewing the situation. It is typically the case that the answers to disputing questions themselves include automatic thoughts, and these must be further disputed. This process, which we have labeled the *Anxious Self/Coping Self Dialogue*, ultimately helps the client arrive at answers to the original disputing questions that are more believable and acceptable to him/her. The output of this dialogue is then summarized into one or two statements that serve as rational responses. A rational response provides a realistic and balanced view of the situation that is typically more positive than that provided by the automatic thoughts. For the next homework assignment, the clients record their automatic thoughts from an anxiety-provoking situation during the week, rate their belief in the automatic thoughts, identify the thinking errors they contain, dispute the automatic thoughts, develop a rational response, and rate their belief in that rational response. As can be seen, these homework assignments build on previous ones, becoming increasingly complex but increasingly empowering.

Toward the end of the final session in this segment, the therapist informs the client that exposures will begin the following week. To the extent that beginning exposures cause the client to feel anxious, the client is encouraged to "avoid avoidance" by coming to the next session and to identify automatic thoughts related to the exposure, challenge them, and arrive at a rational response. The therapist reassures the client that a challenging, but not overwhelming, situation will be used for the first exposure. More experienced therapists often discuss a few possibilities for the first exposure during this session. Therapists new to this treatment approach often discuss details of the exposure with the client the following week, after the therapist has had supervision.

Segment 3: Exposures

Exposures should begin as early as Session 5 but no later than Session 8, depending on the rate at which the earlier material was covered. Chapter 7 from the client workbook reviews the rationale for exposures and introduces the concept of setting achievable behavioral goals. The content of Chapter 7 is briefly touched upon; many of these concepts have been covered earlier (e.g., why exposures are important), and the new material is demonstrated during the exposure itself. Similarly, therapists rarely devote an entire session to discussing Chapter 8 (Ongoing Exposures) or the specific topic chapters (Chapter 9, Interaction Fears; Chapter 10, Observational Fears; Chapter 11, Public Speaking Fears) assigned during this segment. Rather, the content is only briefly addressed during the homework review and an in-session exposure is conducted. During this phase of treatment, therapists strive to complete an exposure almost every session. To follow protocol in our research studies, a minimum of four in-session exposures must be completed. More commonly, at least six in-session exposures are completed, and the more the better. Therefore, although the protocol allows the therapist the freedom to a use a couple of sessions during this segment to do cognitive restructuring alone or to review a topic chapter in detail, our belief is that the time is best devoted to repeated in-session exposures integrating cognitive restructuring.

All exposure sessions follow the same basic format (see Table 3.1). The session begins with a homework review and ends with a homework assignment. The homework assignment typically comprises *in vivo* exposure tasks and associated cognitive restructuring that logically build upon the in-session exposure. The first in-session exposure typically includes a role play with the therapist of a situation that the client assigned a SUDS rating of at least 50. The rule of thumb is that clients should perceive exposures as challenging but not overwhelming or beyond their ability to use cognitive coping skills. Therapists make exposures as realistic

TABLE 3.1. Outline of Exposure Sessions

1. Review homework from previous week.

2. Complete in-session exposure.

   a. Exposure preprocessing
      - Briefly negotiate details of exposure
      - Elicit automatic thoughts
      - Client rates belief in automatic thoughts
      - Client labels thinking errors in automatic thoughts
      - Client disputes one or two automatic thoughts
      - Client develops rational response(s) and rates belief in rational response(s)
      - Client sets nonperfectionistic, behavioral goals

   b. Conduct role play for approximately 10 minutes
      - Request SUDS and the rational response every minute
      - Client uses disputing questions and rational responses as automatic thoughts occur
      - Track client's progress on behavioral goals

   c. Exposure post-processing
      - Review whether goals were attained
      - Review occurrence of automatic thoughts
      - Review use of rational response(s)
      - Discuss any unexpected or new automatic thoughts
      - Client, therapist, and role players react to client's performance
      - Graph and interpret SUDS ratings pattern
      - Examine evidence in relation to automatic thoughts and rational response(s)
      - Client re-rates belief in automatic thoughts and rational response(s)
      - Client summarizes what was learned from the exposure experience

3. Assignment of homework

   a. Related *in vivo* exposures with associated cognitive restructuring

   b. Other assignments as appropriate

as possible by rearranging furniture, using props, and instructing role-play partners (i.e., therapist assistants brought into session to assist with exposures) to behave in particular ways. A bit of effort in making the situation more realistic may mean the difference between an exposure that elicits significant anxiety and one that is too artificial to be relevant. Commonly used props include food or drink for individuals with fears of eating, drinking, or serving food in front of others, and client-prepared notes for presentations. Careful attention should be paid to aspects that make the situation more or less anxiety-provoking. For example, a client who fears eating in front of others may be more anxious when eating something that is easy to spill (e.g., soup) than when eating finger foods.

The essence of the treatment is the coordination between the cognitive restructuring work and the exposure (see Table 3.1). The therapist begins the exposure preprocessing by briefly describing an exposure situation. The client may suggest modifications or alternatives. However, the therapist needs to balance approaching the exposure task collaboratively with being highly vigilant for overly detailed discussions that largely serve to avoid getting started with the exposure. The therapist then elicits the client's automatic thoughts regarding the chosen situation and records the thoughts on the easel. The therapist picks one or two automatic thoughts to dispute rather than attempting to help the client to dispute all automatic thoughts. The client rates his/her belief in the automatic thought and identifies the thinking errors it contains. To the extent possible, the client takes the lead in challenging the thoughts with disputing questions and developing a rational response. The therapist only assists as needed. The rational response is written on a fresh sheet of paper, so that the client may refer to it during the exposure, without being distracted by automatic thoughts listed on the same page.

Next, behavioral goals for the exposure are set. Without guidance, clients with social anxiety disorder tend to set unrealistic, perfectionistic goals (e.g., "I won't get anxious" or "I will never stumble over my words"), or goals that are based on the reactions of other people and not under their control (e.g., to make a good impression). The therapist helps the client to develop two or three measureable and observable goals for the situation (e.g., asking at least three questions to get to know the person better, stating an opinion, talking about three different points during a speech). These goals are recorded below the rational response, so that the client can refer to them during the exposure.

During the exposure, the therapists requests SUDS ratings at 1-minute intervals and whenever anxiety appears to increase or decrease. At each SUDS prompt, the client also reads his/her rational response aloud. Clients quickly adjust to this disruption, particularly if the role player(s) help to reorient them with a verbal cue (e.g., "You were talking about .. . "). The exposure should continue until anxiety has begun to decrease or plateau and the goals have been met, typically around 10 minutes. The therapist should be the one to end the exposure to help the client overcome any tendencies to escape the situation when it becomes difficult.

The postprocessing phase of the exposure includes a review of goal attainment, with the therapist noting the occurrence of automatic thoughts that were the focus of cognitive restructuring before the exposure, a discussion of the usefulness of the rational response, and identification of any unexpected automatic thoughts that should be addressed in the future. Rather than asking the client about how the role play went from his/her perspective, the therapist asks the whether the client's agreed-upon goals were accomplished, providing no opening for the client to revert to a discussion about failure to attain other goals, such as not becoming anxious. The therapist also shares his/her opinion on goal attainment, responding to concerns raised by the client and not allowing the client to disqualify the positive. In later exposures, outside role players may also be asked to share their reactions and answer any questions the client has about how the exposure went. Feedback from the therapist and role players should emphasize information that counters the client's negative beliefs. For example, the client might believe that he blushes bright red, is boring, appears inadequate to others, and cannot carry on a 10-minute conversation. Perhaps, objectively, the client did blush at the beginning of the exposure, only responded to questions from the role player, and reported very high SUDS for the whole 10 minutes (90 or higher). However, the client met his goals of sharing something about himself and staying in the exposure until the therapist said to stop. In this situation, the therapist would point out how the client met his goals and how many of the client's feared consequences (e.g., being too anxious to carry on a conversation) did not occur. Additionally, only in rare cases do clients look as anxious as they think they do, so it is often quite appropriate to acknowledge that the client showed some symptoms of anxiety, but that the anxiety was not as noticeable as the client's SUDS ratings might suggest, the anxiety did not detract from enjoyment of the conversation, and so forth. Therapists who deny seeing any anxiety in a client who was obviously anxious risk damaging their credibility. Especially early in treatment, therapists should think seriously before providing a laundry list of client behaviors that detracted from the quality of the conversation (e.g., the client only responded to questions and did not ask any, the client could have engaged in more eye contact). Many clients discount the positive aspects of the exposure and focus only on the negative feedback. Therefore, it is better to set this information aside temporarily and to make sure that these behaviors are included as goals for the next role play, particularly if the client does not spontaneously suggest one of these problematic behaviors as a goal. For clients who are self-critical during the post-processing for an objectively poor behavior such as never asking any questions, the most common strategy is to share with the client the conceptualization of the problematic behavior as an avoidance response to significant anxiety (rather than as evidence of poor social skills or some other inadequacy within the client). Working from this conceptualization, the therapist may then inquire about automatic thoughts leading to the problematic behavior. The client's responses are often quite illuminating (e.g., "I might inadvertently ask a question about a sensitive subject that will offend the other person"). The therapist would then plan with the client to work on these automatic thoughts and approach the feared social behavior by including it as a goal in a future exposure.

Next, the pattern of SUDS ratings is quickly graphed for the client. Different SUDS patterns may be used to make different points. The most common pattern is for the initial SUDS ratings to be rather high, then to decline over time. In these cases, the therapist can point out that it seems like getting started is the hardest part, and that if the client hangs in there, things seem to get easier. If this pattern holds across future exposures, it can lead to a new rational response (e.g., "It gets easier"; "The hardest part is getting started"). For clients with high SUDS ratings throughout the entire exposure who still meet their goals, the therapist can point out that a person may simultaneously be quite anxious and still do what he/she needs to do in a given social situation (e.g., "I can be anxious and still share my opinion" might be a future rational response). The therapist also inquires about any automatic thoughts that may have interfered with habituation, so that these might be addressed prior to the next exposure. Another common pattern is decreasing or steady SUDS ratings that spike to a high level when the client perceives a difficulty arising during the exposure. Sometimes the therapist is able to observe what led to the spike in anxiety (e.g., a pause in the conversation). At other times, it may not be as obvious, and the client needs to explain what happened (e.g., there was no pause, but the client had an automatic thought that the discussion of the current topic had reached its limits and feared that he/she would be unable to continue the conversation). Such discussions may lead to new goals (e.g., "Allow yourself to pause twice during the conversation, so you learn that you can recover from pauses and not to fear them") and targets

for cognitive restructuring (i.e., the belief that pauses reflect social incompetence might be challenged and lead to a rational response, such as "Pauses are a normal part of conversations" or "I am only 50% responsible for ending a pause"). Clients are then asked to rerate their degree of belief in their automatic thoughts and rational responses, based specifically on their experience of the in-session exposure. Finally, the client is asked what he/she has learned from the exposure that can be applied to life outside of the clinic.

Homework assignments are a very important part of treatment in this segment because the client is asked to enter situations similar to those that have been targeted during in-session exposures. To assist them in engaging in cognitive restructuring prior to the actual conduct of the homework exposure, clients are provided copies of the Be Your Own Cognitive Therapist (BYOCT) worksheet, which is also discussed in session and exemplified in the client workbook. This form leads clients through each of the steps of cognitive restructuring described earlier and is often used for in-session exposures, as well as those assigned for homework. After the homework exposure is completed, the second portion of the BYOCT assists clients in completing a cognitive debriefing and consolidating the learning that has occurred during and after the homework experience.

Segment 4: *Advanced Cognitive Restructuring*

After three or four exposure sessions, the therapist and client should begin to notice common themes in the client's automatic thoughts. This is an indication that it will soon be time to move on to advanced cognitive restructuring (Chapter 12 of the client workbook). This segment assists the client in moving beyond situation-specific automatic thoughts by applying the downward arrow technique (see J. S. Beck, 1995) to thoughts that have frequently recurred over the course of treatment. To accomplish this task efficiently, client and therapist review all previous written homework assignments that involved the recording of automatic thoughts, as well as the thoughts recorded in advance of in-session exposures and work through the Peeling Your Onion worksheet from the client workbook, which provides a systematic approach to questioning automatic thoughts and further probing the responses to these questions, until the client's core belief(s) have been identified.

The beginning of advanced cognitive restructuring does not signal the end to exposures. Rather, the therapist and client create in-session and *in vivo* exposures to challenge core beliefs. For instance, if a client has a core belief along the lines of "I need to be perfect to be accepted by others," the client might be engaged in exposures that involve making mistakes or social missteps (e.g., spilling a drink, turning in a report with an error) and noticing whether others continue to be accepting. Core beliefs may be challenged in other ways as well. For instance, in addition to exposures, the client may be asked to notice instances in which others' mistakes actually make them easy to identify with or more endearing. One session is typically devoted completely to helping the client utilize the downward arrow technique and challenge core beliefs. Additional sessions not only continue to explore core beliefs but also include an in-session exposure.

Segment 5: Termination

As treatment approaches Session 16, the issue of termination and/or reevaluation of the treatment contract will have been raised informally by the therapist several times. After Session 15, Chapter 13 in the client workbook is assigned. Session 16 formally focuses on assessment of progress, relapse prevention, and the issue of termination. The therapist and client go over a worksheet in which the client reports things that he/she has learned during treatment (e.g., how to identify and challenge automatic thoughts, the importance of avoiding avoidance). The therapist asks the client to provide current ratings for all items from the fear and avoidance hierarchy developed earlier in treatment; a discussion follows regarding progress that has been made and where further work is needed. When the therapist and client mutually agree that termination is in order, risk factors for relapse are discussed (e.g., social pressure from others, new situations that arise as improvement continues). Plans to deal with signs of relapse are also made (e.g., the client can review chapters in the client workbook or call the therapist). Mixed emotions (e.g., pride, sadness over the termination of the therapeutic relationship) associated with termination are also processed.

In our clinic, the same measures administered at pretreatment are repeated after Session 16. The client is given feedback on these assessments, with data presented in the context of the initial pretreatment assessment results. At the end of 16 sessions, many clients still experience problematic social anxiety in a few domains. As we stated in the first session, elimination of social anxiety is not the criterion for termination. Instead, if

the client has stopped avoiding key social situations, has experienced a meaningful reduction of anxiety in a few areas, and believes that he/she can use the skills gained in therapy to continue to work independently, then the client is ready to stop treatment. Most individuals who respond to treatment in this way are likely to continue to make progress after termination. Follow-up appointments are recommended to monitor the client's clinical status (e.g., 1- and 6-months posttreatment).

For some individuals, treatment gains will be evident, but the anxiety and avoidance continue to be too severe and pervasive for the client to continue on alone. This phenomenon is most common among clients with severe social anxiety at treatment onset, typically, clients with APD or those who fear many social situations. Clients with significant comorbidities may also take longer to make sufficient treatment gains. In such cases, continued treatment is recommended. The new treatment contract, as with the original one, should be for 16 sessions or less, at which point another assessment should occur. The treatment plan typically consists of more cognitive restructuring and exposures, although new domains are often introduced (e.g., moving from working on friendships to dating relationships).

CASE STUDY

To illustrate better how individual CBT for social anxiety disorder is implemented, a case example is presented. First, background and pretreatment assessment data are given, followed by a description of the client's progress through 16 weeks of treatment and her status 1-year and 5-years posttreatment. Note that treatment was conducted in accordance with the first edition of the client workbook (Hope, Heimberg, Juster, & Turk, 2000) and therapist guide (Hope, Heimberg, & Turk, 2006), resulting in some differences in procedure from the updated version of the protocol presented earlier. We made this decision so that we could present a case example including an examination of longer-term follow-up information.

Josie, age 22, presented to treatment with significant anxiety concerning both social interaction and performance situations. She was a full-time student studying music at a local college and living with a roommate. She was not employed despite significant financial need. Josie described herself as shy and having trouble connecting with others. She socialized with her roommate and her boyfriend, but she often turned down opportunities to socialize with their friends because of anxiety. Josie reported that she had no close friends of her own and that her anxiety kept her from forming close friendships, especially with women her age. Josie's social anxiety had also resulted in occupational and academic impairment. For example, although Josie had gone on numerous job interviews and had even been offered positions, she was currently unemployed because she had difficulty accepting job offers due to her fears that she would get fired. She reported great anxiety in her classes and did not participate unless directly asked a question, even if participation was a significant part of her grade. She often declined to enroll in classes that interested her because of participation requirements. In addition, Josie was required to do recitals and in-class critiques of her music compositions several times a semester. Although she never avoided any of these events, she worried about them for weeks in advance and suffered through them with great anxiety. Josie feared that her social anxiety would cause her even greater difficulty after graduation, when she would need to go on job interviews and auditions.

Pretreatment Assessment

Josie came to the clinic seeking help for social anxiety, but she also had difficulties with general worry and tension, depression, and panic attacks. She was administered the ADIS-IV-L and a series of self-report measures. Based on this information, Josie was assigned a diagnosis of social anxiety disorder, with an ADIS-IV-L CSR of 5, which indicates moderate to severe symptoms. She received additional diagnoses of generalized anxiety disorder, recurrent major depressive disorder of moderate severity, posttraumatic stress disorder related to a recent automobile accident, and panic disorder with agoraphobia.

With regard to measures of social anxiety, Josie's scores indicated significant fear in both social interaction and performance/observation situations (see Table 3.2). Heimberg and colleagues (1992) suggested cutoff scores of 34 for the full 20-item version of the SIAS (interaction fears) and 24 for the SPS (performance/observation fears) to differentiate between individuals with and without social anxiety disorder. Josie's scores on both measures exceeded these cutoffs. Similarly, on the LSAS, Josie reported fear and avoidance of both social interaction and performance situations, and her total score was well above the empirically derived cutoff score for the presence of social anxiety disorder (Mennin et al., 2002).

Ideally, treatment should result in symptom reduction and improved functionality, as well as promote the client's overall sense of well-being and life satisfaction. Safren, Heimberg, Brown, and Holle (1997) reported a mean score of 0.8 on the Quality of Life Inventory for clients with social anxiety disorder, which is significantly lower than the mean score of the nonclinical adult sample reported by Frisch (1994; $M = 2.6$, $SD = 1.3$). Josie's score indicated that her degree of life satisfaction was very low but similar to that of others with social anxiety disorder.

The disruption in functioning caused by social anxiety and the associated poor quality of life frequently results in dysphoria. Josie's score on the BDI-II indicated a level of depression more severe than is typically

TABLE 3.2. Self-Report and Clinician-Administered Assessments at Pretreatment and 1-Year and 5-Year Follow-Ups

Measure	Pretreatment	1-year follow-up	5-year follow-up
Self-report			
Brief Fear of Negative Evaluation Scale	49	23	29
Social Interaction Anxiety Scale	48	22	23
Social Phobia Scale	38	12	24
Beck Depression Inventory–II	25	8	8
Quality of Life Inventory	–0.9	1.1	–0.6
Clinician-rated			
ADIS-IV-L Clinician Severity Rating	5	3	3
Liebowitz Social Anxiety Scale—Total	48	37	31

Note. ADIS-IV-L, Anxiety Disorders Interview Schedule for DSM-IV—Lifetime Version.

seen among individuals in our treatment program (Elting, Hope, & Heimberg, 1997). Josie did not endorse having any thoughts of suicide. Based on clinical interview, we determined that Josie's current low mood was related to recurrent major depression. This most recent depressive episode had begun approximately 6 months prior to her assessment and was associated with negative social experiences while studying abroad. Josie reported that her depressed mood was slightly less distressing and impairing than her social anxiety. Thus, the depression was judged to be secondary to her social anxiety and unlikely to have an adverse impact on her treatment. Similarly, we determined that her other diagnoses, although clinically significant, did not rise to a level of concern that might interfere with or derail the treatment of her social anxiety disorder.

Treatment

Psychoeducational Segment

SESSIONS 1–2

The first four sessions were devoted to laying the groundwork for treatment, establishing rapport, educating Josie about the cognitive-behavioral model of social anxiety disorder, and outlining her goals for treatment.

In the first two meetings, Josie was very soft-spoken, made little eye contact, and expressed feelings of hopelessness about her ability to get better. She asked many questions about how other clients had fared with the treatment program, and the therapist stressed that outcome is often dependent on the client's ability to put in consistent effort throughout treatment. The therapist used some of Josie's own experiences to parallel the challenges and rewards she might face in treatment, such as asking Josie how long she had been playing piano and whether she had noticed any changes over that time. Josie reported that when she started, the process was very effortful, challenging, and even disheartening, but that with ongoing practice and education, she had reached a point where it was enjoyable and easy for her. With this, Josie appeared to be very encouraged about her prognosis, reporting that she was eager to begin treatment and motivated to work very hard. The majority of the first session was spent establishing rapport and introducing psychoeducational material about social anxiety and the components of treatment. To encourage Josie to speak about her own experiences with social anxiety, the therapist employed open-ended questions, asked if the examples sounded familiar to

Josie, and requested that she describe some situations in which her anxiety was better or worse than others. For example, although Josie felt she had a significant amount of anxiety when performing in front of an audience, she felt that this anxiety was typical for most people in that situation. However, her anxiety while interacting with others at receptions before and after performances was severe, and she often avoided these situations by arriving at recitals at the last minute and leaving as soon as she finished. By participating in the session this way, Josie demonstrated an understanding of the important concept that social anxiety exists on a continuum.

SESSION 3

In the third session, the development of Josie's social anxiety and how it was maintained over the years was explored. After asking her mother, Josie learned that she was very shy even as a young child, and that her mother often had to push her to participate in social activities with other children. Josie also reported that her mother tended to keep to herself and limit interactions with others, which Josie may have modeled from a young age. In addition, Josie reported struggling with feelings of falling short from a young age. For example, she reported that she never qualified for elite youth soccer teams, although she was a skilled athlete, and never received more than third place or honorable mention in recitals and competitions. The therapist discussed with Josie how such experiences may have shaped her beliefs that she was not good enough and also highlighted how Josie's tendency to view the negative aspects of situations (e.g., not getting first place) often led her to disqualify other successes (e.g., being among the top five performers in a large competition).

SESSIONS 4–5

In the early part of the fourth session, the therapist and Josie completed a discussion from Session 3 on the role that perfectionistic standards and low self-efficacy played in Josie's experience of social anxiety. The remainder of this session and the next were spent developing and refining Josie's fear and avoidance hierarchy (see Table 3.3). Josie reported that interacting with people in person was easier than talking over the phone because face-to-face contact allowed her to interpret body language and facial expressions to determine how the interaction was going for the other person. In addi-

TABLE 3.3. Fear and Avoidance Hierarchy with Pretreatment, Posttreatment, and 1-Year and 5-Year Follow-Up Ratings

Situation	Pretreatment	Posttreatment	1-year follow-up	5-year follow-up
1 Riding public transportation alone				
Fear	100	20	9	90
Avoidance	100	20	6	85
2 Staying after recitals to socialize				
Fear	95	7	3	55
Avoidance	95	8	0	60
3 Going to recitals				
Fear	90	7	3	45
Avoidance	70	8	0	15
4 Making phone calls to people I used to be close with				
Fear	75	5	3	65
Avoidance	60	5	1	60
5 Class critiques and talking about my compositions in class				
Fear	65	6	1	60
Avoidance	50	1	0	20
6 Talking with professors and authority figures I respect				
Fear	65	4	5	75
Avoidance	50	2	5	60
7 Making/maintaining conversations with friends and people I respect				
Fear	60	3	4	25
Avoidance	60	1	2	10
8 Making the first phone call				
Fear	55	2	4	65
Avoidance	5	0	1	35
9 Hanging out with boyfriend's friends' girlfriends				
Fear	50	6	3	40
Avoidance	85	2	0	15
10 Talking with old friends I've lost touch with				
Fear	40	7	4	30
Avoidance	70	4	2	45

tion, Josie felt that it was easier to interact with males than with females, who she believed were more critical. Josie was also more anxious around individuals she respected and admired than she was with strangers.

Cognitive Restructuring Training Segment

SESSION 6

In this session, Josie was introduced to cognitive restructuring. Though she demonstrated an understanding of the importance of thoughts in producing feelings of anxiety, Josie reported difficulty identifying her own automatic thoughts. Specifically, she tended to identify questions that passed through her mind in anticipation of or during anxiety-provoking situations. For example, when recalling a recent anxiety-provoking situation in which she had to present her work in front of a class, Josie identified the thought, "What will other people think of me?" The therapist helped Josie to restate this question as a statement of what she feared, asking Josie to let her "anxious self" answer the question. She was able to come up with automatic thoughts, such as "Other people will think I'm a moron" and "Other people will think I am unprepared for this presentation." She identified other thoughts, such as "I am wasting their time," "They will get bored with me," and "My professor will be disappointed that I didn't do a better job." Many of the automatic thoughts appeared to be related to a general sense of letting others down. The therapist encouraged Josie that, with continued practice, she would get better at recognizing automatic thoughts.

SESSION 7

In this session, Josie again struggled to identify automatic thoughts, but with prompting, she was increasingly able to do so. She also had some difficulty identifying the thinking errors contained in her automatic thoughts, often insisting that all the thoughts qualified as unhelpful and unproductive thoughts—that is, true but unhelpful. The therapist asked Josie some disputing questions to illustrate that the thoughts were not true or totally accurate, and that other thinking errors could apply. By the end of session, Josie had a better handle on thinking errors and was able to start using some disputing questions successfully. Josie reported that the cognitive restructuring work was much more challenging than she expected, but that she was eager to put the work into action during exposures.

SESSION 8

The therapist decided to take an additional session to continue work on cognitive restructuring before moving onto exposures, so that Josie was maximally prepared. Cognitive restructuring practice was focused on a recent situation in which Josie turned down tickets, offered by a professor at school, to a show by her favorite artist. Josie was much better able to identify her automatic thoughts related to this situation, which included the following:

1. "Other students will be mad at me if I take the tickets."
2. "I will be too scared to go and would waste the tickets."
3. "I will not be able to take public transportation to get there."
4. "If I do take public transportation, I will get lost and miss the show."
5. "Other students want the tickets more than I do."

Josie was able to identify thinking errors such as fortune-telling, mind reading, and catastrophizing, among others. However, there was evidence that Josie was critical of herself and her occasional difficulty grasping the concepts of cognitive restructuring. At first, Josie struggled with labeling the thinking errors in her automatic thoughts and searching for the right rational response. The therapist suggested to Josie that there was no right or wrong way to challenge automatic thoughts or to develop a rational response, but Josie continued to evaluate her suggestions as not good enough. Furthermore, Josie grew extremely frustrated and pessimistic when she used disputing questions to challenge her automatic thoughts. Specifically, she had trouble challenging the thought that getting lost on the subway would have to lead to missing the show entirely. She reported that she doubted her own ability to read the subway map or ask for help and predicted that she would get so lost that she would either turn around and go home or arrive at the show after it had already started. Josie's anxiety about entering the performance late would then, she predicted, lead her to go home anyway. Josie reported that she would feel disappointed, embarrassed, and ashamed if she lost her way on public transportation because it would mean she had failed to attend the performance and in doing so would anger her classmates, who she predicted would feel as though she wasted the opportunity. Josie grew increasingly frustrated with the strength of her anxious thoughts and reported that she felt stupid for not being able to challenge them successfully. This highlighted some patterns noted throughout treatment, including Josie's tendency to rely on perfectionist standards and all-or-nothing thinking (e.g., evaluating her thoughts and behavioral responses as all right or all wrong) and impatience with her own progress in treatment. Despite this, she reported being willing to keep practicing and move on to in-session exposures. The therapist worked with Josie for the remainder of session to challenge her automatic thoughts. It was particularly helpful for Josie to identify that she had no evidence that she would get lost and to recognize that even if she did get lost, it would be important enough for her to attend the performance that she would ask for additional help or directions.

Exposure Segment

SESSION 9

During homework review, Josie reported that she was able to use her cognitive restructuring skills when she ran into an old roommate at a coffee shop. Josie reported that the exchange had gone much more smoothly than she anticipated and this encouraged her to feel more confident in her understanding of and abilities to use cognitive restructuring skills actively in social situations. With regard to the in-session exposure, the therapist wanted to choose a situation that would seem relevant to her treatment goals, elicit a moderate amount of anxiety, and in which Josie was likely to perform reasonably well. The in-session exposure was a follow-up to Josie's recent interaction with her classmate Anne, who mentioned to Josie that some people from class would be getting together one weekend to hang out. However, Anne did not call Josie to make specific plans; neither did Josie follow through with making plans to attend the event, and she ended up missing it. Josie thought that Anne did not call because she might have interpreted Josie's anxiety symptoms (e.g., shyness, quietness, lack of eye contact) as disinterest in socializing. Josie's exposure involved her talking with Anne, whose role was played by the therapist, about this misunderstanding. The following excerpts are from the cognitive restructuring prior to the exposure.

THERAPIST: First, let's go to the BYOCT worksheet and work through the situation before the exposure happens. When you think about this situation happening now? What kind of automatic thoughts come up for you?

JOSIE: I'm not going to talk to her because I won't know what to say. Also, I shouldn't say anything about her not calling me because it would make everything awkward. I should be really friendly and smile the whole time.

THERAPIST: Are you making any predictions about how this interaction will go?

JOSIE: Oh, yeah. I'm going to choke up, and she is going to judge me. I think that's it.

THERAPIST: OK, good job identifying those automatic thoughts. Now what kinds of emotions come up when you think those thoughts?

JOSIE: I feel sad. The anxiousness almost goes away, and I just don't feel like talking to her. I also feel a little bit of anger and frustration at myself because I can't confront her about this and I don't want to make her feel uncomfortable.

THERAPIST: So it sounds like that kind of thinking might lead to you not saying anything at all then, avoiding the interaction?

JOSIE: Yeah, I'd definitely avoid it.

THERAPIST: Well this exposure will allow us to practice confronting those automatic thoughts, but first we need to do some cognitive restructuring practice. Why don't we start by identifying some thinking errors?

JOSIE: Right away I see should statements and fortune-telling. And to think that she's judging me, that's mind reading.

THERAPIST: Good job. Now let's try to dispute some of these thoughts. Let's start with the automatic thought: "I'm not going to talk to her because I won't have anything to say." Do you know this for certain?

JOSIE: (*smiling*) No, actually I do want to talk with her, and I could always ask her little things. I have no evidence that I'll have nothing to say.

THERAPIST: So you could come up with something to say?

JOSIE: Yeah, even if it's just small talk, I could come up with something. I do want to ask her about what happened, but I don't want to come across as too aggressive or confrontational. I feel bad when I confront people.

THERAPIST: So let's figure out some ways you'd feel comfortable asking her to hang out, ways that allow you to get your message across without feeling aggressive or blunt. This can help us start to identify some behavioral goals for the exposure. Let's take a look at what it is you want to ask her or tell her.

JOSIE: Well, I want to ask her if we can hang out some other time, since she didn't call me last time. But I have the automatic thought that I shouldn't say anything because it will make things awkward. I guess if I challenge that, I don't really know that I will make things awkward.

THERAPIST: What might be another outcome if you say something?

JOSIE: She might apologize and ask me if I want to come, and I can tell her that I'd love to come the next time she invites me. She did invite me in the first place. She just never called because she thought I didn't want to go.

THERAPIST: Good. So we identified some automatic thoughts, and you said they made you feel sad and frustrated. Then we challenged them and came up with some coping thoughts. How do those thoughts make you feel?

JOSIE: That's better. I feel a lot better.

THERAPIST: How could we sum these up into a rational response? Does anything stand out to you?

JOSIE: "Saying something might have a positive outcome" really stands out to me. I'd feel better and things might turn out better if I remind myself of that. It will help me to challenge the thought that I'll choke up or run out of things to say.

The therapist selected that automatic thought for cognitive restructuring, because it had been a recurrent one for Josie in homework and seemed relevant to the upcoming exposure. Also, the therapist made an effort to take Josie through the cognitive restructuring relatively quickly because the longer the exposure was delayed, the more anxious she would get and the more difficult it would be for her to focus on the cognitive restructuring because of her anxiety. The next step was to set goals for the exposure. Josie decided that her achievable behavioral goals for this exposure would include telling Anne that she was interested in the last social event, letting Anne know that she would be interested in hanging out some time soon, and giving Anne her phone number.

The exposure began with both Josie and the therapist standing up to simulate more closely the interaction that might occur as they passed each other in the hallway at school. Josie stood where she would be able to see her rational response and behavioral goals written on the easel.

THERAPIST: Josie, what is your initial SUDS rating?

JOSIE: About a 45.

THERAPIST: OK, and what is your rational response?

JOSIE: Saying something might have a positive outcome.

Josie and the therapist began to chat about class, and Josie soon brought up the recently past social event. The therapist let the exposure go on for approximately 5 minutes. Upon being prompted by the therapist, Josie gave SUDS ratings at 1-minute intervals throughout the interaction and read her rational response aloud. After the exposure had ended, post-processing began.

THERAPIST: Did you reach your behavioral goals?

JOSIE: I told her I wanted to hang out and asked her to call me again.

THERAPIST: So you met your goals. Great job. Did any new automatic thoughts come up?

JOSIE: I noticed that I fidgeted a lot. I had the thought "This is scary," but also that she seemed pretty cool about the interaction. I thought I really shouldn't be nervous.

THERAPIST: Did the thoughts we identified earlier come up?

JOSIE: Yeah. I thought I wouldn't know what to say, and there was a pause in the conversation, but it was fine when I said something. I worried that I'd make this awkward for her, but I think it was more awkward for me because I was so nervous.

THERAPIST: How did your rational response work?

JOSIE: It worked pretty well; it got easier to remember and I believed it was true when I said it. It really seemed to help me think more about rational thoughts instead of anxious ones.

THERAPIST: Let's take a look at your SUDS. You started at a 45 and went up to 55 when conversation started. When you said something to her about wishing she'd call you, the SUDS went up to a 60. By the time she told you what happened, the SUDS dropped to 40.

After some small talk, it went down to a 20. That's a pretty significant drop.

JOSIE: It was a lot better after I got over that bump, when I told her I wanted to hang out.

THERAPIST: What thoughts do you remember having then?

JOSIE: "I shouldn't say anything," "I should walk away," "I have to say something."

THERAPIST: So what happened then?

JOSIE: I said my rational response when you asked, right after I asked her about what happened, and I felt a lot better. It felt like things were going to be OK. I feel really good about how it went.

After processing the exposure, the therapist helped Josie to plan an *in vivo* exposure to do on her own that week. She planned to meet her old roommate for coffee, using the BYOCT forms to guide her cognitive restructuring, the exposure, and her own postprocessing of the experience.

SESSION 10

In the 10th session, Josie reported that she had a very challenging but rewarding week. She recalled an in-class critique of her work, and, though her anxiety was intense, she was able to manage it and remain in class by reminding herself of her rational response: "I can learn something from their feedback." Josie also noted that she had completed two *in vivo* exposures, including having coffee with her old roommate and a conversation with her classmate Anne, just as she practiced in last week's session. Josie seemed very encouraged by the outcomes of these situations and her ability to use cognitive restructuring techniques before and during anxiety-provoking events.

For exposure this session, Josie planned to interact with two women playing the roles of her boyfriend's friends' fiancées, to whom Josie felt she could not relate. The therapist anticipated that this exposure would be more difficult for Josie because it involved a fairly unstructured interaction and likely a conversation about topics with which Josie was relatively unfamiliar, such as wedding planning. Josie reported the following automatic thoughts in anticipation of the exposure:

1. "I'm not married yet, so what do I know about relationships and weddings?"
2. "I will offend them with my views."

3. "They are going to think I am weird."
4. "They are going to think I act too young."
5. "I'm not going to give the right answers to their questions."

As with the automatic thoughts in her first exposure, Josie was able to identify thinking errors, including fortune-telling, mind reading, labeling, and all-or-nothing thinking. By using the disputing questions, Josie was able to challenge the automatic thoughts she identified. In response to the first thought, Josie determined that although she was not married, she had been in a relationship for a number of years, so she would be able to relate to the other women on that level. In addition, she had helped her sister plan a wedding, so she was familiar with some aspects of wedding planning. Regarding her fear of being offensive, Josie noted that she was not sure she would offend them with her views and that her different perspective might lead to an interesting conversation. The automatic thought that the other women would think she was weird was more difficult for Josie to challenge, but she was satisfied when she determined that she would be able to live with herself if they thought she was a little unusual and that it was unlikely to affect her relationships with them. In reference to her fears that they would think she acts too young, Josie used the challenge that she was only 2 years younger than these women, but she had chosen a different path for herself that involved continued education and saving marriage until she felt more settled in life, a decision that she felt was very mature. In response to the automatic thought that she would not give the right answer to their questions, Josie argued that perhaps there was no right or wrong answer, and that even if she gave an answer that was inconsistent with the other women's views, she could recover from those mistakes, and differences of opinion could lead to interesting conversation.

Josie decided that an appropriate rational response would be one that helped her feel that she could relate to these women despite their different circumstances. Her rational response for this exposure was "I'm not so different." Josie's goals were to talk about her own interests (e.g., music), ask a question, offer an opinion, and stay in the conversation until the exposure was over. Josie's SUDS ratings started out at 45, decreased to about 20 by the fourth minute of the exposure, and went as low as 15 by the final minute of the 8-minute exposure. Josie met all of her behavioral goals, and though she was quiet compared to the role players early in the conversation, she appeared to grow more at ease as time passed. Josie reported that the exposure went fairly well, and she was pleased that her sharing a story during the conversation led to a change of subject and additional conversation. Although Josie did not share their experiences and opinions, she was able to find a way to relate to them and to participate in the conversation. She reported having thoughts of leaving but convinced herself to stay by reminding herself that she would benefit from staying in the situation. Josie's homework was to call an old music composition classmate, have a conversation over the phone with him, and ask him to listen to her practice a piece she was working on for an upcoming show.

SESSION 11

Prior to this session, Josie was very busy with class work and preparation for an upcoming recital of her compositions as part of a final exam. Consequently, she had missed several sessions. Josie reported that over the course of the past month, she had interviewed for a job at a local bookstore, was offered the position, and accepted it. She said she experienced a significant amount of anxiety on the interview and in the first few days of work, but that she was feeling much more confident about things now. Although she had made dramatic improvements in her self-reported anxiety and continued to improve during the 1-month hiatus from regular treatment, the therapist discussed the importance of completing the remaining 5–6 weeks of the treatment program. Josie committed to following through with treatment and doing her homework more consistently. Though Josie had not formally been doing her homework and an in-session exposure was not conducted, the therapist reviewed her progress so far in relation to her fear and avoidance hierarchy. Socializing with a group of friends and riding public transportation alone were identified as areas for continued work. For homework, Josie was assigned the task of handing out fliers to friends and family for the upcoming recital, which was to involve repeated social interactions and a discussion of her work. She was also given the assignment of reading the chapter in the client workbook related to social interactions and making small talk.

SESSION 12

In the Session 12 homework review, Josie said she interacted with many people on campus and around town while promoting an upcoming show, and that the con-

versations had gone much more smoothly than anticipated. She said it was helpful to remind herself that she was an expert on her own musical compositions, so she could talk at least some about the performance she was advertising. The third in-session exposure, completed in this session, was designed to help Josie work on some of her automatic thoughts related to her upcoming recital that weekend. The therapist had planned an exposure during which Josie was to interact with audience members at a reception following her recital, and staff members from the clinic volunteered to play these roles. Josie agreed that this exposure was very relevant to her current concerns and would make her very anxious. Josie reported the following automatic thoughts in anticipation of the exposure:

1. "I'm going to sound pretentious if I talk confidently about my performance."
2. "They are only talking to me because they feel bad for me."
3. "I have to impress them."
4. "They will think this is boring."
5. "I won't know what to say."

Josie was able to identify thinking errors, including all-or-nothing thinking, labeling, fortune-telling, and mind reading. During the cognitive restructuring, Josie was encouraged to look at her successful experiences in the two previous exposures as evidence that she had things to say that were of interest to others. With the help of the therapist, Josie arrived at this rational response: "I can talk about my performance because I created it."

Josie's goals were to talk slowly, to provide information about herself, to answer questions posed to her, and to stay in a given interaction until the other person ended it. Josie's initial SUDS rating started out at 80, but it had decreased to 30 within 3 minutes. At the end of the 10-minute exposure, Josie's SUDS rating was below 20. Once again, Josie met her behavioral goals, and her performance was objectively skilled. Josie said that in addition to her rational response, it was helpful to tell herself that she did not have to take everything others said to heart. Josie thought the exposure went very well and even reported having fun interacting with the audience members and being the center of attention. She felt that this practice was going to be very helpful when she encountered the real situation at that weekend's recital. Josie's homework was to use the BYOCT worksheet before and after her actual recital to prepare herself to cope with anxious thoughts that might arise before, during, and after the performance.

SESSION 13

Josie came to the session, reporting that her anxiety at the reception following last week's recital was much more manageable than it had been in the past, and that she was actually able to enjoy conversations she had with family, music instructors, and fellow students. She reported feeling confident about her performance, which helped her to feel confident and comfortable while interacting with others at the reception. Though Josie did report experiencing significant anxiety as she began to socialize with family and friends after the recital, she said that her anxiety dropped substantially as she continued to interact with others about her performance, and at no point did she have thoughts of leaving the reception. Josie felt that the recital and reception were a success, and that her anxiety did not prevent her from enjoying these situations as it had in the past.

For an in-session exposure, Josie said it would be helpful to practice receiving feedback, both positive and negative, about her musical and academic performances. This situation was relevant because, as part of a final exam in Josie's music composition course, she was to perform an original composition in front of students and her instructor, then receive their feedback. Though her ability to do this had improved on a smaller scale during her coursework, this particular class critique elicited a considerable amount of anxiety for Josie, and she wanted some direct help with the cognitive restructuring and behavioral practice. The therapist decided to conduct two smaller exposures—one in which Josie received neutral or positive feedback from class members and her instructor, and another in which she received negative feedback. Each exposure was designed to go on for approximately 5–10 minutes to allow Josie to discuss her composition and performance adequately and to receive and respond to feedback. A number of clinic staff members volunteered to assist with this exposure.

Prior to the exposure, Josie identified the following automatic thoughts for both exposures:

1. "I am going to mess this up."
2. "I must appear professional."
3. "I have to perform perfectly to impress them."
4. "I won't know what to say."
5. "I won't understand their questions."

Josie was able to identify thinking errors such as fortune-telling, all-or-nothing thinking, catastrophizing, and should statements. She also noted how her per-

fectionistic standards and feelings of low self-efficacy were quickly elicited by this situation involving overt evaluation of her performance and interaction skills. After challenging her automatic thoughts, Josie decided that a helpful rational response in each of the exposures would be "I know my work because I did it," which she felt would encourage her to continue talking confidently about her own composition and performance, regardless of the feedback she received. Josie's behavioral goals were to answer questions posed to her and to ask follow-up questions, if she needed clarification.

The exposures were set up to take place immediately after a performance and began with Josie saying, "Thank you, I'd like to hear your thoughts about the piece." In the first exposure, she received a mix of neutral and positive feedback about her composition, her performance, and her ability to conduct herself during the critique. Josie's SUDS score started at 45 and dropped down to 15 within 3 minutes. She met all of her behavioral goals. The second exposure began the same way, but this time she received a mix of neutral and negative feedback; listeners pointed out mistakes she made in her performance, told her that she looked nervous, and indicated that they did not like the music she wrote. Josie's SUDS score again started at a 45 and went up as high as 60 when she received her first negative comment. By the fifth minute of the exposure, her SUDS score was 30, and by the end of the exposure, 20. Josie again met her behavioral goals and reported that she handled both situations very well. Josie noted that although her anxiety peaked when she received negative feedback, she felt she responded to the comments politely and was even able to learn from them. She felt the exposure was very helpful in preparing for her upcoming feedback sessions in class. For homework, Josie was asked to read the client workbook chapter on core beliefs and to do an *in vivo* exposure that would involve her taking public transportation to and from school with a friend. She was also asked to complete a BYOCT worksheet before and after her in-class performance and evaluation.

Advanced Cognitive Restructuring Segment

SESSION 14

Josie completed her homework exposure of riding the bus to and from school with a friend and reported that she was not very anxious. She said that next time she would take the bus on her own and work toward going places farther away and less familiar. Josie also reported that things went well with her in-class evaluation, that her performance of the music she composed went well, but that she thought she messed up once or twice. However, she noted that no students gave her feedback indicating that they noticed the mistake. Josie reported feeling incredibly anxious after she finished playing and that right before the feedback session she even had thoughts of excusing herself for a few minutes. Reminding herself of her rational response, "I can learn something from their feedback," encouraged Josie to stay in class and complete the evaluation. Though she received some challenging questions about how she composed the music and who had influenced her, Josie thought she had done a decent job, although she had stumbled over her words a few times. She noted that a few students commented about not particularly liking the style of music she chose, but Josie said she did not take these comments personally. Overall Josie felt that she had learned a lot from the students' and instructor's feedback and that, although anxious, felt it was an acceptable level of anxiety given the performance and evaluation aspects of the situation.

Josie did not read the chapter on core beliefs, so the therapist spent time in session introducing this concept. Josie worked hard in this session to identify her core beliefs, using the Peeling Your Onion worksheet. She realized that her most common automatic thoughts across situations were related to labeling herself, feeling as though she would not live up to others' expectations, and fears that others would judge her negatively because of her social or performance skills. Josie felt that the theme of "not measuring up" was familiar and related potentially to her beliefs about never measuring up to her parents' standards and not doing anything right, which led to more generalized perfectionism. Josie identified the thought, "I'm not measuring up," as related to a fear that she would not be successful in life, and that to be successful, she felt she must be perfect. Identifying this chain of thinking left her feeling sad, frustrated, and disappointed. From here, Josie worked through the worksheet and identified the core belief, "If I'm not perfect, I'm worthless." Time was spent brainstorming exposures Josie could do on her own to test and challenge this core belief. For homework, the therapist asked Josie to mess up intentionally while playing the piano for some family members, so as to challenge her core belief that anything short of perfectionism represents a failure. Josie also identified another situation in which she could intentionally mess up, while using the intercom system at her job. The therapist also

challenged Josie to identify ways that her imperfections might actually contribute to her value as a person. Josie was hesitant to do this but agreed when she reminded herself of the importance of facing feared situations.

SESSION 15

Josie arrived at the 15th session and reported that she had been unable to make a mistake intentionally in her musical performance in front of family members, but she was able to make a mistake while using the intercom system at work. The therapist continued to use cognitive restructuring to explore Josie's core belief, "If I'm not perfect, I'm worthless."

THERAPIST: So, last week we started to talk about some core issues, and I felt like you left here feeling a little overwhelmed. How are you feeling about things now?

JOSIE: It was a difficult session because I was feeling really good about overcoming hard stuff in the beginning, like learning how to pick out automatic thoughts, see how they were wrong, then finding a really good, challenging response to them and actually believing it. I felt good because I can do that now, almost automatically, or at least without too much effort. I felt like I was done, and then we ended up having to face some really scary stuff again. I feel like I took a giant step up, to a harder level of work.

THERAPIST: The things we talked about last week were harder. That's a good sign that we've really worked our way to your core beliefs because it feels so different. But remember all the work and practice that you put into identifying and challenging every other automatic thought or situation that we've worked on. It didn't all happen right away. In terms of core beliefs, we're going to do the same thing. All we've done is identify it. Now we will spend time challenging it and testing out the thought, "If I'm not perfect, I'm worthless." We'll start here in session today, but this is work you'll continue on your own. What might be some thinking errors? What's limiting in thinking that anything less than 100% is a failure?

JOSIE: That's catastrophizing. Probably also a should statement because I feel like I must be perfect. And also maybe fortune-telling because I feel like I'm assuming things will go wrong eventually. That's it.

THERAPIST: What about all-or-nothing thinking?

JOSIE: Oh yeah, definitely. In my mind, it's like there's 0% success or 100% success.

THERAPIST: So what are some ways we can challenge this? It won't be easy, but let's try.

JOSIE: Umm, I guess simple challenges, like "How do I know I'm going to be worthless if I'm not perfect?" I don't know. I guess not being perfect doesn't have to equal being worthless.

THERAPIST: Tell me more about that.

JOSIE: Some things are maybe valuable even when they're not perfect. Like people. Or art.

THERAPIST: So sometimes people's flaws, or quirks, make them more interesting?

JOSIE: Yeah, that's what I like best about my boyfriend. Those things other people are bothered by I find endearing. I like things that are imperfect, that have their own personality to them that's not quite right. I don't really have a problem when the imperfection is with someone else. But with me, it's different.

THERAPIST: Are you a harsher critic of yourself than others?

JOSIE: Definitely. Too bad I can't see myself the way I see others.

THERAPIST: Maybe you can, maybe we can try that. It's hard because you've been looking at yourself critically for a long time. It's going to be a change, and it will take testing and practice. But what might be the reward for trying something besides being a harsher judge of yourself than others?

JOSIE: I guess the work will pay off, like it did with everything else. With practice, I even had fun at my show. I didn't believe that I was going to be a failure. I believed I could do it. It was a huge success.

THERAPIST: Were there any minor flaws with the evening? Things that went wrong, but that you coped with?

JOSIE: Oh, yeah, tons. Like I forgot my friend's name when I was introducing her to my parents. But it didn't ruin the evening. Overall things were good, and I felt good about it. I could skip over those flaws and just enjoy it.

THERAPIST: So when thinking about that situation, how true does it feel that if you are not perfect, you are worthless?

JOSIE: When I came in, I felt overwhelmed by everything; now that we can see all the work I've done, I feel better. I think I can challenge this. I don't think it feels totally true anymore.

THERAPIST: OK, so what's some evidence that this core belief may not be true?

JOSIE: Well, it's OK for everyone else to not be perfect. Maybe a little less OK for me, but I guess it's still somewhat OK. And some people are more valuable to me because of their imperfections. I guess being perfect is boring. Being perfect is impossible.

THERAPIST: So that seems like a high standard to hold yourself to.

JOSIE: (*Laughs.*) Yeah. I don't know anyone who's perfect. Everyone makes mistakes. Even me. Especially me. Everyone in the history of the world has been imperfect.

THERAPIST: Right. Now let's get back to you, not just others. Do we have evidence that you may be valuable even if you're imperfect? Are there upsides of imperfection?

JOSIE: I'll be more unique, more of an individual. It makes for interesting challenges; it could make for a really interesting life. I could learn a lot about different ways to do things, try out all kinds of new things. Make lots of mistakes, and just learn to do things better the next time. Not perfect, but just better. And make room for failure.

THERAPIST: So how much do you believe that if you're not perfect, you're worthless?

JOSIE: Maybe like 20%. Right now, at least, only 20%.

THERAPIST: So how can we sum up some of these challenges that have gotten you to believing this only about 20%? What might be a rational response to this core belief, "If I'm not perfect, I'm worthless."

JOSIE: I don't know; this is hard. If I'm not perfect, I'm worthy? I don't believe it, but it makes me laugh. I guess maybe it's OK if I'm not perfect.

THERAPIST: Does that feel convincing?

JOSIE: Not really. I'm drawing a blank with coming up with the right rational response.

THERAPIST: What if we recognized that this rational response won't be perfect? Maybe we need to find one that's good enough for now. So let's keep at this.

JOSIE: Oh I see, there's the perfectionistic thinking again. I guess really, it is not humanly possible to be perfect. And I don't think I would even want to be that person who finally was perfect.

THERAPIST: So it seems like a lot of work to be chasing perfection when it kind of doesn't exist. It sounds like no matter how hard you try, there would always be the attempt to do better than perfect.

JOSIE: Yeah, like no matter what, I'd never be able to be perfect. It's not humanly possible. I guess if I had to make this a rational response, I'd tell myself something like "There is no such thing as perfect." I like that. I think that will work for now. I'm going to think about this more. This is a challenge, but I want to spend time on this.

THERAPIST: OK, so maybe we can try out this rational response this week by having you do some exposures that will allow you to challenge the core belief, "If I'm not perfect, I'm worthless."

JOSIE: Yeah. I need to do that every day, challenge this, become more accepting of my imperfections. It might be fun to mess up on purpose. But a lot of the time I mess up just naturally, but I guess even then I'm not worthless. Mistakes are going to happen because there is no such thing as perfect.

For homework this session, Josie was assigned the task of intentionally making mistakes in conversation (e.g., "forgetting" people's names, asking them to repeat something they have said), at work (e.g., pressing the wrong button when using the intercom, asking for help with a task), and in performances (e.g., playing the wrong notes while playing the piano for her family and friends).

Termination Segment

SESSION 16

In the final session, Josie and the therapist discussed her progress and the challenges that lay ahead. Josie rerated her fear and avoidance hierarchy, and the decrease in her ratings was considered significant and meaningful (see Table 3.3). She reported that, over the course of treatment, she learned new skills such as recognizing and challenging automatic thoughts and seeing all aspects of herself—including imperfection—as acceptable. The most important change she noted was being able to get and to keep a job at a bookstore, where she must interact with customers and coworkers all day. Josie reported that as a result of her treatment, for the first time she was able to see herself as equal rather than inferior to others, and she was optimistic about her future goals, both personal and professional.

Session-by-Session Assessment

Figure 3.2 displays Josie's session-by-session scores on the SASCI and the BFNE.

Recall that a score of 16 on the SASCI corresponds to no change, with lower scores indicative of increasingly greater improvement relative to baseline levels. Josie started to show modest improvement after Session 3. Her score spiked at Session 8, and then began a steady decline, reaching the minimum score of 4 by Session 12 and remaining there until the end of treatment. For the BFNE, Weeks and colleagues (2005) reported a mean score of 46.91 ($SD = 9.27$) in a large sample with social anxiety disorder and a mean of 26.81 ($SD = 4.78$) among normal controls. Early in treatment, Josie's session scores exceeded the mean of the clinical sample by as much as 10 points. However, her scores declined consistently thereafter, and by the end of treatment were just below the mean of the control sample.

One-Year Follow-Up Assessment

After 1 year with no treatment, Josie showed considerable improvement on all self-report and clinician-administered measures compared to her pretreatment assessment (see Table 3.2). In fact, she no longer met diagnostic criteria for social anxiety disorder. She was considering applications to graduate programs to continue her study of music and had plans to audition for the local orchestra. Josie reported that she had been making friends at her job and felt that she now had a core of social supports on which she could rely.

Five-Year Follow-Up Assessment

Approximately 5 years after the conclusion of her treatment, we had the opportunity to check in with Josie and discuss how things had gone for her since she completed CBT as described herein. She had received no additional therapy, other than a brief period of some premarital counseling with a member of the clergy. Josie had gotten married, moved to a large city, and had a child; she experienced an episode of postpartum depression that resolved without treatment. She had completed a prestigious music fellowship program where she gained additional experience and confidence as a composer and performer. At the time of our check-in, Josie was hoping to devote more time to her music, perhaps as a teacher. Josie was very proud to report that

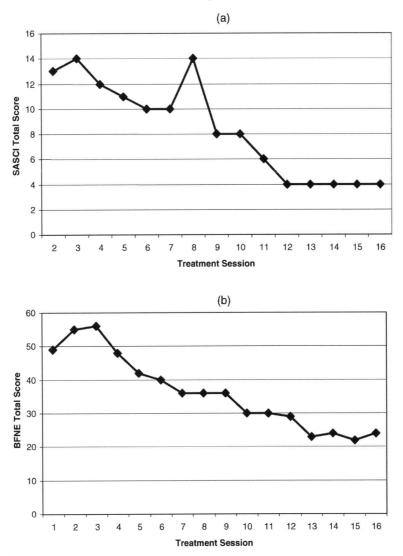

FIGURE 3.2. Weekly scores on the (a) Social Anxiety Session Change Index (SASCI) and (b) Brief Fear of Negative Evaluation Scale (BFNE).

she has been successful in pushing herself to engage in social situations that were difficult at first and that she has learned that things often are not as difficult as she first feared. Josie reported a return of some anxiety symptoms, as reflected in ratings on her fear and avoidance hierarchy, which were higher than those reported at the 1-year follow-up but generally lower than those at the pretreatment assessment (Table 3.3). However, she

reported that this did not significantly interfere with her daily functioning, as reflected in her scores on the majority of self-report and clinician-administered measures (See Table 3.2). As at the 1-year follow-up, Josie did not meet criteria for social anxiety disorder. However, she experienced some distress in social situations that were not relevant to her life at the time of treatment. For instance, socializing with other children's parents at school and church was a new challenge that had led to some anxiety and avoidance in recent years. Josie thought she might benefit from some booster sessions, but she reported that she continues to review her client workbook and therapy notes from time to time to maintain her CBT skills.

CLINICAL PREDICTORS OF SUCCESS AND FAILURE

Josie's treatment turned out well, as it does for many clients. However, treatment response is a variable phenomenon, and researchers have investigated a number of predictors of CBT outcome (see more in the review of this topic by L. Magee, Erwin, & Heimberg, 2009).

Expectancy for improvement, subtype of social anxiety disorder, and comorbidity with other anxiety or mood disorders, as well as APD, have been discussed in other sections of this chapter. Here we briefly review three other variables—adherence to assigned CBT homework, anger, and cognitive change.

Adherence to prescribed homework assignments has been associated with positive treatment outcome, and evidence suggests that adherence to particular components of CBT homework assignments may be differentially predictive of outcome. For instance, adherence to between-session cognitive restructuring and exposure assignments predicts posttreatment outcome better than adherence to assignments related more to psychoeducation early in treatment (Leung & Heimberg, 1996). Other studies have not replicated these effects immediately after treatment (Edelmann & Chambless, 1995; Woody & Adessky, 2002). However, 6-month follow-up assessments revealed that homework-compliant individuals reported fewer avoidant behaviors, less fear of negative evaluation, and less anxiety when giving a speech compared to less compliant clients (Edelman & Chambless, 1995).

Anger is a significant predictor of CBT outcome as well. In a study by Erwin, Heimberg, Schneier, and Liebowitz (2003), individuals with high levels of trait anger were more likely to terminate treatment prematurely. Also, levels of state and trait anger and anger suppression before treatment were significantly correlated with posttreatment severity of social anxiety.

Finally, in a study comparing group CBT, exposure group therapy, and waiting-list control conditions, changes in estimated social cost, or negative cognitive appraisal, mediated pretreatment to posttreatment changes in both active treatment groups (Hofmann, 2004). Furthermore, only the group receiving cognitive techniques, in addition to exposure, continued to show improvement from posttreatment to the 6-month follow-up assessment. Continued benefit was associated with an overall reduction in estimated social cost from pre- to posttreatment assessments, suggesting that the cognitive-behavioral intervention is associated with greater treatment gains that are mediated through changes in estimated social cost (Hofmann, 2004). More recently, Boden and colleagues (2012) demonstrated that changes in interpersonal core beliefs mediated the effect of CBT on social anxiety symptoms, and Goldin and colleagues (2012) showed that increased belief in one's ability to engage in cognitive reappraisal did the same.

SUMMARY AND CONCLUSIONS

Our primary purpose in this chapter was to provide a step-by-step analysis of the conduct of individual CBT for social anxiety disorder from initial assessment to long-term follow-up. Procedural difficulties that may arise in the conduct of CBT for social anxiety disorder were not be discussed in detail here because of space limitations, but they are discussed thoroughly by Heimberg and Becker (2002). Individuals like Josie, who make dramatic improvements in their lives, provide the impetus for continued research on the treatment of social anxiety disorder—a potentially debilitating disorder with an increasingly encouraging prognosis.

REFERENCES

Acarturk, C., de Graaf, R., van Straten, A., ten Have, M., & Cuijpers, P. (2008). Social phobia and number of social fears, and their association with comorbidity, health-related quality of life and help seeking. *Social Psychiatry and Psychiatric Epidemiology, 43*, 273–279.

Aderka, I. M. (2009). Factors affecting treatment efficacy in social phobia: The use of video feedback and individual vs. group formats. *Journal of Anxiety Disorders, 23*, 12–17.

Aderka, I. M., Hofmann, S. G., Nickerson, A., Hermesh, H., Gilboa-Schectman, E., & Marom, S. (2012). Functional impairment in social anxiety disorder. *Journal of Anxiety Disorders, 26*, 393–400.

American Psychiatric Association. (1980). *Diagnostic and statistical manual of mental disorders* (3rd ed.). Washington, DC: Author.

American Psychiatric Association. (2013). *Diagnostic and statistical manual of mental disorders* (5th ed.). Arlington, VA: Author.

Antony, M. M., Coons, M. J., McCabe, R. E., Ashbaugh, A., & Swinson, R. P. (2006). Psychometric properties of the Social Phobia Inventory: Further evaluation. *Behaviour Research and Therapy, 44*, 1177–1185.

Barlow, D. H. (2002). *Anxiety and its disorders: The nature and treatment of anxiety and panic* (2nd ed.). New York: Guilford Press.

Beck, A. T., Steer, R. A., & Brown, G. K. (1996). *Beck Depression Inventory manual* (2nd ed.). San Antonio, TX: Psychological Corporation.

Beck, J. S. (1995). *Cognitive therapy: Basics and beyond.* New York: Guilford Press.

Beidel, D. C., Turner, S. M., Stanley, M. A., & Dancu, C. V. (1989). The Social Phobia and Anxiety Inventory: Concurrent and external validity. *Behavior Therapy, 20*, 417–427.

Blanco, C., Heimberg, R. G., Schneier, F. R., Fresco, D. M., Chen, H., Turk, C. L., et al. (2010). A placebo-controlled trial of phenelzine, cognitive behavioral group therapy and their combination for social anxiety disorder. *Archives of General Psychiatry, 67*, 286–295.

Blanco, C., Xu, Y., Schneier, F., Okuda, M., Liu, S.-M., & Heimberg, R. G. (2011). Predictors of persistence of social anxiety disorder: A national study. *Journal of Psychiatric Research, 45*, 1557–1563.

Boden, M. T., John, O. P., Goldin, P. R., Werner, K., Heimberg, R. G., & Gross, J. J. (2012). The role of maladaptive beliefs in cognitive behavioral therapy: Evidence from social anxiety disorder. *Behaviour Research and Therapy, 50*, 287–291.

Brown, E. J., Heimberg, R. G., & Juster, H. R. (1995). Social phobia subtype and avoidant personality disorder: Effect on severity of social phobia, impairment, and outcome of cognitive-behavioral treatment. *Behavior Therapy, 26*, 467–486.

Brown, E. J., Turovsky, J., Heimberg, R. G., Juster, H. R., Brown, T. A., & Barlow, D. H. (1997). Validation of the Social Interaction Anxiety Scale and the Social Phobia Scale across the anxiety disorders. *Psychological Assessment, 9*, 21–27.

Brown, T. A., Di Nardo, P. A., & Barlow, D. H. (1994). *Anxiety Disorders Interview Schedule for DSM-IV.* New York: Oxford University Press.

Brown, T. A., Di Nardo, P. A., & Barlow, D. H. (2013). *Anxiety and Related Disorders Interview Schedule for DSM-5: Lifetime version (ADIS-5–L).* Manuscript in preparation.

Brown, T. A., Di Nardo, P. A., Lehman, S. L., & Campbell, L. A. (2001). Reliability of DSM-IV anxiety and mood disorders: Implications for the classification of emotional disorders. *Journal of Abnormal Psychology, 110*, 49–58.

Brozovich, F., & Heimberg, R. G. (2008). An analysis of post-event processing in social anxiety disorder. *Clinical Psychology Review, 28*, 891–903.

Bruce, S. E., Yonkers, K. A., Otto, M. W., Eisen, J. L., Weisberg, R. B., Pagano, M., et al. (2005). Influence of psychiatric comorbidity on recovery and recurrence in generalized anxiety disorder, social phobia, and panic disorder: A 12-year prospective study. *American Journal of Psychiatry, 162*, 1179–1187.

Bruch, M. A., Fallon, M., & Heimberg, R. G. (2003). Social phobia and difficulties in occupational adjustment. *Journal of Counseling Psychology, 50*, 109–117.

Bruch, M. A., Gorsky, J. M., Collins, T. M., & Berger, P. (1989). Shyness and sociability reexamined: A multicomponent analysis. *Journal of Personality and Social Psychology, 57*, 904–915.

Carleton, R. N., Collimore, K. C., Asmundson, G. J. G., McCabe, R. E., Rowa, K., & Antony, M. M. (2009). Refining and validating the Social Interaction Anxiety Scale and the Social Phobia Scale. *Depression and Anxiety, 26*, E71–E81.

Chambless, D. L., Fydrich, T., & Rodebaugh, T. L. (2008). Generalized social phobia and avoidant personality disorder: Meaningful distinction or useless duplication? *Depression and Anxiety, 25*, 8–19.

Chambless, D. L., & Ollendick, T. H. (2001). Empirically supported psychological interventions: Controversies and evidence. *Annual Review of Psychology, 52*, 685–716.

Chambless, D. L., Tran, G. Q., & Glass, C. R. (1997). Predictors of response to cognitive-behavioral group therapy for social phobia. *Journal of Anxiety Disorders, 11*, 221–240.

Clark, D. M., Ehlers, A., Hackmann, A., McManus, F., Fennell, M., Grey, N., et al. (2006). Cognitive therapy versus exposure and applied relaxation in social phobia: A randomized controlled trial. *Journal of Consulting and Clinical Psychology, 74*, 568–578.

Clark, D. M., Ehlers, A., McManus, F., Hackmann, A., Fennell, M., Campbell, H., et al. (2003). Cognitive therapy versus fluoxetine in generalized social phobia: A randomized placebo-controlled trial. *Journal of Consulting and Clinical Psychology, 71*, 1058–1067.

Clark, D. M., & Wells, A. (1995). The cognitive model of social phobia. In R. G. Heimberg, M. R. Leibowitz, D. A. Hope, & F. R. Schneier (Eds.), *Social phobia: Diagnosis, assessment, and treatment* (pp. 69–93). New York: Guilford Press.

Collins, K. A., Westra, H. A., Dozois, D. J. A., & Stewart, S. H. (2005). The validity of the brief version of the Fear of Negative Evaluation Scale. *Journal of Anxiety Disorders, 19*, 345–359.

Connor, K. M., Davidson, J. R. T., Churchill, E., Sherwood, A., Foa, E. B., & Weisler, R. H. (2000). Psychometric properties of the Social Phobia Inventory (SPIN): A new self-rating scale. *British Journal of Psychiatry, 176*, 379–386.

Connor, K. M., Kobak, K. A., Churchill, E., Katzelnick, D., & Davidson, J. R. T. (2001). Mini-SPIN: A brief screening assessment for generalized social anxiety disorder. *Depression and Anxiety, 14*, 137–140.

Cox, B. J., Pagura, J., Stein, M. B., & Sareen, J. (2009). The relationship between generalized social phobia and avoidant personality disorder in a national mental health survey. *Depression and Anxiety, 26*, 354–362.

Cox, B. J., Ross, L., Swinson, R. P., & Direnfeld, D. M. (1998). A comparison of social phobia outcome measures in cognitive-behavioral group therapy. *Behavior Modification, 22*, 285–297.

Davidson, J. R. T., Miner, C. M., De Veaugh-Geiss, J., Tupler, L. A., Colket, J. T., & Potts, N. L. (1997). The Brief Social Phobia Scale: A psychometric evaluation. *Psychological Medicine, 27*, 161–166.

Davidson, J. R. T., Potts, N. L., Richichi, E. A., Ford, S. M., Krishnan, R. R., Smith, R. D., et al. (1991). The Brief Social Phobia Scale. *Journal of Clinical Psychiatry, 52*(Suppl. 11), 48–51.

Di Nardo, P. A., Brown, T. A., & Barlow, D. H. (1994). *Anxiety Disorders Interview Schedule for DSM-IV: Lifetime version (ADIS-IV-L)*. New York: Oxford University Press.

Edelmann, R. E., & Chambless, D. L. (1995). Adherence during session and homework in cognitive-behavioral group treatment of social phobia. *Behaviour Research and Therapy, 33*, 537–577.

Elting, D. T., Hope, D. A., & Heimberg, R. G. (1997). Interrelationships among measures commonly used in research on social phobia. *Depression and Anxiety, 4*, 246–248.

Erwin, B. A., Heimberg, R. G., Juster, H. R., & Mindlin, M. (2002). Comorbid anxiety and mood disorders among persons with social phobia. *Behaviour Research and Therapy, 40*, 19–35.

Erwin, B. A., Heimberg, R. G., Schneier, F. R., & Liebowitz, M. R. (2003). Anger experience and expression in social anxiety disorder: Pretreatment profile and predictors of attrition and response to cognitive-behavioral treatment. *Behavior Therapy, 34*, 331–350.

Fergus, T. A., Valentiner, D. P., McGrath, P. B., Gier-Lonsway, S. L., & Kim, H.-S. (2012). Short forms of the Social Interaction Anxiety Scale and the Social Phobia Scale. *Journal of Personality Assessment, 94*, 310–320.

Feske, U., Perry, K. J., Chambless, D. L., Renneberg, B., & Goldstein, A. J. (1996). Avoidant personality disorder as a predictor for severity and treatment outcome among generalized social phobics. *Journal of Personality Disorders, 10*, 174–184.

Fresco, D. M., Coles, M. E., Heimberg, R. G., Liebowitz, M. R., Hami, S., Stein, M. B., et al. (2001). The Liebowitz Social Anxiety Scale: A comparison of the psychometric properties of self-report and clinician-administered formats. *Psychological Medicine, 31*, 1025–1035.

Frisch, M. B. (1994). *Manual and treatment guide for the Quality of Life Inventory*. Minneapolis, MN: National Computer Systems.

Gaston, J. E., Abbott, M. J., Rapee, R. M., & Neary, S. A. (2006). Do empirically supported treatments generalize to private practice?: A benchmark study of a cognitive-behavioural group treatment programme for social phobia. *British Journal of Clinical Psychology, 45*, 33–48.

Gilbert, P. (2001). Evolution and social anxiety: The role of attraction, social competition, and social hierarchies. *Psychiatric Clinics of North America, 24*, 723–751.

Goldin, P. R., Ziv, M., Jazaieri, H., Werner, K., Kraemer, H., Heimberg, R. G., et al. (2012). Cognitive reappraisal self-efficacy mediates the effects of individual cognitive-behavioral therapy for social anxiety disorder in a randomized controlled trial. *Journal of Consulting and Clinical Psychology, 80*, 1034–1040.

Hackmann, A., Clark, D. M., & McManus, F. (2000). Recurrent images and early memories in social phobia. *Behaviour Research and Therapy, 38*, 601–610.

Hackmann, A., Surawy, C., & Clark, D. M. (1998). Seeing yourself through others' eyes: A study of spontaneously occurring images in social phobia. *Behavioural and Cognitive Psychotherapy, 26*, 3–12.

Hambrick, J. P., Turk, C. L., Heimberg, R. G., Schneier, F. R., & Liebowitz, M. R. (2003). The experience of disability and quality of life in social anxiety disorder. *Depression and Anxiety, 18*, 46–50.

Hayes, S. A., Hope, D. A., Van Dyke, M., & Heimberg, R. G. (2007). Working alliance for clients with social anxiety disorder: Relationship with session helpfulness and within-session habituation. *Cognitive Behaviour Therapy, 36*, 34–42.

Hayes, S. A., Miller, N. A., Hope, D. A., Heimberg, R. G., & Juster, H. R. (2008). Assessing client progress session-by-session: The Social Anxiety Session Change Index. *Cognitive and Behavioral Practice, 15*, 203–211.

Heimberg, R. G. (1994). Cognitive assessment strategies and the measurement of outcome of treatment for social phobia. *Behaviour Research and Therapy, 32*, 269–280.

Heimberg, R. G., & Becker, R. E. (2002). *Cognitive-behavioral group therapy for social phobia: Basic mechanisms and clinical strategies*. New York: Guilford Press.

Heimberg, R. G., Brozovich, F. A., & Rapee, R. M. (2010). A cognitive-behavioral model of social anxiety disorder: Update and extension. In S. G. Hofmann & P. M. DiBartolo (Eds.), *Social anxiety: Clinical, developmental, and social perspectives* (2nd ed., pp. 395–422). New York: Academic Press.

Heimberg, R. G., Dodge, C. S., Hope, D. A., Kennedy, C. R., Zollo, L. J., & Becker, R. E. (1990). Cognitive-behavioral group treatment for social phobia: Comparison with a credible placebo control. *Cognitive Therapy and Research, 14*, 1–23.

Heimberg, R. G., & Holaway, R. M. (2007). Examination of the known-groups validity of the Liebowitz Social Anxiety Scale. *Depression and Anxiety, 24*, 447–454.

Heimberg, R. G., Holt, C. S., Schneier, F. R., Spitzer, R. L., & Liebowitz, M. R. (1993). The issues of subtypes in the diagnosis of social phobia. *Journal of Anxiety Disorders, 7*, 249–269.

Heimberg, R. G., Hope, D. A., Dodge, C. S., & Becker, R. E. (1990). DSM-III-R subtypes of social phobia: Comparison of generalized social phobics and public speaking phobics. *Journal of Nervous and Mental Disease, 178*, 172–179.

Heimberg, R. G., Horner, K. J., Juster, H. R., Safren, S. A., Brown, E. J., Schneier, F. R., et al. (1999). Psychometric properties of the Liebowitz Social Anxiety Scale. *Psychological Medicine, 29*, 199–212.

Heimberg, R. G., Liebowitz, M. R., Hope, D. A., Schneier, F. R., Holt, C. S., Welkowitz, L. A., et al. (1998). Cognitive behavioral group therapy vs. phenelzine therapy for social phobia: 12–week outcome. *Archives of General Psychiatry, 55*, 1133–1141.

Heimberg, R. G., Mueller, G. P., Holt, C. S., Hope, D. A., & Liebowitz, M. R. (1992). Assessment of anxiety in social interaction and being observed by others: The Social Interaction Anxiety Scale and the Social Phobia Scale. *Behavior Therapy, 23*, 53–73.

Heimberg, R. G., Salzman, D. G., Holt, C. S., & Blendell, K. A. (1993). Cognitive-behavioral group treatment for social phobia: Effectiveness at five-year followup. *Cognitive Therapy and Research, 17*, 325–339.

Heimberg, R. G., & Turk, C. L. (2002). Assessment of social phobia. In R. G. Heimberg & R. E. Becker (Eds.), *Cognitive-behavioral group therapy for social phobia: Basic mechanisms and clinical strategies* (pp. 107–126). New York: Guilford Press.

Herbert, J. D., Bellack, A. S., & Hope, D. A. (1991). Concurrent validity of the Social Phobia and Anxiety Inventory. *Journal of Psychopathology and Behavioral Assessment, 13*, 357–368.

Herbert, J. D., Hope, D. A., & Bellack, A. S. (1992). Validity of the distinction between generalized social phobia and avoidant personality disorder. *Journal of Abnormal Psychology, 101*, 332–339.

Hofmann, S. G. (2004). Cognitive mediation of treatment change in social phobia. *Journal of Consulting and Clinical Psychology, 72*, 392–399.

Hofmann, S. G., Newman, M. G., Becker, E., Taylor, C. B., & Roth, W. T. (1995). Social phobia with and without avoidant personality disorder: Preliminary behavior therapy outcome findings. *Journal of Anxiety Disorders, 9*, 427–438.

Hope, D. A., Heimberg, R. G., & Bruch, M. A. (1995). Dismantling cognitive-behavioral group therapy for social phobia. *Behaviour Research and Therapy, 33*, 637–650.

Hope, D. A., Heimberg, R. G., Juster, H., & Turk, C. L. (2000). *Managing social anxiety: A cognitive-behavioral therapy approach (client workbook)*. New York: Oxford University Press.

Hope, D. A., Heimberg, R. G., & Turk, C. L. (2006). *Managing social anxiety: A cognitive-behavioral therapy approach (therapist guide)*. New York: Oxford University Press.

Hope, D. A., Heimberg, R. G., & Turk, C. L. (2010a). *Man-*

aging social anxiety: A cognitive-behavioral therapy approach (Client Workbook, 2nd ed.). New York: Oxford University Press.

Hope, D. A., Heimberg, R. G. , & Turk, C.L. (2010b). *Managing social anxiety: A cognitive-behavioral therapy approach* (Therapist Guide, 2nd ed.). New York: Oxford University Press.

Hope, D. A., Herbert, J. D., & White, C. (1995). Diagnostic subtype, avoidant personality disorder, and efficacy of cognitive behavioral group therapy for social phobia. *Cognitive Therapy and Research, 19*, 399–417.

Hope, D. A., Van Dyke, M., Heimberg, R. G., Turk, C. L., & Fresco, D. M. (2002). *Cognitive-behavioral therapy for social anxiety disorder: Therapist adherence scale*. Unpublished manuscript, available from Richard G. Heimberg, Adult Anxiety Clinic, Department of Psychology, Temple University, Philadelphia, PA 19122–6085.

Huppert, J. D., Strunk, D. R., Ledley, D. R., Davidson, J. R. T., & Foa, E. B. (2008). Generalized social anxiety disorder and avoidant personality disorder: Structural analysis and treatment outcome. *Depression and Anxiety, 25*, 441–448.

Kabat-Zinn, J. (1990). *Full catastrophe living: Using the wisdom of your body and mind to face stress, pain, and illness*. New York: Dell.

Katzelnick, D. J., Kobak, K. A., DeLeire, T., Henk, H. J., Greist, J. H., Davidson, J. R. T., et al. (2001). Impact of generalized social anxiety disorder in managed care. *American Journal of Psychiatry, 158*, 1999–2007.

Kendall, P. C., Chu, B., Gifford, A., Hayes, C., & Nauta, M. (1998). Breathing life into a manual: Flexibility and creativity with manual-based treatments. *Cognitive and Behavioral Practice, 5*, 177–198.

Kendall, P. C., Gosch, E., Furr, J. M., & Sood, E. (2008). Flexibility within fidelity. *Journal of the American Academy of Child and Adolescent Psychiatry, 47*, 987–993.

Kessler, R. C., Berglund, P. D., Demler, O., Olga, J. R., Merikangas, K. R., & Walters, E. E. (2005). Lifetime prevalence and age-of-onset distributions of DSM-IV disorders in the National Comorbidity Survey Replication. *Archives of General Psychiatry, 62*, 593–602.

Koszycki, D., Benger, M., Shlik, J., & Bradwejn, J. (2007). Randomized trial of a meditation-based stress reduction program and cognitive behavior therapy in generalized social anxiety disorder. *Behaviour Research and Therapy, 45*, 2518–2526.

Kupper, N., & Denollet, J. (2012). Social anxiety in the general population. Introducing abbreviated versions of the SIAS and SPS. *Journal of Affective Disorders, 136*, 90–98.

Leary, M. R. (1983). A brief version of the Fear of Negative Evaluation Scale. *Personality and Social Psychology Bulletin, 9*, 371–375.

Leary, M. R., Kowalski, R. M., & Campbell, C. D. (1988). Self-presentational concerns and social anxiety: The role of generalized impression expectancies. *Journal of Research in Personality, 22*, 308–321.

Ledley, D. R., Heimberg, R. G., Hope, D. A., Hayes, S. A.., Zaider, T. I., Van Dyke, M., et al. (2009). Efficacy of a manualized and workbook-driven individual treatment for social anxiety disorder. *Behavior Therapy, 40*, 414–424.

Leung, A. W., & Heimberg, R. G. (1996). Homework compliance, perceptions of control, and outcome of cognitive-behavioral treatment for social phobia. *Behaviour Research and Therapy, 34*, 423–432.

Liebowitz, M. R. (1987). Social phobia. *Modern Problems in Pharmacopsychiatry, 22*, 141–173.

Liebowitz, M. R., Heimberg, R. G., Fresco, D. M., Travers, J., & Stein, M. B. (2000). Social phobia or social anxiety disorder: What's in a name? *Archives of General Psychiatry, 57*, 191–192.

Liebowitz, M. R., Heimberg, R. G., Schneier, F. R., Hope, D. A., Davies, S., Holt, C. S., et al. (1999). Cognitive-behavioral group therapy versus phenelzine in social phobia: Long-term outcome. *Depression and Anxiety, 10*, 89–98.

Lincoln, T. M., Rief, W., Hahlweg, K., Frank, M., von Witzleben, I., Schroeder, B., et al. (2003). Effectiveness of an empirically supported treatment for social phobia in the field. *Behaviour Research and Therapy, 41*, 1251–1269.

MacLeod, C., & Mathews, A. (1991). Biased cognitive operations in anxiety: Accessibility of information or assignment of processing priorities? *Behaviour Research and Therapy, 29*, 599–610.

Magee, L., Erwin, B. A., & Heimberg, R. G. (2009). Psychological treatment of social anxiety disorder and specific phobia. In M. M. Antony & M. B. Stein (Eds.), *Handbook of anxiety and the anxiety disorders* (pp. 334–349). New York: Oxford University Press.

Magee, W. J., Eaton, W. W., Wittchen, H.-U., McGonagle, K. A., & Kessler, R. C. (1996). Agoraphobia, simple phobia, and social phobia in the National Comorbidity Survey. *Archives of General Psychiatry, 53*, 159–168.

Mannuzza, S., Schneier, F. R., Chapman, T. F., Liebowitz, M. R., Klein, D. F., & Fyer, A. J. (1995). Generalized social phobia: Reliability and validity. *Archives of General Psychiatry, 52*, 230–237.

Marques, L., Porter, E., Keshaviah, A., Pollack, M. H., Van Ameringen, M., Stein, M. B., et al. (2012). Avoidant personality disorder in individuals with generalized social anxiety disorder: What does it add? *Journal of Anxiety Disorders, 26*, 665–672.

Mattick, R. P., & Clarke, J. C. (1998). Development and validation of measures of social phobia scrutiny fear and social interaction anxiety. *Behaviour Research and Therapy, 36*, 455–470.

Mattick, R. P., & Peters, L. (1988). Treatment of severe social phobia: Effects of guided exposure with and without cognitive restructuring. *Journal of Consulting and Clinical Psychology, 56*, 251–260.

McEvoy, P. M. (2007). Effectiveness of cognitive behavioural group therapy for social phobia in a community clinic: A benchmarking study. *Behaviour Research and Therapy, 45*, 3030–3040.

McEvoy, P. M., Nathan, P., Rapee, R. M., & Campbell, B. N. C. (2012). Cognitive behavioural group therapy for social phobia: Evidence of transportability to community clinics. *Behaviour Research and Therapy, 50*, 258–265.

Mennin, D. S., Fresco, D. M., Heimberg, R. G., Schneier, F. R., Davies, S. O., & Liebowitz, M. R. (2002). Screening for social anxiety disorder in the clinical setting: Using the Liebowitz Social Anxiety Scale. *Journal of Anxiety Disorders, 16*, 661–673.

Mörtberg, E., Clark, D. M., & Bejerot, S. (2011). Intensive group cognitive therapy and individual cognitive therapy for social phobia: Sustained improvement at 5–year follow-up. *Journal of Anxiety Disorders, 25*, 994–1000.

Narrow, W. E., Rae, D. S., Robins, L. N., & Regier, D. A. (2002). Revised prevalence estimates of mental disorders in the United States: Using a clinical significance criterion to reconcile two surveys' estimates. *Archives of General Psychiatry, 59*, 115–123.

Norton, P. J., & Hope, D. A. (2001). Kernels of truth or distorted perceptions: Self and observer ratings of social anxiety and performance. *Behavior Therapy, 32*, 765–786.

Ougrin, D. (2011). Efficacy of exposure versus cognitive therapy in anxiety disorders: Systematic review and meta analysis. *BMC Psychiatry, 11*, 200.

Peters, L., Sunderland, M., Andrews, G., Rapee, R. M., & Mattick, R. P. (2012). Development of a short form Social Interaction Anxiety (SIAS) and Social Phobia Scale (SPS) using nonparametric item response theory: The SIAS-6 and the SPS-6. *Psychological Assessment, 24*, 66–76.

Piet, J., Hougaard, E., Hecksher, M. S., & Rosenberg, N. K. (2010). A randomized pilot study of mindfulness-based cognitive therapy and group cognitive-behavioral therapy for young adults with social phobia. *Scandinavian Journal of Psychology, 51*, 403–410.

Pontoski, K., Heimberg, R. G., Turk, C. L., & Coles, M. E. (2010). Psychotherapy for social anxiety disorder. In D. Stein, E. Hollander, & B. Rothbaum (Eds.), *American Psychiatric Publishing textbook of anxiety disorders* (2nd ed., pp. 501–521). Washington, DC: American Psychiatric Press.

Powers, M. B., Sigmarsson, S. R., & Emmelkamp, P. M. G. (2008). A meta-analytic review of psychological treatments for social anxiety disorder. *International Journal of Cognitive Therapy, 1*, 94–113.

Rapee, R. M., & Heimberg, R. G. (1997). A cognitive-behavioral model of anxiety in social phobia. *Behaviour Research and Therapy, 35*, 741–756.

Rapee, R. M., & Lim, L. (1992). Discrepancy between self- and observer ratings of performance in social phobics. *Journal of Abnormal Psychology, 101*, 728–731.

Ries, B. J., McNeil, D. W., Boone, M. L., Turk, C. L., Carter, L. E., & Heimberg, R. G. (1998). Assessment of contemporary social phobia verbal report instruments. *Behaviour Research and Therapy, 36*, 983–994.

Rodebaugh, T. L. (2009). Social phobia and perceived friendship quality. *Journal of Anxiety Disorders, 23*, 872–878.

Rodebaugh, T. L., Heimberg, R. G., Brown, P. J., Fernandez, K. C., Blanco, C., Schneier, F. R., et al. (2011). More reasons to be straightforward: Findings and norms for two scales relevant to social anxiety. *Journal of Anxiety Disorders, 25*, 623–630.

Rodebaugh, T. L., Woods, C. M., & Heimberg, R. G. (2007). The reverse of social anxiety is not always the opposite: The reverse-scored items of the Social Interaction Anxiety Scale do not belong. *Behavior Therapy, 38*, 192–206.

Rodebaugh, T. L., Woods, C. M., Thissen, D. M., Heimberg, R. G., Chambless, D. L., & Rapee, R. M. (2004). More information from fewer questions: The factor structure and item properties of the original and Brief Fear of Negative Evaluation Scale. *Psychological Assessment, 16*, 169–181.

Roth, D. A., Coles, M. E., & Heimberg, R. G. (2002). The relationship between memories for childhood teasing and anxiety and depression in adulthood. *Journal of Anxiety Disorders, 16*, 149–164.

Rytwinski, N. K., Fresco, D. M., Heimberg, R. G., Coles, M. E., Liebowitz, M. R., Cissell, S., et al. (2009). Screening for social anxiety disorder with the self-report version of the Liebowitz Social Anxiety Scale. *Depression and Anxiety, 26*, 34–38.

Safren, S. A., Heimberg, R. G., Brown, E. J., & Holle, C. (1997). Quality of life in social phobia. *Depression and Anxiety, 4*, 126–133.

Safren, S. A., Heimberg, R. G., & Juster, H. R. (1997). Client expectancies and their relationship to pretreatment symptomatology and outcome of cognitive-behavioral group treatment for social phobia. *Journal of Consulting and Clinical Psychology, 65*, 694–698.

Sanderson, W. C., Di Nardo, P. A., Rapee, R. M., & Barlow, D. H. (1990). Syndrome comorbidity in patients diagnosed with a DSM-III-R anxiety disorder. *Journal of Abnormal Psychology, 99*, 308–312.

Sank, L. I., & Shaffer, C. S. (1984). *A therapist's manual for cognitive behavior therapy in groups.* New York: Plenum Press.

Schneier, F. R., Heckelman, L. R., Garfinkel, R., Campeas, R., Fallon, B. A., Gitow, A., et al. (1994). Functional impairment in social phobia. *Journal of Clinical Psychiatry, 55*, 322–331.

Schneier, F. R., Johnson, J., Hornig, C. D., Liebowitz, M. R., & Weissman, M. M. (1992). Social phobia: Comorbidity and morbidity in an epidemiologic sample. *Archives of General Psychiatry, 49*, 282–288.

Scholing, A., & Emmelkamp, P. M. G. (1993). Exposure with and without cognitive therapy for generalized social phobia: Effects of individual and group treatment. *Behaviour Research and Therapy, 31*, 667–681.

Segal, Z. V., Williams, J. M., & Teasdale, J. D. (2002). *Mindfulness-based cognitive therapy for depression: A new approach to preventing relapse.* New York: Guilford Press.

Stangier, U., Heidenreich, T., Peitz, M., Lauterbach, W., & Clark, D. M. (2003). Cognitive therapy for social phobia: Individual versus group treatment. *Behaviour Research and Therapy, 41*, 991–1007.

Stangier, U., Schramm, E., Heidenreich, T., Berger, M., & Clark, D. M. (2011). Cognitive therapy vs. interpersonal therapy in social anxiety disorder. *Archives of General Psychiatry, 68*, 692–700.

Stopa, L., & Clark, D. M. (1993). Cognitive processes in social phobia. *Behaviour Research and Therapy, 31*, 255–267.

Taylor, S., Woody, S., McLean, P. D., & Koch, W. J. (1997). Sensitivity of outcome measures for treatments of generalized social phobia. *Assessment, 4*, 181–191.

Turner, S. M., Beidel, D. C., Dancu, C. V., & Stanley, M. A. (1989). An empirically derived inventory to measure social fears and anxiety: The Social Phobia and Anxiety Inventory. *Psychological Assessment, 1*, 35–40.

Turner, S. M., Beidel, D. C., & Townsley, R. M. (1992). Social phobia: A comparison of specific and generalized subtype and avoidant personality disorder. *Journal of Abnormal Psychology, 101*, 326–331.

Turner, S. M., Beidel, D. C., Wolff, P. L., Spaulding, S., & Jacob, R. G. (1996). Clinical features affecting treatment outcome in social phobia. *Behaviour Research and Therapy, 34*, 795–804.

Vriends, N., Becker, E. S., Meyer, A., Michael, T., & Margraf, J. (2007). Subtypes of social phobia: Are they of any use? *Journal of Anxiety Disorders, 21*, 59–75.

Vriends, N., Becker, E. S., Meyer, A., Williams, S. L., Lutz, R., & Margraf, J. (2007). Recovery from social phobia in the community and its predictors: Data from a longitudinal epidemiological study. *Journal of Anxiety Disorders, 21*, 320–337.

Wallace, S. T., & Alden, L. E. (1991). A comparison of social standards and perceived ability in anxious and nonanxious men. *Cognitive Therapy and Research, 15*, 237–254.

Watson, D., & Friend, R. (1969). Measurement of social-evaluative anxiety. *Journal of Consulting and Clinical Psychology, 33*, 448–457.

Weeks, J. W., Heimberg, R. G., Fresco, D. M., Hart, T. A., Turk, C. L., Schneier, F. R., et al. (2005). Empirical validation and psychometric evaluation of the Brief Fear of Negative Evaluation Scale in patients with social anxiety disorder. *Psychological Assessment, 17*, 179–190.

Weeks, J. W., Heimberg, R. G., & Rodebaugh, T. L., & Norton, P. J. (2008). Exploring the relationship between fear of positive evaluation and social anxiety. *Journal of Anxiety Disorders, 22*, 386–400.

Weeks, J. W., Spokas, M. E., & Heimberg, R. G. (2007). Psychometric evaluation of the Mini–Social Phobia Inventory (Mini-SPIN) in a treatment-seeking sample. *Depression and Anxiety, 24*, 382–391.

Wenzel, A. (2002). Characteristics of close relationships in individuals with social phobia: A preliminary comparison with nonanxious individuals. In J. H. Harvey & A. Wenzel (Eds.), *A clinician's guide to maintaining and enhancing close relationships* (pp. 199–214). Mahwah, NJ: Erlbaum.

Wlazlo, Z., Schroeder-Hartwig, K., Hand, I., Kaiser, G., & Münchau, N. (1990). Exposure *in vivo* vs. social skills training for social phobia: Long-term outcome and differential effects. *Behaviour Research and Therapy, 28*, 181–193.

Wolpe, J., & Lazarus, A. A. (1966). *Behavior therapy techniques*. New York: Pergamon.

Wong, J., Gordon, E. A., & Heimberg, R. G. (2012). Social anxiey disorder. In P. Sturmey & M. Hersen (Eds.), *Handbook of evidence-based practice in clinical psychology: Volume II, Adult disorders* (pp. 621–649). New York: Wiley.

Woody, S. R., & Adessky, R. S. (2002). Therapeutic alliance, group cohesion, and homework compliance during cognitive-behavioral group treatment of social phobia. *Behavior Therapy, 35*, 5–27.

CHAPTER 4

Obsessive–Compulsive Disorder

MARTIN E. FRANKLIN
EDNA B. FOA

It will not take the reader long to see that successful therapy for obsessive–compulsive disorder (OCD) is markedly different in both structure and content from the usual therapeutic approaches. For this reason, regrettably, few therapists feel self-efficacious enough to undertake this therapy, yet this approach is clearly the treatment of choice for the most beneficial short- and long-term effects in OCD according to clinical trials. The information provided in this detailed chapter should be sufficient for any reasonably well-trained mental health professional to undertake this treatment, particularly if few other options are available. The suffering involved with OCD can be extraordinary, and even imperfect attempts at therapy can relieve much of this suffering. This chapter describes the detailed conduct of intensive daily sessions involving both imaginal and direct *in vivo* practice. Also noticeable is the ingenuity required of therapists (e.g., Where do you find dead animals?). The importance of involving significant others continues a theme first described by Craske and Barlow in Chapter 1 of this volume, in which spouses/partners or other people close to the individual with the problem become an important and integral part of treatment. Finally, this chapter contains an up-to-date review of the current status of psychological and pharmacological approaches to OCD.—D. H. B.

Advances in cognitive-behavioral and pharmacological treatments in the last four decades have greatly improved the prognosis for patients with obsessive–compulsive disorder (OCD). In this chapter we first discuss diagnostic and theoretical issues of OCD and review the available treatments, then describe assessment procedures and illustrate in detail how to implement intensive cognitive-behavioral treatment (CBT) involving exposure and ritual prevention (EX/RP) for OCD. Throughout the chapter, we use case material to illustrate interactions that occur between therapist and patient to demonstrate the process that occurs during treatment.

DEFINITION

In the fifth edition of the *Diagnostic and Statistical Manual of Mental Disorders* (DSM-5; American Psychiatric Association, 2013), OCD is characterized by recurrent obsessions and/or compulsions that interfere substantially with daily functioning. Obsessions are "persistent thoughts, urges, or images that are experienced, at some time during the disturbance, as intrusive and unwanted, and that in most individuals cause marked anxiety or distress" (p. 237). Common obsessions are repeated thoughts about causing harm to others, contamination, and doubting whether one locked the front door. Compulsions are "repetitive behaviors or mental acts that the individual feels driven to perform in response to an obsession or according to rules that must be applied rigidly" (p. 237). Common compulsions include handwashing, checking, and counting. In DSM-5, OCD is categorized among obsessive–compulsive and related disorders (e.g., Stein et al., 2010), which highlights the formal and functional similarity between OCD and several other disorders that involve intense anxiety and associated compulsions (e.g., body dysmorphic disorder), as well as those involving repetitive behaviors that appear to be driven by appetitive urges (e.g., trichotillomania [hair pulling], excoriation [skin picking] disorder; American Psychiatric Association, 2013).

In DSM, the functional link between obsessions and compulsions is emphasized: "Obsessions" are defined as thoughts, images, or impulses that *cause* marked anxiety or distress, and "compulsions" are defined as overt (behavioral) or covert (mental) actions that are performed in an attempt to *reduce* the distress brought on by obsessions or according to rigid rules. This modification is supported by findings from the DSM-IV field trial on OCD, in which over 90% of participants reported that the aim of their compulsions was either to prevent harm associated with their obsessions or to reduce obsessional distress (Foa et al., 1995).

Data from the DSM-IV field study also indicated that the vast majority (over 90%) of individuals with OCD manifest both obsessions and behavioral rituals. When mental rituals are also included, only 2% of the sample report "pure" obsessions (Foa et al., 1995). Behavioral rituals (e.g., handwashing) are equivalent to mental rituals (e.g., silently repeating special prayers) in their functional relationship to obsessions: Both serve to reduce obsessional distress, to prevent feared harm, or to restore safety. Thus, whereas all obsessions are indeed mental events, compulsions can be either mental or behavioral. Identification of mental rituals is an especially important aspect of treatment planning because obsessions and compulsions are addressed via different techniques. For example, we once treated a patient who described himself as a "pure obsessional," who would experience intrusive and unwanted images of harm coming to his girlfriend by an animal attack. The patient would quickly and intentionally insert his own image into the scene to become the victim of the animal mauling, thereby reducing his distress and, in his estimation, reducing the likelihood that some future harm would come to his girlfriend. The substitution

of his own image into the scene constituted a mental ritual, and the success of imaginal exposure exercises required that the patient refrain from this form of compulsion.

A growing consensus about a continuum of insight in individuals with OCD (e.g., Foa et al., 1995; Insel & Akiskal, 1986) led to the inclusion in DSM-IV (American Psychiatric Association, 1994) of a subtype of OCD "with poor insight" to include individuals who indeed have obsessions and compulsions but fail to recognize their senselessness. In DSM-5, individuals are classified as having good or fair insight, poor insight, or absent insight/delusional beliefs, reflecting an even greater recognition of a continuum of insight in OCD (Leckman et al., 2010). Clinically it is important to evaluate the degree of insight prior to initiating CBT because fixed belief about the consequences of refraining from compulsions and avoidance behaviors has been found to be associated with attenuated treatment outcome (e.g., Foa, Abramowitz, Franklin, & Kozak, 1999; Neziroglu, Stevens, Yaryura-Tobias, & McKay, 2000).

To be diagnosed with OCD, obsessions and/or compulsions must be found to be of sufficient severity to cause marked distress, be time-consuming, and interfere with daily functioning. If another Axis I disorder is present, the obsessions and compulsions cannot be restricted to the content of that disorder (e.g., preoccupation with food in the presence of eating disorders).

PREVALENCE AND COURSE OF OCD

Once thought to be an extremely rare disorder, the 12-month prevalence of OCD was estimated at 1.0% in the recent National Comorbidity Survey Replication involving over 9,000 adult participants in the United States (Kessler et al., 2005). Epidemiological studies with children and adolescents suggest similar lifetime prevalence rates in these samples (e.g., Flament et al., 1988; Valleni-Basille et al., 1994). Slightly more than half of adults suffering from OCD are female (Rasmussen & Tsuang, 1986), whereas a 2:1 male to female ratio has been observed in several pediatric clinical samples (e.g., Hanna, 1995; Swedo, Rapoport, Leonard, Lenane, & Cheslow, 1989). Age of onset of the disorder typically ranges from early adolescence to young adulthood, with earlier onset in males; modal onset is ages 13–15 in males, and ages 20–24 in females (Rasmussen & Eisen, 1990). However, cases of OCD have been documented in children as young as age 2 (Rapoport, Swedo, & Leonard, 1992).

Development of the disorder is usually gradual, but acute onset has been reported in some cases. Although chronic waxing and waning of symptoms are typical, episodic and deteriorating courses have been observed in about 10% of patients (Rasmussen & Eisen, 1989). In some cases of pediatric OCD and tic disorders, onset is very sudden and associated with streptococcal infection; treatment of the infection is associated with substantial reduction of symptoms, but recurrence of infection is again associated with symptom exacerbation (Swedo et al., 1998). Presentation of OCD in these cases, which is much more typical in males than in females, came to be known as pediatric autoimmune neuropsychiatric disorders associated with streptococcal infection (PANDAS) and has more recently been revised and broadened under the umbrella term "pediatric autoimmune neuropsychiatric syndrome" (PANS; Swedo, Leckman, & Rose, 2012); the prevalence of PANDAS or PANS has yet to be determined. OCD is frequently associated with impairments in general functioning, such as disruption of gainful employment (Koran, 2000; Leon, Portera, & Weissman, 1995) and interpersonal relationship difficulties (Emmelkamp, de Haan, & Hoogduin, 1990; Riggs, Hiss, & Foa, 1992). Adolescents identified as having OCD (Flament et al., 1988) reported in a subsequent follow-up study that they had withdrawn socially to prevent contamination and to conserve energy for obsessive–compulsive behaviors (Flament et al., 1990). Many individuals with OCD suffer for years before seeking treatment. In one study, individuals first presented for psychiatric treatment over 7 years after the onset of significant symptoms (Rasmussen & Tsuang, 1986). The disorder may cause severe impairment in functioning that results in job loss and disruption of marital and other interpersonal relationships. Marital distress is reported by approximately 50% of married individuals seeking treatment for OCD (Emmelkamp et al., 1990; Riggs et al., 1992).

COMORBIDITY

Convergent epidemiological and clinical data indicate that OCD rarely occurs in isolation: Although the rates of comorbidity differ across studies due to selection of population and methodology, comorbidity is generally high. For example, Weissman and colleagues (1994) found that 49% of individuals diagnosed with OCD suffered from a comorbid anxiety disorder and 27% from comorbid major depressive disorder (MDD). Among studies conducted specifically within anxiety clinics, there is great variability, but comorbid conditions are generally common (for a review, see Ledley, Pai, & Franklin, 2007). In the largest of the studies conducted in the context of an anxiety clinic, Brown, Campbell, Lehman, Grisham, and Mancill (2001) found that 57% of 77 adults with a principal diagnosis of OCD had a current comorbid Axis I condition; the rate rose to 86% for lifetime comorbid Axis I conditions. Notably, when OCD co-occurs with other anxiety disorders, it is typically the principal diagnosis (e.g., the diagnosis of greatest severity; see Antony, Downie, & Swinson, 1998). It also appears to be the case that MDD onset tends to follow that of OCD, suggesting that depression might be a response to OCD symptoms (Bellodi, Sciuto, Diaferia, Ronchi, & Smeraldi, 1992; Diniz et al., 2004).

The data are equivocal with respect to the influence of comorbidity on OCD presentation. In one study, Denys, Tenney, van Megen, de Geus, and Westenberg (2004) found that comorbidity did not influence OCD symptom severity, whereas others (Angst, 1993; Tukel, Polat, Ozdemir, Aksut, & Turksov, 2002) found a relationship between comorbidity and OCD symptom severity. A more consistent finding is that comorbidity is associated with poorer quality of life, particularly in the case of comorbid depression (Lochner & Stein, 2003; Masellis, Rector, & Richter, 2003).

With respect to the effect of comorbid anxiety and depression on treatment outcome, the influence of depression has received more empirical attention to date. Some studies have found that higher levels of depression at pretreatment are related to poorer outcome (e.g., Keijsers, Hoogduin, & Schaap, 1994; Steketee, Chambless, & Tran, 2001), whereas others have found little or no effect (Mataix-Cols, Marks, Greist, Kobak, & Baer, 2002; O'Sullivan, Noshirvani, Marks, Monteiro, & Lelliott, 1991; Steketee, Eisen, Dyck, Warshaw, & Rasmussen, 1999). Some have suggested that, more specifically, the *severity* of the comorbid depression might influence its effects on OCD treatment outcome: Abramowitz, Franklin, Street, Kozak, and Foa (2000) found that only severely depressed patients were less likely to respond to EX/RP therapy for OCD. Similarly, highly depressed patients with OCD seem to be at greater risk for relapse following treatment discontinuation (Abramowitz & Foa, 2000; Basoglu, Lax, Kasvikis, & Marks, 1988). The influence of comorbid anxiety disorders on outcome has received less attention thus far: One study reported that patients with OCD and comorbid generalized anxiety disorder (GAD) terminate OCD treatment at higher rates than other patients (Steketee et al., 2001), and another found that the presence of posttraumatic stress disorder (PTSD) in patients with OCD attenuated response to EX/RP (Gershuny, Baer, Jenike, Minichiello, & Wilhelm, 2002). Within pediatric OCD specifically, comorbidity other than a second anxiety disorder (e.g., externalizing disorder, mood disorder) was associated with poorer acute response to CBT (Storch et al., 2008), and another recent report indicated that comorbid attention-deficit/hyperactivity disorder (ADHD) specifically attenuated CBT outcomes at follow-up among children and adolescents (Farrell, Waters, Milliner, & Ollendick, 2012). Notably, the mechanisms by which these comorbid conditions influence outcome have yet to be explored.

Tourette syndrome and other tic disorders also appear to be related to OCD, although not sufficiently to be grouped within obsessive–compulsive and related disorders in DSM-5. Estimates of the comorbidity of Tourette syndrome and OCD range from 28 to 63% (Comings, 1990; Kurlan et al., 2002; Leckman & Chittenden, 1990; Pauls, Towbin, Leckman, Zahner, & Cohen, 1986). Conversely, up to 17% of patients with OCD are thought to have Tourette syndrome (Comings, 1990; Kurlan et al., 2002; Rasmussen & Eisen, 1989). In a recent report, tic comorbidity was associated with poorer treatment outcome in general (Matsunaga et al., 2005), yet in a recent pediatric study was found to influence pharmacotherapy treatment outcome but not CBT response (March et al., 2007).

DIFFERENTIAL DIAGNOSIS

The high comorbidity of OCD with other disorders noted earlier, as well as the similarity between the criteria for OCD and other DSM disorders, can pose diagnostic quandaries. Below we review some of the more common diagnostic difficulties likely to confront clinicians and provide recommendations for making these difficult diagnostic judgments.

Obsessions versus Depressive Rumination

It is sometimes difficult to differentiate between depressive ruminations and obsessions. The distinction rests primarily on thought content and the patient's reported resistance to such thoughts. Unlike obsessions, ruminations are typically pessimistic ideas about the self or the world, and ruminative content frequently shifts. Additionally, depressive ruminators tend to not make repeated attempts to suppress their ruminations the way individuals with OCD try to suppress obsessions. When depression and OCD co-occur, both phenomena may be present, but only obsessions should be targeted with exposure exercises. We have also found clinically that the generally pessimistic presentation of depressed patients can undermine hopefulness about improvement during EX/RP; thus, these beliefs may require therapeutic intervention even though they are not obsessional.

Anxiety Disorders

OCD was previously classified as an anxiety disorder in DSM-IV, and it often co-occurs with anxiety disorders. Diagnostic criteria are sometimes similar among these related (anxiety) disorders, but the symptoms associated with each diagnosis can usually be distinguished. For example, the excessive worries characteristic of GAD may appear similar to those in OCD but, unlike obsessions, worries are excessive concerns about real-life circumstances and are experienced by the individual as appropriate (ego-syntonic). In contrast, obsessive thinking is more likely to be unrealistic or magical, and obsessions are usually experienced by the individual as inappropriate (ego-dystonic). There are, however, exceptions to this general rule: Individuals with either GAD or OCD may worry about everyday matters, such as their children getting sick. However, when worried about their children catching cold, parents with GAD might focus their concern on the long-term consequences (e.g., falling behind in school, development of a lifelong pattern of debilitation), whereas parents with OCD might focus more on the contamination aspect of illness (e.g., their child being infested with "cold germs"). The problem of distinguishing between obsessions and worries in a particular patient is most relevant when the patient exhibits no compulsions, but, as we mentioned earlier, pure obsessionals comprise only about 2% of individuals with OCD (Foa et al., 1995).

In the absence of rituals, the avoidance associated with specific phobias may also appear similar to OCD. For example, excessive fear of germs and specific phobia both may result in persistent fear of dogs. However, unlike an individual with OCD, a person with a specific phobia can successfully avoid dogs for the most part, or reduce distress quickly by escaping dogs when avoidance is impractical. In contrast, the individual with OCD who is obsessed with "dog germs" continues to feel contaminated even after the dog is gone, and sometimes knowing that a dog was in the vicinity several hours earlier can also produce obsessional distress even if there is no possibility that the dog will return. This distress often prompts subsequent avoidance behaviors (e.g., taking off clothing that might have been near the contaminating dog) not typically observed in specific phobias.

Body Dysmorphic Disorder

The preoccupation with imagined physical defects of body dysmorphic disorder (BDD) is formally similar to the obsessions of OCD, and BDD is grouped with obsessive–compulsive and related disorders in DSM-5. The best way to differentiate between this disorder and OCD is to examine for content specificity of the fear-provoking thoughts. Most individuals with BDD are singly obsessed, whereas most individuals with OCD have multiple obsessions.

Tourette Syndrome and Tic Disorders

To differentiate the stereotyped motor behaviors that characterize Tourette syndrome and tic disorders from compulsions, the functional relationship between these behaviors and any obsessive thoughts must be examined. Motor tics are generally experienced as involuntary and are not aimed at neutralizing distress brought about by obsessions. There is no conventional way to differentiate them from "pure" compulsions, but OCD with "pure" compulsions is extremely rare (Foa et al., 1995). As noted earlier, there appears to be a high rate of comorbidity between OCD and tic disorders (e.g., Pauls et al., 1986); thus, both disorders may be present simultaneously in a given patient. Interestingly, tics were similarly responsive to an EX/RP protocol when compared in a randomized study to habit-reversal training in which a competing response is substituted for the tic; this finding suggests that the conceptual model underlying the treatment of tics might require modification (Verdellen, Keijsers, Cath, & Hoogduin, 2004).

Delusional Disorder and Schizophrenia

Individuals with OCD may present with obsessions of delusional intensity (for a review, see Kozak & Foa, 1994). Approximately 5% of patients with OCD report

complete conviction that their obsessions and compulsions are realistic, with an additional 20% reporting strong but not fixed conviction. Therefore, it is important to consider the diagnosis of OCD "with poor insight" even if these beliefs are very strongly held. The differentiation between delusional disorder and OCD can depend on the presence of compulsions in OCD (Eisen et al., 1998). In OCD, obsessions of delusional intensity are usually accompanied by compulsions.

It is also important to recognize that the content of obsessions in OCD may be quite bizarre, as in the delusions of schizophrenia, but bizarreness in and of itself does not preclude a diagnosis of OCD. For example, one patient seen at our center was fearful that small bits of her "essence" would be forever lost if she passed too close to public trash cans. This patient did not report any other symptoms of formal thought disorder, such as loose associations, hallucinations, flat or grossly inappropriate affect, and thought insertion or projection. Following a course of EX/RP that focused on exercises designed to expose the patient to the loss of her "essence" (e.g., driving by the city dump), her OCD symptoms were substantially reduced. On occasion patients do meet diagnostic criteria for both OCD and schizophrenia, and a dual diagnosis is appropriate under these circumstances. Importantly, EX/RP with such patients should proceed only if the associated treatment exercises do not exacerbate the comorbid thought disorder symptoms.

COGNITIVE AND BEHAVIORAL MODELS

Mowrer's (1939) two-stage theory for the acquisition and maintenance of fear and avoidance behavior has been commonly adopted to explain phobias and OCD. As elaborated by Mowrer (1960), this theory proposes that in the first stage, a neutral event becomes associated with fear by being paired with a stimulus that by its nature provokes discomfort or anxiety. Through conditioning processes, objects, as well as thoughts and images, acquire the ability to produce discomfort. In the second stage of this process, escape or avoidance responses are developed to reduce the anxiety or discomfort evoked by the various conditioned stimuli and are maintained by their success in doing so. Dollard and Miller (1950) adopted Mowrer's two-stage theory to explain the development of phobias and obsessive–compulsive neurosis. As noted earlier, because of the intrusive nature of obsessions, many situations that provoke obsessions cannot readily be avoided. Passive avoidance behaviors, such as those utilized by phobics, are also less effective in controlling obsessional distress. Active avoidance patterns in the form of ritualistic behaviors are then developed and maintained by their success in alleviating this distress.

In light of equivocal empirical support for the two-stage theory and its limitations in explaining the etiology of obsessions, several cognitive explanations were proposed to account for the development and maintenance of OCD symptoms (e.g., Beck, 1976; Carr, 1974). Salkovskis (1985) offered a more comprehensive cognitive analysis of OCD. He posited that intrusive obsessional thoughts are stimuli that may provoke certain types of negative automatic thoughts. Accordingly, an intrusive thought leads to mood disturbances only if it triggers negative automatic thoughts through interaction between the unacceptable intrusion and the individual's belief system (e.g., only bad people have sexual thoughts). According to Salkovskis, exaggerated senses of responsibility and self-blame are the central themes in the belief system of a person with OCD. Neutralization, in the form of behavioral or cognitive compulsions, may be understood as an attempt to reduce this sense of responsibility and to prevent blame. In addition, frequently occurring thoughts regarding unacceptable actions may be perceived by the individual with OCD as equivalent to the actions themselves, so, for example, even if the person has not sinned, the thought of sinning is as bad as sinning itself.

Salkovskis (1985) further proposed that five dysfunctional assumptions characterize individuals with OCD and differentiate them from persons without OCD:

(1) Having a thought about an action is like performing the action; (2) failing to prevent (or failing to try to prevent) harm to self or others is the same as having caused the harm in the first place; (3) responsibility is not attenuated by other factors (e.g., low probability of occurrence); (4) not neutralizing when an intrusion has occurred is similar or equivalent to seeking or wanting the harm involved in that intrusion to actually happen; (5) one should (and can) exercise control over one's thoughts. (p. 579)

Thus, while the obsession may be ego-dystonic, the automatic thought it elicits will be ego-syntonic. By extension, this model suggests that treatment of OCD should largely focus on identifying the erroneous assumptions and modifying the automatic thoughts. This theory paved the way for various elaborations on the cognitive models, experimental studies of the model, and the development of cognitive therapies that derive from the central role of these key cognitive factors.

Salkovskis's (1985) theory sparked examination of the role of responsibility in the psychopathology of OCD (Ladoucer et al., 1995; Rachman, Thordarson, Shafran, & Woody, 1995; Rhéaume, Freeston, Dugas, Letarte, & Ladouceur, 1995). Further attention has been paid to what Rachman (1998) referred to as thought–action fusion (TAF), wherein individuals believe that simply having an unacceptable thought increases the likelihood of the occurrence of a feared outcome, and that thoughts of engaging in repugnant activities are equivalent to actually having done so. Contemporary cognitive theorists would then suggest that obsessive–compulsive beliefs such as TAF, exaggerated responsibility, and intolerance of uncertainty likely result in increased and ultimately futile efforts at thought suppression and other ill-advised mental control strategies, which would then yield increased frequency of such thoughts and associated distress (Purdon & Clark, 2002). Hence, a vicious cycle of avoidance maintains and strengthens the OCD, and the cognitive therapies that derive from these contemporary models would directly target these obsessive–compulsive beliefs in an effort to break the cycle.

In an integrated cognitive-behavioral account, Foa and Kozak (1985) conceptualized anxiety disorders in general as specific impairments in emotional memory networks. Following Lang (1979), they view fear as an information network existing in memory that includes representation about fear stimuli, fear responses, and their meaning. With regard to the fear content, Foa and Kozak suggested that fear networks of individuals with anxiety disorders are characterized by the presence of erroneous estimates of threat, unusually high negative valence for the feared event, and excessive response elements (e.g., physiological reactivity), and are resistant to modification. This persistence may reflect failure to access the fear network because of either active avoidance or because the content of the fear network precludes spontaneous encounters with situations that evoke anxiety in everyday life. Additionally, anxiety may persist because of some impairment in the mechanism of extinction. Cognitive defenses, excessive arousal with failure to habituate, faulty premises, and erroneous rules of inference are all impairments that would hinder the processing of information necessary for modifying the fear structure to reduce fear behavior.

Foa and Kozak (1985) suggested that several forms of fear occur in individuals with OCD. The patient who fears contracting venereal disease from public bathrooms and washes to prevent such harm has a fear structure that includes excessive associations between the stimuli (e.g., bathroom) and the anxiety/distress responses, as well as mistaken beliefs about the harm related to the stimulus. For other individuals with OCD, fear responses are associated with mistaken meaning rather than with a particular stimulus. For example, some patients who are disturbed by perceived asymmetry, and who reduce their distress by rearranging objects, do not fear the objects themselves, nor do they anticipate disaster from the asymmetry. Rather, they are upset by their view that certain arrangements of stimuli are "improper."

Like Reed (1985), Foa and Kozak (1985) proposed that in addition to the pathological content of the obsessions, OCD is distinguished from other disorders by pathology in the mechanisms underlying information processing. Specifically, they suggested that patients with OCD experience impairments in considering the rules for making inferences about harm, often concluding that a situation is dangerous based on the absence of evidence for safety, and that they often fail to make inductive leaps about safety from information about the absence of danger. Consequently, rituals performed to reduce the likelihood of harm can never provide safety and must be repeated. In an elaboration on emotional processing theory and the mechanism by which exposure works, Foa, Huppert, and Cahill (2006) suggested that *in vivo* exposure to the feared stimulus in the absence of the anticipated harm corrects the exaggerated probability estimates; imaginal exposure not only corrects the exaggerated cost but also strengthens the discrimination between "thoughts about harm" and "real harm," thus altering the associations between threat meaning of stimulus and/or response elements in the fear structure.

In contrast to the more general theories of OCD described earlier, some theorists have posed more specific hypotheses to account for the pathology observed in certain OCD subtypes. For example, clinical observations led some investigators to hypothesize that memory deficits for actions underlie compulsive checking (e.g., Sher, Frost, & Otto, 1983). However, the results of experimental investigations of this hypothesis are equivocal. Some support for an action–memory deficit was found in nonclinical individuals with checking rituals (e.g., Rubenstein, Peynircioglu, Chambless, & Pigott, 1993; Sher et al., 1983). In contrast, a study using a clinical sample found that compared to nonpa-

tients, patients with OCD with checking rituals *better* recalled their fear-relevant actions (e.g., plugging in an iron, unsheathing a knife), but not fear-irrelevant actions (e.g., putting paper clips in a box; Constans, Foa, Franklin, & Mathews, 1995). From these data, it appears that checking is not motivated primarily by memory problems; hence, teaching mnemonic strategies to patients with OCD with checking rituals is probably not the optimal clinical strategy; rather, having patients repeatedly confront the low-risk situations that provoke obsessional distress, while simultaneously refraining from checking behavior or mental reviewing of actions, is preferred.

TREATMENTS

Exposure and Ritual Prevention

The prognostic picture for OCD has improved dramatically since Victor Meyer (1966) first reported on two patients who responded well to a treatment that included prolonged exposure to obsessional cues and strict prevention of rituals. This procedure, known at the time as exposure and ritual prevention (EX/RP), was later found to be extremely successful in 10 of 15 cases and partly effective in the remainder. Patients treated with this regimen also appeared to maintain their treatment gains: At a 5-year follow-up, only two of these patients had relapsed (Meyer & Levy, 1973; Meyer, Levy, & Schnurer, 1974).

As was the case with Meyer's program, current EX/RP treatments typically include both prolonged exposure to obsessional cues and procedures aimed at blocking rituals. Exposure exercises are often done in real-life settings (*in vivo*), for example, by asking the patient who fears accidentally causing a house fire by leaving the stove on, to leave the house without checking the burners. When patients report specific feared consequences of refraining from rituals, these fears may also be addressed via imaginal exposure. In fact, *in vivo* and imaginal exposure exercises are designed specifically to prompt obsessional distress. It is believed that repeated, prolonged exposure to feared thoughts and situations provides information that disconfirms mistaken associations and evaluations held by the patients and thereby promotes habituation (Foa & Kozak, 1986). Exposure is usually done gradually by confronting situations that provoke moderate distress before confronting more upsetting ones. Exposure homework is routinely assigned between sessions, and patients are also asked to refrain from rituals.

Since Meyer's (1966) initial positive report of the efficacy of EX/RP, many subsequent studies of EX/RP have indicated that most EX/RP treatment completers make and maintain clinically significant gains. Randomized controlled trials (RCTs) have indicated that EX/RP is superior to a variety of control treatments, including placebo medication (Marks, Stern, Mawson, Cobb, & McDonald, 1980), relaxation (Fals-Stewart, Marks, & Schafer, 1993), and anxiety management training (Lindsay, Crino, & Andrews, 1997). Foa and Kozak's (1996) review of 12 outcome studies ($N = 330$) reporting treatment responder rates indicated that 83% of EX/RP treatment completers were classified as responders at posttreatment. In 16 studies reporting long-term outcome ($N = 376$; mean follow-up interval of 29 months), 76% were responders. Moreover, several studies have now indicated that these encouraging findings for EX/RP are not limited to highly selected RCT samples (Franklin, Abramowitz, Kozak, Levitt, & Foa, 2000; Rothbaum & Shahar, 2000; Valderhaug, Larsson, Gotestam, & Piacentini, 2007; Warren & Thomas, 2001).

In general, EX/RP has been found quite effective in ameliorating OCD symptoms and has produced great durability of gains following treatment discontinuation. In our review of the literature, it also was apparent that among the many variants of EX/RP treatment, some are relevant for outcome and others are not. We review the literature on the relative efficacy of the ingredients that comprise EX/RP to help clinicians decide which EX/RP components are most essential.

EX/RP Treatment Variables

EXPOSURE VERSUS RITUAL PREVENTION VERSUS EX/RP

To separate the effects of exposure and ritual prevention on OCD symptoms, Foa, Steketee, Grayson, Turner, and Latimer (1984) randomly assigned patients with washing rituals to treatment by exposure only (EX), ritual prevention only (RP), or their combination (EX/RP). Each treatment was conducted intensively (15 daily 2-hour sessions conducted over 3 weeks) and followed by a home visit. Patients in each condition were found to be improved at both posttreatment and follow-up, but EX/RP was superior to the single-component treatments on almost every symptom measure at both assessment points. In comparing EX and RP, patients who received EX reported lower anxiety when confronting feared contaminants than did patients who had received RP, whereas the RP group reported greater decreases in urge to ritualize than did the EX patients. Thus, it appears that EX and RP affected different OCD symptoms. The findings from this study clearly suggest that EX and RP should be implemented concurrently; treatments that do not include both components yield inferior outcome. It is important to convey this information to patients, especially when they are experiencing difficulty either refraining from rituals or engaging effectively in exposure exercises during and between sessions.

IMPLEMENTATION OF RITUAL PREVENTION

Promoting abstinence from rituals during treatment is thought to be essential for successful treatment outcome, but the preferred method of RP has changed over the years. In Meyer's (1966) EX/RP treatment program, hospital staff members physically prevented patients from performing rituals (e.g., turning off the water supply in a patient's room). However, physical intervention by staff or family members to prevent patients from ritualizing is no longer typical nor recommended. It is believed that such prevention techniques are too coercive to be an accepted practice today. Moreover, physical prevention by others may actually limit generalizability to nontherapy situations in which others are not present to intercede. Instead, instructions and encouragement to refrain from ritualizing and avoidance are now recommended. As noted earlier, although exposure in itself can reduce obsessional distress, it is not so effective in reducing compulsions. To maximize treatment effects, the patient needs to refrain voluntarily from ritualizing while engaging in systematic exposure exercises. The therapist should strongly emphasize the importance of refraining from rituals and help the patient with this difficult task by providing support, encouragement, and suggestions about alternatives to ritualizing.

USE OF IMAGINAL EXPOSURE

Treatment involving imaginal plus *in vivo* EX/RP at follow-up was superior to an *in vivo* EX/RP program that did not include imaginal exposure (Foa, Steketee, Turner, & Fischer, 1980; Steketee, Foa, & Grayson,

1982). However, a second study did not find that the addition of imaginal exposure enhanced long-term efficacy compared to *in vivo* exposure only (De Araujo, Ito, Marks, & Deale, 1995). The treatment program in the former study differed from that of De Araujo and colleagues on several parameters (e.g., 90-minute vs. 30-minute imaginal exposures, respectively); thus, the source of these studies' inconsistencies cannot be identified.

In our clinical work, we have found imaginal exposure to be helpful for patients who report that disastrous consequences will result if they refrain from rituals. Because many of these consequences cannot be readily translated into *in vivo* exposure exercises (e.g., burning in hell), imaginal exposure allows the patient an opportunity to confront these feared thoughts. Also, the addition of imagery to *in vivo* exposure may circumvent the cognitive avoidance strategies used by patients who intentionally try not to consider the consequences of exposure while confronting feared situations *in vivo*. In summary, although imaginal exposure does not appear essential for immediate outcome, it may enhance long-term maintenance and be used as an adjunct to *in vivo* exercises for patients who fear disastrous consequences. For patients who only report extreme distress as a consequence of refraining from rituals and avoidance behaviors, imaginal exposure may not be needed.

GRADUAL VERSUS ABRUPT EXPOSURES

No differences in OCD symptom reduction were detected in a study comparing patients who confronted the most distressing situations from the start of therapy to those who confronted less distressing situations first, yet patients preferred the more gradual approach (Hodgson, Rachman, & Marks, 1972). However, because patient motivation and agreement with treatment goals are core elements of successful EX/RP, situations of moderate difficulty are usually confronted first, followed by several intermediate steps, before the most distressing exposures are attempted. Thus, we emphasize that exposure will proceed at a pace that is acceptable to the patient, and that no exposure will ever be attempted without the patient's approval. At the same time, it is preferable to confront the highest item on the treatment hierarchy relatively early in treatment (e.g., within the first week of intensive treatment) to allow sufficient time to repeat these difficult exposures over the later sessions.

DURATION OF EXPOSURE

Duration of exposure was once believed to be important for outcome in that prolonged, continuous exposure was found to be more effective than short, interrupted exposure (Rabavilas, Boulougouris, & Perissaki, 1979). Indeed, reduction in anxiety (habitation) across sessions has been associated with improvement following exposure-based treatments for OCD and for PTSD (e.g., Jaycox, Foa, & Morral, 1998; Kozak, Foa, & Steketee, 1988; van Minnen & Hagenaars, 2002). However, several studies have not found a strong relationship between within-session habituation and fear and symptom reduction (Jaycox et al., 1998; Kozak et al., 1988; Mathews, Johnston, Shaw, & Gelder, 1974; Rowe & Craske, 1998). In an elaboration on emotional processing theory, Foa and colleagues (2006) found that the recent deemphasis on the relationship between within-session habituation and outcome is not critical to emotional processing theory because the proposed mechanism underlying symptom reduction is the modification of the relevant erroneous associations through disconfirming information, not through habituation per se. In practical terms, this means patients should be instructed that although, optimally, they should persist with exposure until the anxiety is substantially reduced, the more important factor is repeating the same exposures, to promote reduction of associated anxiety over time. Patients with OCD might be particularly vulnerable to fears of ending exposures "too soon," hence, doing the treatment incorrectly, so this new instruction might help encourage patients to go about their business without ritualizing or avoiding, regardless of whether anxiety still lingers on from an exposure task. The deemphasis on the critical importance of habituation in the moment is more pronounced procedurally when using acceptance and commitment therapy (e.g., Twohig et al., 2010), but generally speaking this viewpoint appears to be gaining acceptance among cognitive-behavioral therapists as well. For example, clinically we often remind patients that whether or not they are anxious is less relevant than what they do (or do not do) when they are anxious, since ritualizing and avoidance will maintain fear down the line.

FREQUENCY OF EXPOSURE SESSIONS

Optimal frequency of exposure sessions has yet to be established. Intensive exposure therapy programs that have achieved excellent results (e.g., Foa, Kozak,

Steketee, & McCarthy, 1992) typically involve daily sessions over the course of approximately 1 month, but quite favorable outcomes have also been achieved with more widely spaced sessions (e.g., Abramowitz, Foa, & Franklin, 2003; De Araujo et al., 1995; Franklin et al., 1998). A recent RCT in pediatric OCD found no difference between intensive and weekly treatment (Storch et al., 2007). Clinically, we have found that less frequent sessions may be sufficient for highly motivated patients with mild to moderate OCD symptoms, who readily understand the importance of daily exposure homework. Patients with very severe symptoms or those who for various reasons cannot readily comply with EX/RP tasks between sessions, are typically offered intensive treatment.

THERAPIST-ASSISTED VERSUS SELF-EXPOSURE

Evaluations of the presence of a therapist during exposure have yielded inconsistent results. In one study, patients with OCD receiving therapist-assisted exposure were more improved immediately posttreatment than those receiving clomipramine and self-exposure, but this difference was not evident at follow-up (Marks et al., 1988). However, these results are difficult to interpret in light of the study's complex design. A second study using patients with OCD also indicated that therapist-assisted treatment was not superior to self-exposure at posttreatment or at follow-up (Emmelkamp & van Kraanen, 1977), but the number of patients in each condition was too small to render these findings conclusive. In contrast to the negative findings of Marks and colleagues (1988) and Emmelkamp and van Kraanen (1977), therapist presence yielded superior outcome of a single, 3-hour exposure session compared to self-exposure for persons with specific phobia (Öst, 1989). Because specific phobias are, on the whole, less disabling and easier to treat than OCD, one may surmise that therapist presence should also influence treatment outcome with OCD. Moreover, using meta-analytic procedures, Abramowitz (1996) found that therapist-controlled exposure was associated with greater improvement in OCD and GAD symptoms compared to self-controlled procedures. A recent study found comparable outcome for patients receiving EX/RP with therapist assistance and those who received teletherapy (Lovell et al., 2006), which further raises the question of whether therapist assistance is required for good outcome. In light of these inconsistent findings, no clear answer is available on the role of thera-

pist assistance with exposure tasks in OCD treatment. However, we have found clinically that the presence of a therapist can be useful in helping patients to remain engaged in exposures while anxiety is high, to avoid subtle rituals or avoidance behaviors during exposure (e.g., distraction, mental rituals), and to remain sufficiently motivated despite distress. Researchers have begun to examine the question of whether telephone therapy or Skype would also be effective, including adapted CBT protocols for Tourette syndrome (Himle, Olufs, Himle, Tucker, & Woods, 2010) and OCD specifically (e.g., Bachofen et al., 1999); such research may provide greater confidence that these methods can be used efficaciously, which will help to address the ongoing problem of the paucity of OCD treatment expertise that plagues most communities.

EX/RP versus Other Treatment Approaches

In this section we review the literature on the efficacy of standard individual EX/RP treatment versus other therapeutic approaches, including group treatment, family-based EX/RP treatment, cognitive therapy, and pharmacotherapy.

INDIVIDUAL VERSUS GROUP EX/RP

Intensive individual EX/RP, although effective, can pose practical obstacles such as high cost for treatment, and scheduling problems for patient and therapist alike. Additionally, because experts in EX/RP treatment are few and far between, patients may need to wait for long periods or travel substantial distances to be treated. Thus, some researchers have begun to examine the efficacy of more affordable and efficient treatment modalities. One such alternative is group treatment. Fals-Stewart and colleagues (1993) conducted a controlled study in which patients with OCD were randomly assigned to individual EX/RP, group EX/RP, or a psychosocial control condition (relaxation). Each of the active treatments was 12 weeks long, with sessions held twice weekly, and included daily exposure homework. Significant improvement in OCD symptoms was evident in both active treatments, with no differences detected between individual and group EX/RP immediately posttreatment or at 6-month follow-up. Profile analysis of OCD symptom ratings collected throughout treatment did indicate a faster reduction in symptoms for patients receiving individual treatment. These results offer evidence for the efficacy of group treatment. However, because patients were excluded from this study if they were diagnosed with *any* personality disorder or with comorbid depression, it may be that the sample was somewhat atypical. In addition, none of the participants had received previous OCD treatment, which is also unusual for this population and suggestive of a less symptomatic sample. Thus, inferences about the broader OCD population merit caution until these results are replicated.

More recently, Barrett, Healy-Farrell, and March (2004) found that individual and group CBT were highly and similarly efficacious for children and adolescents with OCD relative to a wait-list control; this raises the possibility that group interventions might hold particular promise in the treatment of youth with OCD. Also in youth, Asbahr and colleagues (2005) found group CBT and sertraline comparable at post-treatment, but there was less relapse in the former condition. More recently, another Australian research group found comparable outcomes for group treatment compared to individual treatment, both of which were superior to a wait-list control (Anderson & Rees, 2007); not surprisingly, though, individual treatment was associated with more rapid response.

FAMILY INVOLVEMENT
VERSUS STANDARD EX/RP TREATMENT

Emmelkamp and colleagues (1990) examined whether family involvement in treatment would enhance the efficacy of EX/RP for OCD. Patients who were married or living with a romantic partner were randomly assigned to receive EX/RP either with or without partner involvement in treatment. Results indicated that OCD symptoms were significantly lowered following treatment for both groups. No differences between the treatments emerged, and initial marital distress did not predict outcome. However, the reduction in anxiety/distress reported for the sample as a whole was modest (33%), which may have resulted from the relatively short treatment sessions and absence of *in vivo* exposure exercises in treatment sessions.

Mehta (1990) also examined the effect of family involvement on EX/RP treatment outcome. To adapt the treatment to serve the large numbers of young unmarried people seeking OCD treatment and the "joint family system" prevalent in India, Mehta used a family-based rather than spouse-based treatment approach. Patients who did not respond to previous pharmacotherapy were randomly assigned to receive treatment

by systematic desensitization and EX/RP, either with or without family assistance. Sessions in both conditions were held twice per week for 12 weeks; response prevention was described as "gradual." In the family condition, a designated family member (parent, spouse, or adult child) assisted with homework assignments, supervised relaxation therapy, participated in response prevention, and was instructed to be supportive. On self-reported OCD symptoms, a greater improvement was found for the family-based intervention at post-treatment and 6-month follow-up. Although this study had methodological problems that complicate interpretation of findings (e.g., use of self-report OCD measures only, unclear description of treatment procedures), it offers some preliminary evidence that family involvement may be helpful in OCD treatment. Clinically, we routinely enlist the support of family members in EX/RP, providing psychoeducation about the illness and its consequences during the early stages of treatment planning, and advice and encouragement in managing the patient's request for assurances, his or her avoidant behaviors, and violation of EX/RP rules between sessions. We also try to reduce family members' criticism of the patient and unconstructive arguing about OCD and related matters when these issues arise in the therapy.

Published randomized studies of CBT for OCD with youth have each included parents at least to some extent in treatment (Barrett et al., 2004; de Haan, Hoogduin, Buitelaar, & Keijsers, 1998; Pediatric OCD Treatment Study Team, 2004), and a direct comparison of CBT, with and without a family component, using an otherwise identical protocol has yet to be conducted in pediatric OCD. Research on whether family involvement enhances individual CBT outcomes in other anxiety disorders has generally yielded mixed findings, however, and a large, recently completed RCT indicated that both forms of treatment are efficacious and essentially equivalent to one another (Bogels & Bodden, 2005). Higher family dysfunction in general was associated with poorer long-term outcome in a recent study (Barrett, Farrell, Dadds, & Boulter, 2005), as was family accommodation of OCD rituals specifically (Peris et al., 2012), and at this point it might be clinically prudent to include a more comprehensive family component when family members are very directly involved in the patient's rituals (e.g., reassurance seeking) or when family psychopathology threatens generalizability of treatment gains to a chaotic home environment. It also may be that greater family involvement in treatment is needed when the patient is very young (Freeman et al., 2003, 2007).

EX/RP VERSUS COGNITIVE THERAPIES

Increased interest in cognitive therapy (e.g., Beck, 1976; Ellis, 1962), coupled with dissatisfaction with formulations of treatment mediated by processes such as extinction (Stampfl & Levis, 1967) or habituation (Watts, 1973), prompted examination of the efficacy of cognitive procedures for anxiety disorders in general and for OCD in particular. A number of early studies found few differences between standard behavioral treatments and behavioral treatments enhanced with various cognitive approaches (e.g., Emmelkamp & Beens, 1991; Emmelkamp, Visser, & Hoekstra, 1988). Recent advances in cognitive conceptualizations of OCD have apparently yielded more efficacious and durable cognitive treatments. Freeston and colleagues (1997) found a cognitive-behavioral intervention efficacious compared to a wait-list control group for patients with "pure" obsessions. Several other studies (Cottraux et al., 2001; McLean et al., 2001; Vogel, Stiles, & Götestam, 2004; Whittal, Thordarson, & McLean, 2005) have suggested equivalent results for CBT and EX/RP, respectively, although some procedural overlap between the two conditions in these studies makes their findings difficult to interpret. In concert with studies attesting to the utility of cognitively oriented approaches for conditions that are quite similar to OCD, such as hypochondriasis (Barsky & Ahern, 2004; Warwick, Clark, Cobb, & Salkovskis, 1996), it does appear that cognitive therapies hold promise for the treatment of OCD and might be an efficacious potential alternative to EX/RP. More recently, however, Whittal, Woody, McLean, Rachman, and Robichaud (2010) failed to find a difference between cognitive therapy and stress management training (SMT) for a sample with primary obsessions and mental rituals, although this appeared to be due to the fact that SMT yielded substantial and lasting benefit compared to pretreatment rather than because cognitive therapy did not.

The question of whether cognitive therapy improves the efficacy of EX/RP is generally difficult to discern because both exposure therapy and cognitive therapy are intended to modify mistaken cognitions. An RCT that compared "pure" forms of CT or EX/RP, with or without medication, found similar, yet somewhat attentuated, outcomes relative to what might typically be expected from either treatment (van Balkom et al.,

1998). Foa and Kozak (1986) argued that the disconfirmation of erroneous associations and beliefs is a crucial mechanism underlying the efficacy of exposure treatments, hence disputing discussions that mistaken cognitions from EX/RP might be expected to hamper outcome. For example, a patient and therapist sitting on the bathroom floor in a public restroom conducting an exposure to contaminated surfaces routinely discuss risk assessment, probability overestimation, and so forth, as the therapist helps the patient achieve the cognitive modification necessary for improvement. The practical issue of interest is how to maximize efficacy: Is informal discussion of cognitive distortions during the exposure exercises sufficient, or should the therapist engage in formal Socratic questioning of hypothesized distortions, such as inflated responsibility? Notably, in a meta-analytic review, cognitive therapies for OCD that included some form of exposure to feared stimuli were superior to those that did not, suggesting that exposure may be necessary to maximize outcomes (Abramowitz, Franklin, & Foa, 2002).

To expand upon this point further, Hiss, Foa, and Kozak (1994) investigated whether formal relapse prevention techniques following intensive EX/RP enhanced maintenance of gains. Notably, all discussions about cognitive factors typically included during the core treatment (e.g., discussion of lapse vs. relapse, posttreatment exposure instructions, themes of guilt and personal responsibility, and feared consequences) were removed. Patients received this modified EX/RP, followed by either a relapse prevention treatment or a psychosocial control treatment (associative therapy). All patients in both conditions were classified as responders at posttreatment (defined as 50% or greater reduction in OCD symptoms), with treatment gains better maintained in the relapse prevention group than in the associative therapy condition at 6-month follow-up. The percentages of responders at follow-up were 75% in the relapse prevention condition and 33% in associative therapy. The higher than usual observed relapse rate in the associative therapy condition may have resulted from the removal of cognitive techniques typically utilized during the core treatment, such as discussion of feared consequences. These findings, and those discussed earlier, further underscore our belief that blended treatment designed to provide patients the opportunity to disconfirm their erroneous cognitions makes the most sense clinically. Accordingly, our approach clearly incorporates informal cognitive procedures, and discussions of the outcome of exposures are geared toward challenging mistaken beliefs; this is accomplished in the context of a treatment approach that still emphasizes the importance of EX/RP in bringing about such changes.

Serotonergic Medications

Effectiveness of Medications

The use of serotonergic medications in the treatment of OCD has received a great deal of attention in the past 25 years. Of the tricyclic antidepressants, clomipramine (CMI) has been studied most extensively. In controlled trials, CMI has consistently been found to be superior to placebo (e.g., DeVeaugh-Geiss, Landau, & Katz, 1989). Similar results have been obtained with the selective serotonin reuptake inhibitors (SSRIs) fluoxetine, fluvoxamine, and sertraline (see Greist, Jefferson, Kobak, Katzelnick, & Serlin, 1995). Accordingly, each of these medications has been approved by the U.S. Food and Drug Administration (FDA) as treatments for adult OCD. On the whole, these studies suggest that up to 60% of patients show some response to treatment with SSRIs. However, even the average treatment gain achieved by treatment responders is moderate at best (Greist, 1990). In addition, amelioration of obsessive–compulsive symptoms is maintained only as long as the drug is continued: For example, in an early controlled, double-blind discontinuation study, 90% of patients relapsed within a few weeks after being withdrawn from CMI (Pato, Zohar-Kadouch, Zohar, & Murphy, 1988). More recent discontinuation studies with slower taper periods have not yielded such dramatic results, but they nevertheless converge to suggest that maintenance treatment is necessary to sustain achievements attained with pharmacotherapy alone for OCD (Dougherty, Rauch, & Jenike, 2002).

EX/RP versus Pharmacotherapy

Many controlled studies have indicated that serotonergic antidepressants are superior to placebo in ameliorating OCD symptoms (for a review, see Greist et al., 1995). However, only a few controlled studies have directly compared the relative or combined efficacy of antidepressant medications and EX/RP, and several studies that have made such a comparison included complex designs that make it difficult to draw confident conclusions about relative and combined efficacy (e.g., Marks et al., 1980, 1988). Cottraux and colleagues

(1990) compared fluvoxamine (FLV) with antiexposure instructions, FLV plus weekly EX/RP, and pill placebo (PBO) plus EX/RP, and found FLV + EX/RP and FLV + antiexposure instructions superior to PBO + EX/RP; there was a trend toward an advantage for combined treatment, but it failed to reach significance. Hohagen and colleagues (1998) compared EX/RP + FLV to EX/RP + PBO and found that both groups improved significantly and comparably on compulsions, but the patients who received EX/RP + FLV were significantly better at posttreatment on obsessions than those who received EX/RP + PBO. Subanalyses indicated that patients with secondary depression also fared better if they were receiving EX/RP + FLV.

The relative and combined efficacy of CMI and intensive EX/RP was examined in a multicenter, RCT conducted at our center (Penn) and at Columbia University. Findings with both treatment completer and intention-to-treat (ITT) data indicated at posttreatment that the active treatments were superior to placebo, EX/RP was superior to CMI, and the combination of the two treatments was not superior to EX/RP alone (Foa et al., 2005); relapse was more evident following treatment discontinuation in the CMI group than in either treatment that included intensive EX/RP (EX/RP, EX/RP + CMI; Simpson et al., 2004). However, the design used in the Penn–Columbia study may not have optimally promoted an additive effect for CMI because the intensive portion of the EX/RP program was largely completed before patients reached their maximum dose of CMI. In addition, combined treatment effects may be more evident when intensive EX/RP is not used (Foa, Franklin, & Moser, 2002). Notably, an additive effect for combined treatment was found in a recent study in pediatric OCD at Penn, Duke, and Brown (Pediatric OCD Treatment Study Team, 2004), although examination of effect sizes by site indicated that the CBT monotherapy effect at Penn was very large, and no additive effect for combined treatment was found at this site.

In summary, although there is clear evidence that both pharmaceutical treatment with serotonergic medications and EX/RP treatments are effective for OCD, information about their relative and combined efficacy remains scarce because most of the studies that examined these issues have been methodologically limited. Nevertheless, no study has found clear, long-term superiority for combined pharmacotherapy plus EX/RP over EX/RP alone. The absence of conclusive findings notwithstanding, many experts continue to advocate combined procedures as the treatment of choice for OCD (e.g., Greist, 1992). In clinical practice, it is common to see patients in EX/RP treatment who are taking SSRIs concurrently. In uncontrolled examinations of EX/RP treatment outcome for adults (Franklin, Abramowitz, Bux, Zoellner, & Feeny, 2002) and youth (Franklin et al., 1998; Piacentini, Bergman, Jacobs, McCracken, & Kretchman, 2002) treated in OCD outpatient clinics, no posttreatment differences in OCD symptom severity were detected between patients who received EX/RP alone and those who received SSRI medication when receiving EX/RP. From these data we can surmise that concomitant pharmacotherapy is not required for every patient to benefit substantially from EX/RP, and that concomitant pharmacotherapy does not appear to inhibit EX/RP treatment response. With respect to EX/RP augmentation in SSRI partial responders, there is now evidence from randomized trials that EX/RP augmented treatment outcome compared to medication alone in youth (Franklin et al., 2011) and compared to stress management training in adults (Simpson et al., 2010). More definitive conclusions about the effects of augmenting pharmacotherapy with EX/RP await a more carefully controlled examination, however.

ASSESSMENT

Following a diagnostic interview to ascertain the presence of OCD, it is advisable to quantify the severity of the OCD symptoms with one or more of the instruments described below. Quantification of symptom severity assists the therapist in evaluating how successful treatment was for a given patient. In our clinic, we use several assessment instruments. As in most OCD clinical research studies, however, the primary measure of OCD symptom severity used in our center is the Yale–Brown Obsessive–Compulsive Scale (Goodman et al., 1989a, 1989b).

Yale–Brown Obsessive–Compulsive Scale

The Yale–Brown Obsessive–Compulsive Scale (Y-BOCS; Goodman et al., 1989a, 1989b), a standardized, semistructured interview, takes approximately 30 minutes to complete. The Y-BOCS severity scale includes 10 items (five assess obsessions and five, compulsions), each of which is rated on a 5-point scale ranging from 0 (*No symptoms*) to 4 (*Severe symptoms*). Assessors rate the time occupied by the obsessions and compulsions,

the degree of interference with functioning, the level of distress, attempts to resist the symptoms, and level of control over the symptoms. The Y-BOCS has shown adequate interrater agreement, internal consistency, and validity (Goodman et al., 1989a, 1989b). The Y-BOCS served as the primary measure of outcome in most of the published OCD pharmacotherapy and CBT treatment studies conducted during the 1990s.

Self-Report Measures

Obsessive–Compulsive Inventory—Revised

The Obsessive–Compulsive Inventory—Revised (OCI-R; Foa, Huppert, et al., 2002) is an 18-item, self-report measure that assesses the distress associated with obsessions and compulsions. In addition to the total score, six separate subscale scores are calculated by adding the three items that comprise each subscale: Washing, Checking, Ordering, Obsessing, Hoarding, and Neutralizing. Foa, Huppert, and colleagues (2002) reported good internal consistency, test–retest reliability, and discriminant validity in clinical patients with OCD, PTSD, generalized social phobia, and nonanxious controls. The total score ranges from 0 to 72, and each subscale ranges from 0 to 12.

Other Self-Report Measures

A few self-report instruments for assessing OCD symptoms, such as the Leyton Obsessional Inventory (Kazarian, Evans, & Lefave, 1977) and the Lynfield Obsessional/Compulsive Questionnaire (Allen & Tune, 1975), are also available. These instruments are limited in that they assess only certain forms of obsessive–compulsive behavior and/or they include items that are unrelated to OCD symptoms. More recently, Storch and colleagues (2009) have developed the Children's Florida Obsessive–Compulsive Inventory, which is intended primarily for screening purposes.

INITIAL INTERVIEW

After a diagnosis of OCD has been established, and before actually beginning treatment, the therapist should schedule 4–6 hours of appointments with the patient. In these sessions, the therapist needs to accomplish three important tasks. First, the sessions are used to collect the information necessary to develop a treatment plan.

Specifically, the therapist must first identify specific cues that cause the patient distress (threat cues), avoidance, rituals, and feared consequences. Second, the therapist should develop a good rapport with the patient, who will engage in exposure exercises designed to elicit anxiety and distress during intensive EX/RP, and the lack of a good relationship between therapist and the patient may compromise outcome. Third, the therapist needs to explore the patient's beliefs about OCD and the perceived consequences of refraining from rituals and avoidance because this information guides the informal discussions of cognitive processes that take place throughout EX/RP.

Threat cues may be either (1) tangible objects in the environment or (2) thoughts, images, or impulses that the person experiences (for lack of better terms, we have labeled them "external cues" and "internal cues," respectively). Passive avoidance and ritualistic behavior (sometimes called "active avoidance") both serve to reduce the distress associated with the threat cues. Rituals may be further divided into overt or covert (mental) forms. It is essential that patients understand the difference between obsessions and mental compulsions because obsessions are treated with systematic exposure and mental compulsions, with ritual preventions. During treatment, patients should be instructed to report any mental compulsions to the therapist because performing such compulsions during exposure exercises attenuates the effects of these exercises in the same way that behavioral compulsions do.

External Fear Cues

Most individuals with OCD experience fear in reaction to specific environmental cues (objects, persons, or situations), but each patient has his/her own idiosyncratic threat cues. For example, individuals who fear contamination from toilets may differ as to whether they fear all toilets or only those open to the public. One patient may fear only the toilet itself, whereas another may also fear bathroom floors, doorknobs, and faucets. Similarly, two individuals may experience distress at the prospect of a fire burning down their home, but whereas one experiences the distress only when she is the last person to leave the house, the other experiences distress before going to bed at night when his children are present.

The therapist needs to gather specific information about cues that elicit the patient's distress to identify the basic sources of the fear. Identification of the basic

source is important for planning the treatment program. Confronting the source of the fear is essential for successful behavioral treatment of OCD. Often, when such exposure does not take place during treatment, relapse occurs. For example, a patient who feared contamination by her hometown was treated with EX/RP 3,000 miles away from the town. Because of the distances involved, direct exposure to the town was impossible, so treatment comprised exposure to objects contaminated directly or indirectly by contact with the town. Although the patient habituated to the objects used in the exposure sessions, she continued to fear her hometown. Within 1 year after treatment, she had developed fears to new objects related to her hometown. Not until she engaged in repeated exposures to the town itself did she experience lasting improvement.

It is important that the therapist conduct a thorough investigation of objects, situations, and places that evoke obsessional distress for the patient at the time of presentation and at onset. Such information helps to identify the source of the distress. To facilitate communication with the patient about situations that evoke distress, a Subjective Units of Discomfort Scale (SUDS) ranging from 0 to 100 points is introduced. Patients are asked to rate each situation with respect to the level of distress they expect to experience upon exposure. The source of the distress is expected to be 100. The following dialogue between therapist and patient illustrates the process of gathering information about distressing situations.

THERAPIST: When do you get the urge to wash your hands?

PATIENT: In a lot of places. There are so many places.

THERAPIST: Are there any places where the urges are particularly strong?

PATIENT: Well when I am sitting in my living room, particularly near the fireplace. Also in the laundry room, which I never go to. Also, when I walk in the park.

THERAPIST: Let's talk about your living room. How upset are you when you are sitting next to your fireplace?

PATIENT: That's bad. I guess about a 90.

THERAPIST: Can you tell me what makes you so upset in your living room?

PATIENT: Well that is a long story . . . and I know it doesn't make sense.

THERAPIST: Go on. It's important that we understand what makes you uncomfortable and fearful in your living room.

PATIENT: About 2 years ago, I got up in the morning and went into the living room, and I saw a dead squirrel in the fireplace. I guess he got in through the chimney. So, I figured that if the squirrel was dead, he must have been sick. I know that a lot of squirrels have rabies, so I thought that if the squirrel died of rabies, then there are germs all over the chimney.

THERAPIST: Have you tried to have the chimney and the fireplace cleaned?

PATIENT: Yes, we did have a company come in and clean the whole area, but I'm not sure that they can clean away the germs.

THERAPIST: I understand. How about the laundry room, how upsetting is it to be in the laundry room?

PATIENT: That would be a 100; that's why I don't go in there.

THERAPIST: How did the laundry room become dangerous?

PATIENT: Oh, that's another story. Until a year ago, my children used to keep their guinea pigs in the laundry room. One day we found the female guinea pig dead. So I thought that it probably died of rabies, too.

THERAPIST: Oh, I understand. So you are generally afraid you will contract rabies if you come in contact with things that you think are contaminated with rabies germs. Is this true?

PATIENT: Exactly. That's why I don't like to walk in the woods or the park. You know, those places have all kind of animals, and you can never tell where the germs might be.

It is clear from this conversation that it was not living rooms, laundry rooms, or parks per se that the patient feared. Rather, any situation or object that, in her mind, had some probability of being infested with rabies germs became a source of contamination. Some contamination-fearful patients, however, cannot specify feared consequences of coming into contact with stimuli they perceive to be contaminated. For these patients, the primary fear is that they will not be able to tolerate the extreme emotional distress generated by being contaminated. With such patients, it is also important to probe further to discern whether they have fears about the long-term health consequences of experiencing high and unremitting anxiety in response to stimuli that prompt obsessions.

Internal Fear Cues

Anxiety and distress may also be generated by images, impulses, or abstract thoughts that the individual finds disturbing, shameful, or disgusting. Examples of such cues include impulses to stab one's child, thoughts of one's spouse injured in an accident, or images of religious figures engaged in sexual activity. Clearly, internal threat cues may be produced by external situations, such as the sight of a knife triggering the impulse to stab one's child. Some patients may become distressed when they experience certain bodily sensations, such as minor pains triggering the fear of having cancer.

In many cases, patients may be reluctant to express their obsessive thoughts because they are either ashamed of them or fear that expressing them will make the consequence more likely to occur. In these cases, the therapist needs to encourage the expression of these thoughts through direct questioning and a matter-of-fact attitude. Sometimes it helps to tell the patient that many people with and without OCD have unwanted thoughts (as many as 85% of normal individuals; Rachman & DeSilva, 1978). It may also be helpful to remind the patient that talking about the obsessions will be a part of therapy; the evaluation session provides an opportunity to begin this process.

THERAPIST: So tell me, when is it that you feel the urge to count?

PATIENT: It seems like I'm always counting something, but it's mostly when I think about certain things.

THERAPIST: What kind of things?

PATIENT: I don't know. Bad things.

THERAPIST: Can you give me some examples of bad thoughts that will make you want to count?

PATIENT: (brief silence) I really prefer not to talk about them. It makes things worse.

THERAPIST: You mean it makes the counting worse?

PATIENT: Yes.

THERAPIST: All right, I know now that when you think or talk about certain bad things, you have an urge to count, but I still don't know what those bad things are. How about you tell me so that I can help you with them?

PATIENT: I'd really rather not. Can't we talk about something else?

THERAPIST: It is important that I know what the thoughts are to plan your treatment. I'll try to help you. Do the thoughts involve someone being hurt?

PATIENT: Yes.

THERAPIST: Do the thoughts involve only certain people getting hurt or could it be anyone?

PATIENT: Mostly my family.

THERAPIST: OK, what else can you tell me about the thoughts?

PATIENT: I really don't want to say any more.

THERAPIST: I know this is scary, but remember that facing your fears is what this treatment is all about.

PATIENT: OK. It's not always thoughts. Sometimes I see pictures in my mind, where my brother or my mom and dad are killed. I'm afraid when I talk about these thoughts and pictures that they really will die.

THERAPIST: A lot of people have thoughts that they don't like to have. Even people without OCD. Just because you have these thoughts, or talk about them, doesn't mean that bad things will actually happen or that you want them to come true.

It is important to reassure the patient that unpleasant thoughts occur often and to emphasize the distinction between thoughts and reality. Many patients with OCD have magical ideas in which the distinction between "thinking about" and "making things happen" is blurred, a process labeled by Salkovskis (1985) as "thought–action fusion" (TAF). It is important to point out to the patient that thoughts are different from actions. Also, many patients think that if negative thoughts enter their mind, then it means they wish the bad thing will happen. The therapist should assure the patient that thinking about bad things does not mean that one wants them to happen. These sorts of informal discussions of mistaken beliefs are an integral part of correct implementation of EX/RP. Such discussions should accompany the treatment planning process, and be reiterated as needed during exposure exercises. It is, however, important that such discussions accompany EX/RP exercises rather than replace them.

Feared Consequences

Many individuals with OCD are afraid that something terrible will happen if they fail to perform their rituals. Such patients with washing rituals, for example, typically fear that they and/or someone else will become ill or disabled, or die, as a result of being contaminated. Many patients with checking rituals fear that because of their negligence, certain catastrophes will occur, such as their homes burning down, or that they might kill someone while driving. Some patients have only a vague notion of what these negative consequence might be (e.g., "I don't know exactly what will happen, but I feel that if I don't count to seven, something bad will happen to my family"). Others do not fear catastrophes at all, but they cannot tolerate the emotional distress they experience if they do not perform rituals. Some fear that unless they ritualize, anxiety will increase continually, until they have a nervous breakdown. Data from the DSM-IV field trial indicated that approximately two-thirds of patients with OCD could clearly identify consequences other than emotional distress that would result when they refrained from performing rituals, whereas the remainder could report no such consequences (Foa et al., 1995).

It is important to identify the specific details of the patient's feared consequences to plan an effective exposure program. For example, the content of the imaginal exposure of a patient who checks while driving for fear of having hit a pedestrian and being sent to jail differs from that of a patient who fears that hitting a pedestrian will result in punishment by God. Similarly, patients who ritualistically place objects in a specific order may differ with respect to their feared catastrophes. Some perform the ritual to prevent catastrophic consequences (e.g., death of parents), whereas others do so only to reduce distress elicited by disordered objects. The former would benefit from treatment that includes both imaginal and *in vivo* exposure, whereas the latter is likely to profit from *in vivo* exposure alone.

Strength of Belief

Clinical observations have led to suggestions that individuals with OCD who have poor insight do not respond well to exposure and response prevention, although two later studies failed to find a linear relationship between strength of belief in feared catastrophes and improvement following exposure and response prevention (Foa et al., 1999; Lelliott, Noshirvani, Basoglu, Marks, & Monteiro, 1988). Two issues need to be considered in evaluating these collective findings. First, the reliability and validity of the strength of belief measures used in previous studies are unknown. Second, the relationship between overvalued ideation and treatment outcome may not be linear. Clinical observation suggests that only patients who express extreme belief in their obsessional ideation show poor outcome. Indeed, Foa and colleagues (1999) found that only extremely strong belief (fixed belief) was associated with attenuated outcome. Such patients may appear delusional when discussing their feared catastrophes. We hypothesize that the effect of fixed belief on outcome may be mediated by treatment compliance: Patients who are convinced that feared disasters will ensue if they engaged in prescribed exercises probably will not complete the tasks as assigned.

When assessing the strength of belief, it is important to remember that a patient's insight into the senselessness of his/her belief often fluctuates. Some patients readily acknowledge that their obsessional beliefs are irrational, but the beliefs still cause marked distress. A few individuals firmly believe that their obsessions and compulsions are rational. In most patients, though, the strength of belief fluctuates across situations, making it difficult to ascertain the degree to which they believe the obsessions are irrational. The following example is an inquiry into the strength of a patient's belief in her obsessional fear of contracting acquired immune deficiency syndrome (AIDS).

THERAPIST: How likely is it that you will contract AIDS from using a public restroom?

PATIENT: I'm really terrified that I will get AIDS if I use a bathroom in a restaurant.

THERAPIST: I know that you are afraid of getting AIDS, but if you think logically, how likely do you think you are to get AIDS by sitting on a public toilet?

PATIENT: I think I will get AIDS if I use a public toilet.

THERAPIST: So do you mean to say that there is a 100% chance of you getting AIDS if you sit on a public toilet once?

PATIENT: Well, I don't know about once, but if I did it again and again I would.

THERAPIST: What about other people? Will they get AIDS if they use a public toilet?

PATIENT: I guess so. I'm not sure.

THERAPIST: Since most people use public bathrooms, almost everyone should have AIDS by now. How do you explain the fact that a relatively small number of people have AIDS?

PATIENT: Maybe not everybody is as susceptible to AIDS as I am.

THERAPIST: Do you think that you are more susceptible than other people?

PATIENT: I don't know for sure. Maybe the likelihood of my getting AIDS is only 50%.

Based on the interaction just described, the therapist concluded that the patient was not an "overvalued ideator"; thus, the prognosis for this patient is brighter than it would be if she continued strongly to hold her original belief. Accordingly, the implementation of EX/RP for this patient would follow the standard guidelines.

Avoidance and Rituals

To maximize treatment efficacy, all avoidance and ritualistic behaviors, even seemingly minor ones, should be prevented. Therefore, the therapist should gather complete information about all passive avoidance and rituals. When the therapist is in doubt as to whether a particular avoidance behavior is related to OCD, he/she might suggest an "experiment" in which the patient is exposed to the avoided situation. If the patient experiences anxiety or distress, the avoidance behavior should be prevented as part of treatment. Similarly, if it is unclear whether a given action constitutes a ritual, a response prevention "experiment" may be implemented. If refraining from performing the action evokes distress, the action is identified as a ritual and should be addressed in therapy.

Individuals with OCD, like those with specific phobias, often attempt to avoid anxiety-evoking situations. Most passive avoidance strategies are fairly obvious (e.g., not entering public restrooms, not preparing meals, and not taking out the trash). However, the therapist also needs to be attentive to subtle forms of avoidance, such as carrying money in one's pockets to avoid opening a wallet, wearing slip-on shoes to avoid touching laces, and using drinking straws to avoid contact with a glass or a can. Patients with obsessive–compulsive checking rituals also engage in subtle avoidance behaviors that are important to explore, such as arranging their work schedules to ensure that they are rarely, if ever, the last person to leave the business, thus ensuring that the responsibility for checking the safe falls on a coworker.

Active rituals, such as passive avoidance, may be explicit (e.g., prolonged washing, repeated checks of the door, and ordering of objects) and/or subtle (e.g., wiping hands on pant legs, blinking, and thinking "good" thoughts). It is important that the therapist identify both explicit and subtle rituals, so that both may be addressed during treatment.

Although compulsive rituals are intended to reduce the distress associated with obsessions, patients sometimes report that the performance of these rituals is aversive in itself. For example, Ms. S, who was obsessed with the orderliness of objects on her shelves, found reordering the shelves aversive because she was unable to find the "perfect" place for everything. Similarly, Mr. J, who felt contaminated by chemicals, found the act of decontaminating himself by repeated handwashing aversive because he was unable to decide when his hands were sufficiently clean; therefore, he washed until his hands became raw. Rituals may also become aversive because of their intrusion into other aspects of the person's life. For example, Mr. J, who would take 2-hour-long showers to feel adequately clean, was reprimanded repeatedly by his supervisor for arriving late to work.

When certain compulsions become aversive, some patients decrease the time they spend performing the ritual by increasing avoidance behaviors, or by substituting other, less time-consuming rituals. For example, Ms. E, who was obsessed with fears of contamination by funeral-related objects (e.g., cemeteries and people returning from a funeral), responded with hours of showering and handwashing. She eventually retreated into her bedroom and avoided all contact with the outside world. Mr. J, described earlier, avoided taking a shower for days at a time, but between showers he wiped his hands compulsively and avoided touching his wife. In some cases, seemingly "new" rituals may develop during the course of treatment to function in the place of those previously identified and eliminated. For example, Mr. F, who was concerned about his hands becoming contaminated, successfully resisted the urge to wash his hands, but soon after response prevention was implemented, he started to rub his hands together vigorously to "decontaminate" them. When such a substitute ritual is identified, it also needs to be addressed in treatment with ritual prevention. Therapists must not only remain alert to such shifts in ritualistic behaviors but also alert patients to the possibility of such shifts.

History of Main Complaint and Treatment History

Many individuals with OCD are unable to give a detailed account of the onset of their symptoms because the symptoms began subtly, many years ago. Nevertheless, therapists should attempt to collect as much information as possible about the onset and course of the disorder. Such information may provide clues about aspects of the fear network and variables associated with the maintenance of symptoms, and may help to anticipate difficulties that may arise during treatment (e.g., old obsessions or rituals that may resurface as more prominent ones diminish).

Many such individuals also have an extensive history of psychological and pharmacological treatments, and it is important to make a detailed inquiry about the outcome of previous treatments. If the patient has been treated with EX/RP, the therapist should assess whether the treatment was implemented appropriately and the patient was compliant with treatment demands. Knowledge that a patient experienced difficulty complying with response prevention instructions, or that previous therapy failed to provide adequate exposure experiences or response prevention instructions, is important for designing the behavioral program. Other factors that may have prevented successful outcome or caused relapse, such as job stress, death in the family, or pregnancy, should be discussed. At the same time, a prior failed course of EX/RP should not necessarily be viewed as prognostic, especially if the patient recognizes why the therapy was less successful in the past. One of our patients, who had failed multiple trials of less intensive EX/RP, came to our center with the knowledge that his noncompliance with exposure exercises between weekly sessions greatly reduced the effects of treatment. He also noted that the slow progress he observed in these previous therapies demoralized him and caused further disengagement from the treatment. When offered a choice of daily versus twice-weekly sessions, he opted for the daily treatment, noting that the more intensive approach might decrease the chance of similar lapses. He has now successfully completed the intensive regimen.

In our clinic we have observed that a substantial majority of our outpatients have been treated, or are currently being treated, with serotonergic medications. Some seek EX/RP to augment the partial gains they have achieved with the medication. Others wish to discontinue the medication because it was ineffective, it had side effects, or they do not want to continue taking medicine indefinitely. Assessment of the patient's treatment goals is necessary for planning his/her treatment program.

Social Functioning

Obsessive–compulsive symptoms may severely disrupt the daily functioning of patients. Therapists should assess the impact of OCD symptoms on the various areas of functioning. Where appropriate, this information should be used to design suitable exposure exercises. For example, Ms. D experienced difficulties completing assignments at work because she repeatedly checked each task. Treatment included exposures to performing tasks at work without checking. Even if the client is not currently working, exposures simulating work situations may be necessary if symptoms created difficulties in previous jobs.

OCD clearly has a deleterious effect on the intimate relationships of many patients. About half of married individuals seeking treatment for OCD experience marital distress (Emmelkamp et al., 1990; Riggs et al., 1992). Other family and social relationships may also suffer as a result of OCD symptoms. The impairment in social functioning may arise because social contact is either perceived as threatening (e.g., "I may spread germs to other people") or so much of the patient's time and energy is invested in performing rituals and planning ways to avoid distressing situations. Again, information about the relation of social dysfunction to OCD symptoms may lead the therapist to include specific exposures aimed at ameliorating these social difficulties.

The assessment of social functioning should also include an evaluation of what role, if any, other people play in the patient's compulsive rituals. If the patient relies on others for reassurance or compliance with rituals (e.g., family members must remove their shoes before entering the house), the therapist should instruct family members how to respond appropriately when asked to participate in the patient's rituals. A careful analysis of the relationship is called for before specific instructions are given to significant others. Moreover, if family members tend to criticize the patient when obsessional distress arises, it is important to address these negative exchanges in treatment. We have often addressed this issue with a combination of empathic discussion of the frustration experienced by the family member and role playing of more effective responses.

Mood State

Although some patients with serious depression and OCD may benefit from behavioral therapy for OCD (Foa et al., 1992), research suggests that severe depression may limit the extent of reduction of OCD symptoms and the maintenance of those gains (e.g., Abramowitz et al., 2000). Therefore, it is important to assess the mood state of the patient prior to beginning behavioral therapy. Patients with severe depression should be treated with antidepressant medication or cognitive therapy to reduce the depressive symptoms prior to implementing behavioral therapy for the OCD. Treatment with serotonergic antidepressants may reduce OCD symptoms, as well as depression. Because the effects of such medication on OCD symptoms may not be evident until 3 months after treatment begins, the therapist needs to use his/her clinical judgment to decide whether to begin EX/RP when the depression decreases or wait until the effects of the medication on OCD symptoms can be assessed.

Choice of Treatment

How should a therapist determine the most suitable treatment for a given patient? As discussed earlier, exposure and response prevention, as well as serotonergic medications, have demonstrated efficacy for OCD. Therapist and patient are faced with the choice of EX/RP, pharmacotherapy, or a combination of the two. Neither treatment is effective with all patients, and no consistent predictors of who will benefit most from which treatment modality have been identified. Therefore, unless the patient has been particularly successful or unsuccessful with some previous course of treatment, the decision should be based on factors such as availability of treatment, amount of time the patient is able or willing to invest in treatment, and his/her motivation and willingness to tolerate side effects.

The intensive treatment requires a considerable investment of time over a period of several weeks. Many patients are unable, or unwilling, to devote 4–5 hours a day to treatment. These patients should be advised to try pharmacological treatment, which does not require the same extensive time commitment. Recent investigations of the effects of a twice-weekly EX/RP regimen compared to intensive treatment suggested comparable outcomes at follow-up (Abramowitz et al., 2003; Storch et al., 2007); thus, in our center, we routinely offer either program to patients considering EX/RP. Some patients may be unwilling (sometimes expressed as "I can't do that") to experience the temporary discomfort caused by EX/RP. These patients, too, may be advised to try medications. The need to develop "readiness programs" designed to prepare such patients to accept EX/RP treatment is often cited in light of the relatively high refusal rate among patients offered EX/RP. Such programs may include testimonials from previously treated patients, cognitive strategies designed to help the patient calculate objective risks more accurately, psychoeducation about OCD and EX/RP, and a review of the outcome literature for various treatments (Tolin, Maltby, Diefenbach, Hannan, & Worhunsky, 2004). An initial RCT of EX/RP plus motivational interviewing (MI) did not yield outcomes that were superior to EX/RP alone (Simpson et al., 2010), but the study did not specifically recruit patients who were experiencing low motivation. Manualizing programs specifically for those patients and examining the acceptance rate and efficacy of EX/RP infused with MI constitutes the next step in this line of research.

Patients who are concerned about the potential (or have already experienced) side effects of medications or their unknown long-term effects often prefer EX/RP. Other patients are concerned with the prospect of entering an "endless" treatment because, according to present knowledge, relapse occurs when medication is withdrawn (Pato et al., 1988; Thoren, Asberg, Chronholm, Journestedt, & Traskman, 1980). This concern is particularly relevant for women who plan to bear children and need to withdraw from the medication during pregnancy. EX/RP should be recommended to these patients because its effects are more enduring.

As discussed earlier, the long-term effects of combining EX/RP and medication are unclear; therefore, it is premature to recommend treatment programs that combine the two therapies. However, some patients who present for treatment are already on antidepressant medication. Because these medications were found not to interfere with the effectiveness of EX/RP (Franklin et al., 2000), it is recommended that patients continue to take the medication if they have experienced some improvement in either obsessive–compulsive symptoms or depression. However, if the patient has not experienced improvement with medication, withdrawal of the medication before or during EX/RP should be considered. Special consideration should be given to patients with severe depression concurrent with their OCD. It is recommended that these patients be treated with antidepressants or cognitive therapy for the

depression prior to entering intensive EX/RP for the OCD, given recent findings of somewhat attenuated outcome for severely depressed patients (Abramowitz et al., 2000).

INTENSIVE EX/RP

The intensive treatment program comprises four phases: (1) information gathering, (2) intensive EX/RP, (3) a home visit, and (4) maintenance and relapse prevention.

Information Gathering and Treatment Planning

The first stage of information gathering consists of a thorough diagnostic evaluation to determine that the patient's main psychopathology is OCD. The second step is to assess whether the patient is appropriate for EX/RP. We recommend that individuals who are abusing drugs or alcohol should be treated for the substance abuse prior to intensive treatment for OCD. Patients who have clear delusions and hallucinations are also poor candidates for intensive treatment. Individuals with severe MDD should be treated for depression before beginning treatment for OCD. The patient's motivation to comply with the demands of intensive treatment should be carefully evaluated. It is important to describe the treatment program in enough detail that the patient is not surprised when treatment begins. If the patient does not express strong motivation and commitment to treatment, it might be preferable to delay implementation of intensive treatment or to offer alternative treatments, such as medication. As noted earlier, a study of less intensive EX/RP for patients who appear otherwise motivated, yet cannot accommodate the daily regimen into their schedules, suggested an outcome comparable to intensive treatment; future research with much larger samples is needed to determine whether patient factors predict differential outcome to either treatment schedule.

Once a patient is judged to be appropriate for intensive treatment, information gathering for treatment planning begins. This phase typically comprises 4–6 hours of contact with the patient over a period of 2–3 days. During this phase, the therapist collects information about the patient's obsessive–compulsive symptoms, general history, and the history of treatment for OCD, as described earlier. During these sessions, the therapist discusses the rationale for treatment, describes the program in detail, teaches patients to monitor their rituals, and develops a treatment plan.

First Information-Gathering Session

It is very important to discuss the rationale for treatment and to describe the treatment program in detail. The program requires that the patient abandon his/her obsessive–compulsive habits, therefore temporarily experiencing substantial discomfort. If patients do not understand why they are asked to suffer this short-term distress or are not convinced that treatment will work, they are unlikely to comply with treatment instructions. The treatment rationale is explained as follows:

"You have a set of habits that, as you know, are called obsessive–compulsive symptoms. These are habits of thinking, feeling, and acting that are extremely unpleasant, wasteful, and difficult to get rid of on your own. Usually, these habits involve thoughts, images, or impulses that habitually come to your mind, even though you don't want them. Along with these thoughts you have unwanted feelings of extreme distress or anxiety and strong urges to do something to reduce the distress. To try to get rid of the anxiety, people get into the habit of engaging in various special thoughts or actions, which we call 'rituals.'

"Unfortunately, as you know, the rituals do not work all that well, and the distress decreases for a short time only, then comes back again. Eventually, you may find yourself doing more and more ritualizing to try to reduce anxiety, but even then the relief is temporary and you have to do the ritual all over again. Gradually, you find yourself spending so much time and energy ritualizing—which does not work that well anyway—that other areas of your life are seriously disrupted.

"The treatment we are about to begin is called exposure and response prevention. It is designed to break two types of associations. The first association is between sensations of anxiety and the objects, situations, or thoughts that produce this distress. [The therapist uses information collected as examples; e.g., 'Every time you touch anything associated with urine you feel anxious, distressed, or contaminated.'] The second association we want to break is that between carrying out ritualistic behavior and the feeling of less anxiety or less distress. In other words, after you carry out [specifies the identified

rituals], you temporarily feel less distress. Therefore, you continue to engage in this behavior frequently. The treatment we offer breaks the automatic bond between the feelings of discomfort/anxiety/contamination of [specifies the obsession] and your rituals. It will also train you not to ritualize when you are anxious."

After presenting the treatment rationale, the therapist should begin to collect information about the patient's OCD symptoms. The rationale for information gathering and a description of the treatment is presented as follows:

"In the next two sessions, I will ask you specific questions about the various situations and thoughts that generate discomfort or anxiety in you. We will order them according to the degree of distress they generate in you on a scale from 0 to 100, where 0 means *No anxiety* and 100 means *Maximum anxiety or panic*. The exposure treatment program involves confronting you with situations and thoughts that you avoid because they generate anxiety and urges to carry out ritualistic behavior. Why do we want to expose you to places and objects that will make you uncomfortable, situations that you have attempted to avoid even at much cost? We know that when people are exposed to situations that they fear, anxiety gradually declines. Through exposure, then, the association between anxiety and [specifies the obsession] weaken because you are repeatedly exposed to these situations, so that the previously evoked anxiety decreases with time.

"For many people with OCD the obsessions occur within their imagination and rarely take place in reality. This makes it impossible to practice exposure by actually confronting those situations for prolonged periods. For example, if a person fears that her home will burn down, we certainly do not wish to have her house catch on fire in order to practice exposure. Similarly, someone who fears that he has run over a person who is now lying in the road cannot in reality be exposed to such a situation.

"If confrontation with the feared situation is necessary to reduce obsessions, how can you improve without directly confronting the situation? You can confront these fears through imagery, in which you visualize the circumstances that you fear will happen. In imagery practice, you create in your mind detailed pictures of the terrible consequences that you are afraid will occur if you do not engage in the ritualistic behavior. During prolonged exposure to these images, the distress level associated with them gradually decreases.

"When people with OCD encounter their feared situations or their obsessional thoughts, they become anxious or distressed and feel compelled to perform the ritualistic behavior as a way to reduce their distress. Exposure practices can cause this same distress and urge to ritualize. Usually, performing rituals strengthens the pattern of distress and rituals. Therefore in treatment, ritual prevention is practiced to break the habit of ritualizing. This requires that you stop ritualizing, even though you are still having urges to do so. By facing your fears without resorting to compulsions, you gradually become less anxious. Behavior therapists call this process 'habituation.' Therefore, during the 3 weeks of intensive exposure, the association between relief from anxiety and carrying out [specifies the patient's rituals] will become weaker because you will not be allowed to engage in such behaviors; therefore, you will find out that your anxiety decreases even if you do not resort to these activities."

The initial information-gathering session is also used to begin training the patient to monitor his/her rituals accurately. Accurate reports of the frequency and duration of ritualistic behavior are important to evaluate the progress of treatment and to demonstrate the reality of changes to the patient. In some cases, the monitoring also serves an active role in treatment. Patients begin to recognize that rituals do not truly occur "all day long" and the act of monitoring the rituals may decrease their frequency and duration.

"It is very important for the treatment program that we have an accurate picture of the extent to which you engage in obsessive thinking and compulsive behavior. Having a clear picture of how much of your time is taken up by your problem will help us to monitor your progress and adjust the treatment program accordingly. Therefore, during this week, while I am still collecting information to form a treatment program, I would like you to record your symptoms every day. It is not easy to report accurately on how much you engage in your obsessive–compulsive behavior; therefore, we will spend some time now and in the next session going over some rules for how to record your symptoms. Here are some monitoring forms on which you will record your thoughts and rituals."

The therapist should specify which ritual(s) the patient is to record, go over the instructions carefully with the patient, and practice filling out the form with the patient using an "imaginary day" of his/her life. The following rules are helpful in monitoring rituals:

1. Use your watch to monitor the time you spend on your rituals.
2. Do not guess the time of ritualizing; be exact.
3. Write the time immediately on your monitoring form.
4. Do not save the recording to the end of the day or the beginning of the next day.
5. Write a short sentence to describe the trigger for ritualizing.

Prior to beginning treatment, the patient identifies an individual (e.g., parent, spouse, or close friend) who can serve as a support person during the intensive treatment program. The patient is instructed to rely on this person for support during exposures, and the support person is asked to help monitor compliance with response prevention instructions. If the patient experiences difficulty resisting the urge to ritualize, then the support person is contacted for support. Because the support person is involved in the therapy, the therapist allocates time during the information-gathering phase to describe the treatment and discuss its rationale with him or her.

The therapist makes an effort to ensure that the support person and the patient mutually agree that the support person will offer constructive criticism and observations. In making these suggestions, the support person should be sensitive to any difficulties that have arisen in the past. For example, Mr. B, who served as his wife's primary source of reassurance, also criticized her severely when he "caught" her performing her handwashing ritual. To prevent these responses from hampering treatment, to help the husband supervise his wife's response prevention, the therapist spent time with the couple negotiating appropriate, uncritical responses to the wife's requests for reassurance.

The support person is in regular (at least twice weekly) contact with the therapist and is not only informed about the specific homework exposures that the patient has to accomplish but also relays his/her observations about the patient's behavior outside the therapy session.

In addition, with the consent of the patient, the support person should contact the therapist if major treatment violations occur (e.g., refusing to do homework or engaging in ritualistic behavior).

Second Information-Gathering Session

At the beginning of the second information-gathering session, the therapist devotes time to the patient's self-monitoring form, which includes examining the descriptions of situations that trigger ritualistic behavior and offering constructive comments when necessary. The therapist reminds the patient to use short phrases or sentences to describe the trigger situations, assesses the accuracy of the patient's time estimates, and emphasizes the need for accurate measurements.

Generating a Treatment Plan

The bulk of the second information-gathering session is allotted to gathering detailed information about the patient's symptoms and, based on what is learned about the symptoms, developing a treatment with the patient. It is important to explain to the patient how the exposure exercises that comprise his/her treatment will reduce the OCD symptoms. For, example, the patient with religious obsessions is told that the imaginal exposure to burning in hell in excruciating detail is designed to reduce his obsessional distress when a less elaborate image of burning in hell comes into his mind. It is important that patients understand the rationale underlying the central concept in EX/RP, that confronting obsession-evoking stimuli during treatment increases their suffering in the short run but will reduce it in the long run. We often tell patients that the difficulties they experience during the first week of exposure sessions are likely to diminish with proper implementation of EX/RP.

Describing Homework

At the end of the second information-gathering session, the therapist describes the homework assignments included in the treatment program. The homework, which usually requires 2–3 hours, in addition to the 2-hour treatment session, comprises additional exposure exercises to be done between treatment sessions at the patient's home or elsewhere (e.g., a shopping mall or a relative's home). We suggest that the patient monitor his/her SUDS level every 10 minutes during the homework exposures. In some cases, when it is impossible for the patient to maintain an exposure for 45–60 minutes, the therapist works with the patient to develop a plan that allows the exposure to be prolonged. For example, instead of asking the patient to spend 45 minutes sitting in the restroom of a local restaurant, the therapist might suggest that he/she contaminate a handkerchief on the toilet seat and carry this "contamination rag" in a pocket.

Treatment Period

The treatment program at our center typically comprises fifteen 2-hour treatment sessions conducted daily for 3 weeks. Clinical observation suggests that massed sessions produce better results than do sessions spread out over time; therefore, we recommend a minimum of three sessions per week. Each session begins with a 10- to 15-minute discussion of homework assignments and the previous day's ritual monitoring. The next 90 minutes are divided into 45 minutes each of imaginal and *in vivo* exposure. The final 15 minutes are spent discussing the homework assignment for the following day. This format may be adjusted when necessary. For example, if an *in vivo* exposure requires that therapist and patient travel to a local shopping mall to contaminate children's clothing, the entire session is devoted to this activity. Some patients have difficulty engaging emotionally in imaginal exposures (i.e., the images fail to elicit distress). In these cases, treatment should focus exclusively on *in vivo* exercises.

We recommend that the therapist discuss the plan for that session with the patient in the beginning of the session. Barring any unusual circumstances (e.g., patient's stated objection to proceeding with the planned exposure), it is important to limit these discussions to no more than 15 minutes. Patients with OCD are usually very fearful of engaging in exposure tasks, and elaborate discussion of the task at hand may serve as a form of avoidance of going ahead with the exposure. These preexposure discussions are also fertile ground for assurance seeking (i.e., the patient asking the therapist if he/she is certain that the proposed exercise is safe). The therapist should answer such questions carefully, avoiding either extreme (i.e., neither providing compulsive reassurance nor conveying to the patient that the proposed exposure is objectively dangerous).

Imaginal exposure exercises are typically conducted prior to *in vivo* exercises in each session, often as a prelude to the scheduled *in vivo* exercise. During imaginal exposure the patient is seated in a comfortable chair and is given the following instructions:

> "Today you will be imagining [describes scene]. I'll ask you to close your eyes so that you won't be distracted. Please try to picture this scene as fully and vividly as possible, not like you are being told a story, but as if you were experiencing it now, right here. Every few minutes I will ask you to rate your anxiety level on a scale from 0 to 100. Please answer quickly and try not to leave the image."

The imaginal exposure sessions are audiotaped, and the patient is asked to repeat the exposure by listening to the tape as part of that day's homework. The situations included in *in vivo* exposure vary greatly from patient to patient (particularly with patients with prominent checking rituals). Below are some examples of instructions that might be offered to patients during *in vivo* exposure exercises.

For patients with prominent washing rituals:

> "Today, you will be touching [specifies item(s)]. This means that I will ask you to touch it with your whole hand, not just the fingers, and then to touch it to your face, hair, and clothing, all over yourself, so you feel that no part of you has avoided contamination. Then I'll ask you to sit and hold it and repeatedly touch it to your face, hair, and clothes during the rest of the session. I know that this is likely to make you upset, but remember the anxiety will eventually decrease. I also want you to go ahead and let yourself worry about the harm you are afraid will occur—for example, disease—since you won't he washing or cleaning after this exposure. I am sorry that this treatment has to be difficult and cause so much discomfort, but I'm sure you can do it. You'll find it gets easier as time goes on. OK, here it is, go ahead and touch it."

The therapist should give the patient the object to hold, ask him/her to touch it, and then ask the patient to touch the object or the "contaminated" hands directly to his/her face, hair, and clothing. Every 10 minutes the patient should be asked, "What is your level of anxiety or discomfort from 0 to 100 right now as you focus on what you're touching?" This can be shortened to "What is your SUDS?" once the patient understands the question.

For patients with prominent checking rituals:

> "Now, I'd like you to [e.g., write out your checks to pay your monthly bills without looking at them after you've finished; just put them in the envelope and then we will mail them right away, without checking even once after you've done it]. Then we will go on and do [e.g., drive on a bumpy road without looking in the rearview mirror] in the same way. While doing this, I would like you to worry about what harm might occur because you aren't checking your actions, but don't let the thoughts interfere with actually doing those activities."

Patients should be reminded of the specific instructions for response prevention on the first day of treatment and periodically during treatment. We have found that giving patients a printed copy of the rules for response prevention can help them to understand and remember the rules. If the rules as outlined for the patient do not adequately cover the type of ritual(s) the patient exhibits, the therapist should provide a written set of instructions modeled after these forms.

During the last few sessions of treatment, the patient should be introduced to rules of "normal" washing, cleaning, or checking. Response prevention requirements should be relaxed to enable the patient to return to what is considered a normal routine.

Home Visit

It is important to ensure that the patient's gains from the treatment program generalize to the home environment. Usually homework assignments function to produce this generalization, but we have found that visits by the therapist to the patient's home can be quite helpful, especially in cases where the patient is not able to return home daily during the intensive treatment phase (e.g., patients who are from out of town or are hospitalized). The home visit also offers therapist and patient an opportunity to discuss guidelines for "normal" behavior. The therapist should discuss the plans for these visits with the patient and his/her family before the treatment ends. It is also important to note that, in some cases, the majority of the treatment sessions need to be conducted at the patient's home, such as when treating a hoarder. Determining the frequency of home visits during the core treatment should be based on whether the patient's OCD symptoms are readily "transportable" to situations outside the home, or whether they are specific to the home. For patients with prominent washing rituals, with "safe" rooms and areas in their houses, contamination of these areas is imperative and also quite difficult; it is often advisable that the therapist assist directly with these home-based exposures when it is questionable whether the patient can contaminate these "sanctuaries" successfully on his/her own.

Typically, the home visit comprises 4-hour sessions held on each of 2 days at the end of the treatment program. The bulk of the time in these sessions is used to conduct additional exposures to obsessive stimuli in and around the patient's home or workplace. For example, the therapist might accompany the patient as he/she contaminates objects around the house or at the local grocery store. Similarly, the patient might be asked to turn the stove on and off without checking and leave the house with the therapist. Most patients, particularly those who were able to return home during treatment, will report little or no discomfort when doing these exposures because they represent repetition of homework assignments. In some cases, though, the therapist will discover areas that the patient has not contaminated, or some areas at home that continue to generate distress despite previous exposures. The home visit should focus on exposure to situations or objects that remain problematic.

Maintenance Period

In addition to prescribing continued self-exposure tasks to help the patient maintain therapy gains, the therapist may wish to schedule regular maintenance sessions. These sessions may be used to plan additional exposures, to refine guidelines for normal behavior, and to address issues that arise as the patient adjusts to life without OCD.

There is some evidence that patients benefit from continued contact with the therapist following the intensive therapy sessions. In one study, 12 weekly supportive therapy sessions (no exposure exercises) appeared to reduce the number of relapses in a sample of individuals with OCD treated with 3 weeks of intensive EX/RP (Foa et al., 1992). In another study, following the intensive treatment with 1 week of daily cognitive-behavioral sessions followed by eight brief (10-minute) weekly telephone contacts resulted in better long-term outcome than following intensive treatment with 1 week of treatment with free association (Hiss et al., 1994).

Therapeutic Setting

It is advisable for patients to remain in their normal environments during intensive treatment. This is particularly important for patients whose fears are cued mainly by stimuli in their home environment. The hospital may be an artificially protected setting, particularly for patients with prominent checking rituals, who may not feel responsible for their surroundings and as a result do not experience their usual urges to check. If patients live too far away to commute for daily sessions, we recommend that they rent an apartment or hotel room near the clinic. When this is not possible, hospitalization should be considered. Hospitalization is recommended for patients deemed to be at risk for suicide or psychotic breakdown, and for those who need close supervision but lack a support system sufficient to aid them during treatment.

If a patient is employed and his/her OCD symptoms are work related, he/she should be encouraged to continue working, so that relevant exposures can he included in treatment. However, since treatment requires 5 to 6 hours per day, the patient may opt to work half-days during the intensive treatment.

When the patient's symptoms are unrelated to work, he/she may decide not to continue working during intensive treatment. Because of the time-consuming nature of the treatment, we often suggest that patients take some time off from work. If it is not possible for the patient to take 3 full weeks off from work, the therapist might suggest that the patient work half-days or take time off from work during the first and second weeks of the treatment program.

Therapist Variables

Intensive treatment with exposure to feared situations and response prevention of ritualistic behavior provoke considerable stress for patients. Their willingness to undergo such "torture" attests to their strong motivation to rid themselves of the OCD symptoms. The intensive treatment regimen requires that the therapist maintain a delicate balance between pressuring the patient to engage in the treatment and empathizing with his/her distress. Clinical observations and findings from a study by Rabavilas and colleagues (1979) suggest that a respectful, understanding, encouraging, explicit, and challenging therapist is more likely to achieve a successful outcome than a permissive, tolerant therapist. Notably, patients of well-supervised, nonexpert EX/RP

THERAPIST: No other repetitive actions besides washing?

Since this patient did not appear to have multiple types of ritualistic behaviors, the therapist turned to the obsessional content. External cues are usually solicited first.

THERAPIST: What are the things that make you feel you want to wash? For instance, why do you wipe the car seat with alcohol?

JUNE: I think that maybe I got dog dirt on it when I got in from before, or Kenny might have.

THERAPIST: From your shoes?

JUNE: Yes, I also worry about the hem of my dress touching the seat. I've been worrying that my shoe could kick my skirt hem or when I step up a step, like to go in a building, the dress could touch the step.

THERAPIST: A dress like this? June was wearing a dress that came to just below her knee. [The likelihood that it could have touched a curb or sole of her shoe was very slim.]

JUNE: Yes.

THERAPIST: Has your skirt ever had dog dirt on it?

JUNE: I don't think so, but in my mind I think that maybe it could have gotten some on it. I suppose it would be hard for that to happen, wouldn't it?

Thoughts that highly improbable events might have occurred are common in OCD. Such distortions may be the result of intense anxiety. Doubts about "safety" often lead to requests for reassurance or to rituals. Reassuring June that her dress is unlikely to be soiled would have been countertherapeutic because it perpetuates the neurotic fears. Rather, the therapist inquired further about the obsessional content.

THERAPIST: Is dog "dirt" the most upsetting thing that you worry about?

JUNE: Probably. Yes, I think so, but bathroom germs are pretty bad, too.

THERAPIST: What sort of germs?

JUNE: From toilets. You know, when you go to the bathroom.

THERAPIST: Urine and feces?

JUNE: Yes, urine doesn't bother me as much as the other.

THERAPIST: Why?

JUNE: Because I learned in nursing school that it's almost sterile. I had a hard time in the course about microbiology because it upset me to try to learn about bacteria and microorganisms. They make it sound like there are all kinds of germs everywhere that are real dangerous. I didn't learn it very well; I tried to avoid thinking about it.

June's concerns with both dog dirt and bathroom germs suggested that her fear structure includes apprehension about potential illness. The therapist questioned her to better understand the nature of the feared consequences of contamination.

THERAPIST: Are you afraid of diseases that could come from feces?

JUNE: Yes, I guess so. The thing of it is, though, I know other people don't worry about it like I do. To them, you know, they just go to the bathroom and wash their hands and don't even think about it. But I can't get it out of my head that maybe I didn't get clean enough.

THERAPIST: If you didn't wash enough, would you get sick or would you cause someone else to get sick?

JUNE: Mostly I worry that I'll get sick, but sometimes I worry about Kenny, too.

THERAPIST: Do you worry about a particular kind of disease?

JUNE: I'm not sure. Some kind of illness.

It is not uncommon for patients who fear harm that may ensue from not ritualizing to be unable to identify a specific feared consequence. Patients with prominent checking rituals often fear they will forget or throw out something important, but they do not always know exactly what this will be. Repeaters may fear that something bad will happen to loved ones but often cannot specify what particular disaster will befall them. However, many individuals with OCD do fear specific consequences (e.g., blindness or leukemia). At this point, the therapist may choose either to complete the inquiry about external threat cues or pursue the investigation about the feared consequences and the belief that such harm is indeed likely to occur. The latter course was selected here.

THERAPIST: Let's say that you did actually touch dog feces or human feces, and you weren't aware of it, so you didn't wash to remove it. What is the likelihood that you or Kenny would really get seriously ill?

JUNE: Well, I feel like it really could happen.

THERAPIST: I understand that when it happens and you become very distressed, it feels like you will actually become sick, but if I ask you to judge objectively, right now, how likely is it that you will get sick from touching feces and not washing? For example, if you were to touch feces 10 times, how many times would you get sick?

JUNE: Oh, I know it's pretty unlikely, but sometimes it seems so real.

THERAPIST: Can you put a number on it? What's the percent chance that if you touched a small amount of feces and didn't wash that you'd get sick?

JUNE: I'd say low, less than 25%.

THERAPIST: That means that one time in every four you'd get sick.

JUNE: No, that's not right. I guess it's really less than 1%.

From this dialogue it is clear that June did not strongly believe that her feared disasters would actually occur, although her initial estimate of the likelihood was high. A person with poor insight regarding the senselessness of his/her OCD symptoms would have assigned higher probabilities (usually over 80%) and would insist on the accuracy of his/her estimate even in the face of persistent questioning. Note also that this exchange is an example of the informal cognitive restructuring accompanying EX/RP that we discussed earlier. The therapist may need to repeat this discussion during subsequent exposure sessions when June, highly anxious about confronting contaminants, readjusts her likelihood estimates when anxious. Strength of belief can change in a given patient but is stronger when the patient perceives threat.

THERAPIST: OK. Now, besides disease, what else could happen if you got feces on you?

JUNE: I suppose I'm also afraid of what other people might think if I got dog feces on my shoe or on my dress. Somebody would see it or smell it and think it was really disgusting, and I was a dirty person. I think I'm afraid they would think I'm not a good person.

The therapist then questioned June further about this feared consequence, inquiring about the possibility of others evaluating her character negatively because she had feces on her dress. The material regarding feared consequences was collected for later inclusion in the imaginal exposure scenes. To conclude the inquiry about the nature of the obsessions, the therapist further elucidated the external feared stimuli.

THERAPIST: Besides dog and human feces and toilets, what else can "contaminate" you? Is it OK if I use the word "contaminated" to describe how you feel if you handle these things?

JUNE: Yes, it's like I can feel it on my skin, even if I can't see it. Umm, I also get upset if I see "bird doo" on my car.

THERAPIST: Bird droppings? The whitish spots?

JUNE: Yeah, I have to hold my skirt close to me so that I don't touch any of these spots with my clothes.

THERAPIST: OK, bird doo, what else?

JUNE: Dead animals, like on the roadside. I feel like the germs, or whatever it is, get on the tires from the pavement and get on the car. Even if I don't run over it. Like it's spread around the street near it.

THERAPIST: What do you do if you see a dead animal?

JUNE: I swerve wide around it. Once I parked the car and as I got out, I saw this dead cat right behind the car. I had to wash all my clothes and take a shower right away. It was really a mess that day.

THERAPIST: It sounds like that was very difficult for you. Is there anything else besides dead animals that contaminates you?

JUNE: I can't think of any. There are lots of places I avoid now, but that's because of what we just talked about.

The therapist questions June further about other items that are likely to be contaminated because of their potential relationship to the ones she has already noted.

THERAPIST: What about trash or garbage?

JUNE: Yeah, that bothers me. And I also avoid gutters on the street.

THERAPIST: What's in the gutter that upsets you?

JUNE: Dead animals, I guess. And then the rain spreads the germs down the street. Also rotten garbage. It's really dirty. Sometimes the gutters are really disgusting.

THERAPIST: Um hmm. Are you afraid you could get sick from dead animals and garbage?

JUNE: Yes, it's like the toilets or dog dirt.

To prepare for an exposure program in which objects are presented hierarchically with respect to their ability to provoke discomfort, June was asked to rank her major contaminants. Here she also provided information about avoidance behaviors associated with her contaminants.

THERAPIST: Now, let's make a list of the main things that upset you. I'm going to ask you how distressed you would be on a 0- to 100-point scale if you touched the thing I'll name. Zero indicates no distress at all and 100 means you'd be extremely upset, the most you've ever felt.

JUNE: OK.

THERAPIST: What if you touched dog dirt?

JUNE: And I could wash as much as I wanted?

THERAPIST: No, let's say you couldn't wash for a while.

JUNE: 100.

THERAPIST: A dead animal.

JUNE: Also 100.

THERAPIST: Bird doo on your car.

JUNE: That depends on whether it is wet or dry.

THERAPIST: Tell me for both.

JUNE: 100 wet and 95 dry.

THERAPIST: Street gutter.

JUNE: 95.

THERAPIST: Garbage in your sink at home.

JUNE: Not too bad. Only 50. But, the trash can outdoors would be 90.

THERAPIST: Why the difference?

JUNE: Because the inside of the trash can is dirty from lots of old garbage.

THERAPIST: I see. What about a public toilet seat?

JUNE: That's bad. 95.

THERAPIST: Car tires?

JUNE: Usually 90. But if I just passed a dead animal, they'd be 99.

THERAPIST: What about a doorknob to a public bathroom?

JUNE: The outside knob is low, like 40. But the inside knob is 80 because people touch it right after they've used the bathroom, and I've seen that some don't wash their hands.

THERAPIST: I understand. How about grass in a park where dogs are around?

JUNE: If I did walk in the grass, it would be about 80 or 85, but I don't usually do it. I also have a lot of trouble on sidewalks. You know, the brown spots on the concrete. I guess most of it is just rust or other dirt, but I think maybe it could be dog dirt.

THERAPIST: How much does that bother you?

JUNE: To step on a brown spot? About 90. I always walk around them.

The therapist should continue in this manner until a list of 10–20 items is formed. More items may be necessary for patients with multiple obsessional fears or rituals. The items are ordered from low- to high-level fear in preparation for treatment by exposure. Items equivalent with regard to their level of disturbance are grouped together. Moreover, it is important to probe the rationale for one stimulus differing from another because it provides further information about the patient's particular "OCD logic." This information is highly relevant for the construction of the exposure hierarchy and for the informal cognitive discussions about risk assessment, responsibility, and so forth.

Considerable information about avoidance patterns and rituals emerged from the previous interview about external threat cues. More details may be obtained by asking the patient to provide a step-by-step description of a typical day's activities from the time he/she awakens until he/she goes to sleep. Usually, patients are not entirely accurate when describing their compulsive behaviors during the interview because, as one patient told us, they have not "thought of their OCD in that way before." Thus, the self-monitoring tasks assist patients in raising their awareness about the OCD patterns and provide the therapist with more accurate data about rituals and avoidant behaviors.

We were particularly concerned by June's bathroom routines, her shower, use of the toilet, handling of towels and dirty clothes, and dressing and putting on shoes. Additional information about avoidance patterns may be ascertained by inquiring about other routine activities, such as shopping, eating out, housecleaning, preparing meals, working, and so on. The following dialogue exemplifies the degree of detail desired.

THERAPIST: June, for us to plan your treatment carefully, I need to know what you avoid in your daily routine. Why don't you start by describing what you do first when you wake up.

JUNE: I go to use the bathroom first.

THERAPIST: Nightgown on or off?

JUNE: I take off my nightgown because I don't want it to touch the toilet. That way it's clean at night after I shower.

THERAPIST: Go on.

JUNE: I go to the toilet. I suppose I use a lot of toilet paper because I don't want to get anything on my hand. Then I have to shower after a bowel movement.

THERAPIST: How do you get ready to shower?

JUNE: I have to put a new towel on the rod near the shower. I don't like it to touch anything before I use it. Oh, and I put my slippers facing the door, near the shower, so I can put them on without stepping on the bathroom floor when I get out of the shower. Then I get into the shower.

THERAPIST: You said you shower for 45 minutes. Why does it take so long?

JUNE: I have to wash myself in a special order and I count how many times I wash each part. Like I wash my arm four times. That's why it takes so long.

THERAPIST: What is the order you use?

JUNE: First I wash my hands, then my face and hair, and then I go from the top down.

THERAPIST: What about the genital and anal area? [This area should disturb this patient most because she fears contamination from fecal "germs."]

JUNE: Oh yes, those are last, after my feet.

Such a detailed description helps the therapist to anticipate possible avoidance by the patient during treatment and to plan specific exposure instructions. Supervision of normal washing behavior at the end of treatment will address June's tendency to count and to order her washing. During the initial session of information gathering, June was instructed to self-monitor the frequency and duration of her compulsions.

THERAPIST: Between now and our next session, I'd like you to record all the washing and cleaning that you do, including wiping things with alcohol. You can use this form (*Hands her a self-monitoring of rituals form.*) Please write down every time you wash, how long you washed, what made you wash, and how anxious you were before you washed. This kind of record will help us identify any sources of contamination you've forgotten to mention, and we can also use it to measure your progress during treatment.

JUNE: Do you want me to write in each space for each half-hour?

THERAPIST: No, only when you wash or use alcohol.

JUNE: OK.

History of Symptoms and Treatment History

After assessing the patient's current symptoms, the therapist sought information about the onset of the problem, with particular reference to the presence of specific stressors at the time and whether these stressors are still present.

THERAPIST: How long have you been washing like this?

JUNE: It started about 2 years ago in my first year of nursing school. It wasn't real bad right away. It started with the city. I had to go into the city to classes, and the city seemed real dirty.

THERAPIST: Did nursing have something to do with it?

JUNE: Maybe. I was under a lot of tension. I had to quit working as a secretary, and it was pretty hard without an income and a lot of school bills. My mother and dad weren't much help. And then we started to learn all the sterilizing techniques, and I already told you about the course in microbiology.

THERAPIST: Did it gradually get worse?

JUNE: Mostly, but I did notice that it was a lot worse after a rotation on surgery, where I was really worried about germs contaminating the instruments. That's when I started to wash more than usual.

THERAPIST: Did you seek help at that time?

JUNE: I was already seeing Dr. W at the university, and he tried to help.

THERAPIST: You were already in treatment with him? For what reason?

JUNE: He was helping me with an eating problem. I had anorexia. I'd been seeing him for about a year when the washing started.

THERAPIST: Anorexia? Did treatment help?

JUNE: Yes. I was down to 85 pounds and I'm up around 105 now. He mostly asked me to increase my weight every week and he did "cognitive therapy," I think it's called.

THERAPIST: I see. What about the washing problem?

JUNE: He tried the same type of therapy, but it didn't work for that. That's why I'm here. My sister-in-law heard about it, and Dr. W said I should come.

THERAPIST: What about drugs? Were you ever given medication for this problem?

JUNE: Yes, I tried Anafranil [clomipramine] for a while and it helped a little, but it made me dizzy and sleepy, so I decided to stop taking it. Also, I heard that you can't take the medication when you are pregnant, and Kenny and I want to have a baby soon. Before that, I took Xanax [alprazolam]; it calmed me down but didn't stop the washing.

THERAPIST: Have you tried any other treatments?

JUNE: Only for the anorexia. I went to another counseling center at the university for about a year, but that didn't really help at all.

June's history was unusual only in the relatively recent onset of her symptoms. Typically, patients in our clinic present a much longer duration of symptoms, with the mean around 8 years. Other centers in England and Holland report similar figures. June's treatment history of trying various psychotherapeutic and pharmacological treatments prior to seeking EX/RP was quite typical. Since previous failure with nonbehavioral treatments has not been found to influence outcome with EX/RP, the clinician should not be discouraged by such a history. However, because of a possible skeptical attitude about the value of treatment, the therapist should provide the patient with a clear rationale for EX/RP treatment along the lines discussed earlier and demonstrated below.

THERAPIST: Before I continue to collect more information about your problem, let me tell you about our treatment.

JUNE: Well, Dr. F told me something about it, but I'm still not sure what this treatment is going to be like.

THERAPIST: The treatment is called exposure and ritual prevention. I'll be asking you to confront situations and things that frighten you or make you feel contaminated. We will do this gradually, working up to the hardest things. For example, we may begin with the outside door handles of bathrooms and work our way up to toilet seats and bird doo. We'll do this together, and I'll be there to help you. The sessions will last 1½ or 2 hours, and we'll meet every weekday. In addition, I'll assign you homework to do similar things between the therapy sessions.

JUNE: You mean I have to touch them, even dog dirt?

THERAPIST: Yes, to get over these kinds of fears, people must learn to confront what they're afraid of and stay with it until the discomfort decreases.

JUNE: Even if I did, it would probably take me a year to get used to it.

THERAPIST: Remember, you didn't always feel like this about dog dirt. When you were younger, did you ever step in dog dirt and just wipe it off on the grass and go on playing?

JUNE: Yeah, I forget that. It seems such a long time ago. I used to not think twice about this stuff.

THERAPIST: To get you back to how you used to feel, we need to expose you directly to what you're afraid of. Now, there's a second part to treatment. I'm also going to ask you not to wash for 3 days at a stretch. No handwashing or showering for 3 days. Then you can take a shower, but you will have to limit it to 10 minutes. After the shower, you will have to contaminate yourself again, then wait another 3 days for your next shower.

JUNE: I can't believe it! I'll never be able to do that. If I could, I wouldn't be here. How can I not wash? Every day I resolve to stop, but I always give in. You mean I wouldn't be able to wash after I use the bathroom or before I eat? Other people wash after they use the toilet. Why can't I just wash less, like normal people do?

THERAPIST: Other people don't have OCD. Remember, for you, washing makes you feel less "contaminated" and less anxious. Right?

JUNE: Yes.

THERAPIST: If you wash, even briefly, whenever you feel "contaminated," you never get a chance to learn that the feeling of contamination would go away by itself without washing. If you are really very anxious, it might take a while, even several hours, before you feel better, but it will eventually happen. On the other hand, if you wash, even briefly, every few hours, it will reinforce your idea that you have to wash to feel better.

JUNE: But why 3 days? Couldn't I shower once a day like other people?

THERAPIST: For the same reason. You'd still feel relief, even if you waited 24 hours between washings. And that would strengthen your belief that you need to "decontaminate" by washing yourself. You must learn to use soap and water to feel clean and fresh but not to "decontaminate" yourself.

JUNE: I think I understand. I know I shower now to get the things I'm afraid of off my body. I used to shower just to get sweat and dirt off, and feel nice. I'm still not sure I could stand it though, not washing for that long.

THERAPIST: The treatment is very demanding. Before we start the treatment program you will need to make a commitment to yourself that even though you will feel very uncomfortable and even quite upset at times, you won't wash. I'll try to help you as much as I can by planning the treatment so you know what to expect each day and by supporting you whenever you need it. Someone will have to be available to help supervise and support you any time you need it. Between sessions you can always call me here or at home if a problem comes up. I know the treatment won't be easy for you, but I'm sure you can do it if you make up your mind.

At this point, a firm commitment should not be requested. Rather, the patient should be made aware of what will be required so that he/she can adjust to these expectations and plan activities during the treatment period accordingly. The patient should make the arrangements necessary to attend daily treatment sessions for 3 to 4 weeks. As we discussed earlier, two to three sessions per week may be sufficient for patients with less severe symptoms. It is important that the therapist not minimize the difficulty of the treatment regimen, so that the patient is prepared to struggle and enters treatment with a readiness to mobilize inner resources and emotional support from family and friends.

The history of the patient is usually taken in the first session. Because collecting histories of individuals with OCD does not differ from collecting histories of other psychiatric patients, details are not provided here.

Treatment Planning

The therapist began the second session by briefly reviewing the patient's self-monitoring of rituals form. The remainder of the session was devoted to developing a treatment plan.

THERAPIST: OK, now I want to discuss our plan for each day during the first week of therapy. We need to expose you both in imagination and in reality to the things that bother you, which we talked about in our first sessions. As I said already, we'll also limit your washing. The scenes you imagine will focus on the harm that you fear will occur if you do not wash. The actual exposures will focus on confronting the things that contaminate you. Restricting your washing will teach you how to live without rituals. In imaginal exposure, you will picture yourself touching something you're afraid of, like toilet seats, and not washing and then becoming ill. We can have you imagine going to a doctor who can't figure out what's wrong and can't fix it. That's the sort of fear you have, right?

JUNE: Yes, that and Kenny getting sick, and it being my fault.

THERAPIST: OK, so in some scenes you'll be sick, and in others Kenny will get sick. Should I add that other people blame you for not being careful? Is this what you're afraid of?

JUNE: Yes, especially my mother.

THERAPIST: OK. We'll have her criticize you for not being careful enough. Can you think of anything else we should add to the image?

JUNE: No, that's about it.

THERAPIST: We can compose the scenes in detail after we plan the actual exposures. Let's review the list of things you avoid or are afraid to touch and make sure that we have listed them in the right order. Then we'll decide what to work on each day. OK?

JUNE: OK.

June reviewed the list, which included items such as trash cans, kitchen floor, bathroom floor, public hallway carpet, plant dirt, puddles, car tires, dried dog "dirt," and bird "doo." Changes were made as needed.

THERAPIST: Good. Now let's plan the treatment. On the first day we should start with things that you rated below a 60. That would include touching this carpet, doorknobs that are not inside bathrooms, books on my shelves, light switches, and stair railings. On the second day, we'll do the 60- to 70-level items, like faucets, bare floors, dirty laundry, and the things on Kenny's desk. [The therapist continued to detail Sessions 3 to 5, increasing the level of difficulty each day.] In the second week, we will repeat the worse situations like gutters, tires, public toilets, bird doo, and dog dirt, and we'll also find a dead animal to walk near and touch the street next to it.

On rare occasions, direct confrontation with a feared object (e.g., pesticides or other chemicals) may have some likelihood of producing actual harm. In such cases, the therapist's judgment should be exercised to find a middle ground between total avoidance and endangerment. With chemicals, for example, patients are exposed to small quantities that are objectively nonharmful. In June's case the therapist decided that direct contact with a dead animal was not called for, and that stepping on the animal's fur with her shoe and then touching the shoe sole constituted sufficient exposure. In general, the therapist must weigh the level of obsessional distress that will be evoked by a given exposure with the objective risks entailed in completing that exposure. Patients with OCD have difficulty assessing such risks realistically; thus, it is the responsibility of the therapist to evaluate whether exposure is warranted. For example, patients with fears of contracting HIV would certainly be highly distressed if asked to handle a dirty hypodermic needle found in a city gutter, but because exposure to such stimuli is objectively risky, they should not be included on the treatment hierarchy.

THERAPIST: How does this plan sound?

JUNE: The first week is OK, but I'm really scared about the second week. I'm not sure I'll be ready to do the bathrooms and dog dirt by then.

THERAPIST: Many people feel this way at the beginning, but by the end of the first week, you won't be as frightened as you are now about touching tires or public toilets. Remember, I will be here to help you

because it will probably be difficult in the beginning.

JUNE: Yes, I know it. I feel like I don't really have a choice anyhow. This washing is crazy and I'm disgusted with myself. I suppose I'm as ready as I'll ever be.

THERAPIST: Good. Now remember, I'll ask you to keep working on these things for 2 to 3 hours at home after each session, but you will already have done them with me, so I don't think it will be too hard. I take it that you talked to Kenny about assisting us with supervising, since I saw him out in the waiting room.

JUNE: Yes, he said that's fine. He wanted to know what he should do.

THERAPIST: Let's call him in. Did you talk to your sister-in-law about being available when Kenny is at work during the day?

JUNE: Yes, she was really good about it, but she couldn't come today because of the kids.

THERAPIST: If it's difficult for her to come, I could talk to her on the phone. Why don't you go get Kenny now?

Treatment

June was seen for 15 treatment sessions, held every weekday for 3 weeks. During the fourth week the therapist visited her twice at her home for 4 hours each time. During these visits, under the therapist's supervision, June contaminated her entire house and exposed herself to objects at home and in her neighborhood that provoked distress. Thereafter, once-weekly follow-up sessions were instituted to ensure maintenance of gains and to address any other issues of concern to her.

As discussed earlier, treatment begins with exposure to moderately difficult items on the hierarchy and progresses to the most disturbing ones by the beginning of the second week. The most distressing items are repeated during the remainder of the second and third weeks. The following sequence, which occurred on the sixth day of treatment, exemplifies this process.

THERAPIST: How was your weekend?

JUNE: Not that great. I suppose it was as good as I could expect. I took my shower Sunday night and I was so nervous about finishing in time I don't even know if I washed right.

THERAPIST: Most people feel the same way. Remember though, you aren't supposed to wash "right," just to wash. Did Kenny time it?

JUNE: Yes, he called out the minutes like you said, "5, 7, 9," and then "stop."

THERAPIST: You stopped when he said to?

JUNE: Yes, but it still wasn't easy.

THERAPIST: I know. I'm really pleased that you were careful to follow the rules.

JUNE: I have pretty much decided that this is my chance to get better, so I'm trying my best.

THERAPIST: Good. I am glad you feel so positive. How was the homework?

JUNE: I touched the floor and the soles of my shoes and the cement. It is all written on the daily sheet there. On Saturday, I went to my sister's, so I could play with the kids like we said. They stepped on me when I lay on the floor and I tried to touch their bottoms when I held them. On Sunday, Kenny and I went to the park. I didn't sit in the grass but I did walk around and touched my shoes afterward.

THERAPIST: The soles?

JUNE: Yeah. We also went downtown and I threw some things in the trash cans and pushed them down, and tried to touch the sides. It's sort of hard because I felt conspicuous, but I did it anyway.

THERAPIST: That sounds really good. I'm glad to hear it. How about your doormat and going into the garden?

JUNE: I did the doormat and I stood in the garden, but I couldn't touch the dirt. The neighbor's dog always runs all over. I know I should have touched it, but I just couldn't get up the courage.

THERAPIST: Well, you did do many other things. Let's plan to go outside today and do it together, so it will be easier for you to walk in the garden when you go home.

JUNE: OK.

June was very compliant with the treatment regimen. Some patients occasionally lapse on response prevention, particularly during the first week of the treatment program. The therapist should reinforce the patient for partial compliance but emphasize the need to comply fully with treatment instructions. With regard to expo-

sure homework, it is not uncommon for patients to neglect completing some assignments. Again, they should be reinforced for what they have achieved and encouraged to complete all of the assignments.

THERAPIST: How are you and Kenny doing?

JUNE: He got mad on Sunday night after the shower because I started to ask him how he showered and if I was clean enough. I think I nagged him too much, so he lost his temper. We just watched TV, and after a while we talked a bit and he sort of apologized for getting mad. But I understand; I ask too many questions. Otherwise, the rest of the weekend was OK.

THERAPIST: Well, it's unfortunate that Kenny got mad, but it's good that he didn't answer your questions. He's not supposed to reassure you about cleanliness.

JUNE: I think he has a hard time knowing when to answer me and when not to. I am not real sure either. Could you talk to him before Wednesday when I shower again?

THERAPIST: That's a good idea. I'll call him after we're done with today's session. Now, today we'll start with the scene about you driving your car to an appointment with me, and you get a flat tire and have to change it. The cars splash water in the puddle near you, and it lands on the car and on you. Then you notice a dead animal when you walk behind the car, and it's right behind you. You really feel contaminated. You walk to the gas station nearby to see if they can fix the tire and you have to urinate so badly that you have to use their restroom. They agree to fix the tire if you remove it and bring it to them because otherwise they are too busy. Of course, that means you will have to handle the tire that is contaminated by the dead animal. We'll add some bird doo on the street and on the sidewalk, too. Then, later you start to feel sick, and you feel like it's from the dead animal. Sound awful enough?

JUNE: Yeah. Ugh. That one is really bad. Do I have to? Never mind, I know the answer.

THERAPIST: OK. I want you to close your eyes now and imagine that you are driving your car on West Avenue.

Note that the therapist checked the patient's assignment from the previous day to verify that she completed it and did not engage in avoidance and rituals. This provided an opportunity to reinforce efforts at self-exposure. It is important to keep track of completion of homework because patients do not always volunteer information about omissions. They will, however, admit failure to comply if directly asked and are likely to carry out the next assignment if reinforced adequately.

With regard to the conflict between June and Kenny, it is our experience that, like Kenny, most family members are quite willing to help. Difficulty may, however, arise when they are unable to help without becoming upset, thereby increasing the patient's tension. Providing them with an opportunity to ventilate their frustration by contacting the therapist, who also may coach them in alternative reactions, may reduce familial tension.

That same session also included imaginal exposure to do a scenario planned in advance. Since that scenario had already been discussed in detail with the patient, it posed no surprises for her. It is presented for up to 1 hour, or until a substantial decrease in anxiety is evident. Next, the patient is confronted *in vivo* with situations like those included in the fantasized scene.

THERAPIST: It's time to do the real thing now. I looked for a dead animal by the side of the road yesterday and I found one about a mile away. I think we should go there.

JUNE: Yuck, that's terrific. Just for me you had to find it.

THERAPIST: Today's our lucky day. You knew we were going to have to find one today anyhow. At least it's close.

JUNE: Great.

Humor is encouraged and can be quite helpful if the patient is capable of responding to it. At the same time, it is important that the therapist laugh *with* rather than *at* the patient. Patients and therapists often develop a shorthand lexicon for discussing OCD and its treatment that is specific to them and aimed at promoting compliance with treatment. For example, one patient–therapist pair began to discuss exposure homework as "swallowing the frog," based on a proverb that the patient introduced. When the therapist asked the patient if she had "swallowed the frog" that morning, it conveyed the difficulty of the exposure tasks she needed to do between sessions. It is important for the therapist to observe the patient's interpersonal style to determine whether such banter is likely to promote the therapeutic goals.

THERAPIST: (*outside the office*) There it is, behind the car. Let's go and touch the curb and street next to it. I don't think that you need to touch it directly because it's a bit smelly, but I want you to step next to it, then touch the sole of your shoe.

JUNE: Yuck! It's really dead. It's gross!

THERAPIST: Yeah, it is a bit gross, but it's also just a dead cat if you think about it plainly. What harm can it cause?

JUNE: I don't know. Suppose I get germs on my hand?

THERAPIST: What sort of germs?

JUNE: Dead cat germs.

THERAPIST: What kind are they?

JUNE: I don't know. Just germs.

THERAPIST: Like the bathroom germs that we've already handled?

JUNE: Sort of. People don't go around touching dead cats.

THERAPIST: They also don't go running home to shower or alcohol the inside of their car. It's time to get over this. Now, come on over and I'll do it first. (*June follows.*) OK. Touch the curb and the street. Here's a stone you can carry with you and a piece of paper from under its tail. Go ahead, take it.

JUNE: (*looking quite uncomfortable*) Ugh!

THERAPIST: We'll both hold them. Now, touch it to your front and your skirt, and your face and hair. Like this. That's good. What's your anxiety level?

JUNE: Ugh! 99. I'd say 100, but it's just short of panic. If you weren't here, it'd be 100.

THERAPIST: You know from past experience that this will be much easier in a while. Just stay with it and we'll wait here. You're doing fine.

JUNE: (*A few minutes pass in which she looks very upset.*) Would you do this if it weren't for me?

THERAPIST: Yes, if this were my car and I dropped my keys here, I'd just pick them up and go on.

JUNE: You wouldn't have to wash them?

THERAPIST: No. Dead animals aren't delightful, but they're part of the world we live in. What are the odds that we'll get ill from this?

JUNE: Very small, I guess. I feel a little bit better than at first. It's about 90 now.

THERAPIST: Good! Just stay with it now.

The session continued for another 45 minutes, or until anxiety decreased substantially. During this period conversation focused generally on the feared situations and the patient's reaction to them. The therapist inquired about June's anxiety level approximately every 10 minutes. It is important to note that June and the therapist have engaged in conversation throughout the exposure task, discussing issues such as habituation, risk, responsibility, and long-term outcomes. At the same time it is imperative to refocus the patient on the exposure task at hand to ensure that he/she remains engaged with it. Thus, asking for SUDS ratings serves two purposes: It provides data about fear reduction, and it refocuses the patient on the exposure. However, if the informal discussion serves as a distractor, helping the patient "not think about" what he/she is doing, the therapist should limit such conversations.

THERAPIST: How do you feel now?

JUNE: Well, it is easier, but I sure don't feel great.

THERAPIST: Can you put a number on it?

JUNE: About 55 or 60, I'd say.

THERAPIST: You worked hard today. You must be tired. Let's stop now. I want you to take this stick and pebble with you so that you continue to be contaminated. You can keep them in your pocket and touch them frequently during the day. I want you to contaminate your office at work and your apartment with them. Touch them to everything around, including everything in the kitchen, chairs, your bed, and the clothes in your dresser. Oh, also, I'd like you to drive your car past this spot on your way to and from work. Can you do that?

JUNE: I suppose so. The trouble is going home with all of this dirt.

THERAPIST: Why don't you call Kenny and plan to get home after he does, so he can be around to help you. Remember, you can always call me if you have trouble.

JUNE: Yeah. That's a good idea. I'll just leave work after he does. See you tomorrow.

This scenario illustrates the process of *in vivo* exposure. The therapist answered clearly the questions raised without detouring from the essential purpose of the session, exposure to the feared contaminant. After the initial increase, the anxiety may begin to drop rela-tively quickly for some patients and may require longer for others. As noted previously, it is advisable to continue the exposure until the patient appears visibly more at ease and reports a substantial decrease in anxiety (40 or 50%).

After 10–15 sessions, the patient's reported anxiety level is expected to decrease considerably. At the 15th session, June reported a maximum discomfort of 70 SUDs (still somewhat high, although reduced from 99 SUDs), that lasted for a few minutes. Her minimal anxiety was 35 SUDs. Her average anxiety level during this session was 45 SUDs. Ideally, by the end of treatment the highest level should not exceed 50 SUDs and should drop below 20 SUDs at the end of the session. In June's case, more follow-up sessions were required because her anxiety was still quite high.

To facilitate a transition to normal washing and cleaning behavior, the therapist instituted a normal washing regimen during the third week of treatment. The patient was allowed one 10-minute shower daily and no more than five 30-second handwashes when there was visible dirt on her hands or when they were sticky.

When the therapist arrived for a home treatment session the next week, the following conversation ensued:

THERAPIST: How did it go over the weekend?

JUNE: Not too bad. But I got sort of upset Saturday. We went to a picnic and there were several piles of dog dirt around. I had on my flip-flops and I wanted to play volleyball. You can't in flip-flops, so I went barefoot.

THERAPIST: That's great! I'm glad to hear it.

JUNE: Yeah, but then I got really upset about going home and carrying it into the apartment. I did it. I walked all over barefoot and with the flip-flops, but I worried about it for another whole day, until I talked to Kenny about my thoughts on Sunday around noon. I felt better when he said he wouldn't worry about it. It seems like I feel guilty or something, like the house isn't clean enough. But lately if he says it is clean, I've been able to take his word for it.

THERAPIST: Well, in time you'll be able to make this kind of judgment yourself. How about your washing and cleaning?

JUNE: It was all right. I washed for half a minute before I ate because I was dusty from playing volleyball. I deliberately didn't wash when I got home because I felt bad and I knew that if I did, it would be to "decontaminate" myself. I showered Saturday night and I did feel relieved, but I knew I should go and walk around barefoot and touch the floors I'd walked on. So I did that.

THERAPIST: That's great! It sounds like you handled it fine. I'm really pleased. You avoided washing when it would mean reducing feelings of contamination, and you exposed yourself when you felt concerned about germs. That's excellent. Now, let's go over the problem situations that still need work here at home. What things still disturb you?

JUNE: The basement. I haven't done much with the kitty litter box and old shoes that I threw down there a year ago because they got contaminated. The closet still has some contaminated clothes. And I still worry about the backyard some. Also the porch. Pigeons have been perching on the roof and there are droppings on the railing now, so I thought I'd wait until you came to do that.

THERAPIST: OK. Let's start low and work up. Which is easiest?

JUNE: The basement and closets.

THERAPIST: Fine, down we go.

Exposure to contaminants during the home visit is conducted in the same manner as that during treatment sessions. Typically, home sessions last longer, from 2 to 4 hours, until all "dirty" items are touched and "clean" places are contaminated. These visits should be repeated if the patient expresses considerable concern about his/her ability to adopt a permanent regimen of nonavoidance.

Follow-Up Sessions

June was seen weekly for 3 months, until she experienced a setback following the development of a new obsession. She became concerned about hitting a pedestrian while driving. Thoughts that she "might have hit someone" intruded, particularly after turning a corner or glancing in the mirror to change lanes. Once evoked, they persisted for several hours. To overcome this new problem, the therapist directed her to increase her driving and refrain from retracing her path or looking in the mirror to check for casualties. June was told that she could stop her car only if she knew for certain that she hit someone. Thoughts that it "might" have occurred were to be ignored. To reduce June's anxiety about having obsessions (e.g., "Oh, my God, here it is again. This is terrible"), she was advised to expect occasional recurrences of obsessive thoughts. The frequency of obsessions about hitting someone decreased from several each day to once weekly after 3 weeks of self-exposure; the associated anxiety diminished from 95 to 50 SUDs or less.

Of June's germ-related obsessions, only that of dog feces partially recurred. Fears of public bathrooms and dead animals remained low. The therapist felt that June's fear of dog feces had received insufficient attention during treatment. To address this return of fear, June was seen three times a week for 1-hour exposure sessions, in which she touched brown spots on the sidewalk and walked near, and eventually stepped on, dog feces. Homework included going to parks, walking on sidewalks without looking, stepping on dog feces, and stepping on the grass where she thought dogs had been. This treatment continued for 4 weeks and was reduced to twice a week for an additional 3 weeks. Thereafter, June came once weekly for another 6 weeks, during which the therapist assigned self-exposure and dealt with June's everyday concerns. News media coverage of herpes led to a brief concern about public toilets, but this dissipated within a few days.

In the dialogue below, the therapist reviewed with June her progress at a 9-month follow-up.

THERAPIST: I'd like to know how you feel compared to when you first came here 9 months ago.

JUNE: I'm definitely a lot better. But, I still have some bad days when I worry a lot about something, and I get down on myself. But when I remember how upset I was last summer and all that washing I did, it's really a whole lot better. Maybe about 80% better. I'm not ready to be a floor nurse yet, but the job I got after treatment is pretty good for now. Kenny and I are doing fine, except he's real sensitive if I bring up one of my fears. I wish he'd just listen and say "OK" or something instead of looking worried about me. It's like he's afraid I'm going to get upset again. It makes it hard for me to talk freely, but sometimes he does handle it fine. I really can't complain. He's been through a lot, too, when I was really a mess last year and before that.

THERAPIST: I'm glad to hear you feel so much better. You look a lot more at ease. You laugh more now. I don't know if you recall, but you never did in the beginning.

JUNE: I remember.

THERAPIST: What's left now, the other 20%?

JUNE: Obsessions, I guess. I can still work on my fear of driving over someone. Mostly it lasts less than 15 minutes, but now and then it hangs on through an evening.

THERAPIST: How often?

JUNE: Once every week or two, I think. And I still have an urge to avoid walking on the grass in parks. Like I'm hyperalert. I do it pretty often, but I'm self-conscious.

THERAPIST: You mean you have to remind yourself not to avoid dog feces?

JUNE: Yeah. And I tend to see things in black and white, all good or all bad. I catch myself feeling guilty for dumb things like eating dessert after a full meal. I can stop, but it's like I'm out to punish myself or think badly about what I did. I have to watch out for it. Still, the thoughts are nothing like they used to be. I can have fun now. And work is pretty absorbing, so I can go whole days without getting down on myself for something. Will I always do that?

THERAPIST: Maybe to some extent. We know that you have a tendency to obsess. Most people who have had an obsessive–compulsive problem say that the rituals and urges to do them decrease more quickly than the obsessive ideas. You might have disturbing thoughts for a while, but you can expect them to become less frequent if you're careful not to attempt to control them through rituals or by avoiding things. Can you handle that?

JUNE: I suppose so. They're not a lot of fun, but I feel like I'm living a normal life again. I suppose everyone has some problems to deal with.

Rarely do patients report complete remission of all obsessions. It is unrealistic to lead a patient to expect that 4 weeks of treatment will result in a total absence of obsessions and rituals. Patients should expect some continued struggle with obsessions and urges to ritualize. Strategies for coping with such occasional difficulties should be rehearsed.

COMPLICATIONS DURING BEHAVIORAL TREATMENT

Obviously, difficulties may arise during implementation of EX/RP treatment for OCD. Several of these are described below and possible solutions are discussed.

Noncompliance with Response Prevention

Individuals with OCD often report engaging in rituals despite the response prevention instructions. In most cases these represent brief "slips" that the therapist addresses by reiterating the rationale for the treatment regimen and the need to follow the response prevention instructions strictly. The therapist also may offer ways the ritual might be "undone" (e.g., recontaminating or turning the stove on and off again).

Sometimes the patient's support person reports violations of response prevention to the therapist. The therapist should discuss the violations with the patient, emphasizing the fact that continued failure to comply with the response prevention instructions may result in treatment failure. The following is an example of how violations of response prevention may be presented to the patient.

"I understand from your father that on three occasions this weekend he saw you checking the front door lock five or six times before you left the house. As we agreed in the first session, he called to inform me about your checking. I am sure you remember that we agreed that you would check the doors only once, and that if you had a problem, you would discuss it with your father or me right away, so we could help you overcome your urge to ritualize. Will you explain to me what happened?"

If the patient acknowledges the slip and responds with a renewed agreement to follow instructions, the therapist need not pursue the issue further. However, if a second significant infraction of the response prevention instructions occurs, the therapist should again remind the patient of the therapy rules and the rationale for these rules, and "troubleshoot" with the patient how successfully to implement ritual prevention. During the course of this discussion, if it becomes evident that the patient is unwilling to consider these recommendations and remains committed to rituals and avoidance as a means to reduce obsessional distress, then the therapist may broach the subject of discontinuing treatment unless the patient is ready to comply.

> "It seems that right now you aren't able to stop ritualizing. For treatment to be successful, it is essential that you *completely* stop your rituals. Every time that you relieve your discomfort by ritualizing, you prevent yourself from learning that anxiety would have declined eventually without rituals, and you don't permit your obsessional fears to be disconnected from distress and anxiety. Exposing you to feared situations without stopping your rituals won't be helpful. If you cannot follow the no-rituals rule quite strictly, then we ought to stop treatment now and wait until you are really prepared to follow through with all the requirements. It is very hard for people to resist the urge to ritualize, and it may be that you are just not ready yet and will feel more able to do so in the future. It is much better for us to stop treatment now than to continue under conditions where you are unlikely to benefit from treatment. That would only leave you feeling more hopeless about future prospects for improvement."

As discussed earlier, patients sometimes replace identified rituals with less obvious avoidance patterns. For example, a patient may use hand lotion to "decontaminate" the hands instead of the excessive washing that was done originally. If this occurs, the therapist should immediately instruct the patient to stop the new ritual. Other examples of replacement washing rituals include brushing off one's hands or blowing off "germs"; extensive checks are often replaced with quick glances. Direct questioning of the patient to solicit such information should proceed as follows:

> "Now that you've stopped your washing rituals, do you find yourself doing other things to relieve your anxiety? For example, some people start to wipe their hands with paper towels or tissues as a substitute for washing with soap and water. Are you doing anything like this?"

If the answer is "yes," the therapist should identify these new behaviors as rituals and instruct the patient to resist engaging in them in the same manner as he/she resists other compulsions.

Continued Passive Avoidance

Patients who continue to avoid situations likely to evoke obsessional distress are also likely to experience attentuated outcome in EX/RP. For example, a patient may put "contaminated" clothing back in the closet as instructed, but in doing so he/she may ensure that the contaminated clothes do not touch clean garments. Such avoidance reflects an ambivalent attitude toward treatment and hinders habituation of anxiety to feared situations. Because such processes may hinder outcome, the presence of continued and frequent avoidance behavior calls for the therapist and patient to re-evaluate whether the patient should continue treatment.

THERAPIST: Jim, let's make sure that you are doing your homework the right way. I know that you had a problem putting your dirty underwear in with your other dirty clothes. How are you doing with it now?

PATIENT: Well, I was afraid you might ask that. I still haven't mixed them up. I was too scared to do it.

THERAPIST: We discussed this several days ago and you were instructed to do it that night. It would have been better had you told me the next day that you weren't able to. What I'd like you to do for tomorrow is to bring in some dirty clothes. Bring in the underwear and the other clothes in separate bags, and we will mix them here in the office. Are there any other things you have been avoiding that you haven't told me about?

PATIENT: I don't think so.

THERAPIST: I want you to pay careful attention to things you are doing, or not doing, and make a list of anything you are avoiding, particularly things that you are supposed to do for therapy. It is very important that you don't protect yourself by avoiding distressing situations, since if you don't face these situations, your obsessive–compulsive symptoms won't get better. Let's give it another try, but if you can't bring yourself to confront these problematic situations without these little avoidances, perhaps you would be better off delaying your treatment to a later time when you will be more ready to comply with the treatment program.

Arguments

Some individuals who carry out the required exposure without ritualizing may attempt to engage the therapist in arguments about the assignments. It is quite tempting to get involved in arguments with patients over what they will or will not do during treatment. To avoid this, it is important for the therapist and the patient to agree on some ground rules before the intensive program begins. Patients must agree to follow the treatment plan that they developed in conjunction with the therapist, and to expose themselves to the distressing situations without argument. New, feared situations that are discovered should be discussed, and a new exposure program should be developed and agreed to, before exposures to the new situations are carried out. If a patient balks at or attempts to alter a planned exposure, the therapist should acknowledge and empathize with the patient's the discomfort, inquire about the reasons for the hesitation, and encourage the patient to proceed in the following manner:

"I'm sorry to see that you are having so much trouble sitting on the floor. I know it's difficult and that you're frightened, but it won't do you any good if we delay the exposure for another day or let you skip it all together. You really need to touch the floor, so let's go ahead and do it now. We have agreed that today is the 'floor' day, and I wouldn't be doing you a favor if I allowed you to avoid it. Remember, though, I am here to support you as much as I can when you become upset."

In some instances, difficulties may be overcome by first exposing the patient to similar items that generate a lower level of distress. For example, if a patient refuses to touch a toilet seat, then the therapist may ask him/her first to touch the bathroom floor or the door to the bathroom stall. Thereafter, the patient might touch the walls of the stall and the toilet handle before proceeding to the toilet seat itself.

Emotional Overload

Occasionally during treatment a patient will become overwhelmed by fear or another emotion that is not directly related to his/her OCD symptoms. For example, a patient may be upset by a recent event (e.g., the death of a relative) or by fears of facing future plans (e.g., living on one's own or getting a job). Implementing exposure exercises is inadvisable when the patient is extremely upset because it is unlikely that the patient will adequately attend to the exposure stimulus; therefore, anxiety is unlikely to habituate. Instead, the therapist

should discuss the distressing situation with the patient and proceed with exposure only when the patient is calmer. On rare occasions, exposure may be postponed altogether until the next day's session. If this becomes a repetitive pattern, it may be advisable to interrupt treatment until the crisis is over.

Nonanxious Reactions to Exposures

Occasionally patients respond to exposures with emotions other than anxiety or distress, such as anger or depression. Clinical observations suggest that anger often serves as a means for the patient to avoid the distress or anxiety that is the target of exposure. If this happens, the anger should be viewed as an avoidance. The therapist should refocus the patient on the anxiety-evoking aspects of the situation and point out to the patient that the anger only stands in the way of progress.

Sometimes during imaginal exposure, when a patient is exposed to the feared consequences of his/her behaviors, the patient becomes depressed. Such depression and other emotional reactions may reduce the efficacy of treatment, and the therapist needs to help the patient to focus on the anxiety-evoking cues. This may be done by directing the content of the imaginal exposure away from the feared consequences and toward the external threat cues. In some cases, such redirection does not resolve the problem, and the patient continues to display a depressive reaction to the exposure. When this happens, alternative scenarios that do not elicit depression should be developed.

Emergent Fears and Rituals

As mentioned earlier, sometimes patients develop "new" fears or rituals during treatment. Often, the content of these new symptoms is closely related to the original fears and may be treated by extending to these fears the EX/RP instructions given earlier in treatment. For example, following the successful implementation of response prevention for his compulsive handwashing, Mr. F began to rub his hands together to decontaminate them. The therapist identified this as another ritual and instructed Mr. F to resist the urge to rub his hands together. Next, Mr. F began subtly to rub his fingers against the palms of his hands to cleanse his hands and to reduce anxiety. The therapist asked Mr. F to stop this ritual as he had the others and was again successful.

Some emergent fears may not be as clearly connected to the patient's original fears. For example, the fear that June developed of hitting someone while driving was not obviously related to her fears of contamination. Further assessment often results in the discovery of a conceptual link between the two reported fears. In June's case, her fear of being blamed for causing someone to become ill or die, and her concern about being thought of as a "bad person" because she killed someone, or because she smelled of dog feces, may have been the connection between her two identified fears. In such cases, it is important for the therapist to develop exposures that include cues for this more general fear. June's therapist might conduct imaginal exposures that include images of people criticizing June or blaming her for causing someone to die.

Negative Family Reactions

Because family members have typically experienced years of frustration with the patient's symptoms, it is not surprising that some are impatient, expecting treatment to progress smoothly and to result in total symptom remission. It is not uncommon for family members to become disappointed or angry when they perceive that the symptoms are not subsiding quickly enough. In such cases, the therapist should assure family members that occasional strong anxiety reactions are to be expected and do not reflect failure. The family should be encouraged to respond calmly and be supportive should the patient experience a burst of anxiety.

Often, families have developed patterns of behavior designed to reduce the patient's distress. Some family members may continue these patterns either in an attempt to protect the patient from upsetting situations or because it is difficult to break habits established over years of accommodating the patient's requests. For example, Mr. P, who was accustomed to entering his home through the basement, immediately removing his clothes, and showering for his wife's sake, was instructed to enter through the front door and toss his overcoat on the couch. Similarly, family members may find themselves continuing to perform a variety of household activities that they have come to regard as their responsibility because of the patient's wishes to avoid the distress that the activity caused. For instance, Mr. P was responsible for preparing all the family meals because his wife was distressed by the possibility that she might inadvertently contaminate the food. Because such familiar patterns may hinder progress in treatment, the therapist should ask both the patient and family members about such habits and prescribe appropriate alternative behaviors that maximize the patient's exposure and minimize avoidance.

Functioning without Symptoms

At the end of treatment, many individuals with OCD find themselves left with a considerable void in their daily routines. The fact that they no longer need to allocate a large portion of their day to performing rituals leaves them wondering what to do. The therapist should be sensitive to these issues and aid in planning new social or occupational goals to be achieved following therapy. If needed, the therapist should conduct additional sessions or refer the patient to another therapist who will focus on adjustment-related issues. It may also be the case that behavioral treatments such as acceptance and commitment therapy (ACT) are directly applicable to this problem given the explicit focus on functioning; patients with OCD might be especially vulnerable to the belief that they cannot move forward successfully in their lives unless their obsessions are gone, and ACT is particularly well suited to address these kinds of problems. Preliminary evidence from a case series suggested the applicability of ACT to OCD (Twohig, Hayes, & Masuda, 2006), and a randomized controlled trial now provides stronger evidence for the efficacy of ACT (Twhohig et al., 2010).

Because they have spent years performing their rituals, patients may be unsure about what constitutes normal behavior. The therapist should offer guidelines for appropriate washing, checking, repeating, or ordering. If rituals are still present, the therapist needs to instruct patients to continue the response prevention of some behaviors to ensure maintenance of treatment gains. A patient may also develop a fear that the OCD symptoms will return. The therapist should reassure the patient that a single washing of his/her hands does not signal the beginning of a relapse.

CONCLUSION

In this chapter we have reviewed the literature on OCD and its treatment, and provided verbatim dialogue from patient–therapist interactions to demonstrate how EX/ RP is implemented. Our review illustrates clearly that much is already known about CBT and pharmacotherapy for OCD. In our clinical practice with adults, we are guided by the empirical research summarized in this chapter, although not all of our clinical decisions are unequivocally supported by empirical studies. For example, no controlled, direct comparison study has indicated that intensive EX/RP yields superior outcome to less intensive treatment, yet we typically provide intensive treatment to our adult patients with at least moderately severe OCD. Although our clinical experience suggests that weekly sessions are probably insufficient to produce meaningful gains in most adult patients with OCD, it has yet to be established whether two or three weekly sessions would yield results comparable to daily sessions both immediately after treatment and at follow-up. Future research should examine this important issue to establish a "dose–response" curve for EX/RP; in our view clinically the patient's initial severity, comorbidity, and motivational readiness to engage in the treatment influence our recommendations regarding the EX/RP visit schedule . Another important issue is how to best combine EX/RP with medication. Future research will allow us to identify the optimal treatment course for a particular patient.

Empirical results and clinical observations converge to indicate that psychosocial treatment for OCD must involve both exposure and ritual prevention instructions, and that failure to conduct exposures to the most anxiety-evoking situations is likely to compromise outcome. With respect to the therapist-assisted versus self-exposure issue, we routinely choose therapist-assisted exposure in our clinical practice. At present, eliminating therapist assistance with exposure exercises seems premature because existing studies have methodological problems such as insufficient sample sizes, and a recently completed RCT in pediatric OCD indicated that EX/RP with in-session exposure was superior to a brief form of EX/RP that did not include this procedural element (Franklin et al., 2011). With respect to the role of cognitive interventions in the treatment of OCD, the EX/RP program described in this chapter is a "cognitive-behavioral" treatment in that it targets both cognitions and behaviors; however, we do not typically include formal cognitive restructuring. Future research needs to delineate which cognitive and behavioral procedures are most effective for correcting particular pathological emotions. Cognitive procedures may also be utilized in "readiness programs" designed to help patients who are highly ambivalent about EX/RP realize that the treatment is both tolerable and effective. Empirical research to date suggest that although antidepressant medications for OCD do not interfere with the efficacy of CBT, combination treatment is not necessarily more effective than EX/RP alone. However, the partial symptom reduction typically found in pharmacotherapy studies for OCD may render some patients more willing to tolerate the distress associated with EX/RP; thus, premedication may be helpful in promoting readiness in such cases.

What factors seem to enhance long-term efficacy of EX/RP for OCD? Studies suggest that patients with OCD who show great improvement immediately after CBT are more likely to retain their gains at follow-up than those who make only moderate posttreatment gains (e.g., Simpson et al., 2004). Thus, emphasis on procedures that are likely to lead to maximal short-term efficacy also serves to yield superior maintenance of gains. In our clinical experience, understanding of the treatment rationale, active engagement in exposure exercises, strict adherence to ritual prevention instructions, willingness to design and implement exposure exercises between sessions, and willingness to confront even the most difficult tasks on the fear hierarchy are all factors associated with positive treatment outcome. Thus, verbal reinforcement of patients when they accomplish these goals, and reinstruction when they do not, are important in promoting lasting improvement. In addition, relapse prevention techniques designed specifically for OCD have been found effective in promoting maintenance of gains at follow-up (Hiss et al., 1994). In clinical practice we begin discussing relapse prevention procedures long before treatment is completed, and we focus on maintaining gains in the last few active treatment sessions. Some continuing contact with the treating clinician is also thought to be of benefit; thus, brief follow-up sessions are held in the first few months after the active treatment is completed, with contact as needed following the formal follow-up phase. As part of relapse prevention, we often ask our patients to plan EX/RP exercises for hypothetical obsessions they might encounter in the future (e.g., "If you became obsessed in 6 months that touching tree bark would result in your contracting a terrible illness, what exercises should you do?") to encourage them to problem-solve around OCD issues for themselves rather than relying on the therapist's instruction. We also emphasize that the occasional occurrence of obsessions should not be a cause of great alarm, provided that patients implement EX/RP to combat these recurring obsessions and urges to ritualize. The patients who are accepting of this reality are often the ones most able to apply what they have learned in treatment, and this process enables them to keep their OCD symptoms under control long after treatment has terminated.

REFERENCES

Abramowitz, J. S. (1996). Variants of exposure and response prevention in the treatment of obsessive compulsive disorder: A meta-analysis. *Behavior Therapy, 27,* 583–600.

Abramowitz, J. S., & Foa, E. B. (2000). Does major depressive disorder influence outcome of exposure and response prevention for OCD? *Behavior Therapy, 31,* 795–800.

Abramowitz, J. S., Foa, E. B., & Franklin, M. E. (2003). Exposure and ritual prevention for obsessive–compulsive disorder: Effects of intensive versus twice-weekly sessions. *Journal of Consulting and Clinical Psychology, 71,* 394–398.

Abramowitz, J. S., Franklin, M. E., & Foa, E. B. (2002). Empirical status of cognitive-behavioral therapy for obsessive compulsive disorder: A meta-analytic review. *Romanian Journal of Cognitive and Behavior Psychotherapies, 2,* 89–104.

Abramowitz, J. S., Franklin, M. E., Street, G. P., Kozak, M. J., & Foa, E. B. (2000). Effects of comorbid depression on response to treatment for obsessive–compulsive disorder. *Behavior Therapy, 31,* 517–528.

Allen, J. J., & Tune, G. S. (1975). The Lynfield Obsessional/Compulsive Questionnaire. *Scottish Medical Journal, 20,* 21–24.

American Psychiatric Association. (1994). *Diagnostic and statistical manual of mental disorders* (4th ed.). Washington, DC: Author.

American Psychiatric Association. (2013). *Diagnostic and statistical manual of mental disorders* (5th ed.). Arlington, VA: Author.

Angst, J. (1993). Comorbidity of anxiety, phobia, compulsion and depression. *International Clinical Psychopharmacology, 8*(Suppl. 1), 21–25.

Anderson, R. A., & Rees, C. S. (2007). Group versus individual cognitive-behavioural treatment for obsessive–compulsive disorder: A controlled trial. *Behaviour Research and Therapy, 45*(1), 123–137.

Antony, M. M., Downie, F., & Swinson, R. P. (1998). Diagnostic issues and epidemiology in obsessive–compulsive disorders. In R. P. Swinson, M. M. Antony, S. Rachman, & M. A. Richter (Eds.), *Obsessive–compulsive disorder: Theory, research and treatment* (pp. 3–32). New York: Guilford Press.

Asbahr, F. R., Castillo, A. R., Ito, L. M., Latorre, R. D., Moreira, M. N., & Lotufo-Neto, F. (2005). Group cognitive-behavioral therapy versus sertraline for the treatment of children and adolescents with obsessive–compulsive disorder. *Journal of the American Academy of Child and Adolescent Psychiatry, 44*(11), 1128–1136.

Bachofen, M., Nakagawa, A., Marks, I. M., Park, J., Greist, J. H., Baer, L., et al. (1999). Home self-assessment and self-treatment of obsessive compulsive disorder using a manual and a computer-conducted telephone interview: Replica-tion of a UK–US study. *Journal of Clinical Psychiatry, 60,* 545–549.

Barrett, P., Farrell, L., Dadds, M., & Boulter, N. (20050. Cognitive-behavioral family treatment of childhood obsessive–compulsive disorder: Long-term follow-up and predictors of outcome. *Journal of the American Academy of Child and Adolescent Psychiatry, 44,* 1005–1014.

Barrett, P., Healy-Farrell, L., & March, J. S. (2004). Cognitive-behavioral family treatment of childhood obsessive–compulsive disorder: A controlled trial. *Journal of the American Academy of Child and Adolescent Psychiatry, 43,* 46–62.

Barsky, A. J., & Ahern, D. (2004). Interventions for hypochondriasis in primary care: In reply. *Journal of the American Medical Association, 292*(1), 42–43.

Basoglu, M., Lax, T., Kasvikis, Y., & Marks, I. M. (1988). Predictors of improvement in obsessive–compulsive disorder. *Journal of Anxiety Disorders, 2,* 299–317.

Beck, A. T. (1976). *Cognitive therapy and the emotional disorders.* New York: International Universities Press.

Bellodi, L., Scuito, G., Diaferia, G., Ronchi, P., & Smeraldi, E. (1992). Psychiatric disorders in the families of patients with obsessive–compulsive disorder. *Psychiatry Research, 42*(2), 111–120.

Bogels, S. M., & Bodden, D. (2005, November). *Family versus child CBT for childhood anxiety disorders: Short and long-term results of a multicenter study.* In S. M. Bogels (Chair), Family-Based Prevention and Treatment of Childhood Anxiety Disorders Symposium presented at the annual meeting of the Association for Behavioral and Cognitive Therapies, Washington, DC.

Brown, T., Campbell, L., Lehman, C., Grisham, J., & Mancill, R. (2001). Current and lifetime comorbidity of the DSM-IV anxiety and mood disorders in a large clinical sample. *Journal of Abnormal Psychology, 110*(4), 585–599.

Carr, A. T. (1974). Compulsive neurosis: A review of the literature. *Psychological Bulletin, 81,* 311–318.

Comings, D. E. (1990). *Tourette syndrome and human behavior.* Duarte, CA: Hope Press.

Constans, J. I., Foa, E. B., Franklin, M. E., & Mathews, A. (1995). Memory for actions in obsessive compulsives with checking rituals. *Behaviour Research and Therapy, 33,* 665–671.

Cottraux, J., Mollard, L., Bouvard, M., Marks, L., Sluys, M., Nury, A. M., et al. (1990). A controlled study of fluvoxamine and exposure in obsessive–compulsive disorder. *International Clinical Psychopharmacology, 5,* 17–30.

Cottraux, J., Note, I., Yao, S. N., Lafont, S., Note, B., Mollard, E., et al. (2001). A randomized controlled trial of cognitive therapy versus intensive behavior therapy in obsessive compulsive disorder. *Psychotherapy and Psychosomatics, 70*(6), 288–297.

De Araujo, L. A., Ito, L. M., Marks, I. M., & Deale, A. (1995). Does imaginal exposure to the consequences of not ritualising enhance live exposure for OCD?: A controlled study: I. Main outcome. *British Journal of Psychiatry, 167*, 65–70.

de Haan, E., Hoogduin, K. A., Buitelaar, J. K., & Keijsers, G. P. (1998). Behavior thearpy versus clomipramine for the treatment of obsessive–compulsive disorder. *Journal of the American Academy of Child and Adolescent Psychiatry, 37*, 1022–1029.

Denys, D., Tenney, N., van Megen, J. G., de Geus, F., & Westenberg, H. G. (2004). Axis I and II comorbidity in a large sample of patients with obsessive–compulsive disorder. *Journal of Affective Disorders, 80*, 155–162.

DeVeaugh-Geiss, J., Landau, P., & Katz, R. (1989). Treatment of OCD with clomipramine. *Psychiatric Annals, 19*, 97–101.

Diniz, J. B., Rosario-Campos, M. C., Shavitt, R. G., Curi, M., Hounie, A. G., Brotto, S. A., et al. (2004). Impact of age at onset and duration of illness on the expression of comorbidities in obsessive–compulsive disorder. *Journal of Clinical Psychiatry, 65*, 22–27.

Dollard, J., & Miller, N. L. (1950). *Personality and psychotherapy: An analysis in terms of learning, thinking and culture.* New York: McGraw-Hill.

Dougherty, D. D., Rauch, S. L., & Jenike, M. A. (2002). Pharmacological treatments for obsessive compulsive disorder. In P. E. Nathan & J. M. Gordon (Eds.), *A guide to treatments that work* (2nd ed., pp. 387–410). New York: Oxford University Press.

Eisen, J. L., Phillips, K. A., Baer, L., Beer, D. A., Atala, K. D., & Rasmussen, S. A. (1998). The Brown Assessment of Beliefs Scale: Reliability and validity. *American Journal of Psychiatry, 155*, 102–108.

Ellis, A. (1962). *Reason and emotion in psychotherapy.* New York: Lyle Stuart.

Emmelkamp, P. M. G., & Beens, H. (1991). Cognitive therapy with obsessive–compulsive disorder: A comparative evaluation. *Behaviour Research and Therapy, 29*, 293–300.

Emmelkamp, P. M. G., de Haan, E., & Hoogduin, C. A. L. (1990). Marital adjustment and obsessive–compulsive disorder. *British Journal of Psychiatry, 156*, 55–60.

Emmelkamp, P. M. G., & van Kraanen, J. (1977). Therapist-controlled exposure *in vivo*: A comparison with obsessive–compulsive patients. *Behaviour Research and Therapy, 15*, 491–495.

Emmelkamp, P. M. G., Visser, S., & Hoekstra, R. J. (1988). Cognitive therapy vs. exposure *in vivo* in the treatment of obsessive–compulsives. *Cognitive Therapy and Research, 12*, 103–114.

Fals-Stewart, W., Marks, A. P., & Schafer, J. (1993). A comparison of behavioral group therapy and individual behavior therapy in treating obsessive compulsive disorder. *Journal of Nervous and Mental Disease, 181*, 189–193.

Farrell, L. J., Waters, A., Milliner, E., & Ollendick, T. (2012). Comorbidity and treatment response in pediatric OCD: A pilot study of group cognitive-behavioral treatment. *Psychiatry Research, 199*, 115–123.

Flament, M., Koby, E., Rapoport, J. L., Berg, C., Zahn, T., Cox, C., et al. (1990). Childhood obsessive compulsive disorder: A prospective follow-up study. *Journal of Child Psychology and Psychiatry, and Allied Disciplines, 31*, 363–380.

Flament, M., Whitaker, A., Rapoport, J. L., Davies, M., Berg, C., Kalikow, K., et al. (1988). Obsessive compulsive disorder in adolescence: An epidemiological study. *Journal of the American Academy of Child and Adolescent Psychiatry, 27*, 764–771.

Foa, E. B., Abramowitz, J. S., Franklin, M. E., & Kozak, M. J. (1999). Feared consequences, fixity of belief, and treatment outcome in patients with obsessive compulsive disorder. *Behavior Therapy, 30*, 717–724.

Foa, E. B., Franklin, M. E., & Moser, J. (2002). Context in the clinic: How well do CBT and medications work in combination? *Biological Psychiatry, 51*, 989–997.

Foa, E. B., Huppert, J. D., & Cahill, S. P. (2006). Emotional processing theory: An update. In B. O. Rothbaum (Ed.), *Pathological anxiety: Emotional processing in etiology and treatment* (pp. 3–24). New York: Guilford Press.

Foa, E. B., Huppert, J. D., Leiberg, S., Langner, R., Kichic, R., & Hajcak, G., et al. (2002). The Obsessive–Compulsive Inventory: Development and validation of a short version. *Psychological Assessment, 14*(4), 485–495.

Foa, E. B., & Kozak, M. J. (1985). Treatment of anxiety disorders: Implications for psychopathology. In A. H. Tuma & J. D. Maser (Eds.), *Anxiety and the anxiety disorders* (pp. 421–452). Hillsdale, NJ: Erlbaum.

Foa, E. B., & Kozak, M. J. (1986). Emotional processing of fear: Exposure to corrective information. *Psychological Bulletin, 99*, 20–35.

Foa, E. B., & Kozak, M. J. (1996). Psychological treatments for obsessive compulsive disorder. In M. R. Mavissakalian & R. P. Prien (Eds.), *Long-term treatments of anxiety disorders* (pp. 285–309). Washington, DC: American Psychiatric Press.

Foa, E. B., Kozak, M. J., Goodman, W. K., Hollander, E., Jenike, M. A., & Rasmussen, S. (1995). DSM-IV filed trial: Obsessive compulsive disorder. *American Journal of Psychiatry, 152*, 90–96.

Foa, E. B., Kozak, M. J., Steketee, G., & McCarthy, P. R. (1992). Treatment of depressive and obsessive–compulsive symptoms in OCD by imipramine and behavior therapy. *British Journal of Clinical Psychology, 31*, 279–292.

Foa, E. B., Liebowitz, M. R., Kozak, M. J., Davies, S. O., Campeas, R., Franklin, M. E., et al. (2005). Treatment of obsessive compulsive disorder by exposure and ritual prevention, clomipramine, and their combination: A randomized, placebo-controlled trial. *American Journal of Psychiatry, 162*, 151–161.

Foa, E. B., Steketee, G., Grayson, J. B., Turner, R. M., & Latimer, P. (1984). Deliberate exposure and blocking of obsessive–compulsive rituals: Immediate and long-term effects. *Behavior Therapy, 15*, 450–472.

Foa, E. B., Steketee, G., Turner, R. M., & Fischer, S. C. (1980). Effects of imaginal exposure to feared disasters in obsessive–compulsive checkers. *Behaviour Research and Therapy, 18*, 449–455.

Franklin, M. E., Abramowitz, J. S., Bux, D. A., Zoellner, L. A., & Feeny, N. C. (2002). Cognitive-behavioral therapy with and without medication in the treatment of obsessive compulsive disorder. *Professional Psychology: Research and Practice, 33*, 162–168.

Franklin, M. E., Abramowitz, J. S., Furr, J., Kalsy, S., & Riggs, D. S. (2003). A naturalistic examination of therapist experience and outcome of exposure and ritual prevention for OCD. *Psychotherapy Research, 13*, 153–167.

Franklin, M. E., Abramowitz, J. S., Kozak, M. J., Levitt, J., & Foa, E. B. (2000). Effectiveness of exposure and ritual prevention for obsessive compulsive disorder: Randomized compared with non-randomized samples. *Journal of Consulting and Clinical Psychology, 68*, 594–602.

Franklin, M. E., Kozak, M. J., Cashman, L., Coles, M., Rheingold, A., & Foa, E. B. (1998). Cognitive behavioral treatment of pediatric obsessive compulsive disorder: An open clinical trial. *Journal of the American Academy of Child and Adolescent Psychiatry, 37*, 412–419.

Franklin, M., Sapyta, J., Freeman, J., Khanna, M., Compton, S., Almirall, D., et al. (2011). Cognitive behavior therapy augmentation of pharmacotherapy in pediatric obsessive–compulsive disorder: The Pediatric OCD Treatment Study II (POTS II). *Journal of the American Medical Association, 306*, 1224–1232.

Freeman, J. B., Choate-Summers, M. L., Moore, P. S., Garcia, A. M., Sapyta, J. J., Leonard, H. L., et al. (2007). Cognitive behavioral treatment of young children with obsessive compulsive disorder. *Biological Psychiatry, 61*, 337–343.

Freeman, J. B., Garcia, A. M., Fucci, C., Karitani, M., Miller, L., & Leonard, H. L. (2003). Family-based treatment of early-onset obsessive–compulsive disorder [Special issue]. *Journal of Child and Adolescent Psychopharmacology, 13*(2), 71–80.

Freeston, M. H., Ladouceur, R., Gagnon, F., Thibodeau, N., Rhéaume, J., Letarte, H., et al. (1997). Cognitive-behavioral treatment of obsessive thoughts: A controlled study. *Journal of Consulting and Clinical Psychology, 65*, 405–413.

Gershuny, B. S., Baer, L., Jenike, M. A., Minichiello, W. E., & Wilhelm, S. (2002). Comorbid posttraumatic stress disorder: Impact on treatment outcome for obsessive–compulsive disorder. *American Journal of Psychiatry, 159*, 852–854.

Goodman, W. K., Price, L. H., Rasmussen, S. A., Mazure, C., Delgado, P., Heninger, G. R., et al. (1989a). The Yale–Brown Obsessive–Compulsive Scale: II. Validity. *Archives of General Psychiatry, 46*, 1012–1016.

Goodman, W. K., Price, L. H., Rasmussen, S. A., Mazure, C., Fleischmann, R. L., Hill, C. L., et al. (1989b). The Yale–Brown Obsessive–Compulsive Scale: I. Development, use, and reliability. *Archives of General Psychiatry, 46*, 1006–1011.

Greist, J. H. (1990). Treatment of obsessive–compulsive disorder: Psychotherapies, drugs, and other somatic treatments. *Journal of Clinical Psychiatry, 51*, 44–50.

Greist, J. H. (1992). An integrated approach to treatment of obsessive compulsive disorder. *Journal of Clinical Psychiatry, 53*(Suppl.), 38–41.

Greist, J. H., Jefferson, J. W., Kobak, K. A., Katzelnick, D. J., & Serlin, R. C. (1995). Efficacy and tolerability of serotonin reuptake inhibitors in obsessive compulsive disorder: A meta-analysis. *Archives of General Psychiatry, 46*, 53–60.

Hanna, G. L. (1995). Demographic and clinical features of obsessive compulsive disorder in children and adolescents. *Journal of the American Academy of Child and Adolescent Psychiatry, 34*, 19–27.

Himle, M. B., Olufs, E., Himle, J., Tucker, B., & Woods, D. W. (2010). Behavior therapy for tics via Videoconference Delivery: An initial pilot test in children. *Cognitive & Behavioral Practice, 17*, 329–337.

Hiss, H., Foa, E. B., & Kozak, M. J. (1994). A relapse prevention program for treatment of obsessive compulsive disorder. *Journal of Consulting and Clinical Psychology, 62*, 801–808.

Hodgson, R. J., Rachman, S., & Marks, L. M. (1972). The treatment of chronic obsessive–compulsive neurosis: Follow-up and further findings. *Behaviour Research and Therapy, 10*, 181–189.

Hohagen, F., Winkelmann, G., Rasche-Raeuchle, H., Hand, I., Konig, A., Munchau, N., et al. (1998). Combination of behaviour therapy with fluvoxamine in comparison with behaviour therapy and placebo: Results of a multicentre study. *British Journal of Psychiatry, 173*, 71–78.

Insel, T. R., & Akiskal, H. (1986). Obsessive–compulsive disorder with psychotic features: A phenomenologic analysis. *American Journal of Psychiatry, 12*, 1527–1533.

Jaycox, L. H., Foa, E. B., & Morral, A. R. (1998). Influence of emotional engagement and habituation on exposure therapy for PTSD. *Journal of Consulting and Clinical Psychology, 66*, 185–192.

Jenike, M., Baer, L., Minichiello, W., Schwartz, C., & Carey, R. (1986). Concomitant obsessive–compulsive disorder and schizotypal personality disorder. *American Journal of Psychiatry, 143*, 530–532.

Kazarian, S. S., Evans, D. L., & Lefave, K. (1977). Modification and factorial analysis of the Leyton Obsessional Inventory. *Journal of Clinical Psychology, 33*, 422–425.

Keijsers, G. P., Hoogduin, C. A., & Schaap, C. P. (1994). Predictors of treatment outcome in the behavioural treatment of obsessive–compulsive disorder. *British Journal of Psychiatry, 165*, 781–786.

Kessler, R. C., Demier, O., Frank, R. G., Olfson, M., Pincus, H. A., Walters, E. E., et al. (2005). Prevalence and treatment of mental disorders, 1990 to 2003. *New England Journal of Medicine, 352*(24), 2515–2523.

Koran, L. M. (2000). Quality of life in obsessive–compulsive disorder. *Psychiatric Clinics of North America, 23*, 509–517.

Kozak, M. J., & Foa, E. B. (1994). Obsessions, overvalued ideas, and delusions in obsessive compulsive disorder. *Behaviour Research and Therapy, 32*, 343–353.

Kozak, M. J., Foa, E. B., & Steketee, G. (1988). Process and outcome of exposure treatment with obsessive–compulsives: Psychophysiological indicators of emotional processing. *Behavior Therapy, 19*, 157–169.

Kurlan, R., Como, P. G., Miller, B., Palumbo, D., Deeley, C., Andersen, E. M., et al. (2002). The behavioral spectrum of tic disorders: A community-based study. *Neurology, 59*, 414–420.

Ladouceur, R., Rhéame, J., Freeston, M. H., Aublet, F., Jean, K., Lachance, S., et al. (1995). Experimental manipulations of responsibility: An analogue test for models of obsessive–compulsive disorder. *Behaviour Research and Therapy, 33*, 937–946.

Lang, P. J. (1979). A bio-informational theory of emotional imagery. *Psychophysiology, 6*, 495–511.

Leckman, J. F., & Chittenden, E. H. (1990). Gilles de la Tourette syndrome and some forms of obsessive–compulsive disorder may share a common genetic diathesis. *L'Encephale, 16*, 321–323.

Leckman, J. F., Denys, D., Simpson, H. B., Mataix-Cols, D., Hollander, E., Saxena, S., et al. (2010). Obsessive compulsive disorder: A review of the diagnostic criteria and possible subtypes and dimensional specifiers for DSM V. *Depression and Anxiety, 27*, 507–527.

Ledley, D. R., Pai, A., & Franklin, M. E. (2007). Treating comorbid presentations: Obsessive compulsive disorder, anxiety, and depression. In M. M. Antony, C. Purdon, & L. Summerfeldt (Eds.), *Psychological treatment of OCD: Fundamentals and beyond* (pp. 281–293). Washington, DC: American Psychological Association Press.

Lelliott, P. T., Noshirvani, H. F., Basoglu, M., Marks, I. M., & Monteiro, W. O. (1988). Obsessive–compulsive beliefs and treatment outcome. *Psychological Bulletin, 18*, 697–702.

Leon, A. C., Portera, L., & Weissman, M. M. (1995). The social costs of anxiety disorders. *British Journal of Psychiatry, 166*(Suppl.), 19–22.

Lindsay, M., Crino, R., & Andrews, G. (1997). Controlled trial of exposure and response prevention in obsessive compulsive disorder. *British Journal of Psychiatry, 171*, 135–139.

Lochner, C., & Stein, D. J. (2003). Heterogeneity of obsessive–compulsive disorder: A literature review. *Harvard Review of Psychiatry, 11*(3), 113–132.

Lovell, K., Cox, D., Haddock, G., Jones, C., Raines, D., Garvey, R., et al. (2006). Telephone administered cognitive behaviour therapy for treatment of obsessive compulsive disorder: Randomised controlled non-inferiority trial. *British Medical Journal, 333*, 883.

March, J. S., Franklin, M. E., Leonard, H., Garcia, A., Moore, P., Freeman, J., et al. (2007). Tics moderate the outcome of treatment with medication but not CBT in pediatric OCD. *Biological Psychiatry, 61*, 344–347.

Marks, I. M., Lelliott, P., Basoglu, M., Noshirvani, H., Monteiro, W., Cohen, D., et al. (1988). Clomipramine self-exposure, and therapist-aided exposure for obsessive–compulsive rituals. *British Journal of Psychiatry, 152*, 522–534.

Marks, I. M., Stern, R. S., Mawson, D., Cobb, J., & McDonald, R. (1980). Clomipramine and exposure for obsessive–compulsive rituals: I. *British Journal of Psychiatry, 136*, 1–25.

Masellis, M., Rector, N. A., & Richter, M. A. (2003). Quality of life in OCD: Differential impact of obsessions, compulsions, and depression comorbidity. *Canadian Journal of Psychiatry, 48*(2), 72–77.

Mataix-Cols, D., Marks, I. M., Greist, J. H., Kobak, K. A., & Baer, L. (2002). Obsessive–compulsive symptoms dimensions as predictors of compliance with and response to behaviour therapy: Results from a controlled trial. *Psychotherapy and Psychosomatics, 71*, 255–262.

Mathews, A. M., Johnston, D. W., Shaw, P. M., & Gelder, M. G. (1974). Process variables and the prediction of outcome in behavior therapy. *British Journal of Psychiatry, 125*, 256–264.

Matsunaga, H., Kiriike, N., Matsui, T., Oya, K., Okino, K., & Stein, D. (2005). Impulsive disorders in Japanese adult patients with obsessive–compulsive disorder. *Comprehensive Psychiatry, 46*, 43–49.

McLean, P. L., Whittal, M. L., Thordarson, D. S., Taylor, S., Sochting, I., Koch, W. J., et al. (2001). Cognitive versus behavior therapy in the group treatment of obsessive–compulsive disorder. *Journal of Consulting and Clinical Psychology, 69*, 205–214.

Mehta, M. (1990). A comparative study of family-based and patients-based behavioural management in obsessive–compulsive disorder. *British Journal of Psychiatry, 157*, 133–135.

Meyer, V. (1966). Modification of expectations in cases with obsessional rituals. *Behaviour Research and Therapy, 4*, 273–280.

Meyer, V., & Levy, R. (1973). Modification of behavior in obsessive–compulsive disorders. In H. E. Adams & P. Unikel (Eds.), *Issues and trends in behavior therapy* (pp. 77–136). Springfield, IL: Thomas.

Meyer, V., Levy, R., & Schnurer, A. (1974). A behavioral treatment of obsessive–compulsive disorders. In H. R. Beech (Ed.), *Obsessional states*. London: Methuen.

Mowrer, O. H. (1939). A stimulus–response analysis of anxiety and its role as a reinforcing agent. *Psychological Review, 46*, 553–565.

Mowrer, O. H. (1960). *Learning theory and behavior.* New York: Wiley.

Neziroglu, F., Stevens, K. P., Yaryura-Tobias, J. A., & McKay, D. (2000). Predictive validity of the Overvalued Ideas Scale: Outcome in obsessive–compulsive and body dysmorphic disorder. *Behaviour Research and Therapy, 39,* 745–756.

Öst, L. G. (1989). One-session treatment for specific phobias. *Behaviour Research and Therapy, 27,* 1–7.

O'Sullivan, G., Noshirvani, H., Marks, I., Monteiro, W., & Lelliott, P. (1991). Six-year follow-up after exposure and clomipramine therapy for obsessive–compulsive disorder. *Journal of Clinical Archives, 52,* 150–155.

Pato, M. T., Zohar-Kadouch, R., Zohar, J., & Murphy, D. L. (1988). Return of symptoms after discontinuation of clomipramine in patients with obsessive–compulsive disorder. *American Journal of Psychiatry, 145,* 1521–1525.

Pauls, D. L., Towbin, K. E., Leckman, J. F., Zahner, G. E., & Cohen, D. J. (1986). Gilles de la Tourette syndrome and obsessive–compulsive disorder. *Archives of General Psychiatry, 43,* 1180–1182.

Pediatric OCD Treatment Study Team. (2004). Cognitive-behavioral therapy, sertraline, and their combination for children and adolescents with obsessive–compulsive disorder: The Pediatric OCD Treatment Study (POTS) randomized controlled trial. *Journal of the American Medical Association, 292,* 1969–1976.

Peris, T. S., Sugar, C. A., Bergman, L., Chang, S., Langley, A., & Piacentini, J. (2012). Family factors predict treatment outcome for pediatric obsessive-compulsive disorder. *Journal of Consulting and Clinical Psychology, 80,* 255–263.

Piacentini, J., Bergman, R. L., Jacobs, C., McCracken, J. T., & Kretchman, J. (2002). Open trial of cognitive behavior therapy for childhood obsessive–compulsive disorder. *Journal of Anxiety Disorders, 16,* 207–219.

Purdon, C., & Clark, D. A. (2002). The need to control thoughts. In R. Frost & G. Steketee (Eds.), *Cognitive approaches to obsessions and compulsions: Theory, research, and treatment* (pp. 29–43). Oakland, CA: New Harbinger.

Rabavilas, A. D., Boulougouris, J. C., & Perissaki, C. (1979). Therapist qualities related to outcome with exposure *in vivo* in neurotic patients. *Journal of Behavior Therapy and Experimental Psychiatry, 10,* 293–299.

Rachman, S. (1998). A cognitive theory of obsessions: Elaborations. *Behaviour Research and Therapy, 36,* 385–401.

Rachman, S., & DeSilva, P. (1978). Abnormal and normal obsessions. *Behaviour Research and Therapy, 16,* 233–248.

Rachman, S., Thordarson, D. S., Shafran, R., & Woody, S. R. (1995). Perceived responsibility: Structure and significance. *Behaviour Research and Therapy, 33*(7), 779–784.

Rapoport, J. L., Swedo, S. E., & Leonard, H. L. (1992). Childhood obsessive compulsive disorder (144th Annual Meeting of the American Psychiatric Association: Obsessive Compulsive Disorder: Integrating Theory and Practice [1991, New Orleans, LA]). *Journal of Clinical Psychiatry, 53*(Suppl. 4), 11–16.

Rasmussen, S. A., & Eisen, J. L. (1989). Clinical features and phenomenology of obsessive–compulsive disorder. *Psychiatric Annals, 19,* 67–73.

Rasmussen, S. A., & Eisen, J. L. (1990). Epidemiology of obsessive–compulsive disorder. *Journal of Clinical Psychiatry, 51,* 10–14.

Rasmussen, S. A., & Tsuang, M. T. (1986). Clinical characteristics and family history in DSM III obsessive–compulsive disorder. *American Journal of Psychiatry, 1943,* 317–382.

Reed, G. E. (1985). *Obsessional experience and compulsive behavior: A cognitive structural approach.* Orlando, FL: Academic Press.

Rhéaume, J., Freeston, M. H., Dugas, M. J., Letarte, H., & Ladouceur, R. (1995). Perfectionism, responsibility, and obsessive compulsive symptoms. *Behaviour Research and Therapy, 36,* 385–402.

Riggs, D. S., Hiss, H., & Foa, E. B. (1992). Marital distress and the treatment of obsessive–compulsive disorder. *Behavior Therapy, 23,* 585–597.

Rothbaum, B. O., & Shahar, F. (2000). Behavioral treatment of obsessive–compulsive disorder in a naturalistic setting. *Cognitive and Behavioral Practice, 7,* 262–270.

Rowe, M. K., & Craske, M. G. (1998). Effects of an expanding-space vs. massed exposure schedule on fear reduction and return of fear. *Beahviour Research and Therapy, 36,* 701–717.

Rubenstein, C. S., Peynircioglu, Z. F., Chambless, D. L., & Pigott, T. A. (1993). Memory in sub-clinical obsessive–compulsive checkers. *Behaviour Research and Therapy, 31*(8), 759–765.

Salkovskis, P. M. (1985). Obsessional compulsive problems: A cognitive-behavioral analysis. *Behaviour Research and Therapy, 23,* 571–583.

Sher, K. J., Frost, R. O., & Otto, R. (1983). Cognitive deficits in compulsive checkers: An exploratory study. *Behaviour Research and Therapy, 21,* 357–364.

Simpson, H. B., Liebowitz, M. R., Foa, E. B., Kozak, M. J., Schmidt, A. B., Rowan, V., et al. (2004). Post-treatment effects of exposure therapy and clomipramine in obsessive–compulsive disorder. *Depression and Anxiety, 19,* 225–233.

Simpson, H. B., Zuckoff, A. M., Maher, M. J., Page, J. R., Franklin, M. E., & Foa, E. B. (2010). Challenges using motivational interviewing as an adjunct to exposure therapy for obsessive–compulsive disorder. *Behaviour Research and Therapy, 48,* 941–948.

Stampfl, T. G., & Levis, D. J. (1967). Essentials of implosive therapy: A learning-based psychodynamic behavioral therapy. *Journal of Abnormal Psychology, 72,* 496–503.

Stanley, M. A., Turner, S. M., & Borden, J. W. (1990). Schizotypal features in obsessive–compulsive disorder. *Comprehensive Psychiatry, 31*, 511–518.

Steketee, G., Chambless, D. L., & Tran, G. Q. (2001). Effects of Axis I and II comorbidity on behavior therapy outcome for obsessive–compulsive disorder and agoraphobia. *Comprehensive Psychiatry, 42*, 76–86.

Steketee, G., Eisen, J., Dyck, I., Warshaw, M., & Rasmussen, S. (1999). Predictors of course in obsessive-compulsive disorder. *Psychiatry Research, 89*, 229–238.

Steketee, G. S., Foa, E. B., & Grayson, J. B. (1982). Recent advances in the treatment of obsessive–compulsives. *Archives of General Psychiatry, 39*, 1365–1371.

Stein, D. J., Fineberg, N. A., Bienvenu, O. J., Denys, D., Lochner, C., Nestadt, G., et al. (2010). Should OCD be classified as an anxiety disorder in DSM V? *Depression and Anxiety, 27*, 495–506.

Storch, E., Geffken, G., Merlo, L., Mann, G., Duke, D., Munson, M., et al. (2007). Family-based cognitive-behavioral therapy for pediatric obsessive–compulsive disorder: Comparison of intensive and weekly approaches. *Journal of American Academy of Child and Adolescent Psychiatry, 46*, 469–478.

Storch, E. A., Merlo, L. J., Larson, M. J., Geffken, G. R., Lehmkuhl, H. D., Jacob, M. L., et al. (2008). Impact of comorbidity on cognitive-behavioral therapy response in pediatric obsessive–compulsive disorder. *Journal of the American Academy of Child and Adolescent Psychiatry, 47*, 83–92.

Storch, E. A., Khanna, M., Merlo, L. J., Loew, B. A., Franklin, M., et al. (2009). Children's Florida Obsessive Compulsive Inventory: Psychometric properties and feasibility of a self-report measure of obsessive–compulsive symptoms in youth. *Child Psychiatry and Human Development, 40*(3), 467–483.

Swedo, S. E., Leckman, J. F., & Rose, N. R. (2012). From research subgroup to clinical syndrome: Modifying the PANDAS criteria to describe PANS (pediatric acute-onset neuropsychiatric syndrome). *Pediatric Therapeutics, 2*, 2.

Swedo, S. E., Leonard, H. L., Garvey, M., Mittleman, B., Allen, A. J., Perlmutter, S., et al. (1998). Pediatric autoimmune neuropsychiatric disorders associated with streptococcal infections: Clinical description of the first 50 cases. *American Journal of Psychiatry, 155*, 264–271.

Swedo, S. E., Rapoport, J. L., Leonard, H. L., Lenane, M., & Cheslow, D. (1989). Obsessive compulsive disorder in children and adolescents: Clinical phenomenology of 70 consecutive cases. *Archives of General Psychiatry, 46*, 335–341.

Thoren, P., Asberg, M., Cronholm, B., Jornestedt, L., & Traskman, L. (1980). Clomipramine treatment of obsessive–compulsive disorder: I. A controlled clinical trial. *Archives of General Psychiatry, 37*, 1281–1285.

Tolin, D. F., Maltby, N., Diefenbach, G. J., Hannan, S. E., & Worhunsky, P. (2004). Cognitive-behavioral therapy for medication nonresponders with obsessive–compulsive disorder: A wait-list-controlled open trial. *Journal of Clinical Psychiatry, 65*, 922–931.

Tukel, R., Polat, A., Ozdemir, O., Aksut, D., & Turksov, N. (2002). Comorbid conditions in obsessive–compulsive disorder. *Comprehensive Psychiatry, 43*, 204–209.

Twohig, M. P., Hayes, S. C., & Masuda, A. (2006). Increasing willingness to experience obsessions: Acceptance and commitment therapy as a treatment for obsessive compulsive disorder. *Behavior Therapy, 37*, 3–13.

Twohig, M., Hayes, S. C., Plumb, J., Pruitt, L. D., Collins, A. B., Hazlett-Stevens, H., et al. (2010). A randomized controlled trial of acceptance and commitment therapy versus progressive relaxation training for obsessive compulsive disorder. *Journal of Consulting and Clinical Psychology, 78*, 705–716.

Valderhaug, R., Larsson, B., Gotestam, K. G., & Piacentini, J. (2007). An open clinical trial of cognitive-behaviour therapy in children and adolescents with obsessive–compulsive disorder administered in regular outpatient clinics. *Behaviour Research and Therapy, 45*, 577–589.

Valleni-Basille, L. A., Garrison, C. Z., Jackson, K. L., Waller, J. L., McKeown, R. E., Addy, C. L., et al. (1994). Frequency of obsessive–compulsive disorder in a community sample of young adolescents. *Journal of the American Academy of Child and Adolescent Psychiatry, 33*, 782–791.

van Balkom, A. J., de Haan, E., van Oppen, P., Spinhoven, P., Hoogduin, K. A., Vermeulen, A. W. A., et al. (1998). Cognitive and behavioral therapies alone and in combination with fluvoxamine in the treatment of obsessive compulsive disorder. *Journal of Nervous and Mental Disease, 186*, 492–499.

van Minnen, A., & Hagenaars, M. (2002). Fear activation and habituation patterns as early process predictors of response to prolonged exposure treatment in PTSD. *Journal of Traumatic Stress, 15*, 359–367.

Verdellen, C. W., Keijsers, G. P., Cath, D. C., & Hoogduin, C. A. (2004). Exposure with response prevention versus habit reversal in Tourette syndrome: A controlled study. *Behaviour Research and Therapy, 42*, 501–511.

Vogel, P. A., Stiles, T. C., & Götestam, K. G. (20040). Adding cognitive therapy elements to exposure therapy for obsessive–compulsive disorder: A controlled study. *Behavioural and Cognitive Psychotherapy, 32*, 275–290.

Warren, R., & Thomas, J. C. (2001). Cognitive-behavior therapy of obsessive–compulsive disorder in private practice: An effectiveness study. *Journal of Anxiety Disorders, 15*, 277–285.

Warwick, H. M., Clark, D. M., Cobb, A. M., & Salkovskis, P. M. (1996). A controlled trial of cognitive-behavioural treatment of hypochondriasis. *British Journal of Psychiatry, 169*(2), 189–195.

Watts, F. N. (1973). Desensitization as an habituation phenomenon: II. Studies of interstimulus interval length. *Psychological Reports, 33*, 715–718.

Weissman, M. M., Bland, R. C., Canino, G. J., Greenwald, S., Hwu, H. G., Lee, C. K., et al. (1994). The cross national epidemiology of obsessive compulsive disorder: The Cross National Collaborative Group. *Journal of Clinical Psychiatry, 55*(Suppl.), 5–10.

Whittal, M. L., Thordarson, D. S., & McLean, P. D. (2005). Treatment of obsessive–compulsive disorder: Cognitive behavior therapy vs. exposure and response prevention. *Behaviour Research and Therapy, 43*, 1559–1576.

Whittal, M. L., Woody, S. R., McLean, P. D., Rachman, S., & Robichaud, M. (2010). Treatment of obsessions: A randomized controlled trial. *Behaviour Research and Therapy, 48*, 295–303.

CHAPTER 5

An Acceptance-Based Behavioral Therapy for Generalized Anxiety Disorder

LIZABETH ROEMER
SUSAN M. ORSILLO

Generalized anxiety disorder (GAD) has been called the "basic" anxiety disorder, in the sense that generalized anxiety is, by definition, a component of other anxiety and related disorders. Indeed, GAD, although characterized by marked fluctuations, is chronic. Some have even considered that generalized anxiety might be better conceptualized as a personality disorder, since many individuals with this problem cannot report a definitive age of onset; rather, they note that it has been with them all their lives. Psychological and drug treatments, although often evaluated, have not produced the robust results evident with some other anxiety disorders. For this reason, further study of new treatment protocols is all the more pressing. The protocol presented in this chapter, recently developed by Drs. Roemer and Orsillo at our Center, illustrates a cutting-edge, acceptance-based approach to GAD that has achieved a high rate of success in initial trials. This protocol also illustrates, more so than any other chapter in this edition, principles associated with the so-called "third-wave" cognitive-behavioral approach to psychological disorders. Clinicians and students interested in how this approach is actually implemented will find the case study of "Hector" particularly fascinating.—D. H. B.

Generalized anxiety disorder (GAD) is a chronic anxiety disorder, centrally defined in DSM-IV and DSM-5, where criteria are unchanged, by excessive anxiety and worry more days than not over a period of at least 6 months (American Psychiatric Association, 1994, 2013). Clients who meet criteria for GAD also report difficulty controlling the worry they experience, as well as three or more associated symptoms (muscle tension, irritability, restlessness or feeling keyed up, difficulty concentrating or mind going blank, being easily tired, and difficulty sleeping). Epidemiological studies reveal a lifetime prevalence of 5.7% for GAD using DSM-IV criteria (Kessler et al., 2005).

GAD is associated with high levels of comorbidity with other psychological disorders. Over 90% of individuals who meet criteria for GAD during their lifetimes also meet criteria for at least one additional disorder (Bruce, Machan, Dyck, & Keller, 2001), and prospective studies indicate that GAD is a specific risk factor for the development of other mental health disorders, particularly major depression (Bruce et al., 2001). GAD is also associated with significantly reduced quality of life (Hoffman, Dukes, & Wittchen, 2008). Furthermore, individuals with GAD have more annual medical visits than other patients (Belanger, Ladouceur, & Morin, 2005) and are more likely to seek medical, rather than mental health, care for their symptoms (Wang et al., 2005). In fact, GAD is the most common anxiety disorder found among primary care patients (Ballenger et al., 2001), and the mean annual medical cost of GAD is $2,138 higher than for other anxiety disorders (mean = $6,475; Revicki et al., 2012). Given that GAD is associated with a host of physical complaints and conditions, including painful physical symptoms (Romera et al., 2010), gastrointestinal symptoms (Mussell et al., 2008), and cardiological complaints (Logue, Thomas, Barbee, & Hoehn-Saric, 1993), it is not surprising that patients with GAD have a tendency to overutilize medical (Ballenger et al., 2001), and underutilize psychiatric (Kennedy & Schwab, 1997) services.

Although earlier diagnostic criteria for GAD incorporated symptoms of autonomic arousal (e.g., accelerated heart rate), several lines of research converged to support removal of these criteria for DSM-IV. A large-scale study of reported associated symptoms indicated that autonomic symptoms were more rarely endorsed than symptoms of muscle tension, vigilance, and scanning, such as those described earlier (Marten et al., 1993). Furthermore, physiological studies revealed that GAD was more accurately characterized by reduced heart rate variability than by increased autonomic arousal (e.g., Thayer, Friedman, & Borkovec, 1996). Finally, experimental studies of worry revealed that worrying prior to exposure to a feared stimulus leads to less autonomic arousal than relaxation prior to exposure to a feared stimulus (e.g., Borkovec & Hu, 1990). Taken together, these studies suggest that autonomic arousal is not a necessary feature of GAD.

Instead, the central defining feature of GAD is excessive worry, or repeatedly thinking about worst case scenarios involving potential future events. Studies reveal that worry content does not differ between individuals who meet criteria for GAD and those who do not, except that those with GAD report worrying about miscellaneous topics, particularly minor matters, more than those who do not meet criteria (e.g., Roemer, Molina, & Borkovec, 1997). As noted earlier, individuals with GAD report difficulty stopping their worry once it starts, and clients often note that worrying about one topic can lead to worry about another. These findings and observations suggest that worry is a cognitive habit, with clients who meet criteria for GAD getting "stuck"

in cycles of worry about a wide range of topics that are difficult to stop once started. All cognitive-behavioral treatments for GAD emphasize interrupting this cycle, although methods for doing so vary.

Descriptive studies of GAD and worry have revealed affective, cognitive, and interpersonal correlates that may have important treatment implications. Borkovec's seminal research revealed that worry serves an avoidant function, by its perceived association with decreasing the likelihood of already low base rate negative events, and by the reduction in physiological arousal noted earlier (Borkovec, Alcaine, & Behar, 2004), as well as distraction from more emotional topics by self-report (Borkovec & Roemer, 1995). Mennin and others have demonstrated that GAD is associated with both self-reported deficits in emotion regulation (e.g., Mennin, Holaway, Fresco, Moore, & Heimberg, 2007) and limits in implicit regulation of emotional processing (Etkin & Schatzberg, 2011). Studies in this area have also revealed that GAD is associated with the fear or distress of anxiety (and other emotions; Lee, Orsillo, Roemer, & Allen, 2010; Mennin et al., 2007), worry about worry (or metaworry; Wells, 2005), and habitual avoidance of internal experiences (i.e., experiential avoidance; Lee et al., 2010). Furthermore, in a clinical sample, both worry and GAD were uniquely associated with perceived uncontrollability of emotional reactions, beyond shared variance with other known cognitive predictors of GAD (Stapinski, Abbott, & Rapee, 2010). Extensive research also documents an association between GAD and intolerance of uncertainty (the tendency to respond negatively to uncertain events and situations; Gentes & Ruscio, 2011), including an experimental study showing that manipulated uncertainty leads to increased worry (Ladouceur, Gosselin, & Dugas, 2000). GAD is also associated with interpersonal problems (Przeworski et al., 2011), including increased marital distress (Whisman, 2007).

OVERVIEW OF EVIDENCE FOR PSYCHOSOCIAL TREATMENTS OF GAD

Meta-analyses reveal that cognitive-behavioral therapies (CBTs) are efficacious for GAD, with large effect sizes that are maintained over follow-up periods (Borkovec & Ruscio, 2001; Covin, Ouimet, Seeds, & Dozois, 2008), and evidence of comparative efficacy over nondirective therapy (Borkovec & Costello, 1993). Within CBTs, a meta-analysis revealed comparable effects of cognitive therapy and relaxation therapy in treating GAD (Siev & Chambless, 2007). However, GAD remains one of the least successfully treated of the anxiety disorders (Waters & Craske, 2005), with most studies indicating that fewer than 65% of clients meet criteria for high end-state functioning at posttreatment (Ladouceur et al., 2000; Newman et al., 2011).

As briefly reviewed earlier, recent research has refined and expanded our understanding of GAD in an effort to identify causal and maintaining factors to target in therapy and improve its efficacy (see Behar, DiMarco, Hekler, Mohlman, & Staples, 2009, for an extensive review). Recent randomized controlled trials (RCTs) informed by these models indicate that targeting the interpersonal and emotion-focused aspects of GAD (Newman et al., 2011), and intolerance of uncertainty (Dugas et al., 2010), yield effects comparable to existing CBTs for GAD. A small pilot study found that targeting metacognition (e.g., metaworry) in GAD (Wells et al., 2010) produced better outcomes than applied relaxation; however, the very low rates of response to applied relaxation, coupled with the small sample size, indicate a need for further research to confirm this finding. A trial examining the efficacy of emotion regulation therapy for GAD is currently under way (Mennin & Fresco, in press).

We developed the acceptance-based behavioral therapy described in this chapter (which explicitly targets reactivity to [distress about] internal experiences, and experiential and behavioral avoidance, as described below) in an effort to better target GAD and comorbid disorders. We use the term "acceptance-based behavior therapy" (ABBT; Roemer & Orsillo, 2009) to refer to the broad class of therapies based in cognitive-behavioral theory but that explicitly incorporate methods to promote acceptance of internal experiences (e.g., acceptance and commitment therapy [ACT; Hayes, Strosahl, & Wilson, 2012]; dialectical behavior therapy [DBT; Linehan, 1993]; mindfulness-based cognitive therapy [MBCT; Segal, Williams, & Teasdale, 2002]). This ABBT for GAD, which draws from these treatments, as well as Borkovec's CBT for GAD (Borkovec & Sharpless, 2004), has been examined through an open trial and two RCTs. The open trial revealed significant, large effects on clinician-rated GAD severity, self-reported worry, anxiety, and depressive symptoms (Roemer & Orsillo, 2007). A wait-list RCT similarly revealed significant, large effects on clinician and self-reported GAD symptoms, as well as depressive symptoms (Roemer, Orsillo, & Salters-Pedneault, 2008).

Marginally significant, medium effects emerged on clinician-rated additional diagnoses and self-reported quality of life. Significant large effects also emerged on self-reported experiential avoidance and mindfulness, two proposed mechanisms of change in the treatment. All effects were maintained at 9-month follow-up. Of those treated, 77% met criteria for high end-state functioning (falling within normative range on the majority of anxiety measures) at posttreatment; this proportion increased slightly (nonsignificantly) over time. In this trial, ABBT produced a significant increase in engagement in valued, or personally meaningful, activities (Michelson, Lee, Orsillo, & Roemer, 2011). Moreover, ABBT significantly impacted outcome variables proposed in other models to be central to GAD (emotion regulation deficits, intolerance of uncertainty, and perceived control over anxiety-related events; Treanor, Erisman, Salters-Pedneault, Roemer, & Orsillo, 2011). A recently completed RCT comparing ABBT with applied relaxation, an empirically treatment for GAD, revealed comparable effects on clinician-rated and self-reported GAD symptoms, clinician-rated comorbid diagnoses, and self-reported depressive symptoms and quality of life (Hayes-Skelton, Roemer, & Orsillo, 2013). A large proportion of clients in both conditions met criteria for high end-state functioning (some of the highest rates reported in the literature in each condition) and gains were maintained at 6-month follow up. Finally, there is evidence that ABBT works through its proposed mechanisms. Session-by-session changes in acceptance of internal experiences and engagement in meaningful activities predicted outcome above and beyond change in worry (Hayes, Orsillo, & Roemer, 2010).

A recent study that examined the relative efficacy of ACT compared to CBT for a mixed-anxiety sample revealed comparable effects across the full sample (Arch et al., 2012). Although the small size of the GAD subsample precluded within-subgroup analyses, examination of means suggests that ACT was effective in reducing clinician-rated and self-reported GAD symptoms in this study.

Taken together, these findings suggest that psychosocial treatments for GAD are efficacious, and adaptations of CBT that specifically target empirically determined features of GAD are promising. As with all treatments based in behavioral theory, a well-developed case conceptualization is a necessary starting point to use evidence-based treatments effectively with a specific client.

AN ACCEPTANCE-BASED BEHAVIORAL MODEL OF GAD

An acceptance-based behavioral model of GAD is grounded in behavioral learning theory. Consistent with other theories, we propose that individuals with GAD develop the habit of worry, repeatedly anticipating potential dangers and threats. These habits are strengthened through repetition and reinforcing consequences. This worry process is negatively reinforced by both the nonoccurrence of feared outcomes and the reduced physiological activation that is a positive consequence of engaging in worry (Borkovec et al., 2004).

Moreover, individuals with GAD come to associate universal, functional human states such as fear, anxiety, other emotional responses, and even worry with negative personal characteristics. As a result, individuals with GAD respond to anxiety-related thoughts and emotional states with self-criticism and judgment. In an attempt to avoid or escape the uncomfortable, unwanted experience of worry, and the associated negative self-evaluation, individuals with GAD engage in a variety of potentially problematic behaviors. Although these behaviors interfere with quality of life, they provide short-term relief from arousal and negative affect.

Drawing from decades of research on GAD, other anxiety disorders, and broader models of psychopathology (e.g., Hayes et al., 2012), we hypothesize that the following three learned behaviors contribute to the development and maintenance of GAD.

Reacting to Internal Experiences with Distress, Criticism, and Judgment (Leading to Entanglement/Fusion)

One of the most formative, consistent findings to emerge in the field of anxiety disorders has been that the experience of anxiety or fear in and of itself (e.g., sensations of panic, worrisome thoughts, catastrophic images, recurrent painful memories) is not evidence of a disorder. Instead, reactions to these symptoms, or "reaction to our reactions" (Borkovec & Sharpless, 2004) exacerbate their intensity and duration, cause distress, and interfere with quality of life, leading to the anxiety disorder diagnosis. The centrality of "reactions to reactions" to the concept of psychological disorders was recently documented in a treatment trial. Changes in *reactivity* to emotions predicted unique variance in all outcome variables over and above changes in *frequency* of emotional responses in a study of the unified proto-

col for emotional disorders (Sauer-Zavala et al., 2012; see Payne, Ellard, Farchione, Fairholme, & Barlow, Chapter 6, this volume).

A growing body of research documents that individuals with GAD report increased anxiety sensitivity (i.e., fear of anxiety-related bodily sensations; Olatunji & Wolitzky-Taylor, 2009), negative reactivity to their emotional responses (e.g., Lee et al., 2010; Mennin et al., 2007), and worry about their own worry (Wells, 2005). Furthermore, anxiety leads to a narrowed focus of attention (both external and internal) toward potential threat (Cisler & Koster, 2010), which likely both exacerbates these reactions and is strengthened by reactivity, further perpetuating cycles of anxious responding. These reactions can lead individuals to become entangled with (Germer, 2005) or "hooked" on (Chodron, 2007) their experiences of anxiety and worry, so that the anxiety comes to seem self-defining and all-encompassing. Instead of viewing anxiety as a response that is elicited in a particular context, individuals can come to define themselves as "anxious," fusing their identity with these experiences (e.g., Hayes et al., 2012). Thus, negative reactivity to emotions can evolve into negative personal judgments ("I'm so weak!"; "Other people don't worry the way I do"), which in turn can increase anxiety and worry.

Becoming entangled or fused with internal experiences makes it much harder to see the ways that thoughts, feelings, and sensations naturally rise, fall, and change over time. It can also interfere with one's ability to understand and respond effectively to emotional states, leading to diffuse experiences of distress that do not provide clear motivational information. When fear, anxiety, and worry are perceived as distressing, defining, and unrelenting, they naturally elicit attempts to escape and avoid.

Rigid Attempts to Avoid Internal Distress

Trying not to think about or feel or remember something distressing is a natural response.

All people use strategies to turn their attention away from internal distress at times, in order to bring attention to the task at hand. Yet experimental studies show that rigid, repeated efforts to put thoughts, feelings, sensations or memories out of our minds (e.g., experiential avoidance; Hayes, Wilson, Gifford, Follette, & Strosahl, 1996) are often unsuccessful and can actually increase distressing thoughts, feelings, or sensations (e.g., Gross, 2002; Levitt, Brown, Orsillo, & Barlow,

2004; Najmi & Wegner, 2008). Furthermore, instructed effort not to think of situations can increase reported anxiety associated with the target situation (Roemer & Borkovec, 1994), suggesting that experiential avoidance increases distress about thoughts and emotions. Taken together, these studies suggest that rigid efforts to avoid distressing thoughts, feelings, sensations, and memories can increase the frequency of these experiences, as well as the distress associated with them, further strengthening the cycle of reactivity and avoidance. Efforts at experiential avoidance are likely to reduce distress in the short term at least sometimes, leading to immediate negative reinforcement, further strengthening this habitual response.

Reports of experiential avoidance are associated with GAD diagnoses, even beyond shared variance with depressive symptoms (Lee et al., 2010). Furthermore, as described earlier, experimental studies demonstrate that worry itself serves an experientially avoidant function by reducing physiological arousal in response to feared stimuli and distracting individuals from more distressing topics (Borkovec et al., 2004).

Behavioral Avoidance/Constriction

Reactions to internal experiences and rigid experiential avoidance not only feed on each other in a continually escalating cycle, but also naturally lead to avoidance of contexts that elicit anxiety or other experiences of distress. Behavioral avoidance is a core feature of other anxiety disorders, but it has generally been overlooked in GAD. However, individuals with GAD often avoid certain situations, spend extensive time preparing for situations, procrastinate or put off decision making, or seek reassurance, all in an effort to avoid distress, anxiety, and/or uncertainty (Andrews et al., 2010). Clients with GAD report engaging in valued actions (i.e., doing what they find personally meaningful) less than do control participants (Michelson et al., 2011).

Clinically, clients with GAD show a range of avoidance behaviors. Sometimes avoidance is overt, such as when a client does not pursue dating or a promotion at work due to anxiety, fears of being rejected, or worry. Other times, clients who seem to be engaging in a wide range of behaviors that are important (e.g., taking on challenges at work, being involved in activities with their children) may report that they are constantly worrying about what is ahead rather than attending to what they are doing in the moment. Borkovec notes this

focus on the future instead of the present as a core characteristic of GAD (e.g., Borkovec & Sharpless, 2004), and research indicates that GAD and worry are associated with reports of reduced mindfulness (awareness in the present moment; Roemer et al., 2009). This continual focus on what might go wrong in the future can lead clients to feel like spectators in their own lives: behaviorally, but not emotionally, engaged in actions that matter to them.

This conceptual model highlights three targets for intervention when treating clients with GAD and other comorbid disorders: (1) problematic ways of relating to internal experiences, (2) rigid strategies aimed at experiential avoidance, and (3) constriction or avoidance of meaningful actions. Based on this model, the goals of an ABBT for GAD are (1) to cultivate an *expanded* (as opposed to narrowed) awareness and a *compassionate* (as opposed to critical and judgmental), *decentered* (as opposed to entangled and fused) stance toward internal experiences; (2) to increase acceptance of/willingness to have internal experiences; and (3) to engage mindfully in personally meaningful behaviors.

APPLYING ABBT

Context for Therapy

Our first case study of ABBT took place in group format (Orsillo, Roemer, & Barlow, 2003). Although clients benefited from the group context in some ways, they reported that they wanted more individualized focus to help them clarify their values (i.e., what matters to them) and apply the treatment to their specific contexts. As a result, all of our subsequent trials have used individual therapy. However, we think that the modality of treatment can be adjusted to better fit specific settings. In fact, a recent study found that a group version of our protocol led to significant reductions in self-reported anxiety, worry, and GAD symptoms in a community setting (Heatherington et al., 2013). Furthermore, several elements of ABBT (e.g., psychoeducation, mindfulness practice, commitment to valued action) have been effectively conducted in group settings in other, related treatment approaches (e.g., Evans et al., 2008; Kocovski, Fleming, & Rector, 2009).

Given the prevalence of GAD in primary care contexts, we are interested in adapting treatment so it can be used as part of integrative primary care. We wrote a self-help book that may be beneficial in this context (Orsillo & Roemer, 2011), but no studies to date have examined its effectiveness. Briefer workshops (e.g., Blevins, Roca, & Spencer, 2011; Brown et al., 2011) may also be a useful modality for delivery of the conceptual model and suggestions for mindfulness and valued action practices in contexts where individual therapy is less feasible due to economic or time constraints.

Therapist Characteristics

A central aspect of ABBT involves modeling acceptance of intense emotional experiences. Therefore, successful ABBT therapists are able to tolerate intense emotions and convey acceptance to their clients. Similarly, ABBT therapists continually validate and express compassion toward clients in distress, providing for clients an example of how they might respond differently to their own experiences and reduce the cycle of reactivity and avoidance that contributes to maintenance of their symptoms. These characteristics, combined with a clear understanding of the model and how to apply it to specific cases, help therapists to develop a strong, positive working alliance, which significantly predicted outcome in our most recent trial (Sorenson, Hayes-Skelton, Roemer, & Orsillo, 2012).

As we describe more fully below, ABBT is meant to be applied flexibly, with therapists adapting their approach, strategies used, and between-session assignments to meet the presentation and context of clients. As such, flexibility may be an important therapist characteristic. In a small qualitative study, as part of our most recent RCT, we interviewed clients who identified with marginalized backgrounds in terms of race, ethnicity, sexual orientation, socioeconomic status, or religion. Clients identified the flexibility of their therapist as an important factor in how helpful they found treatment and how well it fit with their particular context (Fuchs et al., 2012).

Client Characteristics

In the studies we have conducted on ABBT for GAD, we have had very few exclusion criteria in order to maximize the generalizability of our findings. Clients frequently present with comorbid diagnoses, most commonly major depressive disorder, social anxiety disorder, and other anxiety disorders. Because ABBT targets mechanisms that are likely to underlie these other disorders as well, treatment may positively impact these comorbid conditions (e.g., Roemer et al., 2008). However, outside the constraints of protocol therapy, we would recommend integrating elements of evidence-based methods (e.g., behavioral activation, exposure) when indicated. The disorders we have ruled out in our RCTs, primarily because they warrant specific treatments, include substance dependence, bipolar disorder, schizophrenia, and autism spectrum disorders. Thus, we cannot determine the impact of ABBT on these comorbid presentations.

To date, we have only preliminarily explored potential predictors of response to ABBT. To date, our data suggest that gender, age, GAD severity, frequency and intensity of worry, depressive symptoms, and comorbid diagnoses do not significantly predict outcome (Orsillo, Roemer, & Salters-Pedneault, 2008).

As with most evidence-based treatments, considerably more research is needed to determine the ways an ABBT for GAD might be beneficial for people from marginalized or nondominant cultural backgrounds. A meta-analysis indicated promising results for ABBTs more broadly (Fuchs, Lee, Roemer, & Orsillo, 2013). Our small qualitative study revealed that clients from marginalized backgrounds generally found ABBT helpful (Fuchs et al., 2012). Clients particularly noted that therapist flexibility and the focus on valued living helped them engage in treatment and find it relevant. However, some clients reported that therapist inflexibility or not connecting to specific mindfulness exercises was a barrier.

A commonly expressed concern is that mindfulness may not be accepted by clients who identify strongly with a non-Buddhist religion. However, mindfulness exercises can be adapted to match specific religious practices (Sobczak & West, 2013) because mindfulness is part of many religious traditions, for instance, Western Christian contemplative practice (Dimidjian & Linehan, 2009). More work is needed to explore how best to adapt ABBT for clients from different backgrounds, and also how to use ABBT strategies to address contextual sources of stress such as discrimination and lack of resources (Lee, Fuchs, Roemer, & Orsillo, 2009; Sobczak & West, 2013).

Concurrent Pharmacological Treatment

Although medication is the most common mode of treatment for GAD (Issakidis, Sanderson, Corry, Andrews, & Lapsley, 2004) and is often considered a first-line treatment option (Katzman, 2009), evidence for the sustained clinical impact of pharmacotherapy is limited (Davidson, Bose, Korotzer, & Zheng, 2004; Gelenberg et al., 2000; Rickels et al., 2003). The magnitude of change in GAD symptoms associated with pharmacological treatment ranges from moderate to poor (Hidalgo, Tupler, & Davidson, 2007). Moreover, pharmacological interventions may produce adverse side effects (Katzman, 2009) and are less cost-effective than psychotherapeutic approaches such as CBT (Heuzenroeder et al., 2004).

Clients who were stable on medications were enrolled in our clinical trials. Within ABBT, medications are conceptualized as one of several ways to reduce the intensity of internal reactions, so that it is easier to accept them, have compassion for oneself, and engage in meaningful actions. In this way, a nonexperientially avoidant function for medication can be highlighted (medication helps one to engage more fully in life and accept whatever comes), so that it is consistent with the rest of treatment.

Overview of Treatment Elements

In our clinical trials, we have followed a 16-session, weekly individual protocol for ABBT, with the last two sessions tapered (every other week) and focused on relapse prevention. The first seven sessions focus on psychoeducation and skills building, while the remaining sessions focus on application of skills while the client engages in personally meaningful, valued actions. Here we provide a brief overview of each element of treatment, followed by a composite case example to illustrate the way each element is addressed across the course of therapy. Those interested in more details on our approach should consult our book for therapists (Roemer & Orsillo, 2009) and our self-help book (Orsillo & Roemer, 2011).

Clinical Assessment to Develop an Acceptance-Based Behavioral Conceptualization

To develop a case conceptualization that guides flexible application of treatment elements, we assess symptoms, context, and the three components of the model.

SYMPTOMS

Assessing the client's anxiety and related symptoms provides useful information about targets for change,

while also supporting the therapeutic goal of changing a client's relationship with anxiety. Assessment of anxiety-related thoughts, feelings, physical sensations, and behaviors, the contexts in which anxiety typically occurs, and the frequency and severity of symptoms helps clients begin to observe more accurately specific elements of their anxiety responses. Ongoing self-monitoring of daily anxiety symptoms, as well as guided imaginal recall, can provide a more accurate assessment of specific symptoms than general report given that clients who engage in habitual avoidance or suppression of their anxiety often do not have an accurate perception of its frequency, duration, or variability over time. Brief but specific self-report measures (e.g., the Depression Anxiety Stress Scales; Lovibond & Lovibond, 1995, or the trait and weekly Penn State Worry Questionnaires (Meyer, Miller, Metzger, & Borkovec, 1990; Stöber & Bittencourt, 1998), can also be used, both to obtain baseline measures of symptoms and to track weekly fluctuations in symptoms.

Semistructured clinical interviews such as the Anxiety Disorders Interview Schedule (Di Nardo et al., 1994) can be used to determine both principal and comorbid disorders to guide the selection and emphasis of specific treatment strategies. Depression is an important target of assessment, as are other clinical presentations, such as eating disorders and substance-use disorders, which may indicate specific avoidance strategies that need to be targeted in treatment.

REACTIONS TO INTERNAL EXPERIENCES

Assessing how clients respond to their anxiety symptoms, as well as to internal experiences (e.g., thoughts, emotions, sensations, memories) more generally, contributes to case conceptualization. Therapists may ask questions such as "When you notice you are worrying, what thoughts, feelings and sensations do you experience next?"; "Do you find yourself having critical thoughts about your experiences of anxiety?"; and "What kinds of thoughts do you have?" or use self-report measures that capture these constructs. Self-criticism, judgment, and reactivity that arise for clients in response to their own thoughts and feelings are important targets for intervention. Measures such as the Affective Control Scale (Williams, Chambless, & Ahrens, 1997), a measure of distress in response to anxiety, depression, anger, and positive emotions, and the Self-Compassion Scale (Neff, 2003) can help to identify reactivity to emotions and self-criticism.

EXPERIENTIAL AVOIDANCE

Therapists also assess the strategies that clients use in an attempt to suppress, avoid, or change internal experiences (Hayes et al., 1996). Experiential avoidance strategies may be internal, such as thought or emotion suppression (Gross & Levenson, 1997; Najmi & Wegner, 2008), or external, such as using substances, engaging in self-harm, or restricting eating. Therapist can ask clients what they do to try to manage their distress or anxiety, then listen for avoidant strategies. Efforts in which clients engage automatically or rigidly are most likely to lead to paradoxical increases in distress and symptoms. Therapists need to distinguish between efforts to modulate or regulate emotional distress and rigid efforts to avoid it; often the difference is evident in what happens after the strategy is engaged. The former are likely to be beneficial and may be strengths on which to build in therapy, if used flexibly, whereas the latter are more likely to lead to increased distress and interference. For instance, one client with whom we worked reported going for walks to try to clear her head of worry. When her therapist asked what she did when she returned, she reported that she was more able to focus on being with her children and enjoy their time together. On the other hand, another client who described regularly watching TV in order to distract herself from her worries said that as soon as she turned off the TV, her worried thoughts flooded back, so that she found herself watching TV for hours at a time rather than doing activities she had planned during the day. Whereas the first client's walks might be incorporated into treatment as a way to care for herself and help her engage more effectively with her children, the second client's therapist might help her develop alternative ways of responding to her anxiety. The Acceptance and Action Questionnaire (Bond et al., 2011) can help to identify experientially avoidant strategies; the Difficulties in Emotion Regulation Scale (Gratz & Roemer, 2004) assesses emotion regulation more broadly.

BEHAVIORAL CONSTRICTION

Therapists should also assess how clients are functioning in their daily lives and the ways that anxiety and worry are interfering. Drawing from ACT (Wilson & Murrell, 2004), we focus particularly on the degree to which clients are doing what is important to them (i.e., what they value). We assess this with the Valued Living Questionnaire (Wilson, Sandoz, Kitchens, & Rob-

erts, 2010), while also inviting clients to write about the ways anxiety interferes with their relationships, work–school–household management, self-nourishment, and community involvement. This provides not only important information about current functioning but also a target and motivation for treatment to help clients live fuller, more meaningful lives. This assessment often provides an important first step toward shifting the goal of therapy from anxiety reduction to enhancement of life.

CONTEXT AND HISTORY

As with all treatment approaches, assessing the context surrounding a client is important. Therapists need to learn how the client (as well as family and friends) understands his/her anxiety, in addition to the client's history of anxiety symptoms and other presenting problems. Therapists should also explore the client's cultural identity, with attention to culturally specific sources of coping and strength, as well as contextual stressors that the client may face. This helps to establish rapport and validate the client's experience, and to build the strength of the therapeutic alliance. This information also helps the therapist to ensure that therapy proceeds in a culturally sensitive and responsive way (D. W. Sue & Sue, 2012; S. Sue, 1998).

This comprehensive assessment sets the stage for treatment elements aimed at (1) cultivating an expanded (as opposed to narrowed) awareness and a compassionate (as opposed to critical and judgmental), decentered (as opposed to entangled and fused) stance toward internal experiences; (2) increasing acceptance/willingness to have internal experiences; and (3) mindfully engaging in personally meaningful behaviors.

Therapeutic Relationship

The therapeutic relationship provides an important context for therapeutic change. In ABBT, the therapist provides acceptance and compassion that allows clients to begin to react differently toward their own internal experiences. Therapists explicitly validate the humanness and naturalness of all responses clients share, emphasizing the way one's biological makeup and learning history can easily lead to anxious responses and other emotional reactions, and the way that even apparently "irrational" thoughts can be learned from social and family influences. For instance, when a client noted in session that he knew he should not be anxious about a job interview, his therapist responded that anxiety before an interview is a very natural response given that he really wants the position, and that we are hardwired to fear social rejection. This response modeled a different reaction to his anxiety and was the first step toward cultivating a new, less self-critical response.

It can be challenging to empathize with and validate some clients, particularly when they are hostile or unresponsive. Understanding the learning history and context that produces and maintains these difficult, but also in some ways functional, behaviors helps therapists cultivate compassion. When a therapist expresses genuine compassion toward a client, often the client's reactions change, at least slightly, providing more opportunities for connection, validation, empathy, and further change.

Another challenge to the therapeutic alliance can stem from differences between client and therapist in aspects of identity (e.g., age, gender, race, religion, ethnicity, sexual orientation, immigration status, or social class; Hays, 2008; D. W. Sue & Sue, 2012). Initiating a discussion of potential differences early in therapy provides an opportunity for open communication about potential sources of misunderstanding and may make a client feel more comfortable bringing up any issues that emerge throughout the course of therapy. Therapists take responsibility for learning about a client's cultural context on their own, while remaining sensitive to each client's individual experiences and life contexts, so that he/she can consider how cultural and systemic factors may play a role in the client's responses and can be used to promote growth and positive adaptation. Communicating awareness of, and sensitivity to, the therapist's own areas of relative privilege can also contribute to a stronger therapeutic alliance.

Psychoeducation

Similar to other CBTs, psychoeducation is an important component of this ABBT. Therapists present concepts, using handouts, particularly during the first half of therapy (then revisit these concepts as needed in the second, application phase of treatment). For each concept, therapists draw examples from the client's life (using monitoring forms, assessment material, or asking the client specifically for examples) to ensure that the material is relevant.

Psychoeducation begins with a discussion about the nature of fear, anxiety, and worry (including a discus-

sion of the function of worry), followed by exploration of the function of emotions more broadly, emphasizing the habitual nature of our emotional responding and how repetition strengthens these habits, while interruption can weaken them. Therapists teach clients about the natural inclination to avoid painful or threatening cues, as well as the challenges and costs associated with trying to rigidly control internal experiences and avoid anxiety-eliciting situations. Therapists draw a distinction between clear emotions (that provide information about a response to a current context) and muddy emotions (that may be diffuse, confusing, left over, or longer lasting). Therapists also describe mindfulness skills, specifically noting the ways these skills can be used to clarify emotional responses and enhance participation in valued life activities.

Psychoeducation provides a rationale for the rest of treatment, encouraging engagement in behaviors that take significant time (e.g., mindfulness practice) or effort (e.g., engaging in valued actions). Psychoeducation can also help to promote a new relationship to internal experiences on its own. Realizing how one's emotions become muddy and overwhelming as a result of a series of understandable processes (e.g., not getting enough sleep, still feeling upset about an earlier fight with a partner) can reduce self-criticism and judgment, which in turn can reduce muddiness and reactivity. For some clients, psychoeducation alone leads to engagement in new behaviors and to new learning that promotes accepting responses to internal experiences and increased engagement in life. However, experiential learning is often needed to supplement this clinical strategy.

Many challenges can arise when presenting psychoeducational material. First, it can be difficult to attend to specific client concerns while also presenting extensive new information. Using client examples as you teach and frequently asking clients to share their reactions can help to balance these competing demands. Also, sometimes clients disagree with material being presented. For instance, clients may insist that avoidance is an effective strategy. Arguing with clients is rarely productive, and it can weaken the therapeutic relationship. Furthermore, case conceptualizations are only a hypothesis based on the literature and clinical observation, so it is important not to cling rigidly to them. We find it useful, in this situation, to ask whether clients are willing simply to observe the concept over the next few weeks to see whether they can learn anything new about their experience. This promotes a collaborative approach to treatment and helps to engage clients, while also encouraging valuable feedback on our conceptualization.

Mindfulness Skills Development

"Mindfulness" (Kabat-Zinn, 2003), or attending to the present moment with openness, curiosity, and compassion, is a central skill clients can use to change the nature of their relationship with their internal experiences (e.g., beginning to see thoughts as thoughts, or "decentering"), increase their willingness to have any reactions that arise, and promote engagement in fulfilling, meaningful lives. We use a wide range of methods to help clients bring their awareness to the present moment, and we greet their experiences with curiosity, kindness, and compassion.

SELF-MONITORING

Self-monitoring is a common method used in all CBTs. Similar to these approaches, therapy begins with clients monitoring situations in which worry arises. Each week, based on what is covered in session, new aspects of experience are added (e.g., emotions, efforts to avoid experience, engagement in valued actions). The process of monitoring worry, other internal experiences, and behaviors helps to promote awareness and decentering; clients turn toward their internal experiences rather than habitually turning away, and they see each aspect of their experience rather than blending the components together (e.g., noticing thoughts, emotions, and behaviors separately). As clients begin to notice the distinction between emotion and behavior, they are more able to consider the variety of behavioral options available to them even when strong emotions arise.

Self-monitoring can be challenging for some clients. They may forget to complete monitoring forms, see them as a "homework" requirement done only at the therapist's request, or finish them in the waiting room as opposed to completing them in the moment. Therapists can help clients to see the usefulness of the practice by clearly communicating the rationale for monitoring, underscoring that it is a skill that can be used to clarify emotions, reduce distress, and increase engagement in valued activities, and reviewing the monitoring each session and connecting observations to treatment goals. Therapists can also flexibly adapt monitoring assignments to fit with the client's life while emphasizing the

importance of doing some monitoring in the moment that a reaction occurs to facilitate the development of awareness as anxious habitual patterns unfold. For instance, clients could monitor only one situation a day, or use phones or audio recorders for monitoring rather than paper and pen.

FORMAL MINDFULNESS PRACTICE

Mindfulness is a skill; therefore, practicing it regularly can be extremely helpful. Therapists help clients to determine when that they can set aside some amount of time in which to draw their awareness, again and again, to some aspect of their experience, such as the breath, physical sensations, or thoughts. Mindfulness-based treatments such as MBCT have clients practice for 45 minutes a day; we generally use shorter mindfulness practices and allow clients to choose the length of their practice. We do have all clients practice an adapted progressive muscle relaxation in which clients tense and release a series of muscle groups, noticing the sensations they experience.[1] This gives anxious clients an extended exposure to mindfulness, while providing a focus for attention that may facilitate more prolonged practice. Clients vary in how much they keep up this particular practice versus other, shorter practices.

In our approach, therapists teach clients a progression of practices across the course of treatment, beginning with focus on the breath and body, moving to awareness of taste and sounds, then on to more challenging practices of awareness of emotions and thoughts. Clients and therapists practice together first in session, then discuss the client's experience with the exercise. Initially, clients often label the practice as "good" or "bad," "relaxing" or "stressful." Therapists help clients move toward simply observing and describing their experience during the practice, recognizing that all practice is useful and so-called "bad" practice can teach a lot about how active one's mind is and how repeatedly to bring awareness back to the moment despite a wandering mind.

When discussing in-session practice, therapists draw connections between the practice and clients' presenting problems. For instance, one client reported that when she practiced mindfulness of her breath, her mind kept wandering to her frustration with her roommate, and it was clear that she was bad at mindfulness and was not ever going to get better. Her therapist related these self-critical thoughts and negative predictions to those that often arose when the client took on a new task at work. The therapist suggested that if she practiced observing critical thoughts with compassion and curiosity during formal mindfulness, she might be able to carry these same skills into challenging work situations.

Clients often have trouble setting aside time to practice mindfulness regularly. Traditional problem-solving strategies can be used to find moments (during a subway commute, just after putting the kids to bed) to practice. Therapists also point out that practicing mindfulness may help the client become more efficient and alert throughout the day, so it may be worth some time. Clients can also use mindfulness as an avoidance strategy, particularly if they initially find the practice relaxing. Therapists need to attend to the function of practice behavior to be sure that clients are not using it to avoid unwanted internal experiences.

INFORMAL MINDFULNESS PRACTICE

Although setting aside time to practice can be an excellent way to develop any skill, the goal is always to use the skill while engaging in life. Clients practice mindfulness informally by engaging mindfully in daily tasks such as washing the dishes (Nhat Hanh, 1992), eating, showering, or folding laundry. They gradually begin to practice in more challenging contexts, such as during conversations, dates, meetings at work, or community events. Therapists initially help clients to remember to practice mindfulness during sessions; over time clients begin to remind themselves to come back to the present moment while engaging in therapy, strengthening this skill so they can use it more effectively in their lives.

LANGUAGE CONVENTIONS

Another way to help clients cultivate a decentered awareness of their experiences is to bring attention to their language and introduce a few strategies (drawn from ACT) that help one disentangle from one's thoughts. One is to say (and think) "I'm having the thought that . . . " or "I'm having the feeling that . . . " as opposed to reporting thoughts as facts. Therapists model this and begin to reframe clients' reports using this convention, gradually encouraging clients to make this change themselves. Similarly, therapists encourage clients to consider whether replacing "but" with "and" more accurately captures different situations. For instance, rather than saying, "I would really like to go on this date, but I'm too anxious," a client might say, "I would like to go on this date, and I'm also experiencing anxiety." This highlights that feelings and thoughts do not have to lead to avoidance or escape behaviors.

Engaging in Actions

Finally, therapists help clients turn their attention and effort away from trying to control their internal experiences and instead focus on engaging more fully in their lives. Clients begin exploring what is important to them through a series of writing assignments. First, they describe how anxiety has gotten in the way of their lives in several domains (relationships, work–school–household management, and self-nourishment and community involvement). Next they write about how they would like to be in these areas, if they did not have any anxiety. From there, therapists help clients identify specific areas on which they want to focus. Therapy, then, involves making behavioral plans each week to do something the client values, such as making a social connection, asserting oneself at work, or joining a community organization. For each behavioral action, therapists emphasize the importance of choosing an action regardless of the thoughts and feelings that arise, and clients apply their mindfulness skills, so that they are able to do what matters to them even while anxious.

Shifting from habitual avoidance to engagement is a long, ongoing process. Some clients have difficulty articulating their values because all of their attentional and behavioral resources have been directed toward anxiety management for so long. Once clients have clarified what they find important, approaching these actions can be extremely anxiety provoking and hard to do. However, encouragement from the therapist, cultivation of mindfulness skills, and breaking tasks down into specific manageable pieces (e.g., asking a coworker to lunch, or having one open conversation with a parent) can help a client become willing to make these first important behavioral changes even though anxiety will inevitably be present. Over time, the experience of engaging in valued activities can be naturally reinforcing. Nonetheless, continued awareness and practice is needed so as not to fall back into old, natural patterns of avoidance due to anxiety.

Many challenges arise in pursuing valued actions. First, as Hayes and colleagues (2012) note, clients often think in terms of goals (e.g., finding a partner, losing 15 pounds) as opposed to values (e.g., being emotionally intimate, being physically healthy). Focusing on wanting to lose 15 pounds can lead to self-criticism in the moment, which might interfere with that goal. On the other hand, a person can take actions in the moment that are consistent with wanting to be physically healthy (e.g., going to the gym or eating a healthy lunch) that in turn also help with a goal. Therapists work to help clients identify the values and meaning that underlie any stated goals, so that they can engage in actions in the moment that will be fulfilling and meaningful.

Therapists need to take care not to impose their own values onto clients. Cultural sensitivity is particularly important in this aspect of treatment. For instance, one client we treated with ABBT described a value of being able to provide financially for his parents, leading him to choose a profession that to him was less intrinsically interesting but would allow him to support his family. His therapist came from a more individualistic background and had an initial reaction that choosing a more intrinsically rewarding profession was important. However, the therapist recognized that this would impose his own values on the client rather than help the client to make choices consistent with his own values.

Therapists also need to be sensitive to the real-world constraints that can keep clients from engaging in actions that matter to them. External constraints such as limited resources, inequities, and family contexts need to be validated and accounted for in developing treatment assignments. Relatedly, clients may want others in their lives to act differently. Although this is a very reasonable desire, changing other people is not always possible. Clients can request changes in others or take steps to address injustices in different contexts, but therapists cannot guarantee that these things will lead to the changes for which the client is hoping. Instead, the therapist can help the client make the best choices possible in the face of these constraints, which can certainly include asking for changes and also leaving situations when possible, if necessary.

Relapse Prevention

Anxiety is a natural, habitual response, as is reactivity to internal experiences and experiential avoidance. Therapists help clients develop a plan for maintaining the practices they have found most helpful in treatment, and to prepare for potential "lapses" in the future. Clients are encouraged to refer to their handouts and monitoring sheets when difficulties arise, and to revisit concepts and practices they found helpful in treatment.

CASE STUDY

This composite case is largely based on a single client but with details from other clients added to illustrate certain points. Identifying information is altered to protect confidentiality.

Background Information

Héctor was a 24-year-old Latino man who presented for treatment after being placed on academic probation. Although Héctor had an extremely strong academic record as an undergraduate, he was struggling to keep up with the course demands in his first semester of medical school. Héctor initially sought treatment from his primary care provider for a wide variety of stress-related symptoms, including frequent headaches, muscle tension, and gastrointestinal distress. However, she urged him to seek therapy for what she believed to be an anxiety disorder.

In the initial assessment, Héctor endorsed symptoms consistent with GAD. He described a long history of worry that started in elementary school. His worry focused centrally on his academic demands. He reported worrying constantly about the quality of his work, the sufficiency of his knowledge, and his ability to meet his, and others, academic-related expectations. Héctor was the first person in his family to graduate from college, and his entire extended family was extremely proud of him and significantly invested in Héctor earning a medical degree. Héctor's mother had secured a second job to help meet his rising tuition costs, one of his uncles offered to co-sign on a loan, and his cousin offered him a place to live rent-free. While he was extremely grateful for their support, Héctor constantly worried about disappointing them.

Héctor was also troubled by worries about his mother's health and well-being. He was concerned that she was overextending herself with two jobs, and he worried that she might have a heart attack or fall asleep when driving home and die in a car accident. Héctor also worried a fair amount about his two nephews. In his view, they spent far too much time watching television and playing video games, and needed more structure and guidance than his brother was providing.

Héctor described a number of aches and pains that he attributed to his constant, high level of physical tension. He noted that he had considerable difficulty falling asleep each night, as his mind constantly cycled through a variety of potential, negative outcomes the next day might bring. Not surprisingly, he described having a very difficult time concentrating, especially while he was in class and when he attempted to do his assigned reading. When his anxiety and worry became too severe, he would skip class and head to the gym. In the past, when he exercised long enough he would become so physically fatigued that he would fall asleep immediately when his "head hit the pillow." Unfortunately, that coping strategy recently was becoming less and less effective. First, he found that he was skipping class for the gym more and more frequently, to the point that he was unable to keep up his grades. Moreover, although he was still falling asleep fairly quickly postexercise, recently, he would awaken after only 1 or 2 hours of sleep.

When he was in secondary school and college, Héctor also found that spending time with friends and family kept his GAD symptoms in check. However, 6 months earlier, he had left his support network behind in Miami and relocated to Boston for medical school. Although he initially went to out to eat with some of his classmates and occasionally attended study sessions with them, he never felt entirely comfortable at these events. He worried that his classmates did not think he belonged at such a prestigious medical school, and Héctor was acutely aware that he was one of very few ethnic/minority students.

Engagement Session

In this session, Héctor disclosed that his family did not know that he was in therapy, and that he was too ashamed to tell them about his academic issues. Héctor acknowledged that keeping these secrets was painful and distressing, particularly because it required him to distance himself even further from his main source of social support.

Although Héctor had attended a few counseling sessions in his first semester of college, he had no other history of psychotherapy. Héctor described his brief course of previous therapy as primarily supportive. He noted that meeting a few times with his Latino male therapist, mostly to talk about academic stressors, had been extremely helpful in his transition to college. This experience made him cautiously optimistic about the current course of therapy, although he acknowledged a fear that his problems might now be too severe to overcome completely.

Given the considerable outside-of-therapy demands associated with ABBT, the therapist asked Héctor about

potential barriers to treatment. Although Héctor had a slightly reduced schedule because of his academic probation, he was still taking three courses and working 20–30 hours a week. The therapist validated Héctor's existing commitments, but she also wanted to be realistic in describing the additional time commitment that would be required, particularly in the first six to eight sessions of therapy. The therapist used the training for a marathon analogy to convey the importance of setting aside sufficient time for out-of-therapy assignments. She noted that Héctor's worry habit was deeply ingrained, and that learning new methods of responding would require some commitment to practice. An athlete training for a marathon cannot keep the same work/life schedule while adding in training sessions. Instead, he/she needs to make some temporary accommodations to make time to run. Similarly, a client with GAD cannot develop new habits while maintaining the same busy schedule. Some time and attention must be allocated temporarily to reflecting on the treatment and practicing new ways of responding.

Finally, the (white) therapist explored how her gender and ethnicity might affect treatment.

THERAPIST: It sounds like one of the best things about your previous course of therapy was that you really felt understood by your therapist.

HÉCTOR: Yes, I was surprised that I felt so comfortable with him. I expected that my counselor would be a woman and I was a little hesitant about talking with a man at first. . . . I thought he might think of me as weak for seeking therapy.

THERAPIST: I think most of us go to therapy with expectations about our therapist. We might expect a therapist to be older or younger, male or female, or of a particular ethnicity. Depending on whether or not the therapist meets our expectations, we may be more or less comfortable, feel more or less understood. Did you have any expectations coming in today?

HÉCTOR: Honestly? I knew I was seeing a woman because of your name. And I wasn't sure of your ethnicity. But frankly, I didn't really expect to have a Latina therapist based on the providers I have seen at this center.

THERAPIST: Do you have any thoughts or concerns about working with me that you would like to talk about?

HÉCTOR: Not really . . .

THERAPIST: My hope is that we can work really well together, but it would be understandable if you didn't necessarily trust me or feel comfortable with me right off the bat. You don't know me at all, and it can be really difficult to open up to a stranger. Also, I know that for some people it might matter that I'm not Latina, I'm white. Sometimes that can make someone feel like I can't understand some kinds of experiences, like those related to being a minority or a person of color. But my goal is to do whatever I can to be sensitive to, and understanding of, your unique experiences. I bring some general expertise about anxiety to our work, including ways that experiences with discrimination can relate to anxiety, sometimes in subtle ways, but you are the expert on your own experience. So I will always try to check in with you about the ways in which the things we discuss and the suggestions I make fit with your experience. Please feel free to let me know if I say or do something insensitive, or if you feel like I am not fully understanding what you are telling me. I am definitely not perfect, but my intention is to try and help you as best I can achieve your goals for therapy.

The therapist ended the engagement session by providing some activities for Héctor to complete before the next session. First, she explained a monitoring form used throughout treatment (although the domains to monitor are changed over time as new session material is introduced, this version includes only date, situation, and worry topic as columns) and asked him to begin to notice when he engaged in worry. She also gave him a copy of the Valued Living Questionnaire to complete with the following instructions:

"Sometimes anxiety and worry can prevent us from taking some actions that are consistent with our values. For example, you mentioned that you skip class when you feel too anxious, even though you also noted that you care deeply about being a good student. Anxiety and worry can also make people feel as if they are on automatic pilot, or that their lives are consumed by things they *must* do rather than things they *choose* to do. This questionnaire is a first step toward identifying some of the ways in which anxiety and worry might be interfering with your life. Sometimes it is painful to think about the ways our lives are not as we would wish them to be.

But this awareness is a first step toward making a change. So, notice any feelings that arise as you fill out the forms, and we will be sure to talk about them next week."

Session 1

The goal of Session 1 is to provide an overview of the treatment structure (client and therapist roles, between-session assignments, etc.) and to plan and discuss the rationale for treatment that is informed by a personalized ABBT conceptualization of the client's presenting problems. The therapist asked Héctor to engage in an experiential exercise that involved imagining himself back in one of the anxiety-provoking situations he noted on his monitoring form. Using guided imagery, the therapist helped Héctor to notice that his experience of anxiety was characterized by an interrelated cycle of thoughts (worries), physiological sensations (tightness in his shoulders and chest), and behaviors (leaving class early, heading to the gym).

HÉCTOR: I didn't realize so much was happening when I am anxious. Usually as soon as I notice I am anxious I just do whatever I can to prevent it from escalating.

THERAPIST: That doesn't surprise me. You have developed a strong habit. When you get anxious, you immediately try and distract your attention from your experience and seek out ways to control or dampen your emotions. How difficult was it to imagine yourself back in class on Monday?

HÉCTOR: It was surprisingly easy. I definitely felt just as anxious remembering how I felt as I did sitting in the classroom.

THERAPIST: That is a great thing to notice. Something that is uniquely human is our ability to remember and imagine events vividly. Like other animals, we are hardwired to experience fear in the face of a threat—as if a predator were charging at us. But humans can also simply *imagine* a threat in their minds and experience the same hardwired response to threat. Do you have any idea what you were imagining in class that day?

HÉCTOR: On Monday, my mind just went from 0 to 100—I was barely aware of what I was thinking. But when we went through the exercise today, I noticed a series of pictures in my mind. First I thought, I am not prepared for class. Then I imagined the professor yelling at me, my classmates laughing at me, my family's disappointment . . .

THERAPIST: Hmm . . . if you imagined all those people rejecting you at the same time, it is not surprising that you would feel afraid. We are hardwired to seek social approval. If the entire academic community, your friends, and family all rejected you, you would have a pretty good reason for feeling afraid. Unfortunately, our minds don't distinguish present threats from imagined ones.

The therapist and Héctor discussed the model of fear, anxiety, and worry guiding ABBT for GAD. The therapist explained that fear and anxiety serve adaptive functions. Anxiety allows us to imagine future threats and prepare for them. Fear energizes us to avoid and escape danger. In both of these states, our attention narrowly focuses on the threat and our escape plan, blocking out other information.

Unfortunately, our ability to think, imagine (the future), and remember (the past) allows us to imagine endless threats and to respond with fear even when no threat is present (i.e., our mental representations develop the same emotional properties as the events themselves, leading us to respond to threats that do not exist in the environment). Moreover, although we are hardwired to escape or avoid threat, sometimes in order to do the things that matter to us, we have to approach situations that will likely elicit anxiety (e.g., allow ourselves to be vulnerable in order to gain intimacy, take a risk at work in order to successfully negotiate a challenge). Many of us respond to this conundrum by harshly judging our natural responses and doing everything in our power to avoid experiencing them.

The therapist and Héctor also discussed the function of worry. Although worry is associated with clear negative consequences (interferes with concentration, results in tension and fatigue), it too serves a function.

HÉCTOR: As much as my worry bothers me, in some ways, I am afraid to give it up. Sometimes it feels like the only thing I can do to control the uncontrollable.

THERAPIST: Interesting observation. Tell me more about that.

HÉCTOR: Well, sometimes it feel like if I stop worrying about my mother's health, she will have a heart attack. Or I believe that if I don't worry about a test, I won't actually study.

THERAPIST: Some people notice that worrying about minor, everyday matters takes their mind off more painful thoughts and emotions. Have you ever noticed anything like that?

HÉCTOR: (*beginning to tear up*) Sometimes I think worrying about tests, or being late to class, or what I should wear to a school event is the only thing that keeps me from noticing how lonely I am. Sometimes I feel like if I stopped worrying, I would become so sad and depressed I might never get out of bed.

Near the end of the session, the therapist summed up her conceptualization and plan for treatment.

"Anxiety and worry narrow our focus and pull our attention toward the future. This cycle happens outside of our awareness and can be difficult to change. In this treatment, we will use mindfulness skills to address this habit. Mindfulness increases and expands our present-moment focus and allows us to notice and break this cycle. We also have a tendency to judge and control our emotions because we think they are preventing us from having a satisfying life. In this treatment we will explore whether that reaction to our emotional responses is helpful or harmful, and we will consider alternative ways of responding. Finally, worry is anticipatory; thus, it prevents us from engaging in activities that could be threatening. But sometimes we want to approach these situations—especially if they will help us to live the kind of life we value. In this treatment, we will learn to become more flexible—to consider different behavioral responses—rather than automatically avoiding potentially anxiety-provoking situations."

At the end of Session 1, the therapist led Héctor in a mindfulness of breath exercise. She began by guiding him to notice the way he was sitting in the chair, then drew his attention to where he could feel his breath in his body. The therapist then guided Héctor to gently redirect his awareness back to the sensations of his inhalations and exhalations over the next several minutes, while deepening his breath, no matter how many times his mind wandered to other things. After the therapist and Héctor discussed his experience of this exercise, she asked him to practice it daily between sessions.

Session 2

Session 2 primarily focuses on an introduction to mindfulness. The therapist led Héctor in a mindfulness of breath exercise, then engaged him in a debriefing.

THERAPIST: What did you notice?

HÉCTOR: Well, I am pretty stressed out today. So the exercise didn't work as well as it did when I practiced this week.

THERAPIST: Tell me more about that. How are you defining "worked"?

HÉCTOR: I used the breathing almost every night this week to fall asleep. And it actually seemed to help. At least it calmed me down, so I could get to sleep quicker. But today, I just felt more stressed out.

THERAPIST: What is really interesting about that is that although there is no "goal" to mindfulness, sometimes we do start to expect that it will bring a certain state of being. But actually, this exercise is about noticing and accepting whatever state we are in. So we notice the focus of our attention, guide it to the breath, notice when it wanders, and guide it back. Sometimes that process can be pleasant and calming, but other times it can be frustrating and painful. But observing that process, whatever the process happens to be, is practicing mindfulness.

HÉCTOR: Really? I was certain I was supposed to try and relax.

THERAPIST: We are naturally goal-oriented beings. So our tendency is to look for the goal in mindfulness. Fortunately, mindfulness allows us to give up goals, at least for a moment, and just be. What else did you notice?

HÉCTOR: I couldn't keep my attention on my breath. It was all over the place. I am not sure I have the personality needed to be mindful.

THERAPIST: What a great observation. First, you noticed your attention was pulled in different directions. I'll bet that happens at other times in the day as well. It is useful to get to know just how busy our minds are.

HÉCTOR: I never thought of it like that. I guess it makes sense that I struggle to concentrate in class if I am having so many different thoughts all the time.

THERAPIST: Also, I didn't actually suggest that you should keep your attention on your breath. Just that you should notice where your attention is and continually guide it back to the breath. It is so interesting how quickly our minds judge whether we are doing something "right" or "wrong," isn't it?

HÉCTOR: (*laughing*) I sort of know what you are going to say here, but I also felt like I was breathing the wrong way. I kept breathing out of my mouth and it sounded so loud compared to your breath.

THERAPIST: (*smiling*) Great observation. If our minds are so judgmental about something as simple and natural as breathing, just imagine what judgmental thoughts are present when we are in class, at work, with friends. It sounds like you really used this exercise as an opportunity to get to know the habits of your mind.

The therapist also led Héctor in the Raisin Exercise, which simply involves the practice of eating one raisin mindfully. Following this exercise, she focused on the mindfulness skill of "beginners mind," essentially highlighting the ways in which "knowing" what to expect sometimes prevent us from accurately observing different experiences. The session ended with the therapist leading Héctor through a slightly modified progressive muscle relaxation that was aimed at helping him to practice observing sensations and letting go of tension (rather than reduce anxiety).

Session 3

The therapist began Session 3 with the Mindfulness of Sounds mindfulness exercise. Héctor was able to see the similarity between this practice and the Raisin Exercise in Session 2. Specifically, he noticed that it was difficult for his mind to observe the pitch, tone, and volume of the sounds around him without trying to label (a truck backing up) and judge ("That is loud and annoying") his experience. The therapist was careful to normalize this response and to highlight the utility of becoming aware of what we are all naturally inclined to do.

After reviewing Héctor's monitoring and mindfulness homework, the therapist introduced a new psychoeducational topic—the function of emotions. Héctor quickly provided an example of the ways in which emotions such as fear can serve a communicative function. He described an incident when he was walking home from the library late at night. Although he did not hear or see anything out of the ordinary, Héctor had a sense that he was in danger, so he took a number of precautionary steps: He took his headphones off, crossed the street to be in an environment with more lighting, and called his roommate on his cell phone. The next morning, Héctor read that there was a mugging the previous night on campus, and he was convinced that the fear signals he received protected him from being a victim. The therapist provided an example of the consequences of ignoring the messages our emotions provide.

THERAPIST: Imagine you are experiencing sadness and disappointment because your current job is not fulfilling. That sadness is uncomfortable, so you naturally want to get rid of it. You might spend your evenings zoning out watching television alone, trying to "relax," or you might start staying out late at night with friends, drinking and trying to have a good time so you don't notice that you're feeling sad in that area of your life. You might start finding reasons to miss work or start daydreaming when you're at work. These strategies are all aimed at reducing your sadness. And they might work in the short term, but none of them resolves the problem. What is worse is that those strategies might even create new problems as you start sleeping less, doing less well at work, and running into more conflicts at work. Even though you are doing everything you can to avoid feeling sad, the sadness is there for a reason. The first step to moving forward in that situation is noticing that you are feeling sad and recognizing that your work situation is eliciting these emotions. Only then can you decide what actions to take.

HÉCTOR: That makes sense. But what about the fear I feel when I think about asking a classmate to study with me?

THERAPIST: What do you think your fear is telling you in that situation?

HÉCTOR: That he might think up some excuse to reject me and say no.

THERAPIST: Absolutely. As humans we are hardwired to seek social support and approval. It can absolutely be risky to put ourselves out there to be accepted or rejected. But here is the thing. While it is important to acknowledge the message our emotions are sending, we don't always have to follow their advice. Emotions are associated with action tendencies—when we feel fear, we are prepared to flee, when we feel anger, we are prepared to fight. But our emotions

don't actually control our behavior. And often when we consider taking an action that could be really meaningful—opening up and appearing vulnerable to someone or taking on an academic challenge—our emotions will warn us that such a step is risky. In these cases, we need to acknowledge the message we are receiving, yet we can still choose to take the valued action.

HÉCTOR: I guess that makes sense. I certainly knew that moving away from my family and starting medical school was risky. I felt a lot of fear, but I did it anyways because it is important to my family that I succeed. My abuela [grandmother] always says courage is acting with heart. Being afraid, but doing something anyways, because of love or passion.

However, Héctor also struggled a bit as he tried to determine the function of his emotions in some other contexts.

HÉCTOR: I can see how emotions sometimes can serve a function. But other times the function seems much less clear to me. For example, I know a little test anxiety can be helpful and motivating, but why do I feel terrified some nights when I am studying. I get so scared and anxious that I become paralyzed. My problem is that most of the time I am confused by my emotions and their intensity.

THERAPIST: We make the distinction between what we call "clear" and "muddy" emotions. Clear emotions refer to when we have a very strong emotional response to a particular situation; for instance, we feel strong fear when a car approaches us on the street, which is what we might call a "clear" emotional response. Emotions that are complex, confusing, or too intense and long-lasting for the situation are what we call "muddy."

Together, Héctor and his therapist reviewed how failures in self-care (e.g., not getting enough sleep or eating well, not exercising regularly) increase the likelihood of muddy emotions. They also considered ways that worry (which involves the ability to imagine things that have not yet happened) and rumination (which involves repeatedly remembering past events) both can elicit emotions that are not at all related to whatever is unfolding in the present moment. Finally they discussed the way our "reactions to our reactions" can muddy our emotional responses.

"Another thing that can make our emotions confusing and muddied is that often when we have an emotional response, we don't just have that one response—we have a series of responses that are triggered by that first emotion. For instance, we may feel scared, then angry that we got scared, then afraid the feeling will grow stronger, then ashamed that we are afraid, and so on. We may also have thoughts that come up as responses to a clear emotion, such as "I shouldn't feel this way," "This is a sign that I am a weak person." One reaction that we often have is to try to control emotional responses. We will talk more about that in the next session. Finally, emotional responses can also seem much more intense when we start to feel defined by our emotions—when we see them as stable traits that represent our personality rather than natural human responses to events that come and go."

Normally Session 3 would end with a review of the first completed writing assignment (i.e., writing about how anxiety and worry interferes with relationships, work–school–household management, and self-nourishment and community involvement). However, Héctor admitted that he had not finished it. He noted that it had been a busy week with exams and that he found it hard to set aside time for himself. Together, Héctor and his therapist brainstormed ways he could schedule in the values writing. However, she also noted that sitting down and considering the ways that anxiety is interfering with the things that matter most could be a very painful exercise. The therapist suggested that Héctor recognize that the pain served a function (letting Héctor know that changes were needed for him to live a more personally fulfilling life), and she pointed out that seeking therapy was a sign that he acknowledged that pain and was willing to make some changes. The therapist also gave Héctor new monitoring forms that added a column for emotions, so he could begin to monitor his emotional responses in addition to his worry.

Session 4

Héctor presented to Session 4 visibly upset. He had just returned from a visit back home to Miami, and he was extremely upset over his interactions with his brother. As he began to describe the situation, the therapist gently interrupted.

"Excuse me for interrupting you, Héctor, but I have an important question. I can tell this visit was very upsetting for you and we will be sure to devote a good part of today's session to talking about it. But if you are willing, I would like us to start out our session as we always do, with a brief mindfulness practice. It can really be challenging to practice when you are experiencing a lot of emotions and thoughts, yet it can also be extremely helpful. If you are willing, I would like us to start by becoming aware of the physical sensations we are currently experiencing. I would like to hear about your visit, and then there is another mindfulness exercise that might help us further explore what you are feeling right now. Would that be all right with you?"

Héctor agreed and the therapist introduced a mindfulness exercise that involved increasing awareness of physical sensations. During the debriefing of the practice, Héctor admitted that he found it particularly challenging to keep redirecting his attention from images of his visit to his physical sensations in the moment. However, he noted that it became easier over time. The therapist remarked that Héctor seemed more centered than he had when he first walked in. Héctor replied that he did feel more present and ready to discuss his concerns.

THERAPIST: Did you use your monitoring sheet this weekend to help you work through some of the challenges that arose during your visit home?

HÉCTOR: Absolutely, I was so upset that I needed to get my thoughts down on paper. As I wrote here, on Saturday, when I was at my parent's house but only my brother and his sons were home, I was flooded with worries. My nephews used to be such sweet little boys, but now they will barely make eye contact with me when I greet them. They spend all their time glued to their electronic devices playing violent video games. And my brother completely ignores them—all he wants to do is talk to me about his latest dating adventures.

THERAPIST: Did you notice the specific worries you were experiencing?

HÉCTOR: Yes, I wrote I am worried that my brother and nephews are too much for my mother to handle. I am worried that they are draining her health and finances. I am worried that my nephews will not get a good education, and that they will get involved in the wrong crowd. And I am worried my brother is drinking too much and that he is too selfish.

THERAPIST: Good job observing your responses. How about your emotions? Were you able to identify what emotion or emotions were present?

HÉCTOR: I was very upset. Mostly angry I think. I don't know—this is one of those situations where I felt confused about my feelings.

The therapist suggested that Héctor try a mindfulness practice aimed at observing his emotional responses. She asked him to close his eyes and vividly imagine his interaction with his brother, and she instructed him to notice visual and auditory stimuli, to focus on the physical sensations in his body, to bring his attention to the thoughts running through his mind and finally to his emotions. She reminded him simply to notice his experience, bringing curiousness and compassion to what he was experiencing, observing what happened when he was feeling strong emotions, without altering or judging them. She reminded him to notice whether more than one emotion was present, and to observe any rise and fall in his emotions. After several moments, she asked him to open his eyes.

THERAPIST: What did you notice?

HÉCTOR: At first, all I felt was angry. Then I noticed I was feeling afraid. But what really surprised me is that I felt extremely sad. It's interesting because at the time I thought I was just straight up angry, but thinking back on it I noticed that my emotions seemed to ebb and flow. I guess another thing that was interesting is that I started out just feeling the emotions. But throughout the exercise I started to notice I was observing them. It was really helpful to get some distance—before that I think I just felt consumed with emotion.

THERAPIST: Great observations. Tell me a bit more about your responses to those emotions. And any thoughts you have about their function.

HÉCTOR: I think I felt angry because I disagree with how my brother is raising his sons. But then I got mad at myself for feeling angry. My brother hasn't had the opportunities that I have. Thinking about that made me feel guilty.

THERAPIST: Did you notice any responses to your feelings of guilt?

HÉCTOR: I hate feeling guilty. It feels like a tremendous weight on my chest. I think I tried to distract myself from that feeling and then I just started imagining all the problems that could result from my brother's screwups and I got consumed with fear and worry. But then, when you prompted me, I returned back to observing my emotions. And then the more I focused on my emotions, I started to realize I felt really, really sad. But what was interesting was I think I just accepted it was a sad situation. Usually I can't stand feeling sad, I am afraid it means I am going to get depressed and retreat into my own world. But I think I recognized that this is just a sad situation. I miss my family. I wish I could fix my brother's problems, but I can't.

The therapist tied Héctor's experience to the topic of clear and muddy emotions. She pointed out that anger is a natural response that arises when someone acts against your wishes. And sadness is a normal response to a painful situation. She also helped Héctor identify why his anger was initially so intense. In addition to being angry about the situation on Saturday, he was also having anger about the many times in the past when his brother upset him. Héctor was also imagining that his brother would continue to "screw up," which further fueled his anger. The "reactions to reactions" Héctor experienced also increased the intensity of his response. For example, when Héctor judged the feeling of anger as unacceptable, he started to feel guilty. And when the feeling of guilt was too painful, he distracted himself with multiple worries about the future.

Next, the therapist spent some time on the main concept of the session—the limits and consequence of internal control efforts. She asked Héctor to engage in a number of experiential exercises aimed at demonstrating the often paradoxical effects of efforts to control internal experiences such as thoughts, emotions, and images. For example, the therapist asked Héctor to imagine that he "had to get a good night's sleep" before a big test. She asked him what might happen if, alarmed by the late hour, he purposefully tried to induce a state of sleepiness. Héctor noted that this frequently happened, and the more he tried, the more distressed and awake he became.

Finally, the therapist spent some time going over Héctor's values assignment. Héctor easily identified many ways in which his anxiety was interfering with school and work. He noted that it was harder and harder to concentrate both during class and while doing his homework because his mind was consumed with worries—worries about failing class, about letting down his family, and about his family's health and well-being. Héctor also noted that when his anxiety about his family became too intense, he would call or plan a visit with them. But he found that when he did make the time to talk with or be with his family, he was consumed with worry about the time he was taking away from his schoolwork. Héctor wrote about his fear that he would never find a life partner. He was far too busy with school and his family to date, and he believed it was his destiny to end up alone. He was terrified about this possibility because he described himself as extremely family-oriented.

As the session ended, the therapist gave Héctor a monitoring form that added a column for "efforts to control," so that he could begin to notice these as they occurred throughout the week. She also provided for Héctor a second values assignment to complete for the next session. The therapist noted that often our attempts to avoid anxiety, worry, and stress cause us to make subtle shifts in our behavior, so that we begin doing whatever we are "supposed" to be doing and lose track of what we *want* to be doing, or what *personally matters* to us as individuals. The therapist reviewed the distinction between values and goals, emphasizing the importance of identifying the direction that Héctor wants to move in rather than solely the goals to achieve. The therapist noted that this next assignment was aimed at further exploring three areas of living to see what changes might be necessary to improve Héctor's quality of life.

"Choose two or three relationships that are important to you. You can either pick actual relationships (your relationship with your brother) or relationships you would like to have ("I would like to be part of a couple," "I would like to make more friends"). Briefly write about how you would like to be in those relationships. Think about how you would like to *communicate with others* (e.g., how open vs. private you would like to be, how direct vs. passive you would like to be in asking for what you need and in giving feedback to others). Think about *what sort of support you would like* from other people and *what sort of support you can give* without sacrificing your own self-care. I also would like you to write briefly about the sort of work you would like and *why that appeals to you*. Next write about the *student* you would like to be with respect to your work habits and your *relationships* with your professors and peers.

What is important to you about the *product of your work/studies*. How would you like to *communicate to others* about your work? How would you like to *respond to feedback*? What additional *challenges* would you like to take on? Finally, I would like you to briefly write about the ways in which you would like to spend your free time. What would you like to do to better nourish yourself (e.g., nutrition, exercise, spirituality) or contribute to your community?"

Sessions 5–7

In Sessions 5–7 of treatment, the focus is on encouraging the client to consider moving from a stance of resistance and avoidance to one of willingness. A number of mindfulness and other experiential exercises are used to help clients practice observing their thoughts, emotions, and physical sensations as transient events. For example, Héctor practiced imagining that his thoughts and feelings were going by on a movie screen in front of him. Once clients are able to defuse or decenter from their internal experiences, and they no longer feel defined or threatened by them, they are often more willing to approach and engage in a variety of activities.

Like many clients, Héctor initially struggled a bit with the concept of willingness. At first Héctor thought the therapist was suggesting that he should come to view his anxiety in a more positive light. Or that he should learn to accept his anxiety because it was what a "strong man" needed to do. Using a metaphor adapted from ACT, his therapist tried to clarify the concept of willingness, likening it to one's willingness to wade through a swamp on a journey to a beautiful mountain.

"Taking a stance of willingness suggests that you will accept and move forward with the thoughts and feelings (rational or irrational) that appear as you make your way through life, taking the actions that will help you obtain the things in life that you value. For instance, let's say that you want to ask your classmates if you can join their study group. To do so will likely elicit feelings of fear, thoughts about possible rejection. However, you can be willing to experience those thoughts and feelings, if they are what arise when you take actions consistent with your value to engage in your schoolwork. You may not like the feelings, you may wish it could be another way, but you can be willing to experience whatever comes up in order to take a valued action.

"It is as if you are on a journey to a beautiful mountain. But along the way you come to a disgusting, murky swamp. You don't want to walk through the swamp, and it may not seem fair that you need to do so. But you can choose to walk through if you decide that the journey to the mountain is worth it to you.

"Now if the swamp is to the side of your path, you do not necessarily need to go through it. And, you don't have to dive into the swamp and roll around in it. And you can put on boots, or walk across a plank, in an effort to avoid getting dirty. Yet you might still trip and fall in the swamp, and willingness means you accept that possibility as you move forward on the journey of your choosing."

Several values assignments are used to help clients set their course or mountain "journey." As noted earlier, Héctor was asked to write about his values in three specific domains. This can be a challenging assignment, and often clients confuse values with goals, describe values that suggest the need for control or perfection, or focus on what they perceive to be insurmountable obstacles to living consistently with their values. Thus, often several sessions are devoted to discussing the values assignment, and it is not uncommon for clients to revise their values multiple times in session and for homework. For example, Héctor's initial writing assignment produced some values that could have been problematic for him to pursue.

HÉCTOR: My value in the schoolwork domain is to achieve the highest grades in all of my coursework. I want to be the top student in my graduating class so that I can make my family proud.

THERAPIST: Would aiming to receive a perfect score on an exam be an example of a value or a goal?

HÉCTOR: Right, grades are outcomes, so I guess those are goals.

THERAPIST: Imagine that you are working as a physician. You are surfing the Internet and you stumble upon a webpage where patients rate, and leave comments about, their doctor. What would you want the page to say? My doctor scores well on standardized tests?

HÉCTOR: (chuckling) Well, no. I guess I would want them to say that I was caring and compassionate. And that I was willing to stick with a health problem

until I came up with the right diagnosis and the best treatment I could provide.

THERAPIST: Great, those sound a bit more like values. So, would it be fair to say you want to be engaged with the material you are learning? And that you want to be kind and compassionate toward your patients and committed to their health?

HÉCTOR: Yes, that is what I value. I keep thinking my grades matter most, but I know in my heart that is not why I am in medical school. I am not here to impress my instructors and classmates. I want to be a doctor who makes a difference in the lives of others.

Héctor also struggled a bit with articulating his relationship values:

HÉCTOR: I wrote that I always wanted to be available to my mother, whenever she needed me. I want to be her rock. I get so angry at myself when I am too tired to return her phone calls at night. Or when she needs something to be fixed, like the leaky faucet in the kitchen, and I can't take care of it because I am here in Boston and she is in Miami. Also, I feel bad when she is lonely. I want to prevent her from having to experience any more pain than she already has.

THERAPIST: I know you care deeply for your mother. And I can completely understand your desire to care for her. And yet, much like it is humanly impossible to prevent yourself from feeling emotions, I think it is humanly impossible to ensure that our loved ones are never in pain or in need. Even if you dropped out of medical school and moved back home, there are limits to what you can do for her. And that can be a very difficult and painful thing to accept. It sounds to me like the value is that you want to maintain a strong, caring relationship with your mother. Would you agree?

HÉCTOR: Absolutely.

THERAPIST: And fixing a faucet and returning a call are actions that are consistent with those values. Are there other actions you can take that reflect your values? In other words, if you are in Boston and she is in Miami, can you care for her without fixing her faucet?

HÉCTOR: Well, I could talk to her about it. She appreciates when I listen to her vent about her problems.

THERAPIST: Great, what else?

HÉCTOR: I guess I could call a repair man for her. Or ask my brother to help.

THERAPIST: Wonderful. The point is, there are many actions one can take that are consistent with a value. If we define valued action as just one or two responses, and for whatever reason, we can't respond in those ways, we can end up feeling stuck and miserable. Living consistently with one's values means flexibly considering multiple options to act in ways that are meaningful to us.

Héctor also struggled with articulating his values in relation to his brother and nephews:

HÉCTOR: I want to be close to my brother and his sons, but I can't. It doesn't matter how I treat them, they are selfish and they never want to spend time with me.

THERAPIST: One of the most complicated things about relationship values is that we only have control over half of the relationship. You cannot control how your brother acts; you can only choose how you want to approach him.

HÉCTOR: Are you saying I should just let my brother live his life the way he currently does? Allow him to raise his sons to be disrespectful and rude?

THERAPIST: It is so painful for you to watch your brother make choices that are inconsistent with your values. And I know if you could control his behavior you would. It seems like you keep trying and trying to figure out how to control a situation that just might be out of your control. Sometimes mindfulness skills can help us to clearly accept the reality of a situation. And by "accept" I mean recognize the reality of the situation—I don't mean that you should like or support his approach. But you may need to accept the reality that you only have control over some parts of this very painful situation. It seems to me that you can control how you choose to define your values regarding how you relate to your brother. But you can't control his behavior. If you act lovingly toward him and try to establish a close relationship, your brother may respond in kind. And that bond might allow you to talk with him about your parenting concerns. Or you might end up with a closer relationship and he could continue with his current habits. Or he may completely reject your efforts to become closer. Choosing our actions is like aiming an arrow. We can make choices about how we aim and when we release the arrow. We don't have control over where the arrow lands. However, we may notice where it lands and use that information to inform the way we aim or when we shoot the next time. In a similar way, we can choose the actions we want to take repeatedly, although we don't have control over the consequences of our actions.

Héctor continued to work on defining his values, until he felt that he could clearly articulate what mattered to him in the domains of relationship, schoolwork, self-nourishment, and community involvement. Although it is necessary for clients to achieve this milestone so that they can move into the next phase of treatment, it is important to recognize that values articulation is a dynamic process. Having defined values is helpful in guiding the final nine sessions of treatment, but what is most important is for clients to adopt the general perspective that valuing can provide a compass for directing behavior and improving quality of life.

During these sessions, Héctor was given a final version of the monitoring form that represented an application of the full model. This included columns for date/time, situation, first reactions (thoughts, feelings, sensations), second reactions (efforts to control, muddiness, willingness, acceptance), and actions/responses (e.g., avoidance, valued action, application of mindfulness skills).

Sessions 8–12

The goal of Sessions 8–12 was to personalize the concepts introduced in the first phase of treatment and help Héctor to apply mindfulness and engagement in valued activities to his daily life. At the beginning of each session, Héctor and the therapist worked together to pick a mindfulness practice. Each week they purposely chose exercises, including ones that Héctor found particularly challenging, those he found most useful, and those that seemed to best fit his needs given the particular struggle he was facing (see Table 5.1).

The bulk of these sessions were focused using the mindfulness and acceptance strategies introduced during Phase I to increase Héctor's willingness to engage in his personally articulated valued actions. Héctor continued to monitor valued actions taken, missed opportunities, mindfulness and obstacles to willingness (see Figure 5.1).

TABLE 5.1. Choosing a Mindfulness Practice

Title	Focus of attention	How it can be helpful	Where to find it
Mindfulness of breath	Breath	• Portable • Can be centering • Great introduction to the habits of the mind (busy, judgmental)	MP3 available online at *www.themindful-waythroughanxietybook.com*; Kabat-Zinn (1990); Roemer & Orsillo (2009); Orsillo & Roemer (2011)
Mindfulness of sounds	Sounds	• Helps us to notice our tendency to categorize/judge • Allows us to practice "beginner's mind"—seeing things fully as they are, not as we imagine they will be	MP3 available online; Segal et al. (2002); Roemer & Orsillo (2009); Orsillo & Roemer (2011)
3-minute breathing space	Physical sensations (including breath), thoughts, emotions	• Helps us get centered and present when moving from one activity to another • Useful when we want to "check in" with ourselves	Segal et al. (2002); Roemer & Orsillo (2009); Orsillo & Roemer (2011)
Mindfulness of physical sensations	Physical sensations	• Good practice for bringing curiosity and compassion to physical sensations that are typically feared and avoided • Brings awareness to sensations in the body, without judgment or avoidance	MP3 available online; Orsillo & Roemer (2011)
Mindful progressive relaxation	Muscle tension/ relaxation	• Increases awareness of the sensations of tension and relaxation • Concrete way to practice "letting go" • May elicit a relaxed state	MP3 available online; Orsillo & Roemer (2011)
Mindfulness of emotions and physical sensations	Emotions and/ or accompanying physical sensations	• Increases awareness of the full range of emotions present • Helpful when generally distressed or confused • Useful for evaluating clear and muddy emotions	MP3 available online; Orsillo & Roemer (2011)
Mindfulness of clouds and sky	Thoughts and feelings, imagery	• Allows practice of viewing thoughts and feelings as transient and separate from self • Helps with decentering/defusion	MP3 available online; Roemer & Orsillo (2009); Orsillo & Roemer (2011)
Inviting a difficulty in and working it through the body	Physical sensations related to painful experience	• Helps to cultivate willingness to experience painful emotions • Useful first step when a client is struggling against accepting a painful reality	MP3 available online; Williams et al. (2007); Roemer & Orsillo (2009); Orsillo & Roemer (2011)
Your personal experience with self-compassion/ Mindful observation of self-critical thoughts	Self-critical thoughts	• Brings awareness to experiences of criticism in the past and the present • Helps to identify barriers to self-compassion	MP3 available online; Orsillo & Roemer (2011)

(continued)

TABLE 5.1. *(continued)*

Title	Focus of attention	How it can be helpful	Where to find it
Mountain meditation	Mountain imagery—transience of events external to the mountain	• Uses the image of a mountain to promote the experience of thoughts, feelings, and emotions as changing and impermanent • Particularly helpful for cultivating a sense of inner strength or stability, even in the face of distress and reactivity	MP3 available online; Kabat-Zinn (1995); Roemer & Orsillo (2009); Orsillo & Roemer (2011)

For example, in Session 10, Héctor shared that he had missed an opportunity to engage in a valued action. Specifically, one of his favorite instructors had offered to meet with Héctor to discuss the process of selecting rotations, but Héctor had cancelled the appointment.

THERAPIST: What did you notice about your response to his offer?

HÉCTOR: At first I was excited, but as time went on I became more and more anxious.

THERAPIST: Can you identify the clear emotions that arose?

HÉCTOR: I actually used the Mindfulness of Emotion exercise to sort this out a bit. I felt excited about taking the next step in my education, happy that my in-

---

VALUED ACTIVITY LOG

Please complete this form at the end of each day.

This week, at the end of each day we would like you to think about an action that you took that was consistent with one of your values or an opportunity that you missed to take an action consistent with your value. Briefly describe the action and mark T for taken or M for missed.

On a scale of 0–100 rate how mindful you were during the action or the missed opportunity.

Note any obstacles that you noticed that stopped you from taking action (or could have).

There are no right or wrong answers to this assignment—we all choose not to engage in valued actions for a variety of reasons. This is just a way for us to start to get a better sense of what may be getting in the way for you so that you can make choices as to how you would like to proceed.

Date	Action	Taken (T) or missed (M)	Mindfulness (0–100)	Obstacles

FIGURE 5.1. Values Monitoring Form.

structor singled me out, and nervous about the challenges that lie ahead for me in my career.

THERAPIST: Excellent. Were you also able to observe your reaction to your reactions?

HÉCTOR: Honestly, not until today. I think at the time I just got caught up in my reactions rather than observing them. But during the mindfulness practice today I noticed some of the same old responses I always have. I was afraid to feel good about myself, and my prospects for the future. I had that same sense that worrying about what could go wrong was what I needed to do to ensure that I don't mess up. I also became pretty critical and judgmental about my anxiety.

THERAPIST: What do you think you could have done differently?

HÉCTOR: I have become kind of lax when it comes to filling out the monitoring forms. But I was thinking about what you said last week. I do think that the process of physically completing the form in the midst of my distress can help me to take a pause . . . and remember some of my skills.

Session 11 brought a more challenging issue into therapy. Héctor was extremely distressed over an interaction he had with a university security officer. Héctor was on his way back home from a long night studying when he was approached by a security officer and asked to produce his university identification card. Although it was close to midnight, Héctor observed at least five other students crossing the campus, yet he was the only one who was questioned. Héctor was already sensitive to the fact that he had been the only person of color in the library that night. He was stressed out over exams, missing his family and friends, and frankly tired of dealing with the subtle and obvious discrimination he encountered on a daily basis. Thus, he refused to produce his identification card and reported that he "lost" it and shouted at the officer. Although the situation was eventually sorted out, Héctor was angry, embarrassed over his behavior in the situation, and confused.

HÉCTOR: I am really struggling with this incident. My mind is racing, I feel tense all over and I can't sort out what is clear and what is muddy and, more importantly, what valued action I could have chosen.

THERAPIST: It is natural to experience a rush of conflicting thoughts and emotions in such a painful en-

counter. I am so sorry that, given the racism inherent in our society, you are subjected to differential treatment because of how you look. This structural problem exists outside of you and isn't your fault. And I really understand how the pain and the anger can build up when you have to deal with things like this all the time. I certainly don't want to suggest that you have to change who you are, when the system needs changing. However, I would like us to work with this situation to help you find an effective way of dealing with this kind of thing because we both know that racism isn't going to go away immediately, and that means you have to make choices about how you want to respond. If you are willing, let's spend some time with a mindfulness practice to see if that helps us gain some clarity.

HÉCTOR: I don't feel very open right now, but I do think "Inviting a Difficulty In and Working with It through the Body" (see Figure 5.2) could be a first step.

Following the exercise, Héctor appeared more settled, although he also had tears in his eyes.

THERAPIST: What did you notice?

HÉCTOR: It was pretty easy to locate the tension—it was in the pit of my stomach. But I really struggled with opening up to it. My first response was "I don't want to let go off the struggle against racism. Why should I accept it"? But then I remembered the last time we did this exercise. And I reminded myself that I only had to be open to the present moment. I remembered that acceptance didn't mean resigning myself to a situation. Instead, I focused on accepting that the incident had occurred and that I was rigidly holding tension in my body.

THERAPIST: I am really impressed that you were able to do that. What happened next?

HÉCTOR: I continued to breathe into my stomach and I worked on letting go of my tension. Once my body became more relaxed I turned my attention to my thoughts about the incident.

THERAPIST: And what did you observe?

HÉCTOR: I had thoughts about racism and how unjust it is for people to be treated differently based on their appearance. I felt angry, which I think was a clear emotion, but then I started to feel ashamed of my behavior.

THERAPIST: Was that reaction clear or muddy?

Before you begin this exercise, think of a difficulty you're experiencing right now. It doesn't have to be a significant difficulty, but choose something that you find unpleasant, something that is unresolved. It may be something you are worried about, an argument or misunderstanding you've had, something you feel angry, resentful, guilty, or frustrated about. If nothing is going on right now, think of some time in the recent past when you felt scared, worried, frustrated, resentful, angry, or guilty, and use that.

Noticing the way you are sitting in the chair or on the floor. Noticing where your body is touching the chair or floor. Bringing you attention to your breath for a moment. Noticing the in-breath . . . and the out-breath. . . . Now gently widening your awareness, take in the body as a whole. Noticing any sensations that arise, breathing with your whole body.

When you are ready, bringing to mind whatever situation has been bringing up difficult emotions for you. Bringing your attention to the specific emotions that arise and any reactions you have to those emotions. And as you are focusing on this troubling situation and your emotional reaction, allowing yourself to tune in to any ***physical sensations*** in the body that you notice are arising . . . becoming aware of those physical sensations . . . and then deliberately, but gently, directing your focus of attention to the region of the body where the sensations are the strongest in the gesture of an embrace, a welcoming . . . noticing that this is how it is right now . . . and ***breathing into that part of the body*** on the in-breath and breathing out from that region on the out-breath, exploring the sensations, watching their intensity shift up and down from one moment to the next.

Now, seeing if you can bring to this attention an even deeper attitude of compassion and openness to whatever sensations, thoughts, or emotions you are experiencing, however unpleasant, by saying to yourself from time to time, "It's OK. Whatever it is, it's already here. Let me open to it."

Staying with the awareness of these internal sensations, breathing with them, accepting them, letting them be, and allowing them to be just as they are. Saying to yourself again, if you find it helpful, "It's here right now. Whatever it is, it's already here. Let me be open to it." Softening and opening to the sensation you become aware of, letting go of any tensing and bracing. If you like, you can also experiment with holding in awareness both the sensations of the body and the feeling of the breath moving in and out as you breathe with the sensations moment by moment.

And when you notice that the bodily sensations are no longer pulling your attention to the same degree, simply return 100% to the breath and continue with that as the primary object of attention. And then gently bringing your awareness to the way you are sitting in the chair, your breath, and, when you are ready, opening your eyes.

FIGURE 5.2. Inviting a difficulty in and working with it through the body. From Williams, Teasdale, Segal, and Kabat-Zinn (2007, pp. 151–152). Copyright 2007 by The Guilford Press. Adapted by permission.

HÉCTOR: Well, I think a bit of both. I definitely was able to bring some compassion to myself. No one wants to be treated differently based on his/her appearance.

THERAPIST: That is great. I know it is not easy for you to take a compassionate stance toward your thoughts and actions. What do you think was clear about the response?

HÉCTOR: I am ashamed of my behavior. It is inconsistent with my values to treat anyone the way I treated that officer, even if he/she deserves it. Frankly, I don't care what he thinks of me, but I care what I think about myself.

THERAPIST: It sounds like you said and did some things that were inconsistent with your values. I wonder, though, if you can bring some compassion to yourself for that. Although we intend to behave consistently with our values, we all have lapses. This was a highly charged situation, and you were vulnerable going into it. The important thing is that you are now even more aware of your values. Are there any consistent actions you can take this week?

HÉCTOR: This incident made me realize that my values have been a bit too off balance lately. I have been paying a lot of attention to the schoolwork domain and a pretty good amount of attention to the relationship domain, but I think I need to take some actions consistent with my values regarding self-nourishment and community. At the beginning of the semester I grabbed a flyer for the Latino Medical Student Association, and I think I am going to contact them to see if there are some activities I can get involved with.

THERAPIST: That sounds great.

HÉCTOR: I also think I might try and meet with someone from campus security. I think I want to apologize for my behavior, but I also want to talk to them about cultural sensitivity training. And don't worry, I didn't forget about the arrow thing we talked about a few weeks ago. I can only aim the arrow; I can't control where it lands. I know I might not change their practices, but these actions are consistent with my values.

Sessions 13–16

Héctor completed a treatment reflection writing assignment that set the stage for the final four sessions of therapy. He identified a few specific valued actions that he wanted to take before the end of therapy. He also recognized that although he was maintaining a pretty steady formal mindfulness practice, he had paid less attention to informal mindfulness. Héctor also had made great gains in increasing his self-compassion, but he felt that he needed more practice while he still had the support of therapy.

Thus, Sessions 13–15 continued to follow the structure of Sessions 8–11, but with added attention to issues of maintenance. The therapist become less and less directive throughout this time, allowing Héctor to address obstacles and experience success himself. During this time, Hector began to date and expand his social network, feel more satisfied with his relationships with his family members, and find more success and satisfaction in his schoolwork.

During the final session, the therapist predicted that there would be times when Héctor would feel overwhelmed by emotion, drift away from his mindfulness practice, and lose sight of his values, despite all the notable gains he reported. She described these "lapses" as a natural part of the process of life and helped Héctor to make plans for how to cope. Specifically, she suggested that he review the handouts in his binder, begin self-monitoring again, increase or reengage in mindfulness practice, and consider doing some values writing. The therapist and Héctor collaboratively developed a personalized list of elements that were particularly helpful for him and added that list to his binder. Héctor expressed sadness at saying good-bye to his therapist, and also excitement at feeling able to continue his progress on his own and use the time allocated to therapy to engage in other valued actions moving forward.

CONCLUSION

Evidence suggests that this ABBT for GAD can target symptoms of GAD, comorbid presenting problems, and proposed mechanisms that underlie these clinical presentations, while helping clients to engage in their lives in satisfying ways. This chapter has presented a conceptual basis for this treatment, as well as guidelines for its flexible application, while remaining responsive to the specific context of a given client. More research is needed to better understand mechanisms and processes of change, as well as how to disseminate this treatment in community and primary care settings.

ACKNOWLEDGMENTS

We thank the therapists, students, and clients we have worked with over the years for all they have taught us, as well as National Institutes of Health for funding our work (Grant No. MH074589). We also thank Dave Barlow, Tim Brown, Bonnie Brown, and the staff at the Center for Anxiety and Related Disorders for supporting our research over the past 10 years. We dedicate this chapter to Tom Borkovec, whose seminal work in the treatment of GAD is the sturdy foundation on which our work stands.

NOTE

1. Audio recordings of this exercise, as well as other mindfulness exercises we use, are available at *www.mindfulwaythroughanxietybook.com*. Scripts for many of these mindfulness exercises are available in Roemer and Orsillo (2009) and Orsillo and Roemer (2011).

REFERENCES

American Psychiatric Association. (1994). *Diagnostic and statistical manual of mental disorders* (4th ed.). Washington, DC: Author.

American Psychiatric Association. (2013). *Diagnostic and statistical manual of mental disorders* (5th ed.). Arlington, VA: Author.

Andrews, G., Hobbs, M. J., Borkovec, T. D., Beesdo, K., Craske, M. G., Heimberg, R. G., et al. (2010). Generalized worry disorder: A review of DSM-IV generalized anxiety disorder and options for DSM-V. *Depression and Anxiety, 27*(2), 134–147.

Arch, J. J., Eifert, G. H., Davies, C., Vilardaga, J. C. P., Rose, R. D., & Craske, M. G. (2012). Randomized clinical trial of cognitive behavioral therapy (CBT) versus acceptance and commitment therapy (ACT) for mixed anxiety disorders. *Journal of Consulting and Clinical Psychology, 80*(5), 750–765.

Ballenger, J. C., Davidson, J. R. T., Lecrubier, Y., Nutt, D. J., Borkovec, T. D., Rickels, K., et al. (2001). Consensus statement on generalized anxiety disorder from the international consensus group on depression and anxiety. *Journal of Clinical Psychiatry, 62*, 53–58.

Behar, E., DiMarco, I. D., Hekler, E. B., Mohlman, J., & Staples, A. M. (2009). Current theoretical models of generalized anxiety disorder (GAD): Conceptual review and treatment implications. *Journal of Anxiety Disorders, 23*(8), 1011–1023.

Belanger, L., Ladouceur, R., & Morin, C. M. (2005). Generalized anxiety disorder and health care use. *Canadian Family Physician, 51*(10), 1362–1363.

Blevins, D., Roca, J. V., & Spencer, T. (2011). Life guard: Evaluation of an ACT-based workshop to facilitate reintegration of OIF/OEF veterans. *Professional Psychology: Research and Practice, 42*(1), 32–39.

Bond, F. W., Hayes, S. C., Baer, R. A., Carpenter, K. M., Guenole, N., Orcutt, H. K., et al. (2011). Preliminary psychometric properties of the Acceptance and Action Questionnaire–II: A revised measure of psychological inflexibility and experiential avoidance. *Behavior Therapy, 42*, 676–688.

Borkovec, T. D., Alcaine, O. M., & Behar, E. (2004). Avoidance theory of worry and generalized anxiety disorder. In R. G. Heimberg, C. L. Turk, & D. S. Mennin (Eds.), *Generalized anxiety disorder: Advances in research and practice.* (pp. 77–108). New York: Guilford Press.

Borkovec, T. D., & Costello, E. (1993). Efficacy of applied relaxation and cognitive-behavioral therapy in the treatment of generalized anxiety disorder. *Journal of Consulting and Clinical Psychology, 61*(4), 611–619.

Borkovec, T. D., & Hu, S. (1990). The effect of worry on cardiovascular response to phobic imagery. *Behaviour Research and Therapy, 28*(1), 69–73.

Borkovec, T. D., & Roemer, L. (1995). Perceived functions of worry among generalized anxiety disorder subjects: Distraction from more emotionally distressing topics? *Journal of Behavior Therapy and Experimental Psychiatry, 26*(1), 25–30.

Borkovec, T. D., & Ruscio, A. M. (2001). Psychotherapy for generalized anxiety disorder. *Journal of Clinical Psychiatry, 62*, 37–42.

Borkovec, T. D., & Sharpless, B. (2004). Generalized anxiety disorder: Bringing cognitive-behavioral therapy into the valued present. In S. C. Hayes, V. M. Follette, & M. M. Linehan (Eds.), *Mindfulness and acceptance: Expanding the cognitive-behavioral tradition* (pp. 209–242). New York: Guilford Press.

Brown, L. A., Forman, E. M., Herbert, J. D., Hoffman, K. L., Yuen, E. K., & Goetter, E. M. (2011). A randomized controlled trial of acceptance-based behavior therapy and cognitive therapy for test anxiety: A pilot study. *Behavior Modification, 35*(1), 31–53.

Bruce, S. E., Machan, J. T., Dyck, I., & Keller, M. B. (2001). Infrequency of "pure" GAD: Impact of psychiatric comorbidity on clinical course. *Depression and Anxiety, 14*(4), 219–225.

Chodron, P. (2007). *Practicing peace in times of war.* Boston: Shambhala.

Cisler, J. M., & Koster, E. H. W. (2010). Mechanisms of attentional biases towards threat in anxiety disorders: An integrative review. *Clinical Psychology Review, 30*(2), 203–216.

Covin, R., Ouimet, A. J., Seeds, P. M., & Dozois, D. J. A. (2008). A meta-analysis of CBT for pathological worry among clients with GAD. *Journal of Anxiety Disorders, 22*(1), 108–116.

Davidson, J. R. T., Bose, A., Korotzer, A., & Zheng, H. (2004). Escitalopram in the treatment of generalized anxiety disorder: Double-blind, placebo controlled, flexible-dose study. *Depression and Anxiety, 19*(4), 234–240.

Dimidjian, S., & Linehan, M. M. (2009). Mindfulness practice. In W. T. O'Donohue & J. E. Fisher (Eds.), *General principles and empirically supported techniques of cognitive behavior therapy* (pp. 425–434). Hoboken, NJ: Wiley.

Di Nardo, P. A., Brown, T. A., & Barlow, D. H. (1994). *Anxiety Disorders Interview Schedule for DSM-IV.* Albany, NY: Graywind.

Dugas, M. J., Brillon, P., Savard, P., Turcotte, J., Gaudet, A., Ladouceur, R., et al. (2010). A randomized clinical trial of cognitive-behavioral therapy and applied relaxation for adults with generalized anxiety disorder. *Behavior Therapy, 41*(1), 46–58.

Etkin, A., & Schatzberg, A. F. (2011). Common abnormalities and disorder-specific compensation during implicit regulation of emotional processing in generalized anxiety and major depressive disorders. *American Journal of Psychiatry, 168*(9), 968–978.

Evans, S., Ferrando, S., Findler, M., Stowell, C., Smart, C., & Haglin, D. (2008). Mindfulness-based cognitive therapy for generalized anxiety disorder. *Journal of Anxiety Disorders, 22*(4), 716–721.

Fuchs, C., Lee, J. K., Roemer, L., & Orsillo, S. M. (2013). Using mindfulness- and acceptance-based treatments with clients from nondominant and/or marginalized backgrounds: Clinical considerations, meta-analysis findings, and introduction to the special series. *Cognitive and Behavioral Practice, 20*(1), 1–12.

Fuchs, C., West, L. M., Graham, J. R., Hayes-Skelton, S. A., Orsillo, S. M., & Roemer, L. (2012, April). *Exploring the acceptability of mindfulness-based treatment among individuals from non-dominant cultural backgrounds*. In J. R. Graham (Chair), Examining Mindfulness and Anxiety across Diverse Methods and Contexts Symposium presented at the annual meeting of the Anxiety Disorders Association of America, Arlington, VA.

Gelenberg, A. J., Lydiard, R. B., Rudolph, R. L., Aguiar, L., Haskins, J. T., & Salinas, E. (2000). Efficacy of venlafaxine extended-release capsules in nondepressed outpatients with generalized anxiety disorder: A 6-month randomized controlled trial. *Journal of the American Medical Association, 283*(23), 3082–3088.

Gentes, E. L., & Ruscio, A. M. (2011). A meta-analysis of the relation of intolerance of uncertainty to symptoms of generalized anxiety disorder, major depressive disorder, and obsessive–compulsive disorder. *Clinical Psychology Review, 31*(6), 923–933.

Germer, C. K. (2005). Anxiety disorders: Befriending fear. In C. K. Germer, R. D. Siegel, & P. R. Fulton (Eds.), *Mindfulness and psychotherapy* (pp. 152–172). New York: Guilford Press.

Gratz, K. L., & Roemer, L. (2004). Multidimensional assessment of emotion regulation and dysregulation: Development, factor structure, and initial validation of the Difficulties in Emotion Regulation Scale. *Journal of Psychopathology and Behavioral Assessment, 26*(1), 41–54.

Gross, J. J. (2002). Emotion regulation: Affective, cognitive, and social consequences. *Psychophysiology, 39*(3), 281–291.

Gross, J. J., & Levenson, R. W. (1997). Hiding feelings: The acute effects of inhibiting negative and positive emotion. *Journal of Abnormal Psychology, 106*(1), 95–103.

Hayes, S. A., Orsillo, S. M., & Roemer, L. (2010). Changes in proposed mechanisms of action during an acceptance-based behavior therapy for generalized anxiety disorder. *Behaviour Research and Therapy, 48*(3), 238–245.

Hayes, S. C., Strosahl, K. D., & Wilson, K. G. (2012). *Acceptance and commitment therapy: The process and practice of mindful change* (2nd ed.). New York: Guilford Press.

Hayes, S. C., Wilson, K. G., Gifford, E. V., Follette, V. M., & Strosahl, K. (1996). Experiential avoidance and behavioral disorders: A functional dimensional approach to diagnosis and treatment. *Journal of Consulting and Clinical Psychology, 64*(6), 1152–1168.

Hayes-Skelton, S. A., Roemer, L., & Orsillo, S. M. (2013). A randomized clinical trial comparing an acceptance based behavior therapy to applied relaxation for generalized anxiety disorder. *Journal of Consulting and Clinical Psychology, 81*(5), 761–773.

Hays, P. A. (2008). *Addressing cultural complexities in practice: Assessment, diagnosis, and therapy* (2nd ed.). Washington, DC: American Psychological Association.

Heatherington, L., Harrington, N. T., Harrington, J., Neimeyer, K. F., Weinberg, S. C., & Friedlander, M. L. (2013). *Applying group cognitive behavior therapy for anxiety disorders in community settings: Retention, outcome, and clinical considerations*. Manuscript under review.

Heuzenroeder, L., Donnelly, M., Haby, M. M., Mihalopoulos, C., Rossell, R., Carter, R., et al. (2004). Cost-effectiveness of psychological and pharmacological interventions for generalized anxiety disorder and panic disorder. *Australian and New Zealand Journal of Psychiatry, 38*(8), 602–612.

Hidalgo, R. B., Tupler, L. A., & Davidson, J. R. T. (2007). An effect-size analysis of pharmacologic treatments for generalized anxiety disorder. *Journal of Psychopharmacology, 21*(8), 864–872.

Hoffman, D. L., Dukes, E. M., & Wittchen, H. (2008). Human and economic burden of generalized anxiety disorder. *Depression and Anxiety, 25*(1), 72–90.

Issakidis, C., Sanderson, K., Corry, J., Andrews, G., & Lapsley, H. (2004). Modelling the population cost-effectiveness of current and evidence-based optimal treatment for anxiety disorders. *Psychological Medicine, 34*(1), 19–35.

Kabat-Zinn, J. (1990). *Full catastrophe living: Using the wisdom of your body and mind to face stress, pain, and illness*. New York: Delta.

Kabat-Zinn, J. (1995). *Wherever you go there you are: Mindfulness meditation in everyday life*. New York: Hyperion.

Kabat-Zinn, J. (2003). Mindfulness-based interventions in context: Past, present, and future. *Clinical Psychology: Science and Practice, 10*(2), 144–156.

Katzman, M. A. (2009). Current considerations in the treatment of generalized anxiety disorder. *CNS Drugs, 23*(2), 103–120.

Kennedy, B. L., & Schwab, J. J. (1997). Utilization of medical specialists by anxiety disorder patients. *Psychosomatics, 38*(2), 109–112.

Kessler, R. C., Berglund, P., Demler, O., Jin, R., Merikangas, K. R., & Walters, E. E. (2005). Lifetime prevalence and age-of-onset distributions of DSM-IV disorders in the National Comorbidity Survey Replication. *Archives of General Psychiatry, 62*(6), 593–602.

Kocovski, N. L., Fleming, J. E., & Rector, N. A. (2009). Mindfulness and acceptance-based group therapy for social anxiety disorder: An open trial. *Cognitive and Behavioral Practice, 16*(3), 276–289.

Ladouceur, R., Gosselin, P., & Dugas, M. J. (2000). Experimental manipulation of intolerance of uncertainty: A study of a theoretical model of worry. *Behaviour Research and Therapy, 38*(9), 933–941.

Lee, J. K., Fuchs, C., Roemer, L., & Orsillo, S. M. (2009). Cultural considerations in acceptance-based behavior therapies. In L. Roemer & S. M. Orsillo (Eds.), *Mindfulness- and acceptance-based behavioral therapies in practice* (pp. 215–228). New York: Guilford Press.

Lee, J. K., Orsillo, S. M., Roemer, L., & Allen, L. B. (2010). Distress and avoidance in generalized anxiety disorder: Exploring the relationships with intolerance of uncertainty and worry. *Cognitive Behaviour Therapy, 39*(2), 126–136.

Levitt, J. T., Brown, T. A., Orsillo, S. M., & Barlow, D. H. (2004). The effects of acceptance versus suppression of emotion on subjective and psychophysiological response to carbon dioxide challenge in patients with panic disorder. *Behavior Therapy, 35*(4), 747–766.

Linehan, M. M. (1993). *Cognitive-behavioral treatment of borderline personality disorder.* New York: Guilford Press.

Logue, M. B., Thomas, A. M., Barbee, J. G., & Hoehn-Saric, R. (1993). Generalized anxiety disorder patients seek evaluation for cardiological symptoms at the same frequency as patients with panic disorder. *Journal of Psychiatric Research, 27*(1), 55–59.

Lovibond, S. H., & Lovibond, P. F. (1995). *Manual for the Depression Anxiety Stress Scales.* Sydney: Psychology Foundation of Australia.

Marten, P. A., Brown, T. A., Barlow, D. H., Borkovec, T. D., Shear, M. K., & Lydiard, R. B. (1993). Evaluation of the ratings comprising the associated symptom criterion of DSM-III-R generalized anxiety disorder. *Journal of Nervous and Mental Disease, 181*(11), 676–682.

Mennin, D. S., & Fresco, D. M. (2014). Emotion regulation therapy. In J. J. Gross (Ed.), *Handbook of emotion regulation* (2nd ed., pp. 469–490). New York: Guilford Press.

Mennin, D. S., Holaway, R. M., Fresco, D. M., Moore, M. T., & Heimberg, R. G. (2007). Delineating components of emotion and its dysregulation in anxiety and mood psychopathology. *Behavior Therapy, 38*(3), 284–302.

Meyer, T. J., Miller, M. L., Metzger, R. L., & Borkovec, T. D. (1990). Development and validation of the Penn State Worry Questionnaire. *Behaviour Research and Therapy, 28*(6), 487–495.

Michelson, S. E., Lee, J. K., Orsillo, S. M., & Roemer, L. (2011). The role of values-consistent behavior in generalized anxiety disorder. *Depression and Anxiety, 28*(5), 358–366.

Mussell, M., Kroenke, K., Spitzer, R. L., Williams, J. B. W., Herzog, W., & Löwe, B. (2008). Gastrointestinal symptoms in primary care: Prevalence and association with depression and anxiety. *Journal of Psychosomatic Research, 64*(6), 605–612.

Najmi, S., & Wegner, D. M. (2008). Thought suppression and psychopathology. In A. J. Elliot (Ed.), *Handbook of approach and avoidance motivation* (pp. 447–459). New York: Psychology Press.

Neff, K. D. (2003). The development and validation of a scale to measure self-compassion. *Self and Identity, 2*(3), 223–250.

Newman, M. G., Castonguay, L. G., Borkovec, T. D., Fisher, A. J., Boswell, J. F., Szkodny, L. E., et al. (2011). A randomized controlled trial of cognitive-behavioral therapy for generalized anxiety disorder with integrated techniques from emotion-focused and interpersonal therapies. *Journal of Consulting and Clinical Psychology, 79*(2), 171–181.

Nhat Hanh, T. (1992). *Peace is every step: The path of mindfulness in everyday life.* New York: Bantam Books.

Olatunji, B. O., & Wolitzky-Taylor, K. B. (2009). Anxiety sensitivity and the anxiety disorders: A meta-analytic review and synthesis. *Psychological Bulletin, 135*(6), 974–999.

Orsillo, S. M., & Roemer, L. (2011). *The mindful way through anxiety: Break free from chronic worry and reclaim your life.* New York: Guilford Press.

Orsillo, S. M., Roemer, L., & Barlow, D. H. (2003). Integrating acceptance and mindfulness into existing cognitive-behavioral treatment for GAD: A case study. *Cognitive and Behavioral Practice, 10*(3), 222–230.

Orsillo, S.M., Roemer, L., & Salters-Pedneault, K. (2008, November). *Acceptance-based behavioral therapy for GAD: Predictors of change.* Paper presented at the annual meeting of the Association of Behavioral and Cognitive Therapies, Orlando, FL.

Przeworski, A., Newman, M. G., Pincus, A. L., Kasoff, M. B., Yamasaki, A. S., Castonguay, L. G., et al. (2011). Interpersonal pathoplasticity in individuals with generalized anxiety disorder. *Journal of Abnormal Psychology, 120*(2), 286–298.

Rickels, K., Zaninelli, R., McCafferty, J., Bellew, K., Iyengar, M., & Sheehan, D. (2003). Paroxetine treatment of generalized anxiety disorder: A double-blind, placebo-controlled study. *American Journal of Psychiatry, 160*(4), 749–756.

Revicki, D. A., Travers, K., Wyrwich, K. W., Svedsäter, H., Locklear, J., Mattera, M., et al. (2012). Humanistic and economic burden of generalized anxiety disorder in North America and Europe. *Journal of Affective Disorders, 140*(2), 103–112.

Roemer, L., & Borkovec, T. D. (1994). Effects of suppressing thoughts about emotional material. *Journal of Abnormal Psychology, 103*(3), 467–474.

Roemer, L., Lee, J. K., Salters-Pedneault, K., Erisman, S. M., Orsillo, S. M., & Mennin, D. S. (2009). Mindfulness and emotion regulation difficulties in generalized anxiety disorder: Preliminary evidence for independent and overlapping contributions. *Behavior Therapy, 40*(2), 142–154.

Roemer, L., Molina, S., & Borkovec, T. D. (1997). An investigation of worry content among generally anxious individuals. *Journal of Nervous and Mental Disease, 185*(5), 314–319.

Roemer, L., & Orsillo, S. M. (2007). An open trial of an acceptance-based behavior therapy for generalized anxiety disorder. *Behavior Therapy, 38*(1), 72–85.

Roemer, L., & Orsillo, S. M. (2009). *Mindfulness- and acceptance-based behavioral therapies in practice.* New York: Guilford Press.

Roemer, L., Orsillo, S. M., & Salters-Pedneault, K. (2008). Efficacy of an acceptance-based behavior therapy for generalized anxiety disorder: Evaluation in a randomized controlled trial. *Journal of Consulting and Clinical Psychology, 76*(6), 1083–1089.

Romera, I., Fernández-Pérez, S., Montejo, Á. L., Caballero, F., Caballero, L., Arbesú, J. Á., et al. (2010). Generalized anxiety disorder, with or without co-morbid major depressive disorder, in primary care: Prevalence of painful somatic symptoms, functioning and health status. *Journal of Affective Disorders, 127*(1–3), 160–168.

Sauer-Zavala, S., Boswell, J. F., Gallagher, M. W., Bentley, K. H., Ametaj, A., & Barlow, D. H. (2012). The role of negative affectivity and negative reactivity to emotions in predicting outcomes in the unified protocol for the transdiagnostic treatment of emotional disorders. *Behaviour Research and Therapy, 50*(9), 551–557.

Segal, Z. V., Williams, J. M., & Teasdale, J. D. (2002). *Mindfulness-based cognitive therapy for depression: A new approach to preventing relapse.* New York: Guilford Press.

Siev, J., & Chambless, D. L. (2007). Specificity of treatment effects: Cognitive therapy and relaxation for generalized anxiety and panic disorders. *Journal of Consulting and Clinical Psychology, 75*(4), 513–522.

Sobczak, L. R., & West, L. M. (2013). Clinical considerations in using mindfulness- and acceptance-based approaches with diverse populations: Addressing challenges in service delivery in diverse community settings. *Cognitive and Behavioral Practice, 20*(1), 13–22.

Sorensen, S. M., Hayes-Skelton, S. A., Roemer, L., & Orsillo, S. M. (2012, June). *Working alliance across an acceptance-based behavior therapy and applied relaxation for clients with GAD.* Poster presented at the annual meeting of the Society for Psychotherapy Research, Virginia Beach, VA.

Stapinski, L. A., Abbott, M. J., & Rapee, R. M. (2010). Fear and perceived uncontrollability of emotion: Evaluating the unique contribution of emotion appraisal variables to prediction of worry and generalised anxiety disorder. *Behaviour Research and Therapy, 48*(11), 1097–1104.

Stöber, J., & Bittencourt, J. (1998). Weekly assessment of worry: An adaptation of the Penn State Worry Questionnaire for monitoring changes during treatment. *Behaviour Research and Therapy, 36*(6), 645–656.

Sue, D. W., & Sue, D. (2012). *Counseling the culturally diverse: Theory and practice* (6th ed.). Hoboken, NJ: Wiley.

Sue, S. (1998). In search of cultural competence in psychotherapy and counseling. *American Psychologist, 53*(4), 440–448.

Thayer, J. F., Friedman, B. H., & Borkovec, T. D. (1996). Au-
tonomic characteristics of generalized anxiety disorder and worry. *Biological Psychiatry, 39*(4), 255–266.

Treanor, M., Erisman, S. M., Salters-Pedneault, K., Roemer, L., & Orsillo, S. M. (2011). Acceptance-based behavioral therapy for GAD: Effects on outcomes from three theoretical models. *Depression and Anxiety, 28*(2), 127–136.

Wang, P. S., Lane, M., Olfson, M., Pincus, H. A., Wells, K. B., & Kessler, R. C. (2005). Twelve-month use of mental health services in the united states: Results from the National Comorbidity Survey Replication. *Archives of General Psychiatry, 62*(6), 629–640.

Waters, A. M., & Craske, M. G. (2005). Generalized anxiety disorder. In M. M. Antony, D. R. Ledley, & R. G. Heimberg (Eds.), *Improving outcomes and preventing relapse in cognitive-behavorial therapy* (pp. 77–127). New York: Guilford Press.

Wells, A. (2005). The metacognitive model of GAD: Assessment of meta-worry and relationship with DSM-IV generalized anxiety disorder. *Cognitive Therapy and Research, 29*(1), 107–121.

Wells, A., Welford, M., King, P., Papageorgiou, C., Wisely, J., & Mendel, E. (2010). A pilot randomized trial of metacognitive therapy vs applied relaxation in the treatment of adults with generalized anxiety disorder. *Behaviour Research and Therapy, 48*(5), 429–434.

Whisman, M. A. (2007). Marital distress and DSM-IV psychiatric disorders in a population-based national survey. *Journal of Abnormal Psychology, 116*(3), 638–643.

Williams, J. M. G., Teasdale, J. D., Segal, Z. V., & Kabat-Zinn, J. (2007). *The mindful way through depression: Freeing yourself from chronic unhappiness.* New York: Guilford Press.

Williams, K. E., Chambless, D. L., & Ahrens, A. (1997). Are emotions frightening?: An extension of the fear of fear construct. *Behaviour Research and Therapy, 35*(3), 239–248.

Wilson, K. G., & Murrell, A. R. (2004). Values work in acceptance and commitment therapy: Setting a course for behavioral treatment. In S. C. Hayes, V. M. Follette, & M. M. Linehan (Eds.), *Mindfulness and acceptance: Expanding the cognitive-behavioral tradition* (pp. 120–151). New York: Guilford Press.

Wilson, K. G., Sandoz, E. K., Kitchens, J., & Roberts, M. (2010). The Valued Living Questionnaire: Defining and measuring valued action within a behavioral framework. *Psychological Record, 60*(2), 249–272.

CHAPTER 6

Emotional Disorders
A Unified Transdiagnostic Protocol

LAURA A. PAYNE
KRISTEN K. ELLARD
TODD J. FARCHIONE
CHRISTOPHER P. FAIRHOLME
DAVID H. BARLOW

In this chapter we describe the most recently developed treatment protocol from the Center for Anxiety and Related Disorders at Boston University. In this "unified" transdiagnostic protocol, therapeutic principles common to psychological treatment of the various emotional disorders have been distilled and integrated into a single protocol that is, in theory, applicable to the full range of emotional disorders. Unlike protocols for specific problems or disorders described in other chapters, this new approach is only beginning to benefit from efforts to establish extensive empirical validation. But the components that make up this treatment have achieved wide and deep empirical support, and initial outcomes of this protocol are promising. What is new about this approach is the systematic manner in which the treatment components are applied across disorders, as well as theoretical developments leading to reconceptualization of the principal target of treatment as a common, higher order temperament undergirding disorders of emotion rather than specific DSM-defining system clusters. The major advantage, of course, in addition to greatly simplifying dissemination by eliminating numerous overlapping single-disorder protocols, is that this approach also takes into consideration the extensive comorbidity often found among emotional disorders. This approach is illustrated in the treatment of "Joseph."—D. H. B.

When the first edition of this book was published in 1985 it was the dawn of evidence-based psychological treatments. Descriptions of only those treatments with sufficient empirical support that were broadly applicable to large numbers of individuals with various forms of psychopathology at that time were included. Over succeeding editions of this book some new treatment approaches with wide appeal and strong empirical support have been added, whereas others have been deleted. In addition, the field has matured to the point where public health services around the world have directed that evidence-based psychological treatments become an integral part of health care delivery systems due to their effectiveness, efficiency, and durability (Clark, 2012; Nathan & Gorman, 2007; Ruzek, Karlin, & Zeiss, 2012). It is also a sign of the maturity of a field to examine closely the limitations of existing evidence. Obviously, a considerable number of patients still do not respond as well as would be desirable to our current arsenal of psychological (or drug) treatments, and there is plenty of room for improvement.

Another problem that has become apparent, particularly in the context of emotional disorders, is that there now exists a plethora of treatment protocols for each of the discrete anxiety and mood disorders. Although these protocols, by and large, have proven useful and been well received, it takes a significant amount of training to become sufficiently familiar with the distinct protocols to integrate them into clinical practice (Barlow, Bullis, Comer, & Ametaj, 2013). Unless these treatments become more "user-friendly" as recommended, clinicians are less likely to have a sufficient understanding of, or access to, these evidence-based treatments for the emotional disorders (McHugh & Barlow, 2012). In this chapter, we present a unified protocol (UP) for the transdiagnostic treatment of emotional disorders. "Emotional disorders" in our conception include not only the anxiety, depressive, obsessive–compulsive, and trauma-related disorders but also other classes of disorders in which the experience and regulation of emotion plays a prominent role, such as the somatic disorders, dissociative disorders, and, to some extent, the eating disorders. Borderline personality disorder can also be conceptualized as a disorder of extreme emotional dysregulation (Sauer-Zavala & Barlow, 2013; Neacsiu & Linehan, Chapter 10, this volume) and may fit within our UP conceptualization. Our science and practice have advanced sufficiently that there are now several strong arguments for developing such an approach, in addition to the very practical advantage of substantially reducing the number of existing protocols. We touch on these arguments here before describing the treatment components of the UP in some detail, in keeping with the long-standing format of this book.

RATIONALE FOR A UNIFIED APPROACH

Perhaps the strongest argument for a unified transdiagnostic treatment approach to emotional disorders is an emerging body of evidence supporting commonalities in the etiology of these disorders that we have summarized recently in the form of a new etiological model referred to as "triple vulnerability" (Barlow, 1991, 2000, 2002; Suárez, Bennett, Goldstein, & Barlow, 2009). Of course, it is important to note that shared etiological pathways or pathophysiological processes are not yet firmly established, and that emotional disorders and

their subtypes may each turn out to be associated with unique underlying pathology (reflecting a true categorical organization) with identifiable *taxa*. Yet we believe that the evidence on shared pathological processes is sufficiently strong at present to justify a transdiagnostic treatment approach.

A second argument focuses on conceptions of the major emotional disorders that emphasize their commonalities rather than their differences. The "spectrum" approach is one manifestation of this conception. For example, high rates of comorbidity suggest considerable overlap among disorders. The observed effects of current psychological treatments on comorbid conditions also point to at least a partial nonspecificity of treatment response. From a phenomenological perspective, emerging research on the latent structure of dimensional features of emotional disorders reveals a hierarchical structure that can accommodate these disorders. The sections to follow briefly review evidence relevant to these arguments.

Etiology

We have described in some detail an interacting set of vulnerabilities or diatheses relevant to the development of anxiety, anxiety disorders, and related emotional disorders. This "triple vulnerability" theory encompasses a generalized biological vulnerability, a generalized psychological vulnerability, and a specific psychological vulnerability emerging from early learning (Barlow, 2000, 2002; Suárez et al., 2009). Much of the research on generalized biological and psychological vulnerabilities has focused on a temperament labeled, variously, "neuroticism," "negative affect," "behavioral inhibition," or "trait anxiety." Although the relationships among these closely related traits and temperaments have yet to be worked out fully, it seems that they substantially overlap and represent a common theme associated with a biological vulnerability to develop emotional disorders (Barlow, 2000, 2002; Campbell-Sills, Liverant, & Brown, 2004; Suárez et al., 2009). We have come to refer to this temperament by its most traditional label "neuroticism" (Barlow, Sauer-Zavala, Carl, Bullis, & Ellard, in press; Eysenck, 1947). A generalized biological vulnerability involves nonspecific genetic contributions to the development of neuroticism. Additionally, early life experiences fostering a sense that events, particularly negative events, are unpredictable or uncontrollable, contribute to a generalized psychological vulnerability, or diathesis, to develop neuroticism later on. If a generalized biological and a generalized psychological vulnerability happen to line up and are potentiated by the influence of life stress, the likely result is a development of the two closely related clinical syndromes of generalized anxiety disorder (GAD) and/or depressive disorders. Notice that false alarms (panic attacks) may also occur as a function of stressful life events, facilitated by high levels of baseline anxiety. But these false alarms seem to have a different heritability than anxiety and are not necessarily implicated in a clinical disorder. For that to occur, an additional layer of a more specific psychological vulnerability must be considered. In particular, certain learning experiences seem to focus anxiety on specific life circumstances, and these circumstances or events are associated with a heightened sense of threat or danger. For example, specific early learning experiences seem to determine whether individuals may view somatic sensations, intrusive thoughts, or social evaluation as specifically dangerous (Barlow, 2002; Bouton, Mineka, & Barlow, 2001); that is, to take one example, individuals with social anxiety often have in their background admonitions from parents or family always to be on their best behavior and to look their best, to avoid the dreaded consequence of being negatively evaluated or "disapproved of" by others. It is this specific psychological vulnerability that, when coordinated with the generalized biological and psychological vulnerabilities mentioned earlier, seems to contribute to the development of discrete anxiety disorders such as social anxiety disorder, panic disorder, and specific phobias. This model is also applicable to obsessive–compulsive and trauma and stressor-related disorders. For instance, in obsessive–compulsive disorder (OCD), individuals often report learning from authority figures that having a thought is as bad as engaging in the action (i.e., having the thought about shaking a newborn infant to quiet it is as bad as actually shaking the infant). Existing evidence for this "triple vulnerability" model has been reviewed in detail elsewhere (Bouton et al., 2001; Chorpita & Barlow, 1998; Suárez et al., 2009) and is consistent with the overriding importance of common factors in the genesis and presentation of emotional disorders.

Latent Structure of the Emotional Disorders

Whereas the *Diagnostic and Statistical Manual of Mental Disorders*, fourth and fifth editions (DSM-IV-TR and DSM-5; American Psychiatric Associa-

tion, 2000, 2013) highlight a "splitting approach" to nosology, in an attempt to achieve high rates of diagnostic reliability, this achievement may have come at the expense of diagnostic validity; that is, the current system may be highlighting categories that are minor variations of more fundamental underlying syndromes. Quantitative approaches using latent variable methodology are now capable of examining the full range of anxiety and mood disorders, and their interrelationships, without the constraints of existing (possibly) artificial categories (Brown, Chorpita, & Barlow, 1998; Chorpita, Albano, & Barlow, 1998; Clark, 2005; Clark & Watson, 1991; Watson, 2005). We have been studying this question for a number of years. For example, Brown and colleagues (1998), using a sample of 350 patients with DSM-IV anxiety and mood disorders, confirmed a hierarchical structure to the emotional disorders. In this structure, trait negative affect and trait positive affect were identified as crucial higher-order factors to the DSM-IV disorder factors, with significant paths from negative affect to each of the five DSM-IV disorder factors (GAD, social phobia, panic disorder, OCD, and major depression). Interestingly, low positive affect emerged with significant paths to major depression and social phobia only. In this model, autonomic arousal represents the phenomenon of panic, and this arousal emerges as a lower-order factor with significant paths from panic disorder and GAD (where the relationship was negative).

A separate study followed 606 patients with DSM-IV anxiety and mood disorders over the course of 2 years found further support for this hierarchical model (Brown, 2007). Replicating earlier cross-sectional findings, the two higher-order temperament dimensions of neuroticism/behavioral inhibition/negative affectivity and behavioral activation/positive affectivity accounted for virtually all of the covariance among DSM-IV disorder constructs (GAD, social phobia, and major depression). Furthermore, the rate of change in neuroticism/behavioral inhibition over the study period accounted for virtually all of the covariance among the rate of change in DSM-IV disorder constructs. Findings such as these suggest that commonalities among emotional disorders outweigh the differences. We have concluded from this research that DSM-IV emotional disorder categories are best considered as useful concepts or constructs that emerge as "blips" on a general background of neuroticism/behavioral inhibition but may not be the best way to organize nosology (Brown & Barlow, 2009).

Overlap among Disorders

At the diagnostic level, the overlap among the emotional disorders is most evident in the high rates of current and lifetime comorbidity (e.g., Brown, Campbell, Lehman, Grisham, & Mancill, 2001; Kessler et al., 1996; Roy-Byrne, Craske, & Stein, 2006; Tsao, Mystkowski, Zucker, & Craske, 2002, 2005). Results from Brown, Campbell, and colleagues (2001) indicate that 55% of patients with a principal anxiety disorder had at least one additional anxiety or depressive disorder at the time of assessment. But if one examines for the presence of a disorder over the lifetime of the patient, whether it is present or not at the time of interview, this rate increases to 76%. To take one example, 60% of 324 patients diagnosed with panic disorder with or without agoraphobia (PD/A) were determined to meet criteria for either an additional anxiety or mood disorder, or both. Specifically 47% presented with an additional anxiety disorder and 33% with an additional mood disorder. When lifetime diagnoses are considered, the percentages rise to 77% experiencing any anxiety or mood disorder, breaking down to 56% for any anxiety disorder and 60% for any mood disorder. If posttraumatic stress disorder (PTSD) or GAD were the principal (most severe) diagnoses, comorbidity rates were highest. Merikangas, Zhang, and Aveneoli (2003) followed almost 500 individuals for 15 years and found that relatively few people suffer from anxiety or depression alone. When a single disorder did occur at one point in time, the additional mood state would almost certainly emerge later.

Several possible explanations for these high rates of comorbidity have been reviewed extensively elsewhere (Brown & Barlow, 2002). Among these are relatively trivial issues with overlapping definitional criteria; artifactual reasons, such as differential base rates of occurrence in our setting; and the possibility that disorders are sequentially related, and that the features of one disorder act as risk factors for another disorder. For example, depression seems to follow PDA, and PDA seems to follow PTSD. But the more intriguing explanation, for our purposes, first offered by individuals such as Gavin Andrews and Peter Tyrer (Andrews, 1990, 1996; Tyrer, 1989; Tyrer et al., 1998), is that this pattern of comorbidity argues for the existence of what has been called a "general neurotic syndrome." Andrews and Tyrer have suggested that the difference in the expression of emotional disorder symptoms (individual variation in the prominence of social anxiety,

panic attacks, anhedonia, etc.) is simply a trivial variation in the manifestation of a broader syndrome. This, in turn, is consistent with "triple vulnerability" models mentioned earlier, that anxiety (and mood) disorders emerge from shared psychosocial and biological/genetic diatheses. If this is the case, then a unified treatment protocol cutting across current diagnostic categories to address core features of the anxiety and mood disorders could be a more parsimonious, and, perhaps, powerful option.

We have reviewed the genetic and neurobiological evidence on the commonalities among anxiety and depressive states in some detail elsewhere (Barlow, 2002, Chaps. 3, 6, 7, & 8; Bouton, 2005; Brown, 2007; Suárez et al., 2009). For example, most work on genetic contributions to anxiety and depression supports the early dictum of Ken Kendler (1996; Kendler et al., 1995), "same genes different environment" (Hettema, Neale, & Kendler, 2001; Rutter, Moffit, & Caspi, 2006). Consistent with a theory of an underlying genetic vulnerability, genetic variations have been linked to both trait anxiety and negative emotionality (or neuroticism) (Montag, Fiebach, Kirsch, & Reuter, 2011; Stein, Campbell-Sills, & Gelernter, 2009), and have been found to influence the later development of psychopathology following life stressors (Caspi et al., 2003). Recently, a growing body of literature in genetics has observed links between genetic polymorphisms and both the function and structure of neural pathways implicated in emotional processing, suggesting an association between a genetic predisposition, inefficient or maladaptive emotion processing, and the development of emotion disorders. For example, genetic variations have been associated with hyperactivation in neural structures implicated in emotion generation (Drabant et al., 2012; Lonsdorf et al., 2011; Munafò, Brown, & Hariri, 2008), reduced gray matter volume in limbic regions, and reduced functional connectivity between emotion-generating regions and structures implicated in their inhibitory control (Pezawas et al., 2005).

Increased perceptions of emotions as uncontrollable and intolerable, increased avoidant processing, and increased attempts at emotional control have also been demonstrated across disorders (Campbell-Sills, Barlow, Brown, & Hofmann, 2006a, 2006b; Weinberg & Hajcak, 2010; Weiser, Pauli, Weyers, Alpers, & Mühlberger, 2009). Intolerance of uncertainty and distress has been demonstrated across a full range of disorders, including depression, GAD, social anxiety, and OCD (Boelen, Vrinssen, & van Tulder, 2010; Boswell, Thompson-Holland, Farchione, & Barlow, 2013; Lee, Orsillo, Roemer, & Allen, 2010). In addition, a growing number of studies have shown that individuals with anxiety and mood disorders tend to use maladaptive emotion regulation strategies, including attempts to avoid or dampen the intensity of uncomfortable emotions, that ultimately backfire and contribute to the maintenance of their symptoms (e.g., Campbell-Sills et al., 2006a, 2006b; Liverant, Brown, Barlow, & Roemer, 2008; Mennin, Heimberg, Turk, & Fresco, 2005; Tull & Roemer, 2007). Taken together, the evidence from genetics, neuroscience, behavioral studies, and psychopathology research suggests that a common, overlapping feature across disorders is the propensity toward increased emotional reactivity and inefficient or deficient regulatory control that is coupled with a heightened tendency to view these experiences as aversive and is manifest in attempts to alter, avoid, or control emotional responding.

In summary, the existing literature supports several arguments for stepping back from individual DSM diagnostic categories and associated disorder-specific psychological protocols, and considering a more unified transdiagnostic approach based on new findings on the nature of psychopathology and from the emerging field of emotion science. In addition, current evidence-based cognitive-behavioral therapy (CBT) protocols for emotional disorders have much in common and reduce to three broad principles of change: altering emotion-based misappraisals of salient events; preventing avoidance of negative, emotionally charged internal or external triggers, as well as modifying emotion-driven behaviors (EDBs) and facilitating extinction of fear; and reducing anxiety and distress over the experience of intense emotion. A full explanation of this protocol and a description of its application with a patient follows.

TREATMENT VARIABLES

Setting

All assessments and treatments of patients are conducted in the Center for Anxiety and Related Disorders (CARD) at Boston University. Our clinic receives over 500 new admissions per year, with many patients being offered treatment after their initial intake assessments. CARD, in addition to housing staff psychologists and a psychiatrist, is also a training center for doctoral

students and psychiatric residents. At any given time, numerous National Institutes of Health (NIH)–funded treatment and research studies are ongoing at the Center. Regarding diagnostic breakdown of treatment-seeking patients, the most common diagnosis assigned is GAD, followed by social phobia, PD/A, specific phobia, OCD, and PTSD, but the full range of "neurotic spectrum" disorders are assessed and treated. A small percentage of patients are assigned "coprincipal diagnoses," which refers to cases in which two separate diagnoses are judged to be of equal severity.

Prior to the intake evaluation, each patient is mailed a packet of questionnaires to complete and bring to the assessment, which are scored and interpreted subsequent to the interview. The majority of the intake appointment comprises administration of the Anxiety Disorders Interview Schedule (for DSM-5 [ADIS-5; Brown, Di Nardo, & Barlow, 2014] or for DSM-IV [ADIS-IV; Di Nardo, Brown, & Barlow, 1994]). Following completion of the entire assessment process, consensus diagnoses are determined during a weekly staff meeting, after which the patient is provided diagnostic feedback and treatment recommendations. Based on the information from the interview, the patient may be offered one of several treatment options at the Center, or a referral in the community.

Format

Treatment with the UP is typically conducted in an individual format, although it has been successfully conducted in a group format with patients with mixed principal emotional disorder diagnoses. The treatment described in this chapter reflects the individual treatment protocol, which allows for greater attention to the description and application of treatment components during each session. However, when administered in a group setting, patients are easily able to see the commonalities among their diverse presenting complaints, and this understanding often creates a strong bond among group members. Therefore, it may be useful to adapt the protocol for group treatment as we have done at CARD.

Therapist Variables

The UP has been administered by therapists with varying degrees of clinical experience and expertise with the protocol. To our knowledge, both junior therapists (even therapists who have never had experience with cognitive-behavioral treatments) and senior therapists (i.e., therapists with at least 4 or more years of treatment experience) have been able to adapt to the UP without significant difficulty. Certainly, a background in cognitive-behavioral techniques may be helpful when utilizing the protocol (e.g., facilitating cognitive reappraisal, and designing and conducting exposures). Evidence suggests some benefit to therapist experience, at least when treating PDA with a highly structured CBT protocol (Huppert et al., 2001).

The UP is an emotion-focused treatment approach; that is, the focus of every exercise is on eliciting and changing responses to a variety of emotions and emotional cues. Perhaps one of the most challenging aspects for the therapist is to be able to create and utilize emotion-provoking exposures effectively, which begin early in treatment and continue throughout its course. Most importantly, the therapist must have a sense of when a patient is avoiding the process of experiencing, expressing, or accepting emotions, and this is often signaled by very subtle behavioral cues, such as avoiding eye contact, changing the topic of discussion, arriving late for a session, and not completing (or "overdoing") homework assignments. Each of these behaviors represents attempts to control uncomfortable emotions through either direct avoidance or overcontrol. It is essential that the therapist be able to recognize and address such behaviors when they occur, thereby allowing the opportunity for an effective emotion exposure and discussion of avoidance to facilitate emotional processing.

A second challenge for the therapist is to be able to tolerate and experience the expression of emotion by the patient. It is common for less experienced therapists to quickly "rationalize away" the patient's emotional reactions; however, this only feeds into the cycle of emotions and avoidance. At every step, the therapist should encourage the expression and acceptance of emotion, while guiding the patient in how to "examine" it, without letting the emotion "take over." In such cases, modeling from a senior therapist and/or extensive supervision may be helpful instruction for less experienced therapists in how to allow their patients to be "emotional."

Client Variables

As previously mentioned, the rate of comorbidity among patients with a principal anxiety or mood disorder is approximately 55% (Brown, Campbell, et al., 2001), depending on the principal diagnosis. In most CBT protocols, comorbid diagnoses are never a focus of treatment, although successful treatment of a principal anxiety disorder often results in decreases in comorbidity (e.g., Allen et al., 2010; Brown, Antony, & Barlow, 1995). One advantage of a unified treatment approach is that symptoms related to comorbid diagnoses can be discussed in treatment sessions and may even be the focus of an emotion exposure. For example, a patient with GAD who experiences chronic worry about daily matters may also feel anxious in social situations. Therefore, that patient's in-session emotion exposure might comprise a conversation with a stranger or giving a speech to a small group of people. Contrary to traditional protocols, it is the experience of any emotion that is the target of treatment, which may be particularly beneficial for patients with significant comorbidity or for those who would like to address multiple concerns during the course of treatment.

Concurrent Drug Treatment

Many patients who present for treatment are also taking some form of psychoactive medication. At CARD, patients are required to have stabilized on the dosage of medication prior to the intake interview, so that the therapist has a clear picture of actual symptoms (as opposed to symptoms that may be caused by the initial addition or removal of a medication). Whereas concurrent use of medications such as tricyclic antidepressants and selective serotonin reuptake inhibitors (SSRIs) does not appear to have a negative impact on treatment outcome initially, once the medications are removed, evidence suggests that patients who received medication alone or CBT in addition to medication are more likely to relapse (e.g., Barlow, Gorman, Shear, & Woods, 2000; Heimberg et al., 1998; Liebowitz et al., 1999). The exact mechanisms underlying the return of symptoms are unclear, although some authors have suggested that patients may attribute the success of the treatment to the use of medication and, once it is withdrawn, no longer believe they have the ability to manage their symptoms. However, in a recent investigation using data from a multisite comparative study for the treatment of panic disorder, results indicated that patients who received CBT plus pill placebo were equally likely to believe they had received medication as patients who had actually received the medication (Raffa et al., 2008). Yet those in the CBT plus placebo condition were less likely to relapse compared to those who had received either CBT plus medication or medication alone. Therefore, it appears unlikely that the higher relapse rates in the medication conditions were due solely to this "attribution hypothesis." One other hypothesis to explain greater relapse in patients receiving psychopharmacological treatment is that the medication provides an unintended "protective" effect against increased physiological arousal and anxiety. However, eliciting anxiety and panic is a core component of CBT protocols, so patients taking medication (1) may have experienced greater physical sensations when the medication was removed and/or (2) were never able fully to confront the physiological arousal and panic during the course of treatment. However, these hypotheses have yet to be fully investigated.

One additional consideration is the use of benzodiazepines on a p.r.n., or "as needed," basis during the course of treatment. Following conceptions outlined in the UP, any strategy used to reduce the intensity of emotions in the moment is considered an emotional avoidance strategy, and ultimately contributes to increasing levels of anxiety and emotional reactivity. Therefore, the use of benzodiazepines (or other fast-acting medications) is discouraged, particularly if the medications are carried with the person as a "safety signal."

ASSESSMENT

Case Study

Joseph is a 25-year-old, single man who, at the time of intake, worked as a freelance music teacher and an independent musician, occasionally performing his music at small local venues. Joseph came to our Center seeking help for long-standing, debilitating emotional issues that were standing in the way of his ability to attain personal and professional goals. Joseph reported a long history of struggles with anxiety and depression that were exacerbated and compounded by issues with his physical health.

During his intake interview, Joseph reported significant and oftentimes paralyzing social anxiety, describing significant fear of being evaluated negatively, and of others seeing him as a burden or "in the way." This fear had caused him to avoid important social engagements throughout his life, such as birthday parties or other special occasions, and he often turned down invitations for casual gatherings at bars or at friends' homes. He found himself becoming increasingly iso-

lated because of this, and felt that some of his friends were "giving up" on him. In addition, his fears of being burdensome to others prevented him from asserting himself, which would often cause significant interference. For example, Joseph reported that he wanted to find a job as a music teacher for elementary schoolchildren, but asking others to provide information that was necessary for the completion of job applications, which was nearly impossible for him, would cause Joseph to miss deadlines or promising opportunities. Joseph noted that he has experienced social anxiety his whole life, but that it became more intense for him following a diagnosis of diabetes when he was 9 years old. He described always feeling like a burden on others since that time, and feeling like he was always "in the way." Notably, these feelings extend even to walking down a public sidewalk—one of his most feared situations is inadvertently bumping into someone walking in the other direction, for fear that he has inconvenienced or caused that person to judge him negatively. Joseph reported that his social anxiety currently is more interfering than ever, as it is preventing him from finding work, and his social life is now "nonexistent."

In addition, Joseph described significant embarrassment related to symptoms of irritable bowel syndrome (IBS), which had begun 5 years previously. Specifically, Joseph noted that he avoids any situation from which he cannot leave if he begins to experience stomach problems. He avoids eating all fruits or any type of food that might trigger bloating or loose bowels and reports that he wakes up 3 hours before he needs to leave for work in order to use the bathroom several times before leaving the house, in an attempt to avoid having any unexpected bowel movements while in public situations. He estimated using the bathroom up to five times each morning before leaving for work. In addition, Joseph reported that his fear of having an unexpected bowel movement has prevented him from traveling long distances in cars, attending movies or sporting events, or engaging in any activity where quick access to a restroom is not possible. He reported that his greatest fear related to these symptoms was that he would embarrass himself in front of others, either by becoming flatulent or losing control of his bowels altogether.

Joseph also described significant anxiety and worry about a number of different areas in his life. He worries about making small mistakes in his work, such as grammatical errors. He worries about his potential performance at work should he secure a teaching position, fearing that he would ultimately get fired from his job for some mistake he might make. Joseph worries about his finances and being able to support himself, as well as about the health of his parents and their well-being. He also reported worrying about community and world affairs but noted that he controls these worries by "avoiding the news at all costs." Joseph reports that his worries are difficult to control, and they interfere with his ability to concentrate. He feels restless, tense, irritable, and often has trouble sleeping when he worries. He noted that he spends about 90% of the average day worrying about something, and that these worries have interfered with his social life, his overall well-being, and his ability to find a job.

Joseph also described significant anxiety related to intrusive doubting thoughts, and thoughts that he might cause accidental harm to others. He described difficulty leaving his house in the morning for fear that he might inadvertently leave the stove on or the house unlocked, leaving his roommates vulnerable to fire or burglary. These thoughts drive him to check repeatedly to see that he has locked doors, extinguished candles, or turned off the oven and stove sufficiently, which can take up to an hour. Joseph also notably never received his driver's license for fear that he might accidently run someone over or cause an accident while driving. He reported that his doubting thoughts and thoughts of accidentally causing others harm are extremely distressing to him and make him feel like he is an awful person who cannot be trusted.

Finally, Joseph reported feelings of depression and lack of interest in activities for the past year, since graduating from college. He often has difficulty sleeping at night and reports sleeping too much during the day. He experiences a feeling of "heaviness" and lack of energy, has difficulty concentrating on things. He experiences constant feelings of guilt and worthlessness, and has periodic thoughts of suicide, although he reported no plan or intent. Joseph reported that every few weeks he cuts himself on his legs and chest using a single-edged razor, in order to relieve tension and calm himself down. Joseph stated that although his feelings of depression are "bothersome," he is also "used to them" because they have been present much of his life.

Objective assessment of Joseph's emotional state via self-report questionnaires resulted in a score of 51 on the Social Interaction Anxiety Scale (SIAS; Mattick & Clarke, 1998), reflecting severe social anxiety; a score of 49 on the Beck Depression Inventory–II (BDI-II; Beck, Steer, & Brown, 1996), reflecting severe depression; and a score of 80 on the Penn State Worry Ques-

tionnaire (PSWQ; Meyer, Miller, Metzger, & Borkovec, 1990), reflecting moderate to severe levels of worry. His score on the Work and Social Adjustment Scale (WSAS; a modification of a scale introduced by Hafner & Marks, 1976) suggested that Joseph was experiencing severe interference in his life from these emotional symptoms. A diagnostic interview using the ADIS-IV revealed a principal diagnosis of social anxiety disorder at a clinical severity rating (CSR; described below) of 7, and additional diagnoses of GAD (CSR = 6), OCD (CSR = 5), and major depressive disorder (MDD; CSR = 5).

Interviews

A number of structured and semistructured clinical interviews may be appropriate for diagnosing Axis I disorders. The Structured Clinical Interview for DSM-IV (SCID; First, Spitzer, Gibbon, & Williams, 1996) is widely used and assesses diagnoses. Because this interview is highly structured and focuses only on current symptom count, it achieves a high degree of interrater reliability for many diagnoses. However, this interview does not include dimensional ratings of frequency and severity of symptoms, so it may be less useful for more detailed profiling of emotional disorders.

The Anxiety Disorders Interview Schedules for DSM (ADIS-5; Brown, Di Nardo, & Barlow, 2014), a semistructured, diagnostic clinical interview, focuses on DSM diagnoses of anxiety, OCD and related disorders, and trauma- and stressor-related disorders and their accompanying mood states, as well as somatic symptoms and dissociative disorders, and substance and addictive disorders. The information derived from the interview using the ADIS allows clinicians to determine differential diagnoses and gain a clear understanding of the level and severity of each diagnosis. We refer to the updated DSM-5 version from this point forward. Principal and additional diagnoses are assigned a CSR on a scale from 0 (*No symptoms*) to 8 (*Extremely severe symptoms*), with a rating of 4 or above (*Definitely disturbing/disabling*) passing the clinical threshold for DSM diagnostic criteria. Inquiries about suicidal ideation are part of this interview. The ADIS-IV has demonstrated excellent to acceptable interrater reliability for the anxiety and mood disorders (Brown, Di Nardo, Lehman, & Campbell, 2001).

Two additional clinician-rated measures that provide a wider range of scores are the (1) Structured Interview Guide for the Hamilton Anxiety Rating Scale (SIGH-

A; Shear, Vander Bilt, & Rucci, 2001) and the (2) Structured Interview Guide for the Hamilton Depression Rating Scale (SIGH-D; Williams, 1988). The SIGH-A was developed to create a structured format for administering the Hamilton Anxiety Rating Scale (HARS; Hamilton, 1959). Respondents are asked to indicate the presence and severity of a number of symptoms that may have been present over the past week, including anxious mood, tension, sleep problems, irritability, and so forth. The rater is also asked to rate the interview behavior of the patient. The SIGH-A includes specific instructions on administration and anchor points for assigning severity ratings. This measure demonstrated good interrater and test–retest reliability (Shear et al., 2001). In addition, scores are similar to (although consistently higher than) the HARS.

Similar to the SIGH-A, the SIGH-D was developed to provide more specific instructions for administration and scoring of the Hamilton Depression Rating Scale (HDRS; Hamilton, 1960). Again, patients are questioned about the presence and severity of a range of depressive symptoms over the past week, including depressed mood, suicidal ideation, fatigue, feelings of hopelessness, weight loss, and so forth. The SIGH-D also demonstrated good interrater and test–retest reliability, and produces scores similar to the HDRS (Williams, 1988).

Medical Evaluations

Medical evaluations are generally recommended prior to assignment of diagnoses and initiation of treatment to rule out organic causes for symptoms of emotional disorders. Some conditions, such as hypothyroidism, hyperthyroidism, hypoglycemia, mitral valve prolapse, or alcohol or substance withdrawal, may elicit symptoms similar to those associated with GAD or PDA. Although the diagnosis of such medical conditions does not preclude the need for a psychological treatment, it is generally recommended that such conditions be examined by a physician because an alternative treatment may be clinically indicated.

Self-Monitoring

Self-monitoring forms are an important part of the treatment protocol for several reasons. First, the therapist is able to discuss specific situations or events that occurred over the past week and may have contributed to emotional reactions. Such records can facilitate discussions of concepts presented during the treatment sessions and help the therapist integrate the general treatment components into the patient's specific symptoms. Second, some evidence suggests that patients' retrospective recall of past episodes of anxiety may be inflated, particularly when recalling panic attacks (Margraf, Taylor, Ehlers, Roth, & Agras, 1987; Rapee, Craske, & Barlow, 1990). Self-monitoring forms allow for a prospective, and possibly more accurate, account of anxiety episodes and may therefore be more useful therapeutically. In addition, consistent with the themes outlined in the UP, practicing awareness of emotions in the present moment is believed to be an important component of changing maladaptive patterns of emotional responding. The very nature of self-monitoring requires patients to disengage, even briefly, from the habitual anxious process to write down concrete thoughts, feelings, and behaviors, helping them to begin to adopt a more objective stance toward their own emotional experiences. Developing this habit will ultimately aid patients in beginning to change emotional reactions and resulting behaviors.

Treatment forms used in the UP include self-monitoring forms for emotional awareness, automatic appraisals, emotion avoidance, as well as forms tracking interoceptive and situational exposure. Figure 6.1 illustrates the Monitoring Emotions and EDBs in Context (MEEC) form used in the UP. This form is given for several weeks at the beginning of treatment to begin to orient patients to tracking their own emotional responses. As new skills are introduced (i.e., cognitive reappraisal, changing EDBs), new self-monitoring forms typically replace the MEEC. For instance, once the skill of altering action tendencies associated with emotions is introduced, patients are asked to monitor situations, EDBs, and identify a new response incompatible with the original EDB on the Changing EDBs monitoring form (see Figure 6.2).

Several problems may arise with the introduction and completion of self-monitoring forms. First, some patients may not be compliant with completion of monitoring forms and homework assignments, which is an important issue to be addressed in the therapy session. Adopting a motivation enhancement approach, eliciting reasons underlying the patient's ambivalence regarding completing the homework or monitoring can be a valuable technique (i.e., eliciting reasons why the patient might not wish to complete the homework and perceived benefits to not completing it). This process is crucial as it allows the therapist to identify maladaptive

Date/Time	A's Antecedents		R's Responses			C's Consequences
	Situation/Trigger	Thoughts	Feelings	Behaviors		What happened next?

FIGURE 6.1. Monitoring Emotions and EDBs in Context (MEEC) form.

Situation/Trigger	Emotion	EDB	New (incompatible) response	Consequence

FIGURE 6.2. Changing EDBs monitoring form.

cognitive appraisals and emotional reasons contributing to the lack of completion of monitoring forms. Once such reasons are identified, therapeutic strategies such as cognitive reappraisal may also be used to increase patients' willingness to complete homework forms by addressing some of the reasons for noncompliance raised by the patient. Furthermore, selectively reflecting the benefits of completing the homework and the costs associated with noncompliance can help to build motivation to complete homework forms. In some cases, especially when patient self-efficacy for completion is low, completion of homework forms themselves may become an emotion exposure, and progress toward this goal should be reinforced accordingly.

Another common problem with the completion of self-monitoring may be the tendency for some patients (particularly those with more obsessive or "perfectionistic" features, commonly seen in GAD and OCD) to "overdo" the homework forms; that is, the patient may write an extremely long and involved description of a situation and his/her reactions to it. This is common with patients who feel a need to "unload" every piece of information about the event. Although the patient is doing the homework, his/her overengagement may also be facilitating the anxious/worry process. If this becomes evident, the therapist may want to discuss the tendency to overengage in the homework as an emotional avoidance strategy (or as an EDB) and encourage patients to try to monitor situations and events using one- or two-word descriptions, or even implement a time limit to help ensure that patients do not spend lengthy periods of time generating their descriptions.

Questionnaires

In our research we employ a number of self-report questionnaires over the course of treatment. We describe most of them here, realizing that for purely clinical purposes only a subset would be needed. Two general (diagnosis nonspecific) questionnaires designed to measure symptoms and impairment associated with those symptoms are administered weekly prior to session to track symptoms and impairment across the course of treatment. A larger questionnaire battery is administered pre-, mid-, and posttreatment, and every four sessions during treatment, in order to gain a more comprehensive picture of patients' presenting concern, as well as their overall functioning and quality of life. This battery comprises general questionnaires

(measures designed to assess a range of symptoms associated with anxiety and mood disorders, as well as disorder-specific measures designed to track symptoms associated with specific disorders).

Weekly General Measures

The Overall Anxiety Severity and Impairment Scale (OASIS; Norman, Cissell, Means-Christensen, & Stein, 2006), a brief, five-item questionnaire developed as a continuous measure of anxiety-related symptom severity and impairment, can be used across anxiety disorders, with multiple anxiety disorders, and with subthreshold anxiety symptoms. This measure has good internal consistency, excellent test–retest reliability, and convergent and divergent validity (Campbell-Sills et al., 2009; Norman et al., 2006). The Overall Depression Severity and Impairment Scale (ODSIS; Bentley, Gallagher, Carl, Farchione, & Barlow, 2013), a direct adaptation of the OASIS, is modified to be applicable for depression. It is a brief, five-item questionnaire that assesses dimensional depression-related symptom severity and impairment that can be used across depressive disorders, with varied comorbid presentations, and with subthreshold depressive symptoms. Both measures focus on severity of and impairment associated with particular symptoms over the past week, offering a general, diagnosis nonspecific measure designed to track changes as they occur over the course of treatment.

Additional General Measures

In the Positive and Negative Affect Schedule—Trait version (PANAS; Watson, Clark, & Tellegen, 1988), a brief, reliable, and valid measure of positive and negative affect, individuals rate how frequently they experience 20 feeling or emotion words *in general*. The PANAS assesses core negative affect and deficits in positive affect in those disorders with this characteristic (i.e., agoraphobia, social anxiety disorder, depression) and is useful in determining changes in positive and negative affect over the course of treatment. In an effort to establish degree of interference from symptoms in various domains of living, the WSAS (Hafner & Marks, 1976) includes five items that ask participants to rate the degree of interference caused by their symptoms in work, home management, private leisure, social leisure, and family relationships. The WSAS, a descriptive measure of subjective interference in various domains of living, has been successfully used in previous studies (e.g., Brown & Barlow, 1995).

Quality of Life and Well-Being Measures

The Quality of Life and Enjoyment Satisfaction Questionnaire (QLESQ; Endicott, Nee, Harrison, & Blumenthal, 1993), a 14-item measure that assesses enjoyment and satisfaction across different life areas in the past week, is widely used and has been validated for use in clinical populations and shown to be sensitive to change (Endicott et al., 1993). The Mental Health Continuum—Short Form (MHC-SF; Keyes, 2005, 2006; Keyes et al., 2008; Lamers, Westerhof, Bohlmeijer, ten Klooster, & Keyes, 2011; Westerhof & Keyes, 2009) is a 14-item measure designed to assess social, emotional, and psychological well-being. The measure has shown excellent internal consistency and discriminant validity in both adolescents and adults in the United States, the Netherlands, and South Africa (Keyes, 2005, 2006; Keyes et al., 2008; Lamers et al., 2011; Westerhof & Keyes, 2009).

Diagnosis-Specific Measures

In addition to the general (diagnosis nonspecific) measures, it is important to assess symptoms specific to the individual's specific diagnostic presenting concerns. We use the following measures that assess symptom severity over the past week and can be administered both as self-report and clinician-rated measures, increasing their clinical utility. The Yale–Brown Obsessive–Compulsive Scale–II (Y-BOCS-II; Storch, Larson, Price, Rasmussen, Murphy, & Goodman, 2010) is a revised version of the Y-BOCS (Goodman et al., 1989), designed to assess the presence and severity of OCD symptoms.

The Panic Disorder Severity Scale (PDSS; Shear et al., 1997), a seven-item scale, provides ratings of the core features of panic disorder (panic frequency, distress during panic, anticipatory anxiety, panic-related avoidance of situations and sensations) and the degree of work and social impairment/interference due to PD/A (Shear et al., 1997).

The Liebowitz Social Anxiety Scale (LSAS; Liebowitz, 1987) is a widely used 24-item scale designed to assess the range of social interaction and performance situations that patients with social anxiety may fear and/or avoid (Heimberg et al., 1999; Safren et al., 1999).

The Generalized Anxiety Disorder Severity Scale (GADSS; Shear, Belnap, Mazumdar, Houck, & Rollman, 2006) is a six-item assessment that evaluates the core features of GAD.

The PTSD Symptom Scale (PSS; Foa, Riggs, Dancu, & Rothbaum, 1993) is a 17-item measure designed to assess DSM-IV symptoms of PTSD. Each item, corresponding to the symptoms of PTSD, comprises one brief question that is rated from 0 (*Not at all*) to 3 (*5 or more times per week/Very much*). This measure yields a total PTSD severity score, as well as Reexperiencing, Avoidance, and Arousal subscores (Foa & Tolin, 2000).

Functional Analysis

Regardless of the diagnosis, a clear functional analysis of the patient's behavior is essential prior to beginning treatment. Several components are important to consider when diagnosing a patient based on a functional analysis. These include a close examination of symptom topography (including duration of illness, physical sensations, level of distress and interference from symptoms), triggers (situations, physical symptoms, places, thoughts, etc.), cognitions (beliefs about symptoms and misappraisals), behavioral responses to emotions (including avoidance of situations, places, people, or triggers, as well as escape behaviors), and the consequences of behavioral reactions (limiting quality of life, reduced "comfort zone," etc.).

Joseph, at the diagnostic level, met criteria for several distinct anxiety and mood disorders. His primary concern involved anxiety and avoidance of social situations due to fears of being judged or disliked by others. These fears had been present since Joseph was a young child and clearly fit with a diagnosis of social phobia. However, Joseph also experienced anxiety related to intrusive thoughts about causing potential harm to others. His intrusive doubting thoughts and thoughts of accidental harm to others, coupled with a number of compulsive checking behaviors, which took up at least an hour per day, were consistent with a diagnosis of OCD. Joseph also presented with significant anxiety and uncontrollable worry about his ability to perform well at work, his finances, and the health of his family, along with several associated physical symptoms. These worries, although involving social situations to some degree, also included more diffuse worries related to potential future negative outcomes. These worries were present even outside the context of a depressive episode. Thus, an additional diagnosis of GAD was also assigned. Finally, Joseph's reported symptoms of depression in the past year, along with accompanying lack of interest in activities, sleep difficulties, lack of energy, and poor concentration, resulted in a diagnosis of MDD.

Whereas Joseph's symptoms merited the assignment of multiple co-occurring disorders, it is important to note that at the phenomenological level, these diagnosis-specific symptoms tended to interact and exacerbate one another, such that each disorder-specific cluster of symptoms was not necessarily occurring in isolation. This was an important consideration for treatment, and it provided a strong argument for a unified, transdiagnostic approach. For example, Joseph's low self-esteem, driven by his depressogenic ruminations, fueled his sense of being "less than" and increased the perceived potential to be evaluated negatively by others. This anxiety focused on negative evaluation in turn increased Joseph's more general anxiety and fueled his EDBs, for example, checking, which was often set in motion as a way to control a feared potential outcome of doing something wrong (checking locks to prevent loss of property), causing real harm to others (prevent fire by checking stoves, candles, etc.), or embarrassing himself in public (using the bathroom several times before work to prevent a flare-up of IBS symptoms). These anxieties were in turn congruent with his beliefs about himself as being "in the way" and a "bad person." Joseph's vigilance relative to his IBS symptoms was also fueled by anxiety related to negative evaluation, and an increased focus on his physical symptoms was usually coupled with increased levels of anticipatory anxiety. Joseph's worries about potential future failures at work, his finances, and his family's health were also congruent with a general belief that he would inevitably do something wrong and cause the "bottom to fall out," or that some negative, unexpected outcome was always on the horizon. Joseph linked this sense of unpredictability and uncontrollability to his childhood diagnosis of diabetes, which also was his earliest memory of being "in the way." He recalled several childhood incidents in which the adults in his life appeared "put out" by having to monitor his eating and insulin levels; he recalled developing a sense that he was a burden on others, although he recalled his sense of being "less than" developing much earlier on. Thus, all of these beliefs, behaviors, and physiological responses were interacting in Joseph's emotional experiences, regardless of their specific diagnostic classification, and affecting

his ability to function in an adaptive way. Treatment of Joseph's symptoms with the UP, which focuses on how the interactions of thoughts, feelings and behaviors at any given moment influence overall emotional experiences and subsequent actions, allowed us to target Joseph's phenomenological patterns of dysfunction directly rather than focus on one diagnosis-specific cluster of symptoms at a time.

COMPONENTS OF TREATMENT

The structure of the UP outlines five core treatment modules and three additional modules, designed to be delivered in 12–18, 50- to 60-minute individual treatment sessions, held on a weekly basis. Final sessions may be held every other week to allow patients to consolidate gains and to provide somewhat of a "taper" off the weekly therapy. This format for the final sessions is not a requirement, though, and it may be more beneficial for the patient to continue to have weekly sessions if he/she might potentially have trouble using the treatment concepts consistently without the weekly reinforcement of sessions. Therefore, spacing of the final sessions is determined by the therapist, who takes into consideration the patient's progress and any anticipated difficulties after treatment.

The five core treatment modules designed to target aspects of emotion processing and regulation are as follows: (1) increasing present-focused emotion awareness (Module 3); (2) increasing cognitive flexibility (Module 4); (3) identifying and preventing patterns of emotion avoidance and maladaptive EDBs (Module 5); (4) increasing awareness and tolerance of emotion-related physical sensations (Module 6); and (5) interoceptive and situation-based emotion-focused exposure (Module 7). Preceding these core components is a module focused on enhancing motivation and readiness for change and treatment engagement (Module 1), as well as an introductory module providing psychoeducation about the nature of emotions and a framework for understanding emotional experiences (Module 2). A final module reviews progress over treatment and develops relapse prevention strategies (Module 8). This treatment, which takes place in the context of provoking emotional expression (emotion exposure) through situational, internal, and somatic (interoceptive) cues, as well as through standard mood induction exercises, differs from patient to patient only in the situational cues and exercises utilized. In addition, "exposure" is not conceptualized as a mechanism of action. Rather, successfully provoking emotions creates a setting condition to implement the essential treatment components. Emotion exposures begin with general stimuli (e.g., mood induction and interoceptive provocation) and are later tailored to address each patient's particular concerns and symptoms. Although each session addresses a specific component of the protocol, the expectation is that patients then "carry through" to future sessions the strategies they learn (e.g., patients learn cognitive reappraisal strategies in Module 4 but are expected to continue to use cognitive reappraisal throughout the remainder of treatment).

Module 1: Motivation Enhancement for Treatment Engagement

In this initial treatment module, which is grounded in the principles and therapeutic techniques utilized in motivational interviewing (MI; Miller & Rollnick, 2013), therapists work to increase the patient's readiness and motivation for behavior change, and to foster a sense of self-efficacy, or the patient's belief in his/her ability to change. This module was included in the protocol in reaction to recent research by Westra and colleagues (Westra, Arkowitz, & Dozois, 2009; Westra & Dozois, 2006) suggesting that MI may enhance the efficacy of CBT for anxiety disorders. This module utilizes two specific motivational exercises: (1) a decisional balance exercise, in which the therapist works with the patient to identify and weigh the pros and cons of changing versus staying the same; and (2) a treatment goal-setting exercise that helps patients more clearly articulate achievable and concrete goals for treatment. This module, and the principles and techniques contained therein, are primarily used to help "set the stage" for subsequent learning that takes in the core modules. However, the principles can also be applied throughout the course of treatment to enhance treatment engagement and maintain patient motivation for behavior change.

Module 2: Psychoeducation and Tracking of Emotional Experiences

Following the initial motivation enhancement session, patients are provided with psychoeducation about the nature and function of emotions. This component is common to most CBT protocols, although the focus is expanded to include the function of many different emotions (anger, sadness, etc.), in addition to the function of anxiety. In this module (which typically occurs over the course of one to two sessions), patients are provided information about the cognitive, physiological, and behavioral sequelae of emotional reactions and how these three components interact. It is important that the patient begin to consider that his/her reactions are functional and serve the purpose of providing information about the environment, in addition to protection from harm. This three-component model is then applied to a recent situation or event that the patient experienced, so that he/she may better understand the aspects of each component and how they interact. Patients also learn how to monitor and track more carefully their emotional responses and, as a result, are expected to develop greater awareness of their own patterns of emotional responding, including potential maintaining factors (e.g., common triggers and/or environmental contingencies).

Another important aspect of psychoeducation is the concept of negative reinforcement. Specifically, this is a detailed discussion of how the patient's behavioral response to an emotional episode (usually escape or some form of emotional avoidance) is problematic because it reduces the emotion in the short term (i.e., by removing the person from the emotional stimulus) but reinforces the cycle of emotions in the long term (i.e., by teaching the person that escape/avoidance is the only way to manage these feelings in the future). It is extremely important that the patient understand the connection between behavioral responses and reinforcement of emotion, so that he/she is better able to appreciate the purpose and function of emotion exposures introduced in future sessions.

Module 3: Emotion Awareness Training

The first core module (which typically occurs over the course of one to two treatment sessions) is designed to help patients further identify how they are reacting and responding to their emotions by promoting a more nonjudgmental, present-focused approach to the experience of emotions. Often, patients report feeling that their emotions are confusing, or that they seem to just happen "automatically," and/ or in such way that they are outside of the patient's immediate awareness (i.e., "unconsciously"). Through this module, patients learn to become more aware of the interaction among thoughts, feelings, and behaviors and to view their emotions in a more objective and present-focused manner.

This occurs within the specific context of the situation in which the emotional experience is unfolding. The focus on present-moment experiences is important and is believed to put the patient in a better position to more clearly identify patterns of emotional responding and/or the emotion regulation strategies being employed in the particular situation. In turn, this renders the patient better able to modify the emotional response adaptively to make it more consistent or compatible with ongoing situational or motivational demands. Furthermore, secondary reactions to the patient's emotional experiences are also explored, and the therapist introduces the idea that it is not the emotions per se that are problematic, but rather how the patient reacts to the emotion. As these reactions tend to be judgment-laden (e.g., seeing anxiety as a sign of one's inability to cope an indication of weakness, or a sign of failure) and are often not based on information from the present-moment context, they can prevent the processing of potentially corrective information that would allow for a change in the emotional response. It is expected that as patients develop a more nonjudgmental stance toward their emotions, they will be better able to identify the specific thoughts, physical sensations, and behaviors that may be contributing to their distress, and thus be in a better position to implement strategies for adaptively altering their emotional response. These skills are developed through the practice of brief mindfulness and emotion induction exercises.

Module 4: Cognitive Appraisal and Reappraisal (Increasing Cognitive Flexibility)

Cognitive therapy, initially developed by Aaron T. Beck to treat depression (Beck, 1967; Beck, Rush, Shaw, & Emery, 1979; also discussed in-depth in Young, Rygh, Weinberger, & Beck, Chapter 7, this volume), has become a fundamental part of psychological treatments. Individuals with emotional disorders are likely to have appraisals and interpretations of external events that are characterized by cognitive biases, such as the tendency to overestimate the likelihood of the occurrence of negative events and to underestimate the ability to cope with these events. Thus, the aim of cognitive therapy is to evaluate objectively the likelihood of these negative appraisals and to incorporate more realistic, evidence-based appraisals of the outcome of a situation. On the surface, this technique may appear to be a way to suppress or control negative thoughts by "rationalizing"

them, and occasionally, this is how cognitive therapy is incorrectly used, as noted by Hayes, Strosahl, and Wilson (1999). However, this strategy can also be conceptualized from an emotion regulation perspective, especially if reappraisals are considered one of many possible interpretations of a situation.

The primary aim of this module is to foster greater flexibility in thinking (this module is typically administered in one or two sessions). This is accomplished first by helping patients develop an understanding of how they interpret or appraise situations, and how their appraisals influence patterns of emotional responding, then by teaching them to generate numerous alternative attributions and appraisals when experiencing strong emotional experiences. As their initial interpretations are typically more negative or anxious, patients are encouraged to be more flexible in their thinking (i.e., to generate alternative appraisals) and are taught reappraisal strategies.

As adapted in our usage, the UP focuses on correcting two fundamental misappraisals often found in individuals with emotional disorders: the probability of a negative event happening (probability overestimation) and the consequences if the negative event does happen (catastrophizing) (Barlow & Craske, 2007; Craske & Barlow, 2006). Although a number of other misappraisals are noted in other, traditional CBT protocols, most misappraisals can be condensed into one of the two appraisals listed here.

Module 5: Prevention of Emotion Avoidance and Modifying EDBs

Module 5 generally comprises one to two sessions. The concept of emotion avoidance is likely to be particularly important for patients who do not physically avoid or escape situations but still experience high levels of anxiety without much relief. The therapist should convey that even if the person stays physically in the situation, he/she is likely to engage in a number of other subtle behaviors to prevent full emotional arousal. In the UP, emotional avoidance strategies are behaviors that prevent the full experience of emotion in a situation, as opposed to EDBs, which are behavioral consequences of the experience of emotion (described later in the chapter). Any technique or strategy the patient uses to reduce or to down-regulate emotions may be conceptualized as an emotional avoidance strategy, and it is essential that emotional avoidance be identified and eliminated prior to engagement in emotion exposures, to allow for full emotional processing. Therefore, a very detailed description of individual emotional avoidance strategies must be obtained for each patient.

We have identified three general categories of emotion avoidance strategies: (1) subtle behavioral avoidance, (2) cognitive avoidance, and (3) safety signals (see Table 6.1 for examples). Subtle behavioral avoidance strategies may include a number of different behaviors, with certain behaviors occurring more frequently with particular disorders. For example, the avoidance of caffeine in panic disorder or social phobia (prior to a social engagement) is an attempt to keep physiological symptoms from becoming strong in anxiety-provoking situations. Patients with social phobia may also avoid eye contact or wear sunglasses when interacting in social settings. Individuals with GAD may excessively plan, prepare, or write "to do" lists in an attempt to control

potentially negative outcomes. At the same time, procrastination is also a form of subtle behavioral avoidance, if a particular task or project seems too emotionally arousing for the patient. It is very important to conduct a functional analysis of the subtle behaviors to determine which ones are avoidance strategies, that is, behaviors that serve to reduce or avoid emotional experience and are functional responses to situations. And, notably, what may be an avoidance strategy for one person may be a functional response for another. Cognitive avoidance strategies are typically more difficult to identify because they tend to occur outside of the patient's awareness. Some of these strategies include distraction, "tuning out," and mentally checking lists or reviewing past conversations. However, data also suggest that worry and rumination actually function as a way to down-regulate and avoid emotions (e.g., Borkovec,

TABLE 6.1. Examples of Emotional Avoidance Strategies

Emotional avoidance strategy	Disorder most usually associated
1. Subtle behavioral avoidance	
• Avoid eye contact	Social phobia
• Avoid drinking caffeine	PDA
• Attempt to control breathing	PDA
• Avoid exercise/physiological arousal (interoceptive avoidance)	PDA/depression
• Avoid touching sink/toilet	OCD
• Procrastination (avoiding emotionally salient tasks)	GAD
2. Cognitive avoidance	
• Distraction (reading a book, watching television)	Depression/PDA
• "Tune out" during a conversation	Social phobia
• Reassure self that everything is OK	GAD
• Try to prevent thoughts from coming into mind	OCD
• Distraction from reminders of trauma	PTSD
• Force self to "think positive"	Depression
• Worry	GAD
• Rumination	Depression
• Thought suppression	All disorders
3. Safety signals	
• Carry cell phone	PDA/GAD
• Carry empty medication bottles	PDA
• Hold onto "good luck" charms	OCD
• Carry items that are associated with positive experiences (e.g., teddy bears, pictures)	GAD/depression
• Have mace at all times	PTSD
• Carry water bottle	PDA
• Have reading material/prayer books on hand	GAD
• Carry sunglasses or item to hide face/eyes	Social phobia

1994). The function of worry is to enable the person to prepare for a possible threat. However, when someone experiences chronic worry and associated anxiety, his/her attention is focused on the future as opposed to the present moment. Research has shown that when confronted with an emotionally arousing event, chronic worriers do not experience the full emotional impact of that event because (1) they have been "bracing" themselves for something bad to happen, and (2) their focus has already shifted to other, future negative outcomes (Borkovec, Hazlett-Stevens, & Diaz, 1999). Therefore, the worry functions as a cognitive avoidance strategy and only serves as a maladaptive attempt to gain control over seemingly uncontrollable future events. Obsessions, common to individuals with OCD, may also function in a similar manner.

Safety signals are most common to patients with PDA, although may also be present in individuals with GAD, OCD, or other emotional disorders. Safety signals include any object that the patient carries to feel more safe or "comfortable," particularly if he/she is entering an emotionally arousing situation. Safety signals can range from actual medication (e.g., benzodiazepines for reducing physiological arousal or medications for gastrointestinal distress) to empty medication bottles, to "lucky" objects (a talisman, teddy bear, "lucky" pen, etc.). Regardless of the object itself, if its function is to help the patient reduce emotional arousal in the moment, then it also is problematic because it feeds into the cycle of negative reinforcement.

In addition to changing patterns of emotion avoidance, this module also focuses on helping patients identify and subsequently change EDBs. Data and hypotheses from emotion science suggest that the most efficient and effective way to change emotions is by changing responses to them (Barlow, 1988; Izard, 1971); thus, it is conceivable that the mechanism of change during an exposure is to prevent the action tendency associated with a particular emotional experience. Over the past several decades, research has focused on these action tendencies, and changing action tendencies has become an important treatment component for anxiety, as well as other emotional disorders (Barlow, 1988; Linehan, 1993). For example, Beck and colleagues (1979) based a large part of their treatment for depression on changing the action tendencies of their patients to behave in a "passive, retarded, and apathetic manner" (p. 312). More recently, behavioral activation strategies have become a central feature of newer treatments for de-

pression (Dimidjian et al., 2006; Jacobson, Martell, & Dimidjian, 2001); for a more in-depth discussion, see Dimidjian, Martell, Herman-Dunn, and Hubley (Chapter 9, this volume).

To distinguish action tendencies from avoidance strategies (described earlier), the UP has termed these behavioral responses to emotions as "emotion-driven behaviors" (EDBs). Whereas the function of emotional avoidance strategies is to down-regulate or suppress emotions, EDBs include a specific set of "reactive" behaviors associated with each emotion. For example, the EDB for a panic attack is escape (fight or flight), whereas that for anxiety is hypervigilance. Similarly, the emotion of anger elicits an EDB of attacking–defending, and the EDB for sadness is cognitive, emotional, and physical slowing and withdrawal (see Table 6.2 for examples of EDBs associated with different emotional disorders). It is important to note, however, that the therapist must focus on changing EDBs, in addition to preventing emotional avoidance. For example, a patient with social phobia may be able to maintain eye contact and fully engage in social situations but escape the situation when his anxiety rises to the level of panic. On the contrary, this same patient may be able to stay in the situation as long as needed, but he may be distracting himself the whole time or avoiding conversations with people. Clearly, both scenarios are problematic because the patient is preventing himself from learning that he can experience emotions at their fullest without leaving the situation. It should also be noted that, in practice, avoidance and EDBs may be difficult to distinguish, and this distinction can be downplayed with a given patient, if necessary or clinically relevant.

After the concept of EDBs is introduced, patients begin to track EDBs on the self-monitoring forms and eventually focus on changing EDBs. This can be a very concrete exercise for the patient because he/she is instructed to "do something different than he/she would typically do." The Changing EDBs monitoring form is illustrated in Figure 6.2.

Module 6: Awareness and Tolerance of Physical Sensations

This module (typically one session) was designed to increase patients' awareness of the role of physical sensations as a core component of emotional experiences and to promote increased tolerance of these sensations. In this module, patients are asked to engage in a series

TABLE 6.2. Examples of Emotion-Driven Behaviors and Incompatible Behaviors

EDBs	Disorder most usually associated	Incompatible behaviors
Calling relatives to check on safety	GAD	Restricting contact/calling relatives
Perfectionistic behavior at work or home	GAD	Leaving things untidy or unfinished
Checking locks, stove, or other appliances	OCD	Repeatedly locking–unlocking and turning on–off until memory is unclear
Leaving (escaping from) a theater, religious service, or other crowded area	PDA	Move to the center of the crowd. Smile or produce nonfearful facial expressions
Social withdrawal	Depression	Behavioral activation
Leaving (escaping) a social situation	Social phobia	Staying in situation and approaching people
Verbally/physically attacking someone when in an argument	PTSD	Remove self from situation and/or practice relaxation techniques
Hypervigilance	All disorders	Focus attention on specific task at hand; meditation; relaxation

of interoceptive exposure (IE) exercises designed to induce physical sensations analogous to those typically associated with naturally occurring feelings of anxiety and emotional distress (e.g., shortness of breath, heart palpitations, dizziness), which themselves often become cues for anxiety through interoceptive conditioning (Barlow, 2002). Examples of IE exercises include hyperventilation, spinning (while standing and/or in a chair), running in place, and breathing through a thin straw. The use of IE has largely been confined to the treatment of PDA, and has been shown to be effective in reducing panic attack frequency and the fear of physical sensations that occurs as a primary feature of the disorder (e.g., Barlow et al., 2000; Craske, Rowe, Lewin, & Noriega-Dimitri, 1997). However, given the fact that heightened physiological arousal, and sensitivity to physical sensations, is observed in other emotional disorders, IEs are applied across diagnoses, regardless of whether the physical sensations represent a specific focus of the patient's anxiety.

Module 7: Interoceptive and Situational Exposures

In this final core module, treatment concepts are practiced and extended during in-session emotion expo-sures created by the therapist and individually tailored to the patient's presenting symptoms (this module is the longest; typically lasting four to six sessions). Through exposure to both internal and external cues, patients ultimately increase their tolerance of intense and uncomfortable emotional experiences. In-session exposures can range from an imaginal exposure to a past emotional event (for PTSD or GAD), a conversation with a stranger (for social phobia), going into a dirty bathroom (for OCD), or watching a sad movie or movie clip (for MDD or dysthymia). Furthermore, for some patients, continued engagement in IEs may be indicated to promote greater tolerance of uncomfortable physical sensations. The goal of the exposures is gradually to introduce situations and experiences that serve as external triggers for emotional experiences. By eliciting the emotions that patients have been avoiding, they have the opportunity to practice the techniques taught in treatment (present-focused awareness, cognitive reappraisal, modifying EDBs, and prevention of emotion avoidance). In this sense, exposure to the emotion itself is the necessary mechanism of action for change. Thus, the actual situational context of the exposure becomes less important. Therapists must be creative in the design of the exposure to maximize the emotion provocation for the patient.

Module 8: Relapse Prevention

Treatment concludes with a general review of treatment principles and a discussion of the patient's progress (usually one session). In this module, therapist and patient identify specific strategies for maintaining and extending treatment gains and for responding to future difficulties that may arise. For instance, it is emphasized that a return of anxiety and/or mood difficulties does not reflect relapse and, instead, may be a more natural fluctuation of emotions that can be addressed using the skills developed in treatment.

DETAILED DESCRIPTION OF PROTOCOL

The following session descriptions and accompanying transcripts are from the case of "Joseph," described earlier, treated by one of the authors (K. K. E.).

Introduction: Overview of General Treatment Format and Procedures

During the introductory session, the goals of the treatment program are identified and reviewed. The UP aims to help clients become aware of and better understand emotional experiences and reactions, and to counter maladaptive responses to uncomfortable emotions. Modifying maladaptive responses can help reduce the intensity and frequency of uncomfortable emotions, while still allowing clients to experience them in an adaptive way. It is also important to emphasize that modifying these responses can be challenging, and that change often does not occur in a linear fashion.

Prior to the first treatment module, the therapist also provides a general introduction to treatment logistics, including general session length and structure, the role of therapist and client, and the importance of prioritizing treatment and completing out-of-session practice. The collaborative nature of treatment is emphasized, including the importance of feedback from the patient. Although the UP is ideally delivered in 12–18 sessions of 50–60 minutes each because the UP is based in a modular format, a flexible number of sessions can be used in each module, which may vary the total number of sessions across clients.

Following this introduction to treatment is a detailed review of the presenting complaint. In this review, the therapist focuses on the emotions that result in the most distress and/or interference in the patient's life, the situations and contexts in which those emotions occur, and how the patient has attempted to manage these emotions. Below, Joseph describes anxiety related to a new job opportunity:

THERAPIST: You mentioned you recently were offered an opportunity to teach over the summer. Can you tell me more about that?

JOSEPH: Well, I know I should be excited about it. It's something I really want to do, teaching urban schoolkids music, but it's stressing me out because I know I'm going to screw it up.

THERAPIST: How so?

JOSEPH: Well, in order to teach the class I need to schedule the classrooms and get supplies, but I don't know who I'm supposed to talk to in order to arrange that, and I'm afraid if I send the person who hired me an e-mail, she is going to think I am stupid or incompetent, or that she made a mistake hiring me because I don't know what I'm doing.

THERAPIST: And how are you coping with the anxiety now?

JOSEPH: Well, not very well, I think. I just feel like hiding, like this whole thing was a big mistake. I'm sort of hoping it will just work out somehow, but I don't know how. I've been avoiding e-mailing her, but I haven't talked to anyone else about it either. I keep waking up at night thinking about it, and it feels just like a pit in my stomach.

THERAPIST: So it sounds like it is also affecting your sleep?

JOSEPH: Yes.

THERAPIST: Have you come up with any solutions to your problem yet?

JOSEPH: No, I just feel like a deer in the headlights right now, like I'm frozen, stuck.

THERAPIST: Have you thought about asking someone else at the school for advice?

JOSEPH: No way, I could never do that!

Note that in this early exchange, the therapist has already obtained important information about the patient's emotional experiences and the ways in which he copes with uncomfortable emotions. In this case, Joseph is experiencing a great deal of anxiety related to a new job opportunity. The therapist is already gathering information about some of Joseph's negative automatic appraisals (e.g., Joseph's assumption that by asking for information or help, others will see him as incompetent), anxiety-related physical sensations (e.g., a "pit" in his stomach), and maladaptive behaviors (e.g., worry, rumination, avoidance, procrastination). The therapist is also able to elicit information about how helpful the patient's current ways of responding to uncomfortable emotions are to him. In this case, Joseph is experiencing a great deal of anxiety but has been unable to come up with any solution to his problem, and is "frozen, stuck."

Although the therapist will spend a significant portion of the session reviewing Joseph's presenting complaints and gathering additional information about his responses to emotions, this process will continue across the first several treatment sessions. As the therapist obtains additional information about strategies (adaptive or maladaptive) for managing emotions, emotional or situational avoidance, and engagement in EDBs, this is then integrated into the patient's functional analysis and the treatment plan may be adjusted accordingly.

Module 1: Motivation Enhancement for Treatment Engagement

This module focuses on achieving the goals of preparing and developing each patient's willingness to make identified behavioral changes, based on the MI principals and techniques developed by Miller and Rollnick (2013). Specifically, the principles of (1) expressing empathy, (2) developing discrepancy, (3) rolling with resistance, and (4) supporting self-efficacy are used in this module and throughout the course of treatment to support behavior change. In this module, the therapist explores motivational issues with the patient, through exercises designed to build motivation (through the Decisional Balance Worksheet) and to enhance self-efficacy (using the Treatment Goal-Setting Worksheet). The aim of these exercises is to highlight potential obstacles to change, as well as to identify specific, concrete goals, respectively.

THERAPIST: Let's take a look at your Decisional Balance Worksheet. You noted some pros for change, including being more social and working at a job you enjoy. What about some cons for change?

JOSEPH: Well, sometimes it's easier just to avoid dealing with these situations altogether.

THERAPIST: Right, and it is important to note and be honest with yourself about this because there is part of you here that wants to change, and another part that has learned that, at least in the short-term, it's easier to just stay the same. What about cons for staying the same?

JOSEPH: Well, if I don't ever face my anxiety, I might not ever get to have a social life, or the job I want.

THERAPIST: So, on the one hand, you want to change how you deal with your anxiety so that you can have the life you want, and at the same time, this change is harder than just avoiding?

JOSEPH: Yes, that's right.

THERAPIST: Acknowledging both of these parts of yourself is important because it is actually quite normal to have some apprehension or ambiguity about change. By being open with yourself about this, you are in a much better position to weigh out your decision whether or not to engage in treatment because it will be about weighing out a choice rather than judging yourself for success or failure. If you find yourself wavering during treatment, you will be able to recognize that this may be related to your feelings of apprehension or ambiguity about change, which is quite normal, and not because you are necessarily failing in some way.

Module 2

Understanding Emotions

The therapist begins this module by providing psychoeducation about the nature of emotions and how they become disordered. It is important to highlight the functional, adaptive nature of emotions at the onset of this discussion for two reasons: (1) so the patient can understand why he/she would not simply want to eliminate emotions and (2) to explore the potentially important information provided by adaptive emotions. This second point is illustrated by the introduction of EDBs (behaviors that occur in response to emotions), so that the patient can see how emotion motivates specific responses to internal or external events or situations.

Next, the three-component model of emotional experiences is described as a framework for examining emotions by dividing them into components (cognitions, behaviors, and physiological sensations), thereby making them more manageable. The therapist uses an example relevant to the patient's experience to demonstrate the contribution of each component to his/

her emotional experience. The therapist guides the patient in identifying each component in this example and presents the model as the structural basis for treatment. Each component is addressed separately over the course of treatment as contributing to the overall emotion and interacting with the other components. For homework in this section of the module, the patient is asked to complete a three-component model example in which he/she is asked to break down an emotion from the week into the three-component model presented in session, by recording the thoughts, behaviors, and physiological sensations specific to that example.

THERAPIST: As we talked about, emotions at their core, even ones like anxiety, fear, anger, or sadness, are actually *good* things because they help us to function, and help us to navigate the world around us. The thing is, though, we also have reactions to our emotions. An emotion can trigger all sorts of associated thoughts, memories, physical sensations, and behaviors, oftentimes learned over a lifetime. The problem is, when we experience all of that at once, it can feel overwhelming, and we can get caught up in our emotional responses, and all of sudden these emotions feel like something we can't cope with, that we have to get away from. Suddenly, the anxiety you feel about your new job isn't functioning as a helpful way to motivate you to prepare for the future, which is, at its core, the adaptive function of anxiety. Instead, the anxiety is something paralyzing, something that is waking you in the night and making you feel "frozen."

JOSEPH: Right, and I just want it to go away.

THERAPIST: Right. Instead of feeling helpful and useful, the emotion feels intolerable. So what we need to do is break down these emotional experiences into their component parts to help make them less overwhelming, and to help us identify how an emotion like anxiety goes from something adaptive and useful to something feared and avoided. As I mentioned, emotional experiences are made up of three main parts: thoughts, feelings, and behaviors. What we need to do is get you better at recognizing each of these parts, to make you a better observer of your emotional experiences. Then, throughout treatment, we'll take a closer look at each of these components individually, to see how specific thoughts, feelings

or physical sensations, and behaviors might be influencing your overall experience and causing the experience to go from something helpful and useful to something uncomfortable and unwanted.

Recognizing and Tracking Emotional Responses

An important step to gaining greater understanding of emotional experiences involves more closely monitoring when, where, and why the emotions are occurring. This is done through illustration of the ARC of emotions. In this illustration, it is critical that the therapist clearly work through an example with the patient, focusing on several important points. First, emotions are always triggered by some event or situation (internal or external), even though it may be difficult to identify that trigger initially. However, with repeated practice and awareness, it can get easier to identify specific triggers, and those are known as *antecedents* ("A" in ARC of emotions). Antecedents can occur immediately before the emotion is experienced (e.g., going into an elevator triggers a panic attack), or they may have occurred days or even longer before the emotion is experienced (e.g., an argument with a friend earlier in the week triggering an outburst at a loved one later on). Often, there are multiple antecedents, and may be both immediate and distal. The "R" of ARC of emotions is all *responses* to emotional experiences, including the thoughts, physiological sensations, and behaviors noted in the three-component model. Finally the *consequences*, or "C" of ARC of emotions, signify the short-term and/or long-term results of emotional responding. Consequences are often negative, but it is important that the therapist point out potential positive consequences of emotional responding (e.g., reduction in anxiety after escaping a difficult situation), as this process of negative reinforcement is usually maintaining the cycle of emotions.

Expanding on this discussion, the therapist now introduces the concept of learned behaviors, essentially focusing on how the patient has learned responses to emotions that are usually an attempt to manage or control the emotions, but often end up leading the patient to feeling worse. Habitually responding to emotions prevents any new learning from taking place (i.e., that a situation is not as dangerous as it appears during the experience of a panic attack) and disables the patient from developing a way of coping. This process is what makes adaptive emotions and emotional responses maladaptive.

Module 3: Emotion Awareness Training— Learning to Observe Experiences

The goal of this module is to introduce the patient to the concept of emotion awareness and begin developing a regular practice of this skill. The therapist must convey that the emotion awareness skill is different than the patient's current sense of his/her emotions. This skill allows the patient to see emotions from an objective and nonjudgmental perspective in order to better identify and alter maladaptive thoughts and behaviors. During this introduction, the therapist reviews the difference between *primary emotions*, which are the "first" emotional responses to a situation and memory (usually directly related to the situation or memory itself) and *secondary reactions*, which are reactions to primary emotions that tend to be judgment-laden and not based on the present-moment context. Secondary reactions are problematic because they can prevent receipt of corrective information about the current situation. Additionally, secondary reactions are typically evaluative and critical in nature, which further distances the patient from the potentially helpful or corrective information provided by the current situation or primary emotions, and tend to intensify or prolong the emotional experience. Using personal examples from the patient's own experience to describe both primary emotions and secondary reactions can be very helpful in this discussion.

When reviewing present-focused awareness, it is important that the therapist remind the patient of several important points. First, this type of practice may feel awkward or uncomfortable at first. The goal is not to be "perfect" at the exercise; rather, the patient should focus on becoming an objective observer of emotional experience, and start developing the ability to pay attention mindfully and in the moment. Second, informal, present-focused awareness practice is also important. The therapist can help the patient find a "cue" (e.g., the breath) to shift focus to the present moment, particularly in times of distress. The goal of this more informal practice is repeatedly to pair the patient's chosen cue with a shift in attention and awareness to the present moment, by focusing on a sight, sound, or other sensation, so that engaging this cue will eventually be automatically paired with present-moment awareness. It is important that the therapist note that the breath (or other cue) should *not* be used as distraction—it should only be used as a cue to remind the patient to be mindful of the present moment. Eventually, once the patient has successfully conditioned this cue to help refocus on the present moment, the patient can learn to follow this with a brief "three-point check" of thoughts, physical sensations, and behaviors. By observing what is occurring in the moment within these three domains, the patient can begin to identify how responses in any of these domains may be affecting the overall emotional experience, to compare what is happening in these domains with information from the current context, and ultimately to identify and alter any maladaptive patterns of responding.

These concepts are illustrated in session with the use of a specific nonjudgmental emotion awareness practice during formal mindfulness or awareness exercise. This may be a guided meditation or some other practice that allows the patient to focus on the present moment, while he/she notices and practices letting go of judgments and evaluation. After the patient has had a chance to practice this skill, the next practice involves using the skill to notice slightly stronger emotional experiences. It is often helpful to have the patient identify a salient piece of music to listen to in session; otherwise, the therapist can select a piece of music. At the conclusion of the music, the therapist helps the patient elicit thoughts, feelings, or other reactions and practice discussing this experience in an objective and nonjudgmental way. The following excerpt describes Joseph's reaction to listening to a piece of music:

THERAPIST: What did you notice when you were listening to the music?

JOSEPH: I noticed my mind was sort of jumping from place to place. That was hard—observing my thoughts.

THERAPIST: Although, it sounds like you were able to notice that your thoughts were jumping around a bit and hard to pin down. Since the goal of this exercise is to practice observing, even just noticing your thoughts have taken you somewhere else, even after it has already happened, counts. What about physical sensations—did you notice any of those?

JOSEPH: I noticed when one of the instruments came in, I sort of felt it in my gut.

THERAPIST: So just hearing that new sound brought about a physical sensation?

JOSEPH: Yes.

THERAPIST: And what about behaviors, did you notice any behaviors, or any urges to do something?

JOSEPH: Well, I noticed a couple of times just feeling uncomfortable and sort of wanting to move around.

THERAPIST: And what about the music itself, were you able to listen to the music itself?

JOSEPH: I think I was more sort of lost in my head.

THERAPIST: This is what our emotions can do. An emotion can trigger all sorts of associated thoughts, feelings, and behaviors that have very little to do with what is happening "in the room," yet the initially triggered emotion itself is connected to something occurring in the present moment, just like the music you were listening to, which was really just sounds happening in the present moment. Getting better at observing our reactions to the trigger (in this case, the music), can help us to see how many of our associated thoughts, feelings, and behaviors actually "fit" with the current context, and how many of them are just associations, which may or may not fit the current context at all.

Module 4: Cognitive Appraisal and Reappraisal

Cognitive appraisal first involves discussing the concept that interpretations depend, in large part, on which of the numerous aspects (or stimuli) a person chooses to focus on in any given situation. Focusing only on limited or specific aspects of a situation is critical for our survival. We would be overwhelmed by information if we focused on all stimuli everywhere we went. This process helps us quickly evaluate situations for risk and danger, and allows us to estimate what might happen in the future. This process usually happens outside of awareness. Importantly, the information we focus on and what we perceive as risky or dangerous tends to be the result of learned associations between specific information or stimuli and the affective or threat value of those stimuli. For example, if negative evaluation by others has been associated with threat in the past, an increase in vigilance for negative evaluation may result. Importantly, appraisals can have a powerful impact on our feelings or mood states, and vice versa. The therapist can illustrate this concept by inquiring how appraisals might vary depending on whether the patient was feeling joyful, sad, or angry.

An in-session exercise is used to demonstrate the many possible different appraisals that can be gener-

ated from a situation. The therapist shows the patient an "ambiguous" picture to which many cognitive appraisals can be assigned, instructs the patient to look at the picture for approximately 30 seconds, then elicits both the patient's initial appraisal and at least two or three alternative appraisals. Additionally, the patient is asked what specifically may have contributed to the automatic appraisal (e.g., memories of similar situations, specific details in the picture). This exercise is used to demonstrate the way that situations can be interpreted in many ways, if all available information is considered.

Automatic appraisals, interpretations of situations that happen very quickly, are often negative or pessimistic in nature. *Core* automatic appraisals (e.g., "I am a failure") are appraisals that may be driving many emotional responses. It is helpful if the therapist can identify one or more core automatic appraisals by using the downward arrow technique instead of focusing only on surface-level appraisals related to a specific situation.

Automatic appraisals can lead to a habitual and powerful heuristic that begins to exclude other, possibly more appropriate or realistic appraisals of a situation or event. These automatic appraisals are called "thinking traps," because, over time, a patient may get "stuck" in this way of thinking. As described earlier, two common thinking traps, "probability overestimation" (jumping to conclusions), or the tendency to assume a high likelihood of the occurrence of a negative event, and "catastrophizing" (thinking the worst), or assuming that the consequences of an event will be beyond the individual's ability to cope, are presented as two cognitive biases common to all emotional disorders. The therapist guides the patient in beginning to identify these biases in the context of his experience. Below, the therapist discusses both of these cognitive biases based on a recent situation in which Joseph was nearly hit by a car while crossing the street.

THERAPIST: Tell me what happened when you were nearly hit by the car.

JOSEPH: Well, I was crossing the street, and a car made an illegal right turn and nearly ran me over. My hands hit the hood of her car, and I could see the driver's face yelling at me.

THERAPIST: And what happened next?

JOSEPH: Well, I noticed people on the sidewalk were all looking at me like I was a complete idiot, and I was so embarrassed I just ran home. I didn't go out for the rest of the day, I just couldn't face anyone.

THERAPIST: Can you remember any of your thoughts at the time?

JOSEPH: I just remember feeling like an idiot, like everyone was just staring at me and thinking what a jerk I am.

THERAPIST: You mentioned you were crossing at a crosswalk—was the walk sign on to cross?

JOSEPH: Yes.

THERAPIST: And the driver, you mentioned the driver was taking an illegal turn?

JOSEPH: Yes, there was a "No turn on red" sign.

THERAPIST: So you had the right of way?

JOSEPH: I guess so.

THERAPIST: Let's go back to the reaction of the people on the sidewalk—you said they were staring at you, thinking you were an idiot?

JOSEPH: It seemed like it.

THERAPIST: What evidence did you have to suggest the pedestrians thought you were an idiot?

JOSEPH: I don't know, they were just looking at me and pointing and frowning.

THERAPIST: Do you know for certain that was what they were thinking?

JOSEPH: Well, not for certain.

THERAPIST: Exactly, because we actually don't know what they were thinking. So one possibility is they thought you were an idiot, but can you think of any other possible thoughts that might have been going through their minds? If you were standing on the sidewalk and saw someone almost get run over in a crosswalk, what might some of your thoughts be?

JOSEPH: Well, I guess I might be sort of alarmed, or hoping the person was OK.

THERAPIST: If you saw someone crossing the street and they had the right of way and were nearly hit by a car making an illegal turn, how likely do you think it would be that you would be thinking that person is an idiot?

JOSEPH: Not very likely, I would probably be more concerned.

THERAPIST: But for you, at that moment, how much did it *feel* like that's what the pedestrians were thinking

about you, that you were an idiot, on a scale of 0% or not at all to 100% certain.

JOSEPH: At that moment? Probably 80–90%.

THERAPIST: And sitting here now, how likely do you think it is that the pedestrians were thinking you were an idiot, using the same percentage scale?

JOSEPH: I don't know, maybe 20%?

THERAPIST: And at the time, what emotions were you experiencing?

JOSEPH: Well, when she almost hit me, I think I felt fear.

THERAPIST: Can you remember any physical sensations?

JOSEPH: I think my heart was racing, and I remember feeling hot and shaky.

THERAPIST: So when you were experiencing fear, and all of the associated physical sensations, the thoughts that came with that was that others perceived you as an idiot, in the wrong. And at the time, these thoughts felt like they were true. Now, sitting here, without the experience of fear or the associated physical symptoms, how likely do those thoughts feel?

JOSEPH: Well, sitting here now, it doesn't seem very likely they would be thinking I was an idiot if I almost got run over. It seems sort of extreme.

The therapist discusses the importance of monitoring and recording automatic appraisals, in order to increase the patient's awareness that these automatic appraisals are occurring, and reminds the patient that using the present-focused awareness skills learned in the previous module can help aid in this process—by anchoring in the present moment using the patient's chosen cue (i.e., taking a deep breath and focusing attention on a sound or sensation occurring in the present moment), the patient can use the "three-point check" to observe what thoughts are occurring at that moment. The goal is to notice what automatic thoughts are occurring, then, using information from the current situation, consider other possible interpretations of what is occurring within the current context. In this way, the patient can more flexibly apply information from learned associations (i.e., memory) and information from the current context toward more adaptive appraisals.

As the patient begins to record automatic appraisals, the therapist can help him/her begin to identify patterns in the automatic thoughts. The therapist provides guidance on identifying thinking traps and tries to focus the patient's attention on the "core" appraisal through the use of "downward arrow" Socratic questioning. The excerpt below is from a discussion of Joseph's fears of having a flare-up of his IBS symptoms and needing to use the bathroom in the middle of a party.

THERAPIST: You've talked about how your IBS symptoms have kept you from going to parties. What specifically concerns you about your IBS symptoms and parties?

JOSEPH: Well, that I'll be there at a party and all of a sudden I'll have to run to the bathroom.

THERAPIST: And what concerns you about that?

JOSEPH: Well, people will notice me rushing to the bathroom.

THERAPIST: And what?

JOSEPH: And they'll know I'm in there using the bathroom.

THERAPIST: And what concerns you about that?

JOSEPH: They'll think I'm disgusting.

THERAPIST: And what does that mean to you?

JOSEPH: That I'm gross and worthless. No one will want anything to do with me.

THERAPIST: Now that is what we want, the real core of it, what is driving this interpretation. A lot of these anxious thoughts you've recorded often do come down to feeling worthless. So you think, "If I can't control my bowels, I am going to have to use the bathroom, and if I have to use the bathroom people are going to reject me as disgusting and worthless." Of course, anyone would be anxious about going to a party with that type of appraisal.

As demonstrated earlier, the therapist then engages the patient in a more detailed discussion of this core cognitive reappraisal, focusing on flexible thinking. Countering probability overestimation and decatastrophizing strategies are presented as a way to generate alternative appraisals and to place less focus on the automatic appraisal. Countering probability estimation involves drawing on past evidence to examine how realistic the patient's estimation is when experiencing an emotion. The therapist guides the patient in making concrete estimations and comparing the original estimation to a more realistic one. Decatastrophizing involves helping the patient to identify his/her ability

to cope with the feared situation using past evidence and specific examples (e.g., similar experiences in the past). It is important to communicate that these strategies do not eliminate negative appraisals, but they provide greater flexibility and allow the patient to gain perspective on the feared situations, using more accurate information as a guide rather than being caught up in overlearned automatic appraisals.

Module 5

Emotion Avoidance

The therapist now introduces the concept of emotional avoidance, describing how avoidance is harmful in the long term, despite potentially providing some short-term relief. As noted earlier, types of avoidance, including subtle behavioral (e.g., procrastination), cognitive (e.g., distraction) and safety signals (e.g., carrying a medication bottle), are introduced. It is important that the patient understand why and how avoidance is problematic. The therapist explains that avoidance (1) prevents habituation to a feared stimulus, so that fear levels are maintained at a high or constant level while in contact with the stimulus; (2) interferes with the process of extinction, so that the conditioned association between the cue and fearful response is maintained instead of weakened; and (3) prevents the patient from developing a sense of control or self-efficacy in managing the fear because positive outcomes are attributed to the avoidance strategy. The therapist asks the patient to generate personally relevant examples of avoidance and discusses how those strategies have maintained the cycle of emotions.

THERAPIST: We're going to shift our focus now and look at how behaviors contribute to your emotional experiences. First, let's talk about avoidance. Sometimes you might do things to avoid having to feel an uncomfortable emotion to begin with. For example, you mentioned that having to reach out to your coworkers at the school to get information about something you don't know is very anxiety provoking for you, and brings about appraisals like they will think you are incompetent or stupid, correct?

JOSEPH: Yes, like the supplies I need for my class. I need more music books for the kids but I don't know if I'm supposed to go get them myself, or if I'm supposed to order them through the school, or how I'm supposed to pay for them. I know I should just e-mail [his supervisor], but since she never mentioned anything about ordering supplies I'm afraid she's going to think I'm stupid or asking too much, that I should be taking care of it myself instead of asking her.

THERAPIST: So you avoid asking her, in order to avoid having to feel anxious or "stupid." This is a good example of one of the ways we can actively do things to avoid uncomfortable emotions. There are also some behaviors that can be more subtle, things we aren't even aware we are doing as an avoidance strategy. For example, someone who has panic attacks might avoid caffeine so they don't have to feel the physical sensations of increased arousal. Can you think of any examples of more subtle ways you may be avoiding uncomfortable emotions?

JOSEPH: Well, when you said that, I immediately thought of fruit. I haven't eaten fruit in 2 years because I'm afraid it will make my IBS symptoms flare up.

THERAPIST: So you're trying to avoid bloating and cramping?

JOSEPH: Well that, and probably more important, I'm trying to avoid embarrassing myself in public!

THERAPIST: So you can see, we have subtle and more overt ways of avoiding uncomfortable emotions, but the question is, does it make the problem go away?

JOSEPH: Well no, I still don't know what I'm going to do about ordering books, and I guess I'm still worried about my IBS even without eating fruit.

THERAPIST: So you can see, avoidance might make the problem go away in the short term, but in the long term this strategy is not particularly helpful and may even make the situation worse. In fact, these avoidance behaviors can strengthen the association of fear and anxiety with these situations—the more you avoid e-mailing your supervisor, the more anxiety provoking the thought of contacting her gets.

JOSEPH: True, now it's just looming out there and feels even worse.

Next, in-session exercises to demonstrate the effects of emotional avoidance are conducted. The first exercise involves asking the patient directly to suppress a thought, such as asking the patient to think of anything at all for the next 30 seconds, but not to allow him/ herself to think about a white bear (Wegner, Schneider, Carter, & White, 1987). In this classic example, patients report great difficulty not thinking about a white bear and continually experience recurrent images or thoughts about a white bear throughout the experiment. The effectiveness of suppression strategies is then discussed. Second, the same exercise is conducted but the patient is asked to suppress a personally relevant and distressing memory or thought. Joseph, for example, had been actively trying not to think about an e-mail he had sent to his supervisor, asking for information about how to order supplies for his students. He was worried that he might have come across as incompetent, and that she would respond negatively to his e-mail. The same "white bear" experiment was conducted with this thought: Joseph was asked to think about anything he wanted to for 30 seconds, but not to think about this e-mail. Predictably, Joseph found it extremely difficult to prevent ruminations about his supervisor's potential reactions from coming into his mind. Thus, this exercise presents a poignant and personally relevant demonstration of the futility of active attempts to avoid distressing topics or situations.

Emotion-Driven Behaviors

The concept of EDBs was introduced earlier in treatment (Module 2), and the goal of this module is to focus on EDBs in greater detail and learn to identify and counter maladaptive EDBs. The therapist begins with a review of adaptive and nonadaptive EDBs. Again, an EDB to escape a situation when experiencing panic may be adaptive if a person is encountering a direct threat to his/her safety; however, an EDB to escape when panicking is maladaptive if there is no clear threat present. In the latter example, the panic and resulting EDB is an example of a "false alarm." The therapist can then explain how EDBs are established and maintained through the concept of negative reinforcement. Similar to emotional avoidance, habitual reliance on EDBs does provide some relief in the short term, and can therefore become a powerful learned response that maintains the cycle of emotions. At this point, the patient is asked to generate examples of EDBs from his/her experience and discuss how negative reinforcement may be contributing to emotional distress. In the transcript below, Joseph describes personal examples of EDBs, including repeatedly using the bathroom in an attempt to control his IBS, and engaging in checking behaviors in response to doubting thoughts and fears of disappointing or causing harm to others.

THERAPIST: You mentioned you are getting up several hours before you need to leave for work. Can you tell me what you are doing during that time?

JOSEPH: Well, like I said, once I go to work it is hard for me to use the bathroom, so I want to make sure I have used the bathroom before I leave the house.

THERAPIST: And how many times are you using the bathroom before you leave?

JOSEPH: About five or six times.

THERAPIST: And what caused you to start going five or six times, instead of just the once?

JOSEPH: Well, in the beginning, I'd go once, but then I would start worrying about if I need to go again, so then I'd go again. Then I go back and forth for a while, worrying about if I've gone enough, then go again, then worry .. .

THERAPIST: And how do you know you've gone enough times?

JOSEPH: I never really know for sure, but at some point I just have to leave the house or I'll be late for work. That's why I started getting up earlier, to make sure I have enough time to use the bathroom.

THERAPIST: And what would happen if you went only once?

JOSEPH: That would make me very anxious, I couldn't do that.

THERAPIST: And in that moment when you are experiencing uncertainty about whether or not you have gone enough times, what emotions come with that?

JOSEPH: I start feeling anxious.

THERAPIST: And what do you do when you start to feel anxious?

JOSEPH: I go again.

THERAPIST: And does that make you feel less anxious, at least in the short term?

JOSEPH: Yes, it makes me feel like I have some control over it.

THERAPIST: This is what we refer to as an EDB. What happens is, when you allow yourself to use the bathroom again in response to the worry about not having gone enough, it helps you to feel better temporarily, and that strengthens that relationship—worry, anxiety, use the bathroom again. It's a very powerful concept. So what will you do next time this uncertainty comes along? Something that you know will make you feel better. You have learned that the anxiety you experience resulting from being uncertain as to whether you have dealt with the situation sufficiently to leave the house can be alleviated by just going again, which sets in motion a sort of loop. Can you think of other examples of this kind of relationship, between feeling anxious or uncertain and doing some sort of action?

JOSEPH: Well, I guess it's sort of the same thing when I start worrying about forgetting to turn the stove off or if I've somehow left a candle burning from the night before, and I have to go back and check.

THERAPIST: And can you describe what happens right before you go back and check?

JOSEPH: I start to feel fear. I get an image in my head of the apartment on fire and my roommates still asleep, then I start worrying about it, and thinking what if I left for work and forgot to turn off the stove and the kitchen catches on fire and I end up burning down the apartment, and even worse with my roommates still in the apartment?

THERAPIST: Which is a pretty anxiety-provoking thought. What do you feel physically in that moment?

JOSEPH: I'm not sure, but probably pretty tense and nervous.

THERAPIST: And what do you do?

JOSEPH: I go back and check everything again.

THERAPIST: Once? Or more than once?

JOSEPH: I'll check, then I'll start doubting again, then I'll check again.

THERAPIST: And when you first check, how do you feel?

JOSEPH: At first I feel better.

THERAPIST: So, just like the other example, this EDB of checking gets reinforced each time you do it because it makes you feel better, at least temporarily. When you feel that anxiety, you feel driven to perform the checking as a way of relieving or acting on the anxiety. But these EDBs don't seem to work because the doubting thoughts return, and you end up late for work, or you have to lose out on sleep in order to make time for these behaviors. And just like we talked about with the avoidance behaviors, it seems to make it worse—the doubt and anxiety you feel is so strong that it feels like you couldn't tolerate it if you didn't do these behaviors. What we need to do, just like we did with your thoughts, is start breaking down these associations so you can learn new things about the doubt and anxiety driving these behaviors, like maybe you can tolerate these emotions more than you think, even without engaging in the EDB.

This module concludes with an introduction to countering patterns of avoidance and EDBs through targeting and modifying specific behaviors. The two primary therapeutic strategies are (1) beginning to engage in activities to evoke emotions that are currently being avoided and (2) counteracting maladaptive EDBs by developing and engaging in behaviors that are different, or thatcounteract, these responses.

Module 6: Awareness and Tolerance of Physical Sensations

Module 6 introduces the first opportunity to engage in an exposure that focuses on eliciting physical sensations that often trigger strong emotional reactions, and to begin to build the patient's awareness of the contribution of physical sensations to emotional experiences. Following an introduction to the rationale for provoking physical sensations, therapist and patient work through a list of exercises designed to elicit emotion through physical activation, known as "symptom induction exercises." Some examples include hyperventilating, spinning, and running in place. In addition, any exercises that may be particularly relevant to the patient may be added. Prior to each exercise, the therapist demonstrates the exercise, and following the patient's completion of the exercise asks the patient to rate the intensity, distress, and similarity to physical sensations typically experiences during an emotion, each on a scale of 0 (*Not at all*) to 8 (*Very much*).

THERAPIST: So today we'll do a number of exercises to induce some of these physical sensations that are often present when you experience anxiety, and look at the intensity, distress, and how close the sensations come to your experiences during uncomfortable emotions. The first one I'm going to ask you to do is the hyperventilation exercise. (*following the exercise*) What sensations do you notice?

JOSEPH: I didn't like that at all.

THERAPIST: So you are having thoughts and judgments about the sensations, that you don't like them. What about the actual physical sensations themselves—can you describe them?

JOSEPH: Dizzy, lightheaded, sort of unreal, like I'm disconnected.

THERAPIST: Great. So thinking about those sensations, how would you rate the intensity of those sensations?

JOSEPH: Probably a 7.

THERAPIST: And how about the distress?

JOSEPH: Also a 7.

THERAPIST: And similarity?

JOSEPH: Well, I don't usually get dizzy when I'm anxious, but I guess feeling lightheaded and surreal is closer, so maybe like a 5?

The therapist repeats the exposure two more times, and the last time asks the patient to pay particular attention to any thoughts he is having about the sensations, particularly any negative appraisals, and how these thoughts interact with and either lessen or intensify the physical sensations.

THERAPIST: How would you rate the intensity this time?

JOSEPH: Probably a 5.

THERAPIST: And the distress?

JOSEPH: It was much better that time, probably only a 4.

THERAPIST: What did you notice was different that time?

JOSEPH: Well, I guess I knew what to expect, and I wasn't having the same thoughts as the first time. The first time I kept thinking, "I don't like this," and wondering when it was going to end. This time I just sort of went with it.

THERAPIST: Interesting. So when you just focused on the sensations themselves, without judgment or negative thoughts about them, the intensity was less?

JOSEPH: Yes, definitely.

Following the completion of all the chosen exercises, therapist and patient choose the most relevant exercises to engage in regularly over the next week. The patient is asked to complete one exercise several times a day, until the associated distress decreases. This repeated exposure helps facilitate learning of new information about the dangerousness (or lack thereof) of physical sensations and may help diminish future distress when physical symptoms do occur. See Figure 6.3 for an example of a Symptom Induction Test Form.

Please complete each of the exercises (as described) below. Be sure to engage in each exercise fully, and try to produce at least moderate symptom intensity. After the exercise, please note:

1. the physical symptoms you experienced
2. the **intensity** of the symptoms (0- to 8-point scale; 0 = *No intensity*, 8 = *Extreme intensity*)
3. the level of **distress** you experienced during the task (0- to 8-point scale; 0 = *No distress*, 8 = *Extreme distress*)
4. the degree of **similarity to your naturally occurring symptoms** (0- to 8-point scale; 0 = *Not at all similar*, 8 = *Extremely similar*)

Wait until the symptoms have mostly subsided before attempting the next exercise. Use the other spaces provided to be creative and come up with additional exercises that are specific to you. When you are done, pick three of the exercises that produced the most anxiety for you. Put a star next to those exercises.

Procedure	Symptoms experienced	Intensity	Distress	Similarity
Hyperventilation (60 seconds)				
Breathing through a thin straw (2 minutes)				
Spinning while standing (60 seconds)				
Running in place (60 seconds)				
Other: (____ seconds)				
Other: (____ seconds)				
Other: (____ seconds)				
Other: (____ seconds)				
Other: (____ seconds)				
Other: (____ seconds)				

FIGURE 6.3. Symptom Induction Test Form.

Module 7: Interoceptive and Situational Emotion Exposures

This treatment module allows application of all the skills learned thus far to actual situations, events, or activities that trigger strong levels of emotions that the patient has previously avoided. The therapist begins with a discussion about the rationale for emotion exposures. Although this module in the treatment program is often the most challenging, it is the best opportunity to make lasting behavioral and emotional changes. Emotion exposures serve three critical goals: (1) Interpretations and appraisals about the dangerousness of situations (internal or external) are modified and replaced with newer, more adaptive interpretations and appraisals; and (2) avoidance and related impairment is reversed, EDBs are recognized and modified, and the primary goal of extinguishing anxious and distressing reactions to the experience of intense emotions can proceed.

In addition to engaging in emotion exposures for homework, an important part of this module is practicing emotion exposures in session. This is critical because the therapist can often challenge the patient to engage in more difficult exposures in session and will be able to note any use of avoidance strategies or engagement in EDBs that may be outside the patient's awareness. The particular in-session exposure tasks vary from patient to patient, and it is important that the therapist be able to generate a number of different possible tasks in which to engage. Once the task has been identified, the therapist can discuss any anxious or negative automatic appraisals occurring and help the patient consider other possibilities. The therapist should also remind the patient to use the skills of present-focused awareness and try to prevent any avoidance strategies that would interfere with the exposure. At the end of each session, the therapist helps the patient choose several emotion exposures to engage in outside of session for homework.

For Joseph, several different exposures were designed that targeted a variety of anxiety-provoking situations. Examples included walking straight ahead on a crowded sidewalk, forcing oncoming pedestrians to move aside rather than moving aside himself; engaging in a mock debate with a stranger and sticking to his opinion; eating a piece of fruit and riding on public transportation, and focusing his attention on what is going on around him rather than on any subsequent physical reactions to the fruit (e.g., gas, bloating); going to a party and excusing himself to the restroom, in order to test some of his anticipatory automatic appraisals about what others will think of him; reducing the number of times he uses the bathroom in the morning from five to one; and similarly reducing the number of times he checks stoves, candles, and so forth, before leaving the house.

An exposure near the top of Joseph's hierarchy was to go on a long car trip with some friends and acquaintances to see a concert in a nearby city. This would require him to face several of his fears at once. First, he would have to assert himself and ask his friends if he could come along in the car. Second, he would be traveling with a small group of people, including a few people he does not know well, and might be required to carry on casual conversation. Third, he would be locked in a small, confined space with no easy escape route should his IBS symptoms flare up.

THERAPIST: This was a big exposure assignment for you. Let's start from the beginning, when you had to ask your friend if you could come along on the trip. Do you remember what you were experiencing just before you made that call?

JOSEPH: I noticed I felt shaky. I felt butterflies in my stomach, my face was hot, and my heart was beating fast.

THERAPIST: So, a lot of physical sensations associated with anxiety. What about thoughts?

JOSEPH: I was worried that my friend would be annoyed, like I am putting him out, or that he would be mad I waited so long to ask him. I also noticed I kept procrastinating, looking things up on the Internet, going to the corner store to buy a soda, things like that.

THERAPIST: Good! So you noticed some behaviors, too. And what happened when you called him? Did your anticipatory appraisals come true?

JOSEPH: Not at all, he was actually pretty happy I asked. He said he was hoping I was coming along, sort of like he was expecting it and was happy about it.

THERAPIST: What about the trip itself, how did that go?

JOSEPH: Well, about 10 minutes into it I started to feel some cramping in my stomach and thought, "Oh boy, here we go." Then I remembered the exposure we did with the fruit and decided to try focusing on the music on the stereo, the view out the window, and the conversations that were happening in the car, rather than focusing on my stomach.

THERAPIST: Did that help?

JOSEPH: Well, the cramping was still there, but it wasn't bothering me as much because I wasn't just focusing on that.

THERAPIST: Did you have any urges to use the bathroom?

JOSEPH: I did at one point, and I decided to try what we talked about, and see if I could wait it out and see if it passed, and it did! At one point, though, I did need to use the bathroom.

THERAPIST: What happened then?

JOSEPH: I asked my friend if he could stop at the next rest stop.

THERAPIST: And what was his reaction, or the reaction of the other passengers?

JOSEPH: It was no big deal at all! No one seemed to care, and in fact I think they also wanted to stop, so it was no big deal! I also noticed something else. On the car ride back, I didn't really think about it at all, and my gut started rumbling but I just didn't worry about it and kept focusing on what was going on around me. It wasn't even an issue at all on the way back.

For Joseph, great progress was made through exposures relating to his symptoms of anxiety and management of his IBS symptoms. However, Joseph continued to hold on to a core belief that he was "unworthy" and "unlikable." Additional exposures were designed to target this belief directly.

THERAPIST: You seem to have made some great progress over the last few weeks, would you agree?

JOSEPH: Yes, I definitely feel like I can cope with my anxiety better, and things seem to be going really well at work right now, which helps. The other teachers have even started inviting me out for drinks after work, and I've gone a few times and actually had a lot of fun.

THERAPIST: That's great news. One thing that is interesting—despite these changes, on your weekly questionnaires I notice you are still marking a few items like "I dislike myself" or "I feel utterly worthless."

JOSEPH: Yeah, I still don't think I'm a great person, and I still worry I'm just fooling people, or they are going to find out the "true" me and run the other way.

THERAPIST: I wonder if we can do some exposure work around those?

Using similar techniques learned in Module 4, the therapist helps Joseph generate evidence for and against the statements that he dislikes himself and that he is worthless. He is able to generate some evidence against this belief, for example, the large turnout of friends and supporters at a recent concert he put on. Using this and other evidence, the therapist helps Joseph generate a list of positive self-statements.

THERAPIST: So, what might you say about your recent experiences putting on the concert?

JOSEPH: I don't know, "I am a good musician?"

THERAPIST: That's one, but maybe something even more objective and believable to you, like you work hard on your music?

JOSEPH: That's true. And when I play, people seem to like it.

THERAPIST: So you work hard at your music, and you entertain people with it?

JOSEPH: Yes, that's true. I also am a good listener.

THERAPIST: Tell me more about that.

JOSEPH: Well, I have a friend who is going through a hard time right now, and sometimes he calls me just to talk about it. I usually am pretty good at letting him talk it through.

THERAPIST: So can we add "I am there for people and listen to them" to the list? Maybe even "I am a good friend?"

Once the therapist and Joseph generated a list of statements that are evidence against the core belief of being worthless and disliking himself, Joseph was asked to read these statements aloud and to notice his reactions to them.

THERAPIST: How was that reading those statements?

JOSEPH: Awkward. I felt really uncomfortable. It makes me feel anxious.

THERAPIST: Can you describe that for me?

JOSEPH: Well, I get this weird sort of "zap" of fear and this feeling in the pit of my stomach, and I notice I get these kind of sarcastic thoughts like "That's not true" or "Sure you are."

THERAPIST: So saying nice things about yourself brings on a feeling of fear, and some negative thoughts about yourself?

JOSEPH: Yes. I guess I feel kind of vulnerable, too, like my guard is down.

THERAPIST: That's a very interesting observation. So saying something positive about yourself leaves you feeling a bit vulnerable, exposed maybe? Is it maybe a less familiar feeling to you than the self-criticism?

JOSEPH: Definitely. So is the fear like entering a foreign territory, like I don't know what might jump out at me?

THERAPIST: Maybe something like that! Whereas the negative thoughts are perhaps more familiar and less fearful in a way. What if we made the statements a little less new and unfamiliar by repeating them a few times? (*After Joseph rereads the statements two more times.*) How was it this time?

JOSEPH: Well, a little easier, not quite as foreign, I guess, but still a little strange.

THERAPIST: Good. So exposing yourself to these statements repeatedly seems to have a similar effect as some of the other exposure exercises we've done? A little easier and less foreign each time?

JOSEPH: Yeah, I guess it gets a little easier each time.

THERAPIST: How about continuing with this exposure this week, generating a few more statements, and reading them out loud to yourself each day?

JOSEPH: I could try that.

In future sessions, the therapist revisits the patient's continuing need for emotional exposures. If he/she determines that the patient would benefit from additional emotion exposures, they can be continued both in session and for homework at this time. Additionally, the therapist can focus on any events or emotional reactions over the past week that can be processed in session. Obstacles to exposure completion and reactions to exposures are discussed in session.

Module 8: Accomplishments, Maintenance, and Relapse Prevention

In the final treatment session, the therapist reviews both the major concepts presented in treatment and the patient's progress. The therapist reviews the three-component model of emotions, focusing on cognitive reappraisal, preventing emotional avoidance, and modifying EDBs. The patient is asked for his/her impression of progress made over the course of treatment, and the therapist can highlight areas of improvement and areas in need of continued practice. Reasons for lack of improvement (e.g., initial error in diagnosis, lack of understanding treatment principles, unrealistic goals, and lack of motivation) should also be reviewed. The therapist then discusses the inevitability of future stressors and potential reoccurrence of symptoms. The continuation of informal emotion exposures and use of skills learned are encouraged. The therapist may further assist the patient in staying committed to treatment by establishing long-term goals for the patient.

OUTCOME AND CONCLUSION

Joseph's symptoms were assessed at pre- and posttreatment using a battery of self-report questionnaires, as described earlier. During treatment, Joseph's SIAS score decreased from 51 at pretreatment to 26 at posttreatment. His BDI-II score decreased from 49 at pretreatment to 11 at post-treatment. His PSWQ score decreased from 80 to 35. Functionally, Joseph was able to meet many of his treatment goals over the course of treatment. For example, he was able to find a job he thoroughly enjoyed that matched his career goals. He significantly increased his social interactions and began engaging in activities, such as playing more local concerts, all of which significantly increased his self-confidence and sense of self-worth. He gained control of his IBS symptoms and no longer engaged in avoidance behaviors related to his symptoms. At the time of termination, Joseph noted that he felt "like a completely different person" and was noticeably more positive and confident in his demeanor and presentation. Although Joseph was not part of the research program and, therefore, did not participate in an independent post-treatment clinical interview, his clinician (K. K. E.) estimated that his CSRs for both the social phobia and GAD diagnoses had dropped to a 3 (subclinical), the diagnosis of MDD was in partial remission with a CSR of 2, and although he improved in many of his OCD-related symptoms, the diagnosis of OCD warranted a CSR rating of 4 (just above clinical severity).

Joseph returned to our Center for a follow-up assessment 8 months posttreatment that comprised of readministration of the ADIS and self-report questionnaires. At follow-up, Joseph's self-reported symptom ratings increased slightly from posttreatment. He endorsed somewhat higher scores on the SIAS, particularly on items related to greeting strangers or encountering strangers on the street, with a total follow-up score of 37. His scores on the PSWQ increased slightly, from 35 to 40. Notably, Joseph's BDI score increased from 11 at posttreatment to 35 at follow-up, suggesting a relapse of depressive symptoms. In particular, Joseph indicated increases in pessimistic feelings about the future, guilty feelings, fatigue, and sleep disruption. At the time of his follow-up interview, Joseph reported that he had recently gone through a breakup with his girlfriend at the start of the holiday season, and he attributed his low mood to this breakup and the winter weather. Without further follow-up data, however, it is unclear the degree to which the increase in depressive symptoms is attributable to these situational variables or represents a relapse of his depression. Despite these increases at follow-up, Joseph did show a decrease in WSAS scores from pretreatment to follow-up (from 34, *Severe interference*, to 21, *Moderate interference*), which may reflect that even though his symptoms had returned to some degree, he was able to manage interference from the symptoms much better. However, Joseph did not complete the WSAS at posttreatment, so it is not clear exactly what the trajectory of change is on this measure.

Clinician ratings using the ADIS seemed largely to coincide with Joseph's self-report. He experienced a slight worsening of his GAD and MDD symptoms from posttreatment to follow-up, receiving CSR ratings of 4 and 5, respectively. He was able to maintain his treatment gains for his OCD symptoms, which were again given a CSR of 4. Notably, Joseph's social phobia was given a CSR rating of 2, suggesting that he was able to maintain and possibly even improve on gains made in treatment; whereas he still endorsed some fear and anxiety related to social situations, the interference and distress related to these fears was no longer endorsed at a clinical level.

REFERENCES

Allen, L. B., White, K. S., Barlow, D. H., Shear, M. K., Gorman, J. M., & Woods, S. W. (2010). Cognitive-behavior therapy (CBT) for panic disorder: Relationship of anxiety and depression comorbidity with treatment outcome. *Journal of Psychopathology and Behavioral Assessment, 32*(2), 185–192.

American Psychiatric Association. (2000). *Diagnostic and statistical manual of mental disorders* (4th ed., text rev.). Washington, DC: Author.

American Psychiatric Association. (2013). *Diagnostic and statistical manual of mental disorders* (5th ed.). Arlington, VA: Author.

Andrews, G. (1990). Classification of neurotic disorders. *Journal of the Royal Society of Medicine, 83*(10), 606–607.

Andrews, G. (1996). Current controversies in the anxiety disorders. In R. M. Rapee (Ed.), *Comorbidity in neurotic disorders: The similarities are more important than the difference* (pp. 3–20). New York: Guilford Press.

Barlow, D. H. (1988). *Anxiety and its disorders: The nature and treatment of anxiety and panic.* New York: Guilford Press.

Barlow, D. H. (1991). Disorders of emotion. *Psychological Inquiry, 2*, 58–71.

Barlow, D. H. (2000). Unraveling the mysteries of anxiety and its disorders from the perspective of emotion theory. *American Psychologist, 55*(11), 1247–1263.

Barlow, D. H. (2002). *Anxiety and its disorders: The nature and treatment of anxiety and panic* (2nd ed.). New York: Guilford Press.

Barlow, D. H., Bullis, J. R., Comer, J. S., & Ametaj, A. A. (2013). Evidence-based psychological treatments: An update and the way forward. *Annual Review of Clinical Psychology, 9*, 1–27.

Barlow, D. H., & Craske, M. G. (2007). *Mastery of your anxiety and panic: Client workbook for anxiety and panic* (4th ed.). New York: Oxford University Press.

Barlow, D. H., Gorman, J. M., Shear, M. K., & Woods, S. W. (2000). Cognitive-behavioral therapy, imipramine, or their combination for panic disorder: A randomized controlled trial. *Journal of the American Medical Association, 283*, 2529–2536.

Barlow, D. H., Sauer-Zavala, S. E., Carl, J. R., Bullis, J. R., & Ellard, K. K. (in press). The nature, diagnosis, and treatment of neuroticism: Back to the future. *Clinical Psychological Science.*

Beck, A. T. (1967). *The diagnosis and management of depression.* Philadelphia: University of Pennsylvania Press.

Beck, A. T., Rush, A. J., Shaw, B. F., & Emery, G. (1979). *Cognitive therapy of depression.* New York: Guilford Press.

Beck, A. T., Steer, R. A., & Brown, G. K. (1996). *Beck Depression Inventory manual* (2nd ed.). San Antonio, TX: Psychological Corporation.

Bentley, K. H., Gallagher, M. W., Carl, J. R., Farchione, T. J., & Barlow, D. H. (2013). *Development and validation of an Overall Depression Severity and Impairment Scale.* Manuscript submitted for publication.

Boelen, P. A., Vrinssen, I., & van Tulder, F. (2010). Intolerance of uncertainty in adolescents: Correlations with worry, social anxiety, and depression. *Journal of Nervous and Mental Disease, 198*, 194–200.

Borkovec, T. D. (1994). The nature, functions, and origins of worry. In G. C. L. Davey & F. Tallis (Eds.), *Worrying: Perspectives on theory, assessment, and treatment* (pp. 5–34). New York: Wiley.

Borkovec, T. D., Hazlett-Stevens, H., & Diaz, M. L. (1999). The role of positive beliefs about worry in generalized anxiety disorder and its treatment. *Clinical Psychology and Psychotherapy, 6*, 126–138.

Boswell, J. F., Thompson-Holland, J., Farchione, T. J., & Barlow, D. H. (2013). The intolerance of uncertainty: A common factor in the treatment of emotional disorders. *Journal of Clinical Psychology, 69*, 630–645.

Bouton, M. E. (2005). Behavior systems and the contextual control of anxiety, fear, and panic. In L. Feldman Barrett, P. M. Niedenthal, & P. Winkielman (Eds.), *Emotion and consciousness* (pp. 205–227). New York: Guilford Press.

Bouton, M. E., Mineka, S., & Barlow, D. H. (2001). A modern learning theory perspective on the etiology of panic disorder. *Psychological Review, 108*, 4–32.

Brown, T. A. (2007). Temporal course and structural relationships among dimensions of temperament and DSM-IV anxiety and mood disorder constructs. *Journal of Abnormal Psychology, 116*, 313–328.

Brown, T. A., Antony, M. M., & Barlow, D. H. (1995). Diagnostic comorbidity in panic disorder: Effect on treatment outcome and course of comorbid diagnoses following treatment. *Journal of Consulting and Clinical Psychology, 63*, 408–418.

Brown, T. A., & Barlow, D. H. (1995). Long-term outcome in cognitive-behavioral treatment of panic disorder: Clinical predictors and alternative strategies for assessment. *Journal of Consulting and Clinical Psychology, 63*, 754–765.

Brown, T. A., & Barlow, D. H. (2002). Classification of anxiety and mood disorders. In D. H. Barlow (Ed.), *Anxiety and its disorders: The nature and treatment of anxiety and panic* (2nd ed., pp. 292–327). New York: Guilford Press.

Brown, T. A., & Barlow, D. H. (2009). A proposal for a dimensional classification system based on the shared features of the DSM-IV anxiety and mood disorders: Implications for assessment and treatment. *Psychological Assessment, 21*, 256–271.

Brown, T. A., Campbell, L. A., Lehman, C. L., Grisham, J. R., & Mancill, R. B. (2001). Current and lifetime comorbidity of the DSM-IV anxiety and mood disorders in a large clinical sample. *Journal of Abnormal Psychology, 110*, 49–58.

Brown, T. A., Chorpita, B. F., & Barlow, D. H. (1998). Structural relationships among dimensions of the DSM-IV anxiety and mood disorders and dimensions of negative affect, positive affect, and autonomic arousal. *Journal of Abnormal Psychology, 107*, 179–192.

Brown, T. A., Di Nardo, P. A., & Barlow, D. H. (2014). *Anxiety Disorders Interview Schedule for DSM-5*. New York: Oxford University Press.

Brown, T. A., Di Nardo, P. A., Lehman, C. L., & Campbell, L. A. (2001). Reliability of DSM-IV anxiety and mood disorders: Implications for the classification of emotional disorders. *Journal of Abnormal Psychology, 110*, 49–58.

Campbell-Sills, L., Barlow, D. H., Brown, T. A., & Hofmann, S. G. (2006a). Acceptability and suppression of negative emotion in anxiety and mood disorders. *Emotion, 6*, 587–595.

Campbell-Sills, L., Barlow, D. H., Brown, T. A., & Hofmann, S. G. (2006b). Effects of suppression and acceptance on emotional responses in individuals with anxiety and mood disorders. *Behaviour Research and Therapy, 44*, 1251–1263.

Campbell-Sills, L., Liverant, G. I., & Brown, T. A. (2004). Psychometric evaluation of the behavioral inhibition/behavioral activation scales in a large sample of outpatients with anxiety and mood disorders. *Psychological Assessment, 16*(3), 244–254.

Campbell-Sills, L., Norman, S. B., Craske, M. G., Sullivan, G., Lang, A. J., Chavira, D. A. (2009). Validation of a brief measure of anxiety-related severity and impairment: the Overall Anxiety Severity and Impairment Scale (OASIS). *Journal of Affective Disorders, 112*(1-3), 92–101.

Caspi, A., Sugden, K., Moffitt, T. E., Taylor, A., Craig, I. W., & Harrington, H. (2003). Influence of life stress on depression: Moderation by a polymorphism in the 5-HTT gene. *Science, 301*, 386–389.

Chorpita, B. F., Albano, A. M., & Barlow, D. H. (1998). The structure of negative emotions in a clinical sample of children and adolescents. *Journal of Abnormal Child Psychology, 107*, 74–85.

Chorpita, B. F., & Barlow, D. H. (1998). The development of anxiety: The role of control in the early environment. *Psychological Bulletin, 124*, 3–21.

Clark, D. A. (2012). The English Improving Access to Psychological Therapies (IAPT) program: History and progress. In R. K. McHugh & D. H. Barlow (Eds.), *Dissemination and implementation of evidence-based psychological interventions* (pp. 61–77). New York: Oxford University Press.

Clark, L. A. (2005). Temperament as a unifying basis for personality and psychopathology. *Journal of Abnormal Psychology, 114*, 505–521.

Clark, L. A., & Watson, D. (1991). Tripartite model of anxiety and depression: Psychometric evidence and taxonomic implications. *Journal of Abnormal Psychology, 103*, 103–116.

Craske, M. G., & Barlow, D. H. (2006). *Mastery of your anxiety and worry* (2nd ed.). New York: Oxford University Press.

Craske, M. G., Rowe, M., Lewin, M., & Noriega-Dimitri, R. (1997). Interoceptive exposure versus breathing retraining within cognitive-behavioural therapy for panic disorder with agoraphobia. *British Journal of Clinical Psychology, 36*, 85–99.

Dimidjian, S., Hollon, S. D., Dobson, K. S., Schmaling, K.

B., Kohlenberg, R. J., & Addis, M. E. (2006). Randomized trial of behavioral activation, cognitive therapy, and antidepressant medication in the acute treatment of adults with major depression. *Journal of Consulting and Clinical Psychology, 74*(4), 658–670.

Di Nardo, P. A., Brown, T. A., & Barlow, D. H. (1994). *Anxiety Disorders Interview Schedule for DSM-IV.* Albany, NY: Graywind.

Drabant, E. M., Ramel, W., Edge, M. D., Hyde, L. W., Kuo, J. R., Goldin, P. R. (2012). Neural mechanisms underlying 5-HTTLPR-related sensitivity to acute stress. *American Journal of Psychiatry, 169*, 397–405.

Endicott, J., Nee, J., Harrison, W., & Blumenthal, R. (1993). Quality of Life Enjoyment and Satisfaction Questionnaire: A new measure. *Psychopharmacology Bulletin, 29*(2), 321–326.

Eysenck, H. J. (1947). *Dimension of personality.* London: Routledge & Kegan Paul.

First, M. B., Spitzer, R. L., Gibbon, M., & Williams, J. B. W. (1996). *Structured Clinical Interview for DSM-IV Axis I Disorders—Patient Edition (SCID-I/P, Version 2.0).* New York: Biometrics Research Department, New York State Psychiatric Institute.

Foa, E. B., Riggs, D. S., Dancu, C. V., & Rothbaum, B. O. (1993). Reliability and validity of a brief instrument for assessment post-traumatic stress disorder. *Journal of Traumatic Stress, 6*(4), 459–473.

Foa, E. B., & Tolin, D. F. (2000). Comparison of the PTSD Symptom Scale—Interview Version and the Clinician-Administered PTSD scale. *Journal of Traumatic Stress, 13*(2), 181–191.

Goodman, W. K., Price, L. H., Rasmussen, S. A., Mazure, C., Fleischmann, R. L., & Hill, C. L. (1989). The Yale–Brown Obsessive Compulsive Scale: I. Development, use, and reliability. *Archives of General Psychiatry, 46*(11), 1006–1011.

Hafner, J., & Marks, I. M. (1976). Exposure *in vivo* of agoraphobics: Contributions of diazepam, group exposure, and anxiety evocation. *Psychological Medicine, 6*, 71–88.

Hamilton, M. (1959). The assessment of anxiety states by rating. *British Journal of Medical Psychology, 32*, 50–55.

Hamilton, M. (1960). A rating scale for depression. *Journal of Neurology, Neurosurgery, and Psychiatry, 23*, 56–62.

Hayes, S. C., Strosahl, K. D., & Wilson, K. G. (1999). *Acceptance and commitment therapy: An experiential approach to behavior change.* New York: Guilford Press.

Heimberg, R. G., Horner, K. J., Juster, H. R., Safren, S. A., Brown, E. J., & Schneier, F. R. (1999). Psychometric properties of the Liebowitz Social Anxiety Scale. *Psychological Medicine, 29*(1), 199–212.

Heimberg, R. G., Liebowitz, M. R., Hope, D. A., Schneier, F. R., Holt, C. S., & Welkowitz, L. A. (1998). Cognitive behavioral group therapy vs phenelzine therapy for social phobia: 12-week outcome. *Archives of General Psychiatry, 55*(12), 1133–1141.

Hettema, J. M., Neale, M. C., & Kendler, K. S. (2001). A review and meta-analysis of the genetic epidemiology of anxiety disorders. *American Journal of Psychiatry, 158*, 1568–1578.

Huppert, J. D., Bufka, L. F., Barlow, D. H., Gorman, J. M., Shear, M. K., & Woods, S. W. (2001). Therapists, therapist variables and cognitive-behavioral therapy outcome in a multicenter trial for panic disorder. *Journal of Consulting and Clinical Psychology, 69*, 747–755.

Izard, C. E. (1971). *The face of emotion.* New York: Appleton-Century-Crofts.

Jacobson, N. S., Martell, C. R., & Dimidjian, S. (2001). Behavioral activation treatment for depression: Returning to contextual roots. *Clinical Psychology: Science and Practice, 8*, 255–270.

Kendler, K. S. (1996). Major depression and generalized anxiety disorder: Same genes, (partly) different environments—revisited. *British Journal of Psychiatry, 30*(Suppl.), 68–75.

Kendler, K. S., Walters, E. E., Neale, M. C., Kessler, R. C., Heath, A. C., & Eaves, L. J. (1995). The structure of genetic and environmental risk factors for six major psychiatric disorders in women: Phobia, generalized anxiety disorder, panic disorder, bulimia, major depression, and alcoholism. *Archives of General Psychiatry, 52*, 374–382.

Kessler, R. C., Nelson, C. B., McGonagle, K. A., Lui, J., Swartz, M., & Blazer, D. G. (1996). Comorbidity of DSM-III-R major depressive disorder in the general population: Results from the National Comorbidity Survey. *British Journal of Psychiatry, 168*, 17–30.

Keyes, C. L., Wissing, M., Potgieter, J. P., Temane, M., Kruger, A., & van Rooy, S. (2008). Evaluation of the Mental Health Continuum—Short Form (MHC-SF) in Setswana-speaking South Africans. *Clinical Psychology and Psychotherapy, 15*(3), 181–192.

Keyes, C. L. M. (2005). Mental illness and/or mental health?: Investigating axioms of the complete state model of health. *Journal of Consulting and Clinical Psychology, 73*, 539–548.

Keyes, C. L. M. (2006). Mental health in adolescence: Is America's youth flourishing? *American Journal of Orthopsychiatry, 76*, 395–402.

Lamers, S. M., Westerhof, G. J., Bohlmeijer, E. T., ten Klooster, P. M., & Keyes, C. L. (2011). Evaluating the psychometric properties of the Mental Health Continuum-Short Form (MHC-SF). *Journal of Clinical Psychology, 67*(1), 99–110.

Lee, J. K., Orsillo, S. M., Roemer, L., & Allen, L. B. (2010). Distress and avoidance in generalized anxiety disorder: Exploring the relationships with intolerance of uncertainty and worry. *Behaviour Therapy, 39*, 126–136.

Liebowitz, M. R. (1987). Social phobia. *Modern Problems in Pharmacopsychiatry, 22*, 141–173.

Liebowitz, M. R., Heimberg, R. G., Schneier, F. R., Hope, D. A., Davies, S., & Holt, C. S. (1999). Cognitive-behavioral group therapy versus phenelzine in social phobia: Long-term outcome. *Depression and Anxiety, 10*(3), 89–98.

Linehan, M. M. (1993). *Cognitive behavioral treatment of borderline personality disorder.* New York: Guilford Press.

Liverant, G. I., Brown, T. A., Barlow, D. H., & Roemer, L. (2008). Emotion regulation in unipolar depression: The effects of acceptance and suppression of subjective emotional experience on the intensity and duration of sadness and negative affect. *Behaviour Research and Therapy, 46,* 1201–1209.

Lonsdorf, T. B., Golkar, A., Lindstöm, K. M., Fransson, P., Schalling, M., & Ohman, A. (2011). 5-HTTLPR and COMTval158met genotype gate amygdala reactivity and habituation. *Biological Psychology, 87,* 106–112.

Margraf, J., Taylor, C. B., Ehlers, A., Roth, W. T., & Agras, W. S. (1987). Panic attacks in the natural environment. *Journal of Nervous and Mental Disease, 175,* 558–565.

Mattick, R. P., & Clarke, J. C. (1998). Development and validation of measures of social phobia scrutiny fear and social interaction anxiety. *Behaviour Research and Therapy, 36,* 455–470.

McHugh, R. K., & Barlow, D. H. (Eds.). (2012). *Dissemination and implementation of evidence-baed psychological interventions.* New York: Oxford University Press.

Mennin, D. S., Heimberg, R. G., Turk, C. L., & Fresco, D. M. (2005). Preliminary evidence for an emotion dysregulation model of generalized anxiety disorder. *Behaviour Research and Therapy, 43,* 1281–1310.

Merikangas, K. R., Zhang, H., & Aveneoli, S. (2003). Longitudinal trajectories of depression and anxiety in a prospective community study. *Archives of General Psychiatry, 60,* 993–1000.

Meyer, T. J., Miller, M. L., Metzger, R. L., & Borkovec, T. D. (1990). Development and validation of the Penn State Worry Questionnaire. *Behaviour Research and Therapy, 28,* 487–495.

Miller, W. R., & Rollnick, S. (2013). *Motivational interviewing: Preparing people for change* (3rd ed.). New York: Guilford Press.

Montag, C., Fiebach, C. J., Kirsch, P., & Reuter, M. (2011). Interation of 5-HTTLPR and a variation on the oxytocin recepter gene influences negative emotionality. *Biological Psychiatry, 69,* 601–603.

Munafò, M. R., Brown, S. M., & Hariri, A. R. (2008). Seratonin transporter (5-HTTLPR) genotype and amygdala activation: A meta-analysis. *Biological Psychiatry, 63,* 852–857.

Nathan, P. E., & Gorman, J. M. (Eds.). (2007). *A guide to treatments that work* (3rd ed.). New York: Oxford University Press.

Norman, S. B., Cissell, S. H., Means-Christensen, A. J., & Stein, M. B. (2006). Development and validation of an Overall Anxiety Severity and Impairment Scale (OASIS). *Depression and Anxiety, 23*(4), 245–249.

Pezawas, L., Meyer-Lindenberg, A., Drabant, E. M., Verchinski, B. A., Munoz, K. E., & Kolachana, B. S. (2005). 5-HTTLPR polymorphism impacts human cingulate-amygdala interactions: A genetic susceptibility mechanism for depression. *Nature Neuroscience, 8*(6), 828–834.

Raffa, S. D., Stoddard, J. A., White, K. S., Barlow, D. H., Gorman, J. M., & Shear, M. K. (2008). Relapse following combined-treatment discontinuation in a placebo-controlled trial for panic disorder. *Journal of Nervous and Mental Disease, 196*(7), 548–555.

Rapee, R. M., Craske, M. G., & Barlow, D. H. (1990). Subject described features of panic attacks using a new self-monitoring form. *Journal of Anxiety Disorders, 4,* 171–181.

Roy-Byrne, P. P., Craske, M. G., & Stein, M. B. (2006). Panic disorder. *Lancet, 368,* 1023–1032.

Rutter, M., Moffit, T. E., & Caspi, A. (2006). Gene-environment interplay and psychopathology: Multiple varieties but real effects. *Journal of Child Psychology and Psychiatry, 47,* 226–261.

Ruzek, J. I., Karlin, B. E., & Zeiss, A. (2012). Implementation of evidence-based psychological treatments in the Veterans Health Administration. In R. K. McHugh & D. H. Barlow (Eds.), *Dissemination and implementation of evidence-based psychological interventions* (pp. 78–96). New York: Oxford University Press.

Safren, S. A., Heimberg, R. G., Horner, K. J., Juster, H. R., Schneier, F. R., & Liebowitz, M. R. (1999). Factor structure of social fears: The Liebowitz Social Anxiety Scale. *Journal of Anxiety Disorders, 13*(3), 253–270.

Sauer-Zavala, S. E., & Barlow, D. H. (2013). *The case for borderline personality disorder as an emotional disorder: Implications for treatment.* Manuscript submitted for publication.

Shear, K., Belnap, B. H., Mazumdar, S., Houck, P., & Rollman, B. L. (2006). Generalized anxiety disorder severity scale (GADSS): A preliminary validation study. *Depression and Anxiety, 23*(2), 77–82.

Shear, M. K., Brown, T. A., Barlow, D. H., Money, R., Sholomskas, D. E., & Woods, S. W. (1997). Multicenter collaborative Panic Disorder Severity Scale. *American Journal of Psychiatry, 154,* 1571–1575.

Shear, M. K., Vander Bilt, J., & Rucci, P. (2001). Reliability and validity of a Structured Interview Guide for the Hamilton Anxiety Rating Scale (SIGH-A). *Depression and Anxiety, 13,* 166–178.

Stein, M. B., Campbell-Sills, L., & Gelernter, J. (2009). Genetic variation in 5HTTLPR is associated with emotional resilience. *Neuropsychiatric Genetics, 150B,* 900–906.

Storch, E. A., Larson, M. J., Price, L. H., Rasmussen, S. A., Murphy, T. K., & Goodman, W. K. (2010). Psychometric analysis of the Yale–Brown Obsessive–Compulsive Scale Second Edition Symptom Checklist. *Journal of Anxiety Disorders, 24,* 650–656.

Suárez, L., Bennett, S. M., Goldstein, C., & Barlow, D. H.

(2009). Understanding anxiety disorders from a "triple vulnerability" framework. In M. M. Antony & M. B. Stein (Eds.), *Handbook of anxiety and the anxiety disorders* (pp. 153–172). New York: Oxford University Press.

Tsao, J. C. I., Mystkowski, J. L., Zucker, B. G., & Craske, M. G. (2002). Effects of cognitive-behavior therapy for panic disorder on comorbid conditions: Replication and extension. *Behavior Therapy, 33*, 493–509.

Tsao, J. C. I., Mystkowski, J. L., Zucker, B. G., & Craske, M. G. (2005). Impact of cognitive-behavioral therapy for panic disorder on comorbidity: A controlled investigation. *Behaviour Research and Therapy, 43*, 959–970.

Tull, M. T., & Roemer, L. (2007). Emotion regulation difficulties associated with the experience of uncued panic attacks: Evidence of experiential avoidance, emotional nonacceptance, and decreased emotional clarity. *Behaviour Research and Therapy, 38*, 378–391.

Tyrer, P. J. (1989). *Classification of neurosis.* Chichester, UK: Wiley.

Tyrer, P. J., Seivewright, N., Murphys, S., Ferguson, B., Kingdon, D., & Barczak, B. (1998). The Nottingham study of neurotic disorder: Comparison of drug and psychological treatments. *Lancet, 2*, 235–240.

Watson, D. (2005). Rethinking the mood and anxiety disorders: A quantitative hierarchical model for DSM-V. *Journal of Abnormal Psychology, 114*, 522–536.

Watson, D., Clark, L. A., & Tellegen, A. (1988). Development and validation of brief measures of positive and negative affect: The PANAS scales. *Journal of Personality and Social Psychology, 54*, 1063–1070.

Wegner, D. M., Schneider, D. J., Carter, S. R., III, & White, T. L. (1987). Paradoxical effects of thought suppression. *Journal of Personality and Social Psychology, 53*(1), 5–13.

Weinberg, A., & Hajcak, G. (2010). Electrocortical evidence for vigilance–avoidance in generalized anxiety disorder. *Psychophysiology, 48*(6), 1–10.

Weiser, M., Pauli, P., Weyers, P., Alpers, G., & Mühlberger, A. (2009). Fear of negative evaluation and the hypervigilance–avoidance hypothesis: An eye-tracking study. *Journal of Neural Transmission, 116*, 717–723.

Westerhof, G. J., & Keyes, C. L. (2009). Mental illness and mental health: The two continua model across the lifespan. *Journal of Adult Development, 17*(2), 110–119.

Westra, H. A., Arkowitz, H., & Dozois, D. J. A. (2009). Adding a motivational interviewing pretreatment to cognitive behavioral therapy for generalized anxiety disorder: A preliminary randomized controlled trial. *Journal of Anxiety Disorders, 23*, 1106–1117.

Westra, H. A., & Dozois, D. J. A. (2006). Preparing clients for cognitive behavioural therapy: A randomized pilot study of motivational interviewing for anxiety. *Cognitive Therapy and Research, 30*, 481–498.

Williams, J. B. (1988). A structured interview guide for the Hamilton Depression Rating Scale. *Archives of General Psychiatry, 45*, 742–747.

CHAPTER 7

Cognitive Therapy for Depression

Jeffrey E. Young
Jayne L. Rygh
Arthur D. Weinberger
Aaron T. Beck

One of the most important developments in psychological approaches to emotional problems has been the success of cognitive therapy for depression. Evidence for the powerful efficacy of this approach has increased steadily over the years, particularly in regard to successful long-term outcome. Employing a variety of well-specified cognitive and behavioral techniques, cognitive therapy is also distinguished by the detailed structure of each session with its specific agendas, and by the very deliberate and obviously effective therapeutic style of interacting with the patient through a series of questions (Socratic style). Moreover, the authors underscore very clearly the importance of a collaborative relationship between therapist and patient, and outline specific techniques to achieve this collaborative state, so that patient and therapist become an investigative team. In this chapter, the authors cover not only traditional cognitive therapy but also an expansion of cognitive therapy called "schema-focused" therapy. This approach concentrates on identifying and modifying early maladaptive or "core" schemas thought to develop during childhood in more severely depressed and treatment-resistant patients, often with comorbid personality disorders that may make them vulnerable to relapse. Detailed explication of this expanded treatment will be invaluable to experienced cognitive therapists, as well as to those becoming acquainted with cognitive therapy for depression for the first time. Two compelling cases, Denise, treated with traditional cognitive therapy, and Barbara, treated with schema-focused therapy, illustrate each approach.—D. H. B.

OVERVIEW AND RESEARCH

Depression and the Emergence of Cognitive Therapy

Depression is one of the most common disorders encountered by mental health professionals. Research from the U.S. National Comorbidity Survey Replication (NCS-R; 2005) studies, the Centers for Disease Control and Prevention (CDC; 2010), and the World Health Organization (WHO; 2008), and data provided by the National Institute of Mental Health (NIMH; 2006) indicate the following:

- The lifetime prevalence estimate for major depressive disorder in the United States is 29.9% (Kessler, Petukhova, Sampson, Zaslavsky, & Wittchen, 2012).
- The 12-month prevalence estimate for major depressive disorder in the United States is 8.6% (Kessler et al., 2012).

- Across countries and cultures, the lifetime prevalence estimates for major depressive disorder are 14.6% in high- and 11.1% in low- to middle-income countries; the 12-month prevalence estimates are 5.5% in high- and 5.6% low- to middle-income countries (Bromet et al., 2011).
- Major depressive episodes in the United States are associated with higher rates of substance dependence or abuse among adults ages 18 or older (21.5%) and among youth ages 12–17 (18.9%) than among those without such episodes (8.2% and 6.7%, respectively) (Substance Abuse and Mental Health Services Administration [SAMHSA], 2008).
- Depression increases the risk of heart attacks and is more common in those with chronic conditions such as obesity, diabetes, cardiovascular disease, cancer, asthma, and arthritis (NIMH, 2006; Strine et al., 2008; Chapman, Perry, & Strine, 2005).
- Major depressive disorder in the United States is associated with 27.2 lost workdays and bipolar disorder (I or II) with 65.5 lost workdays for each ill worker per year (Kessler et al., 2006).
- Major depressive disorder is the leading cause of disability in the United States for ages 15–44 (NIMH, 2006), and is a major contributor to the global burden of disease (WHO, 2004).

The high risk of relapse (Scott, 2000), high resource utilization (Howland, 1993), and loss of human capital (Berndt et al., 2000) associated with depression reveal the seriousness of the problem. The WHO (2004) projects that depression will be among the top three causes of the total number of years of life lost to illness, disability, or premature death by 2030. As these reports indicate, depression is widespread, debilitating, costly, and potentially devastating.

No amount of data can adequately capture or convey the personal pain and suffering experienced in depression. Many depressed people do not get professional help (Frank & Thase, 1999; Jarrett, 1995; Wang et al., 2005), and although the number seeking help increased over the last decade, undertreatment remains a serious problem (Olfson et al., 2002; Wang et al., 2005). The cost and/or lack of sufficient coverage by health insurance companies, concerns about confidentiality, continued social stigma, and the lack of information regarding where to go and what type of services to obtain are still obstacles to receiving appropriate and adequate mental health services (SAMHSA, 2008). Obtaining

the right type of help can be at once inhibiting and overwhelming, especially to those already impaired. The following quote remains relevant today:

> Americans who do seek treatment for depressive symptoms must decide where to seek which treatment and from what type of practitioner. . . . The clinician must select a somatic, psychological, or combination of treatment, at a given dose and/or schedule of appointments. . . . Throughout this procedure, the patient decides to what extent he/she will comply with the recommendations, for how long, against recognized and unrecognized economic, practical, physical, and emotional costs. . . . Sadly, the lack of information as well as the continued social stigma of psychiatric illness and treatment influence decision-making. Simultaneously, the decisions occur in an environment filled with social, political, and economic debate, and tension among policy makers, third-party payers, and clinicians, as well as among different types of practitioner guilds. (Jarrett, 1995, p. 435)

When care is provided, it is frequently inadequate or minimally adequate (Wang et al., 2005). Evidenced-based treatments have not been widely adopted in clinical practice (Stirman et al., in press), reflecting a public health crisis (Keller & Boland, 1998). The need for delivery of treatments with proven and rapid efficacy remains paramount.

One of the major developments in the treatment of depression has been the emergence of cognitive therapy, which has expanded exponentially since Beck's publication of a detailed treatment manual for depression in 1979 (Beck, 1967, 1976; Beck, Rush, Shaw, & Emery, 1979). The work of Beck and his colleagues has led to a paradigm shift within psychotherapy (Salkovskis, 1996). Due in part to Beck's development of testable hypotheses and clinical protocols, cognitive therapy has received an enormous amount of professional attention (Hollon, 1998; McGinn & Young, 1996; Rehm, 1990). Of all the cognitive-behavioral treatment approaches to depression, Beck's paradigm (Beck, 1967; Beck et al., 1979) has received the greatest amount of empirical study, validation, and clinical application (Barlow & Hofmann, 1997; de Oliveira, 1998; Dobson & Pusch, 1993; Hollon, 1998; Hollon, Thase, & Markowitz, 2002; Jarrett & Thase, 2010; Rehm, 1990; Roberts & Hartlage, 1996; Scott, 1996a). Cognitive therapy has become the treatment of choice for many disorders (Clark & Beck, 2010; Newman, Leahy, Beck, Reilly-Harrington, & Gyulai, 2002). There are many excellent books for practitioners who teach cognitive therapy procedures (e.g., J. S. Beck, 2011), as well as workbooks and/or guides for clients (e.g., Gilson, Freeman, Yates, & Freeman, 2009; Leahy, 2010; Wright & McCray, 2011).

Along with this attention, however, has come confusion about what is actually meant by the term "cognitive therapy." The actual cognitive therapeutic strategies employed in "cognitive" treatments may differ in many ways from one another and from those explicitly prescribed by Beck and colleagues (1979) in their manual for cognitive therapy of depression. Thus, the reader should be aware that common use of the term "cognitive therapy" does not necessarily imply uniformity in procedures. The therapy described by Beck and colleagues involves the use of both cognitive and behavioral techniques, and can therefore be accurately labeled "cognitive-behavioral"; however, in the literature, both terms have been applied in describing Beck and colleagues' procedures, with some articles utilizing the term "cognitive therapy" (Sacco & Beck, 1995, p. 345).

Research on Treatment of the Acute Phase

Outcome research has found cognitive therapy to be effective with clinical populations in numerous controlled trials (see review by Beck & Alford, 2009; Hollon & Shelton, 2001). Although some early studies (Blackburn, Bishop, Glen, Whalley, & Christie, 1981; Rush, Beck, Kovacs, & Hollon, 1977) suggested that cognitive therapy may be superior to drug treatment for depression at termination, Meterissian and Bradwejn (1989) noted that psychopharmacological interventions often were not adequately implemented. In research in which interventions were adequate, cognitive therapy generally was shown to be equivalent in efficacy to antidepressant medications, including tricyclic antidepressants (TCAs) and selective serotonin reuptake inhibitors (SSRIs) in the treatment of outpatients with nonbipolar depression (DeRubeis et al., 2005; Hollon et al., 1992; Murphy, Simmons, Wetzel, & Lustman, 1984) and a monoamine oxidase inhibitor (MAOI) in the treatment of outpatients with atypical depression (Jarrett et al., 1999). Although many studies did not include pill-placebo conditions, the studies by Jarrett and colleagues and DeRubeis and colleagues (2005) found the active treatments superior to pill-placebos. In a mega-analysis by DeRubeis, Gelfand, Tang, and Simons (1999) of treatment outcome in four studies with

severely depressed outpatients, cognitive therapy was equivalent to antidepressant medication (imipramine or nortriptyline). A study by Bhar and colleagues (2008) found that CBT and pharmacotherapy (paroxetine) produced similar trajectories of change in cognitive and vegetative symptoms of major depression throughout 16 weeks of treatment.

Only two studies that included a pill-placebo found cognitive therapy to be less effective than psychopharmacological intervention. The first was the NIMH Treatment of Depression Collaborative Research Program (TDCRP) with moderate to severe depression in adults. The second was the multisite Treatment for Adolescents with Depression Study (TADS) for reduction of depressive symptoms in adolescents.

The NIMH TDCRP was the first major study to include a pill-placebo condition. The initial results of TDCRP (Elkin et al., 1989) suggested lower rates of improvement with cognitive-behavioral therapy (CBT) than did earlier studies. It also appeared that with more severely depressed patient groups, interpersonal psychotherapy and antidepressant drugs might be superior to CBT. The high visibility and prestige of the NIMH TDCRP study generated a great deal of debate (Hollon, DeRubeis, & Evans, 1996; Wolpe, 1993) because it appeared that the benefits of CBT in the acute treatment phase might have been overestimated in previous studies. However, on later examination of the data, Elkin, Gibbons, Shea, and Shaw (1996) acknowledged Jacobson and Hollon's (1996) observation that the outcome results varied across sites, with cognitive therapy performing as well as medication at one of the three sites with severely depressed clients. Jacobson and Hollon noted that the best results were obtained at the site with the most experienced therapists. Hollon and colleagues (2002, p. 62) "suspect that the explanation is not that cognitive therapy cannot be effective with such patients, but that the therapist's expertise makes a greater difference the more difficult the depression is to treat." Additionally, a study by Albon and Jones (2003) raised the question of the distinctiveness of the two types of psychotherapy treatments in the TDCRP. Albon and Jones, expert therapists in CBT and interpersonal psychotherapy, respectively, developed prototypes of ideal regimens of their own respective treatments. Then, actual transcripts of treatment sessions from the TDCRP were compared to these expert prototypes. Albon and Jones found that both CBT and interpersonal psychotherapy sessions conformed most closely to the cognitive-behavioral prototype, and that closer adherence to the cognitive-behavioral prototype produced more positive correlations with outcome measures across both types of treatment. Perhaps this is why Quilty, McBride, and Bagby (2008) found equivalent outcomes with interpersonal psychotherapy, CBT, and pharmacotherapy, and Peeters and colleagues (2013) found similar remission rates with CBT, interpersonal psychotherapy, and both treatments combined with medication. Similarly, Luty and colleagues (2007) found interpersonal psychotherapy and CBT equally effective overall but (in contrast to the NIMH TDCRP study) they found CBT to be more effective with severe depression.

In further analysis of the same dataset used in the Luty and colleagues (2007) study, Joyce and colleagues (2007) found that comorbidity of personality and major depressive disorders adversely affected the treatment response to interpersonal psychotherapy but not CBT. Bellino, Zizza, Rinaldi, and Bogetto (2007) found interpersonal psychotherapy and CBT (each combined with fluoxetine) equally effective in the treatment of depression in patients with borderline personality and major depressive disorders. Fournier and colleagues (2008) found that at 16 weeks of treatment, CBT was more effective in reducing depression than medication (paroxetine) for patients with moderate to severe depression and no personality disorder, but less effective for those with a personality disorder. This study did not include patients with borderline, schizotypal, or antisocial personality disorders. The efficacy of CBT (alone or as an adjunct to psychopharmacological treatment) with coexisting major depressive and personality disorders is still not clear.

Some writers have argued that the major psychotherapies are essentially equivalent in effectiveness, regardless of the disorder studied. To test this hypothesis, a recent meta-analysis examined whether CBT was superior to other forms of psychotherapy across a range of disorders (Tolin, 2010). The results showed that, *across all disorders included in the study*, CBT was superior to psychodynamic therapy, although not to interpersonal or supportive therapies, at posttreatment and at follow-up. However, the analysis found that CBT was significantly superior to the alternative therapies studied *for depressive and anxiety disorders*. Tolin (2010) concluded that "these results argue against previous claims of treatment equivalence and suggest that CBT should be considered a first-line psychosocial treatment of choice, at least for patients with anxiety and depressive disorders" (p. 710).

The multisite TADS (2004) for reduction of depressive symptoms in adolescents found that the combination of medication (fluoxetine) and CBT produced the most positive outcome, medication alone was superior to pill-placebo, but CBT alone did not significantly differ from pill-placebo. These findings were based on 12-week outcome measures. Analyses (TADS, 2007) on data from outcome measures at Weeks 18, 24, and 36, however, indicated that by Week 36 the effectiveness of CBT significantly increased and was equivalent to medication, and that the combination of medication and CBT was slightly more effective than CBT or medication alone.

Spirito, Esposito-Smythers, Wolff, and Uhl (2011) recently completed an updated review of outcome studies regarding CBT for adolescent depression and suicidality. They summarized the data regarding depression by concluding: "CBT for adolescent depression has received considerable support in the research literature. Individual and group CBT, with and without a parent component, appears to be well established and/or efficacious for the majority of participants." Regarding CBT and suicidality in adolescents, the authors concluded that "the majority of studies of CBT for depressed adolescents have found a reduction in suicidal ideation regardless of CBT format (i.e., individual, group). It should be noted that reductions in suicidality have also been found in response to family therapy, supportive therapy, and pharmacotherapy. Nonetheless, while various forms of therapy resulted in comparable reductions in adolescent suicidality, CBT has shown the most promise in concurrently reducing MDD diagnoses/symptoms and suicidal ideation."

Several studies have not found the combination of CBT and drugs to be superior to either treatment alone with depressed outpatients in the acute phase of treatment (Biggs & Rush, 1999; Evans et al., 1992; Hollon, Shelton, & Loosen, 1991; Scott, 1996a; Shaw & Segal, 1999). The increment in efficacy appears to be modest in the acute phase of treatment at best, with increases in efficacy from 10 to 20% (Conte, Plutchik, Wild, & Karasu, 1986). Studies regarding treatment with depressed inpatients suggest beneficial results when CBT is combined with medication (Bowers, 1990; Miller, Norman, Keitner, Bishop, & Dow, 1989; Stuart & Bowers, 1995; Wright, 1996). Although cognitive therapy appears to be a useful adjunct to standard care with inpatients, it remains unclear whether cognitive therapy alone is sufficient (Hollon et al., 2002).

In attempts to make traditional cognitive therapy more accessible and/or affordable for the general public, Internet-based (ICBT) and group (CBGT) CBTs have been explored. In a review of rapidly accumulating data on ICBT, Johansson and Andersson (2012) concluded that there is mounting support for the effectiveness of guided ICBT (structured self-help materials with therapist contact via e-mail) over unguided ICBT (no therapist contact); the research indicates that guided ICBT is comparable to face-to-face therapy in effectiveness; tailored treatments (which include additional specific techniques for coexisting diagnoses) are superior to nontailored treatments (same material for all patients) with severe depression.

Regarding CGBT, a recent meta-analysis (Feng et al., 2012) on studies published from 2000 to 2010 revealed that CBGT was more effective with mild to moderate depression. The effect decreased as depression severity increased. The optimal length of session was 60–90 minutes. Take-home assignments improved results. Higher turnover rates were related to poorer outcomes. Feng and colleagues (2012) found a small effect on relapse rates at 6 months. The relapse rates were lowest, with no residual symptoms posttreatment.

Research on Relapse Prevention[1]

Even though the vast majority of patients recover from an episode of depression, they nevertheless remain vulnerable to future depression.

Recurrence is a major problem for many individuals suffering from depression: at least 50% of individuals who suffer from one depressive episode will have another within 10 years. Those experiencing two episodes have a 90% chance of suffering a third, while individuals with three or more lifetime episodes have relapse rates of 40% within 15 weeks of recovery from an episode (Kupfer, Frank, & Wamhoff, 1996, p. 293).

Other investigators have estimated that 85% of patients with unipolar depression are likely to experience recurrences (Keller & Boland, 1998, p. 350). Wang (2004), through a 6-year follow-up, found that 49.8% of those treated for major depression developed subsequent major depressive episodes. As these numbers clearly show, there is an urgent need for treatments capable of minimizing and preventing relapse.

What we consider a very exciting finding in the treatment of depression with cognitive therapy is the consistent observation (Paykel, 2007) that patients treated with cognitive therapy alone or with a combination of cognitive therapy and medication fare far better in terms of relapse than do patients treated with medication alone (when both treatments are stopped at termination). Despite differences in sample characteristics and methodologies across studies, cognitive therapy appears to have important prophylactic properties. After a 1-year follow-up, numerous studies have reported lower relapse rates for patients treated with cognitive therapy than for patients treated with antidepressants. Simons, Murphy, Levine, and Wetzel (1986) found relapse rates of 12% with cognitive therapy versus 66% with antidepressants; Bowers (1990) found relapse rates of 20% with cognitive therapy versus 80% with antidepressants; Shea and colleagues (1992) reported 9% relapse with cognitive therapy versus 28% with antidepressants; Hollon and colleagues (2005) reported rates of 31% relapse with cognitive therapy versus 76% with antidepressants. Results from the most extensive meta-analysis to date revealed that "on average, only 29.5% of the patients treated with cognitive therapy relapsed versus 60% of those treated with antidepressants" (Gloaguen, Cottraux, Cucherat, & Blackburn, 1998, p. 68). The prophylactic benefits of cognitive therapy are all the more significant because

there is no evidence that pharmacotherapy confers any protection against the return of symptoms after treatment has been terminated.[2] Since the majority of depressed individuals will experience multiple episodes, the capacity of an intervention to prevent the return of symptoms after treatment may be at least as important as its ability to treat the current episode. (Evans et al., 1992, p. 802)

A related concern—and one of the most salient (but not exclusively associated) with psychotropic agents—is the presence of residual symptoms after treatment: "Treatment of depression by pharmacological means is likely to leave a substantial amount of residual symptoms in most patients" (Fava, Rafanelli, Grandi, Conti, & Belluardo, 1998, p. 820). Inevitably, patients who improve on antidepressants continue to manifest some of the symptoms of depression and, as numerous investigators have concluded, unless patients achieve full recovery, residual symptoms increase the risk of relapse (Evans et al., 1992; Fava, Rafanelli, Grandi, Conti, et al., 1998; Hardeveld, Spijker, de Graaf, Nolen, & Beekman, 2010; Keller & Boland, 1998; Rush et al., 2006).

A group of investigators who were concerned about the risk of relapse associated with residual symptoms looked at the lingering symptoms after treatment with fluoxetine (Prozac). They found that

> even among subjects who are considered full responders to fluoxetine 20 mg for 5 weeks, more than 80% had 1 or more residual DSM-III-R symptoms of major depressive disorder, more than 30% had 3 or more symptoms, and 10.2% met formal criteria for either minor or subsyndromal depression. . . . These findings imply that minimal depressive symptoms are prodromal and increase the risk of developing an initial full-blown episode of major depression. (Nierenberg et al., 1999, pp. 224–225)

Cognitive therapy has been found to be effective in reducing both residual symptoms and relapse after the termination of medication: "Short-term CBT after successful antidepressant drug therapy had a substantial effect on relapse rate after discontinuation of antidepressant drugs. Patients who received CBT reported a substantially lower relapse rate (25%) during the 2-year follow-up than those assigned to [clinical management] (80%)" (Fava, Rafanelli, Grandi, Conti, et al., 1998, p. 818). The protective benefits of cognitive therapy were still noticeable in a 4-year follow-up study, although the benefits faded after a 6-year period (Fava, Rafanelli, Grandi, Canestrari, & Morphy, 1998). Another study found that only 5% of the "CBT treated and recovered" group sought additional treatment compared with 39% of the antidepressant group (see Williams, 1997). Paykel and colleagues (1999) found significantly lower cumulative relapse rates at 68 weeks in patients who received 16 sessions of CBT following a partial response to pharmacotherapy. Bockting and colleagues (2005) compared treatment as usual (TAU, which included continuation of medication) with TAU augmented with brief cognitive therapy and found relapse significantly reduced in patients with five or more previous episodes of depression. The relapse rates were 72% for TAU versus 46% for TAU augmented with brief cognitive therapy.

A preventive strategy used by psychiatrists to deal with high relapse rates associated with antidepressant medication is "continuation medication," which is long-term (and in many cases lifelong) maintenance treatment (Evans et al., 1992; Fava, Rafanelli, Grandi, Conti, et al., 1998; Thase, 1999)—usually at the same dosage provided during the acute phase of treatment. The research comparing relapse rates in patients continuing

medication over the long term versus those treated and then withdrawn from cognitive therapy does not suggest a significant advantage to this practice. For example, DeRubeis and colleagues (2005) found that both groups had equivalent relapse rates (40%); Hollon and colleagues (2005) found that 31% relapsed when treated and then withdrawn from cognitive therapy compared to 47% that relapsed when treated with continuation medication. Fournier and colleagues (2008) found that patients with both major depression and a personality disorder who responded positively to 16 weeks of CBT, with three optional booster sessions over a 12-month period, showed superior sustained improvement with CBT compared to pharmacotherapy withdrawal, and equivalent improvement to pharmacotherapy with continuation over those 12 months. Dobson and colleagues (2008) followed patients who responded to a treatment of CBT, behavioral activation, or pharmacotherapy for acute depression. During a 2-year follow-up, psychotherapy patients received no further treatment and pharmacotherapy patients received either continuation pharmacotherapy or continuation pill-placebo. They found that CBT provided the strongest protection; both psychotherapies were equivalent to pharmacotherapy with continuation; both psychotherapies were superior to continuation pill-placebo.

Some researchers have pointed out the tautological nature of this solution: "Drug treatment results in a higher relapse rate than cognitive-behavioral therapy; therefore patients should be maintained on drugs to prevent relapse" (Antonuccio, Danton, & DeNelsky, 1995, p. 578). Although drugs are still the initial and most frequently prescribed form of treatment for major depression in the United States (Antonuccio et al., 1995; Cipriani et al., 2009), and the most commonly used method to maintain treatment gains (Geddes et al., 2003), three important points need to be considered: premature termination, iatrogenic effects of pharmacotherapy, and cost-effectiveness.

Research has shown that "a sizeable group of patients either chooses not to continue long-term pharmacotherapy in the absence of any depressive symptoms, cannot take medication due to a medical condition that precludes the use of antidepressants, or suffer from side effects that are intolerable to them" (Spanier, Frank, McEachran, Grochocinski, & Kupfer, 1999, p. 250). Although the newer "first-line" medications are more tolerable than older medications, 70% of patients continue to experience significant depressive symptoms with one of these medications, and up to 50% discontinue trials due to unwanted side effects (Connolly & Thase, 2012). Thase (2011) has noted that various combinations of antidepressants are widely prescribed as the result of problems with insufficient or nonresponse, even though properly controlled and adequately powered clinical trials have not yet been conducted on such combinations.

Regarding iatrogenic effects, one group of researchers concluded that "there is much evidence that antidepressant medications are not benign treatments. . . . Many antidepressants are cardiotoxic, have dangerous side effects, and are often used in suicide attempts. . . . [They also] result in relatively poorer compliance than psychotherapy, have a higher dropout rate, and result in as much as a 60% non-response rate with some patient populations" (Antonuccio et al., 1995, p. 581). We should note that psychotherapy also may have unintended and undesirable side effects (Mohr, 1995), but very little is known about negative effects associated with cognitive therapy.

The third consideration is the cost-effectiveness of treatment. The research on this topic is surprisingly limited. Antonuccio, Thomas, and Danton (1997) conducted a cost-effectiveness analysis on several outcome studies on depression and found that over a 2-year period the cost of fluoxetine alone was 33% higher than individual CBT, and that the cost of the combined treatment of fluoxetine with CBT was 23% higher than CBT alone. An Australian study (Vos, Corry, Haby, Carter, & Andrews, 2005) examined the costs and benefits of CBT and drugs in the episodic and maintenance treatment of depression. They found maintenance treatment with SSRIs to be the most expensive option, nearly double that of bibliotherapy, group CBT, individual CBT, and TCAs. Scott, Palmer, Paykel, Teasdale, and Hayhurst (2003) compared the cost-effectiveness of relapse prevention in depression by comparing CBT as an adjunctive treatment to antidepressants and clinical management, and with antidepressants and clinical management alone, over a 17-month period. They found the addition of CBT was more expensive but also more effective in reducing cumulative relapse rates (relapse rates were 29% with adjunctive CBT vs. 47% without adjunctive CBT). Importantly, they noted that the costs associated with adjunctive CBT in their study were a "worst-case" scenario because the follow-up extended only 17 months; other research (as noted in the previous section) has demonstrated maintenance of gains and lowered relapse rates up to 6 years with CBT. Sava, Yates, Lupu, Szentogatai, and David (2009)

conducted a cost comparison of CBT, rational–emotive therapy, and pharmacotherapy (fluoxetine), and found all three treatments equally effective with symptom reduction, but both psychotherapies were more cost-effective than pharmacotherapy for the number of depression-free days/month over a 40-week period. Although Dobson and colleagues (2008) did not conduct a formal statistical comparisons of costs among treatment conditions, they noted that the "cumulative cost of continued medications proved to be more expensive by the end of the first year of follow-up in this study" (p. 471). Scott and colleagues (2003) argued that the incrementally adjusted costs over time to relapse should be considered in decision making on the value of various treatments. These findings suggest that CBT, either alone or in combination with drugs, can enhance cost-effectiveness, particularly when higher short-term costs of combined treatments are balanced against better outcomes and lower marginal costs in the long term.

What is the optimum frequency and duration of sessions for cognitive therapy to be effective, both at termination and at long-term follow-up? According to Sacco and Beck (1995, p. 332):

> General guidelines suggest 15 to 25 (50-minute) sessions at weekly intervals, with more seriously depressed clients usually requiring twice-weekly meetings for the initial 4–5 weeks. To avoid an abrupt termination, a "tapering off" process is recommended, with the last few sessions occurring once every 2 weeks. After termination, some clients may also need a few booster sessions (four or five are common).

Some writers have noted that longer courses of treatment may be necessary for full and more lasting recovery (Elkin et al., 1996; Thase, 1992). Research by Jarrett and colleagues (2001) suggests that relapse rates in high-risk patients with an early age of onset or unstable remission might possibly be reduced further with "continuation-phase cognitive therapy" (C-CT), which consists of 10 sessions (biweekly during the first 2 months and once a month for the following 6 months) following the acute phase of treatment. The focus in the continuation phase is on relapse prevention and the generalization of skills (across responses, settings, stimuli, and times). This strategy is supported by studies (Jarrett et al., 2001; Vittengl, Clark, Dunn, & Jarrett, 2007; Vittengl, Clark, & Jarrett, 2009) aimed at preventing relapse in responders to a variety treatment modalities (pharmacotherapy, interpersonal psychotherapy, and/or CBT) for the acute phase of depression. While more research is being conducted on this strategy (Jarrett & Thase, 2010; Jarrett, Vittengl, and Clark (2008) have suggested using scores on a variety of measures (Hamilton Rating Scale for Depression, Beck Depression Inventory [BDI], Inventory for Depressive Symptomatology, and the Longitudinal Interval Follow-Up Evaluation) to help cognitive therapists decide how many more sessions may be needed to help avoid relapse or recurrence.

Another alternative for relapse prevention is mindfulness-based cognitive therapy (MBCT), developed by Teasdale, Segal, and Williams (1995). MBCT draws from acceptance and meditation strategies that are also central to dialectical behavior therapy for borderline personality (Linehan, 1993a, 1993b). "MBCT aims at developing participants' awareness of, and changing their relationship to, unwanted thoughts, feelings, and body sensations, so that participants no longer avoid them or react to them in an automatic way but rather respond to them in an intentional and skillful manner" (Ma & Teasdale, 2004, p. 32). Teasdale and colleagues (Ma & Teasdale, 2004; Teasdale, 1997a, 1997b; Teasdale et al., 1995, 2002) have argued that the primary mechanism of therapeutic change in cognitive therapy is in distancing or decentering from cognition rather than changing the content of thought. Two studies conducted on MBCT found that TAU followed by MBCT, in comparison with TAU alone, significantly reduced relapse in patients with three or more episodes of depression. In the first study, 66% relapsed with TAU alone versus 37% with TAU followed by MBCT (Teasdale et al., 2000); in the second study, 78% relapsed with TAU alone versus 36% with TAU followed by MBCT (Ma & Teasdale, 2004). Extending the follow-up period to 2 years, Matthew, Whitford, Kenny, and Denson (2010) found TAU followed by MBCT more effective than TAU alone in the "decrease of depressive symptoms, worry and rumination, and improvement in mindfulness skills" (p. 998) but noted a weakening of effects over time that appeared to be related to the amount of formal MBCT practice.

Although prior researchers (Segal, Williams, & Teasdale, 2002) presumed that the difficulty concentrating and negative thinking during a depressive episode would preclude training in attentional control skills with MBCT, van Aalderen and colleagues (2012) recently found that MBCT plus TAU, compared to TAU alone, showed equivalent gains in effectiveness for patients in remission as for those currently depressed.

Manicavasagar, Perich, and Parker (2012) also examined the effectiveness of MBCT in reducing current depression. They compared CBGT and MBCT, and found equivalent improvements in depression. Interestingly, they found no significant differences between the two conditions in mindfulness or rumination scores. The potential for lower costs associated with treatments that can be implemented in a group format suggest that they may be attractive for not only relapse prevention but also recurrent depression.

Research on Chronic Depression

As the previous data demonstrate, CBT has been shown to be an effective treatment across a wide range of depressed populations. Nevertheless, many depressed patients still do not respond to treatment. Depression that is resistant to current treatments remains a major public health problem. Of patients, 40–50% of patients may not complete or respond to CBT treatment for acute depression (DeRubeis et al., 2005; Jarret & Thase, 2010). Fifty percent of patients do not achieve full remission in depressive symptoms after two trials of medication (Mathys & Mitchell, 2011; Rush et al., 2006; Trivedi et al., 2006). Wiersma and colleagues (2008) note from current research that 20% of depressions persist after 2 years and that 25–35% of outpatient mental health patients suffer from chronic depression.

McCullough (2003) has proposed, on the basis of existing research, that there are qualitative differences between chronic and nonchronic forms of depression, and that they require different treatment strategies. According to McCullough, research "shows that the chronic disorders, when compared with acute/episodic major depression (both single and recurrent episodes with interepisode full recovery), differ significantly in terms of age of onset, clinical course patterns, developmental history, modal Axis II comorbidity profiles, characteristic response-to-treatment rates, predictable relapse percentages, and need for long-term treatment" (p. 243). He notes that these differences largely have not been addressed in the treatment literature; consequently, therapeutic work by psychologists, psychiatrists, and social workers has been conducted as if patients with depression are an undifferentiated population. Young, Klosko, and Weishaar (2003) noted that although traditional CBT is highly effective for many patients, there remain a significant number who either are not helped or continue to experience emotional distress and impaired functioning, particularly those with significant character pathology. For those with chronic problems, a more extensive treatment approach may be required.

Before discussing specific treatments for chronic depression, we describe the general characteristics of this population. An early age of onset (usually in midadolescence, before age 20) in the form of dysthymia tends to differentiate between the chronic and nonchronic forms of depression in 70–75% of clinical populations (Keller & Boland, 1998; Keller & Hanks, 1995; McCullough, 2000). Early life trauma or adverse family relations (loss of a parent in childhood; sexual, physical, and/or verbal abuse; neglect; and overprotection) are more evident in those with chronic depression (Chapman et al., 2004; Cong et al., 2012; Dube et al., 2001; Heim & Nemeroff, 2001; Kendler et al., 1995; Lizardi et al., 1995; Randolph & Dykman, 1998; Sachs-Ericsson, Verona, Joiner, & Preacher, 2006). In patients with early-onset dysthymia who experience chronic stress, those with the addition of an adverse family history evidence an increase in depression severity over time, compared to those without such adverse family histories but with familial loadings for dysthymic disorder (Dougherty, Klein, & Davila, 2004). There is a higher prevalence of comorbid disorders, particularly personality disorders (Garyfallos et al., 1999; Pepper et al., 1995). Cluster C personality disorders are associated with chronic depression (Hayden & Klein, 2001).

Five potentially promising treatments that expand on CBT have been developed that can address chronic depression. These treatments are Harley, Sprich, Safren, Jacob, and Fava's (2008) application of Linehan's (1993b) dialectical behavior therapy (DBT) skills training; applications (Barnhofer et al., 2009; Eisendrath et al., 2011) of Segal and colleagues' (2002) MBCT; Wells and colleagues' (2012) metacognitive therapy (MCT); McCullough's (2000) cognitive-behavioral analysis system of psychotherapy (CBASP); and Young and colleagues' (2003) schema therapy (ST).

Harley and colleagues (2008) have provided preliminary evidence that DBT skills training conducted in groups may be an effective alternative for treatment-resistant depression. Patients who had not achieved remission with antidepressant medication were assigned to either a 16-session, once-weekly DBT skills training condition (mindfulness, interpersonal effectiveness, emotion regulation, and distress tolerance) or a wait-list condition. They found significantly greater improvement (with large effect sizes on the Hamilton Rating Scale and BDI) in depressive symptoms in the DBT skills training group. Feldman, Harley, Kerrigan,

Jacobo, and Fava (2009) hypothesized that DBT skills training helps patients process their emotional experience in a way that reduces rather than exacerbates their depressive symptoms.

Another preliminary study (Barnhofer et al., 2009) and one case study (Eisendrath, Chartier, & McLane, 2011) successfully used MBCT to treat chronic depression. Barnhofer and colleagues (2009) compared MBCT plus TAU and TAU alone, and found significantly greater improvement in the MBCT plus TAU group. Eisendrath and colleagues (2011) successfully treated a patient with a modified version of MCBT. They added exercises and metaphors from acceptance and commitment therapy (ACT; Luoma, Hayes, & Walser, 2007; Zettle, 2007) and focused on current depression in their MCBT treatment. These are intriguing initial results, especially since these treatments are of relatively short duration and conducive to a group format.

Wells and colleagues (2012) also conducted a preliminary study in which they used MCT to treat patients with treatment-resistant depression. Attentional control, rumination, worry, and metacognitive beliefs were targeted in eight treatment sessions. They found significant improvements both posttreatment and at 12-month follow-up. This treatment will be of further interest if the positive results can be replicated in a randomized controlled trial.

McCullough's (2000) CBASP is an integrative, time-limited treatment that contains elements of cognitive, behavioral, interpersonal, and psychodynamic psychotherapies. McCullough (2003) states:

> Treatment begins with a cognitive-emotionally retarded adult child who brings a negative "snapshot" view of the world to the session. The chronic patient functions, at least in the social–interpersonal arena, with the structural mindset of a 4–6 year old preoperational (Piaget) child. . . . The patient must be taught to function formally, to perceive that his or her behavior has consequences, be taught to generate authentic empathy, and to learn to assert himself or herself effectively. Psychotherapy begins with an "adult child" who must be assisted to mature developmentally in the cognitive–emotive sphere. (pp. 247, 248)

Change is brought about through a contingency program that relies on negative reinforcement. First, contingencies between behaviors and consequences are exposed. Then, as the result of positive changes in behavior, discomfort and distress are reduced or eliminated. Three techniques are used to bring about change:

situational analysis, interpersonal discrimination exercise, and behavioral skill training/rehearsal. Two studies have used CBASP with chronically depressed outpatients. The first (Keller et al., 2000) compared the effects of CBASP alone, Serzone (nefazodone) alone, and combined treatment after a 12-week acute phase of treatment. The overall response rate was 48% for both monotherapies, compared with 73% for the combined treatment. Among the 76% (519 out of 681) completers of the study, 52% responded to CBASP, 55% responded to Serzone, and 85% responded to combined treatments. The second (Klein et al., 2004), a 1-year follow-up to this initial study, examined relapse and depressive symptoms over time in the CBASP responders by comparing the effects of continuation CBASP therapy (16 sessions over 52 weeks) with assessment only. There were significantly fewer relapses and depressive symptoms for those in the continuation CBASP therapy. A more recent study, however, has provided mixed results. Kocsis and colleagues (2009) compared pharmacotherapy augmented with CBASP, pharmacotherapy augmented with brief supportive therapy, and continued pharmacotherapy alone with nonresponders and partial responders to an initial medication trial. Although 37.5% experienced a partial response or remitted with these three treatments, the researchers did not find significant differences among the three groups. Two more studies currently are in progress (Schramm et al., 2011; Wiersma et al., 2008) to help clarify the specific utility of CBASP for chronic depression.

ST (or schema-focused therapy) also is an integrative therapy (Young et al., 2003), with elements of cognitive, behavioral, interpersonal, and emotion-focused therapies. Hawke and Povencher (2011) note that "Young's schema theory does not attempt to compete with traditional Beckian theory, but rather expands on it for treatment-resistant clientele whose psychological problems are thought to be maintained by complex characterological underpinnings. It does so by placing greater emphasis on the developmental origins of severe psychopathology" (p. 258).

A study by Giesen-Bloo and colleagues (2006) found surprisingly strong and significant results in favor of ST over transference-focused therapy with the chronic disorder of borderline personality. After 3 years of treatment (sessions twice per week), 45% of the patients in schema-focused therapy (vs. 24% in transference-focused therapy) completely recovered. One year later, over half (52%) in ST fully recovered (vs. 29% in transference-focused therapy) and two-thirds (70%) in ST showed significant improvement. In addition, patients in ST were significantly less likely to drop out of therapy (27% dropped out of ST vs. 50% out of transference-focused therapy). Even stronger results were reported (Farrell, Shaw, & Webber, 2009) for group schema-focused therapy (GST; see Farrell & Shaw, 2012) for people with borderline personality disorder. This study compared individual TAU (CBT or psychodynamic) plus adjunct GST with TAU alone. Ninety-four percent receiving TAU plus GST, compared to 16% receiving TAU alone, no longer met criteria for borderline personality disorder at the end of 20 months of treatment. In addition, there was a 0% dropout rate in the TAU plus GST condition compared to 25% in the TAU condition. Given the high degree of similarities between patients with chronic disorders (adverse childhood histories, early-onset depression, and a multitude of schemas), we believe that ST is very likely to be an effective treatment for the chronically depressed population as well. Fritz Renner, at Maastricht University in the Netherlands, is currently conducting a study on the effectiveness of ST with chronic depression (Web link: *clinicaltrials.gov/ct2/show/nct01153867*).

Current Status and Future Research on Treating Depression

There is now a considerable body of research on treatments for depression. Certainly there are enough inconsistencies in the literature to warrant continued debate and research regarding the relative merits of different treatments for depression. Nevertheless, the overall efficacy of cognitive therapy for depression is clearly a replicable and robust finding.

Many important, unanswered questions—along with inconsistent research findings—will probably make it impossible for proponents of any single treatment to make firm recommendations favoring one treatment for depression over another across disorders and populations. In the spirit of Beck's emphasis on testable hypotheses and clinical protocols, we hope that, through more sophisticated research studies, it will eventually be possible to better understand which types of depressed patients benefit most from which type of treatment, or combination of treatments, and in what sequence.

The remainder of this chapter is devoted to describing the cognitive model of depression and schema theory; detailing the basic characteristics of cognitive and schema therapies; and demonstrating applications of cognitive and schema therapies to depression in clinical practice.

COGNITIVE MODEL OF DEPRESSION

The cognitive model assumes that cognition, behavior, and biochemistry are all important components of depressive disorders. We do not view them as competing theories of depression but as different levels of analysis. Each treatment approach has its own "focus of convenience." The pharmacotherapist intervenes at the biochemical level; the cognitive therapist intervenes at the cognitive, affective, and behavioral levels. Our experience suggests that when we change depressive cognitions, we simultaneously change the characteristic mood, behavior, and, as some evidence suggests (Free, Oei, & Appleton, 1998; Joffe, Segal, & Singer, 1996), the biochemistry of depression. Although the exact mechanism of change remains a target of considerable investigation, speculation, and debate (Barber & DeRubeis, 1989; Castonguay, Goldfried, Wiser, Raue, & Hayes, 1996; Crews & Harrison, 1995; DeRubeis et al., 1990; DeRubeis & Feeley, 1990; Hayes & Strauss, 1998; Oei & Free, 1995; Oei & Shuttlewood, 1996; Shea & Elkin, 1996; Sullivan & Conway, 1991; Whisman, 1993), "there are indications that cognitive therapy works by virtue of changing beliefs and information-processing proclivities and that different aspects of cognition play different roles in the process of change" (Hollon et al., 1996, p. 314).

Our focus in this chapter is on the cognitive disturbances in depression. Cognitive science research emphasizes the importance of information processing in depressive symptomatology (Ingram & Holle, 1992). According to these theories, negatively biased cognition is a core process in depression. This process is reflected in the "cognitive triad of depression": Depressed patients typically have a negative view of themselves, of their environment, and of the future. They view themselves as worthless, inadequate, unlovable, and deficient. Depressed patients view the environment as overwhelming, as presenting insuperable obstacles that cannot be overcome, and that continually result in failure or loss. Moreover, they view the future as hopeless: Their own efforts will be insufficient to change the unsatisfying course of their lives. This negative view of the future often leads to suicidal ideation and actual suicide attempts.

Depressed patients consistently distort their interpretations of events, so that they maintain negative views of themselves, their environment, and the future. Beck suggests that much of this distorted cognitive processing takes place outside of conscious awareness, in the form of "automatic thoughts," those thoughts that intervene between life events and the patient's emotional reactions to those events. Automatic thoughts often go unnoticed by the patient because they are out of awareness, they are part of a repetitive or habitual way of thinking, and because they occur so often. Automatic thoughts are often contrary to what a patient logically and consciously knows to be true, and most patients, prior to therapy, cannot stop them through rational thought processes.

This process of cognitive distortion is far more common in depressed patients than in nondepressed individuals. For example, a depressed woman whose husband comes home late one night may conclude that he is having an affair with another woman, even though there is no other evidence supporting this conclusion. This example illustrates an "arbitrary inference," reaching a conclusion that is not justified by the available evidence. Other distortions include all-or-nothing thinking, overgeneralization, selective abstraction, and magnification (Beck et al., 1979).

SCHEMA THEORY

According to subsequent developments within the cognitive model, an important predisposing factor for many patients with depression is the presence of schemas (Stein & Young, 1992; Young, 1990/1999).[3] Beck (1976) emphasized the importance of schemas in depression and provided the following definition:

A schema is a cognitive structure for screening, coding, and evaluating the stimuli that impinge on the organism. . . . On the basis of this matrix of schemas, the individual is able to orient himself in relation to time and space and to categorize and interpret experiences in a meaningful way. (p. 233)

Furthermore, Beck, Freeman, and Associates (1990) noted:

In the field of psychopathology, the term "schema" has been applied to structures with a highly personalized idiosyncratic content that are activated during disorders such as depression, anxiety, panic attacks, and obsessions, and become prepotent. . . . Thus, in clinical depression, for example, the negative schemas are in ascendancy, resulting in a systematic negative bias in the interpretation and recall of experiences as well as in short-term and long-term predictions, whereas the positive schemas become less accessible. It is easy for depressed patients to see the negative aspects of an event, but difficult to see the positive. They can recall negative events much more readily than positive ones. They weigh the probabilities of undesirable outcomes more heavily than positive outcomes. (p. 32)

There has also been increasing recognition that "focusing on core schemas is a key to effective short-term therapy" (Freeman & Davison, 1997, p. 8).

Through clinical observation, Young has identified a subset of schemas that he terms early maladaptive schemas (EMSs): "Early Maladaptive Schemas refer to extremely stable and enduring themes that develop during childhood and are elaborated upon throughout the individual's lifetime and that are dysfunctional to a significant degree" (Young, 1990/1999, p. 9). The 18 EMSs identified by Young are listed in Figure 7.1.[4]

According to Young's (see Young et al., 2003) theory, early schemas[5] result from an interaction between the child's innate temperament and early negative life experiences, especially with significant others. Children gradually construct pervasive, maladaptive views of themselves and others that are filtered through, and consistent with, their schemas.

According to Young, EMSs are (1) a priori truths about oneself and/or the environment; (2) self-perpetuating and resistant to change; (3) dysfunctional; (4) often triggered by some environmental change (e.g., loss of a job or mate); (5) tied to high levels of affect when activated; and (6) as noted earlier, usually result from an interaction of the child's temperament with dysfunctional developmental experiences with family members, caretakers, and peers (Young, 1990/1999). Young goes on to elaborate that when an EMS is triggered, specific early memories, core beliefs, strong emotions, and physiological reactions are also activated. (In Young's model, *core beliefs* represent the cognitive component of schemas.[6])

EMSs are likely to develop when the environment does not meet the child's core needs for safety, stability or predictability, love, nurturance and attention, acceptance and praise, empathy, realistic limits, and validation of feelings and needs. When their core needs are not met, children often internalize attitudes and beliefs

that later prove maladaptive. For example, a child who is criticized repeatedly may develop a Failure schema: a sense that no matter what he/she does, his/her performance will never be good enough.

A schema usually occurs outside of awareness and may remain dormant until a life event (e.g., being fired from a job) activates it. In this example, once the Failure schema has been activated, the patient categorizes, selects, and encodes information in such a way that the schema is maintained. EMSs therefore predispose many depressed patients to distort events in a characteristic fashion, leading to a negative view of themselves, the environment, and the future.

For patients who have a large number of strong and deeply entrenched EMSs, and for patients who cope with their schemas by rigidly avoiding life situations or by overcompensating for them, we have found that the concept of "schema modes" (Young et al., 2003) is very often invaluable in understanding and changing patients' thoughts, feelings, and behaviors. Mode work strengthens and develops healthy modes and weakens dysfunctional modes, thereby increasing control over one's responding.

Young's concept of a mode is similar to that of an ego state. A "mode" is defined as "those schemas or schema operations—adaptive or maladaptive—that are currently active for an individual" (Young et al., 2003, p. 271). Modes include whatever an individual is thinking, feeling, and doing at a given point in time, and may therefore be thought of as states rather than traits. A dysfunctional mode is activated when specific maladaptive schemas have erupted into distressing emotions, avoidance responses, or self-defeating behaviors that take over and control an individual's functioning at a given point in time. An individual may "flip" from one mode to another; as that shift occurs, an individual's cognitions, emotions, and coping responses change as well. Young and colleagues have identified four main types of modes: Child modes (Figure 7.2a), Maladaptive Coping modes (Figure 7.2b), Dysfunctional Parent modes (Figure 7.2c), and the Healthy Adult mode. The Healthy Adult mode is

the healthy, adult part of the self that serves an "executive" function relative to the other modes. The Healthy Adult helps meet the child's basic emotional needs. Building and strengthening the patient's Healthy Adult to work with the other modes more effectively is the overarching goal of mode work in ST (Young et al., 2003, p. 277).

1. ABANDONMENT/INSTABILITY
   The perceived *instability* or *unreliability* of those available for support and connection. Involves the sense that significant others will not be able to continue providing emotional support, connection, strength, or practical protection because they are emotionally unstable and unpredictable (e.g., angry outbursts), or unreliable or erratically present; because they will die imminently; or because they will abandon the patient in favor of someone better.

2. MISTRUST/ABUSE
   The expectation that others will hurt, abuse, humiliate, cheat, lie, manipulate, or take advantage. Usually involves the perception that the harm is intentional or the result of unjustified and extreme negligence. May include the sense that one always ends up being cheated relative to others or "getting the short end of the stick."

3. EMOTIONAL DEPRIVATION
   Expectation that one's desire for a normal degree of emotional support will not be adequately met by others. The three major forms of deprivation are as follows:
   A. *Deprivation of nurturance:* Absence of attention, affection, warmth, or companionship.
   B. *Deprivation of empathy:* Absence of understanding, listening, self-disclosure, or mutual sharing of feelings from others.
   C. *Deprivation of protection:* Absence of strength, direction, or guidance from others.

4. DEFECTIVENESS/SHAME
   The feeling that one is defective, bad, unwanted, inferior, or invalid in important respects; or that one would be unlovable to significant others it exposed. May involve hypersensitivity to criticism, rejection, and blame; self-consciousness, comparisons, and insecurity around others; or a sense of shame regarding one's perceived flaws. These flaws may be *private* (e.g., selfishness, angry impulses, unacceptable sexual desires) or *public* (e.g., undesirable physical appearance, social awkwardness).

5. SOCIAL ISOLATION/ALIENATION
   The feeling that one is isolated from the rest of the world, different from other people, and/or not part of any group or community.

6. DEPENDENCE/INCOMPETENCE
   Belief that one is unable to handle one's *everyday responsibilities* in a competent manner, without considerable help from others (e.g., take care of oneself, solve daily problems, exercise good judgment, tackle new tasks, make good decisions). Often presents as helplessness.

7. VULNERABILITY TO HARM OR ILLNESS
   Exaggerated fear that *imminent* catastrophe will strike at any time and that one will be unable to prevent it. Fears focus on one or more of the following: (A) *medical catastrophes* (e.g., heart attacks, AIDS); (B) *emotional catastrophes* (e.g., going crazy); (C) *external catastrophes* (e.g., elevators collapsing, victimized by criminals, airplane crashes, earthquakes).

8. ENMESHMENT/UNDEVOLOPED SELF
   Excessive emotional involvement and closeness with one or more significant others (often parents), at the expense of full individuation or normal social development. Often involves the belief that at least one of the enmeshed individuals cannot survive or be happy without the constant support of the other. May also include feelings of being smothered by, or fused with, others OR insufficient individual identity. Often experienced as a feeling of emptiness and floundering, having no direction, or in extreme cases questioning one's existence.

(continued)

FIGURE 7.1. Early maladaptive schemas. Copyright 1999 by Jeffrey E. Young. Reprinted by permission.

9. FAILURE

The belief that one has failed, will inevitably fail, or is fundamentally inadequate relative to one's peers, in areas of *achievement* (school, career, sports, etc.) Often involves beliefs that one is stupid, inept, untalented. ignorant, lower in status, less successful than others, and so forth.

10. ENTITLEMENT/GRANDIOSITY

The belief that one is superior to other people; entitled to special rights and privileges; or not bound by the rules of reciprocity that guide normal social interaction. Often involves insistence that one should be able to do or have whatever one wants regardless of what is realistic, what others consider reasonable, or the cost to others; OR an exaggerated focus on superiority (e.g., being among the most successful, famous, and wealthy) in order to achieve *power or control* (not primarily for attention or approval). Sometimes includes excessive competitiveness toward, or domination of others: asserting ones power, forcing one's point of view, or controlling the behavior of others in line with one's own desires—without empathy or concern for others' needs or feelings.

11. INSUFFICIENT SELF-CONTROL/SELF-DISCIPLINE

Pervasive difficulty or refusal to exercise sufficient self-control and frustration tolerance to achieve one's personal goals, or to restrain the excessive expression of one's emotions and impulses. In its milder form, patient presents with an exaggerated emphasis on discomfort avoidance: avoiding pain, conflict, confrontation, responsibility, or overexertion—at the expense of personal fulfillment, commitment, or integrity.

12. SUBJUGATION

Excessive surrendering of control to others because one feels coerced—usually to avoid anger, retaliation, or abandonment. There are two major forms of subjugation:

A. *Subjugation of needs*: Suppression of one's preferences, decisions, and desires.
B. *Subjugation of emotion:* Suppression of emotional expression, especially anger.

Usually involves the perception that one's own desires, opinions, and feelings are not valid or important to others. Frequently presents as excessive compliance, combined with hypersensitivity to feeling trapped. Generally leads to a buildup of anger, manifested in maladaptive symptoms (e.g., passive–aggressive behavior, uncontrolled outbursts of temper, psychosomatic symptoms, withdrawal of affection, "acting cut," substance abuse).

13. SELF-SACRIFICE

Excessive focus on *voluntarily* meeting the needs of others in daily situations at the expense of one's own gratification. The most common reasons are to prevent causing pain to others, to avoid guilt from feeling selfish, or to maintain the connection with others perceived as needy. Often results from an acute sensitivity to the pain of others. Sometimes leads to a sense that one's own needs are not being adequately met and to resentment of those who are taken care of. (Overlaps with concept of codependency.)

14. APPROVAL SEEKING/RECOGNITION SEEKING

Excessive emphasis on gaining approval, recognition or attention from other people or fitting in, at the expense of developing a secure and true sense of self. One's sense of esteem is dependent primarily on the reactions of others rather than on one's own natural inclinations. Sometimes includes an overemphasis on status, appearance, social acceptance, money, or achievements—as a means of gaining *approval, admiration*, or *attention* (not primarily for power or control). Frequently results in major life decisions that are inauthentic or unsatisfying, or in hypersensitivity to rejection.

(continued)

FIGURE 7.1. *(continued)*

15. NEGATIVITY/PESSIMISM

A pervasive, lifelong focus on the negative aspects of life (pain, death, loss, disappointment, conflict, guilt, resentment, unsolved problems, potential mistakes, betrayal, things that could go wrong, etc.), while minimizing or neglecting the positive or optimistic aspects. Usually includes an exaggerated expectation—in a wide range of work, financial, or interpersonal situations—that things will eventually go seriously wrong, or that aspects of one's life that seem to be going well will ultimately fall apart. Usually involves an inordinate fear of making mistakes that might lead to financial collapse, loss, humiliation or being trapped in a bad situation. Because potential negative outcomes are exaggerated, these patients are frequently characterized by chronic worry, vigilance, complaining, or indecision.

16. EMOTIONAL INHIBITION

The excessive inhibition of spontaneous action, feeling, or communication—usually to avoid disapproval by others, feelings of shame, or losing control of one's impulses The most common areas of inhibition involve (A) inhibition of *anger* and aggression; (B) inhibition of *positive impulses* (e.g., joy, affection, sexual excitement, play); (C) difficulty expressing *vulnerability* or *communicating* freely about one's feelings, needs, etc.; or (D) excessive emphasis on *rationality* while disregarding emotions.

17. UNRELENTING STANDARDS/HYPERCRITICALNESS

The underlying belief that one must strive to meet very high *internalized standards* of behavior and performance usually to avoid criticism. Typically results in feelings of pressure or difficulty slowing down and in hypercriticalness toward oneself and others. Must involve significant impairment in pleasure, relaxation, health, self-esteem sense of accomplishment, or satisfying relationships. Unrelenting standards typically present as (A) *perfectionism*, inordinate attention to detail, or an underestimate of how good one's own performance is relative to the norm; (B) *rigid rules* and "shoulds" in many areas of life, including unrealistically high moral, ethical, cultural or religious precepts; or (C) preoccupation with *time and efficiency* so that more can be accomplished.

18. PUNITIVENESS

The belief that people should be harshly punished for making mistakes. Involves the tendency to be angry, intolerant, punitive, and impatient with those people (including oneself) who do not meet one's expectations or standards. Usually includes difficulty forgiving mistakes in oneself or others because of a reluctance to consider extenuating circumstances, allow for human imperfection, or empathize with feelings.

FIGURE 7.1. *(continued)*

Research Related to Schema Theory

A large number of research studies have examined the 18 EMSs, as measured by the Young Schema Questionnaire (YSQ; Young, 2005). While the results have varied somewhat across different populations, all 18 EMSs have generally been supported (Lee, Taylor, & Dunn, 1999; Schmidt, 1994; Schmidt, Joiner, Young, & Telch, 1995).

Numerous studies have looked at EMSs in depressed patients. Hawke and Provencher (2011) provide an excellent review of research on EMSs in both mood (Bailleux, Romo, Kindynis, Radtchenko, & Debray, 2008; Halvorsen et al., 2009; Halvorsen, Wang, Eisemann, & Waterloo, 2010; Riso et al., 2003, 2006; Wang, Halvorsen, Eisemann, & Waterloo, 2010) and anxiety disorders. Elevations across most, if not all,

schema domains have been evident when comparing depressed patients with never-ill controls. In a study specifically comparing EMSs in patients with chronic depression, nonchronic depression, and healthy controls, Riso and colleagues (2003) found that both depressed groups scored higher on all schema domains compared to healthy controls. However, the scores in the chronic depression group were highest on schemas in the disconnection and rejection, impaired autonomy and performance, and overvigilance domains, even when researchers controlled for depressive and personality disorder symptoms. Hawke and Provencher (2011, p. 261) note: "This suggests that chronic depression is associated more strongly with EMSs than the nonchronic form, and that this association is not simply a function of current depressive or Axis II symptoms."

Child Mode	Description	Common associated schemas
Vulnerable Child	Experiences dysphoric or anxious affect, especially fear, sadness, and helplessness, when "in touch" with associated schemas.	Abandonment, Mistrust/Abuse, Emotional Deprivation, Defectiveness, Social Isolation, Dependence/Incompetence, Vulnerability to Harm or Illness, Enmeshment/Undeveloped Self, Negativity/Pessimism.
Angry Child	Vents anger directly in response to perceived unmet core needs or unfair treatment related to core schemas.	Abandonment, Mistrust/Abuse, Emotional Deprivation, Subjugation (or, at times, any of the schemas associated with the Vulnerable Child).
Impulsive/ Undisciplined Child	Impulsively acts according to immediate desires for pleasure without regard to limits or others' needs or feelings (not linked to core needs).	Entitlement, Insufficient Self-Control/Self-Discipline.
Happy Child	Feels loved, connected, content, satisfied.	None. Absence of activated schemas.

FIGURE 7.2A. Child modes. From Young, Klosko, and Weishaar (2003). Copyright 2003 by The Guilford Press. Reprinted by permission.

Maladaptive Coping Modes	Description
Compliant Surrenderer	Adopts a coping style of compliance and dependence.
Detached Protector	Adopts a coping style of emotional withdrawal, disconnection, isolation, and behavioral avoidance.
Overcompensator	Adopts a coping style of counterattack and control. May overcompensate through semiadaptive means, such as workaholism.

FIGURE 7.2B. Maladaptive Coping modes. From Young, Klosko, and Weishaar (2003). Copyright 2003 by The Guilford Press. Reprinted by permission.

Dysfunctional Parent Mode	Description	Common associated schemas
Punitive/Critical Parent	Restricts, criticizes, or punishes the self or others.	Subjugation, Punitiveness, Defectiveness, Mistrust/Abuse (as abuser).
Demanding Parent	Sets high expectations and high level of responsibility toward others; pressures the self or others to achieve them.	Unrelenting Standards, Self-Sacrifice.

FIGURE 7.2C. Dysfunctional Parent modes. From Young, Klosko, and Weishaar (2003). Copyright 2003 by The Guilford Press. Reprinted by permission.

Renner and colleagues (2012) also found EMSs, particularly those in the disconnection and rejection and impaired autonomy and performance domains, to be related to severity of depressive symptoms. They note that, consistent with Beck's theory, "these findings are consistent with the cognitive model of depression, placing schemas or core beliefs in the domains of failure, loss, and worthlessness at the core of depressive symptoms" (p. 587). In their examination of the robustness of EMSs with evidence-based treatments (CBT and interpersonal psychotherapy [IPT], with and without medication) for depression, they found that EMSs remained relatively stable over time (pre- and posttreatment). This finding is consistent with Young and colleagues' (2003) notion of EMSs as stable, trait-like beliefs that remain even after successful treatment of Axis I symptoms. According to the schema model, these results should not be surprising, since none of the treatments in this study specifically targeted change in EMSs.

In a recent study, Eberhart, Auerbach, Bigda-Peyton, and Abela (2011) examined how EMSs and stress impact depressive symptoms by comparing two models of stress: diathesis–stress and stress-generation. The diathesis–stress model posits that EMSs only create vulnerability to depression when interacting with high levels of stressors. The stress generation model posits that EMSs are instrumental in creating stressful conditions which then increase depression. The results supported the stress generation hypothesis. The researchers noted that

> a number of maladaptive schemas in the domains of disconnection and rejection, impaired autonomy and performance, and other-directedness predicted the generation of dependent, interpersonal stressors. These dependent interpersonal stressors, in turn, predicted increases in depressive symptoms. Moreover, there was evidence that these stressors mediated the relationships between maladaptive schemas and depressive symptoms. In particular, mediation effects were observed for subjugation schemas, failure schemas, and a number of schemas related to disconnection and rejection" (p. 96). [body]This research highlights the importance of targeting EMSs in the treatment of chronic depression.

In the following sections we present information about the general characteristics and nature of cognitive therapy, a discussion of the process of cognitive therapy, then two case examples that illustrate cognitive therapy in action. The patient in the first case has a nonchronic form of depression and is treated with "standard" cognitive therapy (as originally outlined in Beck et al.'s 1979 book). The focus of standard cognitive therapy is on changing depressive thinking in the present. The patient in the second case has chronic depression and is treated with both cognitive and schema therapies. The focus of ST, in this case, is on identifying and modifying the patient's underlying schemas through mode work.

CHARACTERISTICS OF THERAPY

Cognitive therapy with adult depressed outpatients is usually undertaken in the therapist's office. It has most frequently been applied in a one-to-one setting. However, group cognitive therapy has also been shown to be successful with many depressed outpatients (Beutler et al., 1987; Jarrett & Nelson, 1987), although it may not be as effective as individual treatment (Wierzbicki & Bartlett, 1987). Additionally, computer-assisted cognitive therapy for depression (50-minute vs. 25-minute sessions with computer assistance) also has been found effective (Wright et al., 2005). It is not unusual to involve spouses, partners, parents, and other family members during treatment. For example, they may provide information that helps patients test the validity of their thinking with respect to how other family members view them. Moreover, couple therapy based on the cognitive model is often very effective in relieving depression related to chronic interpersonal problems (Beck, 1988; O'Leary & Beach, 1990).

In our clinical experience, a number of therapist characteristics contribute to effective cognitive therapy. First, cognitive therapists ideally should demonstrate the "nonspecific" therapy skills identified by other writers (see, e.g., Truax & Mitchell, 1971): They should be able to communicate warmth, genuineness, sincerity, and openness. Second, the most effective cognitive therapists seem to be especially skilled at seeing events from their patients' perspectives (accurate empathy). They are able to suspend their own personal assumptions and biases while listening to depressed patients describe their reactions and interpretations. Third, skilled cognitive therapists can reason logically and plan strategies; they are not "fuzzy" thinkers. In this respect they resemble good trial lawyers, who can spot the sometimes subtle flaws in another individual's reasoning and skillfully elicit a more convincing interpretation of the same events. Skilled cognitive therapists plan strategies several steps ahead, anticipating the desired outcome. Fourth, the best practitioners of this approach are active. They have to be comfortable taking the lead, providing structure and direction to the therapy process.

Although patient characteristics have received some empirical attention (Eifert, Beach, & Wilson, 1998; Padesky, with Greenberger, 1995; Persons, Burns, & Perloff, 1988; Shea et al., 1990), we do not yet have adequate knowledge as to which patient characteristics are related to success in cognitive therapy. Our experience suggests that patients with major depressive disorder (or milder forms of depression) respond well to the cognitive therapy approach described in this chapter. To the extent that the patient is diagnosed with Axis II personality disorders and/or his/her depression is chronic, the combination of cognitive and schema therapies may be significantly longer in duration and more crucial in obtaining a more complete and lasting positive response to treatment.

Cognitive therapy can serve an important adjunctive role to pharmacotherapy for bipolar disorders (Ball et al., 2006; Basco & Rush, 1996; Colom, Vieta, Martinez, Jorquera, & Gastó, 1998; Craighead, Miklowitz, Vajk, & Frank, 1998; Lam, Hayward, Watkins, Wright, & Sham, 2005; Scott, 1996b), and is effective in treating patients with severe endogenous depression (Thase, Bowler, & Harden, 1991; Whisman, 1993). Preliminary evidence also suggests that cognitive therapy is effective in the treatment of women with postpartum depression (Bledsoe & Grote, 2006).

It is advisable to assess patients' suitability for cognitive therapy (Padesky, with Greenberger, 1995; Safran & Segal, 1990; Safran, Segal, Vallis, Shaw, & Samstag, 1993). In our experience, certain patient characteristics are predictive of a more rapid response. "Ideal" cognitive therapy patients are appropriately introspective and can reason abstractly; are well organized, good planners, and conscientious about carrying out responsibilities; are employed or have a history of employment; are not excessively angry at either themselves or at other people; are less dogmatic and rigid in their thinking; can identify a clear precipitating event for the depressive episode; and have close relationships with others. Most patients deviate in some ways from this prototype, and these characteristics are not essential to successful treatment. However, patients with more of these attributes often show faster improvement in depressive symptoms through cognitive therapy.

Age is not an obstacle: Patients across the lifespan seem to benefit from cognitive therapy (Beutler et al.,

1987; Floyd, Scogin, McKendree-Smith, Floyd, & Rokke, 2004; Gallagher-Thompson, Hanley-Peterson, & Thompson, 1990; Harrington, Wood, & Verduyn, 1998; Koder, Brodaty, & Anstey, 1996; Levendusky & Hufford, 1997; Reinecke, Ryan, & DuBois, 1998). Many studies have indicated that children and adolescents show significant clinical improvement following CBT (Curry, 2001). Studies of older patients show that "various forms of cognitive and behavioral psychotherapy can be as effective in treating geriatric depression as depressions occurring earlier in life" (Futterman, Thompson, Gallagher-Thompson, & Ferris, 1995, p. 511).

COLLABORATION

Basic to cognitive therapy is a collaborative relationship between patient and therapist. When therapist and patient work together, the learning experience is enhanced for both, and the cooperative spirit that is developed contributes greatly to the therapeutic process. Equally important, the collaborative approach helps to ensure compatible goals for treatment, and to prevent misunderstandings and misinterpretations between patient and therapist. Because of the importance of the collaborative relationship, we place great emphasis on the interpersonal skills of the therapist, the process of joint selection of problems to be worked on, regular feedback, and the investigative process we call "collaborative empiricism."

Interpersonal Qualities

Because collaboration requires that the patient trust the therapist, we emphasize those interpersonal qualities that contribute to trust. As noted earlier, warmth, accurate empathy, and genuineness are desirable personal qualities for the cognitive therapist, as well as for all psychotherapists. It is important that the cognitive therapist not seem to be playing the *role* of therapist. The therapist should be able to communicate both verbally and nonverbally that he/she is sincere, open, concerned, and direct. It is also important that the therapist not seem to be withholding impressions or information, or evading questions. The therapist should be careful not to seem critical or disapproving of the patient's perspective.

Rapport between patient and therapist is crucial in the treatment of depressed patients. When rapport is optimal, patients perceive the therapist as someone who is tuned in to their feelings and attitudes, who is sympathetic and understanding, and with whom they can communicate without having to articulate feelings in detail or qualify statements. When the rapport is good, both patient and therapist feel comfortable and secure.

A confident, professional manner is also important in cognitive therapy. A therapist should convey relaxed confidence in his/her ability to help a depressed patient. Such confidence can help to counteract the patient's initial hopelessness about the future. Because the cognitive therapist must sometimes be directive and impose structure, especially in the early stages of treatment, it is helpful to maintain a clear sense of professionalism.

Joint Determination of Goals for Therapy

The patient and therapist collaboratively work together to set therapeutic goals, determine priorities among them, and create an agenda for each session. Problems to be addressed over the course of therapy include specific depressive symptoms (e.g., hopelessness, crying, and difficulty concentrating) and external problems (e.g., couple difficulties, career issues, childrearing concerns). Priorities are then jointly determined in accordance with how much distress is generated by a particular problem and how amenable that particular problem is to change. During the agenda-setting portion of each therapy session (discussed in detail in the next section), therapist and patient together determine the items to be covered in that session. Through this collaborative process, target problems are selected on a weekly basis.

The process of problem selection often presents difficulties for the novice cognitive therapist, including failure to reach agreement on specific problems on which to focus, selection of peripheral concerns, and the tendency to move from problem to problem instead of persistently seeking a satisfactory solution to only one problem at a time. Because the problem selection process entails both structuring and collaboration on the part of the therapist, considerable skill is necessary.

Regular Feedback

Feedback is especially important in therapy with depressed patients; it is a crucial ingredient in developing and maintaining the collaborative therapeutic relationship. The cognitive therapist initiates the feedback component early in therapy by eliciting the patient's thoughts and feelings about many aspects of the therapy, such as the handling of a particular problem, the therapist's manner, and homework assignments. Since many patients misconstrue therapists' statements and questions, it is only through regular feedback that the therapist can ascertain whether he/she and the patient are on the same "wavelength." The therapist must also be alert for verbal and nonverbal clues to covert negative reactions.

As part of the regular feedback process, the cognitive therapist shares the rationale for each intervention. This helps to demystify the therapy process and facilitates the patient's questioning of the validity of a particular approach. In addition, when a patient understands how a particular technique or assignment may help solve a particular problem in the patient's life, he/she is more likely to participate conscientiously.

Another key element of the feedback process is for the therapist to check regularly to determine whether the patient understands his/her formulations. Patients sometimes agree with a formulation simply out of compliance, and depressed patients frequently exhibit both compliance and reluctance to "talk straight" with their therapists for fear of being rejected or criticized, or of making a mistake. Therefore, the therapist must make an extra effort to elicit the patient's feelings or wishes relevant to compliance (e.g., anxiety about rejection, wish to please) and be alert for verbal and nonverbal clues that the patient may indeed not understand the explanations.

At the close of each session the cognitive therapist provides a concise summary of what has taken place, and asks the patient to abstract and write down the main points from the session. The patient keeps this summary for review during the week. In practice, the therapist uses capsule summaries frequently during a standard therapeutic interview: in preparing the agenda, in a midpoint recapitulation of the material covered up to that point, and in the final summary of the main points of the interview. Patients generally respond favorably to the elicitation of feedback and presentation of capsule summaries. We have observed that the development of empathy and rapport is facilitated by these techniques.

Collaborative Empiricism

When the collaborative therapeutic relationship has been successfully formed, patient and therapist act as an investigative team. Though we elaborate on the investigative process later, it is appropriate to introduce it in the context of the collaborative relationship. As a team, patient and therapist approach the patient's automatic thoughts and schemas in the same manner that scientists approach questions: Each thought or schema becomes a hypothesis to be tested, and evidence is gathered that supports or refutes the hypothesis. Events in the past, circumstances in the present, and possibilities in the future are the data that constitute evidence, and the conclusion to accept or reject the hypothesis is jointly reached as patient and therapist subject the evidence to logical analysis. Experiments may also be devised to test the validity of particular cognitions. Cognitive therapists need not persuade patients of illogicality or inconsistency with reality because patients "discover" their own inconsistencies. This guided discovery process, a widely accepted educational method, is one of the vital components of cognitive therapy.

THE PROCESS OF COGNITIVE THERAPY

Here we attempt to convey a sense of how cognitive therapy sessions are structured and of the course of treatment. Detailed discussion of particular techniques follows this section.

The Initial Sessions

A main therapeutic goal of the first few sessions is to produce some symptom relief. Reducing the patient's suffering helps to increase rapport, collaboration, and confidence in the therapeutic process. Symptom relief, however, should be based on more than rapport, sympathy, and implied promise of "cure." In the first few sessions, the cognitive therapist starts the process of defining the patient's problems and demonstrating some of the strategies that will be used in the therapy to deal with those problems.

Problem definition is a primary goal in the early stages of therapy. The therapist collaboratively works with the patient to define the specific problems on which they will focus during therapy sessions. The cognitive therapist does this by obtaining as complete a picture as possible of the patient's psychological and life situation difficulties. The therapist also seeks details concerning the depth of depression and particular symptomatology. Cognitive therapists are especially concerned with how patients see their problems.

Once the specific problems have been defined, patient and therapist establish priorities among them.

Decisions are made on the basis of amenability to therapeutic change and centrality of the life problem or cognition to the patient's emotional distress. To help establish priorities effectively, the therapist must see the relationships among particular thoughts, particular life situations, and particular distressing emotions.

Another goal of the initial session is to illustrate the close relationship between cognition and emotion. When the therapist is able to observe the patient's mood change (e.g., crying), he/she points out the alteration in affect and asks for the patient's thoughts just before the mood shift. The therapist then labels the negative thought and points out its relationship to the change in mood. He/she initially gears homework assignments toward helping the patient see the close connection between cognition and emotion.

A frequent requirement in the early stage of therapy is to socialize the patient to cognitive therapy. A patient who has previously undertaken analytically oriented or Rogerian therapies may begin cognitive therapy expecting a more insight-oriented, nondirective therapeutic approach. The cognitive therapist can facilitate the transition to a more active and structured approach by maintaining a problem-oriented stance, which often entails gently interrupting a patient who tends to speculate about the sources of the problems and to seek interpretations from the therapist.

Finally, the therapist must communicate the importance of self-help homework assignments during the initial session by stressing that doing the homework is actually more important than the therapy session itself. The therapist also can enhance motivation by explaining that patients who complete assignments generally improve more quickly. The nature and implementation of self-help homework assignments are considered in further detail in a later section of this chapter.

The Progress of a Typical Therapy Session

Each session begins with the establishment of an agenda for that session. This ensures optimal use of time in a relatively short-term, problem-solving therapeutic approach. The agenda generally begins with a short synopsis of the patient's experiences since the last session, including discussion of the homework assignment. The therapist then asks the patient what he/she wants to work on during the session, and often offers topics to be included.

When a short list of problems and topics has been completed, patient and therapist determine the order in which to cover them and, if necessary, the time to be allotted to each topic. There are several issues to consider in establishing priorities, including stage of therapy, severity of depression, likelihood of making progress in solving the problem, and potential pervasiveness of the effect of a particular theme or topic. The cognitive therapist is sensitive to a patient's occasional desire to talk about something that seems important to him/her at the moment, even if such discussion seems not to be productive in terms of other goals. This kind of flexibility characterizes the collaborative therapeutic relationship.

After these preliminary matters have been covered, patient and therapist move on to the one or two problems to be considered during the session. The therapist begins the discussion of a problem by asking the patient a series of questions designed to clarify the nature of the patient's difficulty. In doing so, the therapist seeks to determine whether early maladaptive schemas, misinterpretations of events, or unrealistic expectations are involved. The therapist also seeks to discover whether the patient had unrealistic expectations, whether the patient's behavior was appropriate, and whether all possible solutions to the problem were considered. The patient's responses suggest to the therapist a cognitive-behavioral conceptualization of why the patient is having difficulty in the area of concern. The therapist by now has discerned the one or two significant thoughts, schemas, images, or behaviors on which to work. When this target problem has been selected, the therapist chooses the cognitive or behavioral techniques to apply and shares their rationale with the patient. The specific techniques used in cognitive therapy are explained in the following sections of this chapter.

At the close of the session, the therapist asks the patient for a summary, often in writing, of the major conclusions drawn during the session. The therapist asks for the patient's reactions to the session to ascertain whether anything disturbing was said and to forestall any delayed negative reactions following the interview. Finally, the therapist gives a homework assignment designed to assist the patient in applying the particular skills and concepts from the session to the problem during the following week.

Progression of Session Content over Time

Although the structure of cognitive therapy sessions does not change during the course of treatment, the content often changes significantly. The first phase of treatment, symptom reduction, focuses on overcoming hopelessness, identifying problems, setting priorities, socializing the patient to cognitive therapy, establishing a collaborative relationship, demonstrating the relationship between cognition and emotion, labeling errors in thinking, and making progress on a target problem. Therapy is initially centered on the patient's symptoms, with attention given to behavioral and motivational difficulties.

In the second phase, which is focused on changing schemas for relapse prevention and chronic cases, therapist and patient turn from specific thoughts about particular problems to core schemas about the self and others, and to the modes associated with those schemas. Therapist and patient explore how the schemas and modes initiate, exacerbate, and maintain many of the patient's problems. Therapist and patient then work collaboratively to restructure and modify the schemas and modes through a variety of techniques, which eventually brings about a broader and more pervasive improvement in life functioning and mood.

Over the course of therapy, the patient assumes increased responsibility for identifying problems, coming up with solutions, and implementing the solutions through homework assignments. The therapist increasingly assumes the role of advisor or consultant as the patient learns to implement therapeutic techniques without constant support. As the patient becomes a more effective problem solver, the frequency of sessions is reduced, and therapy is eventually discontinued.

The remainder of this chapter is devoted to a detailed description of cognitive- and schema-based treatment strategies.

SYMPTOM REDUCTION

Behavioral Techniques

Behavioral techniques are used throughout the course of cognitive therapy, but they are generally concentrated in the earlier stages of treatment. Behavioral techniques are especially necessary for those more severely depressed patients who are passive, anhedonic, socially withdrawn, and unable to concentrate for extended periods of time. By engaging such a patient's attention and interest, the cognitive therapist tries to induce the patient to counteract withdrawal and become more involved in constructive activity. From a variety of behavioral techniques, the therapist selects those that will help the patient cope more effectively with situational and interpersonal problems. Through homework assignments, the patient implements specific procedures for dealing with concrete situations or for using time more adaptively.

The cognitive therapist uses behavioral techniques, with the goal of modifying automatic thoughts. For example, a patient who believes "I can't get anything done any more" can modify this thought after completing a series of graded tasks designed to increase mastery. The severely depressed patient is caught in a vicious cycle, in which a reduced activity level leads to a negative self-label, which in turn results in even further discouragement and consequent inactivity. Intervention with behavioral techniques can change this self-destructive pattern.

The most commonly used behavioral techniques include scheduling activities that include both mastery and pleasure exercises, cognitive rehearsal, self-reliance training, role playing, and diversion techniques. The scheduling of activities is frequently used in the early stages of cognitive therapy to counteract loss of motivation, hopelessness, and excessive rumination. The therapist uses the Weekly Activity Schedule for planning activities hour by hour, day by day (see Figure 7.3). Patients maintain an hourly record of the activities in which they engaged. Activity scheduling also helps patients obtain more pleasure and a greater sense of accomplishment from activities on a daily basis. The patients rate each completed activity (using a 0- to 10-point scale) for both mastery and pleasure. The ratings usually contradict patients' beliefs that they cannot accomplish or enjoy anything anymore. To as-

Note: Grade activities *M* for mastery and *P* for pleasure 0–10.							
	Mon.	Tues.	Wed.	Thurs.	Fri.	Sat.	Sun.
6–7							
7–8							
8–9							
9–10							
10–11							
11–12							
12–1							
1–2							
2–3							
3–4							
4–5							
5–6							
6–7							
7–8							
8–9							
9–10							
10–11							
11–12							
12–6							

Morning / Afternoon / Evening

FIGURE 7.3. Weekly Activity Schedule.

sist some patients in initiating mastery and pleasure activities, the therapist may sometimes find it necessary to subdivide an activity into segments, ranging from the simplest to the most difficult and complex aspects of the activity. We call this the "graded task" approach. The subdivision enables depressed patients to undertake tasks that were initially impossible, thus providing proof of success.

Cognitive rehearsal entails asking a patient to picture or imagine each step involved in the accomplishment of a particular task. This technique can be especially helpful with those patients who have difficulty carrying out a task that requires successive steps for its completion. Sometimes impairment in the ability to concentrate creates difficulties for the patient in focusing attention on the specific task. The imagery evoked by the cognitive rehearsal technique helps the patient to focus and the therapist to identify obstacles that make the assignment difficult for the particular patient.

Some depressed patients rely on others to take care of most of their daily needs. With self-reliance training, patients learn to assume increased responsibility for routine activities such as showering, making their beds, cleaning the house, cooking their own meals, and shopping. Self-reliance involves gaining increased control over emotional reactions.

Role playing has many uses in cognitive therapy. First, it may be used to bring out automatic thoughts through the enactment of particular interpersonal situations, such as an encounter with a supervisor at work. Second, through homework assignments, it may also guide the patient in practicing and attending to new cognitive responses in problematic social encounters. A third use of role playing is to rehearse new behaviors. Thus, role playing may be used as part of assertiveness training and is often accompanied by modeling and coaching.

Role reversal, a variation of role playing, can be very effective in helping patients test how other people might view their behavior. This is well illustrated by a patient who had a "humiliating experience" while buying some clothes in a store. After playing the role of the clerk, the patient had to conclude that she had insufficient data for her previous conclusion that she appeared clumsy and inept. Through role reversal, patients begin to view themselves less harshly as "self-sympathy" responses are elicited.

Finally, the therapist may introduce various distraction techniques to assist the patient in learning to reduce the intensity of painful affects. The patient learns to divert negative thinking through physical activity, social contact, work, play, and visual imagery. Practice with diversion techniques also helps the patient gain further control over emotional reactivity.

Cognitive Techniques

The specific cognitive techniques provide points of entry into the patient's cognitive organization. The cognitive therapist uses techniques for eliciting and testing automatic thoughts, and identifying schemas to help both therapist and patient understand the patient's construction of reality. In applying specific cognitive techniques in therapy, it is important that the therapist work within the framework of the cognitive model of depression. Each set of techniques is discussed in turn.

Eliciting Automatic Thoughts

"Automatic thoughts" are those thoughts that intervene between outside events and the individual's emotional reactions to them. They often go unnoticed because they are part of a repetitive pattern of thinking, and because they occur so often and so quickly. People rarely stop to assess their validity because they are so believable, familiar, and habitual. The patient in cognitive therapy must learn to recognize these automatic thoughts for therapy to proceed effectively. The cognitive therapist and the patient make a joint effort to discover the particular thoughts that precede emotions such as anger, sadness, and anxiety. The therapist uses questioning, imagery, and role playing to elicit automatic thoughts.

The simplest method to uncover automatic thoughts is for therapists to ask patients what thoughts went through their minds in response to particular events. This questioning provides a model for introspective exploration that patients can use on their own, when the therapist is not present, and after the completion of treatment.

Alternatively, when a patient is able to identify those external events and situations that evoke a particular emotional response, the therapist may use imagery by asking the patient to picture the situation in detail. The patient is often able to identify the automatic thoughts connected with actual situations when the image evoked is clear. In this technique, therapists ask patients to relax, close their eyes, and imagine themselves in the distressing situation. Patients describe in detail what is happening as they relive the event.

If a distressing event is an interpersonal one, cognitive therapists also can utilize role playing. The therapist plays the role of the other person in the encounter, while the patient plays him/herself. The automatic thoughts can usually be elicited when the patient becomes sufficiently engaged in the role play.

In attempting to elicit automatic thoughts, the therapist is careful to notice and point out any mood changes that occur during the session, and to ask the patient his/her thoughts just before the shift in mood. Mood changes include any emotional reaction, such as tears or anger. This technique can be especially useful when the patient is first learning to identify automatic thoughts.

Once patients become familiar with the techniques for identifying automatic thoughts, they are asked to keep a Daily Record of Dysfunctional Thoughts (Beck et al., 1979; see Figure 7.4), in which they record the emotions and automatic thoughts that occur in upsetting situations between therapy sessions. In later sessions, patients are taught to develop rational responses to their dysfunctional automatic thoughts and to record

them in the appropriate column. Therapist and patient generally review the daily record from the preceding week, near the beginning of the next therapy session. In sessions, the therapist also teaches chronic patients to recognize modes. Various affective exercises are then used to bring about change in the underlying schemas associated with those modes.

Eliciting automatic thoughts should be distinguished from the interpretation process of other psychotherapies. In general, cognitive therapists work only with those automatic thoughts mentioned by patients. Suggesting thoughts to patients may undermine collaboration and inhibit patients from learning to continue the process on their own. As a last resort, however, when nondirective strategies fail, a cognitive therapist may offer several possible automatic thoughts, then ask the patient whether any of these choices fit.

Even when many efforts to elicit automatic thoughts have been made by the therapist, sometimes the thought remains inaccessible. When this is the case, the cognitive therapist tries to ascertain the particular meaning of the event that evoked the emotional reaction. For ex-

	SITUATION Describe: 1. Actual event leading to unpleasant emotion, or 2. Stream of thoughts, daydream, or recollection, leading to unpleasant emotion.	EMOTION(S) 1. Specify sad/ anxious/ angry, etc. 2. Rate degree of emotion, 1–100.	AUTOMATIC THOUGHT(S) 1. Write automatic thought(s) that preceded emotion(s). 2. Rate belief in automatic thought(s), 0–100%.	RATIONAL RESPONSE 1. Write rational response to automatic thought(s). 2. Rate belief in rational response, 0–100%.	OUTCOME 1. Rerate belief in automatic thought(s), 0–100%. 2. Specify and rate subsequent emotions, 0–100%.
DATE					

Explanation: When you experience an unpleasant emotion, note the situation that seemed to stimulate the emotion. (If the emotion occurred while you were thinking, daydreaming, etc., please note this.) Then note the automatic thought associated with the emotion. Record the degree to which you believe this thought: 0% = not at all; 100% = completely. In rating degrees of emotion: 1 = a trace; 100 = the most intense possible.

FIGURE 7.4. Daily Record of Dysfunctional Thoughts.

ample, one patient began to cry whenever she had an argument with her roommate, who was a good friend. Efforts to elicit automatic thoughts proved unsuccessful. Only after the therapist asked a series of questions to determine the meaning of the event did it become clear that the patient associated having an argument or fight with ending the relationship. Through this process, therapist and patient were able to see the meaning that triggered the crying.

Testing Automatic Thoughts with Nonchronic Patients

When therapist and patient have managed to isolate a key automatic thought, they approach the thought as a testable hypothesis. In this "scientific" approach, which is fundamental to cognitive therapy, the patient learns to think in a way that resembles the investigative process. Through the procedures of gathering data, evaluating evidence, and drawing conclusions, patients learn firsthand that their view of reality can be quite different from what actually takes place. By designing experiments that subject their automatic thoughts to objective analysis, patients learn how to modify their thinking because they learn the *process* of empirical thinking. Patients who learn to think this way during treatment are better able to continue the empirical approach after the end of formal therapy.

The cognitive therapist approaches the testing of automatic thoughts by asking the patient to list evidence from his/her experience for and against the hypothesis. Sometimes, after considering the evidence, the patient immediately rejects the automatic thought, recognizing that it is either distorted or actually false.

When previous experience is not sufficient or appropriate to test a hypothesis, the therapist asks the patient to design an experiment for that purpose. The patient then makes a prediction and proceeds to gather data. If the data contradict the prediction, the patient can reject the automatic thought. The outcome of the experiment may, of course, confirm the patient's prediction. It is therefore very important for the therapist not to *assume* that the patient's automatic thought is distorted.

Some automatic thoughts do not lend themselves to hypothesis testing through the examination of evidence. In these cases, two options are available: The therapist may either produce evidence from his/her experience and offer it in the form of a question that reveals the contradiction or ask a question designed to uncover a logical error inherent in the patient's beliefs. The

therapist might say, for example, to a male patient who is sure he cannot survive without a close personal relationship, "You were alone last year, and you got along fine; what makes you think you can't make it now?"

In testing automatic thoughts, it is sometimes necessary to refine the patient's use of a word. This is particularly true for global labels such as "bad," "stupid," or "selfish." What is needed in this case is an operational definition of the word. To illustrate, a patient at our clinic had the recurring automatic thought, "I'm a failure in math." Therapist and patient had to narrow down the meaning of the word before they could test the thought. They operationalized "failure" in math as "being unable to achieve a grade of C after investing as much time studying as the average class member." Now they could examine past evidence and test the validity of the hypothesis. This process can help patients to see the overinclusiveness of their negative self-assessments and the idiosyncratic nature of many automatic thoughts.

Reattribution is another useful technique for helping the patient to reject an inappropriate, self-blaming thought. It is a common cognitive pattern in depression to ascribe blame or responsibility for adverse events to oneself. Reattribution can be used when the patient unrealistically attributes adverse occurrences to a personal deficiency, such as lack of ability or effort. Therapist and patient review the relevant events and apply logic to the available information to make a more realistic assignment of responsibility. The aim of reattribution is not to absolve the patient of all responsibility but to examine the many factors that contribute to adverse events. Through this process, patients gain objectivity, relieve themselves of the burden of self-reproach, and can then search for ways to solve realistic problems or prevent their recurrence.

Another strategy involving reattribution is for therapists to demonstrate that patients' criteria for assigning responsibility to their own unsatisfactory behavior are stricter than criteria they use in evaluating the behavior of others. Cognitive therapists also use reattribution to show patients that some of their thinking or behavior problems can be symptoms of depression (e.g., loss of concentration) and not signs of physical decay.

When a patient is accurate in identifying a realistic life problem or skills deficit, the cognitive therapist can use the technique of generating alternatives, in which therapist and patient actively search for alternative solutions. Because a depressed person's reasoning often becomes restricted, an effort to reconceptualize the problem can result in the patient's seeing a viable solution that he/she may previously have rejected.

It should be noted that all the cognitive techniques outlined here entail the use of questions by the therapist. A common error we observe in novice cognitive therapists is an exhortative style. We have found that therapists help patients to change their thinking more effectively by using carefully formed questions. If patients are prompted to work their own way through problems and reach their own conclusions, they learn an effective problem-solving process. We next elaborate on the use of questioning in cognitive therapy.

Questioning

As we have stressed throughout this chapter, questioning is a major therapeutic device in cognitive therapy. A majority of the therapist's comments during the therapy session are questions. Single questions can serve several purposes at one time, whereas carefully designed series of questions can help patients consider a particular issue, decision, or opinion. The cognitive therapist seeks through questioning to elicit what patients are thinking, instead of telling patients what he/she believes they are thinking.

In the beginning of therapy, questions are employed to obtain a full and detailed picture of a patient's particular difficulties; to obtain background and diagnostic data; to evaluate the patient's stress tolerance, capacity for introspection, coping methods, and so on; to obtain information about the patient's external situation and interpersonal context; and to modify vague complaints by working with the patient to arrive at specific target problems on which to work.

As therapy progresses, the therapist uses questioning to explore approaches to problems, to help the patient to weigh advantages and disadvantages of possible solutions, to examine the consequences of staying with particular maladaptive behaviors, to elicit automatic thoughts, and to demonstrate EMSs and their consequences. In short, the therapist uses questioning in most cognitive therapeutic techniques.

Although questioning is itself a powerful means of identifying and changing automatic thoughts and schemas, it is important that the questions be carefully and skillfully posed. If questions are used to "trap" patients into contradicting themselves, patients may come to feel that they are being attacked or manipulated by the therapist. Too many open-ended questions can leave patients wondering what the therapist expects of them.

Therapists must carefully time and phrase questions to help patients recognize their thoughts and schemas, and to weigh issues objectively.

Self-Help Homework Assignments

Rationale

Regular homework assignments are very important in cognitive therapy. When patients systematically apply what they have learned during therapy sessions to their outside lives, they are more likely to make significant progress in therapy and to be able to maintain their gains after termination of treatment. Burns and Spangler (2000) found that patients who did the most homework showed larger and more significant decreases in depression than those who were less compliant. Homework assignments are often the means through which patients gather data, test hypotheses, and begin to modify their thoughts and schemas. In addition, the data provided through homework assignments help to shift the focus of therapy from the subjective and abstract to more concrete and objective concerns. When a patient and therapist review the previous week's activities during the agenda-setting portion of the interview, they may do so quickly, and the therapist can draw relationships between what takes place in the session and specific tasks, thereby avoiding tangents and side issues. Homework assignments further patients' self-reliance and provide them with methods to continue working on problems after the end of treatment. Cognitive therapists emphasize the importance of homework by sharing with patients their rationale for assigning homework in therapy. They are also careful to explain the particular benefits to be derived from each individual assignment.

Assigning and Reviewing Homework

The cognitive therapist designs each assignment for the particular patient. The assignment should be directly related to the content of the therapy session, so that the patient understands its purpose and importance. Each task should be clearly articulated and very specific in nature. Near the end of each session, the assignment is written in duplicate, with one copy going to the therapist and the other to the patient.

Some typical homework assignments include reading a book or article about a specific problem, practicing distraction or relaxation techniques, counting automatic thoughts on a wrist counter, rating activities for pleasure and mastery on the Weekly Activity Schedule, maintaining a Daily Record of Dysfunctional Thoughts, and listening to a tape of the therapy session.

During the therapy session, the therapist asks for the patient's reactions to homework assignments. For example, the therapist might ask whether the assignment is clear and manageable. To determine potential impediments, the therapist may ask the patient to imagine taking the steps involved in the assignment. This technique can be especially helpful during the earlier stages of therapy. The patient assumes greater responsibility for developing homework assignments as therapy progresses through the middle and later stages.

It is essential that patient and therapist review the previous week's homework during the therapy session itself. If they do not, the patient may conclude that the homework assignments are not important. During the first part of the therapy sessions, therapist and patient discuss the previous week's assignment, and the therapist summarizes the results.

Difficulties in Completing Homework

When a patient does not complete homework assignments, or does them without conviction, the cognitive therapist elicits automatic thoughts, schemas, or behavioral problems that may help them both understand where the difficulty resides. The therapist does not presuppose that the patient is being "resistant" or "passive–aggressive." When the difficulties have been successfully identified, therapist and patient work collaboratively to surmount them. It is, of course, common for patients to have difficulties in completing homework, and here we consider some of the typical problems and ways to counteract them.

When patients do not understand the assignment completely, the therapist should explain it more fully, specifying his/her expectations in detail. Sometimes using the behavioral technique of cognitive rehearsal (described earlier) can be helpful in such situations.

Some patients believe that they are naturally disorganized and cannot maintain records and follow through on detailed assignments. Therapists can usually help to invalidate such general beliefs by asking patients about other circumstances in which they make lists—for example, when planning a vacation or shopping trip. Therapists can also ask these patients whether they could complete the assignment if there were a substantial reward entailed. This kind of question helps

such patients recognize that self-control is not the problem; rather, they do not believe that the reward is great enough. When patients realize that the problem is an attitudinal one, therapist and patient can proceed to enumerate the advantages of completing the assignment.

More severely depressed patients may need assistance to structure their time, so that homework becomes a regular activity. This can generally be accomplished by setting a specific time each day for the homework assignment. If necessary, patient and therapist can set up a reward system to increase motivation to complete the homework. For example, patients can reward themselves for doing the assignment by making a special purchase.

Some patients are afraid of failing the assignments or of doing them inadequately. In these cases, the therapist can explain that self-help assignments cannot be "failed": Doing an assignment partially is more helpful than not doing it at all, and mistakes provide valuable information about problems that still need work. In addition, because performance is not evaluated, patients cannot lose if they view the activity from a more adaptive perspective.

Sometimes patients believe their problems are too deeply embedded and complex to be resolved through homework assignments. The therapist can explain to these patients that even the most complex undertakings begin with and comprise small, concrete steps. A writer, for example, may resolve "writer's blocks" by taking the attitude, "If I can't write a book, I can at least write a paragraph." When enough paragraphs have been written, the result is a book. Therapist and patient can consider the advantages and disadvantages of the patient's belief that problems cannot be solved by doing homework. Or the therapist can ask the patient to experiment before reaching such a conclusion. In instances in which a patient believes that he/she has not made enough progress and that the homework is therefore not helpful, the therapist can detail the progress the patient has made or help the patient see that it may take more time before substantial change can be perceived.

When patients seem to resent being given assignments, the therapist can encourage them to develop their own assignments. He/she might also offer patients alternative assignments from which to choose, making one of the alternatives noncompliance with homework assignments. If patients choose noncompliance, the therapist can help to examine the consequences of that choice. Still another strategy is to present patients with a consumer model of therapy: Patients have a certain goal (overcoming depression), and the therapist offers a means to achieve that goal; patients are free to use or reject the tools, just as they are free to buy or not to buy in the marketplace.

Some patients believe that they can improve just as readily without homework. In this case, therapists have two options. First, they can offer their own clinical experience (which is supported by existing empirical evidence) that most patients who do not actively engage with and complete therapeutic homework progress more slowly in therapy. The other option is to set up an experiment for a given period of time, during which patients do not have to complete assignments. At the end of the predetermined period, therapists and patients can evaluate patients' progress during that time interval. Once again, it is important for cognitive therapists to keep an open mind: Some patients do indeed effect significant change without formally completing homework assignments.

Special Problems

The novice cognitive therapist often errs by staying with the standard method we have outlined here, even if it is not working very well. The cognitive therapist should be flexible enough to adapt to the needs of patients and to the several special problems that commonly arise in therapy. We have grouped these special problems into two categories: difficulties in the therapist–patient relationship, and problems in which the therapy itself seems not to be working.

Therapist–Patient Relationship Difficulties

The first set of problems concerns the therapist–patient relationship itself. When the therapist first perceives a patient to be dissatisfied, oppositional, angry, or hostile, it is imperative that he/she present these observations to the patient in an empathic manner. It is important that the therapist refrain from responding to the patient simply with an increased and rigid adherence to prescribed techniques or the therapeutic rationale. It also is important that the therapist refrain from self-critical statements. Research indicates that such responses have detrimental effects on the therapeutic relationship (Castonguay et al., 1996; Henry, Strupp, Butler, Schact, & Binder, 1993; Piper et al., 1999). Instead, preliminary research (Castonguay et al., 2004; Safran, Muran, Samstag, & Stevens, 2002) indicates that

the therapist's use of metacommunication skills (open discussion about the patient's negative reaction, exploration of the patient's experience, recognition and acknowledgment of the therapist's contribution to those negative reactions) is significantly more likely to repair and restore—and even improve—the therapeutic bond.

It is essential for therapists to be aware that many interventions can be misinterpreted in a negative way by depressed patients. Therapists approach problems of misinterpretation in the same way that they approach other thoughts: They work with patients to gather data and search for alternative accounts of the evidence. Difficulties in the therapist–patient relationship can generally be resolved through dialogue. There are times when a therapist may need to tailor behavior to the particular needs of an individual patient. For instance, a therapist may become freer with appropriate self-disclosure and personal reactions to meet the needs of a patient who persists in seeing the therapist as impersonal. Similarly, the therapist can make a point of checking formulations of the patient's thoughts more frequently to meet the needs of a patient who continues to believe that the therapist does not understand him/her.

It is imperative in situations like these for the therapist not to assume that the patient is being stubbornly resistant or irrational. Therapeutic reactance ("a motivational state characterized by the tendency to restore or re-assert one's ability to engage in freedoms perceived as lost or threatened" [Arnow et al., 2003, p. 1026]) was found to be a positive predictor of treatment outcome in directive therapy with chronically depressed patients. Arnow and colleagues found that treatment was enhanced when therapists responded in a flexible manner to such patient behaviors. Cognitive therapists collaborate with patients to achieve a better understanding of patients' responses. The reactions themselves often provide data regarding the kinds of distortions patients make in their other social and personal relationships. Therefore, patients' responses give therapists the opportunity to work with them on their maladaptive interpretations in relationships.

Unsatisfactory Progress

A second set of problems occurs when the therapy appears not to be working, even when the patient conscientiously completes homework assignments and the collaborative relationship seems successful. Sometimes problems stem from inappropriate expectations on the part of the patient—or unrealistic expectations on the part of the therapist—regarding the rapidity and consistency of change. When therapy seems not to be progressing as quickly as it "should," both patient and therapist must remember that ups and downs are to be anticipated in the course of treatment. It is important for therapists to keep in mind that some patients simply progress more slowly than others. The therapist or patient, or both, may be minimizing small changes that have indeed been taking place. In this case the therapist can emphasize the small gains that have been made and remind the patient that large goals are attained through small steps toward them.

At times, hopelessness can lead patients to invalidate their gains. Therapists should seek to uncover the maladaptive automatic thoughts, cognitive distortions, and early schemas that contribute to the pervasive hopelessness. In these cases, therapists must work to correct mistaken notions about the process of change and the nature of depression before further progress in therapy can occur.

In some cases in which therapy seems not to be working successfully, it may be that some of the therapeutic techniques have not been correctly used. Problems often arise when patients do not really believe the rational responses or are not able to remember them in times of emotional distress. It is important for a therapist to determine the amount of a patient's belief in the rational responses and help him/her use the new responses as closely as possible to the moment when the automatic thoughts occur. To the patient who does not fully believe a rational response, the therapist can suggest an experimental stance—taking the new belief and "trying it on for size." The patient who cannot think of answers because of emotional upset should be told that states of emotional distress make reasoning more difficult, and that thoughts such as "If this doesn't work, nothing will" can only aggravate the problem. Patients should be assured that they will be able to think of rational responses more readily with practice.

Another problem that derives from the misapplication of cognitive therapy techniques occurs when the therapist uses a particular technique inflexibly. It is often necessary for the therapist to try out several behavioral or cognitive techniques before finding an approach to which a patient responds well. The cognitive therapist must stay with a particular technique for a while to see whether it works, but he/she must also be willing to try an alternative technique when

it becomes apparent that the patient is not improving. To give a specific example, behavioral homework assignments are sometimes more helpful with particular patients, even though the therapist has every reason to predict in advance that cognitive assignments will be more effective.

In some instances in which it appears that little progress is being made in therapy, it turns out that the therapist has selected a tangential problem. The cognitive therapist should be alert to this possibility, especially during the early stages of therapy. When there appears to be little or no significant change in depression level, even when the patient seems to have made considerable progress in a problem area, the therapist should consider the possibility that the most distressing problem has not yet been uncovered. A typical example of this kind of difficulty is the patient who presents difficulty at work as the major problem, when it turns out that relationship problems are contributing significantly to the work difficulties. The real issue may be avoided by the patient because it seems too threatening.

Finally, cognitive therapy is not for everyone. If the therapist has tried all available approaches to the problem and has consulted with other cognitive therapists, it may be best to refer the patient to another therapist with either the same or a different orientation.

Regardless of why therapy is not progressing satisfactorily, cognitive therapists should attend to their own affect and cognitions. They must maintain a disciplined, problem-solving stance. If the cognitive therapist finds him/herself unduly influenced by a patient's despair or begins to notice that his/her own schemas are triggered by therapeutic interactions, then he/she should seek supervision. Hopelessness in patients or therapists is an obstacle to problem solving. If therapists can effectively counteract their own negative self-assessments and other dysfunctional thoughts, then they will be better able to concentrate on helping patients find solutions to their problems.

Case Study of Denise: Nonchronic Depression

In the case study that follows, we describe the course of treatment for a nonchronically depressed woman seen at our Center. Through the case study, we illustrate many of the concepts described earlier in this chapter, including elicitation of automatic thoughts, the cognitive triad of depression, collaborative empiricism, structuring a session, and feedback.

Assessment and Presenting Problems

At the initial evaluation, Denise, a 59-year-old widow, reported that she had been living alone for the last year. Denise's husband had been diagnosed with brain cancer three years earlier and had died approximately 1 year ago. She had two grown, unmarried children (27 and 25 years old) who were pursuing careers in other parts of the country. Denise had an undergraduate degree and had worked until age 30 but stopped after marrying. Denise described her major problems as depression (over the last year and a half), difficulty coping with daily life, and loneliness. She reported one prior episode of major depression around age 25, following the death of her father.

Denise said she had become increasingly socially isolated with the onset of her husband's illness (brain cancer). She reported having had normal friendships as a child, teenager, and young adult. She and her husband had led a relatively quiet life together, with a focus on raising their children and their respective work. When they had free time, they had enjoyed intellectual and cultural activities together (museums, lectures, concerts, and fine restaurants). The few close friends with whom they socialized had retired to Florida and Arizona during the time of the husband's illness.

Denise was diagnosed with a major depressive disorder, recurrent. Her test scores verified the diagnosis of depression. Denise's BDI-II score was 28, placing her in the moderate to severe range of depression. Her most prominent depressive symptoms included loss of pleasure, irritability, social withdrawal, inability to make decisions, fatigue, guilt, difficulty motivating herself to perform daily functions, and loneliness.

Session I

The session began with Denise describing the "sad feelings" she was having. The therapist almost immediately started to elicit Denise's automatic thoughts during these periods.

THERAPIST: What kind of thoughts went through your mind when you had these sad feelings this past week?

DENISE: Well, I guess I'm thinking what's the point of all this. My life is over. It's just not the same. I have thoughts like "What am I going to do?" Sometimes I feel mad at him, you know, my husband. How could he leave me? . . . Isn't that terrible of me? What's wrong with me? How can I be mad at him? He didn't want to die a horrible death. I should have done more. I should have made him go to the doctor when he first started getting headaches. . . . Oh, what's the use?

THERAPIST: It sounds like you are feeling quite bad right now. Is that right?

DENISE: Yes.

THERAPIST: Keep telling me what's going through your mind right now?

DENISE: I can't change anything. It's over. I don't know. . . . It all seems so bleak and hopeless. What do I have to look forward to . . . sickness and then death?

THERAPIST: So one of the thoughts is that you can't change things, and that it's not going to get any better?

DENISE: Yes.

THERAPIST: And sometimes you believe that completely?

DENISE: Yeah, I believe it, sometimes.

THERAPIST: Right now do you believe it?

DENISE: I believe it—yes.

THERAPIST: Right now you believe that you can't change things and it's not going to get better?

DENISE: Well, there is a glimmer of hope, but it's mostly . . .

THERAPIST: Is there anything that you kind of look forward to in terms of your own life from here on?

DENISE: Well, what I look forward to . . . I enjoy seeing my kids, but they are so busy right now. My son is a lawyer and my daughter is in medical school. So, they are very busy. They don't have time to spend with me.

By inquiring about Denise's automatic thoughts, the therapist began to understand her perspective—that she would go on forever, mostly alone. This illustrates the hopelessness about the future that is characteristic of most depressed patients. A second advantage to this line of inquiry is that the therapist introduced Denise to the idea of looking at her own thoughts, which is central to cognitive therapy.

As the session continued, the therapist probed Denise's perspective regarding her daily life. The therapist chose to focus on her inactivity and withdrawal. This is frequently the first therapeutic goal in working with a severely depressed patient.

In the sequence that follows, the therapist guided Denise to examine the advantages and disadvantages of staying in her house all day.

DENISE: Usually I don't want to leave my house. I want to stay there and just keep the shades closed; you know, I don't want to do anything. I just want to keep everything out, keep everything away from me.

THERAPIST: Now, do you feel better when you stay in the house all day trying to shut everything out?

DENISE: Sort of . . .

THERAPIST: What do you mean?

DENISE: Well, I can watch TV all day and just lose myself in these silly shows. I feel better when I see other people and their problems on these shows. It makes me feel less lonely and like my problems aren't so bad.

THERAPIST: And so how much time do you spend doing that?

DENISE: Now, lately? . . . Most of the time. Staying inside and watching TV feels safe, sort of secure, everything . . . like my loneliness, feels more distant.

THERAPIST: Now, after you have spent some time like this, how do you feel about yourself?

DENISE: Afterwards? I usually try not to pay much attention to how I'm feeling.

THERAPIST: But when you do, how do you feel?

DENISE: I feel bad. I feel bad for wasting the day. I don't get to things that I need to take care of . . . like my bills, like cleaning, like taking a shower. I usually end up feeling kind of pathetic . . . and guilty.

THERAPIST: On the one hand you seem to feel soothed and on the other hand, afterwards, you're a bit critical of yourself?

Note that the therapist did not try to debate or exhort Denise to get out of the house or become involved with necessary daily tasks. Rather, through questioning, the therapist encouraged her to examine more closely her assumption that she was really better off watching TV all day in her house. This is the process we call "collaborative empiricism." By the second session, Denise had reexamined her hypothesis about watching TV and remaining in the house all day.

DENISE: About watching TV in the house versus getting out, I thought about that the other day. I remember telling you that it made me feel better to stay there. When I paid attention to what I really felt, it didn't make me feel better. It just kind of blocked out feeling bad, but I didn't feel better.

THERAPIST: It is funny then that when you talked about it, your recollection of the experience was more positive than it actually was, but that sometimes happens with people. It happens to me, too. I think that something is good that's not so hot when I actually check it out.

We now return to the first session. After some probing by the therapist, Denise mentions that it sometimes feels like cognitive therapy "is my last hope." The therapist uses this as an opportunity to explore her hopelessness and suicidal thinking.

THERAPIST: What was going through your mind when you said, "This is my last hope"? Did you have some kind of vision in your mind?

DENISE: Yeah, that if this doesn't work, I feel like I couldn't take living like this the rest of my life.

THERAPIST: If it doesn't work out, then what?

DENISE: Well, I don't really care what happens to me . . .

THERAPIST: Did you have something more concrete in mind?

DENISE: Well, right this minute I don't think I could commit suicide, but if I keep feeling this way for a long time, maybe I could. I don't know, though— I've thought about suicide before, but I have never really thought about how I would do it. I know certain things stop me, like my kids. I think it would really hurt them and some other people, too, like my mother. My mom is in good health now, but she may need me someday. . . . Yeah, those are the two things that stop me, my children, and my mother.

THERAPIST: Now those are the reasons for not committing suicide. Now what are some of the reasons why you might want to, do you think?

DENISE: Because sometimes it just feels so empty and hopeless. There's nothing to look forward to—every day is the same. My life is such a waste, so why not just end it?

The therapist wanted Denise to feel as free as possible to discuss suicidal thoughts; thus, he tried hard to understand both the reasons for her hopelessness and the deterrents to suicide. After determining that she had no imminent plans to make an attempt, the therapist said that he would work with her to make some changes. He then asked her to select a small problem that they could work on together.

THERAPIST: Now are there any small things that you could do that would affect your life right away?

DENISE: I don't know. Well, I guess just calling my friend Diane in Florida. She called about a month ago and then again last week. Both times I told her I was busy and would call her back, but I haven't. I've felt so down. I have nothing to say to her.

THERAPIST: Well, when she lived in the area, what kinds of things did you talk about?

DENISE: We have kids about the same age, so we would talk about our kids. We both like to read and we used to go to a book club together—so we would talk about the books we were reading. Both of us liked art. We used to attend lectures at the museum during the week, so we would talk about art and the lectures. We would spend time making plans to do things together in our free time. It always was very interesting when I spent time and with her. We had so much in common. I do miss her.

THERAPIST: It sounds like you used to be involved in a number of interesting activities. What about now?

DENISE: After my husband got sick and then my friends moved, I just stopped. I haven't done any of those things in quite a while.

THERAPIST: What do you think about attending a lecture series now?

DENISE: I don't know.

THERAPIST: Well, what do you think about that idea?

DENISE: It's an OK idea, but it just seems like too much. I don't think I'll enjoy it . . . the way I feel . . . I don't know.

THERAPIST: Would you be willing to test out that thought that you won't be able to enjoy it now?

DENISE: I don't know . . . I guess so.

THERAPIST: Is that a "yes"?

DENISE: Yes, but I don't see how I'm going to get myself to do it.

THERAPIST: Well, how would you go about finding out about a lecture series?

DENISE: You look online at the museum's website to see what's available.

THERAPIST: OK. Do you have a computer?

DENISE: Yes.

THERAPIST: Is it working?

DENISE: Yes.

THERAPIST: How do you feel about doing that?

DENISE: I guess I could do that. . . . I'm so pathetic, I know what to do. I don't need you to spell it out for me. Why didn't I just do this before?

THERAPIST: Well, you probably had good reasons for not doing it before. Probably you were just so caught up in the hopelessness.

DENISE: I guess so.

THERAPIST: When you are hopeless you tend to deny, as it were, or cut off possible options or solutions.

DENISE: Right.

THERAPIST: When you get caught up in hopelessness then, there is nothing you can do. Is that what you think?

DENISE: Yeah.

THERAPIST: So, then, rather than be down on yourself because you haven't looked this up online before, why don't we carry you right through?

This excerpt illustrates the process of graded tasks that is so important in the early stages of therapy with a depressed patient. The therapist asked the patient a series of questions to break down the process of attending a lecture series into smaller steps. Denise realized that she had known all along what to do, but, as the therapist pointed out, her hopelessness prevented her from seeing the options.

DENISE: Taking this step is going to be hard for me.

THERAPIST: First steps are harder for everybody, but that's why there is an old expression: "A journey of a thousand miles starts with the first step."

DENISE: That's very true.

THERAPIST: It's the first step that is so very important, and then you can ready yourself for the second step, and then the third step, and so on. Eventually, you build up some momentum, and each step begins to follow more naturally. But first, all you have to do is take one small step. You don't have to take giant steps.

DENISE: Well, yeah, I can see that. I guess I was thinking every step was just as hard as the first. Maybe it will get easier.

In the second session, Denise reported success.

DENISE: I checked online about the lecture series and I surprised myself. One actually sounded interesting, and I'm thinking that I might just register for it online. I really didn't think any of those feelings were still there. I'm kind of looking forward to that next step.

At the end of the first session, the therapist helped Denise fill out the Weekly Activity Schedule for the coming week. The activities were quite simple, such as getting up and taking a shower, fixing meals, going out shopping, and checking out the lecture series online. Finally, the therapist asked Denise for feedback about the session and about her hopelessness.

THERAPIST: Do you have any reactions?

DENISE: I'm still feeling down, but I'm also feeling a little better. It's interesting that just the idea of looking at what lectures might be available is making me feel a little lighter. I even had the thought of calling Diane to talk over the options. . . . Is this a sign of better things to come?

THERAPIST: What do you think?

DENISE: Maybe.

Session 2

In the second session, the therapist began by collaborating with Denise to set an agenda. Denise wanted to discuss the fact that she had not been attending to her bills or to her housework and was still spending a good part of the day alone in front of the TV; the therapist utilized this as an opportunity to discuss the issue of activity versus inactivity on the agenda. They then reviewed the previous homework. Denise had carried out all the scheduled activities and had also listed some of her negative thoughts in between sessions. Her BDI-II score had dropped somewhat. (Patients routinely fill out the BDI-II before each session, so that both patient and therapist can monitor the progress of treatment.)

Denise then shared her list of negative thoughts with the therapist. One concern was that she had expressed angry feelings about her husband during the first session.

DENISE: I don't like revealing things about myself, but you told me to write down my thoughts. So here it is. When I went to bed the night after of our first session, I thought about what I said to you, you know, about being angry at my husband. I was thinking that you probably think I am this really harsh and cold person. I mean, here my husband died this horrible death and I have this hard, insensitive reaction. I started thinking that now you probably feel really negatively toward me because of that statement and that you don't want to work with me.

THERAPIST: I'm really glad you're telling me these thoughts. Let me start by asking you who is having these negative thoughts?

DENISE: You? Well, no. Actually, it's me.

THERAPIST: Right. Do you think that someone like me might have another reaction to what you said?

DENISE: I don't know. I mean it is pretty harsh being angry at someone who had no control over what was happening.

The therapist then offered Denise an alternative perspective:

THERAPIST: Do you think that someone might react to your statements with empathy?

DENISE: How could they?

THERAPIST: I imagine it would be very upsetting and annoying to have lost both your husband and your friends—all around the same time. Even though you love and care about all of them, feeling angry is understandable. It sounds like a basic human reaction to some very difficult life events.

DENISE: Yeah, I guess that does make sense. Thanks.

This illustrates how a cognitive therapist can utilize events during the session to teach a patient to identify automatic thoughts and to consider alternative interpretations. In addition, the therapist provided a summary of a key theme he had identified from listening to Denise's automatic thoughts about her husband and about therapy. The theme was her fear of being harshly judged and potentially punished for her statement (punitiveness schema). Cognitive therapists often identify and begin to correct EMSs during the first phase of treatment. More intensive work on changing schemas in a later phase of treatment may be required to inoculate against relapse. We elaborate on this process in the next section of this chapter.

In the segment that follows, the therapist explained how he arrived at the conclusion that punitiveness was an important schema for Denise.

THERAPIST: When you said that you thought I would have a negative opinion about you and not want to work with you because you said you felt angry at your husband, it sounded as though you were really concerned that you would be harshly judged and punished for your statements.

DENISE: Yes, that's right.

THERAPIST: I don't want to make too much out of this at the moment, but you also said that after your friends had moved, you felt angry at them and judgmental of their decision. Even though you knew that each set of friends had to move for specific financial or health reasons and had been in the process of completing their moves over several years, part of you still felt very angry with them. You mentioned that you strongly believe that friends should be there for each other, especially in times of great need, and if a friend lets another friend down, that relationship should end. Is that right?

DENISE: Right.

THERAPIST: So here, you largely have withdrawn from these important relationships and now you're feeling quite lonely. The thought of talking to these friends again brings fears that they will now be angry and punitive with you for your reaction to them. You're caught in a no-win situation. Is that right?

DENISE: Yes, that sounds right.

THERAPIST: So one of the things that can really grab hold of you—and make you feel terrible—is this notion that people, including yourself, should behave in specific ways, and if they or you don't behave the "right" way, then harsh punishment should result. Is that correct?

DENISE: Yes, that sounds right. But hearing you say it makes me realize that it doesn't really sound right.

THERAPIST: What do you mean?

DENISE: It's too extreme. It's too harsh. People are

human and they have limitations, and they make mistakes sometimes.

THERAPIST: It's good that you are starting to notice and evaluate these thoughts rather than just responding to them automatically. What this tells us is that you have to be alert for whenever you have the sense that either you or others should be strongly punished for not behaving in a specified way. The idea that people should not be cut a break, even under very difficult circumstances, may not work very well in real life with real people. You mentioned that both friends told you they felt terrible about leaving you at this time, and both have called you regularly since leaving the area. Do you think that if you begin to respond to and return their calls, they might react differently—in the same way that I reacted differently from what you expected?

DENISE: Yes, that is very likely.

About halfway through the session, the therapist asked the patient for feedback thus far.

THERAPIST: Now, at this point, is there anything that we have discussed today that bothered you?

DENISE: That bothered me?

THERAPIST: Yeah.

DENISE: I feel like I'm a bit of a freak.

THERAPIST: That is important. Can you . . .

DENISE: Well, I'm trying not to feel that way, but I do.

THERAPIST: Well, if you are, you are. Why don't you just let yourself feel like a freak and tell me about it?

DENISE: Well, I'm feeling like I'm just so different from everyone else. Other people don't seem to have my problems. They're still happily married and carrying on with life. I just feel so different from everyone.

This comment led to identification of a third theme, the social isolation/alienation schema. Denise had been viewing herself as increasingly different for the past couple of years. By this point, however, she was beginning to catch on to the idea of answering her thoughts more rationally. After the therapist pointed out the negative thought in the preceding excerpt, the patient volunteered:

DENISE: I know what to do with the thought "I'm a freak."

THERAPIST: What are you going to do with it right this minute?

DENISE: I am going to say to myself, "I'm not so different from other people. Other people have lost their mates. I'm not the only one. I'm just the first one in my group of friends. Eventually, they will all have the same situation as me. It's just a part of life." Seeing you for help doesn't mean I'm a freak. You probably see lots of people and help them with problems like mine.

THERAPIST: Right.

The same automatic thoughts arose later in the session, when Denise noticed the therapist's wedding ring. In the extended excerpt below, the therapist helped her set up an experiment to test the thought "I'm so different from him."

THERAPIST: OK, now let's just do an experiment and see if you yourself can respond to the automatic thought, and let's see what happens to your feeling. See if responding rationally makes you feel worse or better.

DENISE: OK.

THERAPIST: OK. "I'm so different from him." What is the rational answer to that? A realistic answer?

DENISE: You are wearing a wedding ring and that is different from me because I'm alone, without a mate.

THERAPIST: Yes. And?

DENISE: And? . . . I don't really know much about you, other than you're married. I guess from what I do know, that information could also be viewed as a similarity. We both have gotten married and know what it's like to be married. I assume that you've never lost a mate, but maybe that is not true. You may have lost a mate as well.

THERAPIST: So, is it that you're different or that I'm different? Or is it that we just have different situations with respect to our mates at this point in time?

DENISE: We just have different situations right now.

The preceding exchange demonstrates the use of re-attribution. At first, Denise interpreted the therapist's ring as evidence that they were very different. As a result of the guided discovery approach, she reattributed the difference to one of two factors: that either she or the therapist was different or that the situation with re-

spect to mates was different for each. At the end of the experiment, Denise expressed satisfaction that she was finally recognizing this tendency to distort her appraisals.

DENISE: Right now I feel glad. I'm feeling a little better that at least somebody is pointing these things out to me. I never realized I was so judgmental of myself and other people, and that I'm assuming I'm so different from everyone.

THERAPIST: So you feel good that you have made this observation about yourself?

DENISE: Yes.

After summarizing the main points of the second session, the therapist assigned homework for the coming week: to fill out the Daily Record of Dysfunctional Thoughts (see Figure 7.4) and the Weekly Activity Schedule (with mastery and pleasure ratings; see Figure 7.3).

Session 3

By the beginning of the third session, Denise's mood had visibly improved. She had registered for a lecture series at the museum and was looking forward to attending the first lecture. She also had called her friend Diane, with very positive results. She was catching negative and punitive thoughts toward others and herself and challenging these thoughts. The primary agenda item Denise chose to work on was "how I back away from other people," an aspect of her unrelenting standards, punitiveness, and social isolation/alienation schemas.

DENISE: I want to stop withdrawing from people. I want to be more accepting and engaged with others.

THERAPIST: What holds you back?

DENISE: I guess I believe that I have to be a bit removed and strict in relation to others or they'll just behave in whatever way they want. People have to know my rules and abide by them if they want to have a relationship with me.

The therapist continued probing to understand why Denise believed she had to have others adhere to such a strict set of rules to have a relationship. As the discussion progressed, it became obvious that, in the abstract, she could see that such hard-and-fast rules were not necessarily conducive to having a good relationship—in fact, such rules sometimes put others off. But in real-life situations, Denise never felt she was wrong.

The therapist's next task was to help Denise bring her rational thinking to bear on her distorted thinking *in the context of a concrete event*. At the therapist's request, Denise then described a conversation with her friend Diane, and how her intolerance for Diane's deviation from her rules created distance. Denise had wanted Diane and her husband to come for a visit the following summer. Diane, however, told her that their dog had been quite sick, and that if the dog was still alive she could not leave it. Denise thought this was ridiculous. She believed a relationship with a pet should never take precedence over a human relationship. This occurred when Denise actually had wanted and hoped to get closer to Diane again. The therapist helped her use logic to evaluate her maladaptive schema.

THERAPIST: You had the thought "I'm right to set the record straight with her. She can't put me in second place to her dog. She can't do that without consequence." It seems likely that you believed that thought, and that you believed the thought was right. And since you believed that thought was right, you then felt you had to withdraw your affection from her if she didn't abide by your wishes.

DENISE: Right.

THERAPIST: Now, let's look at it. Do you think that thought is correct?

DENISE: Well, yes, it's insulting.

THERAPIST: What's insulting?

DENISE: She's putting her dog in a higher priority position.

THERAPIST: Have you ever had a pet?

DENISE: No.

THERAPIST: Do you think that maybe Diane feels like her dog is a part of her family?

DENISE: I never thought of it that way.

THERAPIST: If you look at the situation from that perspective, how do you feel?

DENISE: I feel like I'm being a little insensitive. . . . That's not right. I'm not allowing for any other perspective. I've never had a pet, so I don't really know what it's like to have a pet. It's not right for me to be

so judgmental of Diane. I need to be more understanding. I wasn't very caring. I am actually behaving in a way that goes directly against my deepest values.

THERAPIST: So, according to your own values, was this right?

DENISE: No, it's not right. I wasn't respecting *her* feelings. I was just demanding that she respect mine. That wasn't right.

THERAPIST: OK, now this is one of the problems. If you want to get over this sense that you should never give in or bend your rules for others, one of the things you can do is look for this thought, "I'm right and you should have a negative consequence for your 'wrong' decision"—and refer back to this conversation we are having now and decide for yourself whether, indeed, you were right. Now, if every time you approach a conflict in a relationship and allow for the possibility that you might not fully understand, but really think underneath, "But I know I'm right," you are going to feel put out, and then you are not going to want to engage with that person. Is that right?

DENISE: Yeah, that sounds right.

THERAPIST: So we have to decide here and now. Do you indeed think that you are right to suspend your initial negative judgment to leave open the possibility of re-evaluating your reaction to her behavior?

DENISE: Yes.

THERAPIST: Now, the next time you get the thought, "I'm right and I'm going to make sure this other person knows it," how are you going to answer that thought?

DENISE: If I'm right? But I'm not necessarily right. I need to consider the other person's perspective. I need to try to understand them and then see if what I'm thinking fits.

THERAPIST: Now are you saying that because that is the correct answer, or because you really believe it?

DENISE: No, I really believe it.

The therapist followed this discussion with a technique called "point–counterpoint" to help Denise practice rational responses to her automatic thoughts even more intensively. In this excerpt, the therapist expressed Denise's own negative thinking as Denise tried to defend herself more rationally.

THERAPIST: Now I am going to be like the prosecuting attorney, and I'll say, "Now I understand you let your friend violate one of your rules of friendship. Is that true?"

DENISE: Yes.

THERAPIST: "Now it seems to me that that was a very bad thing for you to do."

DENISE: No, it wasn't.

THERAPIST: "You don't think it was?"

DENISE: No, I should try to understand her perspective.

THERAPIST: "Well, you can sit there and say you should be more understanding, but I thought you said before that you wanted people to respect you."

DENISE: I do, but I also need to respect others.

THERAPIST: "I know, but now you are saying that you are going to let her get away with this. What's next?"

DENISE: What's next can only be a better understanding of one another. We'll feel closer.

THERAPIST: "But how can you feel closer if she's not respecting your rules of friendship?"

DENISE: Maybe my rules are not appropriate in this situation. I need to learn to be more understanding, flexible, and tolerant of some deviations from my rules.

THERAPIST: "But then you'll lose control of the situation."

DENISE: No, that's an exaggeration. I don't need to control the whole situation. I can still decide what makes sense. I am still in control of what's important.

THERAPIST: "How can that be?"

DENISE: Because I can respect myself and respect my friend as well. I don't have to turn everything into an either–or situation to try to make her see and do it my way. That just makes it difficult for her to get along with me, and I'll lose out on the relationship in the long run if I keep on insisting that she either do it my way or we do nothing.

Finally, the therapist returned to the schema and asked the patient how much she believed the new perspective.

THERAPIST: If you're flexible, you'll lose control. Now do you believe that?

DENISE: No.

THERAPIST: Do you believe it partially?

DENISE: No. In fact, I'm more likely to lose control of any possibility of getting what I want if I'm so inflexible. It's like I lose sight of the importance of the relationship when I get so stuck on thinking that I have to be in control and that the other person has to do it my way.

THERAPIST: OK, so right now, how much do you believe that?

DENISE: Completely.

THERAPIST: 100%?

DENISE: Yes.

THERAPIST: You are sure 100%, not 90 or 80%?

DENISE: No, 100%.

For the remainder of Session 3, Denise and the therapist reviewed other instances in which she noticed that her standards were not flexible and felt the urge to be punitive when her rules were not met. The session ended with a summary of the main issues raised in the first three sessions.

Summary of Initial Sessions

In the first three sessions, the therapist laid the groundwork for the remainder of treatment. He began immediately by teaching Denise to identify her negative automatic thoughts. By doing this, the therapist began to understand her feelings of hopelessness and to explore her isolation. By identifying her thoughts in a variety of specific situations, he was able to deduce several key schemas that later proved central to Denise's thinking: (1) unrelenting standards, (2) punitiveness, and (3) social isolation/alienation. All appeared to be contributing to Denise's social isolation and depression. The therapist made especially skillful use of Denise's thoughts during the second therapy session to help her see that she was distorting evidence about the therapeutic interaction and coming to the inaccurate conclusion that the therapist would be judgmental and punitive with her, and withdraw positive feelings for her, in the same way that Denise tends to respond to others.

Beyond identifying thoughts and distortions, the therapist guided Denise to take concrete steps to overcome her inactivity and withdrawal. He asked her to weigh the advantages and disadvantages of staying in the house all day watching TV; he broke down the task of attending a lecture series at the museum into small, manageable steps; and he worked with her to develop an activity schedule to follow during the week.

Finally, the therapist employed a variety of strategies to demonstrate to Denise that she could test the validity of her thoughts, develop rational responses, and feel better. For example, during the course of the three sessions the therapist set up an experiment, used reattribution, offered alternative perspectives, and practiced the point–counterpoint technique.

One final point we want to emphasize is that the primary therapeutic mode was questioning. Most of the therapist's comments were in the form of questions. This helped Denise to evaluate her own thoughts outside of the session and prevented her from feeling attacked by the therapist.

By the end of these initial sessions, Denise reported being more optimistic that her life could change.

Later Sessions

Denise continued to fill out the Daily Record of Dysfunctional Thoughts and gathered evidence that she could relax her standards and be more tolerant of others' viewpoints and foibles. She discovered that she felt happier, both with herself and others, as a result.

The therapist set up several experiments with Denise to test a series of beliefs: that her friends would become punitive with her when she did not behave perfectly, and that her relationships would become unpleasant and undesirable if she relaxed any of her rigid standards regarding how others should behave in relationships.

Through graded tasks, Denise counteracted her tendency to withdraw by gradually approaching new and sometimes unfamiliar situations. When she noticed herself imposing her standards of behavior on others, or noticed in herself the urge to become punitive, Denise practiced more open and accepting behaviors (by asking open-ended questions that reflected back her understanding of others' responses, and by inhibiting harsh and judgmental statements). She practiced tolerating the discomfort associated with these new behaviors until they began to feel more comfortable and natural.

When Denise terminated therapy, her BDI-II score was in the normal range. The symptom reduction phase of treatment was successfully completed in 20 sessions.

The next section describes and includes a case example of ST for chronic depression.

ST FOR CHRONIC DEPRESSION

ST, developed by Young (1990/1999; Young et al., 2003), can be used with patients who present with recurrent depressive episodes; dysthymic disorder; early age onset of depression; early life trauma or adverse family relations (e.g., the loss of a parent in childhood; sexual, physical or verbal abuse, neglect, and overprotection); comorbid personality disorders; or a large number of EMSs (identified with the YSQ [Young, 2005]). Young and Klosko (1994) have published a self-help book to help patients better understand their schemas.

Beck and colleagues (1990, p. 10) have noted that

> schemas are difficult to alter. They are held firmly in place by behavioral, cognitive, and affective elements. The therapeutic approach must take a tripartite approach. To take a strictly cognitive approach and try to argue patients out of their distortions will not work. Having the patients abreact within the session to fantasies or recollections will not be successful by itself. A therapeutic program that addresses all three areas is essential. A patient's cognitive distortions serve as signposts that point to the schema.

As a result, ST represents a significant expansion of traditional CBT. It places more emphasis on early developmental patterns and origins, long-term interpersonal difficulties, the patient–therapist relationship, and emotion-focused or experiential exercises.

Case Study of Barbara: Chronic Depression

The second case study demonstrates the use of ST with a chronically depressed patient.

History and Presenting Problems

The patient "Barbara" was an extremely attractive, 46-year-old woman who had been married for the past 20 years to George, a functional alcoholic working on Wall Street in investment banking. It was the first marriage for both, but it had been extremely rocky throughout. Barbara had wanted children in the marriage but had been unable to conceive naturally. Although fertility treatments and adoption had been discussed, Barbara reported that George resisted following through on these options because he questioned her ability to be an adequate parent.

At the beginning of George and Barbara's relationship, Barbara reported extremely strong sexual chemistry. However, she stated that the chemistry had been erratic and often disappeared for long periods over the course of their relationship. She said that she had only felt real happiness with George in the first few months of the relationship, when he was extremely generous and attentive. Her decision to marry George was based on a feeling that they were meant for each other. They initially met at a high-end bar, where Barbara had worked as a cocktail waitress. Once their relationship was established, however, George continued to spend most of his free time in cocktail lounges without her, as she did not like to drink.

At the time she came in for her first interview, Barbara was spending most of her time in bed or watching TV. She rarely left the house except to go shopping. Outings with her mom or friends "to lift her spirits" often culminated in shopping sprees, followed by extended verbal berating by George, drunk upon his return home from the bar, because of what he perceived as her lack of taste, judgment, and intelligence regarding purchases. Barbara entered treatment because her husband told her that she "was driving him crazy with all her ridiculous behavior" and that she should "go get fixed." Barbara acknowledged feeling very depressed. She stated that this latest episode of depression started after a particularly upsetting fight with her husband over adopting a child.

Barbara reported having mild to moderate depression most of her life, interspersed with multiple episodes of major depression. She first became aware of feeling moderately depressed around age 11. An only child, she initially described her childhood family as "fine." Barbara described her mother as extremely attentive and devoted, a "very good mother who did everything for me." Barbara stated that her mother lived for her, but she also remembered her mother occasionally falling into depressions. As early as age 6, she recalled that her mother was emotionally unavailable when depressed.

Barbara described her father as a workaholic who was almost never home. When he did come home, he was remote, preferring the solitude of his study over interacting with her and her mother. If Barbara tried to engage him as a child, he would upbraid her by calling her "an annoying simpleton" and demand that she leave him alone.

Barbara described her first major depressive episode, which occurred around age 16, after a breakup with her first serious boyfriend. Later episodes were triggered by other breakups and the fertility problems.

Barbara scored 29 on the BDI-II, placing her in the severe range of depression. She also completed the third edition of the YSQ (Long Form; Young, 2005), and received very high scores on the Emotional Deprivation, Defectiveness, Abandonment, Dependence/Incompetence, Entitlement, Failure, Subjugation, Approval Seeking, and Negativity/Pessimism schemas. Her Schema Mode Questionnaire (Young et al., 2008) indicated that she primarily functioned in the following modes: Detached Protector, Compliant Surrender, Punitive Parent, and Vulnerable Child.

At Barbara's initial consultation, the therapist conducted additional assessment work through imagery (a standard assessment procedure for ST). During this assessment, Barbara was instructed: "Close your eyes and let your mind float to your earliest memories of your mother." Barbara reported painful recollections of being 6 years old with her mother in bed, depressed and emotionally unavailable. She reported feeling very scared and lost at these times. The same imagery exercise was utilized in a subsequent session in which Barbara was asked to retrieve an early memory of her father. In this image, Barbara's father displayed intolerant, demeaning, and rejecting behavior toward her as a child. During the exercise, she reported feeling unacceptable, ashamed of herself, and unwanted by him.

On the Multimodal Life History Inventory (Lazarus & Lazarus, 1991), a 15-page assessment tool covering a wide range of issues dealing with feelings, thoughts, behaviors, and a variety of other psychotherapeutic issues, Barbara reported her main problems as depression, being unhappy with herself, feeling empty and unloved, and feeling unappreciated. She also listed the following behaviors as applicable: procrastination, withdrawal, concentration difficulties, sleep disturbance, crying, and occasional outbursts of temper. She further indicated that she often felt sad, depressed, unhappy, hopeless, useless, and lonely. She endorsed the following statements: "I don't know what to do with my life," "Life is empty, a waste," and "There is nothing to look forward to."

Based on the initial interview, Barbara was diagnosed with major depressive disorder, recurrent episode on Axis I, and dependent personality disorder on Axis II.

Schema Mode Work

This section demonstrates the use of schema mode work—an important component of the ST approach—with Barbara.

The therapist shifted to ST because Barbara's depression was not lifting with standard cognitive therapy. Although Barbara had learned how to challenge her automatic thoughts, identified and challenged her core beliefs with rational responses, and followed through on graded behavioral assignments to test her thoughts and beliefs, she never *emotionally* accepted the rational viewpoint, despite much concrete evidence. Barbara remained convinced that she was worthless, useless, and hopeless. Her EMSs continued to be stubbornly entrenched. The therapist decided that the next step would be to introduce emotion-focused exercises to access Barbara's schemas on a deeper emotional level, utilizing the schema mode approach.

There are seven general steps in schema mode work: (1) Increase awareness of modes by identifying and labeling modes with the patient; (2) explore the origins of modes in childhood and adolescence, and discuss their adaptive value; (3) link current problems and symptoms to the patient's maladaptive modes; (4) uncover the advantages and disadvantages of each mode; (5) use imagery to access the Vulnerable Child mode; (6) conduct dialogues between modes; and (7) generalize the results from mode work in session to the patient's life outside of sessions. The following sections illustrate each step of mode work in helping Barbara.

Step 1: Increase Awareness of Modes by Identifying and Labeling Modes with the Patient

This first step helps both therapist and patient conceptualize the problems in terms of different parts of the self or modes. From the Schema Mode Questionnaire, the therapist already was aware that Barbara primarily functioned in the Detached Protector, Compliant Surrenderer, Punitive Parent, and Vulnerable Child modes. The session reveals how the therapist queries the patient, so that she can begin to recognize and differentiate these parts within herself.

Throughout this section, the patient is encouraged to label modes with terms that feel right—rather than simply applying generic terms from the Schema Mode Questionnaire. Patients are encouraged to find terms that best capture the thoughts, emotions, and/or behaviors associated with each mode. A primary goal with this first step is to help the patient observe these parts, and decenter him/herself from them. This step begins the process of interrupting the automaticity of the modes.

THERAPIST: I'm noticing in our sessions that sometimes you seem very sad and upset and critical of yourself, and other times you seem a bit distracted from what you're feeling, like when you were telling me about the great pair of shoes that you found on your shopping trip.

BARBARA: Yeah, I guess that's true. Talking about my purchases makes me feel better.

THERAPIST: When you say "better," what do you mean?

BARBARA: I feel good.

THERAPIST: Like happy, peaceful, and content?

BARBARA: I feel pleasure.

THERAPIST: In what way is it pleasurable?

BARBARA: I feel pleasure when I look at pretty things with my mom or my friends, and I like buying those things. It takes my mind off of everything else.

THERAPIST: Like you're temporarily distracted from other feelings?

BARBARA: Yeah, that's right.

THERAPIST: What are those other feelings?

BARBARA: Just feeling real bad. I can't stand those feelings.

THERAPIST: So, sometimes there is this one part of you that just wants distance from this other part of you that feels bad?

BARBARA: Yes.

THERAPIST: Are there other things you do besides shopping that help you distance from bad feelings?

BARBARA: Well, yeah, I sleep a lot.

THERAPIST: Anything else?

BARBARA: I watch TV, but TV doesn't always work.

THERAPIST: This part of you that wants distance from feeling bad—what could we call that part of you?

BARBARA: That part of me? I don't know. I don't know what to call it.

THERAPIST: What does it feel like?

BARBARA: It feels like I'm escaping.

THERAPIST: OK. So should we call that part "the Escapist"?

BARBARA: I guess so. . . . That sounds right.

THERAPIST: And the part of you that you've escaped from—can you tell me more about that part of you?

BARBARA: That part feels bad . . . really bad and terrible.

THERAPIST: Let me hear that part speak about those feelings.

BARBARA: I'm just a bad person (*Starts to cry.*) . . . I'm a useless good for nothing. I feel so hopeless. I don't know what to do. I can't figure anything out. I'm such a zero, such a failure. . . . Do we really have to talk about this?

THERAPIST: Barbara, I know that it feels bad to be in touch with this part of yourself, but if you can hang in there for just a bit, it will help me to understand why you're feeling so bad. Do you know what this part of you wants?

BARBARA: I want to feel good.

THERAPIST: What do you think would help you feel better?

BARBARA: I don't know. I really don't know. I just want you to fix me. My husband is right. I am a ridiculous person.

THERAPIST: It sounds like there is one part of you that feels really awful. It sounds like this part is listening and taking in what your husband says about you—that "you're ridiculous." I want you to hold back on agreeing with your husband, and I want to hear more about this part of you that feels awful—the part of you who wants everything fixed. That part . . . do you feel it?

BARBARA: Yes, I feel it.

THERAPIST: Tell me more. What are the things you want to fix?

BARBARA: I don't know. I just want to feel good about myself, proud of myself, but I just don't. I want to have a child, but my husband doesn't think I can handle it. He's probably right. I need so much help with just everyday living. I don't know how to handle anything.

THERAPIST: So this part of you, this part that feels awful and helpless but also wants to feel better, what could we call this part?

BARBARA: I don't know. What do you think?

THERAPIST: Well, what does it feel like?

BARBARA: It feels helpless—ashamed and helpless.

THERAPIST: How old do you feel when you're in touch with this part of yourself?

BARBARA: I feel young, very young.

THERAPIST: Do you want to call that part "Ashamed Little Barbara" [Vulnerable Child mode with associated EMSs of Defectiveness, Dependence/Incompetence, and Enmeshment/Undeveloped Self]?

BARBARA: Sure.

THERAPIST: OK. And now this other part—the one that is agreeing with your husband and calling yourself ridiculous . . .

BARBARA: Well, I am ridiculous and silly. I can't cope with anything.

THERAPIST: Before you agree with that part, I want you to just notice how that part sounds. How does that part sound to you? Does it sound critical?

BARBARA: Yes, but I deserve it. I'm so useless.

THERAPIST: It sounds like you are having a hard time just listening to that part without automatically agreeing with it?

BARBARA: Yeah, I guess that's true.

THERAPIST: So, what do you want to call that part?

BARBARA: I don't know. . . . But . . . you're not going to tell me what to call it, are you?

THERAPIST: Right.

BARBARA: OK. I guess "the Critic" [Punitive Parent mode with associated EMSs of defectiveness and subjugation].

In this part of the session, the therapist has helped Barbara begin to recognize and label the modes: the Detached Protector as "the Escapist," the Punitive Parent as "the Critic," and the Vulnerable Child as "Ashamed Little Barbara." Although not fully illustrated here, the therapist also used a similar sequence of questions to help Barbara identify other modes. From this portion of the session, it is clear that "the Critic" (Punitive Parent mode) is generating a tremendous amount of negative affect in Barbara. Barbara's only apparent way to cope with the onslaught of punitive statements from this mode is "the Escapist" (Detached Protector mode), in which she sleeps away much of her life. Otherwise, Barbara's primary experience of herself rests with "Ashamed Little Barbara" (the Vulnerable Child mode), where she feels defective, useless, hopeless, and helpless.

Step 2: Explore Origins of Modes in Childhood and/or Adolescence

This section illustrates how the therapist helps Barbara recognize the origins of these modes. In addition, the therapist assesses the strength of her Healthy Parent mode.

THERAPIST: Does "the Critic" sound like anyone else you know or have known in your life?

BARBARA: Yes, it sounds like George.

THERAPIST: Anyone else?

BARBARA: Yeah, it also sounds like my Dad . . . just like my Dad.

THERAPIST: In what way?

BARBARA: My Dad used to talk like that to me . . . whenever I tried to get his attention.

THERAPIST: How old were you?

BARBARA: Young, very young . . . 3 or 4 . . . as far back as I remember.

THERAPIST: Can you close your eyes and try to let yourself feel like that young child again with your dad?

BARBARA: (*Closes her eyes.*)

THERAPIST: Tell me what's happening.

BARBARA: He's yelling at me because I pulled on his coat jacket.

THERAPIST: Let me hear what he's saying to you.

BARBARA: "Stop it, you little pest. You're such a simpleton. Can't you find anything better to do than pull on my coat? Get out of here!"

THERAPIST: And how are you feeling as he is yelling these things at you?

BARBARA: I feel stupid, like I'm a jerk. I'm nothing—a useless pest, an annoyance.

THERAPIST: Does it feel like he's right, or are you angry at him?

BARBARA: No. I don't feel angry. I just feel bad (*starts to cry*)—I'm just bad.

THERAPIST: So there is part of you agreeing with him, punishing yourself—like your dad—thinking you're bad.

BARBARA: Yeah.

THERAPIST: And where is your mom?

BARBARA: She's telling me to shush and leave him alone. She says he's tired from working so hard all day.

THERAPIST: And what are you thinking and feeling when she says this?

BARBARA: I'm thinking that I'm a terrible person.

THERAPIST: So, you're getting the message that you are the problem from both of your parents. It feels like both parents are saying you deserve this harsh treatment, and there is a part of you that believes them—you deserve to be punished because you've bothered your father. Is that right?

BARBARA: Yes, that's right.

THERAPIST: So there is also this punishing part of you, this part that accepts that message from your parents—this punitive message that you're bad and a problem, a pest.

BARBARA: Yes.

THERAPIST: What is your mom doing?

BARBARA: After a while, she takes me out. She sees I'm sad and wants me to feel better. She tries to make me feel better by giving me something, like a toy, or something to eat. A lot of times she takes me out shopping and buys me something special.

THERAPIST: And how do you feel when she does this?

BARBARA: I feel a little better while we are out . . . but later, I feel bad. I still feel shame because I'm so bad and useless.

THERAPIST: So there is still the "Ashamed Little Barbara" underneath?

BARBARA: Yes. That is it.

THERAPIST: If you could have rewritten the script for your family, a family with ideal parents, what would you have happen?

BARBARA: I have no idea. They weren't bad. They were doing their best.

THERAPIST: Yes, but what if you had had a daddy who was excited to see you at the end of his work day . . . a daddy who enjoyed coming home to his family . . . who found pleasure in talking with you and getting to know you, and played with you?

BARBARA: You mean . . . a daddy who loved me?

THERAPIST: Yes. I mean a daddy who was able to show you his love through all sorts of actions.

BARBARA: Wow . . . that would have been so different.

THERAPIST: Do you feel any angry feelings at him now as you think about how he spoke to you—this very young child simply trying to get his attention?

BARBARA: No, I was in his way. He worked hard. I had to leave him alone.

THERAPIST: What you just said—does that sound like anyone you know?

BARBARA: Yes. It sounds like my mother.

THERAPIST: And what do you think of that now?

BARBARA: Well. She was just trying to keep the peace and fill in for him.

THERAPIST: But what about you, this sweet innocent little child simply wanting what all children want—love and attention from her father?

BARBARA: It's sad. I feel sad for me.

THERAPIST: Right. It is sad for you. You are a child doing what all children do—children try to get their parents' attention; children want to know they are loved, valued, appreciated. You were no different from any other child, but what is happening here?

BARBARA: (*Cries.*)

THERAPIST: No one's calling your dad on his horrible behavior toward you. Everyone's accommodating *him* and speaking to you as if *you* are the problem, when all that you are doing is what every young child does. And yet your father and your mother are responding as if you are the problem.

BARBARA: Yeah. You're right. Why did they do that?

THERAPIST: Do you think there was something wrong with you, or do you think there was something wrong with the way they were behaving with you?

BARBARA: The way they were behaving with me. . . . It's a problem with the way they treated me.

THERAPIST: Right. They are the ones who should feel shame about their behavior. There was nothing shameful about you or your behavior.

In the preceding section, the therapist helps Barbara to realize the origin of "the Critic," the part of herself that has accepted her "Punitive Parent" message that she was the problem. The therapist's questions and comments also help Barbara realize that the problem was actually her parents' behavior toward her rather than an inherent defect in herself.

The therapist now turns Barbara's attention to the origin of "the Escapist" mode—the part that was seek-

ing relief from these terrible feelings about herself as a child. The therapist also helps Barbara become more aware that "the Escapist" was only able to provide short-term relief.

THERAPIST: Now when you had this bad feeling about yourself as a child, the "Ashamed Little Barbara" feeling, how did you cope with that feeling? What did you do?

BARBARA: A lot of the time, I did nothing. I just sat on my bed in my room daydreaming, wishing everything could be different. I would fantasize being a star, a beautiful person that everyone adored. People would dote on me and give me expensive gifts and clothes that made me look even more beautiful. Sometimes when my mom would take me out and buy me things, it kind of felt like she was making this dream come true.

THERAPIST: Is that "the Escapist" part of you trying to help you feel better?

BARBARA: Yes, it definitely is.

THERAPIST: And then what would happen?

BARBARA: I would feel better, especially as I got older and I got a lot of attention from the way I looked, but eventually my dad always would start yelling again. I remember him yelling at my mom for "spending too much money" simply to turn me into "a pretty Bimbo."

THERAPIST: So the efforts to feel better eventually backfired.

BARBARA: Right. I never felt very good for long. I never felt good inside.

Step 3: Link Current Problems and Symptoms to Maladaptive Modes

In this section, the therapist asks Barbara questions that help her to recognize how these modes that developed in childhood are still operating in the present. Barbara begins to connect these modes with why she is feeling so depressed, and she begins to see the repetitive patterns in her life.

THERAPIST: Let's look at what is happening now in your life. Do you recognize any relationship between what we have been talking about—these different parts of you—and how you are thinking and feeling about yourself and coping with your life now?

BARBARA: Yeah, I'm still trying to feel good—or just not feel—by being "the Escapist." When I go on these shopping sprees and let my mom and my friends dress me up, it still doesn't work any better than it ever did. And sleeping all the time doesn't work either.

THERAPIST: What do you mean?

BARBARA: Well, I only feel good for a short while. Then, instead of my dad coming home, now I'm coming home to George or he's coming home to me. George is just as mean and unavailable as my Dad.

THERAPIST: And then what happens?

BARBARA: I start to feel really bad again, really depressed. I feel like I'm not worth spending time with, like I'm boring and useless. I'm saying all sorts of bad things about myself and I agree with everything George says about me. I'm my worst "Critic." In the end, I still feel like the same old "Ashamed Little Barbara" inside who never ever really feels better. Then, I just want to go to sleep to get away from it all. I'm finally starting to see it more clearly, going around and around the same old circle—nothing has changed and nothing changes. I've been miserable my whole life.

THERAPIST: But there is one very important change.

BARBARA: What is that?

THERAPIST: You're starting to see and understand what's been happening for a long time instead of just being on the treadmill without any awareness.

Step 4: Uncover Advantages and Disadvantages of Each Mode

The therapist now begins to ask Barbara questions regarding the advantages and disadvantages of listening and acting on these different parts of herself. This helps Barbara to gain more distance from the modes and increases her awareness of a choice in how she responds.

THERAPIST: When these different parts of yourself or modes developed, they served a purpose. Why don't we talk about each of them and explore their advantages and disadvantages, both in the past and present? Let's start with "the Escapist."

BARBARA: Well, that part lets me feel good—or at least not feel bad.

THERAPIST: For how long?

BARBARA: For a while.

THERAPIST: And in the long run? Does that part help you feel better?

BARBARA: No, not really. I can't really escape feeling bad. I can't say I feel any better in the long run.

THERAPIST: So, is there any advantage to this part of you—"the Escapist"?

BARBARA: I'm mixed about it.

THERAPIST: Sure. I can understand that. If you don't know of any other way to feel better, any relief is better than no relief at all.

BARBARA: Yeah.

THERAPIST: But sometimes it's good to let yourself feel bad because when you let yourself stay in touch with your feelings, you often can begin to recognize what feels better in the long run . . . like finding activities that are truly interesting to you, or that give you a sense of accomplishment and purpose, or that bring out a feeling of deep enjoyment.

BARBARA: That makes sense, but I have no idea how to find those things.

THERAPIST: Well, that is something we can work on together.

BARBARA: That sounds good.

THERAPIST: And what about "the Critic"? Is there any advantage to listening to "the Critic"?

BARBARA: That part tells me what's wrong with me.

THERAPIST: And what does "the Critic" say is wrong with you?

BARBARA: That I'm stupid and silly, useless and annoying.

THERAPIST: Do you think "the Critic" is right?

BARBARA: Of course.

THERAPIST: But if you put the words of "the Critic" back in your dad's mouth and listen to him speak to little 3-year-old Barbara as she excitedly greets him coming home from work, what do you think?

BARBARA: When you put it that way, I think he's a jerk. I mean, what does he think he is doing to this poor little girl? What's wrong with him?

THERAPIST: Right. So is there any advantage to listening to these critical words?

BARBARA: No . . . no, definitely not.

THERAPIST: Are there any disadvantages of listening to "the Critic"?

BARBARA: Yes. It's getting clearer now why that part is making me feel so bad. I have to stop listening to that part. When I accept what my dad said as the truth, I feel bad, really bad, about myself.

THERAPIST: You mean it brings up that "Ashamed Little Barbara" feeling?

BARBARA: Yes.

THERAPIST: And what about her? What does she need?

BARBARA: She needs to feel good about herself. She needs to hear good things about herself. She needs someone to listen to her and pay attention to her—to love her.

THERAPIST: I agree.

Step 5: Use Imagery to Access the Vulnerable Child Mode

The therapist now begins to engage Barbara in the Vulnerable Child mode. By accessing this mode, the therapist and patient can begin to work on the core schemas that are part of "Ashamed Little Barbara."

THERAPIST: I know it's sometimes unpleasant to let yourself be in touch with "Ashamed Little Barbara," but would you be willing to go there, so that we can get to know that part of you to find out what you need to truly feel better and to find out what is getting in the way?

BARBARA: I guess . . . (*Closes her eyes.*)

THERAPIST: Tell me what you are feeling and thinking right now.

BARBARA: It's the same old feelings—I feel bad . . . and useless. (*Visibly begins to look upset, then opens her eyes.*)

THERAPIST: Can you go back there to "Ashamed Little Barbara," can you let yourself feel her?

BARBARA: OK. (*Closes her eyes again.*)

THERAPIST: Where are you? What are you doing?

BARBARA: I'm sitting on my bed in my room. My daddy just told me to go away.

THERAPIST: And how are you feeling?

BARBARA: Awful.

THERAPIST: And what do you want?

BARBARA: I want my mommy to come in and make me feel better.

THERAPIST: Where is she?

BARBARA: She's in her room, lying on her bed. She doesn't feel good either.

THERAPIST: If you could bring in a healthy mommy to be with you right now, what would she say to you? Let me hear her speak to Little Barbara.

BARBARA: You know he's just tired from work. If you just leave him alone, everything will be all right.

THERAPIST: Let me hear what Little Barbara thinks about this?

BARBARA: That doesn't help much. I still feel upset and bad.

THERAPIST: How about if I come in to help?

BARBARA: OK.

THERAPIST: You are such a loving little girl. So many fathers would relish coming home to such a greeting from their little girl. Something is wrong with your daddy. Why doesn't he recognize that you're offering him something that is precious—so special? . . . How does little Barbara feel as she hears this?

BARBARA: Better.

THERAPIST: Let me talk to your father now.

BARBARA: OK.

THERAPIST: How can you speak to your daughter that way? She's done nothing but welcome you home with joy and love. And look at how you are responding. Your response to her is completely inappropriate. You are so closed off and removed from everything. What is going on with you? Why can't you see that you have a beautiful, creative, and loving daughter? Barbara does not deserve this type of treatment. I'm not going to stand for this and let you hurt her anymore. . . . How does little Barbara feel as she hears this?

BARBARA: A lot better. I wish my mom had spoken to my dad that way. But you know, if you really tried to say anything like that to him, he wouldn't listen. He never listened to my mom. He'd probably just say something mean to you and then shut the door.

THERAPIST: OK. Well if that happened, what would you want to happen next?

BARBARA: I don't know.

THERAPIST: Let me step in again and say this to him

through the door. Whether or not you choose to listen, there is a limit, a limit as to how long we will stay here for you. If you choose not to be here for us, we will not stay here for you.

BARBARA: I don't think he'll change.

THERAPIST: Then you and I, together, will leave him and create a better life.

BARBARA: Is that really possible?

THERAPIST: Do you want to make it happen?

BARBARA: Yes, but what about him? He'll be so lonely.

THERAPIST: Who will be lonely?

BARBARA: He will, unless we stay.

THERAPIST: But if you stay, who will be lonely then?

BARBARA: Me.

THERAPIST: Do you want to continue to be there for someone who chooses not to be there for you?

BARBARA: Well, no—no, that isn't right.

THERAPIST: So what do you want to do?

BARBARA: I want to leave.

In this part of the session, the therapist has taken on the "Healthy Parent" mode for Barbara because she does not have a strong template for this mode. This is one example of what is meant by "limited reparenting." In this role, the therapist temporarily steps in to support the client in relation to unmet basic needs for safety; stability or predictability; love, nurturance, and attention; acceptance and praise; empathy; realistic limits; and validation of feelings and needs. The therapist also counters and challenges any unreasonable messages or beliefs that such needs should remain unfulfilled. As she begins to feel safer and more protected by the "Healthy Parent" through this work, "Little Barbara" no longer feels so ashamed of herself.

Step 6: Conduct Dialogues between Modes

Once patients begin to internalize the Healthy Parent mode demonstrated by the therapist, their own Healthy Adult mode becomes stronger. The patient's Healthy Adult mode can now actively challenge and combat the Punitive Parent mode, thereby supporting, protecting, and healing the Vulnerable Child, with the help of the therapist.

The therapist now addresses the Escapist, or Detached Protector, mode. In the segment that follows,

the therapist sets up a dialogue between the Vulnerable Child and Escapist modes.

THERAPIST: How about having "Little Barbara" talk with "the Escapist" about things that she really enjoys?

BARBARA: OK . . . but how do we do that?

THERAPIST: First, I want you to sit on this side of the couch. When you're on this side of the couch, I want you to let yourself get in touch with and speak for "Little Barbara." Have "Little Barbara" talk about all those things that interest her—those things that interest and excite her and help her feel alive. And then, I want you to get up and sit on the other side of the couch. When you're on this side of the couch, I want you to let yourself get in touch with and speak for "the Escapist." We'll go back and forth between those two parts of yourself to see what comes out. I'll help out "Little Barbara" if she needs me.

BARBARA: [as "Little Barbara"] You know, I once made a dress at school, and I noticed that I really liked sewing. It was a really simple pattern, nothing special, but I had so much fun making it. I think I might want to take a class to try sewing again.

[as "the Escapist"] Why do you want to do that? If it doesn't turn out, you'll just feel bad about yourself. People might think you're ridiculous at this age, trying to learn to sew. Why take the chance that you'll feel bad or stupid? Why don't you just lie down and forget about it?

[as "Little Barbara"] But I might like it. If I don't start trying the things that I think I might enjoy, I'll never know what I like or what makes me happy . . . If I keep listening to you, I'll do nothing but sleep away the rest of my life. I want to have a life.

[as "the Escapist"] I don't know if it's worth the risk of feeling bad.

[as "Little Barbara"] Even if I feel bad at first, it will only be temporary. Either I'll get good at sewing or I can find something else that I'm good at. I'll eventually find something if I just keep at it.

[as "the Escapist"] Well OK, suit yourself.

[as "Little Barbara"] I will.

At this point, the therapist is focused on helping Barbara discover what gives her an inner sense of joy and accomplishment. This task is difficult for Barbara because she spent so many of her early years dependent on her mother, not developing any special skills or talents, and surrendering to what others wanted her to be. Nevertheless, as previous segment illustrates, Barbara has begun to recognize the importance of trying out new activities that interest her, in spite of the temporary discomfort she may feel about the possibility of failing and feeling stupid again. The final step in therapy is to take these lessons she has learned in the sessions and integrate them into her everyday life experiences.

Step 7: Generalize Results from Mode Work to Real Life

Barbara decided to enroll in one sewing class and surprised herself by doing quite well. She then decided to take two more classes—a more advanced sewing class and a course in costume design. Following these classes, she started to volunteer for a local theater group, working on costumes. Barbara received much attention, praise, and appreciation from her teachers and theater friends. At this point in treatment, Barbara commented to her therapist, "You know, I think this is the first time I have ever really felt good and proud of myself."

As Barbara's confidence and her network of friends grew, she became less accepting and less tolerant of George's neglectful and demeaning behaviors toward her. She also became increasingly annoyed with her mother's pattern of excusing George's behavior for the sake of "being financially comfortable." This was in stark contrast to Barbara's unquestioning acceptance of her relationship with George at the beginning of treatment.

As she began to see parallels between how she felt with George and how she felt as a child with her parents, Barbara began to question whether this was a healthy marriage for her. She recognized that many of George's behaviors were damaging to her, just as her parents' behaviors had been. Although Barbara still wanted to adopt a child, she began questioning George's ability to be a good parent.

The following vignette from a later session in Barbara's treatment illustrates how much healthier and assertive she has become in relation to George:

BARBARA: I'm noticing that when George speaks to me in such a condescending tone, I feel like a little girl with my father again. I don't want this. I want to be treated with love and respect, and as an equal. It isn't right for me to accept his behavior—being ignored and demeaned by someone who is supposed to love me.

THERAPIST: So what do you want to do?

BARBARA: I think I'm ready to confront George about his drinking and abusive behavior. I can't even imagine adopting a child and bringing that child into our home if he continues to behave this way.

THERAPIST: What do you want to happen?

BARBARA: I want him to stop drinking and start treating me with love and respect.

THERAPIST: And if he doesn't? Then what?

BARBARA: I guess I'll leave him and seek a divorce.

THERAPIST: And how will that be for you—in the worst case scenario you might imagine?

BARBARA: In the worst case . . . you know, I think I'll be OK. I mean, I have my own life now. I have my own friends. And I have you, if things really get rough.

THERAPIST: I'll be here for you whenever you need my support.

BARBARA: Yeah, I think I'll be OK.

At this point in treatment, Barbara has fully incorporated the Healthy Adult mode and has healed the most damaging schemas that had been part of her Vulnerable Child mode. Along with these changes, Barbara's depression went into full remission. Soon after this session, Barbara confronted her husband. Despite couple therapy, George refused to make any changes, and Barbara filed for divorce.

Barbara did experience one relapse of major depression as her divorce was finalized. "Ashamed Little Barbara" and "the Escapist" temporarily returned during this period. Barbara, however, was able to recognize the reappearance of the Punitive Parent mode and successfully overcame it with her now stronger Healthy Adult mode. She was able to empathize with and forgive herself, and to mourn the lost opportunity to have her own family. She decided to go back to school and succeeded in becoming a certified teacher at the high school level, teaching costume design and drama in the theater department. She also developed a lasting relationship with a caring, emotionally available man who shared her passion for theater. Barbara's chronic depression lifted, and she has, for the most part, been symptom free since.

CONCLUSION

Evidence demonstrating the efficacy of cognitive therapy in the treatment of unipolar and bipolar depression continues to mount. Adolescents, adults, and geriatric patients have all been shown to benefit from cognitive therapy.

Cognitive therapy helps patients understand the relationships among their thoughts, behaviors, and feelings. Cognitions are "put to the test" by examining evidence, setting up *in vivo* experiments, weighing advantages and disadvantages, trying graded tasks, and employing other intervention strategies. Through this process, patients begin to view themselves and their problems more realistically, to feel better, to change their maladaptive behavior patterns, and to take steps to solve real-life difficulties. These changes take place as a direct result of carefully planned, self-help homework assignments—one of the hallmarks of cognitive treatment. Cognitive therapy reduces symptoms by helping patients to identify and modify automatic thoughts, and the behaviors associated with them.

An expansion of cognitive therapy called schema therapy has been developed to deal with the deeper psychological structures that predispose patients to chronic depression. After utilizing interventions aimed at initial symptom reduction, a great deal of subsequent attention and effort are directed toward identifying and modifying the underlying schemas and modes that often predispose individuals to chronic depression.

Following a thorough assessment, an extensive change component is implemented. During this phase of treatment, patients come to understand their own schemas and modes, their developmental origins, and how these dysfunctional schema patterns are triggered, reinforced, and maintained.

Throughout the treatment, cognitive therapists maintain a collaborative alliance with their patients. They are very active in structuring sessions, yet go to considerable lengths to help patients reach conclusions on their own. Cognitive therapists serve as guides, helping patients maneuver through a labyrinth of dysfunctional cognitions and life patterns. As a result, patients develop the psychological tools they need to become more proactive in making the cognitive, affective, interpersonal, and behavioral changes that serve to minimize future episodes of depression.

NOTES

1. Some researchers have found it useful to differentiate between "relapse" (the return of symptoms within 6 months after termination of treatment) and "recurrence" (a whole new episode of depression, occurring at least 12 months after treatment has ended; Gelder, 1994; see also Overholser, 1998). However, this distinction has not been uniformly incorporated into the literature.

2. Reported relapse rates for patients treated with medication have varied depending on the definition of "relapse," the duration of the follow-up period, and the severity of depression within the patient population (Williams, 1997). Because of these differences, some of the estimates have ranged from 34 to 92% (Frank, 1996; Overholser, 1998; Versiani, 1998; Williams, 1997), though lower rates have also been reported (Keller & Boland, 1998).

3. The book by Young (1990/1999) cited here and throughout the chapter, *Cognitive Therapy for Personality Disorders: A Schema-Focused Approach*, refers to the third edition. However, the ideas expressed were developed in 1990, for the original edition. Similarly, the Young Schema Questionnaire was developed in 1990, then reprinted in the third edition.

4. Currently, the concept of a schema domain is not a component of schema theory. Although early factor-analytic research supported the grouping of 18 EMSs into five broader domains, later studies have been inconsistent regarding how schemas cluster together, and some domains have not been supported at all. Nevertheless, we have included research studies that focus on these five domains because the findings do shed light on the relationship between schemas and other constructs. We are in the process of reviewing all of the research available so that we can reexamine the question of how schemas cluster together.

5. For the remainder of the chapter, we use the term "schema" to refer specifically to Young's "early maladaptive schemas."

6. Many cognitive therapists also focus on "underlying assumptions," which represent cognitions that are "deeper" than automatic thoughts but less central than schemas or core beliefs. Underlying assumptions are considered conditional beliefs, whereas most schemas are unconditional. In our own work, we have not found this distinction to be necessary in working with most patients. Thus, conditional and unconditional beliefs that are enduring and pervasive can be merged into the broader construct of a schema.

REFERENCES

Albon, J. S., & Jones, E. E. (2003). Validity of controlled clinical trials of psychotherapy: Findings from the NIMH Treatment of Depression Collaborative Research Program. *American Journal of Psychiatry, 159*(5), 775–783.

American Psychiatric Association. (1987). *Diagnostic and statistical manual of mental disorders* (3rd ed., rev.). Washington, DC: Author.

American Psychiatric Association. (1994). *Diagnostic and statistical manual of mental disorders* (4th ed.). Washington, DC: Author.

American Psychiatric Association. (2013). *Diagnostic and statistical manual of mental disorders* (5th ed.). Arlington, VA: Author.

Antonuccio, D. O., Danton, W. G., & DeNelsky, G. Y. (1995). Psychotherapy versus medication for depression: Challenging the conventional wisdom with data. *Professional Psychology: Research and Practice, 26*(6), 574–585.

Antonuccio, D. O., Thomas, M., & Danton, W. G. (1997). A cost-effectiveness analysis of cognitive behavior therapy and fluoxetine (Prozac) in the treatment of depression. *Behavior Therapy, 28,* 187–210.

Arnow, B. A., Manber, R., Blasey, C., Klein, D. N., Blalock, J. A., Markowitz, J. C., et al. (2003). Therapeutic reactance as a predictor of outcome in the treatment of chronic depression. *Journal of Consulting and Clinical Psychology, 71*(6), 1025–1035.

Bailleux, S., Romo, L., Kindynis, S., Radtchenko, A., & Debray, Q. (2008). Study of the bonds between early maladaptive schemas and strategies of coping (among alcohol-dependent patients and depressed patients). *Journal de Therapie Comportementale et Cognitive, 18*(1), 19–25.

Ball, J. R., Mitchell, P. B., Corry, J. C., Skillecorn, A., Smith, M., & Malhi, G. S. (2006). A randomized controlled trial of cognitive therapy for bipolar disorder: Focus on long-term change. *Journal of Clinical Psychiatry, 67,* 277–286.

Barber, J. P., & DeRubeis, R. J. (1989). On second thought: Where the action is in cognitive therapy for depression. *Cognitive Therapy and Research, 13*(5), 441–457.

Barlow, D. H., & Hofmann, S. G. (1997). Efficacy and dissemination of psychological treatments. In D. M. Clark & C. G. Fairburn (Eds.), *Science and practice of cognitive behaviour therapy* (pp. 95–117). Oxford, UK: Oxford University Press.

Barnhofer, T., Crane, C., Hargus, E., Amarasinghe, M., Winer, R., & Williams, J. M. (2009). Mindfulness-based cognitive therapy as a treatment for chronic depression: A preliminary study, *Behaviour Research and Therapy, 47*(5), 366–373.

Basco, M. R., & Rush, A. J. (1996). *Cognitive-behavioral therapy for bipolar disorder.* New York: Guilford Press.

Beck, A. T. (1967). *Depression: Causes and treatment.* Philadelphia: University of Pennsylvania Press.

Beck, A. T. (1976). *Cognitive therapy and the emotional disorders.* New York: International Universities Press.

Beck, A. T. (1988). *Love is never enough.* New York: Harper & Row.

Beck, A. T., & Alford, B. A. (2009). *Depression: Causes and treatment.* Philadephia: University of Pennsylvania Press.

Beck, A. T., Freeman, A., & Associates. (1990). *Cognitive therapy of personality disorders.* New York: Guilford Press.

Beck, A. T., Rush, A. J., Shaw, B. F., & Emery, G. (1979). *Cognitive therapy of depression.* New York: Guilford Press.

Beck, J. S. (2011). *Cognitive therapy: Basics and beyond* (2nd ed.). New York: Guilford Press.

Bellino, S., Zizza, M., Rinaldi, C., & Bogetto, F. (2007). Combined therapy of major depression with concomitant borderline personality disorder: Comparison of interpersonal and cognitive psychotherapy. *Canadian Journal of Psychiatry, 52*(11), 718–725.

Berger, T., Hammerli, K., Gubser, N., Andersson, G., & Caspar, F. (2011). Internet-based treatment of depression: A randonmized controlled trial comparing guided with unguided self-help. *Cognitive Behavioral Therapy, 40*(4), 251–266.

Berndt, E. R., Koran, L. M., Finkelstein, S. N., Gelenberg, A. J., Kornstein, S. G., Miller, I. M., et al. (2000). Lost human capital from early-onset chronic depression. *American Journal of Psychiatry, 157,* 940–947.

Beutler, L. E., Scogin, F., Kirkish, P., Schretlen, D., Corbishley, A., Hamblin, D., et al. (1987). Group cognitive therapy and alprazolam in the treatment of depression in older adults. *Journal of Consulting and Clinical Psychology, 55*(4), 550–556.

Bhar, S. S., Gelfand, L. A., Schmid, S. P., Gallop, R., DeRubeis, R. J., Hollon, S. D., et al. (2008). Sequence of improvement in depressive symptoms across cognitive therapy and pharmacotherapy. *Journal of Affective Disorders, 110* (1–2), 161–166.

Biggs, M. M., & Rush, A. J. (1999). Cognitive and behavioral therapies alone or combined with antidepressant medication in the treatment of depression. In D. S. Janowsky (Ed.), *Psychotherapy indications and outcomes* (pp.121–172). Washington, DC: American Psychiatric Press.

Blackburn, I. M., Bishop, S., Glen, A. I. M., Whalley, L. J., & Christie, J. E. (1981). The efficacy of cognitive therapy in depression: A treatment trial using cognitive therapy and pharmacotherapy, each alone and in combination. *British Journal of Psychiatry, 139,* 181–189.

Bledsoe, S. E., & Grote, N. K. (2006). Treating depression during pregnancy and the postpartum: A preliminary meta-analysis. *Research on Social Work Practice, 16*(2), 109–120.

Bockting, C. L. H., Schene, A. H., Spinhoven, P., Koeter, M. W. J., Wouters, L. F., Huyser, J., et al. (2005). Preventing relapse/recurrence in recurrent depression with cognitive therapy: A randomized controlled trial. *Journal of Consulting and Clinical Psychology, 73,* 647–657.

Bowers, W. A. (1990). Treatment of depressed in-patients: Cognitive therapy plus medication, and medication alone. *British Journal of Psychiatry, 156,* 73–58.

Bromet, E., Andrade, L. H., Hwang, I., Sampson, N. A., Alonso, J., de Girolamo, G., et al. (2011). Cross-national epidemiology of DSM-IV major depressive episode. *BMC Medicine, 9,* 90.

Burns, D. D., & Spangler, D. L. (2000). Does psychotherapy homework lead to improvements in depression in cognitive-behavioral therapy or does improvement lead to increased homework compliance? *Journal of Consulting and Clinical Psychology, 68*(1), 46–56.

Castonguay, L. G., Goldfried, M. R., Wiser, S., Raue, P. J., & Hayes, A. M. (1996). Predicting the effect of cognitive therapy for depression: A study of unique and common factors. *Journal of Consulting and Clinical Psychology, 64*(3), 497–504.

Castonguay, L. G., Schut, A. J., Aikens, D., Constantino, M. J., Laurenceau, J. P., Bolough, L., et al. (2004). Integrative cognitive therapy: A preliminary investigation. *Journal of Psychotherapy Integration, 14*(1), 4–20.

Centers for Disease Control and Prevention (CDC). (2010). Current depression among adults—United States, 2006 and 2008. *Morbidity and Mortality Weekly Report, 59*(38), 1229–1235.

Chapman, D. P., Perry, G. S., & Strine, T. W. (2005). The vital link between chronic disease and depressive disorders. *Preventing Chronic Disease, 2,* A14. Retrieved from *www.csc.gov/pdc/issues/jan/04_0066.htm.*

Chapman, D. P., Whitfield, C. L., Felitti, V. J., Dube, S. R., Edwards, V. J., & Anda, R. F. (2004). Adverse childhood experiences and the risk of depressive disorders in adulthood. *Journal of Affective Disorders, 82*(2), 217–225.

Cipriani, A., Santilli, C., Furukawa, T. A., Signoretti, A., Nakagawa, A., McGuire, H., et al. (2009). Escitalopram versus other antidepressant agents for depression. *Cochrane Database of Systematic Reviews, 2,* CD006532.

Clark, D. A., & Beck, A. T. (2010). *Cognitive therapy of anxiety disorders: Science and practice.* New York: Guilford Press,

Colom, F., Vieta, E., Martinez, A., Jorquera, A., & Gastó, C. (1998). What is the role of psychotherapy in the treatment of bipolar disorder? *Psychotherapy and Psychosomatics, 67,* 3–9.

Cong, E., Li, Y., Shao, C., Chen, J., Wu, W., Shang, X., et al. (2012). Childhood sexual abuse and the risk of recurrent major depression in Chinese women. *Psychological Medicine, 42,* 409–417.

Connolly, K. R., & Thase, M. E. (2012). Emerging drugs for major depressive disorder. *Expert Opinion on Emerging Drugs, 17*(1), 105–126.

Conte, H. R., Plutchik, R., Wild, K. V., & Karasu, T. B. (1986). Combined psychotherapy and pharmacotherapy for depression. *Archives of General Psychiatry, 43,* 471–479.

Craighead, W. E., Miklowitz, D. J., Vajk, F. C., & Frank, E. (1998). Psychological treatments for bipolar disorder. In P. E. Nathan & J. M. Gorman (Eds.), *A guide to treatments that work* (pp. 240–248). New York: Oxford University Press.

Crews, W. D., Jr., & Harrison, D. W. (1995). The neuropsychology of depression and its implications for cognitive therapy. *Neuropsychology Review, 5*(2), 81–123.

Curry, J. F. (2001). Specific psychotherapies for childhood and adolescent depression. *Biological Psychiatry, 49,* 1091–1100.

de Oliveira, I. R. (1998). The treatment of unipolar major depression: Pharmacotherapy, cognitive behaviour therapy or both? *Journal of Clinical Pharmacy and Therapeutics, 23,* 467–475.

DeRubeis, R. J., & Feeley, M. (1990). Determinants of change in cognitive therapy for depression. *Cognitive Therapy and Research, 14*(5), 469–482.

DeRubeis, R. J., Gelfand, L. A., Tang, T. Z., & Simons, A. D. (1999). Medications versus cognitive behavior therapy for severely depressed outpatients: Mega-analysis of four randomized comparisons. *American Journal of Psychiatry, 156*(7), 1007–1013.

DeRubeis, R. J., Hollon, S. D., Amsterdam, J. D., Shelton, R. C., Young, P. R., Salomon, R. M., et al. (2005). Cognitive therapy vs. medications in the treatment of moderate to severe depression. *Archives of General Psychiatry, 62,* 409–416.

DeRubeis, R. J., Hollon, S. D., Grove, W. M., Evans, M. D., Garvey, M. J., & Tuason, V. B. (1990). How does cognitive therapy work?: Cognitive change and symptom change in cognitive therapy and pharmacotherapy for depression. *Journal of Consulting and Clinical Psychology, 58*(6), 862–869.

Dobson, K. S., Hollon, S. D., Dimidjian, S., Schmaling, K. B., Kohlenberg, R. J., Gallon, R., et al. (2008). Randomized trial of behavioral activation, cognitive therapy, and antidepressant medication in the prevention of relapse and recurrence in major depression. *Journal of Consulting and Clinical Psychology, 76*(3), 468–477.

Dobson, K. S., & Pusch, D. (1993). Towards a definition of the conceptual and empirical boundaries of cognitive therapy. *Australian Psychologist, 28*(3), 137–144.

Dougherty, L. R., Klein, D. N., & Davila, J. (2004). A growth curve analysis of the course of dysthymic disorder: The effects of chronic stress and moderation by adverse parent–child relationships and family history. *Journal of Consulting and Clinical Psychology, 72*(6), 1012–1021.

Dube, S. R., Anda, R. F., Felitti, V. J., Chapman, D. P., Williamson, D. F., & Giles, W. H. (2001). Childhood abuse, household dysfunction, and the risk of attempted suicide throughout the life span: Findings from the adverse childhood experiences study. *Journal of the American Medical Association, 286*, 3089–3096.

Eberhart, N. K., Auerbach, R. P., Bigda-Peyton, J., & Abela, J. R. Z. (2011). Maladaptive schemas and depression: Tests of stress generation and diathesis–stress models. *Journal of Social and Clinical Psychology, 30*(1), 75–104.

Eifert, G. H., Beach, B. K., & Wilson, P. H. (1998). Depression: Behavioral principles and implications for treatment and relapse prevention. In J. J. Plaud & G. H. Eifers (Eds.), *From behavior theory to behavior therapy* (pp. 68–97). Boston: Allyn & Bacon.

Eisendrath, S., Chartier, M., & McLane, M. (2011). Adapting mindfulness-based cognitive therapy for treatment-resistant depression: A clinical case study. *Cognitive Behavioral Practice, 18*(3), 362–370.

Elkin, I., Gibbons, R. D., Shea, M. T., & Shaw, B. F. (1996). Science is not a trial (but it can sometimes be a tribulation). *Journal of Consulting and Clinical Psychology, 64*(1), 92–103.

Elkin, I., Shea, M. T., Watkins, J. T., Imber, S. D., Sotsky, S. M., Collins, J. F., et al. (1989). National Institute of Mental Health Treatment of Depression Collaborative Research Program: General effectiveness of treatments. *Archives of General Psychiatry, 46*, 971–982.

Evans, M. D., Hollon, S. D., DeRubeis, R. J., Piaseki, J. M., Grove, W. M., Garvey, M. J., et al. (1992). Differential relapse following cognitive therapy and pharmacotherapy for depression. In D. S. Janowsky (Ed.), *Psychotherapy indication and outcomes* (pp. 802–808). Washington, DC: American Psychiatric Press.

Farrell, J., & Shaw, I. A. (2012). *Group schema therapy for borderline personality disorder: A step-by-step treatment manual with patient workbook.* Malden, MA: Wiley-Blackwell.

Farrell, J., Shaw, I. A., & Webber, M. (2009). A schema-focused approach to group psychotherapy for outpatients with borderline personality disorder: A randomized control trial. *Journal of Behavior Therapy and Experimental Psychiatry, 40*, 317–328.

Fava, G. A., Rafanelli, C., Grandi, S., Canestrari, R., & Morphy, M. A. (1998). Six-year outcome for cognitive behavioral treatment of residual symptoms in major depression. *American Journal of Psychiatry, 155*(10), 1443–1445.

Fava, G. A., Rafanelli, C., Grandi, S., Conti, S., & Belluardo, P. (1998). Prevention of recurrent depression with cognitive behavioral therapy: Preliminary findings. *Archives of General Psychiatry, 55*(9), 816–820.

Feldman, G., Harley, R., Kerrigan, M., Jacobo, M., & Fava, M. (2009). Change in emotional processing during a dialectical behavior based skills group for major depressive disorder. *Behaviour Research and Therapy, 47*(4), 316–

Feng, C. Y., Chu, H., Chen, C. H., Chang, Y. S., Chen, T. H. Chou, Y. H., et al. (2012). The effect of cognitive behav-

ioral group therapy for depression: A meta-analysis 2000–2010. *Worldviews Evidence Based Nursing, 9*(1), 2–17.

Floyd, M., Scogin, F., McKendree-Smith, N. L., Floyd, D. L., & Rokke, P. D. (2004). Cognitive therapy for depression: A comparison of individual psychotherapy and bibliotherapy for depressed older adults. *Behavior Modification, 28*(2), 297–318.

Fournier, J. C., De Rubeis, R. J., Shelton, R. C., Gallop, R., Amsterdam, J. D., & Hollon, S. D. (2008). Antidepressant medications versus cognitive therapy in depressed patients with or without personality disorder. *British Journal of Psychiatry, 192*(2), 124–129.

Frank, E. (1996). Long-term treatment of depression: Interpersonal psychotherapy with and without medication. In C. Mundt & M. J. Goldstein (Eds.), *Interpersonal factors in the origin and course of affective disorders* (pp. 303–315). London: Gaskell/Royal College of Psychiatrists.

Frank, E., & Thase, M. E. (1999). Natural history and preventative treatment of recurrent mood disorders. *Annual Review of Medicine, 50*, 453–468.

Free, M. L., Oei, T. P. S., & Appleton, C. (1998). Biological and psychological processes in recovery from depression during cognitive therapy. *Journal of Behavior Therapy and Experimental Psychiatry, 29*, 213–226.

Freeman, A., & Davison, M. R. (1997). Short-term therapy for the long-term patient. In L. Vandecreek, S. Knapp, & T. L. Jackson (Eds.), *Innovations in clinical practice: A source book* (pp. 5–24). Sarasota, FL: Professional Resource Press.

Futterman, A., Thompson, L., Gallagher-Thompson, D., & Ferris, R. (1995). Depression in later life: Epidemiology, assessment, etiology, and treatment. In E. E. Beckham & W. R. Leber (Eds.), *Handbook of depression* (2nd ed., pp. 494–525). New York: Guilford Press.

Gallagher-Thompson, D., Hanley-Peterson, P., & Thompson, L. W. (1990). Maintenance of gains versus relapse following brief psychotherapy for depression. *Journal of Consulting and Clinical Psychology, 58*(3), 371–374.

Garyfallos, G., Adarnopoulo, A., Karastergiou, A., Voikli, M., Sotiropoulo, A., Donias, S., et al. (1999). Personality disorders in dysthymia and major depression. *Acta Psychiatrica Scandinavica, 99*(5), 332–340.

Geddes, J. R., Carney, S. M., Davies, C., Furukawa, T. A., Kupfer, D. J., Frank, E., et al. (2003). Relapse prevention with antidepressant drug treatment in depressive disorders: A systematic review. *Lancet, 361*, 653–661.

Gelder, M. G. (1994). Cognitive therapy for depression. In H. Hippius & C. N. Stefanis (Eds.), *Research in mood disorders: An update* (Vol. 1, pp. 115–124). Goettingen, Germany: Hogrefe & Huber.

Giesen-Bloo, J., van Dyck, R., Spinhoven, P., van Tilburg, W., Dirksen, C., van Asselt, T., et al. (2006). Outpatient psychotherapy for borderline personality disorder: A randomized trial of schema-focused therapy vs. transference-focused therapy. *Archives of General Psychiatry, 63,* 649–658.

Gilson, M., Freeman, A. M., Yates, J., & Freeman, S. M. (2009). *Overcoming depression: A cognitive therapy approach* (2nd ed.). New York: Oxford University Press.

Gloaguen, V., Cottraux, J., Cucherat, M., & Blackburn, I. M. (1998). A meta-analysis of the effects of cognitive therapy in depressed patients. *Journal of Affective Disorders, 49,* 59–72.

Halvorsen, M., Wang, C. E., Eisemann, M., & Waterloo, K. (2010). Dysfunctional attitudes and early maladaptive schemas as predictors of depression: A 9-year follow-up study. *Cognitive Therapy Research, 34,* 368–379.

Halvorsen, M., Wang, C. F., Richter, J., Myrland, I., Pedersen, S. K., Eisemann, M, et al. (2009). Early maladaptive schemas, temperament and character traits in clinically depressed and previously depressed subjects. *Clinical Psychology and Psychotherapy, 16*(5), 394–407.

Hardeveld, F., Spijker, J., de Graaf, R., Nolen, W. A., & Beekman, A. T. F. (2010). Prevalence and predictors of recurrence of major depressive disorder in the adult population. *Acta Psychiatrica Scandinavia, 122,*184–191.

Harley, R., Sprich, S., Safren, S., Jacob, M., & Fava, M. (2008). Adaptation of dialectical behavior therapy skills training group for treatment-resistant depression, *Journal of Nervous and Mental Diseases, 196*(2), 136–143.

Harrington, R., Wood, A., & Verduyn, C. (1998). Clinically depressed adolescents. In P. J. Graham (Ed.), *Cognitive-behaviour therapy for children and families* (pp. 156–193). New York: Cambridge University Press.

Hawke, L. D., & Provencher, M. D. (2011). Schema theory and schema therapy in mood and anxiety disorders: A review. *Journal of Cognitive Psychotherapy: An International Quarterly, 25*(4), 257–276.

Hayden, E. P., & Klein, D. N. (2001). Predicting outcome of dysthymic disorder at a 5-year follow-up: The impact of familial psychopathology, early adversity, personality, comorbidity, and chronic stress. *American Journal of Psychiatry, 158,* 1864–1870.

Hayes, A. M., & Strauss, J. L. (1998). Dynamic systems theory as a paradigm for the study of change in psychotherapy: An application to cognitive therapy for depression. *Journal of Consulting and Clinical Psychology, 66*(6), 939–947.

Heim, C., & Nemeroff, C. B. (2001). The role of childhood trauma in the neurobiology of mood and anxiety disorders: Preclinical and clinical studies. *Biological Psychiatry, 49,* 1023–1039.

Henry, W. P., Strupp, H. H., Butler, S. F., Schacht, T. E., & Binder, J. L. (1993). The effects of training in time-limited dynamic psychotherapy: Changes in therapist behavior. *Journal of Consulting and Clinical Psychology, 61,* 434–440.

Hollon, S. D. (1998). What is cognitive behavioural therapy and does it work? *Current Opinion in Neurobiology, 8,* 289–292.

Hollon, S. D., DeRubeis, R. J., & Evans, M. D. (1996). Cognitive therapy in the treatment and prevention of depression. In P. M. Salkovskis (Ed.), *Frontiers of cognitive therapy* (pp. 293–317). New York: Guilford Press.

Hollon, S. D., DeRubeis, R. J., Evans, M. D., Weimer, M. J., Garvey, M. J., Grove, W. M., et al. (1992). Cognitive therapy and pharmacotherapy: Singly and in combination. *Archives of General Psychiatry, 49,* 774–781.

Hollon, S. D., DeRubeis, R. J., Shelton, R. C., Amsterdam, J. D., Salomon, R. M., O'Reardon, J. P., et al. (2005). Prevention of relapse following cognitive therapy vs. medications in moderate to severe depression. *Archives of General Psychiatry, 62,* 417–422.

Hollon, S. D., & Shelton, R. C. (2001). Treatment guidelines for major depressive disorder. *Behavior Therapy, 32,* 235–258.

Hollon, S. D., Shelton, R. C., & Loosen, P. T. (1991). Cognitive therapy and pharmacotherapy for depression. *Journal of Consulting and Clinical Psychology, 59*(1), 88–99.

Hollon, S. D., Thase, M. E., & Markowitz, J. C. (2002). Treatment and prevention of depression. *Psychological Science in the Public Interest, 3,* 39–77.

Howland, R. H. (1993). Chronic depression. *Hospital and Community Psychiatry, 44,* 633–639.

Ingram, R. E., & Holle, C. (1992). Cognitive science of depression. In D. J. Stein & J. E. Young (Eds.), *Cognitive science and clinical disorders* (pp. 187–209). San Diego, CA: Academic Press.

Jacobson, N. S., & Hollon, S. D. (1996). Cognitive-behavior therapy versus pharmacotherapy: Now that the jury's returned its verdict, it's time to present the rest of the evidence. *Journal of Consulting and Clinical Psychology, 64*(1), 74–80.

Jarrett, R. B. (1995). Comparing and combining short-term psychotherapy and pharmacotherapy for depression. In E. E. Beckham & W. R. Leber (Eds.), *Handbook of depression* (2nd ed., pp. 435–464). New York: Guilford Press.

Jarrett, R. B., Kraft, D., Doyle, J., Foster, B. M., Eaves, G. G., & Silver, P. C. (2001). Preventing recurrent depression using cognitive therapy with and without continuation phase. *Archives of General Psychiatry, 58*(4), 381–388.

Jarrett, R. B., & Nelson, R. O. (1987). Mechanisms of change in cognitive therapy of depression. *Behavior Therapy, 18,* 227–241.

Jarrett, R. B., Schaffer, M., McIntire, D., Witt-Browder, A., Kraft, D., & Risser, R. C. (1999). Treatment of atypical depression with cognitive therapy or phenelzine: A double-blind, placebo-controlled trial. *Archives of General Psychiatry, 56,* 431–437.

Jarrett, R. B., & Thase, M. E. (2010). Comparative efficacy and durability of continuation phase cognitive therapy for preventing recurrent depression: Design of a double-blinded, fluoxetine-and pill-placebo-contolled, randomized trial with 2-year follow-up. *Contemporary Clinical Trials, 31*(4), 355–377.

Jarrett, R. B., Vittengl, J. R., & Clark, L. A. (2008). How much cognitive therapy, for which patients, will prevent depressive relapse. *Journal of Affective Disorders, 111*(2–3), 185–192.

Joffe, R., Segal, Z., & Singer, W. (1996). Change in thyroid hormone levels following response to cognitive therapy for major depression. *American Journal of Psychiatry, 153*(3), 411–413.

Johansson, R., & Andersson, G. (2012). Internet-based psychological treatments for depression. *Expert Review of Neurotherapeutics, 12* (7), 861–870.

Joyce, P. R., McKenzie, J. M., Carter, J. D., Rae, A. M., Luty, S. E., Frampton, C. M. A., et al. (2007). Temperament, character and personality disorders as predictors of response to interpersonal psychotherapy and cognitive-behavioural therapy for depression. *British Journal of Psychiatry, 190*, 503–508.

Keller, M. B., & Bolland, R. J. (1998). Implications of failing to achieve successful long-term maintenance treatment of recurrent unipolar major depression. *Biological Psychiatry, 44*(5), 348–360.

Keller, M. B., & Hanks, D. L. (1995). Course and natural history of chronic depression. In J. H. Kocsis & D. N. Klein (Eds.), *Diagnosis and treatment of chronic depression* (pp. 58–72). New York: Guilford Press.

Keller, M. B., McCullough, J. P., Klein, D. F., Arnow, B., Dunner, D. L., Gelenberg, A. J., et al. (2000). A comparison of nefazodone, the cognitive behavioral-analysis system of psychotherapy, and their combination for the treatment of chronic depression. *New England Journal of Medicine, 342*, 1462–1470.

Kendler, K. S., Kessler, R. C., Walters, E. E., MacLean, C., Neale, M. C., Heath, A. C., et al. (1995). Stressful life events, genetic liability, and onset of an episode of major depression in women. *American Journal of Psychiatry, 152*, 833–842.

Kessler, R. C., Akiskal, H. S., Ames, M., Birnbaum, H., Greenberg, P. A., Jin, R., et al. (2006). Prevalence and effects of mood disorders on work performance in a nationally representative sample of U.S. workers. *American Journal of Psychiatry, 163*(9), 1561–1568.

Kessler, R. C., Petukhova, M., Sampson, N. A., Zaslavsky, A. M., & Wittchen, H. U. (2012). Twelve-month and lifetime prevalence and lifetime morbid risk of anxiety and mood disorders in the United States. *Internal Journal of Methods in Psychiatric Research, 21*(3), 169–184.

Klein, D. N., Santiago, N. J., Vivian, D., Blalock, J. A., Kocsis, J. H., Markowitz, J. C., et al. (2004). Cognitive-behavioral analysis system of psychotherapy as a maintenance treatment for chronic depression. *Journal of Consulting and Clinical Psychology, 72*, 681–688.

Kocsis, J. H., Gelenberg, A. J., Rothbaum, B. O., Klein, D. N., Trivedi, M. H., Manber, R., et al. (2009). Cognitive behavioral analysis system of psychotherapy and brief supportive psychotherapy for augmentation of antidepressant nonresponse in chronic depression: the REVAMP Trial. *Archives of General Psychiatry, 66*(11), 1178–1188.

Koder, D. A., Brodaty, H., & Anstey, K. J. (1996). Cognitive therapy for depression in elderly. *International Journal of Geriatric Psychiatry, 11*(2), 97–107.

Kupfer, D. J., Frank, E., & Wamhoff, J. (1996). Mood disorders: Update on prevention of recurrence. In C. Mundt, M. M. Goldstein, K. Hahlweg, & P. Fiedler (Eds.), *Interpersonal factors in the origin and course of affective disorders* (pp. 289–302). London: Gaskell.

Lam, D. H., Hayward, P., Watkins, E. R., Wright, K., & Sham, P. (2005). Relapse prevention in patients with bipolar disorder: Cognitive therapy outcome after 2 years. *American Journal of Psychiatry, 162*(2), 324–329.

Lazarus, A. A., & Lazarus, C. N. (1991). *Multimodal Life History Inventory* (2nd ed.). Champaign, IL: Research Press.

Leahy, R. L. (2010). *Beat the blues before they beat you.* New York: Hay House.

Lee, C. W., Taylor, G., & Dunn, J. (1999). Factor structure of the Schema Questionnaire in a large clinical sample. *Cognitive Therapy and Research, 23*(4), 441–451.

Levendusky, P. G., & Hufford, M. R. (1997). The application of cognitive-behavior therapy to the treatment of depression and related disorders in the elderly. *Journal of Geriatric Psychiatry, 30*(2), 227–238.

Linehan, M. M. (1993a). *Cognitive-behavioral treatment of borderline personality disorder.* New York: Guilford Press.

Linehan, M. M. (1993b). *Skills training manual for treating borderline personality disorder.* New York: Guilford Press.

Lizardi, H., Klein, D. N., Ouimette, P. C., Riso, L. P., Anderson, R. L., & Donaldson, S. K. (1995). Reports of the childhood home environment in early onset dysthymia and episodic major depression. *Journal of Abnormal Psychology, 104*, 132–139.

Luoma, J. B., Hayes, S. C., & Walser R. D. (2007). *Learning ACT: An acceptance and commitment therapy skills-training manual for therapists.* Richmond, BC, Canada: Raincoast Books.

Luty S. E., Carter, J. D., McKenzie, J. M., Rae, A. M., Frampton, C. M. A., Mulder, R. T. et al. (2007). Randomized controlled trial of interpersonal psychotherapy and cognitive-behavioural therapy for depression. *British Journal of Psychiatry, 190*, 496–502.

Ma, S. H., & Teasdale, J. D. (2004). Mindfulness-based cognitive therapy for depression: Replication and exploration of differential relapse prevention effects. *Journal of Consulting and Clinical Psychology, 72*(1), 31–40.

Manicavasagar, V., Perich, T., & Parker, G. (2012). Cognitive predictors of change in cognitive behavior therapy and mindfulness-based cognitive therapy for depression. *Behavioural and Cognitive Psychotherapy, 40*, 227–232.

Mathew, K. L., & Whitford, H. S. (2010). The long-term effects of mindfulness-based cognitive therapy as a relapse prevention treatment for major depressive disorder. *Behavioural and Cognitive Psychotherapy, 38,* 561–576.

Mathys, M., & Mitchell, B. G. (2011). Targeting treatment-resistant depression. *Journal of Pharmacological Practice, 24*(6), 520–533.

Matthew, K. L., Whitford, H. S., Kenny, M. A., & Denson, L. A. (2010). The long-term effects of mindfulness-bassed cognitive therapy as a relapse prevention treatment for major depressive disorder. *Behavioural and Cognitive Psychotherapy, 38,* 561–576.

McCullough, J. P., Jr. (2000). *Treatment for chronic depression: Cognitive behavioral analysis system of psychotherapy (CBASP).* New York: Guilford Press.

McCullough, J. P., Jr. (2003). Treatment for chronic depression: Cognitive behavioral-analysis system of psychotherapy. *Journal of Psychotherapy Integration, 13*(3/4), 241–263.

McGinn, L. K., & Young, J. E. (1996). Schema-focused therapy. In P. M. Salkovskis (Ed.), *Frontiers of cognitive therapy* (pp. 182–207). New York: Guilford Press.

Meterissian, G. B., & Bradwejn, J. (1989). Comparative studies on the efficacy of psychotherapy, pharmacotherapy, and their combination in depression: Was adequate pharmacotherapy provided? *Journal of Clinical Psychopharmacology, 9,* 334–339.

Miller, I. W., Norman, W. H., Keitner, G. I., Bishop, S., & Dow, M. G. (1989). Cognitive-behavioral treatment of depressed inpatients. *Behavior Therapy, 20,* 25–47.

Mohr, D. C. (1995). Negative outcome in psychotherapy: A critical review. *Clinical Psychology: Science and Practice, 2,* 1–27.

Murphy, G. E., Simmons, A. D., Wetzel, R. D., & Lustman, P. J. (1984). Cognitive therapy and pharmacotherapy, singly and together, in the treatment of depression. *Archives of General Psychiatry, 41,* 33–41.

National Institute of Mental Health. (2006). The numbers count: Mental disorders in America (Publication No. 06-4584). Retrieved April 6, 2007, from *www.nimh.nih.gov/publicat/numbers.*

Newman, C. F., Leahy, R. L., Beck, A. T., Reilly-Harrington, N. A., & Gyulai, L. (2002). *Bipolar disorder: A cognitive therapy approach.* Washington, DC: American Psychological Association.

Nierenberg, A. A., Keefe, B. R., Leslie, V. C., Alpert, J. E., Pava, J. A., Worthington, J. J., III, et al. (1999). Residual symptoms in depressed patients who respond acutely to fluoxetine. *Journal of Clinical Psychiatry, 60*(4), 221–225.

Oei, T. P. S., & Free, M. L. (1995). Do cognitive behavior therapies validate cognitive models of mood disorders?: A review of the empirical evidence. *International Journal of Psychology, 30*(2), 145–180.

Oei, T. P. S., & Shuttlewood, G. J. (1996). Specific and non-specific factors in psychotherapy: A case of cognitive therapy for depression. *Clinical Psychology Review, 16*(2), 83–103.

O'Leary, K. D., & Beach, S. R. H. (1990). Marital therapy: A viable treatment for depression and marital discord. *American Journal of Psychiatry, 147*(2), 183–186.

Olfson, M., Marcus, S. C., Druss, B., Elinson, L., Tanielian, T., & Pincus, H. A. (2002). National trends in the outpatient treatment of depression. *Journal of the American Medical Association, 287,* 203–209.

Overholser, J. C. (1998). Cognitive-behavioral treatment of depression, part X: Reducing the risk of relapse. *Journal of Contemporary Psychotherapy, 28*(4), 381–396.

Padesky, C. A., with Greenberger, D. (1995). *A clinician's guide to mind over mood.* New York: Guilford Press.

Paykel, E. S. (2007). Cognitive therapy in relapse prevention in depression. *International Journal of Neuropsychopharmacology, 10,* 131–136.

Paykel, E. S., Scott, J., Teasdale, J. D., Johnson, A. L., Garland, A., Moore, R., et al. (1999). Prevention of relapse in residual depression by cognitive therapy. *Archives of General Psychiatry, 56,* 829–835.

Peeters, F., Huibers, M., Roelofs, J., van Breulkelen, G., Hollon, S. D., Markowitz, J. C., et al. (2013). The clinical effectiveness of evidence-based interventions for depression: A pragmatic trial in routine practice. *Journal of Affective Disorders, 145*(3), 349–355.

Pepper, C. M., Klein, D. N., Anderson, R. L., Riso, L. P., Ouimette, P. C., & Lizardi, H. (1995). DSM-III-R axis II comorbidity in dysthymia and major depression. *American Journal of Psychiatry, 152*(2), 239–247.

Persons, J. B., Burns, D. D., & Perloff, J. M. (1988). Predictors of dropout and outcome in cognitive therapy for depression in a private practice setting. *Cognitive Therapy and Research, 12*(6), 557–575.

Piper, W. E., Ogrodniczuk, J. S., Joyce, A. S., McCallum, M., Rosie, J. S., O'Kelly, J. G., et al. (1999). Prediction of dropping out in time-limited, interpretive psychotherapy. *Psychotherapy, 36,* 114–122.

Quilty, L. C., McBride, C., & Bagby, R. M. (2008). Evidence for the cognitive mediational model of cognitive behavioral therapy for depression. *Psychological Medicine, 38*(11), 1531–1541.

Randolph, J. J., & Dykman, B. M. (1998). Perceptions of parenting and depression-proneness in the offspring: Dysfunctional attitudes as a mediating mechanism. *Cognitive Depressive Disorders, 21,* 401–449.

Rehm, L. P. (1990). Cognitive and behavioral theories. In B. B. Wolman & G. Stricker (Eds.), *Depressive disorders: Facts, theories, and treatment methods* (pp. 64–91). New York: Wiley.

Reinecke, M. A., Ryan, N. E., & DuBois, D. L. (1998). Cognitive-behavioral therapy of depression and depressive symptoms during adolescence: A review and meta-analysis. *Journal of the American Academy of Child and Adolescent Psychiatry, 37*(1), 26–34.

Renner, F., Lobbestael, J., Peeters, F., Arntz, A., & Huibers, M. (2012). Early maladaptive schemas in depressed patients: Stability and relation with depressive symptoms over the course of treatment. *Journal of Affective Disorders, 136,* 581–590.

Riso, L. P., du Toit, P. L., Blandino, J. A., Penna, S., Dacey, S., Duin, J. S., et al. (2003). Cognitive aspects of chronic depression. *Journal of Abnormal Psychology, 112*(1), 72–80.

Riso, L. P., Froman, S. E., Raouf, M., Gable, P., Maddux, R. E., Turini-Santorelli, N., et al. (2006). The long-term stability of early maladaptive schemas. *Cognitive Therapy and Research, 30*(4), 515–529.

Roberts, J. E., & Hartlage, S. (1996). Cognitive rehabilitation interventions for depressed patients. In P. W. Corrigan & S. C. Yudofsky (Eds.), *Cognitive rehabilitation for neuropsychiatric disorders* (pp. 371–392). Washington, DC: American Psychiatric Press.

Rush, A. J., Beck, A. T., Kovacs, M., & Hollon, S. (1977). Comparative efficacy of cognitive therapy and imipramine in the treatment of depressed outpatients. *Cognitive Therapy and Research, 1,* 17–37.

Rush, A. J., Trivedi, M. H., Wisniewski, S. R., Nierenberg, A. A., Stewart, J. W., Warden, D., et al. (2006). Acute and longer-term outcomes in depressed outpatients requiring one of several treatment steps: A STAR*D report. *American Journal of Psychiatry, 163,* 1905–1917.

Sacco, W. P., & Beck, A. T. (1995). Cognitive theory and therapy. In E. E. Beckham & W. R. Leber (Eds.), *Handbook of depression* (2nd ed., pp. 329–351). New York: Guilford Press.

Sachs-Ericsson, N., Verona, E., Joiner, T., & Preacher, K. J. (2006). Parental abuse and mediating role of self-criticism in adult internalizing disorders. *Journal of Affective Disorders, 93*(1–3), 71–78.

Safran, J. D., Muran, J. C., Samstag, L. W., & Stevens, C. (2002). Repairing alliance ruptures. In J. C. Norcross (Ed.), *Psychotherapy relationships that work: Therapists contributions and responsiveness to patients* (pp. 235–254). New York: Oxford University Press.

Safran, J. D., & Segal, Z. V. (1990). *Interpersonal processes in cognitive therapy.* New York: Basic Books.

Safran, J. D., Segal, Z. V., Vallis, T. M., Shaw, B. F., & Samstag, L. W. (1993). Assessing patient suitability for short-term cognitive therapy with an interpersonal focus. *Cognitive Therapy and Research, 17*(1), 23–38.

Salkovskis, P. M. (Ed.). (1996). *Frontiers of cognitive therapy: The state of the art and beyond.* New York: Guilford Press.

Sava, F. A., Yates, B. T., Lupu, V., Szentagotai, A., & David, D. (2009). Cost-effectiveness and cost-utility of cognitive therapy, rational emotive behavioral therapy, and fluoxetine (Prozac) in treating depression: A randomized clinical trial. *Journal of Clinical Psychology, 65* (1), 36–52.

Schmidt, N. B. (1994). The Schema Questionnaire and the Schema Avoidance Questionnaire. *Behavior Therapist, 17*(4), 90–92.

Schmidt, N. B., Joiner, T. E., Young, J. E., & Telch, M. J.

(1995). The Schema Questionnaire: Investigation of psychometric properties and the hierarchical structure of a measure of maladaptive schemata. *Cognitive Therapy and Research, 19*(3), 295–321.

Schramm, E., Zobel, I., Dykierek, P., Kech, S., Brakemeier, E., Kutz, A., et al. (2011). Cognitive behavioral analysis system of psychotherapy versus interpersonal psychotherapy for early-onset chronic depression: A randomized pilot study. *Journal of Affective Disorders, 129,* 109–116.

Scott, J. (1996a). Cognitive therapy of affective disorders: A review. *Journal of Affective Disorders, 37,* 1–11.

Scott, J. (1996b). The role of cognitive behaviour therapy in bipolar disorders. *Behavioural and Cognitive Psychotherapy, 24*(3), 195–208.

Scott, J. (2000). New evidence in the treatment of chronic depression. *New England Journal of Medicine, 342,* 1518–1520.

Scott, J., Palmer, S., Paykel, E., Teasdale, J., & Hayhurst, H. (2003). Use of cognitive therapy for relapse prevention in chronic depression. *British Journal of Psychiatry, 182,* 221–227.

Segal, Z. V., Williams, J. M. G., & Teasdale, J. D. (2002). *Mindfulness-based cognitive therapy for depression: A new approach to preventing relapse.* New York: Guilford Press.

Shaw, B. F., & Segal, Z. V. (1999). Efficacy, indications, and mechanisms of action of cognitive therapy of depression. In D. S. Janowsky (Ed.), *Psychotherapy indications and outcomes* (pp. 173–196). Washington, DC: American Psychiatric Press.

Shea, M. T., & Elkin, I. (1996). The NIMH Treatment of Depression Collaborative Research Program. In C. Mundt, M. J. Goldstein, K. Hahlweg, & P. Fiedler (Eds.), *Interpersonal factors in the origin and course of affective disorders* (pp. 316–328). London: Gaskell/Royal College of Psychiatrists.

Shea, M. T., Elkin, I., Imber, S. D., Sotsky, S. M., Watkins, J. T., Collins, J. F., et al. (1992). Course of depressive symptoms over follow-up: Findings from the National Institute of Mental Health Treatment of Depression Collaborative Research Program. *Archives of General Psychiatry, 49*(10), 782–787.

Shea, M. T., Pilkonis, P. A., Beckham, E., Collins, J. F., Elkin, I., Sotsky, S. M., et al. (1990). Personality disorders and treatment outcome in the NIMH Treatment of Depression Collaborative Research Program. *American Journal of Psychiatry, 147*(6), 711–718.

Simons, A. D., Murphy, G. D., Levine, J. L., & Wetzel, R. D. (1986). Cognitive therapy and pharmacotherapy for depression: Sustained improvement over 1 year. *Archives of General Psychiatry, 43,* 43–48.

Spanier, C. A., Frank, E., McEachran, A. B., Grochocinski, V. J., & Kupfer, D. J. (1999). Maintenance interpersonal psychotherapy for recurrent depression: Biological and clinical correlates and future directions. In D. S. Janowsky (Ed.), *Psychotherapy indications and outcomes* (pp. 249–273). Washington, DC: American Psychiatric Press.

Spirito, A., Esposito-Smythers, C., Wolff, J., & Uhl, K. (2011). Cognitive-behavioral therapy for adolescent depression and suicidality. *Child and Adolescent Psychiatric Clinics of North America, 20*(2), 191–204.

Stein, D. J., & Young, J. E. (1992). Schema approach to personality disorders. In *Cognitive science and clinical disorders* (pp. 271–288). San Diego, CA: Academic Press.

Stirman, S. W., Miller, C. J., Toder, K., Calloway, A., Beck, A. J., Evans, A. C., et al. (in press). Perspectives on cognitive therapy training within community mental health settings: Implications for clinical satisfaction and skill development. *Depression Research and Treatment*.

Strine, T. W., Mokdad, A. H., Balluz, L. S., Gonzalez, O., Crider, R., Berry, J. T., et al. (2008). Depression and anxiety in the United States: Findings from the 2006 Behavioral Risk Factor Surveillance System. *Psychiatric Services, 59*(12), 1383–1309.

Stuart, S., & Bowers, W. A. (1995). Cognitive therapy with inpatients: Review and meta-analysis. *Journal of Cognitive Psychotherapy, 9*(2), 85–92.

Substance Abuse and Mental Health Services Administration (SAMHSA). (2008). Results from 2007 National Survey on Drug Use and Health: National Findings (Office of Applied Studies, NSDUH Series H-34, DHHS Publication No. SMA 08-4343). Rockville, MD: U.S. Department of Health and Human Services.

Sullivan, M. J. L., & Conway, M. (1991). Dysphoria and valence of attributions for others' behavior. *Cognitive Therapy and Research, 15*(4), 273–282.

Teasdale, J. D. (1997a). Assessing cognitive mediation of relapse prevention in recurrent mood disorders. *Clinical Psychology and Psychotherapy, 4*, 145–156.

Teasdale, J. D. (1997b). The relationship between cognition and emotion: The mind-in-place in mood disorders. In D. M. Clark & C. G. Fairburn (Eds.), *Science and practice of cognitive behavior therapy* (pp. 67–93). Oxford, UK: Oxford University Press.

Teasdale, J. D., Moore, R. G., Hayhurst, H., Pope, M., Williams, S., & Segal, Z. V. (2002). Metacognitive awareness and prevention of relapse in depression: Empirical evidence. *Journal of Consulting and Clinical Psychology, 70*(2), 275–287.

Teasdale, J. D., Segal, Z. V., & Williams, J. M. G. (1995). How does cognitive therapy prevent depressive relapse and why should attentional control (mindfulness) training help? *Behaviour Research and Therapy, 33*, 25–39.

Teasdale, J. D., Segal, Z. V., Williams, J. M. G., Ridgeway, V. A., Soulsby, J. M., & Lau, M. A. (2000). Prevention of relapse/recurrence in major depression by mindfulness-based cognitive therapy. *Journal of Consulting and Clinical Psychology, 68*(4), 615–623.

Thase, M. E. (1992). Long-term treatments of recurrent depressive disorders. *Journal of Clinical Psychiatry, 53*(Suppl. 9), 32–44.

Thase, M. E. (1999). How should efficacy be evaluated in randomized clinical trials of treatments for depression? *Journal of Clinical Psychiatry, 60*(Suppl. 4), 23–32.

Thase, M. E. (2011). Antidepressant combinations: Widely used, but far from empirically validated. *Canadian Journal of Psychiatry, 56*(6), 317–323.

Thase, M. E., Bowler, K., & Harden, T. (1991). Cognitive behavior therapy of endogenous depression: Part 2. Preliminary findings in 16 unmedicated inpatients. *Behavior Therapy, 22*, 469–477.

Tolin, D. F. (2010). Is cognitive-behavioral therapy more effective than other therapies? A meta-analytic review. *Clinical Psychology Review, 30*(6), 710–720.

Treatment for Adolescents with Depression Study (TADS) Team. (2004). Fluoxetine, cognitive-behavioral therapy, and their combination for adolescents with depression: Treatment for adolescents with depression study (TADS) randomized controlled trial. *Journal of the American Medical Association, 292*(7), 807–820.

Treatment for Adolescents with Depression Study (TADS) Team. (2007). Long term effectiveness and safety outcomes. *Archives of General Psychiatry, 64*, 1132–1144.

Trivedi, M. H., Fava, M., Wisniewski, S. R., Thase, M. E., Quitkin, F., Warden, D., et al. (2006). Medication augmentation after the failure of SSRIs for depression. *New England Journal of Medicine, 354*, 1243–1252.

Truax, C. B., & Mitchell, K. M. (1971). Research on certain therapist interpersonal skills in relation to process and outcome. In A. E. Bergin & S. L. Garfield (Eds.), *Handbook of psychotherapy and behavior change: An empirical analysis* (pp. 299–344). New York: Wiley.

van Aalderen, J. R., Donders, A. R. T., Giommi, F., Spinhoven, P., Barendregt, H. P., & Speckens, A. E. M. (2012). The efficacy of mindfulness-based cognitive therapy in recurrent depressed patients with and without a current depressive episode: A randomized controlled trial. *Psychological Medicine, 42*, 989–1001.

Versiani, M. (1998). Pharmacotherapy of dysthymic and chronic depressive disorders: Overview with focus on moclobemide. *Journal of Affective Disorders, 51*(3), 323–332.

Vittengl, J. R., Clark, L. A., Dunn, T. D., & Jarrett, R. B. (2007). Reducing relapse and recurrence in unipolar depression: A comparative meta-analysis of cognitive-behavioral therapy's effects. *Journal of Consulting and Clinical Psychology, 75*(3), 475–488.

Vittengl, J. R., Clark, L. A., & Jarrett, R. B. (2009). Continuation-phase cognitive therapy's effect on remission and recovery from depression. *Journal of Consulting and Clinical Psychology, 77*(2), 367–371.

Vocisano, C., Klein, D., Arnow, B., Rivera, C., Blalock, J. A., Rothbaum, B., et al. (2004). Therapist variables that predict symptom change in psychotherapy with chronically depressed outpatients. *Psychotherapy: Theory, Research, Practice and Training, 41*(3), 255–265.

Vos, T., Corry, J., Haby, M. M., Carter, R., & Andrews, G. (2005). Cost-effectiveness of cognitive-behavioural therapy and drug interventions for major depression. *Australian and New Zealand Journal of Psychiatry, 39*(8), 683–692.

Wang, C. E., Halvorsen, M., Eisemann, M., & Waterloo, K. (2010). Stability of dysfunctional attitudes and early maladaptive schemas: A 9-year follow-up study of clinically depressed subjects. *Journal of Behavior Therapy and Experimental Psychiatry, 41*(4), 389–396.

Wang, J. (2004). A longitudinal population-based study of treated and untreated major depression. *Medical Care, 42*(6), 543–550.

Wang, J., Patten, S. D., William, J. V., Currie, S., Beck, C. A., Maxwell, C. J., et al. (2005). Help seeking behaviors of individuals with mood disorders. *Canadian Journal of Psychiatry, 50*(10), 652–659.

Wells, A., Fisher, P., Myers, S., Wheatley, J., Patel, T., & Brewin, C. R. (2012). Metacognitive therapy in treatment-resistant depression: A platform trial. *Behaviour Research and Therapy, 50*(6), 367–373.

Whisman, M. A. (1993). Mediators and moderators of change in cognitive therapy of depression. *Psychological Bulletin, 114*, 248–265.

Wiersma, J. E., van Schaik, D. J. F., van Oppen, P., McCullough, J. P., Schoevers, R. A., Dekker, J. J., et al. (2008). Treatment of chronically depressed patients: A multisite randomized controlled trial testing the effectiveness of "cognitive behavioral analysis system of psychotherapy" (CBASP) for chronic depression versus usual secondary care. *BMC Psychiatry, 8*, 18.

Wierzbicki, M., & Bartlett, T. S. (1987). The efficacy of group and individual cognitive therapy for mild depression. *Cognitive Therapy and Research, 11*(3), 337–342.

Williams, J. M. G. (1997). Depression. In D. M. Clark & C. G. Fairburn (Eds.), *Science and practice of cognitive behaviour therapy* (pp. 259–283). Oxford, UK: Oxford University Press.

Wolpe, J. (1993). Commentary: The cognitivist oversell and comments on symposium contributions. *Journal of Behavior Therapy and Experimental Psychiatry, 24*(2), 141–147.

World Health Organization (WHO). (2004). The Global Burden on Disease 2004 update. Retrieved from *www.who.int/healthinfo/global_burden_disease/GBD_report_2004update_full.pdf*.

Wright, J. H. (1996). Inpatient cognitive therapy. In P. M. Salkovskis (Ed.), *Frontiers of cognitive therapy* (pp. 208–225). New York: Guilford Press.

Wright, J. H., & McCray, L. W. (2011). *Breaking free from depression: Pathways to wellness.* New York: Guilford Press.

Wright, J. H., Wright, A. S., Albano, A. M., Basco, M. R., Goldsmith, L. J., Raffield, T., et al. (2005). Computer-assisted cognitive therapy for depression: Maintaining efficacy while reducing therapist time. *American Journal of Psychiatry, 162*, 1158–1164.

Young, J. E. (1999). *Cognitive therapy for personality disorders: A schema-focused approach* (3rd ed.). Sarasota, FL: Professional Resource Exchange. (Original work published 1990)

Young, J. E. (2005). *Young Schema Questionnaire* (3rd ed.). New York: Cognitive Therapy Center of New York.

Young, J. E., Arntz, A., Atkinson, T., Lobbestael, J., Weishaar, E., van Vreeswijk, M., et al. (2008). *Schema Mode Questionnaire (Version 1.1).* New York: Cognitive Therapy Center of New York.

Young, J. E., & Klosko, J. S. (1994). *Reinventing your life: How to break free of negative life patterns.* New York: Plume.

Young, J. E., Klosko, J. S., & Weishaar, M. E. (2003). *Schema therapy: A practitioner's guide.* New York: Guilford Press.

Zettle, R. (2007). *ACT for depression: A clinician's guide to using acceptance and commitment therapy in treating depression.* Richmond, BC, Canada: Raincoat Books.

CHAPTER 8

Interpersonal Psychotherapy for Depression

KATHRYN L. BLEIBERG
JOHN C. MARKOWITZ

Much evidence has emerged over the past decade supporting the clinical effectiveness of interpersonal psychotherapy (IPT) for a variety of problems, particularly depression. A substantial advantage of IPT is the relative ease with which clinicians can learn to administer this protocol with integrity. In this chapter, the process of IPT is illustrated in some detail in the context of the treatment of "Sara," who was suffering from a major depressive episode associated with grief following the death of her baby girl *in utero* at 27 weeks' gestation, some 2 months earlier. The first author, Kathryn L. Bleiberg, an international authority on training in IPT, was the therapist. Although IPT is relatively easy to comprehend, the twists and turns encountered in the administration of IPT (or any therapeutic approach) are particularly evident in this chapter. Here the therapist skillfully focuses on resolving grief, as well as on the patient's social isolation and conflicts with her husband over emotional reactions to the loss. Also notable about IPT is the finding that the treatment is more successful when administered with fidelity to the goals of IPT and adherence to the protocol. The power of a therapist and patient working well together and staying on task provides some good evidence for the specific effects of an interpersonal focus to psychotherapy.—D. H. B.

Interpersonal psychotherapy (IPT), a time-limited, diagnosis-targeted, pragmatic, empirically supported treatment, was originally developed to treat outpatients with major depression. IPT focuses on current or recent life events, interpersonal difficulties, and symptoms. Through use of the medical model and by linking mood symptoms to recent life events, the IPT therapist helps the patient to feel understood. IPT aids recovery from depression by relieving depressive symptoms, by helping the patient to develop more effective strategies for dealing with current interpersonal problems related to the onset of symptoms, and by mobilizing social support (Bleiberg & Markowitz, 2007). IPT's success as

an individual treatment for major depression has led to its adaptation for subpopulations of patients with mood disorders, including depressed older patients (Reynolds et al., 2006, 2010; Sholomskas, Chevron, Prusoff, & Berry, 1983), depressed adolescents (Mufson, Moreau, & Weissman, 1993; Mufson, Weissman, Moreau, & Garfinkel, 1999; Mufson et al., 2004), and depressed HIV-positive patients (Markowitz, Klerman, Perry, Clougherty, & Mayers, 1992; Markowitz, Kocsis, et al., 1998; Ransom et al., 2008), and patients with antepartum (Spinelli & Endicott, 2003) and postpartum depression (O'Hara, Stuart, Gorman, & Wenzel, 2000), dysthymic disorder (Markowitz, 1998), and bipolar disorder (Frank, 2005). IPT has been adapted for anxiety disorders, including social phobia (Lipsitz, Fyer, Markowitz, & Cherry, 1999), posttraumatic stress disorder (Bleiberg & Markowitz, 2005; Markowitz, Milrod, Bleiberg, & Marshall, 2009), bulimia nervosa (Fairburn, Jones, Peveler, Hope, & O'Connor, 1993; Fairburn et al., 1995) and binge-eating disorder (Wilfley, 2008; Wilson, Wilfley, Agras, & Bryson, 2010), and borderline personality disorder (Markowitz, Skodol, & Bleiberg, 2006). In addition to its adaptation to treat patients with different diagnoses, IPT has been increasingly practiced and studied among patients from different cultures (Markowitz & Weissman, 2012a). Furthermore, IPT's demonstrated efficacy in the treatment of major depression has led to its incorporation into national treatment guidelines (American Psychiatric Association, 2010; Cuijpers et al., 2011).

This chapter describes the principles, characteristics, and techniques of individual IPT for major depression and illustrates how a clinician implements IPT techniques with an actual patient.

MAJOR DEPRESSION

Major depressive disorder (MDD), the most common depressive illness, affects millions of Americans each year. The Global Burden of Disease Study, initiated by the World Health Organization (Murray & Lopez, 1996), estimated that depression is the fourth leading cause of disability and will become the second leading cause worldwide by the year 2020. Epidemiological studies of mood disorders have provided estimates of the prevalence and correlates of MDD. The National Comorbidity Survey Replication (NCS-R; Kessler et al., 2003) found a 16.2% lifetime and 6.6% annual prevalence of MDD in the United States, with the majority of cases of MDD associated with substantial symptom severity and impairment in functioning. National and international studies have consistently found higher prevalence of MDD in women than in men; women are twice as likely as men to experience an episode of MDD. The average age of onset of MDD is between ages 20 and 40 years (Blazer, 2000).

The *Diagnostic and Statistical Manual of Mental Disorders*, fifth edition (DSM-5; American Psychiatric Association, 2013) defines MDD as a mood disorder characterized by one or more major depressive episodes. A major depressive episode entails a period of at least 2 weeks during which a person experiences depressed mood or loss of interest or pleasure in nearly all activities most of the day, nearly every day, accompanied by at least four additional symptoms of depression present nearly every day. Symptoms of depression include the following:

- Significant weight loss (not related to dieting), or weight gain or decrease or increase in appetite.
- Insomnia or hypersomnia.
- Psychomotor agitation or retardation severe enough to be observable by others.
- Fatigue or loss of energy.
- Feelings of worthlessness, or excessive or inappropriate or excessive guilt.
- Diminished ability to think or concentrate, or indecisiveness.
- Recurrent thoughts of death, recurrent suicidal ideation without a specific plan, or a suicide attempt or a specific plan to commit suicide.

To meet full criteria for a major depressive episode, the patient's symptoms must cause clinically significant distress or impairment in social, occupational, or other important areas of functioning. Depression is associated with social withdrawal and difficulty in social and occupational functioning. In some cases, a major depressive episode will be accompanied by symptoms of a manic episode, which is classified in DSM-5 using the specifier *with mixed features*. The symptoms may not be due to the direct physiological effects of a substance or a general medical condition.

THE DEVELOPMENT OF IPT

Klerman, Weissman, and colleagues developed IPT in the 1970s as a treatment arm for a pharmacotherapy study of depression (Markowitz & Weissman, 2012b). Being researchers, they developed a psychotherapy based on research data. Post–World War II research on psychosocial life events and the development of mental disorders had shown relationships between depression and complicated bereavement, role disputes (i.e., bad relationships), role transitions (e.g., losing or getting a new job, or any meaningful life change), and interpersonal deficits. Stressful life events can trigger depressive episodes in vulnerable individuals, and depressive episodes compromise interpersonal functioning, making it difficult to manage stressful life events, and often triggering further negative life events (Bleiberg & Markowitz, 2007).

IPT was also built on the interpersonal theory of Adolph Meyer (1957) and Harry Stack Sullivan (1953), and on the attachment theory of John Bowlby (1973). The interpersonalists broadened the scope of psychiatry by emphasizing social, cultural, and interpersonal factors. Sullivan stressed the role of interpersonal relationships in the development of mental illness and the use of interpersonal relationships to understand, assess, and treat mental illness. Sullivan also indicated that life events and relationships occurring *after* early childhood influenced psychopathology, in contradistinction to the then current focus on pre-Oedipal life events.

Bowlby (1973) posited that the disruption of secure attachments can contribute to the onset of depression, and that psychiatric disorders result from difficulties in forming and maintaining secure attachments. Indeed, social supports protect against depression. In psychiatry, the idea that mental illness was influenced by current life events and not (simply) due to early childhood experiences was novel in an era divided between psychoanalytic and biological approaches (Klerman, Weissman, Rounsaville, & Chevron, 1984).

PRINCIPLES OF IPT: THE IPT MODEL OF DEPRESSION

Two basic principles of IPT explain the patient's depression and situation. These principles are simple enough to grasp, even for a very depressed patient with poor concentration. First, the IPT therapist defines depression as a medical illness and explains that the patient has a common illness that comprises a discrete and predictable set of symptoms, thus making the symptoms seem less overwhelming and more manageable. The IPT therapist assumes that the etiology of depression is complex and multidetermined: The etiology may comprise biology, life experiences, and family history, among other factors. The IPT therapist emphasizes that *depression is a medical illness that is treatable and not the patient's fault.* Explaining that depression is treatable inspires in patients the hope that they can feel better. Hopelessness, a potentially deadly depressive symptom, distorts the generally good prognosis of the illness. Depressed patients often see their symptoms and consequent difficulties in functioning as reflections of a personal failure, character flaw, or weakness.

Defining depression as a blameless illness helps to combat the depressed patient's guilt and self-criticism. The therapist diagnoses depression using DSM-5 or *International Classification of Diseases* (ICD-10; World Health Organization, 1992) criteria and assesses symptoms using rating scales such as the Hamilton Depression Rating Scale (HDRS; Hamilton, 1960) or the Beck Depression Inventory–II (BDI-II; Beck, Steer, & Brown, 1996). IPT's use of the medical model to define depression distinguishes it from other psychotherapies and makes it highly compatible with antidepressant medication in combination treatment.

The second IPT principle is that the patient's depression is connected to a current or recent life event. Stressful life events can precipitate depressive episodes in vulnerable individuals and, conversely, depression can make it difficult for individuals to manage stressful life events. IPT focuses on solving an interpersonal problem in the patient's life, a problem area—complicated bereavement, a role dispute, a role transition, or interpersonal deficits—connected to the patient's current depressive episode. By solving an interpersonal crisis, the patient can improve her[1] life situation and simultaneously relieve depressive symptoms.

CHARACTERISTICS OF IPT

Several characteristics define IPT, sometimes distinguishing it from other psychotherapies.

- *IPT is time-limited and focused.* Acute treatment at the start is set at 12 or 16 weekly sessions. Some studies have included continuation and maintenance phases, which involve biweekly and monthly sessions. IPT's time limit provides hope for patients that their symptoms and life situation can rapidly improve; the time limit encourages patients to stay focused in treatment. It also pressures both patient and therapist to work hard and efficiently within the therapeutic window of opportunity. Therapist and patient agree to focus on one, or at most two, problem areas at the beginning of treatment.

- *IPT is empirically grounded.* Because IPT has shown repeated efficacy in research studies, therapists can offer and deliver the treatment with confidence and optimism, and patients can feel hopeful about the treatment they are receiving.

- *IPT is diagnosis-targeted.* IPT focuses on a specific diagnosis, its symptoms, and how symptoms interfere and interact with social functioning. IPT is not intended for all patients, but it has been tested in a series of randomized controlled trials to determine its efficacy.

- *IPT has a "here-and-now" focus.* IPT focuses on the present and on improving the patient's situation for the future—not on what happened in the patient's past. The IPT therapist relates current symptoms and interpersonal difficulties to recent or current life events. Although past depressive episodes and relationships are reviewed and relationship patterns are identified, treatment focuses on current relationships—building social supports and resolving disputes—and social functioning.

- *IPT focuses on interpersonal problems.* The IPT therapist may recognize intrapsychic defenses but does not see the patient's current difficulties as a function of internal conflict. Instead, the therapist focuses on interpersonal relationships and functioning.

- *IPT focuses on the interrelationship between mood and current life events.* The IPT therapist emphasizes that stressful life events can trigger episodes of major depression and, reciprocally, that depression compromises psychosocial functioning. This makes it difficult to manage life stressors, leading to further negative life events.

- *IPT emphasizes eliciting affect.* Depressed patients often have difficulty understanding, identifying, and articulating what they are feeling. Whereas patients with depression tend to report feeling "bad," they often have difficulty identifying negative feelings more specifically, such as anger, hurt, shame, rejection, disappointment. Furthermore, depressed patients who do recognize such negative affects tend to feel ashamed of having such "bad" emotions. The IPT therapist helps the patient to better identify what she is feeling, validates emotions such as anger and disappointment as normal and useful interpersonal signals, and helps the patient to use such emotion as a guide (Markowitz & Milrod, 2011). Patients in IPT learn to manage their feelings better and to use them in deciding how to behave and what to say in interpersonal encounters.

IPT COMPARED WITH OTHER PSYCHOTHERAPIES

Although IPT has a distinct rationale and is distinguishable from other psychotherapies (Hill, O'Grady, & Elkin, 1992; Weissman, Markowitz, & Klerman, 2000), it is an eclectic psychotherapy that uses techniques seen in other treatment approaches. IPT includes the so-called "common" factors of psychotherapy (Frank, 1971). IPT shares the "here and now" diagnostic focus, time limit, and active approach with cognitive-behavioral therapy (CBT). IPT and CBT both include role playing and skills building. However, IPT is much less structured and assigns no formal homework, although the IPT therapist does encourage activity between sessions to improve mood and as it relates to resolving the interpersonal problem area. Whereas the CBT therapist defines depression as a consequence of dysfunctional thought patterns and attributes the patient's difficulties to them, the IPT therapist emphasizes that depression is a medical illness and relates difficulties to feeling depressed and to recent life events. IPT emphasizes eliciting affect rather than ("hot," affectively charged) automatic thoughts. IPT addresses interpersonal issues in a manner similar to that in marital therapy. Much like a supportive therapist, IPT therapists provide support and encouragement (Bleiberg & Markowitz, 2007).

IPT has been termed a "psychodynamic" psychotherapy on occasion, but it is not (Markowitz, Svartberg, & Swartz, 1998). IPT employs the medical model of depressive illness, whereas psychodynamic psychotherapy uses a conflict-based approach. The IPT therapist does not address unconscious processes, or explore or interpret the transference, but instead focuses on current relationships outside of the treatment room. Childhood experiences are recognized but not emphasized. The IPT therapist relates current symptoms and interpersonal problems to recent life events, not to childhood experiences. IPT acknowledges the influence of past experiences on present difficulties, but only to identify patterns of interpersonal behavior and to empathize with the patient's struggle. Unlike psychodynamic treatment, the goal in IPT is to reduce symptoms and improve social functioning, not to change character or personality. Like the psychodynamic psychotherapist, however, the IPT therapist emphasizes facilitating affect in the treatment room and helping patients become aware of feelings they may not have been aware of previously (Markowitz & Milrod, 2011; Weissman et al., 2000).

THE IPT THERAPIST

The IPT therapist conducts treatment in an office in an academic, hospital, or private practice setting. The therapist typically does not consult with the patient's family or friends.

The IPT therapist takes a non-neutral, active stance, providing psychoeducation about depression, emphasizing the IPT rationale, teaching social skills, and instilling hope. A somewhat directive approach is essential for adhering to the time limit in IPT and keeping the treatment focused on the interpersonal problem area. Taking an active stance may be challenging for therapists with psychodynamic orientations who are used to taking a neutral stance and offering little guidance in the session.

On the other hand, the IPT therapist does not want to reinforce the passivity and dependency that are characteristic of depression. A therapist who solves all problems may reinforce the patient's sense of inadequacy. Hence, the IPT therapist encourages the patient to come up with ideas, explore options, and test them out between sessions. Hence, the patient deserves (and is given) credit for making the life changes that lead to improvement in treatment.

The IPT therapist needs to be supportive, enthusiastic, and optimistic to instill hope that the depression will improve and changes will be forthcoming, and to encourage and inspire the patient to make changes. The structure of the IPT manual (Weissman et al., 2000; Weissman, Markowitz, & Klerman, 2007) and the empirical validation of IPT in randomized controlled studies help to bolster therapist confidence. The IPT therapist frequently congratulates the patient on her progress in treatment and efforts to make changes.

Given the emphasis on helping the patient to identify and express feelings, the IPT therapist needs to feel comfortable encouraging expression of affect and tolerating intense negative affects. The therapist can show by example that feelings are indeed potent, but they are only feelings, and can be understood in an interpersonal context and will pass, if tolerated.

THE IPT PATIENT

Research has demonstrated that a wide range of patients with major depression are good candidates for IPT. IPT has been validated with minor modifications as a treatment for adolescent, adult, peripartum, and geriatric depression. The patient should ideally report some recent life stressor and have some social contacts. Patients with depression who report no recent life events and lack basic social skills tend to do least well in IPT. IPT is not intended for patients with delusional depression, which requires antidepressant and antipsychotic pharmacotherapy or electroconvulsive therapy.

Patients with comorbid moderate or severe personality disorder may be less likely to respond to short-term psychotherapy (Weissman et al., 2000). Accordingly, the recent adaptation of IPT for borderline personality disorder allows up to 32 weeks of treatment (Markowitz et al., 2006).

THE FOUR INTERPERSONAL PROBLEM AREAS

Treatment with IPT focuses on solving one of the following four interpersonal problem areas related to the onset or maintenance of the patient's current depressive episode. The IPT therapist follows strategies specific to each problem area.

Grief

This problem area addresses a patient's complicated bereavement following the death of a significant other. The therapist facilitates the mourning process, encourages catharsis, and ultimately helps the patient to form new relationships and find new activities to compensate for the loss. The therapist explores the relationship and the associated feelings the patient had with the loved one. Patients with complicated bereavement often have had a conflicted relationship with the deceased, reporting unresolved feelings about and anger toward the person, and feeling guilty or uncomfortable with such feelings. Patients may feel guilty about what they did or did not say to or do for the person who died. The therapist encourages exploration of these feelings and validates and normalizes negative feelings, allowing the patient to let go of the guilt she experiences.

The release of negative affects in the therapy office can help to diminish the intensity of such feelings. The therapist also explores positive feelings the patient had for the person she lost and empathizes with the loss. Finally, the therapist helps the patient explore options for forming new relationships and finding new activities to help to substitute for the lost relationship and give the patient a new sense of direction. The loss may provide opportunities to meet people and engage in activities the patient might not otherwise have encountered.

Role Disputes

A "role dispute" is a conflict with a significant other: a spouse, friend, parent, relative, employer, coworker, or close friend. The therapist and patient explore the relationship, the nature of the dispute, and options to resolve it. Patients with depression tend to put other people's needs ahead of their own. They have difficulty asserting themselves, confronting others, and getting angry effectively, which makes it difficult for them to manage interpersonal conflicts. The therapist discusses these depressive tendencies with patients and explains: "It's not your fault. You can learn how to assert yourself."

The therapist validates the patient's feelings in the relationship: recognizing anger as a natural response to someone bothering her, for example. The next question is how to express such feelings. The therapist helps the patient to conceive ways to communicate thoughts and feelings more effectively and role-plays potential interactions with her. If, after exploring and attempting to implement options to resolve the dispute, the conflict has reached an impasse, the therapist helps the patient to consider ways either to live with the impasse or end the relationship.

Role Transitions

A "role transition" is a change in life status, such as beginning or ending a relationship, starting or losing a job, a geographic move, graduation or retirement, becoming a parent, or receiving the diagnosis of a medical illness. The therapist helps the patient to mourn the loss of the old role, to explore positive and negative aspects of the new role, and to determine what positive aspects of the old role, if any, she can retain. Ultimately, the therapist helps the patient adjust to and gain a sense of mastery over the new role. Even if a new role is wanted or positive, the role may be accompanied by unanticipated loss. For example, getting married may involve having to spend less time with one's family of origin due to having to spend time with the spouse's family. Moving to a new, larger house in a better neighborhood may disrupt relationships with friends in the old neighborhood. If a new role is undesired, a patient may discover unseen benefits in therapy. A patient who has lost a job may come to see the loss as an opportunity to pursue a better job.

Interpersonal Deficits

Interpersonal deficits, the least developed of the four problem areas, are the focus of IPT for major depression only when a patient reports no recent life events and, therefore, lacks any of the first three problem areas. Patients in this category tend to be socially iso-

lated, and to have few social supports and a history of difficulty forming and sustaining relationships or finding relationships unfulfilling. The goal of treatment in this problem area is to reduce the patient's isolation. Because the patient lacks current relationships, treatment focuses on patterns in past relationships and starting to form new ones. The therapist reviews past significant relationships, exploring positive and negative aspects and identifying recurrent problems. The therapist helps the patient to explore options for meeting people and participating in activities that she used to enjoy.

Unlike treatment for the other problem areas, treatment for interpersonal deficits may focus on the relationship with the therapist. In the absence of other relationships, and with the understanding that the patient is likely to feel uncomfortable in the therapeutic situation, the therapist encourages the patient to discuss her feelings about the therapist and work on interpersonal problems that arise in their relationship. Ideally, the relationship with the therapist serves as model for the patient to form other relationships. Given that IPT usually focuses on a life event, it is not surprising that patients who lack such life events have been shown to respond least well to IPT. It is important to identify patients who have underlying dysthymic disorder because such patients often describe few recent life events. There is an IPT protocol adapted to the treatment of patients who are dysthymic (Markowitz, 1998; Weissman et al., 2000).

THE PROCESS OF IPT TREATMENT

Acute IPT treatment for major depression comprises initial, middle, and termination phases. IPT techniques help the patient to pursue the goals of treatment for each interpersonal problem area. This section leads into a case example illustrating the implementation of these techniques.

The Initial Phase (Sessions 1–3)

Tasks of the initial sessions of IPT for major depression include eliciting the patient's chief complaint; reviewing her symptoms and establishing a diagnosis; determining the interpersonal context for the current depressive episode; forming a therapeutic alliance; and setting the frame of the treatment, including the treatment goals and strategies. Although these tasks are common to other psychotherapeutic interventions, the techniques and process for accomplishing them are specific to IPT.

Diagnosing Major Depression

To diagnosis MDD, the therapist reviews current symptoms of depression using either DSM-5 or ICD-10 criteria, inquiring about each symptom and about any past history of depression. The therapist may administer a symptom severity scale such as the HDRS (Hamilton, 1960) or the BDI-II (Beck et al., 1996) and repeat the instrument every few weeks to monitor the patient's progress. The therapist rules out other diagnoses, such as bipolar illness, depression due to general medical condition or substance, and other psychiatric disorders. If the patient meets criteria for MDD, the therapist tells her, describing explicitly each of the symptoms she reported:

> "You have an illness called major depression. The symptoms you describe having had for the past couple of months—feeling down most of the time, having difficulty enjoying things, feeling like you have to push yourself to get things done, difficulty sleeping, loss of appetite, trouble concentrating, and feeling very self-critical and down on yourself and pessimistic about your future—are all symptoms of depression. Depression is a treatable illness. It is not your fault that you feel this way and have had difficulty functioning, any more than it would be your fault if you had asthma or high blood pressure, or any other medical problem. And although you're feeling hopeless, that's just a depressive symptom. Your prognosis with treatment is quite good. You can feel better."

In the initial phase, and as needed throughout the treatment, the therapist provides psychoeducation about depression and how it affects social functioning. The therapist helps the patient to identify and understand her depressive symptoms and how better to manage them, and to distinguish between the illness and premorbid strengths and capabilities. The therapist determines the need for medication based on symptom severity, past response to medications, and patient preference.

The "Sick Role"

The IPT therapist gives the patient the "sick role" (Parsons, 1951), a temporary role intended to help the patient recognize that she suffers from an illness that comprises a distinct set of symptoms that compromise

functioning. Assuming the sick role relieves the patient of self-blame and exempts her from responsibilities that the depression compromises until she recovers. The therapist educates the patient about how depression can impair social functioning and how to explain the illness to family and friends to gain support. The sick role also gives the patient the responsibility of working on improving her symptoms in treatment.

The Interpersonal Inventory

In IPT the psychiatric history includes the "interpersonal inventory," a thorough review of the patient's past and current social functioning, close relationships, relationship patterns, expectations of others within relationships, and the perceived expectations that others have of the patient. The interpersonal inventory should give the therapist a sense of how the patient interacts with other people. It should also illuminate how relationships may have contributed to the current depressive episode and, conversely, how depressive symptoms may be affecting current relationships. Furthermore, the interpersonal inventory assesses actual and potential social support. To glean this information, the IPT therapist asks detailed questions about the patient's past and current relationships. An inquiry about current relationships might include the following questions:

> "Who is in your life currently? . . . Do you have a significant other? . . . Girlfriend/boyfriend? . . . What is your relationship like with him/her? . . . What do you like about him/her? . . . What don't you like? . . . Do you and your spouse argue? . . . What do you argue about? . . . What happens when you argue—what do you do/say? . . . What do you expect of him/her? . . . What do you think he/she expects of you?"

Identification of Interpersonal Problem Areas

The primary goal of the interpersonal inventory is to determine which interpersonal issues are most related to the patient's current depressive episode. The therapist should identify major interpersonal problem areas that can become the treatment focus. The therapist inquires about any changes in the patient's life that occurred around the onset of current depressive symptoms: "What was going on in your life when you became depressed?" The therapist explores different areas in the patient's life: home, work, relationships with significant others, family members, and friends. The therapist should pick one problem area on which to focus, or at most two; too many treatment foci yield an unfocused treatment. The therapist relates the depression to a problem area and presents this to the patient in a formulation:

> "It seems from what you have been telling me that the main problem has been your difficulty in getting along with your husband. Although the causes of depression are complex and not fully known, we do know that conflicts with significant others can be related to depression. Furthermore, depression can make it difficult to handle conflicts with other people. I suggest that we meet for the next 12 weeks to figure out how you can better deal with the problems with your husband you've described. In IPT, we call that conflict a 'role dispute.' As you solve your role dispute, both your life and your depression should improve. Does this make sense to you?"

Only with the patient's explicit agreement to work on the chosen interpersonal problem area does the therapist proceed to the middle phase of treatment. The patient's agreement on the focus allows the therapist to bring her back to this theme thereafter, maintaining a thematic flow for the treatment.

Explanation of the Treatment Contract and the IPT Approach

In addition to agreeing on a treatment focus in the initial sessions, the therapist and patient discuss and come to an understanding about other aspects of the treatment. The therapist discusses practical issues, including the time limit, the length and frequency of sessions, termination date, appointment time, fee, and so forth. The therapist explains that IPT is one of several empirically supported antidepressant treatments and describes the basic IPT principles. The therapist emphasizes the "here and now," and the social and interpersonal focus of the treatment, explaining:

> "We'll work together to try to understand how current stresses and relationships may be affecting your mood. We will work on helping you to better manage these stresses and the problems you may be having in relationships. We'll explore what you want and need in your relationships and help you figure out how to get what you want and need.

> "I'll be interested in hearing each week about what's going on in your relationships with other people, how those interactions make you feel, and also how your feelings influence what happens with other people."

The therapist encourages the patient to bring up any discomforts she has about the sessions.

> "If anything bothers you, please bring it up. I do not intend to do anything to make you uncomfortable, but if you feel that way, please tell me, so that we can address the issue. It's just the sort of interpersonal tension that we need to focus on in your outside life as well."

The Middle Phase (Sessions 4–9)

Having made the treatment contract and chosen an interpersonal problem area as the focus of treatment, the therapist can proceed to the middle phase of sessions, in which the goal is to work on resolving the focal problem area.

Each session begins with the question, "How have you been feeling since we last met?" This question elicits an interval history of mood, events, and interpersonal interactions that transpired between sessions. It also keeps the patient focused on current mood and situation. The patient is likely to respond by describing a mood ("I felt really down") or an event ("My husband and I had a huge fight"). After further inquiry, the therapist links the patient's mood to a recent event, or an event to her mood ("No wonder you felt depressed after the fight you had with your husband!").

Inquiring about emotionally laden interpersonal interactions, the therapist uses "communication analysis"—the reconstruction and evaluation of affectively charged interactions—to help the patient understand how she felt in the situation and what she might have done to communicate more effectively. The therapist *explores the patient's wishes and options*, helping her to decide what she wants and exploring the options for achieving it.

> "What did you want to happen in that situation? . . . What could you have done to get what you wanted in that situation? What other options do you have?"

Depressed patients often have difficulty seeing that they have options, and their tendency to deem their own needs to be less important than others' contributes to difficulty in asserting themselves. The therapist explains this to the patient and offers empathy, blaming the depressive syndrome for the patient's difficulties where appropriate. To help the patient choose which options to pursue, the therapist uses *decision analysis*. The case example presented later in this chapter elaborates these techniques.

The therapist *role-plays* potential interactions with the patient to prepare her for interpersonal interactions in real life. Rather than supplying words for the patient during role play, the therapist instead encourages her to come up with her own words. This empowers the patient, fostering her independence from the therapist. The therapist points out that the patient is able to figure out what to say and do in interpersonal interactions, despite depression making her feel unable to do so. The therapist asks the patient how she felt during role play, whether the content and tone of voice felt comfortable, and how she imagines it will feel to say the words in reality. When a patient communicates effectively during role play—and, ultimately, in real life—the therapist reinforces the adaptive behavior with congratulations and encouragement. Real-life successes not only improve mood but also inspire patients to try to assert themselves in subsequent situations.

Depressed patients withdraw socially and to lose interest in activities they previously found pleasurable. The therapist encourages the patient to resume social activity and to explore options for new activities and opportunities to form new relationships, if applicable. The therapist empathizes with difficulty the patient feels in pushing herself to engage with others, but stresses that, once engaged, she will likely feel better. Indeed, the IPT therapist asks the patient to take risks—both in asserting herself with others and in pushing herself to reengage in social activities. The therapist explicitly acknowledges that he/she is asking the patient to take risks, yet assures her that these risks will likely lead to improvement of her mood and life situation. The therapist will be there to discuss anything that goes right or wrong.

The Termination Phase (Sessions 10–12)

In the final sessions, the therapist reviews the patient's progress in symptom improvement, as well as the extent to which the patient has resolved the focal problem area. By reviewing why the patient is better, through the actions she has taken to resolve the interpersonal

focus, the therapist reinforces the patient's growing self-esteem by pointing out that the patient's actions have led to her gains. The therapist congratulates the patient on her progress and hard work, and expresses optimism that the patient can maintain that progress independent of the therapist.

The therapist addresses nonresponse in patients whose moods and life situations do not improve, or only partially improve. The therapist should explain that it is the *treatment* that failed—*not* the patient. The therapist gives the patient hope by emphasizing that depression is treatable and many other effective treatments exist, and by encouraging her to explore alternative treatments.

The therapist explores the patient's feelings about the treatment and termination, acknowledging not only his/her own sadness to be ending their relationship but also happiness about the patient's improvement and confidence that she will be able to maintain the progress she made in treatment. Should symptoms recur, the patient has gained tools to manage symptoms of depression on her own. Furthermore, the patient can return to IPT for "booster" sessions as needed.

Using the IPT medical model, the therapist provides psychoeducation about relapse and recurrence of major depression and prepares the patient about potential for relapse. Patients who have experienced one or more episodes of major depression unfortunately remain vulnerable to future episodes. The therapist explains this and advises that given the link between stressful life events and mood, the patient can anticipate that she may have difficulty with future, stressful life events. Fortunately, the patient can use the coping skills gained in treatment to ward off a worsening of symptoms. If the patient has improved in IPT but has either significant residual symptoms or a history of multiple episodes, therapist and patient may contract for continuation or maintenance IPT, which has also demonstrated efficacy in forestalling relapse (Frank et al., 2007).

CASE STUDY

The following case demonstrates how a clinician (K. L. B.) implemented IPT for major depression in a 12-week acute treatment and illustrates how one works with the problem area of grief. In IPT, grief (complicated bereavement) is considered as a focal problem area when the onset of depression is related to the death of a significant other and the patient is experiencing an abnormal grief reaction (Weissman et al., 2000). Although cases that focus on the grief problem area usually address complicated bereavement related to the death of a person who has actually lived, the following case involves complicated bereavement related to a stillbirth (Bleiberg, 2012). Indeed, the IPT problem areas can apply to a wide range of cases. IPT treatment goals and techniques specific to working with the grief problem area are demonstrated.

Background Information

Sara, a 35-year-old, married, childless woman, was referred for treatment of major depression 2 months after the death of her baby girl *in utero* at 27 weeks' gestation. Her doctor considered a bacterial infection the most likely cause of the stillbirth. Sara's chief complaint was "I feel like I should be over it."

At 27 weeks, after not having felt the baby move for several hours, Sara called her doctor, who told her to come to the hospital. The doctor found no heartbeat and told Sara that he needed to deliver the fetus. Sara recalled feeling shocked, numb, and unable to cry at first. She was given medication to induce labor and an epidural, and delivered the baby vaginally. Despite efforts to revive her, the baby girl was pronounced dead shortly after delivery. Sara said that she wanted to hold her and was given the baby to hold, swaddled in a white-and-pink blanket. She recalled that she and her husband had cried uncontrollably while they took turns holding the baby, and for a long time after giving the baby back to the doctor. She remembered that the baby was "very cute" and looked like her husband. She was given pictures of the baby and footprints to take home. Sara and her husband decided not to have a funeral or memorial service for the baby.

Sara reported that since the stillbirth 2 months earlier, she had been feeling sad and irritable most of the day, nearly every day, and unable to enjoy previous pleasures such as reading fiction, cooking, going to the movies, and exercise. She worked as a nurse on an inpatient medical floor in a New York City hospital, and prior to the stillbirth had very much enjoyed her work. She now felt unable to enjoy work because of her mood, and she feared having to talk about her loss with coworkers who knew she had been pregnant. She was crying frequently, socially withdrawn, had low energy and difficulty concentrating, experienced decreased appetite, and felt very bad about herself. She denied ever having thoughts of suicide or feeling that life was not worth living.

Sara reported that despite trying not to think about the baby's death, she nonetheless was frequently bothered by thoughts about the baby, often wondering what her life would have been like had she survived. Sara had returned to work 3 weeks after the stillbirth, hoping that work would distract her and help her "get over" her loss. She reported feeling very angry at and avoiding other pregnant women, including close friends and women with newborns, in addition to other reminders of her pregnancy. She felt angry at having had to go through pregnancy, labor, and delivery without gaining the pleasure of having a child.

Sara was plagued by inappropriate guilt. She felt guilty because she feared that she had done something to cause her loss, despite the doctor telling her that she could have done nothing to prevent it. He explained that when bacterial infections cause fetal death, they often cause no symptoms in the mother and go undiagnosed until they cause serious complications. Nevertheless, Sara felt that she should have recognized the infection, and she felt guilty about having waited until age 35 to try to conceive. She felt like a failure for having had a stillbirth. Sara felt guilty that she had disappointed and upset her husband by losing the baby, and she did not want to burden him with her feelings about the loss.

Sara had never sought treatment prior to her current evaluation. She described one prior episode of major depression in her late 20s, lasting 4–6 weeks, precipitated by a breakup with a boyfriend of several years, but reported feeling much worse since losing the baby. She reported that her mother had been treated for depression with antidepressant medication with good results.

Sara was an attractive woman of average height and weight who looked her stated age. She was casually but neatly dressed in jeans and a large sweater. Sara's movements were slightly slowed; her speech was fluent. Her mood was depressed and anxious, and her affect, congruent and tearful. She denied current or past suicidal ideation and any history of substance abuse or psychotic symptoms. She denied current or past medical conditions, including thyroid dysfunction. She reported no known prior pregnancies, pregnancy losses, or fertility issues prior to the stillbirth. In fact, she had conceived after just a couple of months of trying to get pregnant.

Sara was good candidate for IPT: She met criteria for major depression and had experienced a recent life event proximate to the onset of her symptoms. Furthermore, IPT could address the interpersonal problems she was experiencing related to the onset of her symptoms. Sara was also a potential candidate for CBT, pharmacotherapy, or (evidence-based antidepressant) psychotherapy combined with medication. She was uninterested in doing written homework and resistant to taking medication because she was hoping to conceive again in the near future.

IPT Treatment with Sara

Acute Phase (Sessions 1–3)

Treatment with Sara followed the IPT format for acute treatment. In the first three sessions, the therapist obtained a thorough psychiatric history and set the treatment framework. In the first session, she obtained a chief complaint and a history of Sara's present illness. Because treatment occurred prior to the release of DSM-5, the therapist used DSM-IV criteria to determine that Sara met criteria for major depressive disorder. She administered the HDRS to assess the severity of Sara's symptoms.

The therapist offered Sara empathy for her pregnancy loss, saying: "I am *so* sorry. You've suffered a terrible loss. No wonder you have been feeling so badly and having such a difficult time." The therapist gave Sara her diagnosis of major depression, reviewed her specific symptoms, and gave her the "sick role," and offered her hope:

> "The symptoms you've described having in the past couple of months—depressed mood, not being able to enjoy things and your loss of interest in things, feeling very badly about yourself and guilty, your difficulty eating and sleeping, and difficulty concentrating—are all symptoms of major depression. Major depression is an *illness* that is *treatable*. It is *not* your fault that you have been feeling this way. And you have a very good chance of recovering."

The therapist explained that Sara's HDRS score of 24 indicated moderately severe depression and that she would readminister the HDRS at regular intervals to monitor Sara's progress. Given the severity of Sara's symptoms, her willingness to participate in psychotherapy, and her reluctance to take medication in anticipation of trying to conceive again, the therapist did not think medication was needed.

The therapist described IPT and the treatment rationale:

THERAPIST: I am trained in interpersonal psychotherapy, which I think could be helpful to you. Interpersonal psychotherapy—often called IPT—is a time-limited treatment that focuses on how recent life events and stresses—such as losing a baby—affect your mood, and how mood symptoms make it difficult to current life events and stresses, particularly problems in relationships. Although we will take the first few sessions to review your history, our sessions will focus on the here and now, on your *current* difficulties and relationships, not on the past. Does this make sense to you?

SARA: Yes.

THERAPIST: Often, people respond to treatment with IPT in 12 weekly sessions. I propose that we meet once a week for a 50-minute session for the next 12 weeks. If it's helpful, at the end of the 12 sessions, we can discuss whether it might be useful to have additional sessions to work on issues and maintain your progress. How does that sound to you?

SARA: It sounds good. I hope I can feel better in 12 weeks.

THERAPIST: You *can* feel better in 12 weeks. IPT has been shown in numerous research studies to effectively treat symptoms like the ones you have described.

After the first session Sara felt somewhat more hopeful but stated that she did not like the idea that she had a diagnosis of major depression. Although she could understand that there was a relationship between her stillbirth and her mood, Sara still felt she should be feeling better after 2 months and did not want to think of herself as depressed, like her mother, and in need of help. Sara stated that she was always the "strong one" and was used to functioning at a very high level. The therapist was not surprised by Sara's initial skepticism, as it can take time for patients to accept the medical model. Furthermore, patients with depression often feel uncomfortable about seeking help because they fear burdening others. Nevertheless, therapist and patient agreed to work together for 12 weeks, then decide whether further sessions were needed.

In obtaining Sara's psychiatric history, the therapist conducted an *interpersonal inventory*, carefully reviewing Sara's past and current social functioning and close relationships. She started the inventory by asking about Sara's family.

"Where did you grow up? . . . Who was in your family? . . . How would you describe your relationship with your mother? . . . With your brother?"

Sara had grown up in Canada with her parents, now in their early 60s, and her younger brother, now age 33, all of whom still lived near Toronto where she had been raised. Her father had worked a lot while Sara was growing up, and although she was fond of him, she did not feel so close to him. Sara felt closer to her mother and spoke with her weekly but was easily irritated by her. It bothered Sara that her mother was not assertive and was intermittently depressed. She spoke weekly with her brother, who lived with his wife and 2-year-old son. She described her relationship with her brother as fairly close. She reported speaking to her brother less often since the stillbirth because she felt jealous that he had a child. When they did speak, Sara avoided asking about her nephew.

After exploring Sara's relationships with family members, the therapist asked about other important people in her life and about her relationship with her husband. At age 33, Sara met her husband, Steve, who was 1 year her junior. She described Steve as warm and charming, and reported that he took great care of her. She felt she did not "deserve him" because he was "such a good guy." She described her previous boyfriends as less emotionally available and "not very nice." Both Sara and Steve had originally came from Canada but met in New York City, where mutual friends introduced them. Sara had moved to New York in her early 20s, whereas her husband had moved there 2 years before they met.

Since the stillbirth, Sara felt distant from Steve and argued with him about "little things." She reported feeling guilty that she had let him down by losing the baby and feared that he blamed her for the baby's death. She did not want to burden him further by sharing her own distress about the loss. She also felt that Steve would not be able to understand her fears about trying to conceive again.

Sara reported having a few close girlfriends who lived in the tristate area and, until the pregnancy loss, had spoken with them about once per week. She had several friends at work with whom she had chatted almost daily until the loss. She described herself as "independent," "outgoing," and "not one to lean on other people" prior to becoming depressed. Rather, her friends turned to her when they had problems. Sara said

that before the depression, her friends would describe her as hardworking and energetic. She rarely argued with friends because she felt "uncomfortable" with conflict. She avoided confronting friends and coworkers when she disagreed or felt angry with them.

The therapist asked Sara if there was anyone to whom she had turned for comfort after her loss because it is important to have someone in whom to confide after such a terrible loss or any stressful experience. Sara replied that she had been avoiding her friends and family since the loss. She had felt uncomfortable talking to friends, family, and coworkers about her pregnancy when she was pregnant because she did not like being the center of attention and felt guilty that she did not enjoy the first trimester of her pregnancy. She felt even more uncomfortable discussing her pregnancy loss. Her parents and in-laws came to see Sara and her husband after the loss, but she felt unable to talk with them about what had happened and how she was feeling. Her coworkers knew that she had been pregnant, and Sara felt obligated to say something to them about what had happened. The therapist noted that it sounded like Sara could trust no one with her feelings about the stillbirth. Sara did not want to reach out to family or friends, or let them know how bad she felt; she explained: "I don't want to bother people with my problems. I don't want to be weak."

The therapist reframed Sara's difficulty in reaching out to others, using the medical model to explain how depression affects social functioning:

THERAPIST: You are not weak—you are *depressed*—and that's not your fault. People with depression tend to minimize their own needs and avoid seeking help from their friends, as you have, because they fear being a burden. However, it is not only appropriate to seek support from others but it also can be *really* helpful to get their support. In fact, support from others has been shown to help in recovery from depression. I appreciate your dilemma. Your depression makes you feel uncomfortable seeking support, yet support from others has been shown to reduce depression and protect people from becoming depressed. Does this make sense to you?

SARA: Yes, but I also don't want to hear what they have to say. It just makes me more upset. They don't understand what I have been through.

THERAPIST: What kinds of things have people said to you?

Sara replied that it bothered her when people said things like "You'll get pregnant again" or "I know someone who also lost a baby." These statements made her feel angry. She felt that others could not understand what she had experienced. One close friend had recently given birth to her first child, and Sara had avoided calling and seeing her. It felt unfair that her friend had a baby when she did not. A coworker had been pregnant at the same time but had a relatively easy pregnancy. Sara felt that her coworker was not sympathetic to her physical discomfort during pregnancy.

By the end of the first phase of treatment, the therapist had connected Sara's major depressive episode to her interpersonal situation in a *formulation* centered on an IPT focal problem area. Sara's chief complaint reflected that she was still grieving the loss of her baby and unable to resume her normal level of functioning. Her situation was a clear example of the grief problem area: Sara was suffering from complicated bereavement. While it is normal to grieve for months after losing a loved one, the severity of Sara's depressive symptoms—especially the excessive guilt, low self-esteem, and social isolation—and her avoidance of thoughts, feelings, and reminders of the baby and the baby's death, reflected an abnormal grief reaction. She had not sought emotional support after the stillbirth and had not really mourned the loss of her baby. In fact, people often develop complicated bereavement when they lack or have not used their social network to help them mourn the loss of their loved one.

The therapist presented this formulation to Sara:

THERAPIST: From what you are telling me, it's clear that the loss of your baby triggered your current depression. You have suffered a terrible loss and you are having trouble grieving. No wonder you are having such a hard time. This is not your fault. Furthermore, your loss and your depression have affected your relationships with people in your life, like your husband, your friends and coworkers, and you're having difficulty expressing your feelings to them. I suggest that we focus our sessions on handling your grief over this terrible event. Grief is one of the problem areas that IPT has been shown to treat. I suggest we work on helping you to mourn the loss and to improve your relationships that have been affected by your loss. How does this sound to you?

SARA: It sounds good.

With Sara's explicit agreement about the treatment focus, the therapist began the middle phase of treatment.

Middle Phase (Sessions 4–9)

During the middle phase, therapist and patient worked on resolving Sara's interpersonal problem area. In IPT, the strategy for working with grief is to help the patient to tolerate and manage the affect of loss, and to gather social support to help the patient through mourning. In addition, the therapist helps the patient to use existing social supports, to reestablish interests and relationships, and to form new relationships and explore new activities to compensate for the loss (Weissman et al., 2000, 2007).

The therapist continued providing psychoeducation about complicated bereavement and how depression affects social functioning, and repeatedly linked Sara's depression to the identified problem area. She began each session with the *opening question*, "How have things been since we last met?" This question elicited affect and a history of Sara's mood and events between sessions, and kept Sara focused on her current mood and life events.

To facilitate the mourning process, the therapist encouraged Sara to think about the loss. In fact, this process had begun during the initial phase, while the therapist took a history of the events related to the onset of Sara's depression. The therapist asked Sara to describe the events prior, during, and after the baby's death—often a source of patient guilt—and explored Sara's feelings associated with these events. In helping a patient mourn the loss of a loved one, the IPT therapist asks the patient to describe her feelings about the death and about the person who died. The therapist explores what the patient and the deceased did together, what the patient liked and did not like about the person, and what the patient wished they had done together but did not have a chance to do. The therapist asks the patient to describe how the deceased died and how she learned about the death, and explores the patient's related feelings. Because Sara's baby died *in utero*, the therapist modified this inquiry somewhat by encouraging Sara to talk about her experience of being pregnant, about the baby, and what she imagined the baby would be like. The therapist asked Sara what she liked about carrying the baby, what she did not like, and what she had hoped to do with the baby.

Sara tearfully described having had mixed feelings about her pregnancy. She reported that she and Steve started trying to conceive 6 months after getting married and, to her surprise, she got pregnant after 2 months. When she discovered she was pregnant, Sara felt really happy but scared about becoming a parent. She questioned whether she was "ready." Sara reported that she made a great effort to practice good prenatal care: She ate healthy, pregnancy-safe foods, took prenatal vitamins, and started prenatal yoga classes. Practicing good prenatal care made her feel good, "as if I was already a mom taking care of my baby."

Sara quickly began to experience terrible fatigue and unrelenting nausea, which lasted for the first 12 weeks of the pregnancy. She described feeling as if she had been "taken over" by the pregnancy. She complained that she loved to cook but did not want to cook because she felt so sick. Despite the nausea, she ensured that she got the nutrients the baby needed. The fatigue and nausea were so debilitating that Sara could no longer meet the physical demands of her job as a nurse. As a result, she was unable to hide her pregnancy from her coworkers; she told her supervisor, who was happy to accommodate Sara by giving her more administrative responsibilities in lieu of patient care until she felt better. Sara resented having to give up clinical work with patients, which was the part of her job she enjoyed. She felt self-conscious about her symptoms and very guilty that her coworkers had to absorb her patient load, despite their being very supportive. It bothered her that others idealized pregnancy, whereas she found it so unpleasant. At the same time, she felt guilty and selfish that she had complained about the pregnancy: Sara felt that she should have just been grateful she was pregnant.

The therapist empathized with Sara's discomfort during her first trimester and validated her need to complain:

THERAPIST: The first trimester of pregnancy can be really difficult and disruptive. Give yourself a break! It can be hard to appreciate being pregnant when you are feeling so terrible. It sounds like you did appreciate being pregnant—you made a great effort to take care of yourself. You watched your diet carefully and rearranged your work situation.

SARA: I don't know . . . I guess that's true.

When the exhaustion and nausea subsided in her second trimester, Sara began to feel more optimistic and excited about having a child. Seeing sonograms made the baby seem "more real" and helped Sara feel connected to the baby. At Week 16, Sara learned that the baby was a girl. Excited, she immediately began considering names and envisioning what the baby would look like. Sara imagined her as a combination of herself and her husband, with blue eyes and blond, curly hair. She thought the baby would be a kind person, like her husband. She imagined walking the baby to the park in a stroller and playing with her. At Week 20, Sara began to feel the baby move, which she very much enjoyed. When the baby moved, Sara would stop whatever she was doing to watch and feel her abdomen. She described feeling the movements as "some of the happiest moments in my life." Neither she nor her husband had thought of a name for the baby, but referred to her as "Sweetie" *in utero*.

For weeks after the stillbirth, Sara struggled with physical reminders of the baby. After the delivery, she had leaky breasts for a few days and vaginal bleeding for several weeks. She reported that she still looked pregnant for weeks after delivering the baby, as her uterus slowly returned to its prepregnancy size. At the time of her initial evaluation, Sara reported that she still had to lose 5 pounds to return to her prepregnancy weight. Sara missed being pregnant and described feeling "empty" and "alone" without the baby inside her. She was eager and ready to be a parent, yet felt frightened about conceiving again because she feared losing another baby.

A couple of weeks after the stillbirth, Sara's doctor determined that an undetected bacterial infection caused the stillbirth. The doctor explained that there was nothing Sara or her husband could have done to prevent the loss, and that this kind of loss was very rare. Despite her doctor's explanation, Sara blamed herself for her baby's death and feared that her husband blamed her too, although he repeatedly denied this. The therapist explored Sara's guilt further:

THERAPIST: What could you have done to prevent your baby's death?

SARA: (*tearfully*) I don't know. . . . I should have been able to do something.

The therapist offered Sara empathy and support, and related her guilt to depression:

THERAPIST: It would be great if there were something you could have done to prevent this tragedy, but there is generally nothing parents can do to prevent a pregnancy loss. It sounds like you did everything you could—you took very good care of yourself. You are struggling with inappropriate and excessive guilt—a symptom of depression. You are blaming yourself for something you didn't do. Perhaps when you find yourself feeling guilty, you can try to label this as a symptom of depression.

SARA: Yes. I guess I can try.

Talking about the pregnancy, the baby, and the baby's death, and exploring related feelings enabled Sara to develop a more balanced and realistic perception of her relationship with the baby and her role in the baby's death. She realized that she had not taken her pregnancy for granted. In fact, she had done everything she could to manage a difficult first trimester and take care of her baby. In addition, her experience with the pregnancy and the baby made Sara realize that, despite her initial anxiety, she was ready and excited to become a parent. By the end of the first month of treatment, Sara's mood was somewhat improved and her HDRS score had fallen to 18. She was less self-critical and more hopeful.

An important part of treating grief is facilitating the expression of affect related to the loss of the loved one. The therapist explored Sara's feelings as she spoke about the baby and her loss, giving Sara time to articulate what she was feeling and to cry. Although IPT therapists generally take an active stance, when facilitating the expression of painful feelings, it is important to allow for silences. By listening silently, the therapist showed that she could tolerate Sara's painful feelings, and that catharsis was an important part of mourning her loss. Sara was able to express not only feelings she had been avoiding but also feelings of which she had previously been unaware.

Sara had avoided looking at the pictures and footprints of the baby from the hospital, which had been stored in a box under her bed. She and the therapist explored what it would be like for her to look at these items. Sara feared it would be scary, and that she would feel really bad. The therapist gently encouraged Sara to take a risk and look because it might make her feel better to experience the feelings she had been avoiding:

"Your feelings are not going to hurt you. You might actually feel better if you allow yourself to let out some of the feelings you have been trying to keep

inside. I know I am asking you to take a risk, but you might be pleasantly surprised."

Between sessions, Sara looked at the pictures and the footprints. The therapist asked what it was like for her.

SARA: I cried a lot. She was so cute. It wasn't as hard as I thought it would be. It felt like a release. I was surprised that I felt a little better afterwards.

THERAPIST: I am *so* glad you took a risk and looked. It sounds like it made you feel better.

In fact, every few weeks before the end of treatment, Sara looked at the pictures and the footprints. She explained that the pictures were sort of comforting because they made her feel a connection to her baby.

In addition to encouraging catharsis, the therapist encouraged Sara to work on her interpersonal interactions, to reconnect with the people in her life, and to consider opportunities to form new relationships and start new activities to compensate for the loss. The therapist explained that people with depression tend to isolate themselves and stop engaging in previously pleasurable activities, both of which can perpetuate depression. Sara reported not wanting to talk to people because she feared that she would have to talk about the loss, or that things people said would make her feel worse. In fact, as Sara and the therapist discussed, *she* could guide the conversation in a way that made her feel comfortable. They explored and role-played options for maintaining control of such conversations. Furthermore, Sara could tell people what would be helpful to her. The therapist explained:

"People with depression often have difficulty asserting their needs. If you communicate your needs to others—like your husband, friends, coworkers, and your family—you might improve those relationships *and* your mood. The people in your life may not know what you need. If you tell them, you might not only get support from them, but you might enjoy their company again and feel better."

Using *communication analysis*, the therapist asked Sara to recount arguments and unpleasant interactions with others: what she was feeling during the interaction, what she said or did, and what the other person said or did. They explored what Sara wished other people would say or do, what *options* she had for asking them to do these things, and they *role-played* Sara asking for what she wanted. Sara reported that she hated running into people who knew she had been pregnant but did not know about the stillbirth. In fact, she avoided going places because she feared having to answer questions about the stillbirth. Sara and the therapist explored these interactions and how Sara could handle them more effectively:

THERAPIST: What kinds of things have people asked, or what are you afraid they will ask?

SARA: People have asked "How's your baby?" or "Weren't you pregnant?"

THERAPIST: How does that make you feel?

SARA: Awful!

THERAPIST: How do you handle it?

SARA: I don't know. . . . Sometimes I say "It didn't work out" or "My baby died."

THERAPIST: That sounds good. How does it feel for you to say that?

SARA: It feels OK, but then they want to know what happened and say stupid things like "At least you know you can get pregnant" or "You can have another one."

THERAPIST: What would you like them to say or do?

SARA: I would like them to just say "I'm sorry," and not ask any questions. I don't want to talk about what happened.

THERAPIST: How could you convey that?

SARA: I guess I could say, "I'm sorry, but I'd rather not talk about it."

THERAPIST: How does that sound? How did it feel to say that?

SARA: It felt OK. Don't you think that is rude to say that?

THERAPIST: No. You said it politely and it's appropriate for you to assert your needs. It is an uncomfortable situation for both you and the person who asked the question. If you are polite and direct with people, they are likely to understand. But why not try it and see?

Sara reported that she had avoided returning calls from old friends. She explained that she felt uncomfortable seeing her friends who had babies because it would remind her of the baby she had lost. Sara also did not want to have to talk about the loss. She did not want to tell them how she felt because she feared hurting their feelings. Sara and the therapist role-played Sara telling her friends about her discomfort and explaining that she did not want to offend them. Role play helped Sara feel prepared and less anxious about going to work, walking around her neighborhood, and talking to old friends. As a result, she gradually starting going out more and began returning phone calls. She returned to the yoga studio where she had taken prenatal yoga and started taking regular yoga classes, which helped her mood and provided an opportunity to be among other people. By midtreatment Sara's HDRS had fallen to 13, consistent with mild depression.

Since the stillbirth, Sara had been bickering with her husband Steve "over stupid things" and felt "distant from him." The therapist asked her to describe a recent incident. Sara said that Steve came home from work and told her that his friend's wife had just had a baby. She felt it was insensitive for him to tell her about other people's positive pregnancy experiences. It bothered her that Steve did not seem as uncomfortable as she was with this information, and that he no longer seemed as upset as she about the loss. The interaction made her feel "alone." She had responded to him by saying, "That's nice," then leaving the room and ruminating for the rest of the evening about his insensitivity.

Sara reported that they often had similar interactions. The therapist once again related Sara's difficulty in asserting herself with her husband to depression, and noted that keeping her feelings inside might actually be making Sara feel worse. They explored interpersonal options for handling this situation in a way that might make Sara feel better. The therapist helped Sara to explore what her husband's intentions might have been in the situation she described. She wondered whether he was trying to make her feel better because his friend's wife had experienced several miscarriages. They role-played Sara telling her husband how she felt. Subsequently, when Sara was able to express her feelings to him, she learned that Steve was, in fact, telling her these stories to give her hope. Furthermore, her husband revealed that he was still upset about the loss of their baby but did not want to upset *her* by sharing his feelings. Sara was relieved that she and Steve were "on the same page" and felt good that she was able to feel close to him again. They subsequently were able to share more of their mixed feelings about the pregnancy experience.

Termination Phase (Sessions 10–12)

During the final sessions, the therapist and Sara reviewed the progress Sara had made. She reported her mood was much improved. Her HDRS was now a 5, consistent with euthymia and remission. Sara's affect was brighter, and she was less preoccupied with the loss of her baby: "I still get upset when I think about my baby, but I don't get as upset. It doesn't ruin my entire day. I am actually able to enjoy things again." Furthermore, Sara no longer blamed herself for her baby's death. She felt good about her ability to communicate her feelings more effectively with her husband, friends, and others, and to enjoy socializing and other activities again.

The therapist congratulated Sara on her hard work and achievements, and told her how happy she was that Sara felt so much better. They discussed the potential for relapse and how Sara could maintain her progress. Given Sara's history of depression, the therapist explained that Sara was, unfortunately, vulnerable to future episodes; however, Sara could anticipate that she would be vulnerable in the setting of stressful life events—role disputes, role transitions, deaths—and use the coping skills she had learned during their work together. Sara anticipated trying to conceive again, and, she hoped, getting pregnant again—both role transitions. The therapist explored with Sara ways that she could take care of herself during this potentially stressful time. They discussed Sara's reaching out to others for support, communicating with her husband about how she was feeling, and forgiving herself if she found herself having a hard time.

In the final session, Sara told the therapist that she had reread her diary entries from the days before beginning treatment and could not believe how far she had come, that her pregnancy loss had forced her to seek treatment for depression that she now realized had been a lifelong problem; in retrospect, she had suffered numerous episodes of mild to moderate depression. Sara admitted that she initially had felt very resistant to the medical model. Defining depression as a medical illness ultimately relieved Sara of her shame and guilt about her difficulty in functioning. Furthermore, being able to see depression as a set of discrete symptoms made it seem more manageable. Sara reported that she was getting along better with her mother; now that she understood depression, she felt more sympathy for her mother's struggle with depression. She was grateful for the opportunity to learn coping skills that she felt

confident about maintaining. In addition, Sara said that she would not hesitate to seek treatment in the future should she find herself becoming depressed again.

The therapist's frequent encouragement, the time limit, and the brief duration of IPT helped keep Sara motivated. Sara said that she appreciated the opportunity to talk about her feelings about her pregnancy, her baby, and her baby's death, and that she felt the therapist understood and supported her. She recognized that her feelings, while powerful, made sense in context and had subsided with discussion. Sara confessed that she appreciated the therapist's "pushing" her to reconnect with others. She had not thought she could handle socializing with others but was pleasantly surprised.

Although each patient is unique, Sara's therapy resembled other IPT treatments for major depression and is a good example of working with the problem area of grief. The exploration and normalization of affect, communication analysis, exploration of options, use of role play, encouragement to take social risks, and other techniques employed in Sara's treatment are characteristic of working with interpersonal difficulties related to any of the four IPT problem areas.

COMMON PROBLEMS THAT ARISE DURING TREATMENT

The problems that typically arise during IPT treatment for major depression are (1) those inherent to working with depressed patients and (2) those related to the therapeutic frame. Although these problems are not unique to IPT, how the therapist views and treats these issues distinguishes IPT from other psychotherapies. In keeping with important IPT themes, the therapist attributes problems to depression, and to the patient's difficulties handling interpersonal interactions and communicating effectively outside of the treatment. The therapist continues to maintain an optimistic, supportive, and nonjudgmental stance and avoids transference interpretations.

For example, patients with major depression superimposed on dysthymic disorder ("double depression") and their therapists are often discouraged by the chronicity of their depression. In these cases, the therapist should remain hopeful and optimistic. Some depressed patients feel that their depression is incurable despite reassurances from the therapist. In these cases, the IPT therapist employs the medical model, labeling the hopelessness as a symptom of depression, and emphasizes that patients need not feel hopeless since depression is treatable. Depressed patients often view seeking treatment as a personal failure. The IPT therapist frames seeking treatment as the appropriate and smart way to treat a medical illness, and a positive step toward gaining mastery over their problems (Weissman et al., 2000, 2007).

The most serious problem to arise in any treatment for depression is when a patient expresses suicidal ideation. As in any treatment, the therapist determines whether hospitalization is necessary, based on the seriousness of the intent and the availability of the patient's social supports. The therapist is as available as possible to the patient and schedules extra sessions as needed. The therapist assesses the circumstances in which the suicidal ideation developed, what the patient hoped to accomplish by ending her life, and reviews how the patient imagines others would react to her suicide. The therapist helps the patient explore alternative ways of expressing what she intended to communicate by committing suicide. The therapist provides psychoeducation about suicide, explaining that it is the most deadly symptom of depression, and that therapist and patient have to work together to keep the patient alive long enough to get through successful treatment—at which point the patient will again want to live. Augmenting the therapy with medication treatment should be considered for severely suicidal patients. The therapist remains optimistic that the patient's depression will improve, and that she will no longer feel that life is not worth living (Weissman et al., 2000, 2007).

Problems may arise in the relationship with the therapist. For example, a patient who has poor social supports may come to view the therapeutic relationship as a substitute for relationships outside of the therapy. Because IPT focuses on relationships *outside* of the treatment, the therapist gently refocuses the patient to outside relationships. Whereas the therapist notes that the patient's ability to connect within the treatment relationship reflects her ability to form intimate relationships, he/she clarifies that they are not friends or family and emphasizes the importance of the patient's life outside of the treatment. The therapist helps the patient explore options for connecting with others in ways similar to the way she connected with the therapist (Weissman et al., 2000, 2007).

Missed and late sessions are also considered to be symptomatic of depression. The therapist calls attention to and empathizes with the fact that the patient has missed or is late to a session, and notes that difficulty getting to sessions may reflect functioning that is characteristic of depression. It is likely that the patient is late to appointments outside of the therapy. The therapist can remind the patient of the time limit of IPT to motivate her to come to sessions. In the event that the patient misses or comes late to sessions because she is uncomfortable with the material being discussed in session, or because she has some other negative feeling about the treatment or the therapist, the therapist empathizes with the patient's feelings and helps her to explore ways to express these feelings directly.

When a patient is silent to the extent that it seems she refrains from sharing thoughts and feelings, or when she changes or avoids subjects, or has problems with self-disclosure, the therapist notes this behavior and explores the patient's feelings related to the behavior. These behaviors are particularly problematic in a time-limited, focused treatment such as IPT because they make it difficult to work on the chosen problem area. The patient may feel uncomfortable and ashamed to share her thoughts and feelings with the therapist. The therapist assures the patient that there is little that can surprise him/her, and that she does not have to talk about everything.

PREDICTORS OF RESPONSE

Although there is strong evidence that IPT is an efficacious treatment for major depression and other disorders, there are fewer data on factors that predict response to IPT. Data from comparative treatment studies involving IPT suggest some clinical predictors of response. In the multisite National Institute of Mental Health Treatment of Depression Collaborative Research Program (NIMH TDCRP; Elkin et al., 1989), 250 outpatients with major depression were randomly assigned to 16 weeks of imipramine (IMI), IPT, CBT, or placebo. The TDCRP dataset has been examined for predictors of response by several researchers. Sotsky and colleagues (1991) found that TDCRP subjects with low-baseline-level social dysfunction responded well to IPT, whereas those with interpersonal deficits responded less well. These findings support the discussion earlier in this chapter that IPT works least well for patients with few or no social contacts, who report no recent life events, and whose treatment, therefore, focuses on the IPT problem area of interpersonal deficits. High initial symptom severity and impaired functioning predicted superior response to IPT and to IMI compared to CBT

(Sotsky et al., 1991; Weissman et al., 2000). In another analysis, TDCRP subjects with symptoms of atypical depression, such as mood reactivity and reversed neurovegetative symptoms, responded better to IPT and CBT than to IMI or to placebo (Stewart, Garfinkel, Nunes, Donovan, & Klein, 1998).

Barber and Muenz (1996) found that among patients who completed treatment in the TDCRP study, IPT had greater efficacy than CBT for patients with obsessive–compulsive personality disorder, whereas CBT was better for patients with avoidant personality disorder, as measured by the HDRS. However, another study examining the relationship between personality traits and outcome in the same dataset found no significant differences among personality traits (Blatt, Quinlan, Pilkonis, & Shea, 1995; Weissman et al., 2000).

In another study, Thase and colleagues (1997) found that among 91 patients with depression, patients who had abnormal electroencephalographic (EEG) sleep profiles had significantly poorer response to IPT than did patients with normal profiles. In this study, unlike the Sotsky and colleagues (1991) study, symptom severity did not significantly predict response to IPT (Weissman et al., 2000). Additional potential predictors of response appear in the earlier section in this chapter describing the IPT patient Sara.

CONCLUSION

IPT is a time-limited, diagnosis-targeted treatment with demonstrated efficacy for patients with major depression and other mood disorders. It has been adapted for the treatment of anxiety disorders, eating disorders, and, most recently, personality disorders. Although there is substantial evidence of IPT's efficacy for the treatment major depression and other mood and psychiatric disorders, further evidence of predictors of response to IPT is warranted. This chapter has focused on the original IPT protocol: IPT as an individual treatment for major depression.

IPT employs the medical model and focuses on *current* or recent life events, interpersonal difficulties, and symptoms. IPT emphasizes the interrelationship between mood and life events: Negative or stressful life events affect mood and, conversely, mood symptoms affect how people manage negative or stressful life events. Treatment with IPT focuses on one of four interpersonal problem areas—grief, role disputes, role transitions, and interpersonal deficits. The therapist

helps patients recover from depression by relieving depressive symptoms and by helping them to resolve the chosen interpersonal problem area. The IPT therapist takes an active, optimistic, and supportive stance.

The case of Sara demonstrates the techniques used and the process of treatment with IPT. IPT is an eclectic treatment with proven efficacy that uses techniques employed by other psychotherapies. The combination of IPT's main principles, techniques, strategies, and therapist and patient characteristics distinguishes it from other antidepressant treatments.

For further information about IPT and its adaptations, readers may consult the *Comprehensive Guide to Interpersonal Psychotherapy* by Weissman and colleagues (2000), the *Clinician's Quick Guide to Interpersonal Psychotherapy* (2007), and the *Casebook of Interpersonal Psychotherapy* (Markowitz & Weissman, 2012a).

NOTE

1. For stylistic simplicity, patients are referred to in the feminine. Indeed, most depressed patients are women.

REFERENCES

American Psychiatric Association. (2000). *Diagnostic and statistical manual of mental disorders* (4th ed., text rev.). Washington, DC: Author.

American Psychiatric Association. (2010). Practice guideline for the treatment of patients with major depressive disorder, third edition. *American Journal of Psychiatry, 167*(Suppl.), S1–152.

American Psychiatric Association. (2013). *Diagnostic and Statistical manual of mental disorders* (5th ed.). Arlington, VA: Author.

Barber, J. P., & Muenz, L. R. (1996). The role of avoidance and obsessiveness in matching patients to cognitive and interpersonal psychotherapy: Empirical findings from the Treatment for Depression Collaborative Research Program. *Journal of Consulting and Clinical Psychology, 64,* 951–958.

Beck, A. T., Steer, R. A., & Brown, G. K. (1996). *Beck Depression Inventory manual* (2nd ed.). San Antonio, TX: Psychological Corporation.

Blatt, S. J., Quinlan, D. M., Pilkonis, P. A., & Shea, M. T. (1995). Impact of perfectionism and need for approval on the brief treatment of depression: The National Institute of Mental Health Collaborative Research Program revisited. *Journal of Consulting and Clinical Psychology, 63,* 125–132.

Blazer, D. G., II. (2000). Mood disorders epidemiology. In B. J. Sadock & V. A. Sadock (Eds.), *Kaplan and Sadock's comprehensive textbook of psychiatry* (7th ed., Vol. 1, pp. 1298–1308). Philadelphia: Lippincott/Williams & Wilkins.

Bleiberg, K. L. (2012). Interpersonal psychotherapy for peripartum depression. In J. C. Markowitz & M. M. Weissman (Eds.), *Casebook of interpersonal therapy* (pp. 224–242). New York: Oxford University Press.

Bleiberg, K. L., & Markowitz, J. C. (2005). Interpersonal psychotherapy for posttraumatic stress disorder. *American Journal of Psychiatry, 162*, 181–183.

Bleiberg, K. L., & Markowitz, J. C. (2007). Interpersonal psychotherapy and depression. In C. Freeman & M. Power (Eds.), *Handbook of evidence-based psychotherapies: A guide for research and practice* (pp. 41–60). Oxford, UK: Oxford University Press.

Bowlby, J. (1973). *Attachment and loss.* New York: Basic Books.

Cuijpers, P., Geraedts, A. S., van Oppen, P., Andersson, G., Markowitz, J. C., & van Straten, A. (2011). Interpersonal psychotherapy of depression: A meta-analysis. *American Journal of Psychiatry, 168*, 581–592.

Elkin, I., Shea, M. T., Watkins, J. T., Imber, S. D., Sotsky, S. M., Collins, J. F., et al. (1989). National Institute of Mental Health Treatment of Depression Collaborative Research Program: General effectiveness of treatments. *Archives of General Psychiatry, 46*, 971–982.

Fairburn, C. G., Jones, R., Peveler, R. C., Hope, R. A., & O'Connor, M. (1993). Psychotherapy and bulimia nervosa: Longer-term effects of interpersonal psychotherapy, behavior therapy, and cognitive behavior therapy. *Archives of General Psychiatry, 50*, 419–428.

Fairburn, C. G., Norman, P. A., Welch, S. L., O'Connor, M. E., Doll, H. A., & Peveler, R. C. (1995). A prospective study of outcome in bulimia nervosa and the long-term effects of three psychological treatments. *Archives of General Psychiatry, 52*, 304–312.

Frank, E. (2005). *Treating bipolar disorder: A clinician's guide to interpersonal and social rhythm therapy.* New York: Guilford Press.

Frank, E., Kupfer, D. J., Buysse, D. J., Swartz, H. A., Pilkonis, P. A., Houck, P. R., et al. (2007). Randomized trial of weekly, twice-monthly, and monthly interpersonal psychotherapy as maintenance treatment for women with recurrent depression. *American Journal of Psychiatry, 164*, 761–767.

Frank, J. (1971). Therapeutic factors in psychotherapy. *American Journal of Psychotherapy, 25*, 350–361.

Hamilton, M. (1960). A rating scale for depression. *Journal of Neurology, Neurosurgery, and Psychiatry, 2*, 56–62.

Hill, C. E., O'Grady, K. E., & Elkin, I. (1992). Applying the Collaborative Study Psychotherapy Rating Scale to rate therapist adherence in cognitive-behavior therapy, interpersonal therapy, and clinical management. *Journal of Consulting and Clinical Psychology, 60*, 73–79.

Kessler, R. C., Berglund, P., Demler, O., Koretz, D., Merikangas, K. R., Rush, A. J., et al. (2003). The epidemiology of major depressive disorder: Results of the National Comorbidity Survey Replication (NCS-R). *Journal of the American Medical Association, 289*, 3095–3105.

Klerman, G. L., Weissman, M. M., Rounsaville, B. J., & Chevron, E. S. (1984). *Interpersonal psychotherapy of depression.* New York: Basic Books.

Lipsitz, J. D., Fyer, A. J., Markowitz, J. C., & Cherry, S. (1999). An open trial of interpersonal psychotherapy for social phobia. *American Journal of Psychiatry, 156*, 1814–1816.

Markowitz, J. C. (1998). *Interpersonal psychotherapy for dysthymic disorder.* Washington, DC: American Psychiatric Press.

Markowitz, J. C., Klerman, G. L., Perry, S. W., Clougherty, K. F., & Mayers, A. (1992). Interpersonal therapy of depressed HIV-seropositive patients. *Hospital and Community Psychiatry, 43*, 885–890.

Markowitz, J. C., Kocsis, J. H., Fishman, B., Spielman, L. A., Jacobsberg, L. B., Frances, A. J., et al. (1998). Treatment of HIV-positive patients with depressive symptoms. *Archives of General Psychiatry, 55*, 452–457.

Markowitz, J. C., & Milrod, B. (2011). The importance of responding to negative affect in psychotherapies. *American Journal of Psychiatry, 168*, 124–128.

Markowitz, J. C., Milrod, B., Bleiberg, K. L., & Marshall, R. D. (2009). Interpersonal factors in understanding and treating posttraumatic stress disorder. *Journal of Psychiatric Practice, 15*, 133–140.

Markowitz, J. C., Skodol, A. E., & Bleiberg, K. (2006). Interpersonal psychotherapy for borderline personality disorder: Possible mechanisms of change. *Journal of Clinical Psychology, 62*, 431–444.

Markowitz, J. C., Svartberg, M., & Swartz, H. A. (1998). Is IPT time-limited psychodynamic psychotherapy? *Journal of Psychotherapy Practice and Research, 7*, 185–195.

Markowitz, J. C., & Weissman, M. M. (Eds.). (2012a). *Casebook of interpersonal psychotherapy.* New York: Oxford University Press.

Markowitz, J. C., & Weissman, M. M. (2012b). IPT: Past, present, and future. *Clinical Psychology and Psychotherapy, 19*, 99–105.

Meyer, A. (1957). *Psychobiology: A science of man.* Springfield, IL: Thomas.

Mufson, L., Dorta, K. P., Wickramaratne, P., Nomura, Y., Olfson, M., & Weissman, M. M. (2004). A randomized effectiveness trial of interpersonal psychotherapy for depressed adolescents. *Archives of General Psychiatry, 61*, 577–584.

Mufson, L., Moreau, D., & Weissman, M. M. (1993). *Interpersonal psychotherapy for depressed adolescents.* New York: Guilford Press.

Mufson, L., Weissman, M. M., Moreau, D., & Garfinkel, R. (1999). Efficacy of interpersonal psychotherapy for depressed adolescents. *Archives of General Psychiatry, 56*, 573–579.

Murray, C. L., & Lopez, A. D. (1996). *The global burden of disease* (Vol. 1). Cambridge, MA: Harvard University Press.

O'Hara, M. W., Stuart, S., Gorman, L. L., & Wenzel, A. (2000). Efficacy of interpersonal psychotherapy for postpartum depression. *Archives of General Psychiatry, 57*, 1039–1045.

Parsons, T. (1951). Illness and the role of the physician: A sociological perspective. *American Journal of Orthopsychiatry, 21*, 452–460.

Ransom, D., Heckman, T. G., Anderson, T., Garske, J., Holroyd, K., & Basta, T. (2008). Telephone-delivered interpersonal psychotherapy for HIV-infected rural persons with depression: A pilot trial. *Psychiatric Services, 50*, 871–877.

Reynolds, C. F., III, Dew, M. A., Martire, L. M., Miller, M. D., Cyranowski, J. M., Lenze, E., et al. (2010). Treating depression to remission in older adults: A controlled evaluation of combined escitalopram with interpersonal psychotherapy versus escitalopram with depression care management. *International Journal of Geriatric Psychiatry, 25*, 1134–1141.

Reynolds, C. F., III, Dew, M. A., Pollock, B. G., Mulsant, B. H., Frank, E., Miller, M. D., et al. (2006). Maintenance treatment of major depression in old age. *New England Journal of Medicine, 354*, 1130–1138.

Sholomskas, A. J., Chevron, E. S., Prusoff, B. A., & Berry, C. (1983). Short-term interpersonal therapy (IPT) with the depressed elderly: Case reports and discussion. *American Journal of Psychotherapy, 36*, 552–566.

Sotsky, S. M., Glass, D. R., Shea, M. T., Pilkonis, P. A., Collins, J. F., Elkin, I., et al. (1991). Patient predictors of response to psychotherapy and pharmacotherapy: Findings in the NIMH Treatment Of Depression Collaborative Research Program. *American Journal of Psychiatry, 148*, 997–1008.

Spinelli, M., & Endicott, J. (2003). Controlled clinical trial of interpersonal psychotherapy versus parenting education program for depressed pregnant women. *American Journal of Psychiatry, 160*, 555–562.

Stewart, J. W., Garfinkel, R., Nunes, E. V., Donovan, S., & Klein, D. F. (1998). Atypical features and treatment response in the National Institute of Mental Health Treatment of Depression Collaborative Research Program. *Journal of Clinical Psychopharmacology, 18*(6), 429–434.

Sullivan, H. S. (1953). *The interpersonal theory of psychiatry.* New York: Norton.

Thase, M. E., Buysse, D. J., Frank, E., Cherry, C. R., Cornes, C. L., Mallinger, A. G., et al. (1997). Which depressed patients will respond to interpersonal psychotherapy?: The role of abnormal EEG profiles. *American Journal of Psychiatry, 154*, 502–509.

Weissman, M. M., Markowitz, J. C., & Klerman, G. L. (2000). *Comprehensive guide to interpersonal psychotherapy.* New York: Basic Books.

Weissman, M. M., Markowitz, J. C., & Klerman, G. L. (2007). *Clinician's quick guide to interpersonal psychotherapy.* New York: Oxford University Press.

Wilfley, D. E. (2008). *Interpersonal psychotherapy for binge eating disorder (BED) therapist's manual.* Unpublished manuscript.

Wilson, G. T., Wilfely, D. E., Agras, W. S., & Bryson, S. W. (2010). Psychological treatments of binge eating disorder. *Archives of General Psychiatry, 67*, 94–101.

World Health Organization. (1992). *The ICD-10 classification of mental and behavioral disorders: Clinical descriptions and diagnostic guidelines.* Geneva, Switzerland: Author.

CHAPTER 9

Behavioral Activation for Depression

SONA DIMIDJIAN
CHRISTOPHER R. MARTELL
RUTH HERMAN-DUNN
SAMUEL HUBLEY

The behavioral activation (BA) approach to treating depression has received very strong empirical support in the past few years, with results as good or better than cognitive therapy and antidepressant medications, even for the most severe cases of depression. Seemingly counterintuitive at first blush, this treatment does not focus on the notion of "just do it" but takes a comprehensive look at contingent relationships in the patient's life across the full range of behavior, cognition, and affect that may be maintaining the depression. As such, this very idiographic approach does not prescribe a set number of sessions to accomplish certain goals but is very adaptable to the individual with depression. In the detailed and very human description of the treatment of "Mark," readers will also note a very up-to-date focus on the role of rumination in depression (or worry in anxiety) as a fundamentally avoidant technique. The illustration of creative therapeutic strategies for activating patients, and the very adaptable and flexible nature of BA will be of interest to all therapists treating depression, since it may be one of the easiest to learn and most disseminable of evidence-based psychological treatments for depression.—D. H. B.

Behavioral activation (BA) is a structured, brief psychosocial approach that aims to alleviate depression and prevent future relapse by focusing directly on behavior change. BA is based on the premise that problems in vulnerable individuals' lives, and their behavioral responses to such problems, reduce their ability to experience positive reward from their environment. The treatment aims to increase activation systematically in ways that help clients to experience greater contact with sources of reward in their lives and to solve life problems. The treatment procedures focus directly on activation, and on processes that inhibit activation, such as escape and avoidance behaviors and ruminative thinking, to increase experiences that are pleasurable or productive and improve life context. We believe that

BA is an important new treatment for depression for two main reasons. First, its efficacy is supported by recent empirical research; second, it is based on simple and easily grasped underlying principles and utilizes a small set of straightforward procedures.

BEHAVIORAL MODELS OF DEPRESSION

Basic Concepts

The central premise in virtually all behavioral models is the assumption that depression is associated with particular behavior–environment relationships that evolve over time in a person's life. "Behavior" is a very broad construct in these models and includes everything from taking a walk to grieving over the loss of a loved one. Behaviors can be fairly circumscribed (e.g., lying on the couch watching television after dinner) or they can be part of a more general repertoire (e.g., avoidance of asserting one's own needs and desires in conflictual interactions).

"Environment" is also a broad construct that can best be thought of as the settings in which behaviors currently occur, as well as those in which behaviors have evolved over time. The temporal nature of environments is crucial for understanding behavioral approaches to depression. Often, behavior that appears to serve no function in a person's current environment has served a very important function in the past. Thus, when practitioners wonder why a depressed person is engaging in a particular set of behaviors, such as remaining in an unsatisfying job, it is often necessary to consider how particular repertoires (e.g., avoiding potential losses) have evolved over time.

Finally, all behavioral models of depression emphasize the importance of contingent relationships between behaviors and the environments in which they occur. Contingent relationships are "if–then" relationships between human activities and their (often interpersonal) environmental consequences. For example, practitioners working within a behavioral framework are probably less interested in the *fact* that a depressed client stays in bed each morning worrying, for example, about the future of a troubled marriage, than they are about the consequences of this behavior. What happens as a result? Does the client become more or less depressed? By staying in bed, does the client avoid something aversive, such as confronting a spouse about an issue in the marriage, or going to work and facing a pile of uncompleted tasks? Understanding contingent relationships is a central feature of behavioral models of depression and a requisite skill of BA therapists.

Behavioral Roots of BA

These general behavioral concepts were developed and refined into specific conceptual frameworks and treatments for depression by both Ferster (1973, 1981) and Lewinsohn and colleagues (Lewinsohn, 1974; Lewinsohn, Antonuccio, Steinmetz-Breckenridge, & Teri, 1984; Lewinsohn, Biglan, & Zeiss, 1976). Ferster's primary assumption was that depression is the result of a learning history in which the actions of the individual do not result in positive reward from the environment,

or in which the actions are reinforced because they allow the individual to escape from an aversive condition. Over time, behavior that would typically produce positive consequences ceases to do so. For example, for a variety of different reasons, a person's efforts to form close relationships with others might gradually fade away because they are not followed by positive reinforcement (e.g., reciprocal efforts from others).

Ferster (1973, 1981) reasoned that this decrease in response-contingent positive reinforcement produces two additional consequences that facilitate depression. First, when people's efforts do not result in reward, they often become more focused on responding to their own internal state than to potential sources of positive reinforcement in the external environment. This is the classic "turning inward" that is often seen in depression, and that makes sense from a behavioral perspective; when individuals learn that their own behavior is an unreliable predictor of positive consequences in their environment, they naturally spend less time attending to contingencies in that environment.

The second consequence of decreased rates of positive reinforcement that Ferster (1973, 1981) observed was a narrowing of individuals' repertoire of adaptive behaviors. This makes logical sense as well because fewer and fewer behaviors are being maintained by positive reinforcement. Individuals may adopt extremely passive repertoires (e.g., "doing nothing") because their active attempts to become engaged in life are not rewarded.

Finally, Ferster (1973, 1981) observed that increases in aversive consequences following behavior typically lead depressed individuals to become preoccupied with escape and avoidance. In effect, more energy is expended attempting to avoid or escape from anticipated aversive consequences than attempting to contact potential positive reinforcers in the environment.

Lewinsohn's (1974) early behavioral model of depression was very compatible with many of the ideas proposed by Ferster's (1973) behavioral analysis of depression. Lewinsohn and colleagues similarly emphasized the importance of response-contingent reinforcement and conceptualized that its rate was influenced by three factors: the number of potentially reinforcing events for an individual; the availability of reinforcement in the environment; and the instrumental behavior of the individual required to elicit the reinforcement. Lewinsohn also identified social avoidance as a core part of his model. Importantly, Lewinsohn, Sullivan, and Grosscup (1980) developed the first stand-alone behaviorally oriented treatment for depression. Later, Lewinsohn, Hoberman, Teri, and Hautzinger (1985) proposed an integrated model that was intended to explain the interactive and complex nature of depression, including dispositional factors such as cognition, with environmental factors. This model did not overemphasize or give precedence to either cognitive factors or environmental factors in the etiology and maintenance of depression; rather it attempted to account for the complexity of depression. Research initiated in Lewinsohn's laboratory has continued through the work of former students and colleagues across diverse settings and populations (Dimidjian, Barrera, Martell, Muñoz, & Lewinsohn, 2011).

Beck, Rush, Shaw, and Emery (1979) also pioneered early work on BA. Incorporating BA strategies as a core component of cognitive therapy (CT) for depression, Beck and colleagues formalized and widely disseminated some of the principal BA strategies utilized within a larger framework emphasizing the importance of cognition in etiology and treatment of depression.

Contemporary BA

The work of Ferster, Lewinsohn, and Beck strongly influenced the development of contemporary BA in important ways. They were a direct influence on Jacobson and colleagues' initial research and clinical development of BA (Jacobson, Martell, & Dimidjian, 2001; Martell, Addis, & Jacobson, 2001; Martell, Dimidjian, & Herman-Dunn, 2010). Their work similarly formed the context of other investigators, such as the team of Lejuez, Hopko, LePage, Hopko, and McNeil (2001; Lejuez, Hopko, Acierno, Daughters, & Pagoto, 2011), who articulated a BA approach that is convergent in both theory and clinical emphasis on targeting behavior change. This approach, BA treatment for depression, has been supported in multiple studies by their group (e.g., Hopko, Lejuez, LePage, Hopko, & McNeil, 2003).

With respect to a conceptual model of depression, the current conceptualization draws heavily on the work of Ferster (1973, 1981) and Lewinsohn (1974) in emphasizing the central importance of context and activity in understanding depression. While acknowledging that genetic, biological, and other distal factors may be causally related to depression, the current behavioral conceptualization focuses on the aspects of a person's life context that may have triggered depression, and particular ways of responding to this context

that may be maintaining depression. Specifically, the model assumes that one reason people get depressed is because changes in the context of their lives provide low levels of positive reinforcement and high levels of aversive control. Lives that are "less rewarding" can lead to feelings of sadness and depressed mood. And when people get depressed, they often pull away from the world in important ways, and the basic routines of their lives become easily disrupted. Both of these processes can increase depressed mood and make it difficult to solve problems effectively in one's life. In fact, these processes are conceptualized as "secondary problem behaviors," because they frequently prevent people from (1) connecting with aspects of their lives that may provide some improvement in mood and (2) solving problems that may help to decrease stress and improve life context.

The BA approach to therapy addresses both of the factors that may be contributing to depression: those aspects of one's life that need to be changed to reduce depression and the ways withdrawal from the world may be maintaining or increasing depression. BA accomplishes these aims through "guided activation," which is the use of a series of behavior change strategies that the therapist and client develop together on the basis of a careful examination of what activities will be reinforcing for a given client and help to disrupt the relationships that are maintaining the depression. The point of BA is not to engage in increased activation at random or activities that are "generally" thought to be pleasing or to improve mood (e.g., seeing a movie); in contrast, activation strategies are highly individualized and "custom tailored." The role of the BA therapist is to act as a "coach" while the client implements the activation strategies, providing expert help in setting achievable goals, breaking difficult tasks down into manageable units, troubleshooting problems that arise, and maintaining motivation during the process of change.

EMPIRICAL CONTEXT

The first study to revitalize interest in a purely behavioral approach to treating depression was conducted by Jacobson and colleagues (1996), who proposed a simple but provocative question: Could the behavioral component of CT account for the efficacy that CT has demonstrated in previous clinical trials? Adults with major depression were randomly assigned to one of three treatment conditions, including BA only, BA plus interventions designed to modify automatic thoughts, and the full CT package. Results suggested that BA was comparable to the full CT package in both acute efficacy (Jacobson et al., 1996) and prevention of relapse over a 2-year follow-up period (Gortner, Gollan, Dobson, & Jacobson, 1998).

On the basis of these findings, BA was developed into a more fully articulated behavioral intervention that included the behavioral aspects of CT and incorporated the early behavioral work of Ferster (1973, 1981) and Lewinsohn (1974), as described earlier. This expanded BA model has been articulated in published reports (Jacobson et al., 2001; Martell et al., 2001, 2010) and in a patient-oriented self-help manual (Addis & Martell, 2004). BA was further tested in a large, randomized, placebo-controlled clinical trial that compared its acute and long-term efficacy to both CT and antidepressant medication (ADM). Two hundred forty-one patients were randomly assigned to BA, CT, ADM, or pill-placebo, and severity was used as a stratification variable during randomization. The findings suggested that BA is a particularly promising treatment for depression (Dimidjian et al., 2006). Among more severely depressed patients, its performance was comparable to the current standard of care, ADM, and demonstrated better retention. Both BA and ADM were superior to CT among more severely depressed patients. Moreover, follow-up results indicate that BA appears to have promising enduring effects (Dobson et al., 2008). Finally, BA may demonstrate an important cost-effectiveness advantage compared to continuing patients on medication.

These results were consistent with a range of other studies suggesting that activation interventions are particularly important components of cognitive-behavioral treatments. In a classic study, Zeiss, Lewinsohn, and Muñoz (1979) reported comparable outcomes for depressed patients who received treatment focused on interpersonal skills, pleasant activities, or cognitive change. In addition, in a study with depressed older adults, Scogin, Jamison, and Gochneaur (1989) found no differences in outcome between a cognitive bibliotherapy treatment and a behavioral bibliotherapy treatment among mildly and moderately depressed older adults. The importance of behavioral strategies has also been reported in other studies across multiple diagnostic categories (e.g., Borkovec, Newman, Pincus, & Lytle, 2002; Foa, Rothbaum, & Furr, 2003; Gloaguen, Cottraux, Cucherat, & Blackburn, 1998). Other process-oriented research has similarly emphasized the

importance of BA components of CT (Bennett-Levy et al., 2004) and has suggested the possibility of negative outcomes when therapists work on changing clients' thoughts about interpersonal relationships as opposed to changing actual interpersonal relationships (Hayes, Castonguay, & Goldfried, 1996).

In addition, Ferster's early focus on avoidance has also been underscored by contemporary behavior therapists. Specifically, Linehan (1993) incorporated the use of "opposite action" for sadness as a means to target depression in dialectical behavior therapy. And Hayes and colleagues (1996) have emphasized the role of experiential avoidance in the development of a wide range of psychopathologies and in the conceptualization of acceptance and commitment therapy (ACT; Hayes, Strosahl, & Wilson, 1999). A study on an early precursor to ACT found significant treatment benefits for depressed clients in comparison to standard CT (Zettle & Rains, 1989).

Some preliminary studies also suggest that patient activation is an important element of the change process. In a substance use treatment study in which one condition was augmented with BA interventions, pre- to posttreatment increases in environmental reward were associated with reductions in depressive and anxiety symptoms for such patients, but not for those receiving substance use treatment only (Daughters et al., 2008). In a study of cognitive-behavioral therapy (CBT) for depression, increases from baseline in activation predicted posttreatment depression improvement (Christopher, Jacob, Neuhaus, Neary, & Fiola, 2009).

Recent enthusiasm for BA is fueled in large part by the broad dissemination potential of a straightforward, parsimonious intervention such as BA. The application of BA in novel settings and with diverse populations is a focus of much recent research (see below for detailed discussion of settings and client variables). Technology is playing an increasingly important role in the expansion of BA. Teletherapy over the phone and with videoconferencing technology has been shown to be effective for adolescent and late-life depression (Lazzari, Egan, & Rees, 2011; Quijano et al., 2007) as well as computerized adaptations of BA delivered via the Internet (Spates, Kalata, Ozeki, Stanton, & Peters, 2012; Spek et al., 2007, 2008; Van Voorhees et al., 2009; Warmerdam, Van Straten, Twisk, Riper, & Cuijpers, 2008). Finally, novel training methods are also being enhanced with technology. Based on pilot data from a preliminary computerized BA training program (Hubley, Woodcock, Dimeff, & Dimidjian, in press), our group is currently testing a fully developed computer-assisted therapy program to train therapists in BA.

In summary, research on BA provides a strong foundation for clinical application with depressed patients and for extension to novel populations (Dimidjian et al., 2011). These conclusions are consistent with other meta-analyses that incorporate clinical trial data from over 30 studies (Cuijpers, van Straten, & Warmerdam, 2007; Ekers, Richards, & Gilbody, 2007; Mazzucchelli, Kane, & Rees, 2009) and with influential treatment guidelines (e.g., National Institute of Health and Clinical Excellence, 2009).

ASSESSING DIAGNOSTIC, CLINICAL, AND FUNCTIONAL DOMAINS

The application of BA is based on a comprehensive diagnostic, clinical, and functional assessment. Some of these assessment activities are completed as a precursor to the initiation of therapy, and others are ongoing throughout the course of therapy.

In our treatment outcome research, we have used a number of structured diagnostic interview instruments to assess *Diagnostic and Statistical Manual of Mental Disorders* (DSM) diagnoses, including the Structured Clinical Interview for DSM-IV Axis I Disorders (SCID-I; First, Spitzer, Gibbon, & Williams, 1997), and the Structured Clinical Interview for DSM-IV Axis II Personality Disorders (SCID-II; First, Spitzer, Gibbons, Williams, & Benjamin, 1996). In addition, we have used measures of depressive severity, including the clinician-administered Hamilton Depression Rating Scale (HDRS; Hamilton, 1960), the client self-reported Beck Depression Inventory–II (BDI-II; Beck, Steer, & Brown, 1996), and the nine-item Patient Health Questionnaire Depression Scale (PHQ-9; Kroenke, Spitzer, & Williams, 2001).

In routine clinical practice, we recommend conducting a baseline diagnostic interview (although it can be administered using a less structured format than a research-based interview), and the ongoing use of a measure to assess depressive severity is important. Typically, the most easily administered measure is a self-report measure (e.g., BDI-II; Beck et al., 1996). Also, a number of self-report instruments may serve as useful assessment measures of patient activity level and of the reward available in a client's environment. The Behavioral Activation for Depression Scale (BADS; Kanter, Mulick, Busch, Berlin, & Martell, 2007; Kant-

er, Rusch, Busch, & Sedivy, 2009), a 29-item measure of client activation, has been used in several studies (e.g., Weinstock, Munroe, & Miller, 2011) to measure changes in levels of activation and avoidance over the course of BA. The BADS has been validated in European Spanish (Barraca, Pérez-Álvarez, & Lozano Bleda, 2011), Persian (Mohammadi & Amiri, 2010), and Dutch (Raes, Hoes, Van Gucht, & Kanter, 2010). A recently developed nine-item short form of the BADS demonstrated improved psychometric properties compared to the original, and good internal consistency and predictive validity in the validation study (Manos, Kanter, & Luo, 2011).

In addition, self-report questionnaires have been developed to measure the construct of response-contingent positive reinforcement, including the Environmental Reward Observation Scale (EROS; Armento & Hopko, 2007) and the Reward Probability Index (RPI; Carvalho et al., 2010). Both of these measures are brief, and initial psychometric studies indicate promising psychometric properties. Clinicians who want a nomothetic measure of pleasurable activities to augment the idiographic behavioral assessment (described in more detail below) can use the Pleasant Events Schedule (Lewinsohn & Graf, 1973). These measures may prove to be useful clinical tools that can be administered periodically throughout the course of treatment to assess change in activity and reward. For a full discussion of measures available and issues related to measuring the BA model, see Manos, Kanter, and Busch (2010).

Because functional capacity is such a key component of BA treatment, it is important to gather detailed information about the impact of the client's depression on functional status across multiple life domains, including work, family, social activity, and so forth. These domains can be assessed using clinical interview or standard assessment instruments (e.g., the Social Adjustment Scale [Weissman & Bothwell, 1976] and the Medical Outcomes Study 36-Item Short Form Health Survey [Ware & Sherbourne, 1992]).

COURSE OF TREATMENT

BA is a theory-driven as opposed to a protocol-driven treatment and, as such, is highly idiographic in its application. Treatment does not follow a required session-by-session format; however, it does follow a general course over time. This general course comprises the following activities, which are described in greater detail below:

- Orienting to treatment
- Developing treatment goals
- Individualizing activation and engagement targets
- Repeatedly applying and troubleshooting activation and engagement strategies
- Reviewing and consolidating treatment gains

Orienting to Treatment

BA begins with orienting the client to the treatment, a process that is typically the focus of the first two sessions. The primary tasks to accomplish during this initial phase of treatment include discussing the BA model of depression and primary treatment strategies, and providing information about the structure of treatment, and the roles and responsibilities of the client and therapist.

The presentation of the treatment model includes describing the behavioral approach to depression and the process of change during treatment, discussing the specific ways the model fits with the client's experiences, and encouraging and responding to questions and concerns about the model. The model is presented both verbally during the first session and in a brief, written description that is given to the client at the end of the first session. In addition, many clients find the illustration provided in Figure 9.1 to be a helpful adjunct when orienting to the model. A detailed transcript illustrating the presentation of the treatment rationale is included in the case study below, and the key points to address are summarized in Table 9.1.

During the second session, therapist and client again discuss the treatment model and the client's reactions, including questions that may have arisen following the first session. It is essential that the therapist obtain "buy in" from the client with the basic elements of the treatment model. Therapy works best if the client accepts and buys into the rationale for treatment and the case conceptualization (Addis & Carpenter, 2000). The therapist is advised to guard against moving too quickly if the client does not express agreement with the key tenets of the model. Thus, during the initial sessions, it is essential that the therapist encourage the client to ask questions and elicit the client's potential doubts and concerns.

For instance, some clients may find it difficult to accept the idea that changing behavior directly is an effective way to work with depression. Often, clients are strongly committed to a biological explanation for their

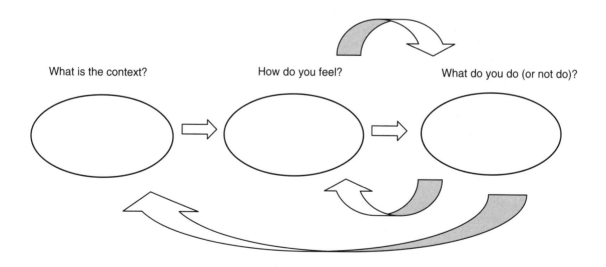

What is the context?   How do you feel?   What do you do (or not do)?

Have any problems started, continued, or worsened?

FIGURE 9.1. The behavioral activation treatment model.

TABLE 9.1. 10 Key Points to Address When Presenting the Treatment Model

1. Behavioral activation is based on the idea that the events in your life and how you respond to such events influence how you feel.

2. BA assumes that one reason people get depressed is that their lives are providing too few rewards and too many problems. Sometimes it is possible to identify easily stressors or problems; other times there are no clearly identifiable stressors but there is still not adequate reward from the environment.

3. When one's life context is difficult, it is common to experience feeling sad, down, discouraged, anxious, fatigued, drained, and so forth.

4. When feeling these ways, it is also common to do (or not do) particular actions. People often pull away from the world around them and find that basic routines in their lives become disrupted.

5. Pulling away from the world when feeling down is natural and understandable. The problem is that it also can initiate downward spirals with how you feel (e.g., the less you do, the worse you feel, and the worse you feel, the less you do).

6. Acting (or not acting) in such ways also can maintain depression by making it hard to solve life problems effectively; this initiates another downward spiral in which what you do or don't do makes the context of life harder or keeps you from improving it.

7. In this treatment, we will work together to focus on specific things you can do to help shift these downward spirals and help you become more active and engaged in your life.

8. BA is not just about "doing more." If feeling better were that easy, you would have already done it. We can work together to identify the activities that would be most helpful *and* the small and manageable steps you can take to get started. You can think of me as a your coach or a consultant in the process of change.

9. Each session will involve developing practical and do-able steps to engage in activities that improve mood and to solve specific life problems. Between sessions, you will work on homework assignments that we develop together; these assignments are an essential part of therapy and will focus on re-connecting or building parts of your life that increase feelings of pleasure or accomplishment and bring you closer to important life goals.

10. Activating and engaging in specific ways can help you experience more reward and effectively solve life problems. When you are active, engaged, and solving problems effectively, it is likely that you will be moving toward important life goals and feeling better.

depression. It is not advisable for therapists to debate this position; instead, therapists can explain that there are many sources of vulnerability to depression, and that one of the effective ways to change depression is by changing what one does. At times, clients also may think that the emphasis on behavioral change means that all they need to do is exercise more, go to a few more movies, or take a few more walks, and their depression will remit. If clients understand BA in this way, then it is not surprising when they feel that the treatment invalidates their degree of distress and the difficulty they face in overcoming depression. We often find it helpful to talk to clients about two points. First, behavior can have a powerful effect on our moods, and people are often unaware of this link, particularly when they are depressed. For example, subtly shifting the way someone approaches interactions with family members may not rid that person of depression, but it can reduce the severity of depressed mood, thereby setting the stage for other changes that collectively help to reverse the depression. The second point is that behavior change is not easy; if it were, we would all behave exactly as we think we should all the time (and we know this is not the case!). Changing behavior requires knowing what to change, and this can take some serious and sustained "detective work" in therapy. The therapist can again emphasize his/her role as a coach in helping the client to figure out what to change and how to do it.

In addition to presenting and discussing the treatment model, it is also important to discuss thoroughly the structure of treatment and the roles of therapist and client. It is necessary to emphasize three key elements: between-session practice, collaboration, and the structure of sessions.

1. It is important early in treatment to highlight the active nature of BA and establish the importance of between-session practice. The therapist sets the tone of therapy and expectations by highlighting that BA is a very action-oriented and problem-focused treatment in which the majority of the "work" of therapy goes on between sessions, as the client implements plans that therapist and client devise in session. Subsequent sessions examine what the client has learned, highlight relevant consequences of activities, and identify barriers and troubleshoot to maximize the likelihood of success on future attempts. The assignment of homework begins in the very first session, when the therapist asks the client to read the brief pamphlet that reviews the key ideas of the BA approach (see Martell et al., 2001).

2. It also is important to emphasize that BA is a collaborative approach to therapy, in which therapist and client work together in the service of the client's goals.

3. It is also helpful to orient clients to the structured nature of each treatment session. Although the specific foci of each session vary across clients and across time, each session nonetheless follows a similar general outline. Specifically, as in cognitive therapy for depression (Beck et al., 1979), each session begins with therapist and client setting an agenda in a collaborative fashion. The aim of the agenda is to organize the time effectively and to ensure that sessions address the client's most important topics and have maximal likelihood of helping the client reach key goals. Because the goal of treatment is activation, the more control given to the client in setting the agenda, the better. In addition, given the integral role of homework in BA, the majority of each session is devoted to reviewing homework from the previous session and assigning homework for the next session. The ending of each session includes asking the client to reiterate a "take-home message" from the session, verifying that the client has a clear understanding of the assigned homework, and reviewing the time for the next scheduled session and methods to reach the therapist, if needed, in the interim.

In attending to each of these specific tasks, the therapist establishes his/her credibility as an expert who can help the client and conveys a sense of hope. By establishing at the outset of treatment a strong foundation of collaboration, client and therapist can begin working together toward the client's goals.

Developing Treatment Goals

The ultimate goal of BA is to help clients modify their behavior to increase contact with sources of positive reinforcement in their lives. Typically, this process involves first addressing basic avoidance patterns and areas of routine disruption and, second, addressing short- and long-term goals. A good deal of the therapist's time in BA is spent helping clients to increase awareness of their escape and avoidance repertoires and to practice active coping responses. Often, part of this process also involves changing basic routines (e.g., sleeping, eating, and social contact). Thus, short-term goals are set to specify concrete accomplishments that can help clients shift their life situations in a less depressing direction. Often, therapists are uncertain about

how to sequence treatment targets; generally, we focus initially on behavior change that has the greatest likelihood of success, which may be based on ease of accomplishment or level of importance to client values and priorities. Common examples might include getting the house cleaned, spending time with friends and family, making headway on a large pile of paperwork on which the client has procrastinated, exercising more frequently, and so on. Often, behaviors necessary for progress on short-term goals can be scheduled and structured in such a way that they substitute for maladaptive avoidant or withdrawal responses. A therapist works with a client to make progress on short-term goals *regardless of how the client is feeling*. In other words, one of the therapist's primary goals is to help the client change the pattern of having his/her behavior governed by mood. Rather, the objective is to make progress on goals regardless of how one feels at a particular point in time, under the assumption that progress on life goals is itself antidepressive. This is a crucial point because clients often judge the success of a particular behavior change based on how it makes them feel in the moment. Thus, it is important for therapists to remain mindful of the consequence of different behaviors specifically with respect to whether they help clients move toward or achieve treatment goals.

Once the short-term goals relating to avoidance, withdrawal, and routine disruption have been addressed, clients are assisted in addressing larger life circumstances that may be related to depression. Larger life goals are those shifts that take time to accomplish but have the potential to alter a person's life situation in substantial ways. Common examples include finding a new job, getting out of a distressing relationship, starting a new relationship, or moving to a new city or town. BA can be helpful in teaching and encouraging clients to continue to make progress toward these goals even though their actual realization may take some time to accomplish. Essentially, in BA, clients learn basic change strategies that can be used to accomplish short-term and larger life goals.

Individualizing Activation and Engagement Targets

No two people are the same, and no person is exactly the same from situation to situation. In the context of treating depression, this means that the particular activation strategies that work for one person may not work for another, and they may work for the same person sometimes, but not always. Whether activity–environment transactions shift someone's mood in a positive or negative direction is an empirical question, and one that requires careful attention and assessment to answer. Much of the skill of doing competent BA relies on just this kind of careful examination. In BA, this process is referred to as "functional analysis," which is the key to individualizing activation targets and the heart of BA. Functional analysis involves identifying for each client the variables that maintain the depression and are most amenable to change. This understanding forms the basis of the case conceptualization and guides the idiographic application of specific activation strategies. In general, the therapist must engage the client in a detailed examination of the following:

- What is maintaining the depression?
- What is getting in the way of engaging in and enjoying life?
- What behaviors are good candidates for maximizing change?

This process sounds simple, yet in practice, it can be complicated given that we all frequently lack awareness of the contingencies that control our behavior. Given this reality, early in treatment, we talk explicitly about the goal (and the challenge!) of identifying these relationships.

Two key steps are involved in identifying the contingencies that control behavior. First, therapist and client must clearly and specifically define the behavior of interest; this includes defining the frequency, duration, intensity, and setting of the behavior. The behaviors of greatest interest are those most closely tied to changes in mood. For clients who are familiar with antidepressant treatment, we often explain that we want to identify the ingredients of a behavioral antidepressant that works for them. In order to do so, we need to define specifically the activities that maintain depression (e.g., "down activities") and those that improve mood and functioning (e.g., "up activities"). For instance, for one client, difficulty completing basic household tasks was maintaining and exacerbating his experience of depression. It was important to specify the problems of (1) filling and closing bags of household trash, then leaving them in the pantry room rather than taking them to the dumpster behind the house for the past 6 weeks, and (2) receiving bills in the mail and placing them unopened in a file drawer for the past 4 months. Treatment with this client began with a series of graded tasks to

accomplish the goal of taking out the trash. This was identified specifically as a potential "up" activity (even though it was, admittedly, not a pleasurable one) and selected as an initial focus because therapist and client decided it was more easily accomplished than addressing the bills, which the client experienced as more overwhelming.

Second, therapist and client can begin to identify the antecedents and consequences of the behavior, with the goal of specifying variables that elicit or reinforce depression. In terms of the BA model, this is parallel to identifying the links between context and mood, between action and mood, and the downward spirals that can maintain depression over time. Understanding basic behavioral principles can often be of great value in identifying these contingent relationships. What does this mean in practical terms? For depressed clients, a number of contingent relationships are often observed. As we discussed earlier, negative reinforcement contingencies are often pervasive. "Negative reinforcement" means that the likelihood of a behavior occurring is increased by the removal of something from the environment, typically an aversive condition. Negative reinforcement contingencies can be a very adaptive part of human behavior. For instance, putting on a warm coat to avoid getting cold, stopping at stop signs to avoid getting in accidents, and being extra nice to a parent after crashing the car to avoid being punished are all examples of ways that negative reinforcement can serve one well. Unfortunately, however, when an individual becomes depressed, his/her behavioral repertoires can become dominated by escape and avoidance behaviors that temporarily allow a person to escape from painful feelings or difficult interpersonal situations. In this way, many avoidant and escape behaviors may be understood as secondary coping responses—efforts to cope with the experience of depression that, unfortunately, make it worse. For example, a person might attempt to escape from feelings of hopelessness and fatigue by taking a long nap in the middle of the afternoon. This might, as a consequence, temporarily remove the person from an aversive context, but it can also prevent him/her from taking the steps necessary to shift into a less depressive context overall (exercising, applying for jobs, cleaning the house, etc.). Substance abuse, excessive sleeping, watching too much television, and general inactivity are all common examples of secondary coping responses that can be maintained by negative reinforcement. These types of negative reinforcement contingencies are often central in preventing people from coming into contact with potentially reinforcing environments that contribute to leading a more adaptive and engaged life. Careful assessment is required to identify whether and how specific negative reinforcement contingencies are active in a client's life. Positive reinforcement contingencies may also be problematic for clients. In these cases, the likelihood of a behavior is increased because it is contingently associated with positive consequences. For instance, going to bed early may be positively reinforced by family members offering empathy and support. Some behaviors, such as overeating and substance abuse, can also provide immediate positive reinforcement but detract from long-term goals, thereby maintaining the depression.

How do we conduct functional analyses in BA? There exist two primary supports for the BA therapist doing functional analyses: the BA model and activity monitoring. First, the BA model used to orient clients at the outset of treatment can be used throughout treatment to guide assessment of specific events that arise in a client's life to help identify key links between activity and mood. For example, if a client begins to talk in session about feeling troubled by a difficult interaction with her son, the therapist can suggest that they use the model to understand the components of the interaction. Together, they can discuss and write down specifically what happened (e.g., "My son said that he was failing math"), how the client felt (e.g., "I felt sad about how hard our lives always seem to be and afraid that he would not graduate"), and what the client did (e.g., "I left dinner, went to my room, and thought about how I'm failing as a parent"). These components can then be linked to identify the downward spiral that maintains negative mood (e.g., isolating and ruminating increases anxiety and sadness) and the downward spiral that prohibits effective problem solving (e.g., "I didn't talk directly with him, and he got angry, went out with his friends, and didn't come home until the middle of the night"). This process of assessment helps to identify targets of activation for that difficult event (e.g., generate and practice alternatives to leaving the interaction and ruminating; identify and implement steps to solving the problem of her son's poor performance in math). Repeated application of the model in sessions and for use as homework between sessions also will help therapist and client identify patterns of maladaptive actions over time and place. Finally, repeated use of the model in such ways teaches the client a method to guide his/her actions long after therapy has ended.

Second, activity monitoring in the context of daily life is the heart of the assessment process in BA. Through detailed and ongoing activity monitoring that the client completes between sessions, therapist and client can work together to develop an understanding of the questions listed earlier. Given the role of activity monitoring, it is important early in treatment for the therapist to set the stage to explain clearly how to do it, defining both what to monitor and when to do it. Also, therapists must carefully and skillfully review monitoring tasks to reinforce the client's efforts to begin developing activation and engagement assignments.

Therapists may elect to use a number of different formats for activity monitoring, the most basic form of which includes recording both an activity and a mood rating for each hour of the client's waking day. Therapists also may elect to have clients monitor mastery (sense of accomplishment) or pleasure (enjoyment) associated with specific activities. Generally, we advise clients to record enough information about activities that we can begin to identify links between what they were doing and how they were feeling, but not so much information that the task is overly burdensome. It also is helpful to identify at what intervals during the day the client will write down the observations (e.g., morning, lunch, dinner, before bed). If recording for each hour is too taxing for a client, time sampling procedures may also be used. In such a procedure, client and therapist agree on a specified number of hours when activities will be monitored during the week between sessions. Time sampling procedures need to include a variety of situations in which the client functions during the week. In general, therapists will want to encourage clients to complete entries at regular intervals throughout the day and are advised to work with clients to develop plans for recording that take advantage of natural cues and rhythms in their lives to facilitate such regular recording.

Therapists can provide clients with a simple weekly Activity Record for monitoring assignments (e.g., see Figure 9.2). However, as is often emphasized in BA, the function of the behavior is more important than its form; thus, clients may eschew monitoring on an Activity Record but be comfortable using personal calendars, smartphones, or other idiosyncratic recording methods. Adapting the monitoring assignment to a form that is compatible with the client's normal daily routine is highly encouraged. For instance, clients who spend a lot of time in their car may keep their records above the visor; others may find it helpful to keep it

Instructions: Record your activity for each hour of the day, and record a mood rating associated with each activity. Use the scale below with the anchors that you and your therapist develop to guide your mood rating. Aim to make entries on your Activity Record at least every 3–4 hours each day.

	Monday	Tuesday	Wednesday	Thursday	Friday	Saturday	Sunday
5–6							
6–7							
7–8							
8–9							
9–10							
10–11							
11–12							
12–1							
1–2							
2–3							
3–4							
4–5							
5–6							
6–7							
7–8							
8–9							
9–10							
10–11							
11–12							
12–1							
1–2							
2–3							
3–4							
4–5							

Mood Ratings: 0: Description, with examples of associated activities: _____

_____

5: Description, with examples of associated activities: _____

_____

10: Description, with examples of associated activities: _____

_____

FIGURE 9.2. Activity Record (hourly).

taped to the refrigerator or bathroom mirror; still others find it useful to carry it with them in a pocket, purse, backpack, or briefcase.

When a client has completed an activity monitoring assignment, it is essential for the therapist to review it in detail. Failing to review activity monitoring records may mean missed opportunities to reinforce the client's behavior and to develop the case conceptualization. Much of competent BA lies in skillfully reviewing a completed Activity Record. What does the competent therapist attend to when reviewing the records? In general, the therapist will want to keep the case conceptualization questions listed earlier in the forefront of his/ her mind when reviewing a completed activity log. The therapist reviews the Activity Record to understand the client's activities, routines, and life context, and to begin to identify patterns that may be maintaining or exacerbating depressed mood.

Specific questions that therapists can use to guide their review of activity schedules are listed below:

- What would the client be doing if he/she were not depressed (working, managing family responsibilities, exercising, socializing, engaging in leisure activities, eating, sleeping, etc.)?
- Is the client engaging in a wide variety of activities, or have his/her activities become narrow?
- What is the relationship between specific activities and mood?
- What is the relationship between specific life contexts/problems and mood?
- In what ways are avoidance and withdrawal maintaining or exacerbating depression? What does the client avoid or from what is he/she pulling away? In what specific ways?
- Are there routine disruptions?
- Where has contact with reinforcers been lost?
- Are there deficits in coping skills and strategies?

To answer these questions, it is essential to focus on the parts of the client's activity and context that change and the parts that are consistent over time. It is not uncommon for depressed clients to report that their mood is always low, no matter what they are doing or where they are doing it. They may describe that they simply feel "blah" all the time or that, perhaps, their mood changes, but such changes are minor or irrelevant. A central premise of BA, however, is that variability is everywhere, though sometimes it is difficult to detect.

Moreover, the variability is not random. Instead, *variations in behavior and its settings have a direct effect on a person's mood* and, as such, provide critical information about central contingencies. When clients report that they feel depressed "all the time," it is either because they are inaccurately reporting on their mood retrospectively, their behavioral repertoires are extremely narrow (e.g., lying in bed all day long), or they have not learned to discriminate between subtle differences in mood. This last point is a critical one. One of the key tasks for therapists is to help clients understand that their moods are intimately linked to what they are doing, where they are doing it, and the resulting consequences. Treating depression requires making a series of strategic changes in each of these domains, all of which are based on understanding the basic contingent relationships.

Repeatedly Applying and Troubleshooting Activation and Engagement Strategies

Given the idiographic nature of BA, the course of treatment may look quite different across a range of clients. Despite this diversity, we discuss below a few straightforward behavioral methods that are frequently used.

Activity Scheduling and Self-Monitoring

The major work of therapy in BA occurs between treatment sessions. It is uncommon for clients to leave a session without some specific activities with which to experiment during the week. Thus, activity scheduling and monitoring of outcome are standard methods used throughout treatment. At the end of each session, the client should clearly understand the specific activity assignment and have a clear strategy for implementing it during the week (including a plan for overcoming likely obstacles to implementation).

Specifically scheduling the activity is a useful tool for having the client commit to times when he/she will do the homework. When the assignment is listed in writing on a particular day of the week, at a particular hour, the client has the benefit of an external aid to motivate behavior change (i.e., working from the "outside-in" as opposed to the "inside-out"). Activity scheduling is also used frequently for clients with significant routine disruptions. Schedules can be an aid in the effort to develop and follow regular routines for eating, working, sleeping, exercising, and maintaining social contact. Depending on the activity, the client may not specifically schedule the time but may instead record its completion on a daily log.

A key part of scheduling activities frequently involves careful attention to contingency management. As social psychologists have long known, "The correlations between intention and behavior are modest . . . the weak intention–behavior relation is largely due to people having good intentions but failing to act on them" (Gollwitzer, 1999, p. 493). Given this reality, it is essential for BA therapists to consider ways they can help clients structure their environment so as to maximize success with treatment assignments and goals.

One helpful method of contingency management is the use of public commitment to enhance the likelihood of completing assignments (Locke & Latham, 2002). Often, we explore whether friends, coworkers, or family members are available to be included in activation plans. For instance, one of our clients learned in treatment that when his depression was more severe, it was essential for him to tell his wife each morning the primary tasks he intended to complete that day. For him, "keeping his word" was an effective reinforcer that helped to increase his activation.

In addition, we work with clients to structure their environments in other ways that will enhance activation. Thus, for a client who works on an exercise plan during the week, putting on her exercise clothes before she leaves work at the end of the day is an essential part of the plan.

Finally, clients may also experiment with the use of arbitrary reinforcers for specific behavior change tasks. Although the emphasis of BA is heavily on increasing contact with natural reinforcers in one's environment, the selective use of arbitrary reinforcers can at times be helpful. The client we noted earlier planned a special dinner with his wife at the end of a week of adherence with activation tasks; the client who was working on the exercise program bought a new shirt for exercising after she started her new program.

Occasionally, therapists may suggest the use of aversive contingencies to help promote behavior change; for instance, one client found it useful to agree to call his therapist if he was going to stay in bed and miss work for the day. We have described to other clients the method of writing donation checks to their least favored charities, which are then cashed if they do not complete scheduled activities (Watson & Tharp, 2002). Often, simply the suggestion of an aversive contingency

is sufficient to motivate change. For instance, the client who agreed to call his therapist did, in fact, call early one Monday morning; when he was halfway through leaving a message, he stated, "This is ridiculous. Forget it, I am going to work."

When clients do activity scheduling, it is also essential to build in a monitoring component such that they record the context and consequences of activation. This provides both information about the specific activation assignment, and regular and ongoing practice in noticing contingent relationships between activity and mood. It is essential for the therapist to discuss what the client learned from the activation and self-monitoring tasks in each session. In addition, the therapist needs to provide regular feedback about progress and to highlight areas of improvement or troubleshoot problems that may have arisen.

It is essential for the therapist not to shy away from asking about homework that is incomplete or not done. Attending to these domains is exactly the job of the BA therapist. Repeated and persistent focus on a small set of activation tasks often occupies a great deal of the course of treatment. Asking about what prevented the completion of homework gives therapist and client essential information about important barriers and possible examples of avoidance patterns. The purpose of such discussions is not to punish or shame the client, so it is important to approach homework review with a direct and nonjudgmental attitude. At the same time, discussing incomplete or partially completed homework may be experienced as aversive by the client, which may help to facilitate his/her doing the homework next time (i.e., through being negatively reinforced by escaping from the therapist's uncomfortable questioning). If this occurs naturally, it is not a problem and can in fact enhance treatment progress. However, the therapist should never use shame or criticism, however subtly, to enhance homework completion.

Graded Task Assignment

Graded task assignment, which is a core part of CT for depression (Beck et al., 1979), is also a hallmark of BA and a key part of most activity scheduling efforts. Thus, it is important for therapists to help clients break down behaviors into specific, achievable units to facilitate successful behavior change. Knowing how to break down tasks and grade them appropriately in a stepwise progression from simple to complex requires therapists to use a broad array of basic self-management and problem-solving skills. Toward this end, it is also important for therapists to help clients learn the method of grading tasks during therapy, so that they can apply this skill to new contexts and tasks after therapy has ended. In explaining the tool of graded task assignment, it is often important to remind clients that the goal is not to accomplish all parts of the activity; rather, the goals are to get started on important tasks, increase activation, and disrupt avoidance. Therapists can also explain to clients that breaking tasks down helps to ensure success with subtasks, and such success experiences can in turn reinforce and motivate work on successive components of the larger task.

It is very important to break down tasks in such a way that early success is guaranteed. If clients experience difficulty with tasks, therapists may want to revisit explicitly whether the task was broken down and graded sufficiently. Clients also can be asked to envision the steps involved in a given task before attempting it outside of therapy, and to anticipate any obstacles that might arise. If this process suggests that certain components may be difficult to master, therapist and client can grade that task into smaller and more achievable components.

Avoidance Modification and Problem Solving

This is perhaps one of the most rich and varied aspects of BA. As noted earlier, clients may be addressing avoidance of concrete tasks at work or home, avoidance of painful emotions such as grief or fear, avoidance of interpersonal conflict, and so forth. The specific methods used to address these areas are tied to the specific nature of the avoidance. For instance, a client who avoids the experience of grief over a lost relationship may be assisted in spending time each day reviewing photos of the former partner, reminiscing about times they shared, and so forth. A client who avoids tasks at work may be assisted in breaking down tasks, making specific to-do lists, asking others for help, and so forth. A client who avoids interpersonal conflict may be assisted in practicing assertive communication in role plays in sessions, experimenting with discussions with friends, bringing a family member to a therapy session, and so forth. That said, within this broad domain, a number of basic strategies may be helpful in planning treatment.

First, it is essential when addressing avoidance to start from a collaborative stance with the client. It is important to understand and to communicate an understanding of the discomfort that a client may experience in a particular situation, which is then followed by some action on the part of the client to end the aversive experience. Therapists can emphasize the ways that avoidance may serve an adaptive function in the short term but be problematic in the long term. Given that many avoidant behaviors may be under the control of immediate contingencies, it is often helpful to highlight repeatedly the long-term consequences of particular behaviors. Returning to the BA model to highlight such patterns is often helpful.

Second, basic problem-solving methods are frequently used to address avoidance. Although we rarely teach problem-solving steps in a structured and formal manner, addressing avoidance typically involves figuring out how to approach and solve problems. Thus, it is essential for therapists to maintain a problem-solving mind-set with respect to avoidance and to work with clients to generate a range of options for possible alternative coping behaviors. Problem-solving strategies include defining and assessing the problem, generating alternative solutions, managing environmental contingencies, and troubleshooting the solution when needed. It should be noted that all of the other basic strategies are also frequently used in the service of avoidance modification and problem solving (activity scheduling and monitoring, graded task assignment, etc.).

Third, to help maintain a consistent focus on avoidance, clients may be assisted by several mnemonic devices. These devices help to organize a method of examining, "What is the function of a behavior; what are its consequences?" We have used the acronym AC-TION to identify the general approach that we ask clients to take (Martell et al., 2001):

- Assess—Is this behavior approach or avoidance? Will it be likely to make me feel better or worse?
- Choose—Either choose to continue this behavior, even if it makes me feel worse, or try a new behavior.
- Try—Try the behavior chosen.
- Integrate—Any new behavior needs to be given a fair chance, so integrate a new behavior into a routine before assessing whether it has been helpful or not.
- Observe the Results—Pay close attention and monitor the effects of the new behavior.
- Never Give Up—Remember that making changes can often require repeated efforts and attempts.

When clients demonstrate behavioral patterns characterized by avoidance behaviors, therapists may use the acronym of being in a TRAP (Martell et al., 2001):

- Trigger—usually something in the environment (e.g., criticized by employer)
- Response—usually an emotional reaction (e.g., feels shame and sadness)
- Avoidance Pattern—The avoidance behavior(s) used to cope with the emotional response (e.g., leaves work early, complains to partner about displeasure with job)

Therapists then ask the client to get out of the TRAP and back on TRAC; that is, under the same trigger and response conditions, they are asked to experiment with "alternative coping" behaviors.

Engagement Strategies

Research has well documented the frequency and negative consequences of ruminative behavior among people with depression (Nolen-Hoeksema, 2000). The BA approach considers ruminating as a behavior that frequently prevents people from engaging fully with their activities and environments. BA therapists are on alert for client reports of ruminating and are also careful to assess whether ruminating is a problem when clients return to sessions reporting that an activation assignment "didn't work." If, for example, a client reports that she experienced little mood improvement while playing with her son in the park, the therapist will want to examine whether she was only partially engaged with the task of playing because her mind was focused on why her former partner did not want to continue their relationship, what that meant about her value as a woman, and so forth.

In addressing rumination in BA, we are less interested in the particular content of ruminative thoughts than in the context and consequences of rumination. For instance, in working with a client who frequently ruminated about a job that he regretted having declined, the BA therapist asked him to examine the following types of questions: What were you doing while you were thinking about the other job? How engaged were you with the activity of the moment and with your surroundings? What happened during and after your thinking about the other job? In examining these questions, therapist and client identified that the client was more likely to ruminate when he was working on

aversive tasks in his current job, about which he felt significant anxiety; thus, ruminating was negatively reinforced by distracting the client from anxiety and decreasing his focus on the aversive tasks. BA therapists may ask clients who ruminate frequently to experiment with "attention to experience" practice, in which they deliberately focus their attention on their current activity and surroundings. For instance, they may be asked to bring their full awareness to physical sensations (colors, sounds, smells, tastes, physical movements, etc.). These strategies are akin to mindfulness practices (Segal, Williams, & Teasdale, 2002) and are also very consistent with the dialectical behavior strategy of "opposite action all the way" (Linehan, 1993).

Reviewing and Consolidating Treatment Gains

As therapist and client agree that there has been sufficient improvement and termination seems indicated, remaining sessions should focus on relapse prevention, which largely involves reviewing and consolidating gains the client has made. Toward the end of therapy, it is often wise to focus on anticipating situations in the client's life that may trigger depressive feelings and behaviors, and to generate plans for coping with such situations. Upcoming life events that can be anticipated as challenges for the client (e.g., the death of a parent, a career change) should be discussed in detail, and the client can draft a self-help plan to activate in the face of the stressor. In addition, it is also very important to review the basic BA model and the methods used in therapy to ensure that the client is leaving with a solid understanding of how to apply these as tools in the future. For instance, therapists will want to review how to identify links between what one does and how one feels, how to set specific and concrete goals, how to use graded task assignment, and how to identify and target primary avoidance patterns (noticing that one is ruminating more at work, noticing that one is starting to fail to return phone calls of friends, etc.).

The Therapy Setting

Initial research on BA primarily focused on the context of outpatient individual psychotherapy settings; however, recent studies are examining application across a broad array of settings and delivery modes. For example, several groups have found creative ways to transport BA to settings outside of specialty mental health clinics. Preliminary trials have documented the promise of treating adult primary care patients with depression using BA (Gros & Haren, 2011; Uebleacker, Weisberg, Haggarty, & Miller, 2009), and Ekers and colleagues have provided confirmation showing that nonspecialists can learn and effectively deliver BA in primary care settings (Ekers, Dawson, & Bailey, 2013; Ekers, Richards, McMillian, Bland, & Gilbdoy, 2011). Similarly, Hopko and colleagues (2011) recently conducted a successful randomized controlled trial (RCT) of BA for depressed cancer patients in oncology clinics. Dimidjian and colleagues are also currently testing BA in a multisite RCT for antenatal depression with a flexible delivery format, and obstetric nurses and behavioral health providers as study clinicians. Group therapy appears to be a viable format for delivering BA to larger numbers of clients (Houghton, Curran, & Saxon, 2008; Porter, Spates, & Smitham, 2004). There is also growing interest in integrating BA into university settings (e.g., Cullen, Spates, Pagoto, & Doran, 2006; Gawrysiak, Nicholas, & Hopko, 2009; Reynolds, MacPherson, Tull, Baruch, & Lejuez, 2011).

Treatment duration has ranged from 12- to 24-session formats. Limitations of client resources, insurance reimbursement, and other factors may necessitate particular treatment durations. In our studies and clinical work, we often schedule brief phone contacts between sessions to reinforce the interpersonal connection to the therapist and the importance of completing the between-session assignments, and to provide an opportunity to address questions or problems with the between-session assignments.

Although BA is most often delivered as an individual treatment modality, significant others in clients' lives are often included in sessions across the course of treatment. Decisions about whether to include significant others in treatment follow from the functional analysis; thus, they are determined on an idiographic basis. Conjoint sessions can be helpful in assessing patterns that may be maintaining the client's depression, providing information and education to the family member about the treatment rationale and approach, and providing opportunities for the client and family member to practice new interpersonal behaviors with the therapist's direct and immediate feedback.

Therapist Qualities

In our experience, a number of structural and stylistics qualities are important for BA therapists to bring to their clinical work. Briefly, the structured nature of

BA is maintained through the use of agendas to guide session foci; therapists engage clients in the process of collaborative agenda setting at the outset of each session. Typically, the agenda includes some review of progress through administration of a depression inventory (e.g., BDI-II or HRSD), review of homework, discussion of target problems, assignment of new homework, and a session summary. In addition, the structure is guided by a steadfast focus on nurturing activation. From a stylistic standpoint, essential qualities of the BA therapist include an emphasis on collaboration or learning together as a team. In so doing, the therapist is mindful of pacing to support active collaboration and of soliciting information to ensure that the client understands information presented in session (e.g., specific targets or interventions, the overall BA model, or other "take-home" points from the session). All of the BA strategies also require the basic skill of being a good problem solver. Therapists approach most matters that arise in treatment simply as problems to be solved. Thus, therapists must be naturally curious about factors that maintain problems and be skilled at generating a range of more functional alternative behaviors. Toward this end, it is important to be comfortable with a direct, matter-of-fact, and nonjudgmental manner of communication, particularly in the face of challenges such as not doing assigned activation plans or not attending scheduled sessions. Therapists must also balance a genuine sense of empathy and understanding for the suffering and struggles of their clients with an optimistic and dogged commitment to the possibility of change. BA therapists validate the struggles clients experience and seek out occasions to encourage progress, even if seemingly minimal. Finally, understanding basic behavioral concepts and principles can help therapists conceptualize cases according to a behavioral model of depression and present a coherent framework to clients.

The acronym ENLIVEN (Dimidjian, 2011) captures the structural and stylistic strategies necessary for the competent BA therapist in an easily remembered mnemonic:

- Establishes and follows agenda
- Nurtures activation
- Learns together with client
- Is nonjudgmental
- Validates
- Encourages
- Naturally expresses warmth

In our treatment outcome research, we have used ongoing clinical supervision and therapist consultation teams to assist therapists in adhering to and refining these important therapist qualities. Therapists typically meet together weekly for 1–2 hours. The teams help therapists increase skills with basic treatment strategies (conceptualizing treatment plans, doing functional analysis, effectively grading tasks, etc.). In the context of a focus on specific cases and strategies, the team also provides essential reinforcement for the therapist qualities of empathy, nonjudgment, problem solving, curiosity and persistence, and optimism about change. Although we have not tested this hypothesis empirically, we strongly suspect that it would be difficult for many therapists to maintain these qualities particularly in their work with clients struggling with severe, complicated, or chronic depression without the support of an effective consultation team.

Client Variables

Our treatment outcome research suggests that depressed adults can experience acute and enduring clinical benefit from a course of BA. Our clinical impressions are that engagement with the basic treatment rationale and willingness to complete homework assignments are both important predictors of outcome in BA. Moreover, it is important to note that we used a number of client characteristics as exclusionary criteria in our treatment research. For instance, if a client were acutely suicidal, such that his/her risk could not be managed on an outpatient basis, then we would refer him/her for more acute and intensive treatment. In addition, if a client had a comorbid diagnostic disorder that was more severe and prominent (more interfering and the primary focus of the client), and necessitated another evidence-based treatment (e.g., obsessive–compulsive disorder), then we would also refer him/her to a more specifically appropriate treatment. We also carefully evaluated any potential medical problems that may have contributed to depression and referred clients for appropriate concurrent medical treatment, if necessary.

Recent clinical research also highlights the potential of BA as a treatment option for patients across the lifespan, including adolescents (McCauley, Schloredt, Gudmundsen, Martell, & Dimidjian, 2011; Ritschel, Ramirez, Jones, & Craighead, 2011; Ruggiero, Morris, Hopko, & Lejuez, 2007; Van Voorhees et al., 2009). This work is in line with earlier work by Lewinsohn and colleagues (1984) in the development of the Cop-

ing with Depression Course for adolescents. This treatment program includes activity scheduling, relaxation training, assertiveness and social skills training, and cognitive restructuring. Admittedly, the inclusion of cognitive restructuring in the Coping with Depression Course places this program in the broader area of CBT rather than specific BA, but the emphasis is on scheduling pleasant events. Evidence also supports the use of BA with older adults (Acierno et al., 2012; Meeks, Looney, van Haitsma, & Teri, 2008; Meeks, Teri, van Haitsma, & Looney, 2006; Snarski et al., 2011; Sood, Cisek, Zimmerman, Zaleski, & Fillmore, 2003; Teri, Logsdon, Uomoto, & McCurry, 1997), ethnically diverse patients (Kanter, Hurtado, Rusch, Busch, & Santiago-Rivera, 2008; Kanter, Santiago-Rivera, Rusch, Busch, & West, 2010), patients with anxiety and borderline symptoms (Hopko, Lejuez, & Hopko, 2004; Hopko, Sanchez, Hopko, Dvir, & Lejuez, 2003), patients with posttraumatic stress disorder (Jakupcak et al., 2006; Mulick & Naugle, 2004; Wagner, Zatzick, Ghesquiere, & Jurkovich, 2007), substance users with elevated depressive symptoms (Daughters et al., 2008; MacPherson et al., 2010), patients with schizophrenia (Mairs, Lovell, Campbell, & Keeley, 2011), inpatients (Curran, Lawson, Houghton, & Gournay, 2007; Hopko, Lejuez, et al., 2003), patients with cancer (Armento & Hopko, 2009; Hopko, Bell, Armento, Hunt, & Lejuez, 2005; Hopko et al., 2011) and other medical comorbidities such as obesity (Pagoto, Bodenlos, Schneider, Olendzki, & Spates, 2008) and diabetes (Schneider et al., 2011). Although many of these studies are preliminary, reporting data from small open-trial designs, the breadth of this work suggests that BA may be adapted as a treatment framework for a wide variety of clients struggling with depression and comorbid problems.

CASE STUDY

Background Information

The following section presents the treatment of Mark, a 43-year-old man with a long history of depression. Mark was in treatment for 19 sessions across 4 months. The description here is presented to illustrate the implementation of core BA principles and strategies. Earlier sessions are described in greater detail to provide the reader with "how-to" information regarding the primary principles and strategies. Later sessions emphasize a thematic focus for which the same types of principles and strategies are applied. It is important to emphasize at the outset that this case description is not intended to communicate a prescriptive course of treatment, and readers are advised against following the sequence of strategies in a lockstep fashion. BA is a highly idiographic treatment, in which the choice of specific activation strategies is driven by functional analysis; given this, the reader is encouraged to attend to the ways the therapist conceptualizes Mark's difficulties and implements treatment strategies over the course of therapy. It is our hope that this detailed illustration will inspire readers to apply the basic principles and core strategies in a flexible and idiographic manner.

Mark sought treatment at the urging of his primary care physician. His recent episode of depression had lasted without remission for 3 years. Mark also had a history of alcohol abuse. His early alcohol abuse had caused significant problems in Mark's first marriage, which ended in divorce when he was in his early 20s; however, problems with alcohol were not a cause of current concern. He had been in therapy previously, during his separation and divorce 4 years earlier. However, Mark described it as unstructured and unfocused, and reported that he stopped going after a few sessions. He lived alone, although he had joint custody of his twin adolescent daughters; Mark and his ex-wife alternated parenting every other week.

Mark reported that he had had periods of depression for "as long as I can remember." In particular, he recalled his first episode of depression at age 12, shortly after his father abruptly left and severed all contact with Mark and his family. Mark reported that he had believed his parents were happily married and, at that time, blamed himself for his father's departure. Mark reported that his mother and older siblings never discussed his father. In describing his mood during adolescence and adulthood, he reported, "I have periods when I'm able to function OK. I go to work and all that, but I'm never really happy." Mark's primary depressive symptoms included depressed mood, loss of pleasure in nearly all activities, excessive guilt, fatigue, difficulty concentrating, and occasional passive thoughts of death.

Mark had had a social network that revolved primarily around his former marriage, but he had withdrawn from that network since his separation and divorce. Currently, he spent most of his time alone, with the exception of caring for his daughters. Mark was college educated and worked as an accountant for a local manufacturing company. He also wrote children's stories and, prior to his most recent episode of depression, was working on a number of stories as a member of a local writer's group.

Case Conceptualization and Overview of Treatment

Mark's depression was conceptualized as occurring in the context of his divorce and the changes that ensued following that process; in addition, vulnerabilities related to his family history also formed a context for his current experience. Mark experienced intense grief and anxiety following his divorce to which he responded with patterns of interpersonal avoidance, which in turn were negatively reinforced by reductions in the grief and anxiety. Mark had trouble fully engaging in his significant relationships and instead avoided intimacy in various ways in both overt ways (e.g., refusing social contacts) and subtle (e.g., ruminating about mistakes he made in the past, failing to express commitment to the relationship and what he thought or felt about various topics on a regular basis). Over the course of treatment, the therapist and Mark hypothesized that avoiding close interpersonal connections in his adult life kept Mark detached enough that he would not feel subsequent losses as acutely as those he felt as a child. However, these patterns of avoidance also maintained Mark's depression by limiting his experience of reward in many of his current contexts. Treatment focused initially on increasing activation and addressing many secondary problems and routine disruptions that had become established. Treatment sought to reverse the downward spirals of depression by scheduling and structuring activities. Although Mark increased his activation relatively quickly, his mood did not improve significantly. This led to a primary focus on Mark's rumination and the ways it functioned to avoid intimacy in his relationships, and experimentation with new behaviors designed to move Mark closer to his goal of having a close intimate relationship and feeling better.

Session 1

Session 1 focused on reviewing the results from the assessment process, presenting the treatment model, encouraging questions and feedback, and tailoring the model to Mark's specific experiences. The review of the assessment process is typically brief; in this part of the session, the aim of the therapist is to ensure that he/she has a solid understanding of the client's presenting problems, relevant history, and previous experience with treatment, if any. The therapist also reviews the basic diagnostic formulation to ensure that the assessment outcome matches the client's subjective experience of his/her current problems. Discussion of the treatment typically forms the bulk of the early sessions. The following transcript provides an example of the therapist presenting the treatment model and responding to frequently asked questions about the etiology of depression. Specifically, the therapist puts forth the idea that depression is treated behaviorally, regardless of etiology.

THERAPIST: Let me tell you a little about the basic model that guides BA. The first idea is that there are often things that happen in people's lives that make it hard for them to connect with the kinds of experiences that would normally help them feel good. These shifts can be clear and easy-to-detect changes like major losses or disruptions in life. And they can also be smaller things, like the kind of things that just bug you a little but they keep happening, or you have a bunch of them happen all around the same period of time. The most important part is the idea that the effect of these events is that it's harder to connect with the kinds of experiences that could give you a sense of pleasure or accomplishment in your life, and that could help you feel better. Does that sound like it fits for you?

MARK: I would say that is true for me. Definitely getting divorced was a big one. I think that did set things off, but even now, there isn't much that helps me feel better. Even things that I think should help me feel better don't do much. I just don't have the energy at this point.

THERAPIST: Yes, exactly. It's very normal to feel a whole range of things in the context of such events. Often sadness or grief is central, but so are feelings of fatigue and a sense of not having energy or interest in anything. All of these are parts of the experience of depression.

MARK: That describes it.

THERAPIST: I'm going to draw that out here on this form. In the first circle, we can list some of the events we've already talked about, like the divorce, sharing custody of your girls, and your move. Those reactions of fatigue and low energy that follow are very normal, and we'll write them in here in the second circle. What we find often happens is that people can

respond to these changes by pulling away from their lives even more. This pulling away can happen sometimes in obvious ways, like staying in bed or calling in sick to work, or canceling social engagements, and sometimes in more subtle ways, like being focused more on your thinking than on the activities you are engaged in. Does that make sense for you?

MARK: Yes, absolutely. I do all of those things.

THERAPIST: It makes total sense that you would pull away when you are feeling so down. The problem with pulling away like this is that it tends to keep people stuck in feeling depressed, and the pulling away can become a problem in its own right. So that is the arrow that links what you do and how you feel in a kind of downward spiral. The more you pull away or the more you are caught in your thoughts, the worse you actually feel, the less energy you have.

MARK: Yes. That sums it up.

THERAPIST: And, actually, for many people, there is also a second downward spiral. So the more the first downward spiral is set in motion, it actually can lead to new problems, like your boss gets frustrated with you or your friends stop calling, or it can keep you from solving some of the problems that triggered the depression in the beginning. So the ultimate goal of our work together is to figure out new actions you can take here (*pointing to the third circle on the diagram*) that can help to reverse this downward spiral. We will want to learn together what sorts of activities may have a positive effect on your mood, and then help you activate and engage in those specific ways. And we will figure out how to solve the problems that are creating stress or dissatisfaction in your life. How do you see this fitting with your experience? Do you have questions about what I've said? Parts that fit or don't fit?

MARK: I understand what you are saying, and I think some of it fits, but I guess I don't understand why I get so depressed. I mean, other people have stressful things in their lives and they seem to function. Other people get divorced or have crappy jobs, and they move on. I mean, come on, I've been divorced for 4 years now. I think depression runs in my family. My older brother has been depressed forever, and I sometimes wonder if my dad was depressed when he took off. Sometimes, I can't really identify anything that has happened in my life. I mean, I am never really happy and then, it's just like a switch goes in my brain and I'm back in that dark hole again. How does that fit with what you are saying?

THERAPIST: That is an excellent question. What I mean as I talk about depression is that some people are more vulnerable than others. And, there are many ways that you may be vulnerable to depression—through genetics, biology, or experiences in your history. In fact, we can add some of these things you are talking about now to the first circle as part of the context for you. (*Writes in family history.*) What this treatment emphasizes is that it's possible to change depression by making changes in what you do.

MARK: That makes sense to me. One part of what you said definitely fits for me—the part about pulling away more. I definitely do that. Sometimes I don't talk to another person or get out of bed all weekend. I know it makes it all worse. But I still do it. I don't seem to be able to do anything else when I feel that way.

As the therapist replies to these very common questions, she seeks to normalize avoidant responses to depression. It is essential for the client to experience the therapist as someone who understands and has sincere empathy for his/her struggle. The therapist must communicate that the client's behaviors make sense, even though they may not serve the client well in the long term. In this way, the client is more likely to experience the therapist as an ally in the change process as opposed to someone who oversimplifies or "doesn't get" the challenges of making changes. Additionally, the therapist also emphasizes to Mark the importance of guided activity, highlighting her own role as an expert and the importance of careful assessment. She emphasizes the difference between assignments based on a superficial understanding of depression and those that are guided by functional analysis, a key aspect of the treatment, to which the therapist will return many times.

THERAPIST: Those are great observations and are really on target with what I have noticed for a lot of people as well. What many people experience is that when they start to activate and engage, they can actually feel worse initially! The troubling fact about pulling away or avoiding is that it does provide some short-term relief. But in the long term, that downward spiral can keep you trapped in depression.

MARK: That makes a ton of sense to me. I just don't want to do anything. Making a meal makes me tired.

I feel irritated by the sound of silverware scratching on plates. It's kind of crazy, but I just want to crawl in a hole, to turn out a light in my head and make it all go away. Then, I end up feeling worse when I do stay in bed. I used to drink, too. I knew it would make it worse, and I don't do it much anymore, but it helped in the moment, even though I knew it didn't *really* help. I guess I felt better temporarily and that was enough.

THERAPIST: Yes, exactly. Avoidance is a perfectly natural response. What unfortunately happens, though, is that you are not in touch with all those things that can give you pleasure and a sense of accomplishment, *and* you are not engaged in solving the problems that create stress in your life.

MARK: That's the first and second downward spirals you were talking about, right? I get it but it just all feels so overwhelming. Just the thought of it . . .

THERAPIST: Yes, I know. That is where I come in. It's important to emphasize that this treatment is not just about me saying you should "do more" in general. Sometimes I tell people that it's not the Nike approach to therapy, where I tell you each week to "just do it." You have probably received feedback like that from other people in your life, and you may even say something similar to yourself.

MARK: Yeah, guilty as charged.

THERAPIST: My assumption is that if this were easy to figure out, you would already have done it. It's a simple treatment but that doesn't mean it's easy. The reason that you are here is that it's not easy, and that is where my expertise comes in. A major part of this treatment is the idea of *guided activation*. This means that you and I will be working together to identify specific ways in which you can experiment with activation. My expertise lies in figuring out, first, where the places are that would be the most helpful in increasing your activation and engagement, *and* second, what small and manageable steps you can take to get started. You can think of me as a coach or consultant to you in the process of change. We will work together, as a team, in small steps, all along the way. How does that sound?

MARK: The idea of it sounds good. I guess it's worth trying.

THERAPIST: I'd like to ask you to read a short pamphlet about this treatment, between now and the next time that we meet. It will provide you with more information. When we meet next time, we can talk more about how we will put the ideas into practice.

With this initial session, the therapist has begun to teach Mark about the treatment model and is getting him actively involved in and on board with the rationale. The therapist has oriented Mark to their respective roles in treatment and has given him this first homework assignment (reading the treatment rationale pamphlet). These critical tasks of the first session set the stage for additional discussion in Session 2.

Session 2

In Session 2, the therapist carefully follows up on a number of the key orienting tasks, which includes ensuring that Mark is on board with the basic treatment model and explaining the structure of the therapy. The therapist attends to these topics in opening the session:

THERAPIST: It's great to see you today, Mark.

MARK: Thanks. It's good to be back here.

THERAPIST: That's great. You know, when I was thinking about our session last time, I realized that there were a couple of points I wanted to emphasize more. One of the important ones is that this is a very collaborative approach to therapy, and one that is also fairly structured. So each time we meet, we will start out by setting an agenda for the session, and we will do this collaboratively. In fact, over time, you will set the agenda more and more, though I may have more to say about it in the beginning. The idea is that I'm the expert on how to get over depression, and you are the expert on yourself and your life, and what things help or don't help.

MARK: That sounds reasonable to me.

THERAPIST: Great. So in terms of the agenda for today, I have a couple of things. I'd like to talk more about the treatment approach and your reaction, and more about how we put some of the ideas into practice. Do you have items you want to be sure we address today?

MARK: No, that sounds good. I did read the pamphlet, and it really hit home. It was like they wrote it about me, basically. I thought, "Thank goodness somebody has figured this out."

THERAPIST: That's great. I think one of the core ideas of the model is things happen that tend to trigger depressed mood, and then people tend to do things, or not do things, that make the depression worse. For you, my understanding is that the main trigger was your divorce and that occurred in the context of your history of important losses, too, in your family growing up.

MARK: Yeah, both are true. I've really pulled back on a lot, like not exercising and not doing things with other people or even with my girls. We used to cook these great dinners together and now it's like an effort to get organized to order pizza. It's kind of like that everywhere—at work, too. I'm just managing the minimum and, honestly, a lot of times I'm not even doing that.

THERAPIST: I know. It can be very hard to keep doing the sort of things that will keep you feeling well. And that is where this therapy comes in. From our session last time and from your reading, what is your understanding of what we are going to be doing in here, and how I am going to be helpful? If you were to tell a friend of yours what we were going to do in this therapy, what would you say?

MARK: I guess I would say that we are going to pinpoint the activities that give me some pleasure or help me feel like I'm handling things well. Then, we will figure out how to help me get into the position of being more involved in some of those things.

THERAPIST: Yes, that is a big part of it. Sometimes in people's lives something that is completely beyond their control triggers depression, and then what I call secondary problem behaviors get triggered or made worse. These are the behaviors that involve pulling away or avoiding, as you were saying, like stopping fun activities with your girls or withdrawing at work. And in those cases we work on the secondary problem behaviors, and that is the core of the therapy. Other times, we also need to address larger problems in your life that may be related to what makes you vulnerable to depression. In those cases, therapy can involve *both* directly addressing the secondary problem behaviors *and* working directly on the problems, after we have kind of cleared the path for doing some problem solving by getting you activated and engaged.

MARK: That sounds like it's probably the case for me because I know I had a lot of problems relating to Diane that were part of our divorce, and those are not any better.

THERAPIST: Yes, we will talk more as we go along about what set off the depression for you. In a global sense, we know now that it was the divorce. But, as we start following your mood and activities day to day, we will see the ways that your mood has ups and downs. We will work together and look at that carefully, asking what set that off, how you responded to your mood hitting that point, and whether it would help if you tried something different.

The therapist has now stated twice that generally a contextual event triggers depression, while earlier acknowledging that several things can contribute to vulnerability. This is a subtle but important point because clients sometimes believe their depression came "out of the blue" or that it is simply "biological" and not modifiable by behavioral means. By emphasizing an environmental antecedent (e.g., a loss of positive reinforcement), the therapist sets up the idea that rather than depression being completely beyond patients' control, their depressive response makes sense, and more importantly, it is possible to make behavioral changes to regain or establish new reinforcers in their lives. Moreover, the therapist has continued to emphasize the importance of carefully monitoring and assessing the relationships among mood, activity, and context as a key part of designing effective behavior change plans. The therapist then builds on this foundation as she moves into the other main focus of Session 2—the initiation of activity monitoring. Here, the therapist explains to Mark why activity monitoring is important, begins to teach him how to complete an Activity Record (see Figure 9.3), and links it directly to some of his recent experiences.

THERAPIST: One of the main tools that we use in this therapy is called an Activity Record. This is one example. (*Hands Mark the record.*) As you can see, it has blocks for each hour of the day. I'd like you to use this to start recording your activity and your mood. It's basically a way to keep track of how you are spending your time during the day and how you are feeling. We want to learn what you are doing on an hour-by-hour and day-to-day basis. What things in your life help you feel better, and what things make you feel worse? You and I will review these very carefully together, focusing on how you are spending your time and how you feel. Sometimes the Activity Record tells us right away where changes need to be

made, and other times we have to look at it over a couple of weeks.

MARK: OK.

THERAPIST: Is there anything you have been doing since you started to feel more depressed that is different from what you normally do?

MARK: Yes, exercising less, watching more TV, and just the amount of time I spend thinking about all this. It's just crazy.

THERAPIST: It's not crazy at all, but I agree that it's not helping you very much. And it's very difficult, which is why you are here. We can start to figure this out together. It's great that you are already aware of those patterns, and those are good examples of looking concretely at what you are doing. This therapy is about increasing your awareness of how your mood is affected subtly from activity to activity and increasing those that tend to be more rewarding. It's like we are on a detective mission for the "up" and "down" activities in your life, those that are linked with feeling improved mood and those are that not.

MARK: Makes sense. So, should I write all this down? Do you really want me to do this every hour?

THERAPIST: Here's the guideline that I use: I want people to record their activity frequently enough that they are not relying heavily on memory. The problem with memory when you are depressed is that your awareness can be dulled or biased by the depression. So you don't have to do it every hour. We have to be realistic about the rest of your life! But you may want to experiment with doing it every 3–4 hours. Sometimes, people like to do it at breakfast, lunch, dinner, and before bed.

MARK: That might work for me.

THERAPIST: Let's go over what to write down. You put your activity down for each hour block and then for each hour block you also assign a mood rating from 0 to 10. Let's look at today as an example. What were you doing in the hours before you came here?

MARK: I was at work.

THERAPIST: Okay, great. What were you doing at work?

MARK: I was teaching a new employee how to use our computer system. It was really frustrating because she wasn't picking it up and I didn't have much patience.

THERAPIST: That's great information to record. Why

Instructions: Record your activity for each hour of the day, and record a mood rating associated with each activity. Use the scale below with the anchors that you and your therapist develop to guide your mood rating. Aim to make entries on your Activity Record at least every 3–4 hours each day.

	Monday	Tuesday	Wednesday	Thursday	Friday	Saturday	Sunday
5–6							
6–7			Awake thinking in bed (9)				
7–8							
8–9		At work (7)					
9–10			Getting ready for work (8)				
10–11			At work (7)				
11–12							
12–1							
1–2							
2–3							
3–4	Working/ teaching employee (5)	Home (7)					
4–5							
5–6							
6–7	Therapy (5)	Making Dinner (6)					
7–8		TV (9)	TV (9)				
8–9							
9–10							
10–11							
11–12							
12–1							
1–2							
2–3							
3–4							
4–5							

Mood Ratings: 0: Description, with examples of associated activities: *writing; playing with my kids*

5: Description, with examples of associated activities: *doing a work task that is only moderately interesting but I'm focused and concentrating*

10: Description, with examples of associated activities: *thinking about how I've screwed everything up*

FIGURE 9.3. Sample completed Activity Record (hourly) (assigned on Monday and reviewed on Thursday).

don't you write down "working–teaching new employee." Now, I also want you to record your mood on a 0- to 10-point scale, so let's see if we can get some anchors here. What would be 0 mood for you? We can track this in whatever way will be most useful for you, so we could consider that 0 might be feeling really good, with no depression or feeling down at all. If so, we would then consider 10 to be when you feel your absolute worst, the worst you could possibly feel. It might be helpful to think of some activities that are a 5 or in between, when you're not feeling your best but you're not feeling particularly bad either. Which activities might be associated with each?

The therapist and Mark then worked together to identify activities that were associated with the low, middle, and high ends of the scale. Some clients prefer to use the low end of the scale to indicate feeling negative mood, whereas others (like Mark) prefer to anchor the low end as indicating feeling positive mood ("really good" for Mark). Allowing such flexibility can be helpful as long as therapist and client are clear about the anchors that will be used when the client completes the monitoring at home. It should also be noted that therapists may ask clients to rate other dimensions, such as the degree to which activities were associated with mastery and pleasure (Beck et al., 1979) or a sense of being nourished or depleted (Segal et al., 2002). These may be rated instead of or in addition to mood. Often we begin by asking clients to record mood ratings given that this is an easier starting place for many clients because it requires less discrimination of subjective experience; moreover, the mood rating provides essential information about potential antidepressant activities. For some clients, it is helpful to build on this by teaching them how to distinguish between mastery and pleasure, and the ways in which both can be helpful in regulating mood. In the case of rating mood or mastery–pleasure, it is important to review carefully the method and scale we want clients to use. For other clients, the dimensions of nourishing and depleting are helpful to identify activities that are antidepressant.

THERAPIST: Given this scale, what was your mood rating for the 2 hours of "working" today?

MARK: Probably a 5.

THERAPIST: That's exactly it. Now, sometimes what happens is that people don't fill it out because they

think, "I wasn't doing anything." It's important to realize that even if you are not doing an activity, we want to know that, too.

MARK: What do you mean?

THERAPIST: Well, when people think "activities," they often think of things like "going to the store," "watching a movie," "picking up my child from school." But, we are conceptualizing activity more broadly. It might be driving by Diana's house or having a significant phone conversation with someone, or even lying in bed, spending time thinking about Diana.

MARK: That would be true on a lot of days.

THERAPIST: Yes, and you can write that down. Those are some of the most important things. In some ways, the more detail, the better. We want to start noticing subtle changes. We want to build on those times that you feel just a little better, and we want to figure out what the problem is when you feel worse.

MARK: I think I got it.

THERAPIST: Great! People usually come away from this thinking that it sounds really simplistic. And it does. It sounds simple, but in practice it is not that simple. It can be difficult to do in the beginning, to really look at all your activities and figure out how your mood is related to them. It takes skill and hard work on both our parts. Is there anything that we can think of now that might get in the way of your doing this monitoring this week?

The therapist ended the session by discussing with Mark potential barriers to doing the assignment, encouraging him to make contact by phone if any questions arose, and offering encouragement about the likelihood that she could be helpful to him.

Session 3

As noted earlier, one of the necessary competencies of a BA therapist is the ability to review an Activity Record and glean information that will help to customize activation and engagement strategies. Session 3 focused heavily on reviewing Mark's Activity Record (see Figure 9.3) and using the information collected as a springboard for more detailed assessment of key problem behaviors. Again, the therapist's focus in these early sessions is on increasing activation in areas that will improve Mark's mood; this work will set the foundation for later work on avoidance modification and problem solving.

THERAPIST: Shall we go over your Activity Record?

MARK: OK. (*Hands the therapist the record.*)

THERAPIST: Why don't you walk me through it? What did you learn? (*Hands the record back to Mark.*)

MARK: I'm not sure if this is what you had in mind. I started the next day after our last session. I went to work that day, but I was feeling so lousy that I left early and came home. I was just kind of fiddling around the house until dinner. I felt really down all day up to that point; I rated my mood as a 7. I did make dinner, which was a little better for me. I used to love to cook for Diana and myself, and we would make these big feasts sometimes with the girls. Since the divorce, though, sometimes I just grab a bag of chips or something like that, or on a good night I might order a pizza. When I was cooking, I felt a little better then, about a 5.

THERAPIST: This is terrific. You did a really great job with this. You completed the record exactly as we talked about—writing down your activities and also your mood rating—and all of this information is extremely useful. I want to ask you some more questions about specific parts of the day in a minute, but right now let me just get an overall sense of things.

Notice how the therapist is careful to reinforce the client's efforts early in the review process. Clients are often uncertain about how to complete the record, and it is not uncommon for them to return with partially or improperly completed records. In such cases, therapists must balance the need to provide corrective feedback and to reinforce the client's efforts. Frequent client errors include writing down activities very globally (e.g., "at work" for 6 hours), failing to record mood ratings, or failing to record anything because they did "nothing." In such cases, the therapist should address these problems in a straightforward and matter-of-fact manner.

THERAPIST: What happened after you made dinner?

MARK: Well, after dinner, I started watching TV, and everything kind of tanked from there. I sat and watched TV until 2:00 in the morning. I guess it helped in that it kept my mind off of worries about work and just feeling lousy about Diana, but I was really depressed the whole time. In fact, I rated my mood as a 9.

THERAPIST: That is really important information. I see that you were also up the next night watching TV until 1:00 A.M. Is this true of a lot of nights for you, or are these two more like exceptions?

MARK: I wish they were exceptions, but no, it's been more the rule. And then what happens is that I just can't get up in the morning. Well, I guess I do wake up, but I just lie there in bed. I've been getting to work pretty late, and some days I just call in sick.

THERAPIST: So we'll use this log to pick up themes of specific activities that can help you feel good and those that may be contributing to your depression, like we talked about last time, the "up" and "down" activities. It seems like there are a few that might be important. I'm thinking that the watching TV and going to bed late is one big one, and the other two are cooking and how you are doing at work.

MARK: I think the TV is a really big one.

Notice here that the therapist identified a few broad areas that appear to be related to the maintenance of the client's depression. The BA therapist is also alert to disruptions in the client's normal routines; in Mark's case, both eating and sleeping routines appear to have been significantly altered. The therapist then works collaboratively with Mark to target a specific area for further assessment and problem solving (i.e., nighttime TV watching). At this point, the therapist begins the more explicit process of functional analysis.

THERAPIST: OK, why don't we start there? Let's get clear first about what the problem is because it doesn't sound like it's watching TV in general.

MARK: That's true. Normally, I would watch some TV, like I might watch for an hour. But, actually, come to think of it, I was more involved in my writing then, too. So, normally, I might watch TV until about 9:00 P.M. and then turn off the TV and write for another hour. Or, if I had the girls, we might watch a show together and then turn off the TV and read or play a game, or just hang out together, or maybe I'd be on a phone call or something.

THERAPIST: So, this is different for you. The problem, then, is that you don't turn off the TV at 9:00 P.M. and instead watch it for an additional 4–5 hours.

MARK: Yes, that's the problem.

THERAPIST: Are you doing this every night of the week or just on work nights?

MARK: I hate to admit it, but it's pretty much all nights, not always so late, but pretty much always later than is good for me.

To this point, the therapist has successfully defined the problem in specific and behavioral terms. With a clear and mutual understanding of the problem, therapist and client can begin to consider the contingencies that may be maintaining the problem and what may be amenable to change.

THERAPIST: We should probably look at what gets in the way of turning the TV off, since it does not seem to have a great effect on your mood. If you were to turn off the TV at 9:00 P.M. now, what do you think would happen?

MARK: I thought about turning it off last night, but I just didn't want to think about all of this stuff.

THERAPIST: By "all this stuff," do you mean the divorce and the pressures at work?

MARK: Yes, both of them.

THERAPIST: So, that is what you are actively avoiding. And the TV helps you to distract?

MARK: Yes, I just don't have the mental awareness now to start writing. I can't focus on it, and I'm just not interested.

THERAPIST: I think you have the right idea in terms of distraction, but the problem is that you are distracting yourself with something that doesn't give you much pleasure and not much accomplishment.

MARK: And meanwhile the house is a mess. I haven't paid my bills in months, and . . .

THERAPIST: Yes, that makes sense. That's the second downward spiral we talked about. What do you think about working together on the problem of watching TV? Then, we can tackle some of those other things you are raising. The TV problem might be simple to solve, but my guess is that there is more to understand about it.

Notice how easily the client can become overwhelmed and hopeless in response to the myriad problems in his life. The therapist is alert to this possibility during sessions and is careful to refer back to the BA model as a way to understand the client's experience and to refocus the client on the problem at hand. In addition, the therapist also takes a keen interest in the "minutiae" of the client's day-to-day behavior, particularly if such behavior is related to mood. This detailed level of interest is critical. Its intent is twofold: First, such discussions guide the choice of activation targets and specific assignments; second, it is the intent that such discussions will teach Mark to take a similar interest and begin to notice patterns that are more and less helpful in working his way out of depression.

THERAPIST: Let's understand better what happens with the TV. Does it come into your mind, the thought that you might be better off if you turned off the TV?

MARK: Typically, I think, "I should go to bed." But I know that if I go to bed, I'll just lie there awake anyway, thinking about what Diana is doing, thinking about how much I am going to hate being at work the next day. So, then I think I might as well watch TV.

THERAPIST: Is that what happens in bed? You lie there and ruminate about Diana or things you have done or haven't done at work?

MARK: Pretty much exactly.

In this transcript, the therapist has effectively identified a number of key relationships. Nighttime TV watching is associated with (1) deteriorated mood; (2) poor performance at work; and (3) a process of negative reinforcement in which negative affect (specifically, grief and anxiety) potentially is reduced when the client is watching TV. The therapist has done so in a collaborative and nonjudgmental manner, and the client is on board. At this point, the therapist explicitly examines her hypothesis with Mark about the relationship between TV and mood. On the basis of this understanding, they can then consider possible activation strategies.

THERAPIST: I'm wondering if part of what is happening is that watching TV is helpful in the short run because it takes your mind away from these topics that are connected to a lot of potential sadness and also anxiety about the future.

MARK: Yeah, that's true.

THERAPIST: But the tough part is that while it works in the short run, it's that same downward spiral or vicious cycle in the long run because watching TV gives you almost no pleasure and it keeps you from doing activities that you previously got a lot out of, and it sets you up for having problems at work.

MARK: Yes, exactly. It's crazy, I know, but it's such an easy way out when I'm just beaten by the day.

THERAPIST: Absolutely! So we have to take that into account when we think about making any changes here. I'm thinking that you could try going to bed in spite of that, and we could work on the ruminating. Or, if you are going to be up, you could do things that are better than the TV. Which do you lean toward?

The therapist attends to the function (distraction) of the problem behavior (TV watching), while engaging in problem solving in a very collaborative manner.

MARK: Probably finding other things, better than the TV. I used to go to a book group one night a week. It was made up of other writers and I liked a few of the people a lot, so when I was doing that, I was also doing reading in the evenings, too.

THERAPIST: OK, does reading seem more of a way you could start getting back into some of your writing, versus jumping in with writing itself?

MARK: Yes, there is no way I could write now. I would just be staring at a blank page, feeling like crap.

THERAPIST: OK, that makes sense. So what about starting with this? One option is that you could have a limit for yourself of 9:00 P.M. for TV and we could work on identifying a book that you could read instead.

MARK: It's a good idea. It's more a question of my doing it.

It is very important that the therapist not gloss over comments such as Mark's final statement. When clients express doubt about how or whether they will implement an activation strategy, it is essential to attend to this in detail. Additionally, it is helpful for the therapist to be attentive to statements such as "I'll just have to make myself do it," which generally indicate that therapist and client have not sufficiently identified the contingencies that control the behavior. In our experience, use of sheer willpower is unlikely to meet with great success, and suggestions of such signal that further assessment is required, as the therapist illustrates.

THERAPIST: So we need to be sure we are getting at the real problem, instead of just saying, "Oh, you are going to do this," and leaving it at that. What kind of reader are you? Are you someone who can get really involved in a book?

MARK: I do get really involved. In fact, I'll think about the book a lot during the day, if I'm already into it.

THERAPIST: But getting yourself to do it is hard.

MARK: Yes, it's getting started on things.

THERAPIST: That is great to know. So, we have to somehow get you involved in the book so that when 9:00 P.M. rolls around, you are already involved, so it will be easier to turn off the TV.

MARK: That would make it easier.

THERAPIST: What if you were to buy a book on the way back from our session and begin reading it in the café of the bookstore.

MARK: Oh, yeah, that is right on the way back. I can do that.

THERAPIST: Mark, I think the trick with all of this is to figure out what is going to help you move toward the things that will be beneficial for your mood. And this is what is really hard—getting yourself to go back to the things that you used to enjoy, when you have no interest in them right now. When you feel good, you take it for granted that it's easy to do things like reading, spending time with friends or your girls, and even writing. When you don't feel good, you really notice it. The problem is that you're in this vicious cycle again. The longer you do not do things, the more badly you feel and the less you want to do. The trick for us is to figure out ways to help you start to do some of the things that will give you pleasure again.

The therapist acknowledges to the client that the new behavior will be hard to initiate because of mood, and that it is necessary to do so anyway. Many times, clients employ an "inside-out" or mood-dependent approach to their depression; that is, they passively wait for their mood to improve before making behavioral changes. BA therapists teach clients that when they feel down, they cannot afford to wait for a better mood to strike them. The goal is to get active when they feel down (as hard as that is). Increasing activation will eventually improve mood, even if not immediately, and it will interrupt the pattern of secondary problems created by withdrawal and avoidance. Addressing mood-dependent behavior (or talking about an outside-in vs.

inside-out approach) is a sensitive point in therapy, in which a *great* deal of empathy for the experience of feeling depressed is required. *The therapist must skillfully balance encouragement of action with validation of the difficulty of activating when depressed.* In addition, strongly encouraging even the smallest signs of increased activation (frequently with the use of significant praise) is essential in supporting the process of change.

MARK: Yeah, I know. A lot of the time I might know what I need to do, but I have no idea how to get myself to do it. I've just dropped a lot of stuff, like anything social in the evenings. I don't try to make plans. And, like I said, for almost a year I was going to that writer's book group every Thursday. But then I said to myself, I'm not writing. This whole divorce is wiping me out. What is the point of going? I have nothing to add." But it's true that when I went, I used to get a lot out of it. I'm just not interested now, though.

THERAPIST: Yes, exactly. That's where you and I will work together. I want to come back to the social connections and the routines around writing, but let's stick with the reading and nighttime TV for a bit longer first, if that's OK?

MARK: Yeah, that makes sense.

THERAPIST: Let's think through this book plan again. Is there anything that might come up between here and the bookstore that would derail that plan?

At this point, the therapist and Mark spend the remainder of the session discussing particular books he could purchase that would maximize his engagement, and they discuss potential barriers that might arise to derail him from the intended plan. They also continued to review the Activity Record to identify other key problems, including ruminating at work, withdrawing from social networks, and experiencing disruptions in routines that previously brought him pleasure (e.g., cooking, exercise). In each case, the therapist uses a similar method that she used with the problem of TV watching: defining the problem, identifying the antecedent and consequences, and checking out hypotheses about how the activity is related to mood with the client. The therapist also frequently returns to the overall BA model to help explain links between activities and mood. In each case, they work to learn together what possible targets will be most promising for activation.

Also, the therapist continues to emphasize that simply deciding to "make myself do it" is not likely to be an effective activation strategy for Mark, and that it is essential to tie the activation plan to a clear understanding of the function of the problem behaviors. The therapist employs a combination of gentle questioning, consistent validation of the roles of withdrawal and avoidance through reliance on the BA model, and repeated discussion of potential barriers to activation plans. Importantly, the therapist also highlights for Mark that compliance with the homework assignments may not bring immediate relief.

"What will be really good this week is to see what effect these things have on your mood. Even if they have just a little bit of a positive effect, then we know that we are on the right track. And, Mark, they might not have an immediate positive effect on your mood. It might be that the act of getting yourself to do it is the success itself, and that you need to keep doing it for a while before you start to feel better. But, it's my guess that some of this stuff will help your mood a little bit, even in the short run."

The session concluded with the therapist and Mark reviewing the homework assignments, which included purchasing a new book, starting to read it in the café, and turning off the TV every night at 9:00 P.M. and reading. In addition, they agreed that Mark would return a telephone call of an old friend, Mary, who lived in his neighborhood and had been trying to contact him recently.

Session 4

Mark arrived at to Session 4 with little improvement in the severity of his depression. He reported that he had increased his social contact but was not feeling any better. Mark also had delayed the task of purchasing the new book and continued to watch TV late at night. The therapist addressed both of these problems in a direct, matter-of-fact way with curiosity and interest.

MARK: It was a really bad weekend. I did call Mary and ended up going to this kind of cocktail party at the community pool that she had organized. I was kind of shocked that I went, but I thought being outside would do me good. I was thinking about what we were talking about, and I thought about how much I used to love swimming. I was actually a lifeguard during summers in college. But I think I felt worse after I went. I suppose there were moments that were fun, but I was so frustrated by it all. I just spent the rest of the weekend holed up in my apartment.

THERAPIST: Would that be good to put on the agenda? Doing things that you used to enjoy and not enjoying them?

MARK: Sure.

THERAPIST: And I want to make sure we check in about how it went with the book versus the TV, too. Which do you want to talk about first—calling Mary and the party or the TV?

MARK: I guess we can do the TV first. I just bought the book today. On Friday, I was at that party, so I didn't get home and in bed until midnight.

THERAPIST: Did you watch TV then?

MARK: No, I do think I was more tired from being outside all night, so I just fell asleep when I got back.

THERAPIST: And what about Saturday and last night?

MARK: It was kind of par for the course. I stayed up late both nights.

Given the importance of attending consistently and regularly to the completion of homework, here the therapist assesses what interfered with Mark's full completion of the previous assignment.

THERAPIST: I'm glad you bought the book. That's terrific! I'm curious, too, though, about what got in the way of getting it sooner. Am I recalling correctly that you were going to buy it on the way back from the session last week?

MARK: Yeah, I was, but when I left, someone called me from work about needing to meet, so I didn't have as much time as I thought. But I thought I could do it after work, and then in the evening, I thought, "I'll get it on the weekend because I'll have more time." I don't know.

THERAPIST: If you go back to your leaving the session last time, when you got the phone call from work, was there anything else that derailed the plan?

MARK: No, that was really it. I was still pretty optimistic about getting the book. It was just that I didn't have as much time as I thought I would, and I had to get to work.

THERAPIST: OK, that is good to know. So your plan was

to get the book on the weekend, and you just bought it today. On the weekend, did you think about getting it, or did it just come up again today?

MARK: I did, but I felt so bad after the party I just couldn't get myself to do it.

THERAPIST: It sounds like you were really down. Do you remember that diagram we used in our first session to understand the big picture of depression? I think it fits here, too.

MARK: How so?

THERAPIST: So, if we think about the party as what happened, then you felt really down and discouraged, right? (*Pulls out the model and writes in this situation.*)

MARK: Definitely.

THERAPIST: And you pulled away by staying at home over the weekend and not buying the book. My guess is that this fueled feeling more discouraged. Is that right?

MARK: Totally. I thought, good heavens, I can't even do a simple thing like buy a damn book.

THERAPIST: That's it, so there is that downward spiral getting set into motion.

MARK: It's it exactly. I wanted to do less and less and I felt worse and worse.

THERAPIST: It's great that you can see how these are all connected. I'm curious how it was that you got yourself to get the book today. Are you feeling better, or is it something else?

MARK: I'm not feeling quite as bad, and given that I was already out, it was easier to go get the book. Plus I knew that we were going to meet and you were probably going to ask me about it.

THERAPIST: That is so great to know! So one thing we know is that I have got to keep following up about these things because it helps you do them.

MARK: (*laughing a little*) True, not that I enjoyed imagining being called to task on it, but it did help, I guess.

THERAPIST: And getting yourself out of the house to buy a book this weekend was a lot harder than getting yourself out this morning, since you were already leaving to go to work. Being out already made it easier to accomplish your task.

MARK: Right. That sort of thing seems to happen a lot lately.

THERAPIST: So one solution would be to not wait for the weekend when you've got a specific task to do because that seems to be a harder time for you to accomplish things. The other thing would be for us to set up a system of phone check-ins when you are feeling particularly down, since it seems to help to know that we will be following up on these tasks when we meet. The other issue, though, is to figure out what brought you down so much this weekend, and what to do about that.

MARK: I think that is the biggest thing.

THERAPIST: Shall we talk a bit about the party and the weekend in order to figure out what is going to help most? How does that sound? And we'll make sure to come back to the TV and reading plan.

MARK: OK. I would like not to feel as lousy as I was feeling.

THERAPIST: Why don't we take a look at your Activity Record? (*Reviews the record.*) It looks like your mood ratings were moderate on Thursday and Friday after we met. Then, Friday, at the party and for the rest of the weekend, they were high—7's, 8's, and 9's, too.

MARK: I'm not sure this is for me, honestly. I think I gave it a fair shot, calling Mary, going to the party. I didn't want to do either, but I did. And I felt worse afterwards.

When clients report that they are increasing activation and their mood is not improving, it is important to assess a number of possible explanations. First, therapists may consider whether the activation assignments were too ambitious and did not incorporate successful grading. In such cases, it is important for therapists to acknowledge responsibility for this and recommend an assignment based on smaller components of the task. Second, therapists want to consider whether the functional analysis was accurate. Is it possible that they are activating the client in a domain that is unlikely to yield improvements in mood? Third, therapists want to consider whether ruminative thinking is interfering with activation. In such cases, clients "physically" engage in the activation assignments, whereas "mentally" they remain disengaged from their context and are less likely to have an opportunity to experience reward. Fourth, it is possible that although activation may not immediately improve mood, it may still be "on the right track," because clients are taking active steps toward solving problems and addressing important life goals.

In Mark's case, the therapist decided initially to pursue the possibility that rumination was interfering with activation, based on Mark's comments in earlier sessions about frequently ruminating about Diana and their divorce.

THERAPIST: I guess one thing we could explore together is what was on your mind during the party. When you were standing by the pool talking to other people, or even swimming in the water, what was on your mind?

MARK: You know, when I was diving into the water, I do remember that those were the pleasurable moments of the party. The sound of the water splashing, the coolness, the silence under the water, that was all great. That is what I used to love about swimming too. But the other part—I think I was mentally checking out. I was with a lot of people I really like. Mary is great, and her whole family was back visiting from the East Coast. I haven't seen them in years and I really enjoy all of them. They are great people. But, it didn't really matter. I just wasn't there.

THERAPIST: Were you thinking about Diana or yourself in relation to her?

MARK: Yeah, that was mainly it.

THERAPIST: Were the other folks there conversing with you?

MARK: Yes, and I was talking with them. I mean, I could hear the words coming out of my mouth, but I was just not there.

THERAPIST: So you have one rating on this record for the party, a 7. But, if we were to break these different pieces apart—the swimming, when you were fully engaged with the activity, and the talking, when your mind was elsewhere—what would you rate each?

MARK: The swimming . . . it was good. I guess that would be a 3, if 0 is feeling good; I mean it didn't take it all away. But the talking . . . that was terrible, a 9.

The therapist has successfully identified the problem that was interfering with the potential benefits of activation. She continues to assess the nature and scope of the problem.

THERAPIST: I'm trying to figure out if when you are actively engaged in an activity that kind of requires some attention to it, are those the times that are more enjoyable?

MARK: Yeah, that's true.

THERAPIST: Is this a problem that also interferes with your mood and accomplishment of tasks at work?

MARK: Yes, exactly. I go into my office and it's like where does the time go? Hours go by and I haven't done a damn thing. I'm just wandering over and over things that happened with Diana, what I said, what I could have said. It's awful.

THERAPIST: OK, so we know this is an important problem to address. It's interfering with your enjoyment of times that have the potential to improve your mood, and it's interfering with managing your job well. Can we spend a little more time on what happened at the party?

MARK: OK.

THERAPIST: How would you normally be when talking with Mary's family, if you were not thinking about all these things? What would I see differently in those times than what I might have observed on Friday?

MARK: I'd be talking to everyone. I wouldn't be feeling so bad.

THERAPIST: Yes, that is exactly true. What I'm really curious about is, when you are not feeling so bad, what would you be doing differently? Would you be asking them more questions? Making more eye contact? Responding differently?

MARK: Yeah, all of those things. I'd be more active in the conversation.

THERAPIST: So you would be more engaged.

MARK: Yes, more engaged. Less of that heavy feeling; you know, that "this really sucks" feeling.

In the preceding portion of the session, the therapist has begun to define behaviorally what Mark does in interpersonal interactions when he is not depressed. Carefully specifying these behaviors is an important step in developing some possible plans for targeted change in how Mark approaches similar situations.

THERAPIST: Do you think that if you could practice talking, when you weren't feeling down, more like you normally would with these people that you might feel better?

MARK: I don't know.

THERAPIST: I think the key is to notice what you do in response to the ruminating and to see whether that is

helping or not helping your mood, and then for us to begin to explore what you may need to do differently. It seems that at the party, what you were doing when your mood was better, was to be more engaged.

MARK: It's true. But, when I'm like this, I don't have much to say.

THERAPIST: Yes, when you are depressed, you are more quiet and withdrawn.

MARK: Yes, because it's painful. I see Mary's parents and I think, "They've been married for 30 years. I could have had that with Diana." Then, I start thinking that she is with someone else. It just goes downhill from there.

THERAPIST: You are absolutely right. There is a lot of pain there. And what's happened is that in response to that pain, you have narrowed activity in your life. So you not only feel the pain of being reminded of that loss, but also there is not a lot else going on in your life. And even when you are doing things, you are not as engaged because you are feeling so much pain. I think we need to get you back to doing the things you did before you had the breakup, and before the two of you got together. We need to get you back to your baseline, and once we do that, we can figure out how to get you feeling even better than that.

MARK: It sounds good.

THERAPIST: I know you are thinking this is like pie in the sky, but we can figure out how to do this. The key is to figure out some concrete and manageable steps to help you engage more when you are doing some of these activities, like going to the party. You are right. It's worlds harder to do when you are not feeling well, but these behaviors are partly why you enjoyed those occasions more in the past. We know that you enjoyed Mary and her family in the past, and we know that you got a lot of pleasure from swimming when your mind was fully present with the activity. So the trick is not only to call your friends, like you did so wonderfully with Mary, but also to go to the gathering, and to get yourself really to interact instead of just being there at the party. For times when you find yourself withdrawing into your thoughts, we need to develop specific strategies to help you do less of that. Can you think of anything that would help you do that?

MARK: I don't know. I just don't seem to have much to say these days.

THERAPIST: I know it's hard. There are a variety of things you could try, such as asking more questions, and then closely attending to the response. Or you could focus on something more specific, such as voice or facial expression, to keep your mind from wandering. Sometimes it works just to notice that you've drifted and to take a deep breath to refocus on your goal in that moment.

MARK: I suppose I could try it. My mind just seems to keep wandering.

THERAPIST: I know. So your job here would be to practice being more vigilant as to when that happens because it will happen. The more you notice you're drifting, the more you can practice refocusing yourself back on your friend. Does your mind wander in here?

MARK: I guess a little.

THERAPIST: Why don't we try it in here? Let's pick something to focus on, and then you can practice here.

MARK: OK. What do I do?

THERAPIST: I'm going to time us for the next 5 minutes and, as we talk, I want you to practice fully engaging in our discussion. Your mind is going to wander, particularly if we are talking about something that reminds you of Diana, I would guess. So let's pick something you can focus on to bring your attention back to our conversation. How about the sound of my voice, like changes in tone, how I articulate words, the pace of my speech?

MARK: I can try.

THERAPIST: Great. So, let's talk about some options for social connections that you could make this weekend.

The therapist and Mark continued this discussion for the next few minutes, at which time, the therapist interrupted their conversation to ask Mark for feedback about his experience.

THERAPIST: What did you notice?

MARK: I don't know, maybe you are talking kind of softly.

THERAPIST: How engaged were you with our discussion? Why don't you give me a rating, with 0 being not engaged at all and 10 being totally engaged?

MARK: I guess maybe 7. It wasn't that hard here because I was really focused. I guess I did start to think about Diana a little when we were talking about my calling Mary. I did remind myself to pay attention to your voice, and I guess you just sounded so interested. It made it harder for me to wander off in my thoughts when you seemed to be paying so much attention to what we were talking about.

THERAPIST: That was my impression, too, that your engagement was generally high, and that you did appear to refocus your attention a couple times. That is terrific!

MARK: Yeah, but it was a little strange. I mean, usually people aren't that focused when they are just talking about usual stuff.

THERAPIST: That is very true. I might have been paying closer attention to what you were doing and saying than other folks are in typical social interactions. And this may feel pretty artificial now in general. My guess, though, is that once you get more engaged in social interactions, it won't be necessary to concentrate so hard. It will just come automatically again.

MARK: That makes sense.

In this way, the therapist generates a strategy to block avoidance (rumination) by substituting a new behavior in the form of attending to direct and immediate experience. Although, in this case, Mark experimented with directing his attention to interpersonal stimuli, clients may also be directed to experiment with attention to other aspects of sensory stimuli, such as sights, smells, and so forth. The in-session behavioral rehearsal is very important in that it allows the client to practice and receive direct feedback from the therapist, both of which increase the likelihood of success outside of the session. The therapist then returns to the specific task of reviewing and developing behavioral assignments for the next session.

THERAPIST: Let's go back to your not getting out all weekend. Do you think going out to buy the book was too hard? Is there something easier you could've done to help you get a little more engaged this weekend?

MARK: I'm not sure. How hard is it to go out and buy a book?

THERAPIST: Very hard, when you're really down. Let's think about smaller steps. If you can do a smaller step and get a little reinforcement for it, then it becomes easier to move toward your goal.

The therapist and client continue along these lines with graded task assignment. Given that Mark has previously enjoyed socializing, he and the therapist came up with a plan that on the weekend, he would start by returning some phone calls from friends and inviting Mary for lunch. During lunch, he would focus specifically on attending to their conversation. The therapist also raised the possibility of swimming as an exercise activity. Mark reported that he thought his plate was full with the assignments they had already developed, and they decided to table further discussion of swimming. The therapist then uses the final moments of the session to review the homework, to encourage progress, to validate the difficulty of change, and to reinforce the basic treatment model.

Session 5

At the outset of the session, Mark reports improvement in his mood and the therapist includes this as an item on the agenda. Their discussion allows the therapist to emphasize an important point about maintaining new behaviors in consistent and regular routines. In this session, the therapist continues to emphasize the pattern of social connections and to assess factors that increase Mark's vulnerability to exacerbated mood when alone.

THERAPIST: Let's understand in more detail how it is that you are feeling better?

MARK: I think the reading plan is helping. I finished the book.

THERAPIST: Great! So you probably need another book.

MARK: (*laughing*) I guess that's true. You don't think just the one cured the problem?

THERAPIST: (*laughing*) Oh, how I wish that were the case! Seriously, though, Mark, I think that is such an important question. There is a real temptation when you start feeling a little better to back off from some of the very things that are helping. It makes sense because making these changes requires so much effort, I know. But maintaining the routines are so important.

MARK: It's true. I actually think I've been doing pretty well with that this week. I've been reaching out more to other people.

THERAPIST: This is fantastic.

MARK: And Mary called me again. So, I guess I didn't do what we talked about in terms of calling her, but

I did ask her about lunch when she called. I didn't really want to because I was feeling down when she called. I had just gotten a letter from the lawyer about some new money stuff with Diana. But, I did ask Mary, and I took the girls, too. I think they enjoyed it a lot. I did really focus on asking them all a lot of questions during lunch. I think that helped, too.

THERAPIST: Mark, you have definitely had more social contact in the last few days! You are doing a huge part of this treatment, which is acting in accordance with the goals and plans that we are setting here, as opposed to being directed by how you feel in the moment.

MARK: I tried.

THERAPIST: You did it! You talked about having lunch with your coworker. Did you do that?

MARK: I did do that.

THERAPIST: You did a lot! That's great. OK, I may be pushing our luck here, but what do you think about adding swimming to our agenda?

MARK: I knew you were going to ask about that again.

THERAPIST: (*laughing*) You know me too well. What's your thought about it?

MARK: It's probably a good idea. There is actually a swim lesson that the girls like to do on the weekends, and I could take them and do laps at the same time in the other pool.

THERAPIST: Fantastic! Do you have them with you this weekend? Could we schedule that for the weekend?

MARK: Yeah, I think that would help.

THERAPIST: Mark, do you think that reconnecting with people and some of these activities, like reading, are connected with your improved mood?

MARK: Yes, that definitely had a lot to do with it. I am still not sure that we are getting to the real problem with all of this, but you are right that it does help.

THERAPIST: So we should talk about that, too. Before we move to that, is there anything else that you think is contributing to your positive mood, or is it mostly having more social contact, which you find reinforcing?

MARK: It's the social contact and trying to distract myself with the reading.

THERAPIST: That is so great! Good reminder, too. Let's talk some about another book and how to keep up that schedule.

At this point, the therapist and Mark focus on developing a specific plan for selecting and purchasing a new book to continue the reading routine. Next, the therapist returns to Mark's comments about whether the interventions are addressing what is most important.

THERAPIST: What you mentioned before about the real problem . . . I'm curious what you meant.

MARK: I guess I'm still thinking about Diana a lot. I think that there is a part of me that has to let go, yet just isn't letting go. I am thinking, just asking myself, "Is there still a chance for us? What did I do to screw it all up so badly?" And then I start thinking, "Is this all I have now—having lunch with people, reading by myself at night?" You know, the kind of stuff we've been focusing on . . . I don't know. Is it really going to fix anything?

THERAPIST: Mark, I know it feels like this stuff isn't really getting at the real problem in terms of your thinking about Diana, and I agree that is really important to talk about. At the same time, I don't want us to lose sight of the fact that this other stuff makes a huge difference. It's important for you to reconnect with ways to buoy up your mood before you start to tackle some of the past problems and those that still come up with Diana. Also, I think we will find that there are some similar patterns, so maybe the ways you have tended to pull away from other people since you've been down might have some connections with what happened with Diana.

MARK: That's true. I guess they are not totally separate.

THERAPIST: Are you saying that it's time now to start focusing our time more directly on those topics?

MARK: I think so. Maybe I'm more aware of it because I'm feeling a little better. I guess I'm asking more often, "Is this all there is now?" It just seems like a damn lonely life to be leading, if this is it.

The therapist and Mark end the session by reviewing the assignments. In addition, they agree on a plan to return to Mark's important questions in the next session.

Sessions 6–9

In this next series of sessions, the therapist and Mark return to Mark's question from Session 5. In repeated sessions, he reports improvements in mood related to making progress on projects at home, exercising, and becoming more socially connected in casual and friendship circles. These areas of progress are reflected consistently on his Activity Record forms, which now specifically target the areas of social engagement, reading, and swimming (see Figure 9.4). (This version of the Activity Record can be considered when the activation targets are clear and well developed, and the detailed information gained via hour-by-hour monitoring is not as necessary. It can also be used for clients who have difficulty with the more detailed Activity Record.)

Even with clear areas of improved activation and mood, Mark also reports that his mood is vulnerable to his tendency to ruminate frequently about his ex-wife. The therapist and Mark begin to explore the potential function of rumination about his ex-wife. As they did with respect to both TV watching and rumination dur-

Task	Monday	Tuesday	Wednesday	Thursday	Friday	Saturday	Sunday
Reading	✓	✓	✓	✓			✓
Reaching out to other people	✓	✓	✓			✓	✓
Swimming						✓	✓
Mood	5	5	5	6	8	3	3

FIGURE 9.4. Sample completed Activity Record (daily).

ing social interactions, they develop some initial hypotheses about the consequences of Mark's ruminating about his ex-wife.

THERAPIST: Is it possible that ruminating might be a form of avoidance itself? It's like your mind gets stuck in a broken record format. You keep replaying what you did wrong, what you could have done, and one of the effects is that you are actually avoiding the painful emotions about the loss of the relationship, and maybe also avoiding exploring new relationships?

MARK: It feels like I can't stand the loss of it. That's what I can't accept—that it is lost. I keep thinking maybe there is a way to recapture it, even though I know there simply is not. We can't even communicate about the kids' health care without a lawyer.

THERAPIST: So, in a way, ruminating may be a way to avoid feeling grief and sadness. I wonder if part of this comes from what you learned about how to cope with major loss after your dad left. It seems like no one talked about that and you got pretty caught up in thinking about how you might have been responsible. I wonder if it's hard to know what to do emotionally right now.

MARK: It's certainly true about what happened when I was a kid.

THERAPIST: So one possibility we could experiment with is taking time specifically to experience the sadness and loss.

MARK: I don't know. Thinking about her and what I've lost seems overwhelming. I just want to be done with it and move on.

THERAPIST: I know. Exactly! The problem is that ruminating seems to have the effect of keeping you from moving on. Instead of moving onto other relationships or pursuits in your life, your mind keeps replaying what happened and didn't happen with Diana.

MARK: I just don't know if I'm ready for other relationships.

THERAPIST: So, if you weren't ruminating as much, do you think you might experience more fear?

MARK: When I think about getting into another relationship. . . . You know, I think that there is actually a person at work who is interested in dating, but that's been part of the reason that I've kind of held back

from doing things with her. She's asked me to lunch a couple of times. I just don't want to be back in the same place again 2 years from now. I can't take this whole thing again, and I don't want to subject my kids to it either.

THERAPIST: So, it may be possible that ruminating has the effect of keeping at bay not only feelings of loss about Diana but also fears about future loss.

The therapist also emphasized the importance of continuing with activation plans developed in earlier sessions to maintain adaptive routines and improve mood. In particular, they highlight the need for consistent attention to social contact, exercise, and reading. In addition, the therapist and Mark discuss his return to the writers' group into more detail, beginning to break down that larger task into manageable pieces. Work on these targets forms the majority of the middle of the course of treatment. As Mark begins to address feelings of loss more directly and continues his work on social connections, exercise, and limiting TV watching, he also begins to express interest in dating again.

Sessions 10–15

In this section of treatment, the therapist and Mark begin to address directly the prospect of his developing new intimate relationships in his life, specifically with a woman at work to whom he is attracted. They explore what is necessary to approach rather than avoid Mark's fear of starting a new relationship, and the therapist hypothesizes in particular that Mark's ruminative style may have functioned to avoid learning from patterns in past relationships. The therapist used the TRAP/TRAC acronym as a simple way to help Mark recognize the conditions under which he was likely to avoid (the TRAP), and to then engage in more adaptive coping behavior to get back on "TRAC." For example, Mark reported that he would see the woman at work (trigger), begin to feel nervous (response), and either not talk with her or restrict his conversation to perfunctory work issues (the avoidance pattern). His alternative coping under the same conditions involved asking her if she would like to have coffee. Sessions then focus heavily on examining in detail what Mark might learn from his former marriage that would be instructive in future relationships. The following dialogue provides an example of the types of foci that these sessions target.

MARK: One of the things that happened a lot with Diana is I never felt like I was really present with her or the girls. It was like they were in this little world together and I was always on the outside somehow. I often thought that I should put myself more in the center, like say more of what I thought, but I just didn't. I never did.

THERAPIST: Did that cause conflict with her?

MARK: Yes, absolutely. It was one of things that she said when she ended things. Being on the outside is a big thing for me.

THERAPIST: What does being on the outside involve specifically? How would I know if you were doing that?

MARK: It's just not being willing to speak up about things. She always said it was like I wasn't really in or out on anything, just kind of on the fence the whole time.

THERAPIST: Can you think of a specific example when that was an issue?

MARK: Well, my mother and brothers never really liked Diana very much, but I didn't do much to stand up for her with them. I just kind of let things unfold. . . .

THERAPIST: So, that might have been a TRAP with her? Was it a trigger that you thought she wanted something from you in terms of your commitment?

MARK: Yes, it was, because I ended up feeling really overwhelmed by that.

THERAPIST: And the avoidance pattern was withdrawing.

MARK: I did. I just backed off, and she had to handle the whole scene with my family.

THERAPIST: So with your coworker, if you were to take a stand with her now, what would that look like? What would alternative coping be?

MARK: I have no idea.

THERAPIST: Do you think there is a similar trigger?

MARK: Maybe, because I think she is wondering what's up with me? Like am I interested or not?

THERAPIST: Have you been clear with her about being interested in dating her?

MARK: Not really. We talk often at work, but I can't say that I've really said much about it.

THERAPIST: Would you like to ask her out?

MARK: Yes, I guess I would.

THERAPIST: Why don't we think of some specific things you could say as alternatives to withdrawing and practice with some of them?

In these sessions, the therapist and Mark define, in very specific and concrete terms, the types of behaviors associated with decreased satisfaction and quality in his former marriage. For instance, the therapist's following question to Mark is a central question asked repeatedly over the course of BA: "What does being on the outside involve specifically? What does it look like? How would I know if you were doing that?" The therapist emphasizes identifying clear, specific, and observable behaviors when analyzing behaviors and defining goals. Then, the therapist and Mark work to identify specific strategies that he can use to practice alternative behaviors in pursuing a future relationship. They continue to use the TRAP/TRAC framework to examine situations that arise and Mark's response, and to guide him toward a more engaged approach to intimate interpersonal relationships. As Mark begins dating, they have ample opportunity to revise and refine strategies through activation assignments that target being direct and present in intimate interactions.

Sessions 16–19

By Session 16, the therapist and Mark agree that the bulk of the work of understanding and problem-solving Mark's depression in terms of his unique life context and avoidant response patterns that maintain his depression has been completed. Mark has successfully activated in terms of his secondary problem behaviors (e.g., increased reading, exercise, social contacts, and projects around the house; decreased TV watching) and he has taken steps toward solving the problems of grief and fear of intimacy via initiating a new relationship.

Thus, the final sessions of treatment focused on reviewing and consolidating primary themes and methods used in therapy. Specifically, the therapist and Mark identified the importance of continuing to practice his new skills of blocking rumination by attending to immediate goals and to his direct and immediate experience, and being more direct and expressive with his new partner. In addition, the therapist carefully reviewed with Mark the ways he had learned to use the BA fundamentals himself. Together they reviewed ways that Mark would know when he was starting to feel depressed or to engage in avoidance response patterns. They also reviewed specific steps he could take to begin self-monitoring his mood and activities, and to problem-solve alternative coping behaviors. They also specifically identified a number of alternative behaviors that were uniquely helpful in breaking the vicious cycle of depression, avoidance, and withdrawal; these antidepressant behaviors included, for example, exercise, calling a friend, and reading. Mark reported that he felt well equipped with these tools and the opportunities he had had to practice them in therapy. He also reported feeling encouraged about the positive changes he had already made in his life. He ended treatment expressing optimism about his future and warmly thanked the therapist for all of their work together. Over time, Mark continued to maintain the gains he made in treatment. He established a new relationship with a woman, and they became engaged over the course of the following year. He continued to practice many of the skills he had learned in therapy in the context of this new relationship, with his children, and with his coworkers and friends.

Case Summary

The course of treatment with Mark provides an example of many of the core principles and strategies of BA. The treatment followed from careful and ongoing functional analysis of key problems that Mark presented, which in turn allowed the therapist to develop the organizing case conceptualization. This work was completed in collaboration with Mark during sessions and was also a focus of the ongoing clinical consultation team meetings, of which Mark's therapist was a member. During treatment, the therapist used a range of specific strategies, including goal setting, self-monitoring, graded task assignment, problem solving, behavioral rehearsal, and attention to experience. She also addressed a number of important treatment targets frequently observed in BA, including interpersonal avoidance, rumination, and routine disruption.

Overall, the therapist worked as a coach throughout therapy, helping Mark to problem-solve specific steps to overcome patterns of avoidance and to engage in activities. She also taught Mark to identify links between activity and mood so that they could learn together where to focus time and attention. She used the EN-LIVEN strategies within each session. She maintained the structure of each session and the overall course of treatment, with a sustained focus on learning together and taking action. She maintained a matter-of-fact, nonjudgmental, problem-solving approach to the chal-

lenge of treating depression and the difficulties that arose during the course of Mark's therapy, responding with warmth, encouragement, and understanding. She relied consistently on the BA model, acknowledging the difficulty of change when depressed and the importance of action, especially when mood is low. She returned regularly and persistently to an activation focus on the selected targets of change and worked as a team with Mark to support him in learning how to build a life that was rich and rewarding.

CONCLUSION

This chapter provides the conceptual basics and the how-to specifics that are required to use BA with depressed clients. Evolving from the seminal foundation established by the work of Ferster, Lewinsohn, and Beck, BA highlights the power of direct and sustained attention to behavior change. BA aims to help clients become active and engaged in their lives in ways that reduce current depression and help to prevent future episodes. BA therapists help depressed clients to increase activities that bring greater reward and to solve important problems. Both outcome research and other converging lines of empirical inquiry suggest that BA holds promise as an efficacious treatment for depression (Dimidjian et al., 2011). Future research will examine in greater detail the process of change in BA and the ease with which BA can be transported to a wide range of clinical practice settings.

REFERENCES

Acierno, R., Rheingold, A., Amstadter, A., Kurent, J., Amella, E., Resnick, H., et al. (2012). Behavioral activation and therapeutic exposure for bereavement in older adults. *American Journal of Hospice and Palliative Medicine, 29*(1), 13–25.

Addis, M. E., & Carpenter, K. M. (2000). The treatment rationale in cognitive behavioral therapy: Psychological mechanisms and clinical guidelines. *Cognitive and Behavioral Practice, 7*(2), 147–156.

Addis, M. E., & Martell, C. R. (2004). *Overcoming depression one step at a time: The new behavioral activation approach to getting your life back.* Oakland, CA: New Harbinger.

American Psychiatric Association. (2013). *Diagnostic and statistical manual of mental disorders* (5th ed.). Arlington, VA: Author.

Armento, M. E. A., & Hopko, D. R. (2007). The Environmental Reward Observation Scale (EROS): Development, validity, and reliability. *Behavior Therapy, 38,* 107–119.

Armento, M. E. A., & Hopko, D. R. (2009). Behavioral activation of a breast cancer patient with coexistent major depression and generalized anxiety disorder. *Clinical Case Studies, 8*(1), 25–37.

Barraca, J., Pérez-Álvarez, M., & Lozano Bleda, J. H. (2011). Avoidance and activation as keys to depression: Adaptation of the Behavioral Activation for Depression Scale in a Spanish sample. *Spanish Journal of Psychology, 14*(2), 998–1009.

Beck, A. T., Rush, A. J., Shaw, B. F., & Emery, G. (1979). *Cognitive therapy of depression.* New York: Guilford Press.

Beck, A. T., Steer, R. A., & Brown, G. K. (1996). *Manual for the BDI-II.* San Antonio, TX: Psychological Corporation.

Bennett-Levy, J., Butler, G., Fennell, M., Hackman, A., Mueller, M., & Westbrook, D. (2004). *Oxford guide to behavioural experiments in cognitive therapy.* Oxford, UK: Oxford University Press.

Borkovec, T. D., Newman, M. G., Pincus, A. L., & Lytle, R. (2002). A component analysis of cognitive-behavioral therapy for generalized anxiety disorder and the role of interpersonal problems. *Journal of Consulting and Clinical Psychology, 70,* 288–298.

Carvalho, J. P., Gawrysiak, M. J., Hellmuth, J. C., McNulty, J. K., Magidson, J. F., Lejuez, C. W., et al. (2010). The reward probability index: design and validation of a scale measuring access to environmental reward. *Behavior Therapy, 42*(2), 249–262.

Christopher, M. S., Jacob, K. L., Neuhaus, E. C., Neary, T. J., & Fiola, L. A. (2009). Cognitive and behavioral changes related to symptom improvement among patients with a mood disorder receiving intensive cognitive-behavioral therapy. *Journal of Psychiatric Practice, 15*(2), 95–102.

Cuijpers, P., van Straten, A., & Warmerdam, L. (2007). Behavioral activation treatments of depression: A meta-analysis. *Clinical Psychology Review, 27,* 318–326.

Cullen, J. M., Spates, C. R., Pagoto, S. L., & Doran, N. (2006). Behavioral activation treatment for major depressive disorder: A pilot investigation. *Behavior Analyst Today, 7,* 151–166.

Curran, J., Lawson, P., Houghton, S., & Gournay, K. (2007). Implementing behavioural activation in inpatient psychiatric wards. *Journal of Mental Health Training, Education and Practice, 2*(2), 28–35.

Daughters, S. B., Braun, A. R., Sargeant, M. N., Reynolds, E. K., Hopko, D. R., Blanco, C., et al. (2008). Effectiveness of a brief behavioral treatment for inner-city illicit drug users with elevated depressive symptoms: The Life Enhancement Treatment for Substance Use (LETS Act!). *Journal of Clinical Psychiatry, 69*(1), 122–129.

Dimidjian, S. (2011, July). *Behavioral activation.* Workshop presentation at Sangath, Goa, India.

Dimidjian, S., Barrera, M., Jr., Martell, C., Muñoz, R. F., & Lewinsohn, P. M. (2011). The origins and current status of behavioral activation treatments for depression. *Annual Review of Clinical Psychology, 7,* 1–38.

Dimidjian, S., Hollon, S. D., Dobson, K. S., Schmaling, K. B., Kohlenberg, R. J., Addis, M., et al. (2006). Randomized trial of behavioral activation, cognitive therapy, and antidepressant medication in the acute treatment of adults with major depression. *Journal of Consulting and Clinical Psychology, 74,* 658–670.

Dobson, K. S., Hollon, S. D., Dimidjian, S., Schmaling, K. B., Kohlenberg, R. J., Gallop, R., et al. (2008). Randomized trial of behavioral activation, cognitive therapy, and antidepressant medication in the prevention of relapse and recurrence in major depression. *Journal of Consulting and Clinical Psychology, 76*(3), 468–477.

Ekers, D. M., Dawson, M. S., & Bailey, E. (2013). Dissemination of behavioural activation for depression to mental health nurses: training evaluation and benchmarked clinical outcomes. *Journal of Psychiatric and Mental Health Nursing, 20*(2), 186–192.

Ekers, D., Richards, D., & Gilbody, S. (2008). A meta-analysis of randomized trials of behavioural treatment of depression. *Psychological Medicine, 38*(5), 611–623.

Ekers, D., Richards, D., McMillan, D., Bland, J. M., & Gilbody, S. (2011). Behavioural activation delivered by the non-specialist: Phase II randomised controlled trial. *British Journal of Psychiatry, 198*(1), 66–72.

Ferster, C. B. (1973). A functional analysis of depression. *American Psychologist, 28,* 857–870.

Ferster, C. B. (1981). A functional analysis of behavior therapy. In L. P. Rehm (Ed.), *Behavior therapy for depression: Present status and future directions* (pp. 181–196). New York: Academic Press.

First, M. B., Spitzer, R. L., Gibbon, M., & Williams, J. B. W. (1997). *User's guide for the Structured Clinical Interview for DSM-IV Axis I Disorders.* Washington, DC: American Psychiatric Press.

First, M. B., Spitzer, R. L., Gibbons, M., Williams, J. B. W., & Benjamin, L. (1996). *User's guide for the Structured Clinical Interview for DSM-IV Axis II Personality Disorders (SCID-II).* New York: Biometrics Research Department, New York State Psychiatric Institute.

Foa, E. B., Rothbaum, B. O., & Furr, J. M. (2003). Augmenting exposure therapy with other CBT procedures. *Psychiatric Annals, 33,* 47–53.

Gawrysiak, M., Nicholas, C., & Hopko, D. R. (2009). Behavioral activation for moderately depressed university students: Randomized controlled trial. *Journal of Counseling Psychology, 56*(3), 468–475.

Gloaguen, V., Cottraux, J., Cucherat, M., & Blackburn, I. M. (1998). A meta-analysis of the effects of cognitive therapy in depressed patients. *Journal of Affective Disorders, 49,* 59–72.

Gollwitzer, P. M. (1999). Implementation intentions: Strong

effects of simple plans. *American Psychologist, 54*, 493–503.

Gortner, E. T., Gollan, J. K., Dobson, K. S., & Jacobson, N. S. (1998). Cognitive-behavioral treatment for depression: Relapse prevention. *Journal of Consulting and Clinical Psychology, 66*, 377–384.

Gros, D. F., & Haren, W. B. (2011). Open trial of brief behavioral activation psychotherapy for depression in an integrated Veterans Affairs primary care setting. *Primary Care Companion to CNS Disorders, 13*(4).

Hamilton, M. A. (1960). A rating scale for depression. *Journal of Neurology, Neurosurgery, and Psychiatry, 23*, 56–61.

Hayes, A. M., Castonguay, L. G., & Goldfried, M. R. (1996). Effectiveness of targeting the vulnerability factors of depression in cognitive therapy. *Journal of Consulting and Clinical Psychology, 64*(3), 623–627.

Hayes, S. C., Strosahl, K. D., & Wilson, K. G. (1999). *Acceptance and commitment therapy: An experiential approach to behavior change.* New York: Guilford Press.

Hopko, D. R., Armento, M. E. A., Robertson, S., Ryba, M. M., Carvalho, J. P., Colman, L. K., et al. (2011). Brief behavioral activation and problem-solving therapy for depressed breast cancer patients: Randomized trial. *Journal of Consulting and Clinical Psychology, 79*(6), 834–849.

Hopko, D. R., Bell, J. L., Armento, M. E. A., Hunt, M. K., & Lejuez, C. W. (2005). Behavior therapy for depressed cancer patients in primary care. *Psychotherapy, 42*(2), 236–243.

Hopko, D. R., Lejuez, C. W., & Hopko, S. D. (2004). Behavioral activation as an intervention for coexistent depressive and anxiety symptoms. *Clinical Case Studies, 3*(1), 37–48.

Hopko, D. R., Lejuez, C. W., LePage, J. P., Hopko, S. D., & McNeil, D. W. (2003). A brief behavioral activation treatment for depression: A randomized pilot trial within an inpatient psychiatric hospital. *Behavior Modification, 27*, 458–469.

Hopko, D. R., Sanchez, L., Hopko, S. D., Dvir, S., & Lejuez, C. W. (2003). Behavioral activation and the prevention of suicidal behaviors in patients with borderline personality disorder. *Journal of Personality Disorders, 17*(5), 460–478.

Houghton, S., Curran, J., & Saxon, D. (2008). An uncontrolled evaluation of group behavioural activation for depression. *Behavioural and Cognitive Psychotherapy, 36*(2), 235–239.

Hubley, S., Woodcock, E. A., Dimeff, L. A., & Dimidjian, S. (in press). Disseminating behavioural activation for depression via online training: Preliminary steps. *Behavioural and Cognitive Psychotherapy.*

Jacobson, N. S., Dobson, K. S., Truax, P. A., Addis, M. E., Koerner, K., Gollan, J. K., et al. (1996). A component analysis of cognitive-behavioral treatment for depression. *Journal of Consulting and Clinical Psychology, 64*, 295–304.

Jacobson, N. S., Martell, C. R., & Dimidjian, S. (2001). Behavioral activation treatment for depression: Returning to contextual roots. *Clinical Psychology: Science and Practice, 8*, 255–270.

Jakupcak, M., Roberts, L. J., Martell, C., Mulick, P., Michael, S., Reed, R., et al. (2006). A pilot study of behavioral activation for veterans with posttraumatic stress disorder. *Journal of Traumatic Stress, 19*(3), 387–391.

Kanter, J. W., Hurtado, G. D., Rusch, L. C., Busch, A. M., & Santiago-Rivera, A. (2008). Behavioral activation for Latinos with depression. *Clinical Case Studies, 7*(6), 491–506.

Kanter, J. W., Mulick, P., Busch, A. M., Berlin, K. S., & Martell, C. (2007). The Behavioral Activation for Depression Scale (BADS): Psychometric properties and factor structure. *Journal of Psychopathology and Behavioral Assessment, 29*(3), 191–202.

Kanter, J. W., Rusch, L. C., Busch, A. M., & Sedivy, S. K. (2009). Validation of the Behavioral Activation for Depression Scale (BADS) in a community sample with elevated depressive symptoms. *Journal of Psychopathology and Behavioral Assessment, 31*(1), 36–42.

Kanter, J. W., Santiago-Rivera, A. L., Rusch, L. C., Busch, A. M., & West, P. (2010). Initial outcomes of a culturally adapted behavioral activation for Latinas diagnosed with depression at a community clinic. *Behavior Modification, 34*(2), 120–144.

Kroenke, K., Spitzer, R., & Williams, J. (2001). The PHQ-9: Validity of a brief depression severity measure. *Journal of General Internal Medicine, 16*, 606–613.

Lazzari, C., Egan, S. J., & Rees, C. S. (2011). Behavioral activation treatment for depression in older adults delivered via videoconferencing: A pilot study. *Cognitive and Behavioral Practice, 18*(4), 555–565.

Lejuez, C. W., Hopko, D. R., Acierno, R., Daughters, S. B., & Pagoto, S. L. (2011). Ten year revision of the brief behavioral activation treatment for depression: Revised treatment manual. *Behavior Modification, 35*(2), 111–161.

Lejuez, C. W., Hopko, D. R., LePage, J. P., Hopko, S. D., & McNeil, D. W. (2001). A brief behavioral activation treatment for depression. *Cognitive and Behavioral Practice, 8*(2), 164–175.

Lewinsohn, P. M. (1974). A behavioral approach to depression. In R. M. Friedman & M. M. Katz (Eds.), *The psychology of depression: Contemporary theory and research* (pp. 157–185). New York: Wiley.

Lewinsohn, P. M., Antonuccio, D. O., Steinmetz-Breckenridge, J., & Teri, L. (1984). *The Coping with Depression Course: A psychoeducational intervention for unipolar depression.* Eugene, OR: Castalia.

Lewinsohn, P. M., Biglan, A., & Zeiss, A. S. (1976). Behavioral treatment of depression. In P. O. Davidson (Ed.), *The behavioral management of anxiety, depression and pain* (pp. 91–146). New York: Brunner/Mazel.

Lewinsohn, P. M., & Graf, M. (1973). Pleasant activities and depression. *Journal of Consulting and Clinical Psychology, 41*, 261–268.

Lewinsohn, P. M., Hoberman, H., Teri, L., Hautzinger, M. (1985). An integrative theory of depression. In S. Reiss & R. Bootzin (Eds.) *Theoretical issues in behavior therapy,* (pp. 331–359). New York: Academic Press.

Lewinsohn, P. M., Sullivan, J. M., & Grosscup, S. J. (1980). Changing reinforcing events: An approach to the treatment of depression. *Psychotherapy: Theory, Research, Practice, and Training, 17*, 322–334.

Linehan, M. M. (1993). *Cognitive-behavioral treatment of borderline personality disorder.* New York: Guilford Press.

Locke, E. A., & Latham, G. P. (2002). Building a practically useful theory of goal setting and task motivation: A 35-year odyssey. *American Psychologist, 57*, 705–717.

MacPherson, L., Tull, M. T., Matusiewicz, A. K., Rodman, S., Strong, D. R., Kahler, C. W., et al. (2010). Randomized controlled trial of behavioral activation smoking cessation treatment for smokers with elevated depressive symptoms. *Journal of Consulting and Clinical Psychology, 78*(1), 55–61.

Mairs, H., Lovell, K., Campbell, M., & Keeley, P. (2011). Development and pilot investigation of behavioral activation for negative symptoms. *Behavior Modification, 35*(5), 486–506.

Manos, R. C., Kanter, J. W., & Busch, A. M. (2010). A critical review of assessment strategies to measure the behavioral activation model of depression. *Clinical Psychology Review, 30*, 547–561.

Manos, R. C., Kanter, J. W., & Luo, W. (2011). The Behavioral Activation for Depression Scale–Short Form: Development and validation. *Behavior Therapy, 42*(4), 726–739.

Martell, C. R., Addis, M. E., & Jacobson, N. S. (2001). *Depression in context: Strategies for guided action.* New York: Norton.

Martell, C. R., Dimidjian, S., & Herman-Dunn, R. (2010). *Behavioral activation for depression: A clinician's guide*: Guilford Press.

Mazzucchelli, T., Kane, R., & Rees, C. (2009). Behavioral activation treatment of depression in adults: A meta-analysis and review. *Clinical Psychology: Science and Practice, 16*, 383–411.

McCauley, E., Schloredt, K., Gudmundsen, G., Martell, C., & Dimidjian, S. (2011). Expanding behavioral activation to depressed adolescents: Lessons learned in treatment development. *Cognitive and Behavioral Practice, 18*(3), 371–383.

Meeks, S., Looney, S. W., Van Haitsma, K., & Teri, L. (2008). BE-ACTIV: A staff-assisted behavioral intervention for depression in nursing homes. *The Gerontologist, 48*(1), 105–114.

Meeks, S., Teri, L., Van Haitsma, K., & Looney, S. (2006). Increasing pleasant events in the Nursing Home Collaborative Behavioral Treatment for Depression. *Clinical Case Studies, 5*(4), 287–304.

Mohammadi, A., & Amiri, M. (2010). Behavioral Activation for Depression Scale: Psychometric properties and confirmatory factor analysis for Persian version. *Iranian Journal of Psychiatry and Clinical Psychology, 16*, 65–73.

Mulick, P. S., & Naugle, A. E. (2004). Behavioral activation for comorbid PTSD and major depression: A case study. *Cognitive and Behavioral Practice, 11*(4), 378–387.

National Institute of Health and Clinical Excellence. (2009). *Depression: The treatment and management of depression in adults.* London: Author.

Nolen-Hoeksema, S. (2000). The role of rumination in depressive disorders and mixed anxiety/depressive symptoms. *Journal of Abnormal Psychology, 109*, 504–511.

Pagoto, S., Bodenlos, J. S., Schneider, K. L., Olendzki, B., & Spates, C. R. (2008). Initial investigation of behavioral activation therapy for co-morbid major depressive disorder and obesity. *Psychotherapy Theory Research and Practice, 45*, 410–415.

Porter, J. F., Spates, C. R., & Smitham, S. (2004). Behavioral activation group therapy in public mental health settings: A pilot investigation. *Professional Psychology: Research and Practice, 35*(3), 297–301.

Quijano, L. M., Stanley, M. A., Petersen, N. J., Casado, B. L., Steinberg, E. H., Cully, J. A., et al. (2007). Healthy IDEAS: A depression intervention delivered by community-based case managers serving older adults. *Journal of Applied Gerontology, 26*(2), 139–156.

Raes, F., Hoes, D., Van Gucht, D., & Kanter, J. W. (2010). The Dutch version of the behavioral activation for depression scale (BADS): Psychometric properties and factor structure. *Journal of Behavior Therapy and Experimental Psychiatry, 41*, 246–250.

Reynolds, E. K., MacPherson, L., Tull, M. T., Baruch, D. E., & Lejuez, C. W. (2011). Integration of the brief behavioral activation treatment for depression (BATD) into a college orientation program: Depression and alcohol outcomes. *Journal of Counseling Psychology, 58*(4), 555–564.

Ritschel, L. A., Ramirez, C. L., Jones, M., & Craighead, W. E. (2011). Behavioral activation for depressed teens: A pilot study. *Cognitive and Behavioral Practice, 18*(2), 281–299.

Ruggiero, K. J., Morris, T. L., Hopko, D. R., & Lejuez, C. W. (2007). Application of behavioral activation treatment for depression to an adolescent with a history of child maltreatment. *Clinical Case Studies, 6*(1), 64–78.

Schneider, K. L., Pagoto, S. L., Handschin, B., Panza, E., Bakke, S., Liu, Q., et al. (2011). Design and methods for a pilot randomized clinical trial involving exercise and behavioral activation to treat comorbid type 2 diabetes and major depressive disorder. *Mental Health and Physical Activity, 4*(1), 13–21.

Scogin, F., Jamison, C., & Gochneaur, K. (1989). Comparative efficacy of cognitive and behavioral bibliotherapy for mildly and moderately depressed older adults. *Journal of Consulting and Clinical Psychology, 57,* 403–407.

Segal, Z. V., Williams, J. M. G., & Teasdale, J. D. (2002). *Mindfulness-based cognitive therapy for depression.* New York: Guilford Press.

Snarski, M., Scogin, F., DiNapoli, E., Presnell, A., McAlpine, J., & Marcinak, J. (2011). The effects of behavioral activation therapy with inpatient geriatric psychiatry patients. *Behavior Therapy, 42*(1), 100–108.

Sood, J. R., Cisek, E., Zimmerman, J., Zaleski, E. H., & Fillmore, H. H. (2003). Treatment of depressive symptoms during short-term rehabilitation: An attempted replication of the DOUR project. *Rehabilitation Psychology, 48*(1), 44–49.

Spates, C. R., Kalata, A. H., Ozeki, S., Stanton, C. E., & Peters, S. (2012). Initial open trial of a computerized behavioral activation treatment for depression. *Behavior Modification, 36*(6), 1–39.

Spek, V., Cuijpers, P. I. M., Nyklicek, I., Riper, H., Keyzer, J., & Pop, V. (2007). Internet-based cognitive behaviour therapy for symptoms of depression and anxiety: A meta-analysis. *Psychological Medicine, 37*(3), 319–328.

Spek, V., Cuijpers, P., Nyklicek, I., Smits, N., Riper, H., Keyzer, J., et al. (2008). One-year follow-up results of a randomized controlled clinical trial on internet-based cognitive behavioural therapy for subthreshold depression in people over 50 years. *Psychological Medicine, 38*(5), 635–640.

Teri, L., Logsdon, R. G., Uomoto, J., & McCurry, S. M. (1997). Behavioral treatment of depression in dementia patients: A controlled clinical trial. *Journals of Gerontology: Psychological Sciences, 52,* 59–66.

Uebelacker, L. A., Weisberg, R. B., Haggarty, R., & Miller, I. W. (2009). Adapted behavior therapy for persistently depressed primary care patients: An open trial. *Behavior Modification, 33*(3), 374–395.

Van Voorhees, B. W., Fogel, J., Reinecke, M. A., Gladstone, T., Stuart, S., Gollan, J., et al. (2009). Randomized clinical trial of an internet-based depression prevention program for adolescents (Project CATCH-IT) in primary care: 12-week outcomes. *Journal of Developmental and Behavioral Pediatrics, 30*(1), 23–37.

Wagner, A. W., Zatzick, D. F., Ghesquiere, A., & Jurkovich, G. J. (2007). Behavioral activation as an early intervention for posttraumatic stress disorder and depression among physically injured trauma survivors. *Cognitive and Behavioral Practice, 14*(4), 341–349.

Ware, J. E., & Sherbourne, C. D. (1992). The MOS 36-Item Short-Form Health Survey (SF-36), I: Conceptual framework and item selection. *Medical Care, 30,* 473–483.

Warmerdam, L., Van Straten, A., Twisk, J., Riper, H., & Cuijpers, P. (2008). Internet-based treatment for adults with depressive symptoms: Randomized controlled trial. *Journal of Medical Internet Research, 10,* e44.

Watson, D. L., & Tharp, R. G. (2002). *Self directed behavior.* Belmont, CA: Wadsworth/Thomson Learning.

Weinstock, L. M., Munroe, M. K., & Miller, I. W. (2011). Behavioral activation for the treatment of atypical depression: A pilot open trial. *Behavior Modification, 35*(4), 403–424.

Weissman, M. M., & Bothwell, S. (1976). Assessment of social adjustment by patient self-report. *Archives of General Psychiatry, 33*(9), 1111–1115.

Zeiss, A. M., Lewinsohn, P. M., & Muñoz, R. F. (1979). Nonspecific improvement effects in depression using interpersonal skills training, pleasant activity schedules, or cognitive training. *Journal of Consulting and Clinical Psychology, 47,* 427–439.

Zettle, R. D., & Rains, J. C. (1989). Group cognitive and contextual therapies in treatment of depression. *Journal of Clinical Psychology, 45*(3), 436–445.

CHAPTER 10

Borderline Personality Disorder

Andrada D. Neacsiu
Marsha M. Linehan

This chapter presents one of the more remarkable developments in all of psychotherapy. Few therapists are willing to undertake the overwhelmingly difficult and wrenching task of treating individuals with "borderline" characteristics, yet these people are among the neediest encountered in any therapeutic setting. They also impose an enormous burden on the health care system. Over the past several decades, Linehan and her colleagues have developed a demonstrably effective treatment for individuals with borderline personality disorder (BPD) that constitutes one of the most substantial contributions to the armamentarium of the psychotherapist in recent times. What is even more interesting is that this approach blends emotion regulation, interpersonal systems, and more traditional cognitive-behavioral approaches into a coherent whole. To this mix Linehan adds her personal experience with Eastern philosophies and religions, yet the authors remain true to the empirical foundations of their approach. The fascinating case study presented in this chapter illustrates Linehan's therapeutic expertise and strategic timing in a way that will be invaluable to all therapists who deal with personality disorders. The surprising and tragic outcome underscores the enormous burden of clinical responsibility inherent in any treatment setting, as well as the practical issues that arise when treatment ultimately fails.—D. H. B.

Clinicians generally agree that clients with a diagnosis of borderline personality disorder (BPD) are challenging and difficult to treat. As a result, BPD has become a stigmatized disorder resulting in negative attitudes, trepidation, and concern with regard to providing treatment (Aviram, Brodsky, & Stanley, 2006; Lequesne & Hersh, 2004; Paris, 2005). Perhaps of greatest concern is the generally high incidence of suicidal behavior among this population. Approximately 75% of clients who meet criteria for BPD have a history of suicide attempts, with an average of 3.4 attempts per individual (Soloff, Lis, Kelly, Cornelius, & Ulrich, 1994). Suicide threats and crises are frequent, even among those who never engage in any suicidal or nonsuicidal self-injurious behavior (NSSI). Suicidal ideation is also frequent and contributes to the onset and maintenance of daily negative mood (Nisenbaum, Links, Eynan, & Heisel, 2010). Although much of this behavior is without lethal consequence, follow-up studies of individuals with BPD have found suicide rates of about 7–8%, and the percentage who eventually commit suicide is estimated at 10% (for a review, see Linehan, Rizvi, Shaw-Welch, & Page, 2000). Among all individuals who have committed suicide, from 7 to 38% meet criteria for BPD, with the higher incidence occurring primarily among young adults with the disorder (e.g., Brent et al., 1994; Isometsa et al., 1994). Lethality and frequency of suicidal behavior seem to be strongly related to impulsivity (Chesin, Jeglic, & Stanley, 2010) and poor psychosocial functioning (Soloff & Chiappetta, 2012), which may make it difficult to decide what to prioritize in treatment. Individuals with BPD also have difficulties with anger and anger expression. Not infrequently, intense anger is directed at their therapists. The frequent coexistence of BPD with both Axis I conditions (e.g., mood or anxiety disorders) and other personality disorders clearly complicates treatment further. In particular, comorbid posttraumatic stress disorder (PTSD) results in greater impairment in individuals with BPD (Harned, Rizvi, & Linehan, 2010).

The criteria for BPD, as defined in the fifth edition of the *Diagnostic and Statistical Manual of Mental Disorders* (DSM-5; American Psychiatric Association, 2013), reflect a pervasive pattern of instability and dysregulation across all domains of functioning. An additional popular measure for BPD is Zanarini's Rating Scale for BPD (ZAN-BPD; Zanarini, 2003). Other assessment measures used to diagnose BPD include the International Personality Disorders Examination (IPDE; Loranger, 1995) and the Diagnostic Interview for DSM-IV Personality Disorders (DIPD-IV; Zanarini, Frankenburg, Sickel, & Yong, 1996). The Borderline Symptom List (BSL; Bohus et al., 2001, 2007) and the McLean Screening Instrument for Borderline Personality Disorder (MSI-BPD; Zanarini et al., 2003) are additional screening measures for BPD.

Linehan (1993a), followed by additional theorists, proposed BPD to be a disorder of pervasive emotion dysregulation (see also Conklin & Westen, 2005; Livesley, Jang, & Vernon, 1998). Indeed, most DSM-5 BPD criterion behaviors can be defined either as a direct consequence of emotion dysregulation or as responses that function to modulate the aversive emotional states (Linehan, 1993b; McMain, Korman, & Dimeff, 2001).

More recent research is finding that problems with emotion dysregulation are common in many other DSM disorders (Kring & Sloan, 2010). Individuals diagnosed with a variety of other mental health disorders appear to have emotion dysregulation patterns that are similar to those seen in BPD. Increased sensitivity and reactivity, when compared to controls, has been connected to generalized anxiety disorder (GAD; Mennin, Heimberg, Turk, & Fresco, 2005), substance dependence (Thorberg & Lyvers, 2006), and social anxiety disorder (SAD) and specific phobias (Etkin & Wager, 2007). Furthermore, the transaction between vulnerability and an insufficient coaching environment is

similar to the etiological theories presented in panic disorder (Barlow, Allen, & Choate, 2004), GAD (Mennin, 2004), and some specific phobias (Cisler, Olatunji, Feldner, & Forsyth, 2010). Thus, pervasive emotion dysregulation is likely relevant to many other clinical populations beyond BPD.

This chapter focuses primarily on describing dialectical behavior therapy (DBT), as a treatment of BPD (Linehan, 1993a, 1993b) and of pervasive emotion dysregulation. Before describing DBT, we first review other treatments for BPD and provide information on their theoretical rationales and supporting data (when such data are available). We then present the empirical support for DBT as a treatment for BPD and for emotion dysregulation. This is followed by a more in-depth description of DBT—its philosophical roots, underlying theory, and treatment protocols.

OVERVIEW OF OTHER TREATMENT APPROACHES

Various approaches have been applied to the treatment of BPD. Although it is not our purpose to present a scholarly review of all the many treatments for BPD, we believe it helpful to review briefly the status of other treatments before presenting DBT in detail.

Psychodynamic

Psychodynamic approaches currently receiving the most attention include those of Kernberg (1984; Kernberg, Selzer, Koenigsberg, Carr, & Appelbaum, 1989), Adler and Buie (1979; Adler, 1981, 1993; Buie & Adler, 1982), and Bateman and Fonagy (2004). Among these, Kernberg's (1984) theoretical contributions are clearly prominent. His object relations model is comprehensive as to theory and technique and has had considerable influence on the psychoanalytic literature. His expressive psychotherapy for clients with "borderline personality organization" (BPO) or BPD, transference-focused psychotherapy (TFP), emphasizes three primary factors: interpretation, maintenance of technical neutrality, and transference analysis. The focus of the therapy is on exposure and resolution of intrapsychic conflict. Treatment goals include increased impulse control and anxiety tolerance, ability to modulate affect, and development of stable interpersonal relationships. TFP also uses a target hierarchy approach in the first year of treatment. The targets are (1) containment of suicidal and self-destructive behaviors, (2) therapy-destroying behaviors, and (3) identification and recapitulation of dominant object relational patterns, as experienced in the transference relationship (Clarkin, Levy, Lenzenweger, & Kernberg, 2007). Kernberg (1984) has also distinguished a supportive psychotherapy for more severely disturbed clients with BPO or BPD. Like expressive psychotherapy, supportive psychotherapy also places great emphasis on the importance of the interpersonal relationship in therapy (transference); however, interpretations are less likely to be made early in treatment, and only the negative responses to the therapist and to therapy (negative transference) are explored. Both expressive and supportive psychotherapy are expected to last several years, with primary foci on suicidal behaviors and therapy-interfering behaviors. The data supporting the use of TFP are not extensive. Clarkin and colleagues (2007) conducted a multisite randomized controlled trial (RCT) comparing TFP with the leading evidence-based treatment (DBT) and with an additional psychodynamic psychotherapy treatment designed to exclude elements considered to be the mechanism of change in TFP. A sample of mixed-gender individuals with BPD was randomized to DBT ($N = 30$), TFP ($N = 30$), and dynamic supportive treatment (ST; $N = 30$). Research therapists were supervised on a weekly basis, and adherence ratings were assessed although not reported. Results indicated that all three treatments demonstrated improvement in depression, anxiety, global functioning, and interpersonal adjustment. Only DBT and TFP were associated with significant improvement in suicidality (small effect sizes); similarly, only the psychodynamic treatments resulted in significant reductions in anger (medium effect sizes). According to the Clarkin and colleagues, irritability, physical and verbal assault, and impulsivity only changed in TFP. These results represent within-condition changes, as there were no differences between conditions. TFP was superior to control conditions in a secondary analysis including several measures of psychodynamic constructs, such as metacognitive and social-cognitive capacities, and reflective functioning (Levy & Scala, 2012). These results must be interpreted with caution. While positive changes were evident in all conditions, the mechanism of change proposed for TFP was not supported, and the comparison condition was questionable given that it is unclear whether the DBT therapists were adherent to the model.

Doering and colleagues (2010), followed up with an independent RCT comparing TFP with treatment by behavioral and nonbehavioral community experts. One hundred and four women diagnosed with BPD underwent 1 year of treatment. The authors reported that TFP was superior in reducing suicidality, dropout, borderline psychopathology, use of services, and poor global functioning. Participants in TFP on average received twice as many sessions. When researchers controlled for the number of sessions attended, group differences on suicide attempts and use of services were no longer significant, although all other results remained significant (Doering et al., 2010). This study has been criticized for including all participants in the analyses (regardless of whether they attended any therapy session) and for choosing post hoc a statistical test that did not accurately reflect the findings on suicidal behavior (Kleindienst, Krumm, & Bohus, 2011).

Mentalization therapy, developed by Bateman and Fonagy (2004), is an intensive therapy grounded in attachment theory (i.e., BPD is viewed as an attachment disorder), with a focus on relationship patterns and nonconscious factors inhibiting change. "Mentalization" refers to one's perception or interpretation of the actions of others and oneself as intentional. The treatment is based on the theory that individuals with BPD have an inadequate capacity for mentalization. Treatment, therefore, focuses on bringing the client's mental experiences to conscious awareness, facilitating a more complete, integrated sense of mental agency. The goal is to increase the client's capacity for recognizing the existence of the thoughts and feelings he/she is experiencing. Mentalization-based therapy (MBT) has been successfully offered as an 18-month partial hospitalization followed by 18-month biweekly therapy (Bateman & Fonagy, 1999) or as an 18-month outpatient individual and group intervention (Bateman & Fonagy, 2009). MBT as a treatment for BPD has been tested with two RCTs.

The first RCT compared 18 months of treatment as usual (TAU) with MBT for 18 months in a partial hospitalization setting, followed by 18 months of outpatient MBT (Bateman & Fonagy, 1999). Clients were randomly assigned to either standard psychiatric care without individual psychotherapy (control condition) or to partial hospitalization, a treatment program with the following goals of therapy: (1) psychoanalytically informed engagement of clients in treatment; (2) reduction of psychopathology, including depression and anxiety; (3) reduction of suicidal behavior; (4) improvement in social competence; and (5) reduction in lengthy hospitalizations. The experimental treatment group received once-weekly individual psycho-therapy provided by psychiatric nurses, once-weekly psychodrama-based expressive therapy, thrice-weekly group therapy sessions, a weekly community meeting, a monthly meeting with a case administrator, and a monthly medications review. At the end of the 18-month partial-hospitalization treatment, those receiving MBT showed significant reductions in suicidal behavior (suicide attempts and self-mutilation), inpatient hospitalization stays, measures of psychopathology (including depression and anxiety), and social functioning relative to the control group. These gains were maintained and increased during an 18-month follow-up period consisting of twice-weekly group therapy (Bateman & Fonagy, 2001). The researchers noted that their program contains three characteristics they hypothesize to be related to treatment effectiveness: a consistent theoretical rationale for treatment, a relationship focus, and consistent treatment over time. Gains were maintained at a 5-year follow-up, although participants in MBT continued to have impairments in general social function (Bateman & Fonagy, 2008).

The second RCT (Bateman & Fonagy, 2009) compared 18 months of outpatient MBT with a structured clinical management (SCM) control condition. MBT included individual and group psychotherapy, as well as crisis phone coaching. SCM developed by the authors to mirror best practices in the treatment of BPD was primarily a supportive intervention, with case management including both group and individual therapy. It was unclear from the study description whether participants in both conditions were offered a similar amount of time in therapy. Assessments were conducted at pretreatment, at 6 and 12 months during treatment, and at the end of treatment. One hundred and thirty-four men and women with a diagnosis of BPD and a recent history of suicidal behavior were included in the study. Analyses were conducted at each assessment time point, and not longitudinally, which makes results difficult to interpret. Nevertheless, substantial improvements in both conditions was reported, with MBT being superior to SCM in reducing suicide attempts in the last 6 months, self-injury episodes in the last 12 months, and hospitalization throughout the treatment year. SCM was superior to MBT in reducing self-harm episodes in the first 6 months of treatment. MBT was also significantly better than SCM at increasing general assessment of functioning, depression, and social adjustment (Bateman & Fonagy, 2009).

Psychopharmacological

Reviews of the literature regarding drug treatments for BPD highlight a dilemma for the prescribing pharmacotherapist: BPD involves dysregulation in too many domains for a single drug to serve as a panacea (Dimeff, McDavid, & Linehan, 1999; Lieb, Zanarini, Linehan, & Bohus, 2004; Nose, Cipriani, Biancosino, Grassi, & Barbui, 2006). In general, results indicate that several agents may be useful for improving global functioning, cognitive-perceptual symptoms (e.g., suspiciousness, ideas of reference, transitory hallucinations), emotion dysregulation, or impulsive–behavioral dyscontrol (for reviews, see Lieb et al., 2004; Nose et al., 2006).

Lieb, Völlm, Rücker, Timmer, and Stoffers (2010) conducted a meta-analysis of 27 RCTs and organized the evidence based on class of medications. They found that for first-generation antipsychotics, evidence supports the effectiveness of haloperidol in the reduction of anger and flupentixol in the reduction of suicidal behavior. Thiothixene was found not to be effective. For second-generation antipsychotics, evidence supports aripiprazole's effectiveness in reducing pathological symptoms of BPD, as well as comorbid psychopathology. Olanzapine is accumulating increased evidence with regard to its positive effect in reducing affective instability, anger, and psychotic symptoms, although findings for its effect on suicidal behavior are mixed (Lieb et al., 2010). In addition to superiority to placebo, olanzapine has been shown to decrease impulsive aggression and chronic dysphoria more effectively than fluoxetine (Zanarini, Frankenburg, & Parachini, 2004). Olanzapine is consistently found to have a weight gain side effect. Ziprasidone was found not to be effective (Lieb et al., 2010).

With regard to mood stabilizers and antidepressants, valproate semisodium was found to have a significant effect in reducing interpersonal problems and depression in clients with BPD, including those with aggressive and impulsive behavior (Stein, Simeon, Frenkel, Islam, & Hollander, 1995). Lamotrigine is more effective than placebo in reducing impulsivity, and topiramate was found to reduce associated psychopathology and anger. Topiramate was found to have a significant side effect of weight loss. Antidepressants evidenced limited effectiveness in the treatment of BPD problems. Finally, omega-3 fatty acids were found to reduce suicidality and depression above and beyond placebo (Lieb et al., 2010).

In summary, some drug treatments may be effective in treating aspects of the BPD psychopathology. Nevertheless, caution is in order when considering pharmacotherapy for BPD. Clients with BPD are notoriously noncompliant with treatment regimens, may abuse the prescribed drugs or overdose, and may experience unintended effects of the drugs. With these caveats in mind, carefully monitored pharmacotherapy may be a useful and important adjunct to psychotherapy in the treatment of BPD.

Cognitive-Behavioral

Treatment of BPD has received increasing attention from cognitive and behavioral theorists. The cognitive approach views the problems of the client with BPD as residing within both the content and the process of the individual's thoughts. Beck's approach to treating BPD (Beck & Freeman, 1990) is representative of cognitive psychotherapy generally, with the focus of treatment on restructuring thoughts and on developing a collaborative relationship through which more adaptive ways of viewing the world are developed. More specifically, it focuses on decreasing negative and polarized beliefs that result in unstable affect and destructive behaviors (Brown, Newman, Charlesworth, Crits-Christoph, & Beck, 2004). In an open clinical trial of cognitive therapy for clients with BPD, decreases in problems associated with BPD including depression, hopelessness, and suicide ideation were found at the end of treatment and during follow-up.

An RCT compared 1 year of cognitive therapy (CT) and Rogerian supportive therapy (RST) for 65 men and women who met diagnostic criteria for BPD. In this study, participants were offered one session weekly in each condition for 6 months, followed by 12 sessions aimed at maintaining gains over the subsequent 6 months. Cottraux and colleagues (2009) found that CT was superior to RST in retaining clients in therapy. No additional differences between conditions were found, although CT led to reductions in hopelessness and impulsivity faster than RST. Follow-up analyses, nevertheless, showed a significant difference between conditions, with participants who underwent CT demonstrating higher clinical global improvement than participants treated with RST. Given the small sample size and the large number of dropouts from this study, the effectiveness of CT is still unclear (Cottraux et al., 2009).

The cognitive-behavioral therapies of Young, Klosko, and Weishaar (2003; Kellogg & Young, 2006), Pretzer (1990), Blum, Pfohl, St. John, Monahan, and Black (2002), and Schmidt and Davidson (as cited in Weinberg, Gunderson, Hennen, & Cutter, 2006) attempt to address some of the difficulties experienced in applying traditional cognitive approaches to the treatment of BPD. Pretzer's approach emphasizes modifying standard CT to address difficulties often encountered in treating clients with BPD, such as establishing a collaborative relationship between therapist and client, maintaining a directed treatment, and improving homework compliance. Blum and colleagues developed a twice-weekly outpatient group treatment that uses a psychoeducational approach to teaching cognitive-behavioral skills (e.g., distancing, goal setting, and problem solving) to clients with BPD and to their support systems (e.g., family, friends, other care providers). The treatment is offered in a group setting and has been tested under the acronym STEPPS (Systems Training for Emotional Predictability and Problem Solving). The treatment focuses on destigmatization of BPD, emotional control, and behavioral control. Bos, van Wel, Verbraak, and Appelo (2011) conducted the most recent RCT on STEPPS. In their study, participants loosely diagnosed with BPD, representative of routine clinical practice, were randomized to either STEPPS and individual therapy ($N = 84$) or TAU ($N = 84$). At the end of the 18-week treatment, as well as at 6-month follow-up, participants treated with STEPPS reported less general and BPD-specific psychopathology, and more improvements in quality of life. Treatment was offered weekly for 18 sessions and also included a one-time follow-up session within the third and sixth months in the study. These findings, coupled with prior studies comparing STEPPS and TAU with rigorously selected BPD samples (Blum et al., 2008; Bos, van Wel, Verbraak, & Appelo, 2010) supports the effectiveness and efficacy of this intervention.

Young's schema-focused therapy (SFT; Young et al., 2003; also see Young, Rygh, Weinberger, & Beck, Chapter 7, this volume) postulates that stable patterns of thinking ("early maladaptive schemas") can develop during childhood and result in maladaptive behavior that reinforces the schemas. SFT includes a variety of interventions aimed at challenging and changing these early schemas through the identification of a set of dysfunctional schema modes that control the individual's thoughts, emotions, and behaviors (i.e., detached protector, punitive parent, abandoned/abused child, angry/impulsive child). Giesen-Bloo and colleagues (2006) completed the first RCT of TFP and SFT. TFP was compared to SFT in a study in which 86 participants received 3 years of twice-weekly individual sessions of either SFT or TFP. Study results indicated an overall decrease in BPD symptoms for both treatments; however, participants who received SFT had significantly greater improvements overall and a lower attrition rate. Suicide and NSSI behaviors were not assessed as an outcome measure in this study. A follow-up secondary analyses study also demonstrated that SFT's cost to implement was 20% lower than the cost needed to implement TFP (van Asselt et al., 2008). In addition, Farrell, Shaw, and Webber (2009) demonstrated the effectiveness of SFT in an 8-month group format. In their study, the authors tested the effect of augmenting TAU with an SFT group. When compared to TAU alone, TAU–SFT resulted in significantly higher remission from BPD.

An effectiveness trial was also conducted in 2009. Nadort and colleagues (2009) tested a disseminated version of SFT in regular health care centers with or without afterhours crisis support by phone. Data from 62 participants suggested that the added phone availability did not result in additional improvement, and that across conditions SFT was successful, leading to 42% recovery from BPD after 1.5 years of treatment.

Weinberg and colleagues (2006) completed an RCT of manual-assisted cognitive treatment (MACT) and TAU. MACT is a brief cognitive-behavioral treatment that incorporates strategies from DBT, CT, and bibliotherapy. The treatment targets NSSI behaviors in participants diagnosed with BPD. MACT was provided as an adjunctive treatment to TAU for study participants ($N = 30$). Participants were 30 women diagnosed with BPD, with a history of NSSI behaviors and at least one in the last month; however, suicide was considered one of the exclusionary criteria for study participation. Participants were randomly assigned to MACT plus TAU or to TAU-alone conditions. Upon completion of the 6-week treatment and at the 6-month follow-up, participants who received MACT had significantly fewer and less severe NSSI behaviors than those in the TAU-alone condition. These results should be interpreted with caution due to small sample size and the use of self-report measures only in assessment of NSSI behaviors.

EVIDENCE FOR DBT AS AN EFFECTIVE BPD TREATMENT

DBT evolved from standard cognitive-behavioral therapy as a treatment for BPD, particularly for recurrently suicidal, severely dysfunctional adults. The theoretical orientation to treatment is a blend of three theoretical positions: behavioral science, dialectical philosophy, and Zen practice. Behavioral science, the principles of behavior change, is countered by acceptance of the client (with techniques drawn both from Zen and from Western contemplative practice); these poles are balanced within the dialectical framework. Although dialectics was first adopted as a description of this emphasis on balance, dialectics soon took on the status of guiding principles that have advanced the therapy in directions not originally anticipated. DBT is based within a consistent behaviorist theoretical position. However, the actual procedures and strategies overlap considerably with those of various alternative therapy orientations, including psychodynamic, client-centered, strategic, and cognitive therapies.

Efficacy

Although, as described earlier, several treatments have demonstrated efficacy in the treatment of people diagnosed with BPD, DBT has the most empirical support at present and is generally considered the frontline treatment for the disorder. DBT as a treatment for BPD has been evaluated in a number of controlled trials (see Table 10.1). Four of the RCTs specifically recruited clients with suicidal behaviors (Linehan et al., 1999, 2006; Linehan, Armstrong, Suárez, Allmon, & Heard, 1991; McMain et al., 2009). Two RCTs included DBT in both conditions, with the addition of medication in one condition (Linehan, McDavid, Brown, Sayrs, & Gallop, 2008; Soler et al., 2005). The results in general have shown DBT to be highly effective. In adults diagnosed with BPD who are at high risk for suicide, 1 year of DBT yielded significantly higher improvements on anger outbursts, suicidal behavior, and hospitalization compared to TAU (Linehan et al., 1991; Linehan, Heard, & Armstrong, 1993), client-centered therapy (CCT, Turner, 2000), and community treatment by non-behavioral experts (CTBE; Linehan et al., 2006) but not to a dynamic emotion-focused treatment plus protocol-based pharmacotherapy program (McMain et al., 2009). One study showed that participants treated with DBT were half as likely to engage in suicidal behaviors compared to participants in the CTBE condition, further indicating that DBT is an effective treatment for reducing suicidal behavior. During the 1 year of treatment, depression, hopelessness, and suicidal ideation improved in both DBT and control treatments (Linehan et al., 1991, 2006; McMain et al., 2009). Furthermore, there was similar remission from major depressive disorder (MDD) and anxiety disorders in the DBT and in the control condition (Harned et al., 2008), although remission from substance dependence was significantly higher in DBT.

Treatment superiority was maintained when participants in the DBT condition were compared to only those control subjects who received stable individual psychotherapy during the treatment year, and even after researchers controlled for number of hours of psychotherapy and telephone contacts (Linehan & Heard, 1993; Linehan et al., 1999). Superiority was also maintained when comparing DBT with a treatment that had equal prestige, and was administered by expert therapist with allegiance to the treatment model (CTBE; Linehan et al., 2006). These studies suggest that the efficacy of DBT is due to specific treatment factors and not general factors or the expertise of the treating psychotherapists.

In BPD samples selected regardless of their suicide risk, findings are mixed with regard to suicidal behavior; nevertheless DBT outperforms control conditions in improving indices of emotion regulation (Koons et al., 2006; Verheul et al., 2003). DBT is also effective for adults diagnosed with BPD and a comorbid drug dependence disorder (Linehan et al., 1999, 2002).

Evidence also suggests that DBT adaptations are successful in treating people diagnosed with BPD. Soler and colleagues (2009) found a 13-week DBT skills-only intervention to be more successful in reducing problematic emotions than a psychodynamically informed standard group therapy (SGT) for participants meeting diagnostic criteria for BPD.

Bohus and colleagues (2004) compared a 12-week inpatient DBT adaptation with TAU for females diagnosed with BPD who reported a history of suicidal behavior. In a self-harming subsample, significantly more patients in DBT than in TAU abstained from NSSI at posttreatment (62 vs. 31%). Roepke and colleagues (2011) also found that a 12-week inpatient course of DBT resulted in significant improvement in depression and self-esteem when compared to TAU for women diagnosed with BPD.

Beyond BPD, studies have demonstrated the effectiveness of DBT with older depressed adults (Lynch et al., 2007; Lynch, Morse, Mendelson, & Robins, 2003), with adults with binge-eating disorder (Safer & Joyce, 2011; Safer, Robinson, & Jo, 2010), with suicidal adolescents (Barnoski, 2002; Katz, Cox, Gunasekara, & Miller, 2004; McDonell et al., 2010; Rathus & Miller, 2002) and suicidal college students (Pistorello, Fruzzetti, MacLane, Gallop, & Iverson, 2012), and with adults with a cluster B personality disorder (Feigenbaum et al., 2012).

EVIDENCE FOR DBT AS AN EFFECTIVE TREATMENT FOR EMOTION DYSREGULATION

As noted earlier, many mental disorders, including BPD, can be conceptualized as disorders of emotion regulation with deficits in both emotion up-regulation and down-regulation. For example, theorists have proposed that MDD should be conceptualized as an emotion dysregulation disorder based partly on a deficit in up-regulating and maintaining positive emotions (see Kring & Bachorowski, 1999, for a review). Similarly, literature reviews have demonstrated that anxiety disorders, schizophrenia, and even bipolar disorders are directly linked to emotion dysregulation (Kring & Werner, 2004). Once one realizes that emotions include both actions and action tendencies, one can see the link between emotion dysregulation and many disorders defined as behavior dyscontrol (e.g., substance dependence). As previously discussed, difficulties with emotion dysregulation, similar to those seen in BPD, are common in other disorders. Specifically problems with recognizing emotions, describing and labeling emotions, knowing what to do when an emotion is on the scene, and emotional avoidance are common in many Axis I disorders. Therefore, an important theoretical premise in DBT is that people who exhibit emotion dysregulation lack the skills needed for successful regulation. DBT includes a set of skills aimed at improving emotion regulation in BPD in particular, and in people who report emotion dysregulation in general.

An increasing number of RCTs suggest that DBT skills training alone is a promising intervention for a variety of populations (see Table 10.1). The majority of these studies offered only the skills training component of DBT. Therefore, although skills training was originally developed to be part of a comprehensive intervention, the number of studies suggests that DBT skills training by itself can be a successful intervention for a variety of populations with emotion regulation difficulties. Furthermore, DBT skills use (the product of skills training) has been shown to be an active mechanism of change for emotion regulation outcomes in treatment for BPD (Neacsiu, Rizvi, & Linehan, 2010).

TABLE 10.1. Table of Randomized Control Trials and Controlled Trials for DBT

Citation	Design	Methodology	N/condition	DBT variant offered	General outcomes reported	Emotion regulation outcomes reported	Study inclusion criteria	Study exclusion criteria
Barnoski (2002)	Controlled trial	DBT vs. TAU (historical controls), 12-month FU assessment	DBT = 42 TAU = 116	rDBT (standard)—1 year	DBT < TAU in number of reconvictions for a felony offense in the 12 months following discharge	None	Adolescents at a juvenile rehabilitation institution	None
Bohus et al. (2013)	RCT	iDBT-PTSD vs. TAU-WL; assessments at pre- and posttreatment and at 6-week FU	iDBT-PTSD = 36 TAU-WL = 38	iDBT adapted for PTSD—3 months	iDBT-PTSD >TAU-WL in PTSD remission and PTSD interview and self-report assessments	None	Females 17–65 years old, referred for childhood sexual abuse	Schizophrenia, mental retardation, requiring immediate other treatment, recent life-threatening suicide attempt, medical condition contraindicated for exposure
Bohus et al. (2004)	RCT	iDBT vs. WL + TAU; assessments at pre- and posttreatment; at 1- and 3-month FU	iDBT = 40 TAU = 20	Inpatient DBT (iDBT)—3 months	iDBT > TAU on abstinence from NSSI (62% vs. 31%)	DBT = TAU on anger; DBT > TAU on decrease in depression and anxiety	Female, BPD, suicide attempt (SA) or two NSSI episodes in last 2 years	Lifetime schizophrenia, mental retardation, bipolar I, current substance abuse
Bradley & Follingstad (2003)	RCT	DBT-ST vs. no treatment (control)—9 weeks	DBT-ST = 24 Control = 25	DBT-ST adapted	No significant differences between conditions	DBT-ST > control in decrease in depression across and trauma symptoms	Self-reported childhood abuse and significant trauma and depression	None
Carter et al. (2010)	RCT	DBT vs. TAU + WL; assessments at pretreatment, 3 months, and 6 months	DBT = 38 TAU + WL = 35	DBT (standard)—6 months	DBT = TAU in NSSI, hospital admissions or length of stay in hospital, quality of life, disability	None	Female, BPD, 18–65; multiple episodes of NSSI, at least three in the last year	Not a fit/unmotivated, presence of a disabling organic condition, schizophrenia, bipolar disorder, psychotic depression, florid antisocial behavior, developmental disability

(continued)

TABLE 10.1. (continued)

Citation	Design	Methodology	N/condition	DBT variant offered	General outcomes reported	Emotion regulation outcomes reported	Study inclusion criteria	Study exclusion criteria
Cavanaugh, Solomon, & Gelles (2011)	RCT	Dialectical psychoeducational workshop (DPEW) vs. anger management workshop (AMW); assessments at pre- and posttreatment	DPEW = 28 AMW = 27	DBT-ST modified for interpersonal violence (DPEW)—8 weeks	DPEW > AMW (at posttreatment) in adaptive coping skills, empathy skills, and in decreasing potential risk for interpersonal violence	DPEW > AMW (at posttreatment) in anger management skills	Males, 18 or older, never engaged in intimate partner violence, endorsed violent urges	None
Clarkin, Levy, Lenzweger, & Kernberg (2007)	RCT	DBT vs. TFP vs. supportive treatment (ST); assessments at pretreatment, 4, 8, and 12 months	DBT = 17 TFP = 23 ST = 22	DBT (standard) adapted to include medication management	DBT = TFP = ST in improving global functioning and social adjustment; TFP = DBT (not ST) in reducing suicidality (analyses only included people with ≥ 3 assessments)	DBT = TFP = ST in improving depression and anxiety; TFP = ST (not DBT) in reducing anger and impulsivity; only TFP significantly changed irritability and assault behaviors	BPD, 18–50	Comorbid psychotic disorders, bipolar I disorder, delusional disorder, delirium, dementia, amnestic and other cognitive disorders; active substance dependence
Courbasson, Nishikawa, & Dixon (2012)	RCT	DBT vs. TAU; assessments at pretreatment, 3, 6, 9, 12, 15, and 18 months (last two are FU time points)	TAU = 8 DBT = 13	DBT (standard)—1 year	DBT < TAU in dropout; DBT posttreatment > pretreatment in dysfunctional eating behaviors and attitudes; severity and use of substances	DBT posttreatment > pretreatment in ability to cope and regulate negative emotions	Women ≥ 18; any eating disorder and substance abuse/dependence, agreed not to change medication	Organic brain syndrome; mental retardation; psychosis; and chronic suicidality; in treatment for an eating disorder or substance use
Evershed et al. (2003)	Controlled trial	rDBT vs. TAU; assessments at pre-, mid-, and posttreatment, and at 6-month FU	rDBT = 8 TAU = 9	Residential DBT adapted for forensic sample—18 months	DBT > TAU in seriousness of violence incidents	DBT > TAU in self-reported hostility and anger	Male, inpatient in a high security hospital, having borderline features	None
Feigenbaum et al. (2012)	RCT	DBT vs. TAU; assessments at pretreatment, 6 months, and 1 year	DBT = 26 TAU = 16	DBT (standard)—1 year	DBT < TAU in decrease of self-rated risk	DBT = TAU in aggression, anger expression,	Age range = 18–65, diagnosed with a	Extensive forensic history that suggests immediate danger to

402

Study	Design	Comparison	N	Intervention			Inclusion	Exclusion
					behavior DBT = TAU in NSSI reductions, use of services	depression, irritability (significant decrease in both conditions)	cluster B personality disorder	others: schizophrenia, bipolar disorder; primary substance use disorder, severe cognitive impairment
Harley et al. (2008); Feldman et al. (2009)	RCT	TAU + DBT-ST vs. TAU + WL; assessments at pre- and posttreatment and at a 6-month FU	TAU + DBT-ST = 13, TAU + WL = 11	DBT-ST group intervention adapted for treatment-resistant depression—16 weeks	See next column	TAU + DBT-ST > TAU + WL at improving depression from Week 0 to Week 16	Diagnosis of depression, 18–65, on stable medication	BPD, bipolar, psychotic spectrum disorders, active substance abuse/dependence, mental retardation, pervasive developmental disorder, active suicidality, unstable medical conditions, exposure to CBT
Hill, Craighead, & Safer (2011)	RCT	DBT-AF vs. WL	DBT-AF = 18, WL = 14	DBT-ST—modified for AF	DBT-AF = WL in improvement in number of bingeing and purging episodes	DBT-AF > WL in decreasing depression, emotion dysregulation	Recent BED behavior, vomiting as primary compensatory behavior. Stable psychotropic medication.	Male, 18 or older, current diagnosis of anorexia nervosa, in psychotherapy, current suicidal ideation, substance dependence, present psychosis
Hirvikoski et al. (2011)	RCT	DBT-ST vs. loosely structured discussion group (control)	DBT-ST = 26, Control = 25	Adapted DBT-ST for Swedish population—14 sessions	DBT-ST = Control in satisfaction	None	Meets diagnostic criteria for ADHD, adult, on stable dose of medication	Substance abuse; IQ ≤ 70; diagnosed brain injury; autism spectrum disorder; suicidality; homelessness; severe depression, psychosis, or bipolar without stable medication
Katz et al. (2004)	Controlled trial	rDBT vs. TAU residential unit; assessments at pre- and posttreatment and at 1-year FU	rDBT = 31, TAU = 31	rDBT—average stay is 18 days	rDBT < TAU in incidents on the ward; rDBT = TAU in emergency room visits and hospitalizations after discharge; in NSSI, and in suicidal ideation	rDBT = TAU in depression reduction and hopelessness (significant decrease in both conditions)	Inpatients, 14–17, admitted for suicide attempts, or suicidal ideation	Mental retardation, psychosis, bipolar disorder, severe learning disability

(continued)

TABLE 10.1. *(continued)*

Citation	Design	Methodology	N/condition	DBT variant offered	General outcomes reported	Emotion regulation outcomes reported	Study inclusion criteria	Study exclusion criteria
Koons et al. (2001)	RCT	DBT vs. TAU	DBT = 10 TAU = 10	DBT (standard)—6 months	DBT < TAU in NSSI, hospitalizations, suicidal ideation, and dissociation	DBT > TAU on hopelessness, depression, anger suppression, and expression	Women veterans, BPD	Schizophrenia, bipolar, substance dependence and antisocial personality disorder
Koons et al. (2006)	RCT	DBT vs. TAU; assessments at pretreatment, 3, and 6 months	DBT = 10 TAU = 10	DBT (standard)—6 months	Trend for DBT to reduce NSSI more than TAU (p < .10), DBT = TAU on reduction of services use; DBT > TAU in reduction of suicidal ideation	DBT > TAU in reduction of depression (self-report) and hopelessness; DBT = TAU in reduction of depression (interview), anxiety, anger suppression; DBT > TAU in reduction of anger expression	Women veterans, BPD	Schizophrenia, bipolar disorder, substance dependence, antisocial personality disorder
Linehan et al. (1991, 1993, 1994)	RCT	DBT vs. TAU; assessments every 4 months, including during a 1-year FU	DBT = 22 TAU = 22	DBT (standard)—1 year	DBT > TAU in reducing risk for suicidal behavior and decreasing use of services; DBT < TAU in reducing dropout; DBT = TAU in decreasing suicidal ideation	DBT = TAU in reduction of depression and hopelessness (significant decrease in both conditions)	BPD, women, 18–45 with current and past suicidal behavior (at least one episode in the last 8 weeks)	Lifetime psychotic disorder, lifetime bipolar disorder, mental retardation, seizure disorder requiring medication, mandate to treatment, need for primary treatment for a debilitating condition
Linehan et al. (1999)	RCT	DBT vs. TAU; assessments every 4 months; 4 month FU	DBT = 12 TAU = 16	DBT (standard)—1 year	DBT > TAU in substance abuse	DBT = TAU in anger outcomes (significant decrease in both)	BPD, female, current drug dependence	Psychotic disorder, bipolar disorder, mental retardation
Linehan et al. (2002)	RCT	DBT + LAAM vs. comprehensive validation therapy with 12-step (CVT-	DBT = 11 CVT-12S = 12	DBT (standard)—1 year	DBT participants maintained reductions in opiate use	None	Females 18–45, BPD, with current opiate dependence	Bipolar disorder, psychosis, seizure disorder, mental retardation,

404

Study	Design	Conditions (N)	Treatment	Procedure	Outcomes	Additional outcomes	Population	Exclusion criteria
				12s) + LAAM; assessments every 4 months, including one FU assessment	throughout the 12-month treatment; CVT-12S participants attained the same reductions but increased their use of opiates in the last 4 months; similar decreases in psychopathology			pregnancy, medical condition for which the use of opiate replacement medication was contraindicated, indications of treatment coercion
Linehan et al. (2006); Harned et al. (2008); Bedics, Atkins, Comtois, & Linehan (2012)	RCT	DBT = 52 CTBE = 49	DBT (standard)—1 year	DBT vs. community treatment by experts (CTBE); assessments every 4 months and during a 1-year FU	DBT < CTBE in suicide attempts, use of crisis services, dropout; DBT led to a significant reduction in substance use disorders; DBT = CTBE in reduction of suicidal ideation, remission from major depression, anxiety, and eating disorders; DBT > CTBE in introject affiliation increases	DBT = CTBE in reduction of depression (significant decrease in both conditions; DBT showed significant change in self-affirming, self-loving, self-protecting, and less self-attacking through treatment and FU; CTBE showed significant treatment interaction for therapist affirm/therapist protect	BPD, women, 18–45 with current and past suicidal behavior (at least one episode in the last 8 weeks)	Lifetime psychotic disorder, lifetime bipolar disorder, mental retardation, seizure disorder requiring medication, mandate to treatment, need for primary treatment for a debilitating condition
Linehan et al. (2008)	RCT	DBT + placebo = 12 DBT + olanzapine = 12	DBT (standard)—6 months	DBT + placebo vs. DBT + olanzapine	Placebo > olanzapine in reduction of NSSI	Olanzapine was faster than placebo at reducing irritability and physical aggression	18–60, BPD, dysregulated anger, scored high on irritability	Schizophrenia, bipolar I, schizoaffective, psychotic disorder, mental retardation, seizure disorder, substance dependence within last 6 month, NSSI in the prior 8 weeks from screening, pregnant

(continued)

TABLE 10.1. (continued)

Citation	Design	Methodology	N/condition	DBT variant offered	General outcomes reported	Emotion regulation outcomes reported	Study inclusion criteria	Study exclusion criteria
Lynch et al. (2007)	RCT	8-week medication trial followed by RCT for nonresponders: standard DBT + medication (DBT-MED) vs. medication only (MED); assessments at pretreatment, 2, 6, 9, and 15 months	DBT + MED = 21 MED = 14	DBT (standard)—6 months	DBT + MED achieves remission from major depressive disorder faster than MED only	None	Over 55 years of age; meets criteria for at least one personality disorder; scores high on depression	Bipolar disorder, psychotic symptoms, signs of cognitive impairment, current ECT
Lynch et al. (2003)	RCT	Antidepressants (MED) vs. DBT-ST + MED; assessments at pretreatment, posttreatment, and 6-month FU	MED = 15 DBT-ST + MED = 16	DBT-ST adaptation (skills and 30-minute phone coaching/week)—7 months	Remission from depression (DBT > MED) gap even wider at FU; dependency & adaptive coping improved in DBT only	Self-reported depression (DBT > MED)	Current MDD, age 60+; scores high on two depression measures	Bipolar disorder, psychotic symptoms, signs of cognitive impairment, current ECT
McDonell et al. (2010)	Controlled trial	rDBT vs. residential TAU (historical matches)	rDBT = 106 TAU = 104	rDBT (varied intensity of DBT therapy in residential setting)	With DBT, significantly fewer NSSI episodes during 1 year of treatment than with TAU	None	Youth ages 12–17	Admissions for legal competence restoration
McMain et al. (2009)	RCT	DBT vs. general psychiatric management (GPM); assessments every 4 months and during 1-month FU	DBT = 90 GPM = 90	DBT (standard)—1 year	DBT = GPM in decreasing suicidal behavior, use of crisis services (significant decrease in both conditions)	DBT = GPM in decreasing depression, anger, symptom distress (significant decrease in both conditions)	BPD, ages 18–60, at least two episodes of suicidal or NSSI episodes in the past 5 years, at least one of which was in the 3 months preceding enrollment	Psychotic disorder, bipolar I disorder, delirium, dementia, mental retardation, substance dependence in the last month, medical condition that precluded psychiatric medications, serious medical condition, plans to leave in the next 2 years

Study	Design	Comparison	N	Treatment	Outcome	Secondary outcome	Inclusion	Exclusion
Neacsiu, Eberle, Kramer, Weismann, & Linehan (2013)	RCT	16-week DBT-ST vs. 16-week Activities Support Group (ASG); assessment every 2 months including a 2-month FU	DBT-ST = 22 ASG = 22	DBT-ST condensed to 16 weeks	DBT-ST= ASG in improvements in depression severity; DBT-ST > ASG in improvements in anxiety severity, increase in skills use	DBT-ST >ASG in improvements in difficulties with emotion regulation and affect control DBT-ST = ASG in alexithymia decrease	Adults, ages 18–65, high emotion dysregulation, meets criteria for a DSM-IV-TR diagnosis for a depressive or anxiety disorder	Current psychotic disorder, Bipolar I, BPD, had DBT before, mandated to treatment, severe suicidality, not willing to discontinue ancillary psychotherapy
Pistorello et al. (2012)	RCT	DBT vs. supervision by experts in psychodynamic treatment (SBE); assessment every 3 months and during 6-month FU	DBT = 31 SBE = 32	DBT (standard)—7 months to 1 year	DBT > SBE in decreasing NSSI, use of psychotropic medication, and suicidality and in increasing quality of life	DBT > SBE in decreasing depression (self-report)	Ages 18–25, current suicidal ideation, past history of at least one NSSI or one suicide attempt	Psychosis, had individual or group DBT
Rakfeldt (2005)	Controlled trial	rDBT vs. no treatment—17 weeks; assessments at pre- and posttreatment	rDBT = 7 Control = 8	rDBT adapted to include two 1-hour sessions/ week	rDBT = Control in functioning index; rDBT > Control in interpersonal relationships, social networks, intentionality, and global functioning	None	Living in the young adult services residential program; has serious emotional disturbance	None
Rathus & Miller (2002)	Controlled trial	rDBT vs. TAU (assignment to TAU for less severe clients)	rDBT = 29 TAU = 82	rDBT adapted—12 weeks, twice weekly	DBT > TAU in reducing psychiatric hospitalizations DBT = TAU in suicide attempts (1 in DBT, 7 in TAU)	None	Adolescents in DBT: suicide attempt in last 16 weeks, at least three BPD criteria	None
Roepke et al. (2011)	Controlled trial	iDBT vs. WL + TAU; assessments at pretreatment and at 10 weeks	iDBT = 40 TAU = 20	iDBT—3 months	DBT > TAU in increasing self-esteem	With DBT, significant improvement in depression; with TAU, no change in depression	Female, BPD	Lifetime diagnosis of schizophrenia, bipolar I or II, substance abuse within last 6 months, mental retardation

(continued)

TABLE 10.1. (continued)

Citation	Design	Methodology	N/condition	DBT variant offered	General outcomes reported	Emotion regulation outcomes reported	Study inclusion criteria	Study exclusion criteria
Safer, Telch, & Agras (2001)	RCT	DBT-ST vs. WL	DBT-ST = 14 WL = 15	DBT-ST—20 weeks	DBT > WL at significantly reducing rates of bingeing–purging		Ages 18–65, at least one binge–purge episode per week	None
Safer, Robinson, & Jo (2010); Safer & Joyce (2011)	RCT	(DBT-ST BED) vs. active comparison group therapy (ACGT)—20 weekly sessions; assessments at pre- and posttreatment, and at 3-, 6-, and 12-month FU	DBT-ST BED = 50 ACGT = 51	DBT skills training adapted for BED (DBT-ST BED)—20 weeks	DBT-ST BED = ACGT in binge-eating abstinence posttreatment (64% in DBT and 36% in ACGT); DBT < ACGT in binge days post-treatment but not at FU; moderate effect size favoring DBT for self-reports on restraining and eating concerns; DBT more likely to produce rapid responders who do better at FU	No differences in emotion-regulation measures, eating-related depression, anxiety or anger, depression, or self-esteem	Men and women over age 18; binge-eating disorder; within commuting distance from study	Body mass index < 17.5 kg/m2; in psychotherapy; unstable medications; regular use of compensatory behaviors; psychosis; current alcohol/drug abuse or dependence; severe depression with suicide attempts; use of weight-altering medications; severe medical condition; current pregnancy or breast feeding; planning gastric bypass
Salbach-Andrae et al. (2009)	RCT	25 weeks CBT vs. 25 weeks DBT-AN/BN vs. 12 weeks waitlist	CBT = 19 DBT-AN/BN = 16 WL = 15	DBT adapted for adolescents with anorexia/bulimia nervosa	57.9% in CBT, 62.5% in DBT-AN/BN, and 0% in waitlist remitted from DSM-IV-TR criteria for eating disorders; DBT-AN/BN=CBT	Small positive effect sizes in emotion regulation	AN or BN adolescent females (ages 12–21), IQ >85	Unable to speak/understand German; psychotic disorder

Study	Design	Comparison	N	Treatment length	Outcomes		Population	Exclusions
Soler et al. (2005)	RCT	DBT-ST + placebo vs. DBT-ST + olanzapine	DBT-ST+ placebo = 30 DBT-ST + olanzapine = 30	DBT-ST adapted—12 weeks, with phone coaching added	>WL in calorie avoidance, meal frequency, and psychological distress / Olanzepine > placebo in reducing weight gain and cholesterol levels; olanzepine = placebo in decreases of psychopathology	Olanzapine < placebo in frequency of impulsivity and aggressive behavior. olanzapine > placebo in decreasing depression and anxiety	BPD, ages 18–45, no Axis I disorder, high clinical severity, not in psychotherapy	None
Soler et al. (2009)	RCT	DBT-ST vs. sychodynamically oriented standard group therapy (SGT); assessments every 2 weeks	DBT-ST = 29 SGT = 30	DBT-ST adapted—3 months	See next column	DBT > SGT in reductions of depression, anxiety, irritability, anger, and affect instability	BPD, ages 18–45, Clinical Global Impression of Severity score = 4, no current psychotherapy	Schizophrenia, drug-induced psychosis, organic brain syndrome, substance dependence, bipolar, mental retardation, current depression
Telch, Agras, & Linehan (2001)	RCT	DBT-ST vs. WL; assessments at pre- and posttreatment and at 6-month FU	DBT-ST = 22 WL = 22	DBT skills training adapted for BED	DBT = WL on all outcomes	DBT women reported less desire to eat when angry	Females, ages 18–65, meet criteria diagnostic criteria for BED	Current psychotherapy, weight loss program, or using psychotropic medication; current substance use disorder, current suicidality, psychosis, pregnancy
Trupin, Stewart, & Beach, & Boesky (2002)	Controlled trial	rDBT vs. TAU; assessments pre and posttreatment	rDBT = 45 TAU = 45	rDBT—variable length	Behavioral problems significantly decreased in DBT cottages but not in TAU cottage	None	Adolescents in a Washington State JRA, in three different cottages	None

(continued)

TABLE 10.1. *(continued)*

Citation	Design	Methodology	N/condition	DBT variant offered	General outcomes reported	Emotion regulation outcomes reported	Study inclusion criteria	Study exclusion criteria
Turner (2000)	RCT	DBT vs. TAU; assessments at 6 and 12 months	DBT = 12 TAU = 12	DBT (standard)—1 year, adapted to reduce therapy time and incorporate psychodynamic techniques	DBT > TAU in mental health functioning; DBT > TAU in amount of suicidal behavior, although significant improvement in both	DBT = TAU in improvement of emotional functioning	BPD, willing to be randomized	Schizophrenia, schizoaffective, bipolar, organic mental disorder, and/or mental retardation
Van den Bosch et al. (2002); Verheul et al. (2003)	RCT	DBT vs. TAU; assessments at pretreatment, at 11, 22, 33, 44, and 52 weeks, and at 18-month FU	DBT = 27 TAU = 31	DBT (standard)—1 year	DBT < TAU in reducing suicide attempts (DBT = 2, TAU = 8); NSSI significantly decreased in DBT and increased in TAU; effects moderated by severity of suicidal behavior; DBT = TAU in substance use	DBT > TAU in reducing impulsive acts	BPD, female; ages 18–70	Psychotic disorder, bipolar disorder, mental retardation; not living in the area
Van Dijk, Jeffrey, & Katz (2013)	RCT	DBT-ST vs. WL	DBT-ST = 13 WL = 13	DBT-ST adapted for bipolar disorders—12 weeks	DBT-ST=WL in reducing depression, mindfulness (both improved)	DBT-ST=WL in improving affect control (both improved)	BPD, age 18 or older	Currently in a manic state, developmental delay, ongoing violent or aggressive behaviors, unable to understand English

Study	Design	Intervention	N	Description	Outcome	Findings	Inclusion criteria	Exclusion criteria
Waltz et al. (2009)	RCT	DBT skills video vs. control (informational video), alternating viewing order	N = 30	DBT video on "opposite action"	Of those who participated in the FU, 80% had used opposite action at least once	DBT video viewers showed significant decrease in emotional intensity.	18 or older, literate, BPD, IQ > 90, aware of diagnosis, in treatment	Previous formal DBT experience, actively psychotic
Wasser, Tyler, McIlhaney, Taplin, & Henderson (2008)	Controlled trial	rDBT vs. STM (Standard Therapeutic Milieu); one primary match (exact match on age, gender, & having an Axis I disorder), one secondary match (similar match in age, gender)	Primary: rDBT = 7 STM = 7 Secondary: rDBT = 12 STM = 12	rDBT adapted due to lack of resources (conducted by non-DBT clinicians)	STM > rDBT for psychomotor excitation at discharge; rDBT > STM psychopathology	DBT = STM in reducing depression (both reduced it significantly).	Adolescents at KidsPeace	None
Wolf et al. (2011)	RCT	DBT-ST vs. DBT-ST + Computer-Based Skills Training (CBST)	DBT-ST = 11 DBT-ST + CBST = 13	DBT-ST—6 months with or without adjunct CD-ROM–based self-help program	DBT-ST + CBST > DBT-ST in improvement of skills acquisition and knowledge	None	BPD, in therapy	Schizophrenia, current substance dependence, severe cognitive dysfunction

Note. > denotes significantly greater than; < denotes significantly less than; = denotes no significant difference between; AF, appetite-focused; FU, follow-up; iDBT, inpatient DBT; RCT, randomized controlled trial; TAU, treatment as usual; TFP, transference-focused psychotherapy; WL, wait list; NSSI, nonsuicidal self-injury; LAAM, levomethadyl acetate hydrochloride; PTSD, posttraumatic stress disorder; rDBT, residential DBT; ECT, electroconvulsive therapy; DBT-ST, DBT skills training; DBT-ST BED, DBT-ST for binge-eating disorder; ADHD, attention-deficit/hyperactivity disorder.

DBT: TREATMENT OVERVIEW

Philosophical Basis: Dialectics

The term "dialectics" as applied to behavior therapy refers both to a fundamental nature of reality and to a method of persuasive dialogue and relationship. (See Wells [1972, cited in Kegan, 1982] for documentation of a shift toward dialectical approaches across all the sciences during the last 150 years; more recently, Peng & Nisbett [1999] discussed both Western and Eastern dialectical thought.) As a worldview or philosophical position, dialectics guides the clinician in developing theoretical hypotheses relevant to the client's problems and to the treatment. Alternatively, as dialogue and relationship, "dialectics" refers to the treatment approach or strategies used by the therapist to effect change. Thus, central to DBT are a number of therapeutic dialectical strategies.

Dialectics as a Worldview

DBT is based on a dialectical worldview that emphasizes wholeness, interrelatedness, and process (change) as fundamental characteristics of reality. The first characteristic, the Principle of Interrelatedness and Wholeness, provides a perspective of viewing the system as a whole and how people relate to the system, rather than seeing people as if they exist in isolation. Similar to contextual and systems theories, a dialectical view argues that analysis of parts of any system is of limited value unless the analysis clearly relates the part to the whole. The second characteristic is the Principle of Polarity. Although dialectics focuses on the whole, it also emphasizes the complexity of any whole. Thus, dialectics asserts that reality is nonreducible; that is, within each single thing or system, no matter how small, there is polarity. For example, physicists are unable to reduce even the smallest of molecules to one thing. Where there is matter, there is antimatter; even every atom is made up of both protons and electrons: A polar opposite is always present. The opposing forces are referred to as the "thesis" and "antithesis," present in all existence. Dialectics suggests that the thesis and antithesis move toward a "synthesis," and inherent in the synthesis will be a new set of opposing forces. It is from these opposing forces that the third characteristic is developed. This characteristic of the dialectical perspective refers to the Principle of Continuous Change. Change is produced through the constant synthesis of the thesis and the an-

tithesis, and because new opposing forces are present within the synthesis, change is ongoing. These dialectical principles are inherent in every aspect of DBT and allow for continuous movement throughout the therapy process. A very important dialectical idea is that all propositions contain within them their own oppositions. Or, as Goldberg (1980, pp. 295–296) put it, "I assume that truth is paradoxical, that each article of wisdom contains within it its own contradictions, that truths stand side by side. Contradictory truths do not necessarily cancel each other out or dominate each other, but stand side by side, inviting participation and experimentation." One way that client and therapist address this is by repeatedly asking: "What is being left out?" This simple question can assist in finding a synthesis and letting go of an absolute truth, a nondialectical stance.

Dialectics as Persuasion

From the point of view of dialogue and relationship, dialectics refers to change by persuasion and by making use of the oppositions inherent in the therapeutic relationship rather than by formal impersonal logic. Through the therapeutic opposition of contradictory positions, both client and therapist can arrive at new meanings within old meanings, moving closer to the essence of the subject under consideration. The spirit of a dialectical point of view is never to accept a proposition as a final truth or an undisputable fact. Thus, the question addressed by both client and therapist is "What is being left out of our understanding?" Dialectics as persuasion is represented in the specific dialectical strategies we describe later in this chapter. As readers will see, when we discuss the consultation strategies, dialectical dialogue is also very important in therapist consultation meetings. Perhaps more than any other factor, attention to dialectics can reduce the chances of what psychodynamic therapists have labeled "staff splitting," that is, the frequent phenomenon of therapists' disagreeing or arguing (sometimes vehemently) about how to treat and interact with an individual client who has BPD. This "splitting" among staff members is often due to one or more factions within the staff deciding that they (and sometimes they alone) know the truth about a particular client or clinical problem.

Dialectical Case Conceptualization

Dialectical assumptions influence case conceptualization in DBT in a number of ways. First, dialectics suggests that a psychological disorder is best conceptualized as a systemic dysfunction characterized by (1) defining the disorder with respect to normal functioning, (2) assuming continuity between health and the disorder, and (3) assuming that the disorder results from multiple rather than single causes (Hollandsworth, 1990). Similarly, Linehan's biosocial theory of BPD assumes that BPD represents a breakdown in normal functioning, and that this disorder is best conceptualized as a systemic dysfunction of the emotion regulation system. The theory proposes that the pathogenesis of BPD results from numerous factors: Some are genetic–biological predispositions that create individual differences in susceptibility to emotion dysregulation, known as "emotion vulnerability"; others result from the individual's interaction with the environment, referred to as the "invalidating environment." Assuming a systemic view compels the theorist to integrate work from a variety of fields and disciplines.

A second dialectical assumption that underlies the biosocial theory is that the relationship between the individual and the environment is a transaction between the person and the environment. Within social learning theory, this is the principle of "reciprocal determinism." Besides focusing on reciprocal influence, a transactional view also highlights the constant state of flux and change of the individual–environment system. Therefore, BPD can occur in multiple environments and families, including chaotic, perfect, and even ordinary families.

Both transactional and interactive models, such as the diathesis–stress model of psychopathology, call attention to the role of dysfunctional environments in bringing about disorder in the vulnerable individual. A transactional model, however, highlights a number of points that are easy to overlook in an interactive diathesis–stress model. For example, a person (Person A) may act in a manner stressful to an individual (Person B) only because of the stress Person B is putting on Person A. Take the child who, due to an accident, requires most of the parents' free time just to meet survival needs. Or consider the client who, due to the need for constant suicide precautions, uses up much of the inpatient nursing resources. Both of these environments are stretched in their ability to respond well to further stress. Both may invalidate or temporarily blame the victim if any further demand on the system is made. Although the system (e.g., the family or the therapeutic milieu) may have been predisposed to respond dysfunctionally in any case, such responses

may have been avoided in the absence of exposure to the stress of that particular individual. A transactional, or dialectical, account of psychopathology may allow greater compassion because it is incompatible with the assignment of blame, by highlighting the reality of the situation rather than judgments about each person. This is particularly relevant with a label as stigmatized among mental health professionals as "borderline" (for examples of the misuse of the diagnosis, see Reiser & Levenson, 1984).

A final assumption in our discussion regards the definition of behavior and the implications of defining behavior broadly. Linehan's theory, and behaviorists in general, take "behavior" to mean anything an organism does involving action and responding to stimulation (*Merriam-Webster's New Universal Unabridged Dictionary*, 1983, p. 100). Conventionally, behaviorists categorize behavior as motor, cognitive/verbal, and physiological, all of which may be either public or private. There are several points to make here. First, dividing behavior into these three categories is arbitrary and is done for conceptual clarity rather than in response to evidence that these response modes actually are functionally separate systems. This point is especially relevant to understanding emotion regulation given that basic research on emotions demonstrates that these response systems are sometimes overlapping, somewhat independent, but definitely not wholly independent, thus remaining consistent with the dialectical worldview. A related point here is that in contrast to biological and cognitive theories of BPD, biosocial theory suggests that there is no a priori reason for favoring explanations emphasizing one mode of behavior as intrinsically more important or compelling than others. Rather, from a biosocial perspective, the crucial questions are under what conditions a given behavior–behavior relationship or response system–response system relationship holds, and under what conditions these relationships enter causal pathways for the etiology and maintenance of BPD.

BIOSOCIAL THEORY

Emotion Dysregulation

Linehan's biosocial theory suggests that BPD is primarily a dysfunction of the emotion regulation system. Behavioral patterns in BPD are functionally related to or are unavoidable consequences of this fundamental dysregulation across several, perhaps all, emotions, including both positive and negative emotions. From Linehan's point of view, this dysfunction of the emotion regulation system is the core pathology; thus, it is neither simply symptomatic nor definitional. Emotion dysregulation is a product of the combination of emotional vulnerability and difficulties in modulating emotional reactions. Emotional vulnerability is conceptualized as high sensitivity to emotional stimuli, intense emotional responses, and a slow return to emotional baseline. Deficits in emotion modulation may be due to difficulties in (1) inhibiting mood-dependent behaviors; (2) organizing behavior in the service of goals, independently of current mood; (3) increasing or decreasing physiological arousal as needed; (4) distracting attention from emotionally evocative stimuli; and/or (5) experiencing emotion without either immediately withdrawing or producing an extreme secondary negative emotion (see Crowell, Beauchaine, & Linehan, 2009, for a further discussion).

Conceptually, the deficit in the emotion regulation system leads to not only immense emotional suffering but also multiple behavioral problems in people diagnosed with BPD. When clinicians' ratings of characteristics associated with psychopathology are examined, tendencies toward being chronically anxious and unhappy, depressed, or despondent are the most highly descriptive of the BPD (Bradley, Zittel, & Westen, 2005). Dysfunction leads the individual to attempt to escape aversive emotions, often leading to further suffering. For example, a female client experiencing intense anger after a fight with her partner may, in an effort to escape the anger, engage in cutting behaviors. She begins to feel relief from her anger for a short period of time. However, once her anger begins to subside, shame in response to the cutting behavior begins to increase and the cycle of emotion escape behavior continues. Although the mechanisms of the initial dysregulation remain unclear, it is likely that biological factors play a primary role. Siever and Davis (1991) hypothesized that deficits in emotion regulation for clients with BPD are related to both instability and hyperresponsiveness of catecholamine function. The etiology of this dysregulation may range from genetic influences to prenatal factors, to traumatic childhood events affecting development of the brain and nervous system. Furthermore, adoption studies of monozygotic (MZ) twins (Davison & Neale, 1994) suggest a genetic vulnerability. However, researchers do not claim that genetic or biological factors account for all pathology. If pathology were solely determined by genetics, then 100% of the MZ twins would presumably share the same pathology. Because this does not occur, we can explain the differences through the transactions between biology, as described earlier, and the environment.

Invalidating Environments

Most people with an initial temperamental vulnerability to emotion dysregulation do not develop BPD. Thus, the theory suggests further that particular developmental environments are necessary. The crucial developmental circumstance in Linehan's theory is the transaction between emotion vulnerability and the presence of the "invalidating environment" (Linehan, 1987,1993a), which is defined by its tendency to negate, punish, and/or respond erratically and inappropriately to private experiences, independent of the validity of the actual behavior. Private experiences, and especially emotional experiences and interpretations of events, are not taken as valid responses to events by others; are punished, trivialized, dismissed, or disregarded; and/or are attributed to socially unacceptable characteristics, such as over reactivity, inability to see things realistically, lack of motivation, motivation to harm or manipulate, lack of discipline, or failure to adopt a positive (or, conversely, discriminating) attitude. The invalidating environment can be any part of an individual's social environment, including immediate or extended family, school, work, or community. Within each of these environments are even more specific idiosyncrasies that may impact the environment, such as birth order, years between siblings, teachers and peers, and/or coworkers. It is important to note that because two children grew up in the same home does not mean that they were raised in identical environments. Furthermore, people are often not aware of their invalidating behaviors and are not acting with a malicious intent.

There are three primary characteristics of the invalidating environment. First, the environment indiscriminately rejects communication of private experiences and self-generated behaviors. For example, a person may be told, "You are so angry, but you won't admit it" or "You can't be hungry, you just ate." Second, the invalidating environment may punish emotional displays and intermittently reinforce emotional escalation. For example, a woman breaks up with her partner and is feeling depressed. Her friends and family begin telling her "Get over it," "He wasn't worth it," and "Don't feel sad." Over the course of the next week, she becomes more depressed and is beginning to withdraw from daily activities. Again, her environment responds in an invalidating manner. Finally after another 3 days of high emotional arousal she makes a suicide attempt. At that moment the environment jumps in and provides support by taking care of her. Unfortunately, this type of pattern often results in inadvertent reinforcement of extreme dysfunctional behavior. Finally, the invalidating environment may oversimplify the ease of problem solving and meeting goals for an individual.

The high incidence of childhood sexual abuse reported by adults diagnosed with BPD (e.g., Herman, 1986; Herman, Perry, & van der Kolk, 1989) suggests that sexual abuse may be a prototypical invalidating experience for children. The relationship of early sexual abuse to BPD, however, is quite controversial and open to many interpretations. On the one hand, Silk, Lee, Hill, and Lohr (1995) reported that the number of criterion BPD behaviors met was correlated with severity of childhood sexual abuse in a group of clients with BPD. On the other hand, a review by Fossati, Madeddu, and Maffei (1999) suggested that sexual abuse is not a major risk factor for BPD.

The overall results of this transactional pattern between the emotionally vulnerable individual and the invalidating environment are the emotional dysregulation and behavioral patterns exhibited by the borderline adult. Such an individual has never learned how to label and regulate emotional arousal, how to tolerate emotional distress, or when to trust his/her own emotional responses as reflections of valid interpretations of events, resulting in self-invalidation (Linehan, 1993a). In more optimal environments, public validation of one's private, internal experiences results in the development of a stable identity. In the family of a person with BPD, however, private experiences may be responded to erratically and with insensitivity. Thus, the individual learns to mistrust his/her internal states, and instead scans the environment for cues about how to act, think, or feel. This general reliance on others results in the individual's failure to develop a coherent sense of self. Emotional dysfunction also interferes with the development and maintenance of stable interpersonal relationships, which depend on both a stable sense of self and a capacity to self-regulate emotions. The invalidating environment's tendency to trivialize or ignore the expression of negative emotion also

shapes an expressive style later seen in the adult with BPD—a style that vacillates from inhibition and suppression of emotional experience to extreme behavioral displays. Behaviors such as overdosing, cutting, and burning have important affect-regulating properties and are additionally quite effective in eliciting helping behaviors from an environment that otherwise ignores efforts to ameliorate intense emotional pain. From this perspective, the dysfunctional behaviors characteristic of BPD may be viewed as maladaptive solutions to overwhelming, intensely painful negative affect.

DIALECTICAL DILEMMAS

Linehan (1993a) describes "dialectical dilemmas" as behavioral patterns of the client that often interfere with therapy. These behavioral patterns, also referred to as "secondary targets" in treatment (compared to other targets we describe later), represent six behaviors that are dichotomized into a set of three dimensions of behavior defined by their opposite poles (see Figure 10.1). At one end of each dimension is the behavior that theoretically is most directly influenced biologically via deficits in emotion regulation. At the other end is behavior that has been socially reinforced in the invalidating environment. These secondary targets are characteristics of people diagnosed with BPD that often interfere with change, thus interfering with therapy.

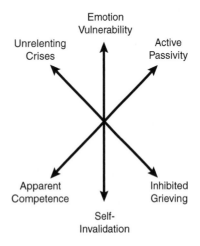

FIGURE 10.1. Dialectical dilemmas in DBT.

Emotion Vulnerability–Self-Invalidation

One dialectical dilemma is represented by biologically influenced emotional vulnerability on the one hand (e.g., the sense of being out of control or falling into the abyss) and by socially influenced self-invalidation on the other (e.g., hate and contempt directed toward the self, dismissal of one's accomplishments). Along this dimension of behavior, clients with BPD often vacillate between acute awareness of their own intense, unbearable, and uncontrollable emotional suffering on the one hand, and dismissal, judgment, and invalidation of their own suffering and helplessness on the other.

Emotion vulnerability here refers to the client's acute experience and communication of emotional vulnerability and excruciating emotional pain. "Vulnerability" here means the acute experience of vulnerability rather than the sensitivity to emotional cues that defines the term when discussing the emotion dysregulation difficulties of the person diagnosed with BPD. Three reactions to emotional vulnerability are common in BPD: (1) freezing or dissociating in the face of intense emotion; (2) rage, often directed at society in general or at people who are experienced as invalidating; and (3) intense despair. Suicide here can function to communicate to others the depth of one's suffering ("I'll show you") and/or as an escape from an unendurable life.

On the other side of this polarity is self-invalidation. What is invalidated, in essence, is one's own emotional experiencing and dysregulated responses. The most typical pattern here is a reaction to emotional pain with intense self-blame and self-hate. These people identify themselves as perpetrators, which results in intense levels of shame and contempt toward the self ("There is nothing wrong with me, I'm just a bad person"). Mood-dependent perfectionism is also common. Here, the individual belittles, ignores, or discounts the difficulty of his/her own life or may overestimate the ease of solving current problems. Unfortunately, this may initiate a cycle that may eventually end in death. Extreme perfectionism often ultimately leads to failure, especially in people who overestimate their abilities; the failure then results in self-hatred, which cues suicidal behaviors in these people. Finally, self-invalidation can also be expressed through willful suppression, meaning that the individual actively denies the experience of all emotion. Often clients who come into our offices simply state, "I don't do emotions." As with emotion vulnerability, self-invalidation needs to be attended to actively and directly, due to the lethal consequences of these behaviors.

Active Passivity–Apparent Competence

A second dimension of behavior is a tendency toward active passivity versus the socially mediated behavior of apparent competence. Either pole of this dimension can lead to anger, guilt, or shame on the part of the client, and a tendency for the therapist to either under- or overestimate the client's capabilities.

"Active passivity" may be defined as passivity in solving one's own problems, while actively engaging others to solve one's problems. It can also be described as passivity that appears to be an active process of shutting down in the face of seeing problems coming in the future. In a sense, people diagnosed with BPD do not appear to have the ability to regulate themselves internally, particularly when the regulation required is non-mood-dependent behaviors. people diagnosed with BPD appear to be "relational selves" rather than "autonomous selves"; that is, they are more highly regulated by their environment than by internal dialogues, choices, and decisions. Their best form of self-regulation is to regulate their environment, such that it then provides the regulation they need. The problem here is that managing one's environment and getting the support one needs requires a good deal of emotional consistency and regulation, characteristics that ordinarily are difficult for people diagnosed with BPD. Lorna Benjamin has described this characteristic as "My misery is your command" (1996, p. 192).

On the opposite side of the polarity is "apparent competence," which refers to the tendency of other people to overestimate the capabilities of the individual with BPD. Thus, this characteristic is defined by the behavior of the observer rather than the behavior of the individual with BPD. This failure to perceive their difficulties and "disability" accurately has serious effects on people diagnosed with BPD. Not only do they not get the help they need, but also their emotional pain and difficulties may easily be invalidated, leading to a further sense of being misunderstood. A number of behavioral patterns can precipitate this overestimation of the competence of the individual with BPD. Often, as a result of a significant discrepancy between the individual's verbal and nonverbal presentations, the individual with BPD believes that he/she has sufficiently communicated his/her level of distress, when in fact the observer interprets the individual as effectively managing a difficult situation. An example would be a woman speaking nonchalantly and without emotion about urges toward suicide after a fight with her husband. People diagnosed with BPD also frequently have difficulty generalizing behaviors across situations, especially in relationships. For example, the person may be able to cope well in the presence of one person, such as a therapist, but be unable to cope when he/she is alone or with someone other than the therapist. The therapist, understandably, may then fail to predict the dysregulation that occurs as the client walks away from the therapy session. Additionally, there may be a difficulty in generalizing coping behaviors across different moods. In one mood, a problem is solvable; in another, it is not. This may not be so difficult to figure out if mood changes are readily apparent to the observer, but often they are not. Thus, accurate estimates of the person's competence actually require the observer, such as the therapist, constantly to anticipate mood changes that might occur to be able to predict what a client might or might not do. It is this characteristic, more than any other, that leads so often to a client walking out of a session, with the therapist believing that all is well, only to end up in the emergency department with a suicide attempt 2 hours later. At times, client failures are nothing more than failures of the therapist (and often the client, also) to predict future behavior accurately.

Unrelenting Crisis–Inhibited Grieving

The third dimension of behavior is the tendency of the client with BPD to experience life as a series of unrelenting crises as opposed to the behavior of "inhibited grieving" (i.e., an inability to experience emotions associated with significant trauma or loss). The client experiences each of these extremes in a way that facilitates movement to the other extreme; for example, attempting to inhibit emotional experiences related to current crises may result in problem behaviors that add to existing crises. As with all of these dialectical dilemmas, the solution is for therapist and client to work toward a more balanced position that represents a synthesis of the opposing poles.

People diagnosed with BPD who experience unrelenting crises have lives that are often characterized as chaotic and in crisis. "Crisis" is defined as the occurrence of problems that are extreme, with significant pressure to resolve them quickly. The consequence of the unrelenting crisis is that the individual with BPD, as well as the person's environmental resources, such as family, friends, coworkers, and even the therapist, slowly wear down. There are three typical scenarios that result in a pattern of unrelenting crisis. First, people with extreme impulsivity and emotion dysregulation engage in behaviors that result in crisis situations. Poor judgment is a key element to assess when analyzing the impulsive behaviors of people diagnosed with BPD. Second, situations that do not start out as crises can quickly become critical due to the lack of resources available to many people with a BPD diagnosis. This may be due to socioeconomic status, or to lack of family or peer support. Finally, unrelenting crises can be due simply to fate or bad luck at a given moment, a phenomenon that is out of the person's control. For example, an unexpected disaster in a client's apartment due to the neighbors running the water in their sink for an extended period of time, might occur. The floors in the client's apartment are damaged by the water and he/she does not have the financial resources to pay for renter's insurance or to replace the carpet in the apartment. His/her apartment is now uninhabitable, but he/she does not have any place else to stay. This problem is out of the person's control, but it is still that person's responsibility to solve.

At the other extreme, and often precipitated by a crisis, is the phenomenon of "inhibited grieving." In this context, "grief" refers to the process of grieving, which includes experiencing multiple painful emotions associated with loss, particularly traumatic loss, not just the one emotion of deep sadness or grief. People with a BPD diagnosis may not be able to experience or process the grief related to loss of the life they had expected for themselves, and ordinarily they do not believe they will recover from the grief if they actually try to experience or to cope with it on their own. As one client said to us, "I don't do sadness." Another said, "I feel sad, I die." People diagnosed with BPD may not recognize their own emotional avoidance and shutdown. Thus, it is crucial for the therapist to attend to emotional avoidance, particularly of sadness and grief, and to assist clients through the grief process. Areas that must be confronted, grieved, and finally accepted include an insurmountably painful childhood, a biological makeup that makes life harder rather than easier, inability to "fit in" in many environments, absence of loving people in the current environment, or loss of hope for a particular future for which one had ardently hoped. What must be confronted by the therapist is that egregious losses can be real and clients might be right: They really cannot get out of the abyss if they fall into it. Regardless of the situation to be grieved, avoidance of these situations may lead to increased shame. The shame is a result of believing that one is unloved, being alone, or fearing that one will not be able to cope in the face of emotional situations. Many of our clients believe that if they begin to address any of these areas, they will not be able to function in their lives, and often this is true. They do not have the skills or resources to assist them with the process of experiencing emotions. We often tell clients that managing grief or processing emotions requires going to the cemetery to pay tribute to what is lost, but building a house at the cemetery and living there is not a good idea. It is a place to visit, experience the sadness of the loss, and then leave. The use of this metaphor has helped many of our clients to experience emotion without falling into the abyss.

STAGES OF THERAPY AND TREATMENT GOALS

In theory, treatment of all clients with BPD can be organized and determined based on their levels of disorder, and is conceptualized as occurring in stages. "Level of disorder" is defined by the current severity, pervasiveness, complexity, disability, and imminent threat presented by the client. Clients can enter into five stages of treatment based on their current level of disorder. First, a pretreatment stage prepares the client for therapy and elicits a commitment to work toward the various treatment goals. Orientation to specific goals and treatment strategies, and commitment to work toward goals addressed during this stage, are likely to be important throughout all stages of treatment.

In Stage 1 of therapy, the primary focus is on stabilizing the client and achieving behavioral control. Out-of-control behaviors constitute those that are disordered due to the severity of the disorder (e.g., as seen in an actively psychotic client) or severity combined with the complexity of multiple diagnoses (e.g., as seen in a suicidal client who has BPD with comorbid panic disorder and depression). Generally, the criteria for putting a client in Stage 1 are based on level of current functioning, together with the inability of the client to work on any other goals before behavior and functioning come under better control. As Mintz (1968) suggested in discussing treatment of the suicidal client, all forms of

psychotherapy are ineffective with a dead client. In the subsequent stages (2–4), the treatment goals are to replace "quiet desperation" with nontraumatic emotional experiencing (Stage 2); to achieve "ordinary" happiness and unhappiness, and to reduce ongoing disorders and problems in living (Stage 3); and to resolve a sense of incompleteness and to achieve freedom (Stage 4). In summary, the orientation of the treatment is first to get action under control, then to help the client to feel better, to resolve problems in living and residual disorder, and to find freedom (and, for some, a sense of transcendence). Most research to date has focused on the severely or multiply disordered clients who enter treatment at Stage 1. The construct of stages aids in treatment planning and conceptualization with the client, and in identifying the appropriate level of care needed.

Pretreatment: Orienting and Commitment

Specific tasks of orientation are twofold. First, client and therapist must arrive at a mutually informed decision to work together. Typically, the first one to four sessions are presented to the client as opportunities for client and therapist to explore this possibility. Diagnostic interviewing, history taking, and formal behavioral analyses of high-priority, targeted behaviors can be woven into initial therapy sessions or be conducted separately. Second, client and therapist must negotiate a common set of expectancies to guide the initial steps of therapy. Client and therapist discuss, outline, and agree specifically on what they can expect from each other. When necessary, the therapist attempts to modify the client's dysfunctional beliefs regarding the process of therapy. Issues addressed include the rate and magnitude of change that can reasonably be expected, the goals of treatment and general treatment procedures, and various myths the client may have about the process of therapy in general. The dialectical/biosocial view of BPD is also presented. Orientation covers several additional points. First, DBT is presented as a supportive therapy requiring a strong collaborative relationship between client and therapist. DBT is not a suicide prevention program, but a life enhancement program in which client and therapist function as a team to create a life worth living. Second, DBT is described as a cognitive-behavioral therapy with a primary emphasis on analyzing problematic behaviors and replacing them with skillful behaviors, and on changing ineffective beliefs and rigid thinking patterns. Third, the client is told that DBT is a skills-oriented therapy, with special emphasis on behavioral skills training. The commitment and orienting strategies, balanced by validation strategies described later, are the most important strategies during this phase of treatment. The therapist places a strong effort into getting the client to commit to not engaging in suicidal or NSSI behaviors for some specified period of time before allowing the client to leave the session; it can be for 1 year, 6 months, until the next session, or until tomorrow.

Stage 1: Attaining Basic Capacities

The primary focus of the first stage of therapy is attaining behavioral control in order to build a life pattern that is reasonably functional and stable. Furthermore, DBT does not promote itself as a suicide prevention program; instead, it focuses on "building a life worth living." Therefore, the primary treatment goal in DBT and in Stage 1 specifically is to assist clients in building a life they will experience as worth living. DBT attains this goal by focusing the treatment on specific behavioral targets agreed upon by both therapist and client. Specific targets in order of importance are to reduce life-threatening behaviors (e.g., suicide attempts, suicide ideation, NSSI behaviors, homicidal threats and behaviors), therapy-interfering behaviors (e.g., late to session, missing sessions, not following treatment plan, hostile attacks on the therapist), and quality-of-life–interfering behaviors (e.g., substance abuse, eating disorder, homelessness, serious Axis I disorders), and to increase behavioral skills. These targets are approached hierarchically and recursively as higher-priority behaviors reappear in each session. However, this does not mean that these behaviors must be addressed in this specific order during a session; it means that, based on the hierarchy, all relevant behavior must be addressed at some point within the session. For example, if a client is 30 minutes late to session (therapy-interfering behavior) and has attempted suicide within the last week (life-threatening behavior), the therapist may choose to address the therapy-interfering behavior first, then move on to address the life-threatening behaviors.

With severely dysfunctional and suicidal clients, significant progress on Stage 1 targets may take up to 1 year or more. In addition to these therapy targets, the goal of increasing dialectical behaviors is universal to all modes of treatment. Dialectical thinking encourages clients to see reality as complex and multifaceted, to hold contradictory thoughts simultaneously and learn to integrate them, and to be comfortable with incon-

sistency and contradictions. For people with a BPD diagnosis, who are extreme and dichotomous in their thinking and behavior, this is a formidable task indeed. A dialectical emphasis applies equally to a client's patterns of behavior because the client is encouraged to integrate and balance emotional and overt behavioral responses. In particular, dialectical tensions arise in the areas of skills enhancement versus self-acceptance, problem solving versus problem acceptance, and affect regulation versus affect tolerance. Behavioral extremes, whether emotional, cognitive, or overt responses, are constantly confronted while more balanced responses are taught.

Life-Threatening Behaviors

Keeping a client alive must, of course, be the first priority in any psychotherapy. Thus, reducing suicide crisis behaviors (any behaviors that place the client at high and imminent risk for suicide or threaten to do so, including credible suicide threats, planning, preparations, obtaining lethal means, and high suicide intent) is the highest priority in DBT. The target and its priority are made explicit in DBT during orientation and throughout treatment, simply because suicidal behavior and the risk of suicide are of paramount concern for clients with BPD. Similarly, any acute, intentional NSSI behaviors share the top priority. The priority here is due to the risk of suicidal and NSSI behavior as the single best predictor of subsequent suicide. Similarly, DBT also targets suicide ideation and client expectations about the value and long-term consequences of suicidal behavior, although these behaviors may not necessarily be targeted directly.

Therapy-Interfering Behaviors

Keeping clients and therapists working together collaboratively is the second explicitly targeted priority in DBT. The chronic nature of most problems among clients with BPD, including their high tendency to end therapy prematurely and the likelihood of therapist burnout and iatrogenic behaviors when treating BPD, requires such explicit attention. Both client and therapist behaviors that threaten the relationship or therapeutic progress are addressed directly, immediately, consistently, and constantly—and most importantly, before rather than after either the therapist or the client no longer wants to continue. Interfering behaviors of the client, including those that actually interfere with receiving the therapy (e.g., lateness to sessions, missed sessions, lack of transportation to sessions, dissociating in sessions) or with other clients benefiting from therapy (in group or milieu settings; e.g., selling drugs to other clients in the program), and those that burn out or cross the personal limits of the therapist (e.g., repeated crisis calls at 3:00 A.M., repeated verbal attacks on the therapist) are treated within therapy sessions. Behaviors of the therapist include any that are iatrogenic (e.g., inadvertently reinforcing dysfunctional behaviors), as well as any that cause the client unnecessary distress or make progress difficult (e.g., therapist arriving late to sessions, missing sessions, not returning phone calls within a reasonable time frame). These behaviors are dealt with in therapy sessions, if brought up by either the client or the therapist, and are also discussed during the consultation/supervision meeting.

Quality-of-Life–Interfering Behaviors

The third target of Stage 1 addresses all other behaviors that interfere with the client having a reasonable quality of life. Typical behaviors in this category include serious substance abuse, severe major depressive episodes, severe eating disorders, high-risk and out-of-control sexual behaviors, extreme financial difficulties (uncontrollable spending or gambling, inability to handle finances), criminal behaviors that are likely to lead to incarceration, employment- or school-related dysfunctional behaviors (a pattern of quitting jobs or school prematurely, getting fired or failing in school, not engaging in any productive activities), housing-related dysfunctional behaviors (living with abusive people, not finding stable housing), mental health–related patterns (going in and out of hospitals, failure to take or abuse of necessary medications), and health-related problems (failure to treat serious medical disorders). The goal here is for the client to achieve a stable lifestyle that meets reasonable standards for safety and adequate functioning.

When necessary, DBT incorporates evidence-based behavioral interventions to address specific quality-of-life–interfering behaviors. Because DBT is a principle-based treatment, it allows seamless integration of other evidence-based protocols as long as they are compatible with the basic assumptions and philosophy of DBT. For example we have recently added to DBT a prolonged exposure protocol to treat PTSD among highly suicidal BPD clients (Harned, Korslund, Foa, & Linehan, 2012). Following Harned and colleagues' (2012) guidelines for client readiness and implementation of

the protocol within standard DBT, a pilot study was conducted with 13 women diagnosed with comorbid BPD and PTSD, and at high risk for suicide. Outcomes showed 70% with reliable improvement in PTSD symptoms and a 60% remission rate, results similar to PE findings in the standard PTSD literature.

Behavioral Skills

The fourth target of Stage 1 is for the client to achieve a reasonable capacity for acquiring and applying skillful behaviors in the areas of distress tolerance, emotion regulation, interpersonal effectiveness, self-management, and the capacity to respond with awareness without being judgmental ("mindfulness" skills). In our outpatient program, the primary responsibility for skills training lies with the weekly DBT skills group. The individual therapist monitors the acquisition and use of skills over time, and aids the client in applying skills to specific problem situations in his/her own life. Additionally, it is the role of the individual therapist, not the skills group leader, to provide skills coaching to the client as needed when problems arise.

Stage 2: Quiet Desperation

Stage 1 of DBT takes a direct approach to managing dysfunctional behavioral and regulating emotional patterns. Although the connection between current behavior and previous traumatic events (including those from childhood) may be explored and noted, the focus of the treatment is distinctly on analyzing the relationship among current thoughts, feelings, and behaviors, and on accepting and changing current patterns. The aim of Stage 2 DBT is to reduce "quiet desperation," which can be defined as extreme emotional pain in the presence of control of action (Linehan et al., 1999). A wide range of emotional experiencing difficulties (e.g., avoidance of emotions and emotion-related cues) are targeted in this stage, with the goal of increasing the capacity for normative emotional experiencing (i.e., the ability to experience a full range of emotions without either severe emotional escalation or behavioral dyscontrol). Stage 2 addresses four goals: remembering and accepting the facts of earlier distressing and/or traumatic events; reducing stigmatization and self-blame often associated with traumatic social invalidation; reducing oscillating denial and intrusive response syndromes; and resolving dialectical tensions regarding placement of blame for past difficulties.

Stage 3: Resolving Problems in Living and Increasing Respect for Self

In the third stage, DBT targets the client's unacceptable unhappiness and problems in living. At this stage, the client with BPD has either done the work necessary to resolve problems in the prior two stages or was never severely disordered enough to need it. Although problems at this stage may still be serious, the individual is functional in major domains of living. The goal here is for the client to achieve a level of ordinary happiness and unhappiness, as well as independent self-respect. To this end, the client is helped to value, believe in, trust, and validate him/herself. The targets here are the abilities to evaluate one's own behavior nondefensively, to trust one's own responses, and to hold on to self-evaluations, independent of the opinions of others. Ultimately, the therapist must pull back and persistently reinforce the client's independent attempts at self-validation, self-care, and problem solving. Although the goal is not for clients to become independent of all people, it is important that they achieve sufficient self-reliance to relate to and depend on others without self-invalidating.

Stage 4: Attaining the Capacity for Freedom and Sustained Contentment

The final stage of treatment in DBT targets the resolution of a sense of incompleteness and the development of a capacity for sustained contentment. The focus on freedom encompasses the goal of freedom from the need to have one's wishes fulfilled, or one's current life or behavioral and emotional responses changed. Here the goals are expanded awareness, spiritual fulfillment, and the movement into experiencing flow. For clients at Stage 4, insight-oriented psychotherapy, spiritual direction or practices, or other organized experiential treatments and/or life experiences may be of most benefit.

STRUCTURING TREATMENT: FUNCTIONS AND MODES

Functions of Treatment

Standard DBT is structured around five essential functions: (1) to enhance behavioral capabilities by expanding the individual's repertoire of skillful behavioral patterns; (2) to improve the client's motivation to change by reducing reinforcement for dysfunctional behaviors and high-probability responses (cognitions, emotions, actions) that interfere with effective behaviors; (3) to ensure that new behaviors generalize from the therapeutic to the natural environment; (4) to enhance the motivation and capabilities of the therapist, so that effective treatment is rendered; and (5) to structure the environment so that effective behaviors, rather than dysfunctional behaviors, are reinforced.

Modes of Treatment: Who Does What and When

Responsibility for performing functions and meeting target goals of treatment in standard DBT is spread across the various modes of treatment, with focus and attention varying according to the mode of therapy. The individual therapist (who is always the primary therapist in DBT) attends to the order of targets and is also, with the client, responsible for organizing the treatment so that all goals are met. In skills training, a different set of goals is targeted; during phone calls, yet another hierarchy of targets takes precedence. In the consultation/supervision mode, therapists' behaviors are the targets. Therapists engaging in more than one mode of therapy (e.g., individual, group, and telephone coaching) must stay cognizant of the functions and order of targets specific to each mode, and switch smoothly from one hierarchy to another as the modes of treatment change.

Individual Therapy

DBT assumes that effective treatment must attend both to client capabilities and behavioral skills deficits, and to motivational and behavioral performance issues that interfere with use of skillful responses (function 2). Although there are many ways to effect these principles, in DBT the individual therapist is responsible for the assessment and problem solving of skill deficits and motivational problems, and for organizing other modes to address problems in each area.

Individual outpatient therapy sessions are scheduled on a once-a-week basis for 50–90 minutes, although twice-weekly sessions may be held as needed during crisis periods or at the beginning of therapy. The priorities of specific targets within individual therapy are the same as the overall priorities of DBT discussed earlier. Therapeutic focus within individual therapy sessions is determined by the highest-priority treatment target relevant at the moment. This ordering does not change over the course of therapy; however, the relevance of a target does change. Relevance is determined by either the client's most recent, day-to-day behavior (since the last session) or by current behavior during the therapy session. If satisfactory progress on one target goal has been achieved or the behavior has never been a problem, or if the behavior is currently not evident, then the therapist shifts attention to another treatment target according to the hierarchy. The consequence of this priority allocation is that when high-risk suicidal behaviors or intentional self-injury, therapy-interfering behaviors, or serious quality-of-life–interfering behaviors occur, at least part of the session agenda is devoted to each of these topics. If these behaviors are not occurring at the moment, then the topics to be discussed during Stages 1, 3, and 4 are set by the client. The therapeutic focus (within any topic area discussed) depends on the stage of treatment, the skills targeted for improvement, and any secondary targets. During Stage 1, for example, any problem or topic area can be conceptualized in terms of interpersonal issues and skills needed, opportunities for emotion regulation, and/or a necessity for distress tolerance. During Stage 3, regardless of the topic, the therapist focuses on helping the client decrease problems in living and achieve independent self-respect, self-validation, and self-acceptance both within the session and in everyday life. (These are, of course, targets all through the treatment, but the therapist pulls back further during Stage 3 and does less work for the client than during the two preceding stages.) During Stage 2, the major focus is on reducing pervasive "quiet desperation," as well as changing the extreme emotions and psychological meanings associated with traumatizing cues.

For highly dysfunctional clients, it is likely that early treatment will necessarily focus on the upper part of the hierarchy. For example, if suicidal or NSSI behavior has occurred during the previous week, attention to it takes precedence over attention to therapy-interfering behavior. In turn, focusing on therapy-interfering behaviors takes precedence over working on quality-of-life–interfering behaviors. Although it is often possible to work on more than one target (including those generated by the client) in a given session, higher-priority targets always take precedence, but all relevant targets must be addressed adequately during the session. Again, targets do not need to be addressed in sequential order; they just have to be addressed during the session. Determining the relevance of targeted behaviors is assisted by the use of diary cards, filled out by the client

during at least the first two stages of therapy and brought to weekly sessions. Failure to complete or to bring in a card is considered a therapy-interfering behavior and should be openly addressed as such. Diary cards record daily instances of suicidal and NSSI behavior, urges to self-harm or to engage in suicide behaviors (on a 0- to 5-point scale), "misery," use of substances (licit and illicit), and use of behavioral skills. Other targeted behaviors (bulimic episodes, daily productive activities, flashbacks, etc.) may also be recorded on the blank area of the card. The therapist doing DBT must develop the pattern of routinely reviewing the card at the beginning of each session. The card acts as a road map for each session; therefore, a session cannot begin until a diary card has been completed. If the card indicates that a life-threatening behavior has occurred, it is noted and discussed. If high suicide or self-harm urges are recorded, or there is a significant increase (e.g., an increase of 3 points or higher on the 0- to 5-point scale for urges) over the course of the week, they are assessed to determine whether the client is at risk for suicide. If a pattern of substance abuse or dependence appears, it is treated as a quality-of-life–interfering behavior.

Work on targeted behaviors involves a coordinated array of treatment strategies, described later in this chapter. Essentially, each session is a balance among structured, as well as unstructured, problem solving (including simple interpretive activities by the therapist) and unstructured validation. The amount of the therapist's time allocated to each—problem solving and validating—depends on (1) the urgency of the behaviors needing change or problems to be solved, and (2) the urgency of the client's needs for validation, understanding, and acceptance without any intimation of change being needed. However, there should be an overall balance in the session between change (problem solving) and acceptance (validation) strategies. Unbalanced attention to either side may result in a nondialectical session, in addition to impeding client progress.

Skills Training

The necessity of crisis intervention and attention to other primary targets makes skills acquisition within individual psychotherapy very difficult. Thus, a separate component of treatment directly targets the acquisition of behavioral skills (function 1). In DBT this usually takes the form of separate, weekly, 2- to 2½-hour group skills training sessions that clients must attend, ordinarily for a minimum of 6 months and preferably for a year. Skills training can also be done individually, although it is often more difficult to stay focused on teaching new skills in individual than in group therapy. After a client has gone through all skills modules twice (i.e., for 1 year), remaining in skills training is a matter of personal preference and need. Some DBT programs have developed graduate groups for clients who have acquired the skills but still need weekly consultation in applying the skills effectively to everyday difficulties. It is important to note that there is no research to date on the effectiveness of graduate groups. In adolescent programs, family members are usually invited. Some programs include a separate friends and families skills training group as well.

Each group typically has a leader and a co-leader. Whereas the primary role of the leader is to teach the skills, the co-leader focuses on managing group process by keeping members both focused and attending to the material being taught, as well as processing the information (e.g., ensuring that everyone is on the correct page, noticing when the leader's invalidation has led to a member shutting down, waking someone up, sitting next to a member who is crying during group). We have found that it is difficult to keep the group focused and the leader on schedule for teaching the skills if the leader attempts to manage both roles on his/her own. Oftentimes, the co-leader role is more difficult to learn.

Skills training in DBT follows a psychoeducational format. In contrast to individual therapy, in which the agenda is determined primarily by the problem to be solved, the skills training agenda is set by the skill to be taught. As mentioned earlier, skills training also uses a hierarchy of treatment targets to keep the group focused: (1) therapy-destroying behaviors (e.g., using drugs on premises, which could lead to the clinic being shut down; property damage; threatening imminent suicide or homicidal behavior to a fellow group member or therapist); (2) increasing skills acquisition and strengthening; and (3) decreasing therapy-interfering behaviors (e.g., refusing to talk in a group setting, restless pacing in the middle of sessions, attacking the therapist and/or the therapy). However, therapy-interfering behaviors are not given the attention in skills training that they are given in the individual psychotherapy mode. If such behaviors were a primary focus, there would never be time for teaching behavioral skills. Generally, therapy-interfering behaviors are put on an extinction schedule, while a client is "dragged" through skills training and simultaneously soothed. In DBT, all skills training clients are required to be in concurrent individual psycho-

therapy. Throughout group or individual skills training, each client is urged to address other problematic behaviors with his/her primary therapist; if a serious risk of suicide develops, the skills training therapist refers the problem to the primary therapist.

Although all of the strategies described below are used in both individual psychotherapy and skills training, the mix is decidedly different. Skills acquisition, strengthening, and generalization strategies are the predominant change strategies in skills training. In addition, skills training is highly structured, much more so than the individual psychotherapy component. Half of each skills training session is devoted to reviewing homework practice of the skills currently being taught, and the other half is devoted to presenting and practicing new skills. Except when interpersonal process issues seriously threaten progress, the agenda and topics for discussion in skills training are usually predetermined.

Four skills modules are taught on a rotating basis over the course of 6 months. In standard DBT, mindfulness skills are taught for 2 consecutive weeks at the beginning of each of the subsequent modules. New members join a group during either the 2 weeks of mindfulness or the first 2 weeks of the subsequent module.

Mindfulness skills are viewed as central in DBT; thus, they are labeled the "core" skills. These skills represent a behavioral translation of meditation (including Zen and contemplative prayer) practice and include observing, describing, spontaneous participating, being nonjudgmental, focusing awareness, and focusing on effectiveness. Unlike standard behavioral and cognitive therapies, which ordinarily focus on changing distressing emotions and events, a major emphasis of DBT is on learning to manage pain skillfully. Mindfulness skills reflect the ability to experience and to observe one's thoughts, emotions, and behaviors without evaluation, and without attempting to change or control them. Distress tolerance skills comprise two types of skills. First, crisis survival skills are used to regulate behavior, in order to manage painful situations without making them worse (e.g., without engaging in life-threatening behavior) until the problem can be solved. Second, "accepting reality" skills are used to tolerate the pain of problems that cannot be solved in either the short-term future or that may have occurred in the past and, therefore, cannot be changed ever.

Emotion regulation skills target the reduction of emotional distress and include affect identification and labeling, mindfulness of current emotions (i.e., experiencing nonjudgmentally), identifying obstacles to changing emotions, increasing resilience, and acting opposite to the emotion. Interpersonal effectiveness skills teach effective methods for deciding on objectives within conflict situations (either asking for something or saying "no" to a request) and strategies that maximize the chances of obtaining those objectives without harming the relationship or sacrificing self-respect.

It is important to highlight here one skill that is essential in the DBT emotion regulation module: the skill of opposite action. This emotion regulation skill encourages clients to act opposite to their emotional urge in order to reduce their emotional arousal. The theoretical premise behind opposite action is that acting in accordance with the action urge associated with an emotion increases the likelihood that that emotion will fire again (Linehan, Bohus, & Lynch, 2007). Clients are taught that reversing expressive (e.g., facial expression, posture, voice tone) and action components of emotion responses is common to many treatments that address emotional disorders and, in essence, can be one of the main mechanisms of change in effective psychotherapy. For example, effective treatments for anxiety are based on principles of exposure and response prevention that encourage active replacement of an emotion-consistent behavior with an emotion-inconsistent behavior (e.g., Foa & Kozak, 1986). The skill of opposite action expands this principle to be applicable all emotions, not just to fear. It also provides specific guidelines for how exactly to implement opposite actions for each problematic emotion. Therefore, if an emotion is not justified in the situation or is not effective, opposite action involves (1) exposure to the stimuli or cues evoking the emotion, (2) blocking of the behavior prompted by the emotion's action urge, and (3) acting in a way that is opposite or inconsistent with the emotional response (Linehan, 1993b). For example, the action urge of fear is to avoid; therefore, the opposite action is to fully approach the situation. For anger, the action urge is to attack physically or emotionally, clench fists, and to judge the situation. The opposite action to anger therefore involves gently removing oneself from the situation, unclenching the fists, and opening the palms of hands, relaxing the shoulders, making empathic statements, and actively working to generate empathy for the person or situation with whom one is angry (Linehan, 1993b, 2013).

The skill of opposite action is very similar to the recommendation to change action tendencies in order to change anxiety, which was proposed by Barlow in 1988. According to Barlow and colleagues (2004), negative emotionality is a latent factor underlying depression and anxiety disorders; therefore they proposed a unified treatment protocol for mood and anxiety disorders. Barlow and colleagues' unified protocol suggests that difficulties with negative emotions can be treated through altering antecedent cognitive reappraisals (i.e., the probability of an event to happen and the likelihood of a catastrophic outcome), preventing emotional avoidance, and facilitating action tendencies that are not associated with the emotion. For this last strategy, they highlight that a crucial step is to prevent action tendencies associated with the emotion and to facilitate different action tendencies, encouraging approach when emotions says avoidance. The examples given are similar to opposite action (e.g., asking an individual diagnosed with GAD to engage in nonperfect behavior; encouraging someone with an anger problem to act detached and passive; asking someone diagnosed with depression to act active and not withdraw).

Self-management skills are taught in conjunction with the other behavioral skills; however, there is not a specific module allocated to these skills because behavioral principles are inherent in all of DBT. Self-management skills include knowledge of the fundamental principles of learning and behavior change, and the ability to set realistic goals, to conduct one's own behavioral analysis, and to implement contingency management plans.

Telephone Consultation

Telephone calls between sessions (or other extratherapeutic contact when DBT is conducted in other settings; e.g., inpatient units) are an integral part of DBT. Telephone consultation calls also follow a target hierarchy: (1) to provide emergency crisis intervention and simultaneously break the link between suicidal behaviors and therapist attention; (2) to provide coaching in skills and promote skills generalization; and (3) to provide a timely context for repairing the therapeutic relationship. With respect to calls for skills coaching, the focus of a phone call varies depending on the complexity and severity of the problem to be solved and the amount of time the therapist is willing to spend on the phone. It is important to note that these calls are not considered therapy sessions and should not be used as such. With easy or already clear situations, in which it is reasonably easy to determine what the client can or should do in the situation, the focus is on helping the client use behavioral skills (rather than dysfunctional behaviors) to address the problem. Alternatively, with complex problems, or with problems too severe for the client to resolve soon, the focus is on ameliorating and tolerating distress, and inhibiting dysfunctional problem-solving behaviors until the next therapy session. In the latter case, resolving the crisis is not the target of telephone coaching calls.

With the exception of taking necessary steps to protect the client's life when he/she has threatened suicide, all calls for help are handled as much alike as possible. This is done to break the contingency between suicidal and NSSI behaviors, and increased phone contact. To do this, the therapist can do one of two things: refuse to accept any calls (including suicide crisis calls), or insist that the client who calls during suicidal crises also call during other crises and problem situations. As Linehan (1993b) notes, experts on suicidal behaviors uniformly say that therapist availability is necessary with suicidal clients. Thus, DBT chooses the latter course and encourages (and at times insists) on calls during nonsuicidal crisis periods. In DBT, calling the therapist too infrequently, as well as too frequently, is considered therapy-interfering behavior. Through orientation to coaching calls during pretreatment the client learns what to expect during the calls. For example, a therapist may communicate to the client in session what he/she will ask during the call: "What's the problem? What skills have you used? Where is your skills book? Go get it, and let's figure out what other skills you can use to get through this situation." It is important to highlight that clients and therapists can easily fall into the trap of considering the act of calling for phone consultation a skill. Although asking for help may be a current target of treatment, it is not considered a skill to be used when the client is in distress. A therapists wants to reinforce the client for effectively reaching out; however, he/she does not want to reinforce the client who does not try using actual skills to manage the problem at hand prior to calling the therapist.

Additionally, the therapist is balancing the change-focused strategies with validation throughout the call. It is important that the therapist be aware of contingency management principles that may be occurring during the phone calls to avoid inadvertently reinforcing crisis behaviors and to increase contact between sessions.

A skills trainer uses phone calls only to keep a client in therapy (including, of course, when necessary, to keep the client alive). All other problems, including suicidal crises, are turned over to the primary therapist as soon as possible. We have learned that this can be one of the most difficult distinctions for group leaders to uphold. Clients may call for a variety of reasons, and it is the role of the group leader consistently to refer the client back to the individual therapist.

The final priority for phone calls to individual therapists is relationship repair. Clients with BPD often experience delayed emotional reactions to interactions that have occurred during therapy sessions. From a DBT perspective, it is not reasonable to require clients to wait up to a whole week before dealing with these emotions, and it is appropriate for a client to call for a brief "heart-to-heart" talk. In these situations, the role of the therapist is to soothe and to reassure. In-depth analyses should wait until the next session.

Consultation Team

DBT assumes that effective treatment of BPD must pay as much attention to the therapist's behavior and experience in therapy as it does to the client's. Treating clients with BPD is enormously stressful, and staying within the DBT therapeutic framework can be tremendously difficult (function 4). Thus, an integral part of the therapy is the treatment of the therapist. Every therapist is required to be on a consultation team either with one other person or with a group. DBT consultation meetings are held weekly and attended by therapists currently providing DBT to clients. At times, the clinical setting may require that the team be part of an administrative meeting due to time and space restraints. When this occurs, it is important to set a specific agenda and time limitations on each part of the meeting (administration, DBT) to ensure that therapist consultation issues are addressed. The roles of consultation are to hold the therapist within the therapeutic framework and to address problems that arise in the course of treatment delivery. Thus, the fundamental target is increasing adherence to DBT principles for each member of the consultation group. The DBT consultation team is viewed as an integral component of DBT; that is, it is considered peer group therapy for the therapists, in which each member is simultaneously a therapist to other members and a client. The focus is on applying DBT strategies to increase DBT-adherent behaviors and decrease non-DBT behaviors.

There are three primary functions of consultation to the therapist in DBT. First, a consultation team helps to keep each individual therapist in the therapeutic relationship. The role here is to cheerlead and to support the therapist. Second, the supervisor or consultation team balances the therapist in his/her interactions with the client. In providing balance, consultants may move close to the therapist, helping him/her maintain a strong position. Or consultants may move back from the therapist, requiring the therapist to move closer to the client to maintain balance. Third, within programmatic applications of DBT, the team provides the context for the treatment.

JOINING THE CONSULTATION TEAM

Each team comprises therapists who are currently treating a DBT client or are available to take on a DBT client. The consultation team is a community of therapists treating a community of clients. Prior to joining the team, it is important that the therapist be completely aware of his/her commitment. As with clients during the pretreatment phase of DBT, therapists must make a commitment to the team (see Table 10.2). The team member conducting the commitment session will use the same strategies and techniques used in a first session with a DBT client (e.g., devil's advocate, pros and cons, troubleshooting). New therapists must commit to doing the behaviors listed in Table 10.2), to working actively toward increasing their own effectiveness and adherence when applying DBT principles and to being responsible for treatment and outcomes of all clients treated by the team. For example, members of the team are agreeing that if a client being treated by any member of the team commits suicide, then all members will say "Yes" when asked if they have ever had a client commit suicide.

CONSULTATION MEETING FORMAT

There are multiple ways to run a DBT team meeting. The following is the way we conduct our meetings at the University of Washington (although it is important to note that even this format could change as needs of members change). Each of our DBT teams has an identified team leader. This person is typically the most experienced DBT therapist on the team, and his/her role is to articulate the DBT principles when necessary for overseeing the fidelity of the treatment provided. Additionally, a team may have an observer who rings a bell whenever team members make judgmental comments (in content or tone) about themselves, each other, or a client; stay polarized without seeking synthesis; fall out of mindful-

TABLE 10.2. DBT Consultation Team Commitment Session

1. To keep the agreements of the team, especially remaining compassionate, mindful, and dialectical.

2. To be available to see a client in whatever role one has joined the team for (e.g., individual therapist, group skills trainer, clinical supervisor, pharmacotherapist).

3. To function as a therapist in the group (to the group) and not just be a silent observer or a person that only speaks about his or her own problems.

4. To treat team meetings in the same way one treats any other group therapy session (i.e., attending the weekly meetings [not double scheduling other events or clients], on time, until the end, with pagers, PDAs, and phones out of sight and off or, if necessarily on, on silent).

5. To come to team meetings adequately prepared.

6. To be willing to give clinical advice to people who have more experience (especially when it's hard to imagine yourself as being able to offer anything useful).

7. To have the humility to admit your mistakes/difficulties and the willingness to have the group help you solve them.

8. To be nonjudgmental and compassionate of your fellow clinicians and clients. To ring the bell of nonjudgmentalness to remind yourself to not be judgmental or unmindful, but not to ring it as a proxy for criticizing someone. The bell is a reminder, not a censor.

9. To properly assess the problem before giving solutions (do unto others as you wish they would more often do unto you).

10. To call out "Elephant in the room" when others are ignoring or not seeing the elephant.

11. To be willing to go through a chain analysis even though you were only 31 seconds late and you would have been there on time if it were not for that traffic light that always takes all day to change.

12. To participate in team by sharing the roles of Leader, Observer, Note Taker or other tasks critical to team functioning.

13. If you feel that the consult team is not being useful or don't like the way it is being run, then say something about it rather than silently stewing in frustration.

14. To repair with the team in some way when team meetings are missed, because the team is only as strong as the weakest link. Therefore, the absence of any team member is felt.

15. To carry on even when feeling burnt out, frustrated, tired, overworked, underappreciated, hopeless, ineffective (easier committed to than done, of course).

ness by doing two things at once; or jump in to solve a problem before assessing the problem. The point of these observations is not to lay blame but to focus the team's awareness on the behavior and move past it.

A team may begin with a mindfulness practice. There are several functions of mindfulness on a team. First, it helps members transition into the team by participating fully and focusing on only one thing in the moment, using a DBT mind-set. Second, it can provide an opportunity for team members to enhance their skills in leading and providing feedback about the practice with other team members. Consultation team agreements (see Table 10.3) have been developed to facilitate a DBT frame and help to create a supportive environment for managing client–therapist and therapist–therapist difficulties. Therefore, a team may elect to read one or all of the team agreements during the team meeting. Most importantly, an agenda is set by the team following the DBT hierarchy of targets, with a specific focus on the needs of the therapist rather than the problems of the clients. Our agenda uses the following format; however, the following items can be prioritized differently based on the needs of an individual team: (1) the therapists' need for consultation around clients' suicidal crises or other life-threatening behaviors; (2) therapy-interfering behaviors (including client absences and dropouts, as well as therapist therapy-interfering behaviors); (3) therapist team-interfering behaviors and burnout; (4) severe or escalating deterioration in quality-of-life behaviors; (5) reportage of good news and therapists' effective behaviors; (6) a summary of the work of the previous skills group and graduate group by group leaders; and (7) discussion of administrative issues (requests to miss team or be out of town, new client contacts; changes in skills trainers or group time, format of consultation group, etc.). This agenda spans the 1-hour consultation meeting. Although the agenda may look impossibly long, therapists ordinarily manage the time by being explicit about their need for help and consultation from the team.

Ancillary Care

When problems in the client's environment interfere with functioning or progress, the therapist moves to the case management strategies. There are three case management strategies: the consultant-to-the-client strategy, environmental intervention, and the consultation/supervision team meeting (described earlier). Because DBT is grounded in dialectics and avoids becoming

TABLE 10.3. DBT Consultation Team Agreements

1. *Dialectical agreement*: We agree to accept a dialectical philosophy: There is no absolute truth. When caught between two conflicting opinions, we agree to look for the truth in both positions and to search for a synthesis by asking questions such as "What is being left out?"

2. *Consultation to the client agreement*: We agree that the primary goal of this group is to improve our own skills as DBT therapists, and not serve as a go-between for clients to each other. We agree to not treat clients or each other as fragile. We agree to treat other group members with the belief that others can speak on their own behalf.

3. *Consistency agreement*: Because change is a natural life occurrence, we agree to accept diversity and change as they naturally come about. This means that we do not have to agree with each others' positions about how to respond to specific clients, nor do we have to tailor our own behavior to be consistent with everyone else's.

4. *Observing limits agreement*: We agree to observe our own limits. As therapists and group members, we agree to not judge or criticize other members for having different limits from our own (e.g., too broad, too narrow, "just right").

5. *Phenomenological empathy agreement*: All things being equal, we agree to search for nonpejorative or phenomenologically empathic interpretations of our clients', our own, and other members' behavior. We agree to assume that we and our clients are trying our best and want to improve. We agree to strive to see the world through our clients' eyes and through one another's eyes. We agree to practice a nonjudgmental stance with our clients and with one another.

6. *Fallibility agreement*: We agree ahead of time that we are each fallible and make mistakes. We agree that we have probably either done whatever problematic things we're being accused of, or some part of it, so that we can let go of assuming a defensive stance to prove our virtue or competence. Because we are fallible, it is agreed that we will inevitably violate all of these agreements, and when this is done, we will rely on each other to point out the polarity and move to a synthesis.

rigid, a therapist intervenes in the client's environment only under very specific conditions: (1) The client is unable to act on his/her own behalf and outcome is extremely important; (2) a key person in the environment will only speak with someone who is in high power (e.g., the therapist instead of the client); (3) when the client's or others' lives are in imminent danger; (4) when it is the humane thing to do and will cause no harm; and (5) when the client is a minor.

CONSULTATION-TO-THE-CLIENT STRATEGY

The consultation-to-the-client strategy was developed with three objectives in mind. First, clients must learn how to manage their own lives and care for themselves by interacting effectively with other people in the environment, including health care professionals. The consultation-to-the-client strategy emphasizes clients' capacities and targets their ability to take care of themselves. Second, this strategy was designed to decrease instances of "splitting" between DBT therapists and other people interacting with clients, which occurs when different providers in a client's network hold differing opinions on how to treat the client. A fundamental tenet of this strategy is that therapists do not tell others, including other health care professionals, how to treat the client. The therapist may suggest but may not demand. What this means in practice is that the therapist is not attached to others treating a client in a specific way. By remaining in the role of a consultant to the client, the therapist stays out of such arguments. Finally, the consultation-to-the-client strategy promotes respect for clients by imparting the message that they are credible and capable of performing interventions on their own behalf.

As mentioned previously, it is the responsibility of the individual DBT therapist to coordinate and organize care with ancillary treatment providers (function 5; e.g., case managers, pharmacotherapists). The consultation-to-the-client strategy balances the consultation-to-the-therapist strategy described earlier, primarily by providing direct consultation to the client in how to interact with other providers rather than consulting with people in the client's environment on how to interact with the client. Except for special circumstances listed earlier, DBT therapists do not discuss clients with ancillary providers, or other providers in the client's environment, without the client present. The therapist works with the client to problem-solve difficulties he/she has with his/her network, leaving the client to act as the intermediary between the therapist and other professionals.

ENVIRONMENTAL INTERVENTION

The bias in DBT is toward teaching the client how to interact effectively with his/her environment. Thus, the consultation-to-the-client strategy is the dominant case management strategy and is used whenever possible. There are times, however, when intervention by the therapist is needed. In general, the environmental intervention strategy is used over the consultation-to-the-client strategy when substantial harm may befall the client if the therapist does not intervene. The general rule for environmental intervention is that when clients lack abilities that they need to learn or that are impossible to obtain, or are not reasonable or necessary, the therapist may intervene.

Client Variables

DBT was developed to treat the multidiagnostic, difficult-to-treat clients. Therefore, there are a number of requisite client characteristics for Stage 1 DBT. Of these, voluntary participation and a commitment to a specified time period (e.g., 16 weeks, 6 months to 1 year) are critical. The effective application of DBT requires a strong interpersonal relationship between therapist and client. The therapist must first work to become a major reinforcer in the life of the client, then use the relationship to promote change in the client. Continuing the relationship can only be used as a positive contingency when a client wants to be in treatment; thus, contingency management is seriously compromised with involuntary clients. Court-ordered treatment is acceptable, if clients agree to remain in therapy even if the order is rescinded. A client characteristic necessary for group therapy is the ability to control overtly aggressive behavior toward others. DBT was developed and evaluated with perhaps the most severely disturbed portion of the population with BPD; all clients accepted into treatment had histories of multiple suicidal and NSSI behaviors. However, the treatment has been designed flexibly and is likely to be effective with less severely disturbed clients.

Therapist Variables

In comparison to other aspects of therapy, the therapist characteristics that facilitate DBT have received little attention. However, evidence supports the assumption that effective therapy for clients with BPD requires the proficient balancing of acceptance and change strategies (Shearin & Linehan, 1992). This research also found that therapists' nonpejorative perceptions of clients were associated with less suicidal behavior.

Linehan (1993b) describes requisite therapist characteristics in terms of three bipolar dimensions that must be balanced in the conduct of therapy. The first dimension represents the balance of an orientation of acceptance with an orientation of change. The therapist must be able to inhibit judgmental attitudes (often under very trying circumstances) and to practice acceptance of the client, of the self, and of the therapeutic process exactly as these are in the current moment. Nevertheless, the therapist remains cognizant that therapy implies necessity to change, and he/she assumes responsibility for directing the therapeutic influence. Second, the therapist must balance unwavering centeredness with compassionate flexibility. "Unwavering centeredness" is the quality of believing in oneself, the therapy, and the client. "Compassionate flexibility" is the ability to take in relevant information about the client and to modify one's position accordingly by letting go of a previously held position. In balancing these two dimensions, the therapist must be able to observe his/her own limits without becoming overly rigid. Finally, the DBT therapist must be able to balance a high degree of nurturing with benevolent demanding. "Nurturing" refers to teaching, coaching, assisting, and strengthening the client, whereas "benevolent demanding" requires the therapist to recognize existing capabilities, to reinforce adaptive behavior, and to refuse to "do" for the client when the client can "do" for him/herself. Above all, the ability to demand requires willingness to believe in the client's ability to change.

TREATMENT STRATEGIES

"Treatment strategies" in DBT refer to the role and focus of the therapist, as well as to a coordinated set of procedures that function to achieve specific treatment goals. Although DBT strategies usually comprise a number of steps, use of a strategy does not necessarily require the application of every step. It is considerably more important that the therapist apply the intent of the strategy than that he/she should inflexibly lead the client through a series of prescribed maneuvers.

DBT employs five sets of treatment strategies to achieve the previously described behavioral targets: (1) dialectical strategies, (2) core strategies, (3) stylistic strategies, (4) case management strategies (discussed earlier), and (5) integrated strategies. DBT strategies are illustrated in Figure 10.2. Within an individual session and with a given client, certain strategies may be used more than others, and all strategies may not be necessary or appropriate. An abbreviated discussion

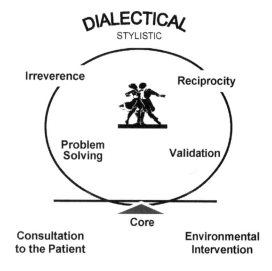

FIGURE 10.2. Treatment strategies in DBT. From Linehan (1993b). Copyright 1993 by The Guilford Press. Reprinted by permission.

of the first three types of DBT treatment strategies follows.

Dialectical Strategies

Dialectical strategies permeate the entire therapy, and their use provides the rationale for adding the term "dialectical" to the title of the therapy. There are three types of dialectical strategies: those having to do with how the therapist structures interactions; those pertaining to how the therapist defines and teaches skillful behaviors; and certain specific strategies used during the conduct of treatment.

Dialectics of the Relationship: Balancing Treatment Strategies

"Dialectical strategies" in the most general sense of the term have to do with how the therapist balances the dialectical tensions within the therapy relationship. As noted earlier, the fundamental dialectic within any psychotherapy, including that with a client who has BPD, is that between acceptance of what is and efforts to change what is. A dialectical therapeutic position is one of constant attention to combining acceptance and change, flexibility and stability, nurturing and challenging, and focusing on capabilities and on limitations and deficits. The goals are to bring out the opposites, both in therapy and in the client's life, and to provide conditions for syntheses. The presumption is that change may be facilitated by emphasizing acceptance, and acceptance, by emphasizing change. The emphasis on opposites sometimes takes place over time (i.e., over the whole of an interaction), rather than simultaneously or in each part of an interaction. Although many, if not all, psychotherapies, including cognitive and behavioral treatments, attend to these issues of balance, placing the concept of balance at the center of the treatment ensures that the therapist remains attentive to its importance.

Three primary characteristics are needed to maintain a dialectical stance in the therapeutic relationship: movement, speed, and flow. "Movement" refers to acting with certainty, strength, and total commitment on the part of the therapist. If the therapist only moves halfheartedly, the client will only move halfheartedly. "Speed" is of the essence and entails keeping the therapy moving, so that it does not become rigid or stuck. Finally, "flow" refers to being mindful of the moment-to-moment unfolding of a session and responding smoothly, and with apparent effortlessness.

Teaching Dialectical Behavior Patterns

Dialectical thinking is emphasized throughout the entire treatment. Not only does the therapist maintain a dialectical stance in his/her treatment of the client but he/she also focuses on teaching and modeling dialectical thinking to the client. The therapist helps the client move from an "either–or" position to a "both–and" position, without invalidating the first idea or its polarity when asserting the second. Behavioral extremes and rigidity—whether cognitive, emotional, or overtly behavioral—are signals that synthesis has not been achieved; thus, they can be considered nondialectical. Instead, a "middle path" similar to that advocated in Buddhism is advocated and modeled. The important thing in following the path to Enlightenment is to avoid being caught and entangled in any extreme and always follow the Middle Way (Kyokai, 1966). This emphasis on balance is similar to the approach advocated in relapse prevention models (e.g., Marlatt & Gordon, 1985) for treating addictive behaviors.

Specific Dialectical Strategies

There are eight specific dialectical treatment strategies: (1) entering and using paradox, (2) using metaphor, (3) playing the devil's advocate, (4) extending, (5) activating the client's "wise mind," (6) making lemonade out of lemons (turning negatives into positives), (7) allowing natural change (and inconsistencies even within the therapeutic milieu), and (8) assessing dialectically by always asking the question "What is being left out here?" Due to space limitations, a selection of these strategies is included in the following sections. For a complete review, the interested reader is referred to the DBT treatment manual (Linehan, 1993a).

ENTERING THE PARADOX

Entering the paradox is a powerful technique because it contains the element of surprise. The therapist presents the paradox without explaining it and highlights the paradoxical contradictions within the behavior, the therapeutic process, and reality in general. The essence of the strategy is the therapist's refusal to step in with rational explanation; the client's attempts at logic are met with silence, a question, or a story designed to shed a small amount of light on the puzzle to be solved. The client is pushed to achieve understanding, to move toward synthesis of the polarities, and to resolve the dilemma him/herself. Linehan (1993b) has highlighted a number of typical paradoxes and their corresponding dialectical tensions encountered over the course of therapy. Clients are free to choose their own behavior but cannot stay in therapy if they do not work at changing their behavior. They are taught to achieve greater independence by becoming more skilled at asking for help from others. Clients have a right to kill themselves, but if they ever convince the therapist that suicide is imminent, they may be locked up. Clients are not responsible for being the way they are, but they are responsible for what they become. In highlighting these paradoxical realities, both client and therapist struggle with confronting and letting go of rigid patterns of thought, emotion, and behavior, so that more spontaneous and flexible patterns may emerge.

USING METAPHOR: PARABLE, MYTH, ANALOGY, AND STORYTELLING

The use of metaphor, stories, parables, and myth is extremely important in DBT and provides alternative means of teaching dialectical thinking. Stories are usually more interesting, are easier to remember, and encourage the search for other meanings of events under scrutiny. Additionally, metaphors allow clients to distance themselves from the problem. In general, the idea of metaphor is to take something the client does understand and use it as an analogy for something the client does not understand. Furthermore, metaphors and stories can be developed collaboratively over the course of treatment. When therapist and client relate to a metaphor, it can be a powerful tool to use throughout the treatment, reminding the client what he/she is working on. For example, changing behavior by learning new skills can be compared to building a new hiking trail in the woods. At first, the current trail is defined and easy to navigate; however, it always leads to a dead end (old dysfunctional behavior). To build a new trail (skillful behaviors), the hiker must repeatedly go through a new, undefined area until it becomes worn in. This takes time, and the hiker moves slowly and deliberately, clearing away the brush. Additionally, while the new path is developing, the old path is slowly becoming grown over. The therapist can return to this story each time the client begins to struggle between trying new skills and returning to old dysfunctional behavior.

PLAYING DEVIL'S ADVOCATE

The devil's advocate technique is quite similar to the argumentative approach used in rational–emotive and cognitive restructuring therapies. With this strategy, the therapist presents a propositional statement that is an extreme version of one of the client's own dysfunctional beliefs, then plays the role of devil's advocate to counter the client's attempts to disprove the extreme statement or rule. For example, a client may state, "Because I'm overweight, I'd be better off dead." The therapist argues in favor of the dysfunctional belief, perhaps by suggesting that because this is true for the client, it must be true for others as well; hence, all overweight people would be better off dead. The therapist may continue along these lines: "And since the definition of what constitutes being overweight varies so much among people, there must be an awful lot of people who would be considered overweight by someone. That must mean they'd all be better off dead!" Or "Gosh, I'm about 5 pounds overweight. I guess that means I'd be better off dead, too." Any reservations the client proposes can be countered by further exaggeration, until the self-defeating nature of the belief becomes apparent. The devil's ad-

vocate technique is often used in the first several sessions to elicit a strong commitment from the client and in commitment sessions with new therapists joining the DBT team. The therapist argues to the client that since the therapy will be painful and difficult, it is not clear how making such a commitment (and therefore being accepted into treatment) could possibly be a good idea. This usually has the effect of moving the client to take the opposite position in favor of therapeutic change. To employ this technique successfully, it is important that the therapist's argument seem reasonable enough to invite counterargument, and that the delivery be credible, made in a naive but offbeat manner.

EXTENDING

The term "extending" has been borrowed from *aikido*, a Japanese form of self-defense. In that context, extending occurs when the student of *aikido* waits for a challenger's movements to reach their natural completion, then extends a movement's endpoint slightly further than what would naturally occur, leaving the challenger vulnerable and off balance. In DBT, extending occurs when the therapist takes the severity or gravity of what the client is communicating more seriously than the client intends. This strategy is the emotional equivalent of the devil's advocate strategy. It is particularly effective when the client is threatening dire consequences of an event or problem to induce change in the environment. Take the interaction with the following client, who threatens suicide if an extra appointment time for the next day is not scheduled. The following interchange occurred after attempts to find a mutually acceptable time failed.

CLIENT: I've got to see you tomorrow, or I'm sure I will end up killing myself. I just can't keep it together by myself any longer.

THERAPIST: Hmm, I didn't realize you were so upset! We've got to do something immediately if you are so distressed that you might kill yourself. What about hospitalization? Maybe that is needed.

CLIENT: I'm not going to the hospital! Why won't you just give me an appointment?

THERAPIST: How can we discuss such a mundane topic as session scheduling when your life is in danger? How are you planning to kill yourself?

CLIENT: You know how. Why can't you cancel someone or move an appointment around? You could put an appointment with one of your students off until another time. I can't stand it anymore!

THERAPIST: I'm really concerned about you. Do you think I should call an ambulance?

The aspect of the communication that the therapist takes seriously (suicide as a possible consequence of not getting an appointment) is not the aspect (needing an extra appointment the next day) that the client wants taken seriously. The therapist takes the consequences seriously and extends the seriousness even further. The client wants the problem taken seriously, and indeed is extending the seriousness of the problem.

MAKING LEMONADE OUT OF LEMONS

Making lemonade out of lemons is similar to the notion in psychodynamic therapy of utilizing a client's resistances; therapeutic problems are seen as opportunities for the therapist to help the client. The strategy involves taking something that is apparently problematic and turning it into an asset. Problems become opportunities to practice skills; suffering allows others to express empathy; weaknesses become one's strengths. To be effective, this strategy requires a strong therapeutic relationship; the client must believe that the therapist has a deep compassion for his/her suffering. The danger in using this strategy is that it is easily confused with the invalidating refrain repeatedly heard by clients with BPD. The therapist should avoid the tendency to oversimplify a client's problems, and refrain from implying that the lemons in the client's life are really lemonade. While recognizing that the cloud is indeed black, the therapist assists the client in finding the positive characteristics of a situation—thus, the silver lining.

Core Strategies

Validation

Validation and problem-solving strategies, together with dialectical strategies, make up the core of DBT and form the heart of the treatment. Validation strategies are the most obvious acceptance strategies, whereas problem-solving strategies are the most obvious change strategies. Both strategies are used in every interaction with the client, although the relative frequency of each depends on the particular client, the current situation, and the vulnerabilities of that client. However, through-

out an entire session, there should be an overall balance between the acceptance and change strategies. We discuss validation strategies in this section and problem-solving strategies in the next.

Clients with BPD present themselves clinically as people in extreme emotional pain. They plead, and at times demand, that their therapists do something to change this state of affairs. It is very tempting to focus the energy of therapy on changing the client by modifying irrational thoughts, assumptions, or schemas; critiquing interpersonal behaviors or motives contributing to interpersonal problems; giving medication to change abnormal biology; and reducing emotional overreactivity and intensity; and so on. In many respects, this focus recapitulates the invalidating environment by confirming the client's worst fears: The client is the problem and indeed cannot trust his/her own reactions to events. Mistrust and invalidation of how one responds to events, however, are extremely aversive and can elicit intense fear, anger, and shame, or a combination of all three. Thus, the entire focus of change-based therapy can be aversive because the focus by necessity contributes to and elicits self-invalidation. However, an entire focus of acceptance-based therapy can also be invalidating when it appears to the client that the therapist does not take his/her problems seriously. Therefore, once again, a dialectical stance focuses on a balance between the two poles.

Validation (according to the *Oxford English Dictionary*; Simpson & Weiner, 1989) refers to identifying the validity of an object or making something valid. It also encompasses activities such as corroborating, substantiating, verifying, and authenticating. The act of validating includes providing support from an authoritative source about the truth or validity of something (Merriam-Webster, 2006). Communicating that something is valid implies that objective evidence and reputable authority support or justify the response given (Simpson & Weiner, 1989). These are precisely the meanings associated with the term when used in the context of psychotherapy in DBT.

The essence of validation is this: The therapist communicates to the client that her [*sic*] responses make sense and are understandable within her [*sic*] current life context or situation. The therapist actively accepts the client and communicates this acceptance to the client. The therapist takes the client's responses seriously and does not discount or trivialize them. Validation strategies require the therapist to search for, recognize, and reflect to the client the validity inherent in her [*sic*] response to events. With unruly children, parents have to catch them while they're good in order to reinforce their behavior; similarly, the therapist has to uncover the validity within the client's response, sometimes amplify it, and then reinforce it. (Linehan, 1993b, pp. 222–223, original emphasis)

Two things are important to note here. First, "validation" means the acknowledgment of that which is valid. It does not mean "making" valid. Nor does it mean validating that which is invalid. The therapist observes, experiences, and affirms, but he/she does not create validity. Second, "valid" and "scientific" are not synonyms. Science may be one way to determine what is valid, logical, sound in principle, and/or generally accepted as authority or normative knowledge. However, an authentic experience or apprehension of private events (at least, when similar to the same experiences of others or when in accord with other, more observable events) is also a basis for claiming validity. Validation can be considered at any one of six levels. Each level is correspondingly more complete than the previous one, and each depends on the previous levels. They are definitional of DBT and are required in every interaction with the client. These levels are described most fully in Linehan (1997), and the following definitions are taken from her discussion.

LISTENING AND OBSERVING (V1)

Level 1 validation requires listening to and observing what the client is saying, feeling, and doing, as well as a corresponding active effort to understand what is being said and observed. The essence of this step is that the therapist is staying awake and interested in the client, paying attention to what the client says and does in the current moment. The therapist notices the nuances of response in the interaction. Validation at Level 1 communicates that the client per se, as well as the client's presence, words, and responses in the session have "such force as to compel serious attention and [usually] acceptance" (see earlier definitions of validation; pp. 360–361)

ACCURATE REFLECTION (V2)

The second level of validation is the accurate reflection back to the client of his/her own feelings, thoughts, assumptions, and behaviors. The therapist conveys an understanding of the client by hearing what the client has said and seeing what the client does, and how he/she responds. Validation at Level 2 sanctions, empowers, or authenticates that the individual is who he/she actually is (p. 362).

ARTICULATING THE UNVERBALIZED (V3)

In Level 3 of validation, the therapist communicates understanding of aspects of the client's experience and response to events that have not been communicated directly by the client. The therapist "mind-reads" the reason for the client's behavior and figures out how the client feels and what he/she is wishing for, thinking, or doing just by knowing what has happened to the client. The therapist can make the link between precipitating event and behavior without being given any information about the behavior itself. The therapist can also articulate emotions and meanings the client has not expressed (p. 364).

VALIDATING IN TERMS OF PAST LEARNING OR BIOLOGICAL DYSFUNCTION (V4)

At Level 4, behavior is validated in terms of its causes. Validation here is based on the notion that all behavior is caused by events occurring in time; thus, in principle, it is understandable. The therapist justifies the client's behavior by showing that it is caused by past events. Even though information may not be available to determine all the relevant causes, the client's feelings, thoughts, and actions make perfect sense in the context of the client's current experience, physiology, and life to date. At a minimum, what "is" can always be justified in terms of sufficient causes; that is, what is "should be," in that whatever was necessary for it to occur had to have happened (p. 367).

VALIDATION IN TERMS OF PRESENT CONTEXT OR NORMATIVE FUNCTIONING (V5)

At Level 5, the therapist communicates that behavior is justifiable, reasonable, well grounded, meaningful, and/or efficacious in terms of current events, normative biological functioning, and/or the client's ultimate life goals. The therapist looks for and reflects the wisdom or validity of the client's response and communicates that the response is understandable. The therapist finds the relevant facts in the current environment that support the client's behavior. The therapist is not blinded by the dysfunctionality of some of the client's response patterns to those aspects of a response pattern that may be either reasonable or appropriate to the context. Thus, the therapist searches the client's responses for their inherent reasonableness (as well as commenting on the inherent dysfunctionality of much of the response, if necessary) (pp. 370–371).

RADICAL GENUINENESS (V6)

In Level 6, the task is to recognize the client as he/she is, seeing and responding to his/her strengths and capacities, while keeping a firm empathic understanding of his/her actual difficulties and incapacities. The therapist believes in the client and his/her capacity to change and move toward ultimate life goals just as the therapist may believe in a friend or family member. The client is responded to as a person of equal status, due equal respect. Validation at the highest level is the validation of the individual as "is." The therapist sees more than the role, more than a "client" or "disorder." Level 6 validation is the opposite of treating the client in a condescending manner or as overly fragile. It is responding to the individual as capable of effective and reasonable behavior rather than assuming that he/she is an invalid. Whereas Levels 1–5 represent sequential steps in validation of a kind, Level 6 represents change in both level and kind (p. 377).

Cheerleading strategies constitute another form of validation and are the principal strategies for combating the active passivity and tendencies toward hopelessness in clients with BPD. In cheerleading, therapists communicate the belief that clients are doing their best and validate clients' ability to eventually overcome their difficulties (a type of validation that, if not handled carefully, can simultaneously invalidate clients' perceptions of their helplessness). In addition, therapists express a belief in the therapy relationship, offer reassurance, and highlight any evidence of improvement. Within DBT, cheerleading is used in every therapeutic interaction. Although active cheerleading should be reduced as clients learn to trust and to validate themselves, cheerleading strategies always remain an essential ingredient of a strong therapeutic alliance.

Finally, functional validation, another form of validation used regularly in DBT, is a form of nonverbal or behavioral validation that at times may be more effective than verbal validation. For example, a therapist drops a 50-pound block on the client's foot. It would be considered invalidating for the therapist simply to respond verbally, saying, "Wow, I can see that really hurts! You must be in a lot of pain." Functional validation would entail the therapist removing the block from the client's foot.

Problem Solving

We have previously discussed how clients with BPD typically experience therapies with a primary focus on change as invalidating. However, therapies that focus exclusively on validation can prove equally problematic. Exhortations to accept one's current situation offer little solace to an individual who experiences life as painfully unendurable. Within DBT, problem-solving strategies are the core change strategies, designed to foster an active problem-solving style. For clients with BPD, however, the application of these strategies is fraught with difficulties. The therapist must keep in mind that in clients with BPD the process will be more difficult than that with many other client populations. In work with clients who have BPD, the need for sympathetic understanding and interventions aimed at enhancing current positive mood can be extremely important. The validation strategies just described, as well as the irreverent communication strategy described later, can be tremendously useful here. Within DBT, problem solving is a two-stage process that concentrates first on understanding and accepting a selected problem, then generating alternative solutions. The first stage involves (1) behavioral analysis, (2) insight into recurrent behavioral context patterns, and (3) giving the client didactic information about principles of behaviors, norms, and so on. The second stage specifically targets change through (4) analysis of possible solutions to problems, (5) orienting the client to therapeutic procedures likely to bring about desired changes, and (6) strategies designed to elicit and strengthen commitment to these procedures. The following sections describe in more detail some of these procedures.

Behavioral Analysis

Behavioral analysis is one of the most important strategies in DBT. It is also the most difficult. The purpose of a behavioral analysis is first to select a problem, then to determine empirically what is causing it, what is preventing its resolution, and what aids are available for solving it. Behavioral analysis addresses four primary questions:

1. Are ineffective behaviors being reinforced, are effective behaviors followed by aversive outcomes, or are rewarding outcomes delayed?
2. Does the client have the requisite behavioral skills to regulate his/her emotions, respond skillfully to conflict, and manage his/her own behavior?
3. Are there patterns of avoidance, or are effective behaviors inhibited by unwarranted fears or guilt?
4. Is the client unaware of the contingencies operating in his/her environment, or are effective behaviors inhibited by faulty beliefs or assumptions?

Answers to these questions guide the therapist in the selection of appropriate treatment procedures, such as contingency management, behavioral skills training, exposure, or cognitive modification. Thus, the value of an analysis lies in helping the therapist assess and understand a problem fully enough to guide effective therapeutic response. The first step in conducting a behavioral analysis is to help the client identify the problem to be analyzed and describe it in behavioral terms. Identifying the problem can be the most difficult task for the therapist, and if not done accurately and specifically, can lead therapist and client astray. Problem definition usually evolves from a discussion of the previous week's events, often in the context of reviewing diary cards. The assumption of facts not in evidence is perhaps the most common mistake at this point. An identified problem is further assessed with a chain analysis—an exhaustive, blow-by-blow description of the chain of events leading up to and following the behavior. In a chain analysis, the therapist constructs a general road map of how the client arrives at dysfunctional responses, including where the road actually starts (highlights vulnerability factors and prompting events), and notes possible alternative adaptive pathways or junctions along the way. Additional goals are to identify events that automatically elicit maladaptive behavior, behavioral deficits that are instrumental in maintaining problematic responses, and environmental and behavioral events that may be interfering with more appropriate behaviors. The overall goal is to determine the function of the behavior (i.e., the problem the behavior was instrumental in solving).

Chain analysis always begins with a specific environmental event. Pinpointing such an event may be dif-

ficult because clients are frequently unable to identify anything in the environment that set off the problematic response. Nevertheless, it is important to obtain a description of the events co-occurring with the onset of the problem. The therapist then attempts to identify both environmental and behavioral events for each subsequent link in the chain. Here the therapist must play the part of a very keen observer, thinking in terms of very small chunks of behavior, and repeatedly identifying what the client was thinking, feeling, and doing, and what was occurring in the environment from moment to moment. The therapist asks the client, "What happened next?" or "How did you get from there to there?" Although, from the client's point of view, such links may be self-evident, the therapist must be careful not to make assumptions. For example, a client who had attempted suicide once stated that she decided to kill herself because her life was too painful for her to live any longer. From the client's point of view, this was an adequate explanation for her suicide attempt. For the therapist, however, taking one's life because life is too painful was only one solution. One could decide life is too painful, then decide to change one's life. Or one could believe that death might be even more painful and decide to tolerate life despite its pain. In this instance, careful questioning revealed that the client actually assumed she would be happier dead than alive. Challenging this assumption, then, became a key to ending her persistent suicide attempts. It is equally important to pinpoint exactly what consequences are maintaining the problematic response. Similarly, the therapist should also search for consequences that serve to weaken the problem behavior. As with antecedent events, the therapist probes for both environmental and behavioral consequences, obtaining detailed descriptions of the client's emotions, somatic sensations, actions, thoughts, and assumptions. A rudimentary knowledge of the rules of learning and principles of reinforcement is crucial.

The final step in behavioral analysis is to construct and test hypotheses about events that are relevant to generating and maintaining the problem behavior. The biosocial theory of BPD suggests several factors of primary importance. For example, DBT focuses most closely on intense or aversive emotional states; the amelioration of negative affect is always suspected as being among the primary motivational variables for dysfunctional behavior in BPD. The theory also suggests that typical behavioral patterns, such as deficits in dialectical thinking or behavioral skills, are likely to be instrumental in producing and maintaining problematic responses.

Solution Analysis

Once the problem has been identified and analyzed, problem solving proceeds with an active attempt at finding and identifying alternative solutions. DBT posits that there are five responses to any one problem: (1) Solve the problem; (2) change the emotional reaction to the problem; (3) tolerate the problem; (4) stay miserable, or (5) make things worse. These five options are presented as needed prior to problem solving to ensure that therapist and client are consistently working toward the same goal.

At times, solutions are discussed throughout the behavioral analysis, and pointing to these alternative solutions may be all that is required, rather than waiting until the behavioral analysis is completed. The therapist may ask, "What do you think you could have done differently here?" Throughout this process, the therapist is actively modeling effective problem solving and solution generation, with a heavier emphasis on modeling and guiding the client early on in treatment. At other times, a more complete solution analysis is necessary. Here the task is to "brainstorm" or generate as many alternative solutions as possible. Solutions should then be evaluated in terms of the various outcomes expected. The final step in solution analysis is to choose a solution that will somehow be effective. Throughout the evaluation, the therapist guides the client in choosing a particular behavioral solution. Here, it is preferable that the therapist pay particular attention to long-term over short-term gain, and that chosen solutions render maximum benefit to the client rather than benefit to others.

Problem-Solving Procedures

DBT employs four problem-solving procedures taken directly from the cognitive and behavioral treatment literature. These four—skills training, contingency procedures, exposure, and cognitive modification—are viewed as primary vehicles of change throughout DBT, since they influence the direction that client changes take from session to session. Although they are discussed as distinct procedures by Linehan (1993b), it is not clear that they can in fact be differentiated in every case in clinical practice. The same therapeutic sequence may be effective because it teaches the client

new skills (skills training), provides a consequence that influences the probability of preceding client behaviors occurring again (contingency procedures), provides nonreinforced exposure to cues associated previously but not currently with threat (exposure procedures), or changes the client's dysfunctional assumptions or schematic processing of events (cognitive modification). In contrast to many cognitive and behavioral treatment programs in the literature, these procedures (with some exceptions noted below) are employed in an unstructured manner, interwoven throughout all therapeutic dialogue. Thus, the therapist must be well aware of the principles governing the effectiveness of each procedure in order to use it strategically. The exceptions are in skills training, where skills training procedures predominate.

Skills Training

An emphasis on skills building is pervasive throughout DBT. In both individual and group therapy, the therapist insists at every opportunity that the client actively engage in the acquisition and practice of behavioral skills. The term "skills" is used synonymously with "ability" and includes, in its broadest sense, cognitive, emotional, and overt behavioral skills, as well as their integration, which is necessary for effective performance. Skills training is called for when a solution requires skills not currently in the individual's behavioral repertoire, or when the individual has the component behaviors but cannot integrate and use them effectively. Skills training in DBT incorporates three types of procedures: (1) skills acquisition (modeling, instructing, advising); (2) skills strengthening (encouraging *in vivo* and within-session practice, role playing, feedback); and (3) skills generalization (phone calls to work on applying skills; taping therapy sessions to listen to between sessions; homework assignments).

Contingency Procedures

Every response within an interpersonal interaction is potentially a reinforcement, a punishment, or a withholding or removal of reinforcement. Contingency management requires therapists to organize their behavior strategically, so client behaviors that represent progress are reinforced, while unskillful or maladaptive behaviors are extinguished. or punished. Natural over arbitrary consequences are preferred. An important contingency in DBT is the therapist's interpersonal behavior with the client, which is contingent on alliance.

Effective contingency management requires that the therapist orient the client to the principles of learning. The therapist must attend to the client's behaviors and use the principles of shaping to reinforce those behaviors that represent progress toward DBT targets. Equally important is that the therapist take care not to reinforce behaviors targeted for extinction. In theory, this may seem obvious, but in practice, it can be quite difficult. The problematic behaviors of clients with BPD are often quite effective in obtaining reinforcing outcomes or in stopping painful events. Indeed, the very behaviors targeted for extinction have been intermittently reinforced by mental health professionals, family members, and friends. Contingency management at times requires the use of aversive consequences, similar to "setting limits" in other treatment modalities. Three guidelines are important when using aversive consequences. First, punishment should "fit the crime," and a client should have some way of terminating its application. For example, in DBT, a detailed behavioral analysis follows a suicidal or NSSI act; such an analysis is an aversive procedure for most clients. Once it has been completed, however, a client's ability to pursue other topics is restored. Second, it is crucial that therapists use punishment with great care, in low doses, and very briefly, and that a positive interpersonal atmosphere be restored following any client improvement. Third, punishment should be just strong enough to work. Although the ultimate punishment is termination of therapy, a preferable fallback strategy is putting clients on "vacations from therapy." This approach is considered when all other contingencies have failed, or when a situation is so serious that a therapist's therapeutic or personal limits have been crossed. When utilizing this strategy, the therapist clearly identifies what behaviors must be changed and clarifies that once the conditions have been met, the client can return. The therapist maintains intermittent contact by phone or letter, and provides a referral or backup while the client is on vacation. (In colloquial terms, the therapist kicks the client out, then pines for his/her return.)

Observing limits constitutes a special case of contingency management involving the application of problem-solving strategies to client behaviors that threaten or cross a therapist's personal limits. Such behaviors interfere with the therapist's ability or willingness to conduct the therapy. Therapists must take responsibility for monitoring their own personal limits

and for clearly communicating them to clients. Therapists who do not do this eventually burn out, terminate therapy, or otherwise harm their clients. DBT favors natural over arbitrary limits. Thus, limits vary among therapists, over time and over circumstances. Limits should also be presented as for the good of the therapist, not for the good of the client. What the client argues is in his/her best interests may not ultimately be good for the therapists.

Cognitive Modification

The fundamental message given to clients in DBT is that cognitive distortions are just as likely to be caused by emotional arousal as to be the cause of the arousal in the first place. The overall message is that, for the most part, the source of a client's distress is extremely stressful life events rather than a distortion of benign events. Cognitive restructuring procedures, such as those advocated by Beck, Brown, Berchick, Stewart, and Steer (1990) and Ellis (1973), are used and taught in DBT, although they do not hold a dominant place. In contrast, contingency clarification strategies described earlier are used relentlessly, highlighting contingent relationships operating in the here and now.

Exposure

All of the change procedures in DBT can be reconceptualized as exposure strategies. The principles of exposure used in DBT have been developed for anxiety disorders (see Foa & Kozak, 1986) and expanded in DBT to address all problematic emotions. These strategies work by reconditioning dysfunctional associations that develop between stimuli (e.g., an aversive stimulus, hospitalization, may become associated with a positive stimulus, being nurtured; a client may later work to be hospitalized) or between a response and a stimulus (e.g., an adaptive response, expression of emotions, is met with an aversive consequence, rejection by a loved one; a client may work to suppress emotions). As noted earlier, the DBT therapist conducts a chain analysis of the eliciting cue, the problem behavior (including emotions), and the consequences of the behavior. Working within a behavior therapy framework, the therapist operates according to three guidelines for exposure in DBT: (1) Exposure to the cue that precedes the problem behavior must be nonreinforced (e.g., if a client is fearful that discussing suicidal behavior will lead to his/her being rejected, the therapist must not reinforce the client's shame by ostracizing him/her); (2) dysfunctional responses are blocked in the order of the primary and secondary targets of treatment (e.g., suicidal or NSSI behavior related to shame is blocked by getting the client's cooperation in throwing away hoarded medications); and (3) actions opposite to the dysfunctional behavior are reinforced (e.g., the therapist reinforces the client for talking about painful, shame-related suicidal behavior).

Formal and informal exposure procedures involve first orienting the client to the techniques and to the fact that exposure to cues is often experienced as painful or frightening. Thus, the therapist does not remove the cue to emotional arousal, and at the same time he/she blocks both the action tendencies (including escape responses) and the expressive tendencies associated with the problem emotion. In addition, a crucial step of exposure procedures is teaching the client some means of titrating or ending exposure when emotions become unendurable. The therapist and client collaborate in developing positive, adaptive ways for the client to end exposure voluntarily, preferably after some reduction in the problem emotion has occurred.

Stylistic Strategies

DBT balances two quite different styles of communication that refer to how the therapist executes other treatment strategies. The first, reciprocal communication, is similar to the communication style advocated in CCT. The second, irreverent communication, is quite similar to the style advocated by Whitaker (1975) in his writings on strategic therapy. Reciprocal communication strategies are designed to reduce a perceived power differential by making the therapist more vulnerable to the client. In addition, they serve as a model for appropriate but equal interactions within an important interpersonal relationship. Irreverent communication is usually riskier than reciprocity. However, it can facilitate problem solving or produce a breakthrough after long periods when progress has seemed thwarted. To be used effectively, irreverent communication must balance reciprocal communication, and the two must be woven into a single stylistic fabric. Without such balancing, neither strategy represents DBT.

Reciprocal Communication

Responsiveness, self-disclosure, warm engagement, and genuineness are the basic guidelines of reciprocal communication. Responsiveness requires attending to the client in a mindful (attentive) manner and taking the client's agenda and wishes seriously. However, this does not mean that the therapist gives priority to the client's agenda over the treatment hierarchy. It refers to the therapist validating the importance of the client's agenda openly. It is a friendly, affectionate style reflecting warmth and engagement in the therapeutic interaction. Self-involving self-disclosure is the therapist's immediate, personal reactions to the client and his/her behavior. This strategy is used frequently throughout DBT. For example, a therapist whose client complained about his coolness said, "When you demand warmth from me, it pushes me away and makes it harder to be warm." Similarly, when a client repeatedly failed to fill out diary cards but nevertheless pleaded with her therapist to help her, the therapist responded, "You keep asking me for help, but you won't do the things I believe are necessary to help you. I feel frustrated because I want to help you, but I feel that you won't let me." Such statements serve both to validate and to challenge. They constitute both an instance of contingency management because therapist statements about the client are typically experienced as either reinforcing or punishing, and an instance of contingency clarification because the client's attention is directed to the consequences of his/her interpersonal behavior.

Self-disclosure of professional or personal information is used to validate and model coping and normative responses. The key point here is that a therapist should only use personal examples in which he/she has successfully mastered the problem at hand. This may seem like an obvious point, but it is very easy to fall into this pit by trying actively to validate the client's dilemma. For example, when working with a client whose goal is to wake up early each morning to exercise, but who is having difficulty getting out of bed, the therapist may attempt to validate the behavior as normative by stating, "Yeah, I struggle with getting up every morning, too, even though I tell myself every night that I am going to exercise in the morning." However, this self-disclosure is only useful to the client if the therapist continues by stating what skillful behavior he/she uses to get up each morning and exercise successfully.

Irreverent Communication

Irreverent communication is used to push the client "off balance," get the client's attention, present an alternative viewpoint, or shift affective response. It is a highly useful strategy when the client is immovable, or when therapist and client are "stuck." It has an "off-beat" flavor and uses logic to weave a web the client cannot escape. Although it is responsive to the client, irreverent communication is almost never the response the client expects. For irreverence to be effective it must be both genuine (vs. sarcastic or judgmental) and come from a place of compassion and warmth toward the client. Otherwise, the client may become even more rigid. When using irreverence the therapist highlights some unintended aspect of the client's communication or "reframes" it in an unorthodox manner. For example, if the client says, "I am going to kill myself," the therapist might say, "I thought you agreed not to drop out of therapy." Irreverent communication has a matter-of-fact, almost deadpan style that is in sharp contrast to the warm responsiveness of reciprocal communication. Humor, a certain naiveté, and guilelessness are also characteristic of the style. A confrontational tone is also irreverent, communicating "bullshit" to responses other than the targeted adaptive response. For example, the therapist might say, "Are you out of your mind?" or "You weren't for a minute actually believing I would think that was a good idea, were you?" The irreverent therapist also calls the client's bluff. For the client who says, "I'm quitting therapy," the therapist might respond, "Would you like a referral?" The trick here is to time the bluff carefully, with the simultaneous provision of a safety net; it is important to leave the client a way out.

CASE STUDY

Background

At the initial meeting, "Cindy," a 30-year-old, white, married woman with no children, was living in a middle-class suburban area with her husband. She had a college education and had successfully completed almost 2 years of medical school. Cindy was referred to one of us (M. M. L.) by her psychiatrist of 1½ years, who was no longer willing to provide more than pharmacotherapy following a recent hospitalization for a near-lethal suicide attempt. In the 2 years prior to referral, Cindy had been hospitalized at least 10 times (once for 6 months) for psychiatric treatment of suicidal ideation; had engaged in numerous instances of both NSSI behavior and suicide attempts, including at least 10 instances of drinking Clorox bleach, multiple deep cuts, and burns; and had had three medically severe or near-

ly lethal suicide attempts, including cutting an artery in her neck. At the time of referral, Cindy met DSM-III-R (American Psychiatric Association, 1987) and Gunderson's (1984) criteria for BPD. She was also taking a variety of psychotropic drugs. Until age 27, Cindy was able to function well in work and school settings, and the marriage was reasonably satisfactory to both partners, although her husband complained about Cindy's excessive anger. When Cindy was in the second year of medical school, a classmate she knew only slightly committed suicide. Cindy stated that when she heard about the suicide, she immediately decided to kill herself also, but had very little insight into what about the situation actually elicited her inclination to kill herself. Within weeks she left medical school and became severely depressed and actively suicidal. Although Cindy self-presented as a person with few psychological problems before the classmate's suicide, further questioning revealed a history of severe anorexia nervosa, bulimia nervosa, and alcohol and prescription medication abuse, originating at the age of 14 years. Indeed, she had met her husband at an Alcoholics Anonymous (AA) meeting while attending college. Nevertheless, until the student's suicide in medical school, Cindy had been successful at maintaining an overall appearance of relative competence.

Treatment

At the initial meeting, Cindy was accompanied by her husband, who stated that he and Cindy's family considered his wife too lethally suicidal to be out of a hospital setting. Consequently, he and Cindy's family were seriously contemplating the viability of finding long-term outpatient care. However, Cindy stated a strong preference for inpatient treatment, although no therapist in the local area other than M. M. L. appeared willing to take her into outpatient treatment. The therapist agreed to accept Cindy into therapy, contingent on the client's stated commitment to work toward behavioral change and to stay in treatment for at least 1 year. (It was later pointed out repeatedly that this also meant the client had agreed not to commit suicide.) Thus, the therapist began the crucial first step of establishing a strong therapeutic alliance by agreeing to accept the client despite the fact that no one else was willing to do so. She pointed out, however, that acceptance into therapy did not come without a cost. In this manner, the therapist communicated acceptance of the client exactly as she was in the current moment, while concomitantly making clear that Cindy's commitment toward change was the foundation of the therapeutic alliance. At the fourth therapy session, Cindy reported that she felt she could no longer keep herself alive. When reminded of her previous commitment to stay alive for 1 year of therapy, Cindy replied that things had changed and she could not help herself. Subsequent to this session, almost every individual session for the next 6 months revolved around the topic of whether (and how) to stay alive versus committing suicide. Cindy began coming to sessions wearing mirrored sunglasses and would slump in her chair or ask to sit on the floor. Questions from the therapist were often met with a minimal comment or long silences. In response to the therapist's attempts to discuss prior self-injurious behavior, Cindy would become angry and withdraw (slowing down the pace of therapy considerably). The client also presented with marked dissociative reactions, which would often occur during therapy sessions. During these reactions, Cindy would appear unable to concentrate or hear much of what was being said. When queried by the therapist, Cindy would describe her experience as feeling "spacey" and distant. The client stated that she felt she could no longer engage in many activities, such as driving, working, or attending school. Overall, the client viewed herself as incompetent in all areas.

The use of diary cards, which Cindy filled out weekly (or at the beginning of the session, if she forgot), assisted the therapist in carefully monitoring Cindy's daily experiences of suicidal ideation, misery, and urges to harm herself, as well as actual suicide attempts and NSSI behaviors. Behavioral analyses that attempted to identify the sequence of events leading up to and following Cindy's suicidal behavior soon became an important focus of therapy. At every point the therapist conceptualized self-injurious behavior as to be expected, given the strength of the urge (but considered it ultimately beatable), and pointed out repeatedly that if the client committed suicide, therapy would be over, so they had better work really hard now, while Cindy was alive.

Over the course of several months, the behavioral analyses began to identify a frequently recurring behavioral pattern that preceded suicidal behaviors. For Cindy, the chain of events would often begin with an interpersonal encounter (almost always with her husband), which culminated in her feeling threatened, criticized, or unloved. These feelings were often followed by urges either to self-mutilate or to kill herself, depending somewhat on the covarying levels of hope-

lessness, anger, and sadness. Decisions to self-mutilate and/or to attempt suicide were often accompanied by the thought, "I'll show you." At other times, hopelessness and a desire to end the pain permanently seemed predominant. Both are examples of emotional vulnerability. Following the conscious decision to self-mutilate or to attempt suicide, Cindy would then immediately dissociate and at some later point cut or burn herself, usually while in a state of "automatic pilot." Consequently, Cindy often had difficulty remembering specifics of the actual acts. At one point, Cindy burned her leg so badly (and then injected it with dirt to convince the doctor that he should give her more attention) that reconstructive surgery was required. Behavioral analyses also revealed that dissociation during sessions usually occurred following Cindy's perception of the therapist's disapproval or invalidation, especially when the therapist appeared to suggest that change was possible. The therapist targeted in-session dissociation by immediately addressing it as it occurred.

By several months into therapy, an apparently long-standing pattern of suicidal behaviors leading to inpatient admission was apparent. Cindy would report intense suicidal ideation, express doubts that she could resist the urge to kill herself, and request admission to her preferred hospital; or, without warning, she would cut or burn herself severely and require hospitalization for medical treatment. Attempts to induce Cindy to stay out of the hospital or to leave the hospital before she was ready typically resulted in an escalation of suicidality, followed by her pharmacotherapist's (a psychiatrist) insistence on her admission or the hospital's agreement to extend her stay. Observation of this behavioral pattern led the therapist to hypothesize that the hospitalization itself was reinforcing suicidal behavior; consequently, she attempted to change the contingencies for suicidal behaviors. Using didactic and contingency clarification strategies, the therapist attempted to help Cindy understand how hospitalization might be strengthening the very behavior they were working to eliminate. This issue became a focal point of disagreement within the therapy, with Cindy viewing the therapist's position as unsympathetic and lacking understanding of her phenomenal experience. In Cindy's opinion, the intensity of her emotional pain rendered the probability of suicide so high that hospitalization was necessary to guarantee her safety. She would buttress her position by citing frequently her difficulties with dissociative reactions, which she reported as extremely aversive and which, in her opinion, made her unable to function much of the time. From the therapist's perspective, the deleterious long-term risk of suicide created by repeated hospitalization in response to suicidal behavior was greater than the short-term risk of suicide if hospitalization stays were reduced. These differences in opinion led to frequent disagreements within sessions. It gradually became clear that Cindy viewed any explanations of her behavior as influenced by reinforcement as a direct attack; she implied that if hospitalization was reinforcing her suicidal behavior, then the therapist must believe that the purpose of her suicidality was for admission into the hospital. This was obviously not the case (at least some of the time), but all attempts to explain reinforcement theory in any other terms failed. The therapist compensated somewhat for insisting on the possibility that she (the therapist) was correct by doing three things. First, she repeatedly validated the client's experience of almost unendurable pain. Second, she made certain to address the client's dissociative behavior repeatedly, explaining it as an automatic reaction to intensely painful affect (or the threat of it). Third, she frequently addressed the quality of the relationship between Cindy and herself to strengthen the relationship and maintain Cindy in therapy, even though to do so was a source of even more emotional pain. By the fifth month, the therapist became concerned that the current treatment regimen was going to have the unintended consequence of killing the client (via suicide). At this point, the therapist's limits for effective treatment were crossed; therefore, she decided to employ the consultation-to-the-client strategy to address Cindy's hospitalizations. The first-choice strategy would have been to get Cindy to negotiate a new treatment plan with her preferred hospital and admitting psychiatrist. Cindy refused to go along, however, because she disagreed with the wisdom of changing her current unlimited access to the inpatient unit. The therapist was able to get Cindy to agree to a consultation meeting with all of her treatment providers, and, with some tenacity, the therapist actually got Cindy to make all the calls to set up the meeting (including inviting her insurance monitor, who was coordinating payment for treatment).

At the case conference, the therapist presented her hypothesis that contingent hospitalization was reinforcing Cindy's suicidal behavior. She also assisted Cindy in making the case that she (the therapist) was wrong. Using reciprocal communication and contingency management, the therapist stated that she simply could not conduct a therapy she thought might kill the client

(and she had to go along with what she thought was best even if she were wrong—"to do otherwise would be unethical"), and she requested that a new system of contingencies be agreed upon to disrupt the functional relationship between Cindy's suicidal behavior and hospitalization. Therefore, a plan was developed wherein the client was not required to be suicidal to gain hospital admittance. Under this new set of contingencies, Cindy could elect, at will, to enter the hospital for a stay of up to 3 days, at the end of which time she would always be discharged. If she convinced people that she was too suicidal for discharge, she would be transferred to her least-preferred hospital for safety. Suicidal and NSSI behaviors would no longer be grounds for admission except to a medical unit, when required. Although there was some disagreement as to the functional relationship between suicidal behavior and hospitalization, this system was agreed upon. Following this meeting, Cindy's husband announced that he was no longer able to live with or tolerate his wife's suicidal behavior, and that the constant threat of finding her dead had led to his decision to file for divorce. The focus of therapy then shifted to helping Cindy grieve over this event and find a suitable living arrangement. Cindy alternated between fury that her husband would desert her in her hour of need (or "illness," as she put it) and despair that she could ever cope alone. She decided that "getting her feelings out" was the only useful therapy. This led to many tearful sessions, with the therapist simultaneously validating the pain; focusing on Cindy's experiencing the affect in the moment, without escalating or blocking it; and cheerleading Cindy's ability to manage without going back into the hospital. Due to Cindy's high level of dysfunctionality, she and her therapist decided that she would enter a residential treatment facility for a 3-month period. The facility had a coping skills orientation and provided group but not individual therapy. Cindy saw her therapist once a week and talked to her several times a week during this period. With some coaching, Cindy looked for and found a roommate to live with and returned to her own home at the end of 3 months (the ninth month of therapy). Over the course of treatment, the therapist used a number of strategies to treat Cindy's suicidal, NSSI, and therapy-interfering behaviors. In-depth behavioral chain and solution analysis helped the therapist (and sometimes the client) gain insight into the factors influencing current suicidal behavior. For Cindy, as for most clients, performing these analyses was quite difficult because the process usually generated intense feelings of shame, guilt, or anger. Thus, behavioral analysis also functioned as an exposure strategy, encouraging the client to observe and experience painful affect. It additionally served as a cognitive strategy in helping to change Cindy's expectancies concerning the advantages and disadvantages of suicidal behavior, especially as the therapist repeatedly made statements such as "How do you think you would feel if I got angry at you and then threatened suicide if you didn't change?" Finally, behavioral analysis served as contingency management, in that the client's ability to pursue topics of interest in therapy sessions was made contingent on the successful completion of chain and solution analysis.

Cindy presented early in therapy with exceedingly strong perceptions as to her needs and desires, and with a concomitant willingness to engage in extremely lethal suicidal behavior. As previously mentioned, several of these acts were serious attempts to end her life, whereas others functioned as attempts to gain attention and care from significant others. This client also presented with an extreme sensitivity to any attempts at obvious change procedures, which she typically interpreted as communicating a message about her incompetence and unworthiness. Although Cindy initially committed herself to attending weekly group skills training for the first year of therapy, her attendance at group meetings was quite erratic, and she generally tended either to miss entire sessions (but never more than three in a row) or to leave during the break. Cindy answered the therapist's attempts to address this issue by stating that she could not drive at night due to night blindness. Although considered a therapy-interfering behavior and frequently addressed over the course of therapy, missing skills training was not a major focus of treatment due to the continuing presence of higher-priority suicidal behavior. The therapist's efforts to engage the client in active skills acquisition during individual therapy sessions were also somewhat limited and were always preceded by obtaining Cindy's verbal commitment to problem solving. The stylistic strategy of irreverent communication was of value to the therapeutic process. The therapist's irreverence often served to "shake up" the client, resulting in a loosening of dichotomous thinking and maladaptive cognitions. The result of this was Cindy's increased willingness to explore new and adaptive behavioral solutions. Finally, relationship strategies were heavily employed as tools to strengthen the therapeutic alliance and to keep it noncontingent on suicidal and/or dissociative behaviors. Included here were between-session therapist-initiated telephone calls to check in,

the therapist routinely giving out phone numbers when she was traveling, and sending the client postcards when she was out of town.

By the 12th month of therapy, Cindy's suicidal and self-injurious behavior, as well as urges to engage in such behavior, receded. In addition, her hospital stays were reduced markedly, with none occurring after the eighth month. While living at home with a roommate, Cindy was readmitted to medical school. Part of the reason for returning to school was to turn her life around, so that she could try to regain her husband's love and attention, or at least his friendship. As the therapy continued to focus on changing the contingencies of suicidal behavior, reducing both emotional pain and inhibition, and tolerating distress, a further focus on maintaining sobriety and reasonable food intake was added. During the first months of living in her home without her husband, Cindy had several alcoholic binges, and her food intake dropped precipitously. These behaviors became immediate targets. The therapist's strong attention to these behaviors also communicated to Cindy that the therapist would take her problems seriously even if she were not suicidal. Therapy focused as well on expanding her social network. As with suicidal behaviors, attention to these targets served as a pathway to treating associated problems. As crisis situations decreased in frequency, greater attention was paid to analyzing family patterns, including experiences of neglect and invalidation, that might have led to Cindy's problems in later life. Cindy did not report a history of sexual or physical abuse. Thus, the explicit goal of Stage 2 was to understand Cindy's history and its relationship to her current problems.

In other cases, especially when there has been sexual and/or physical abuse in childhood, movement to Stage 2 before Stage 1 targets have been mastered is likely to result in retrogression to previously problematic behaviors. For example, Terry, another client treated by the same therapist (M. M. L.), had been quite seriously abused physically by her mother throughout childhood and sexually abused by her father, beginning at age 5. The sexual advances were nonviolent at first but became physically abusive at approximately age 12. Prior to this therapy, Terry had not disclosed the incidents of abuse to anyone.

After successful negotiation of Stage 1 targets, the therapist proceeded to expose Terry to trauma-related cues by simply having her begin to disclose details of the abuse. These exposure sessions were intertwined with work on current problems in Terry's life. Following one exposure session focused on the sexual abuse, Terry reverted to some of her previously problematic behaviors, evidenced by withdrawal and silence in sessions, suicidal ideation, and medication noncompliance. The appearance of such behavior marked the necessity of stopping Stage 2 discussions of previous sexual abuse to address Stage 1 targets recursively. Three sessions were devoted to a behavioral analysis of Terry's current suicidal, therapy-interfering, and quality-of-life–interfering behaviors; these were eventually linked both to fears about how the therapist would view her childhood emotional responses to her father, and to holiday visits with her father that precipitated conflicts over how Terry should be feeling about him in the present. This two-steps-forward, one-step-back approach is common to therapy for clients with BPD, and in particular may mark the transition between Stage 1 and Stage 2.

As previously mentioned, Stage 3 targets the client's self-respect, regardless of the opinions of others. Betty, who was also in treatment with the same therapist (M. M. L.), had successfully negotiated Stages 1 and 2, and had become a highly competent nurse with training and supervisory responsibilities. Therapy with Betty was then focused on maintaining her self-esteem in the face of very powerful significant others (e.g., her supervisor) who constantly invalidated her. Components of the treatment included the therapist's noting and highlighting Betty's tendency to modify her self-opinion in accordance with that of others, persistent attempts to extract from Betty self-validation and self-soothing, and imagery exercises wherein Betty imagined and verbalized herself standing up to powerful others. Much of the therapy focus was on Betty's interpersonal behavior within the therapy session, with attention to relating this behavior to her interactions with other important people. Thus, treatment at that point was very similar to the functional-analytic psychotherapy regimen developed by Kohlenberg and Tsai (1991). Overall, this third stage of therapy involved the movement to a more egalitarian relationship between the client and the therapist, in which emphasis was placed on the client's standing up for her own opinions and defending her own actions. This approach required that the therapist both reinforce the client's assertions, and step back and refrain from validating and nurturing the client in the manner characteristic of Stages 1 and 2. In addition, therapy sessions were reduced to every other week, and issues surrounding eventual termination were periodically discussed.

Stage 4 of DBT targets the sense of incompleteness that can preclude the experience of joy and freedom. Sally started Stage 1 treatment with the same therapist (M. M. L.) 15 years ago. Stage 1 lasted 2 years; this was followed by a break of 1 year, after which treatment resumed for several years of bimonthly sessions leading to monthly sessions, and currently comprising four or five sessions a year. Sally has been married for 30 years to an irregularly employed husband who, though devoted and loyal, is quite invalidating of her. Although apparently brilliant, he is usually dismissed from jobs for his interpersonal insensitivity. She has been employed full-time at the same place for years, working with children. The son Sally felt closest to died in a plane accident 2 years ago; her mother died last year, and her father is very ill. Despite having a stable marriage, working in a stable and quite fulfilling job, having raised two well-adjusted sons, and still being athletic, life feels meaningless to Sally. In the past she was very active in spiritual activities; following meditation retreats or extended periods of daily meditation, she would report contentment and some sense of joy. Since her son died, Sally has let go of most of her spiritual activities. Following a 2-year focus on grieving, she is now ready for Stage 4. Treatment planning is focused on actively practicing and keeping track of progress in radical acceptance (or "letting go of ego," in Zen terminology), either alone or with group support.

TRANSCRIPTS

The following (composite) transcripts represent actual examples of the process of therapy occurring over several sessions with different clients. These particular dialogues between therapist and client have been chosen to provide the reader with comprehensive examples of the application of a wide range of DBT treatment strategies. The session targets in the following transcript were orienting and commitment. The strategies used were validation, problem solving (insight, orienting, and commitment), dialectical (devil's advocate), and integrated (relationship enhancement).

Obtaining the client's commitment is a crucial first step in beginning therapy with clients who have BPD. As illustrated in the following transcript, the dialectical technique of devil's advocate can be highly effective when used as a commitment strategy. In this first therapy session, the therapist's ultimate goal was to obtain the client's commitment to therapy, as well as a commitment to eliminate suicidal behavior. She began by orienting the client to the purpose of this initial session.

THERAPIST: So are you a little nervous about me?

CLIENT: Yeah, I guess I am.

THERAPIST: Well, that's understandable. For the next 50 minutes or so, we have this opportunity to get to know each other and see if we want to work together. So what I'd like to do is talk a little bit about the program and how you got here. So tell me, what do you want out of therapy with me, and what are you doing here?

CLIENT: I want to get better.

THERAPIST: Well, what's wrong with you?

CLIENT: I'm a mess. (*Laughs.*)

THERAPIST: How so?

CLIENT: Umm, I don't know. I just can't even cope with everyday life right now. And I can't even .. . I'm just a mess. I don't know how to deal with anything.

THERAPIST: So what does that mean exactly?

CLIENT: Umm, well, everything I try these days just seems overwhelming. I couldn't keep up on my job, and now I'm on medical leave. Plus everyone's sick of me being in the hospital so much. And I think my psychiatrist wants to send me away because of all my self-harming.

THERAPIST: How often do you self-harm?

CLIENT: Maybe once or twice a month. I use my lighter or cigarettes, sometimes a razor blade.

THERAPIST: Do you have scars all over?

CLIENT: (*Nods yes.*)

THERAPIST: Your psychiatrist tells me you've also drunk Clorox. Why didn't you mention that?

CLIENT: I guess it didn't enter my mind.

THERAPIST: Do things just not enter your mind very often?

CLIENT: I don't really know. Maybe.

THERAPIST: So maybe with you I'm going to have to be a very good guesser.

CLIENT: Hmm.

THERAPIST: Unfortunately, though, I'm not the greatest guesser. So we'll have to teach you how to have things come to mind. So what is it exactly that you want out of therapy with me? To quit harming yourself, quit trying to kill yourself, or both?

CLIENT: Both. I'm sick of it.

THERAPIST: And is there anything else you want help with?

CLIENT: Um, well, I don't know how to handle money, and I don't know how to handle relationships. I don't have friends; they don't connect with me very often. I'm a former alcoholic and a recovering anorexic/bulimic. I still have a tendency toward that.

THERAPIST: Do you think maybe some of what is going on with you is that you've replaced your alcoholic and anorexic behaviors with self-harm behaviors?

CLIENT: I don't know. I haven't thought about it that way. I just feel that I don't know how to handle myself, and—you know, and I guess work through stuff, and that is obviously getting to me because if it wasn't, I wouldn't be trying to kill myself.

THERAPIST: So from your perspective, one problem is that you don't know how to do things. A lot of things.

CLIENT: Yeah, and a lot of it is, I do know how, but for some reason I don't do it anyway.

THERAPIST: Um hmm.

CLIENT: You know, I mean I know I need to save money, and I know that I need to budget myself, and I do every single month, but every single month I get in debt. But, um, you know, it's really hard for me. You know, it's like sometimes I know it, or I know I shouldn't eat something and I do it anyway.

THERAPIST: So it sounds like part of the problem is you actually know how to do things; you just don't know how to get yourself to do the things you know how to do.

CLIENT: Exactly.

THERAPIST: Does it seem like maybe your emotions are in control—that you are a person who does things when you're in the mood?

CLIENT: Yes. Everything's done by the mood.

THERAPIST: So you're a moody person.

CLIENT: Yes. I won't clean the house for 2 months, and then I'll get in the mood to clean. Then I'll clean it immaculately and keep it that way for 3 weeks—I mean, just immaculate—and then when I'm in the mood I go back to being a mess again.

THERAPIST: So one of the tasks for you and me would be to figure out a way to get your behavior and what you do less hooked up with how you feel?

CLIENT: Right.

The therapist used insight to highlight for the client the observed interrelationship between the client's emotions and her behavior. She then began the process of shaping a commitment through the dialectical strategy of devil's advocate.

THERAPIST: That, of course, is going to be hell to do, don't you think? Why would you want to do that? It sounds so painful.

CLIENT: Well, I want to do it because it's so inconsistent. It's worse, you know, because when I'm .. . I know that, like with budgeting money or whatever, I know I need to do it, and then when I don't do it, it makes me even more upset.

THERAPIST: Why would you ever want to do something you're not in the mood for?

CLIENT: Because I've got to. Because I can't survive that way if I don't.

THERAPIST: Sounds like a pretty easy life to me.

CLIENT: Yeah, but I can't afford to live if I just spend my money on fun and stupid, frivolous things that I . . .

THERAPIST: Well, I guess maybe you should have some limits and not be too off the wall, but in general, I mean, why clean the house if you're not in the mood?

CLIENT: Because it pisses me off when it's a mess. And I can't find things, like I've lost bills before and then I end up not paying them. And now I've got collection agencies on my back. I can't deal with all this, and I end up self-harming and going into the hospital. And then I just want to end it all. But it still doesn't seem to matter because if I'm not in the mood to clean it, I won't.

THERAPIST: So the fact that it makes horrible things happen in your life so far hasn't been enough of a motivation to get you to do things against your mood, right?

CLIENT: Well, obviously not (*laughs*) because it's not happening.

THERAPIST: Doesn't that tell you, though? This is going to be a big problem, don't you think? This isn't going to be something simple. It's not like you're going to walk in here and I'm going to say, "OK, magic wand," and then all of a sudden you're going to want to do things that you're not in the mood for.

CLIENT: Yeah.

THERAPIST: Yeah, so it seems to me that if you're not in the mood for things, if you're kind of mood-dependent, that's a very tough thing to crack. As a matter of fact, I think it's one of the hardest problems there is to deal with.

CLIENT: Yeah, great.

THERAPIST: I think we could deal with it, but I think it's going to be hell. The real question is whether you're willing to go through hell to get where you want to get or not. Now I figure that's the question.

CLIENT: Well, if it's going to make me happier, yeah.

THERAPIST: Are you sure?

CLIENT: Yeah, I've been going through this since I was 11 years old. I'm sick of this shit. I mean, excuse my language, but I really am, and I'm backed up against the wall. Either I need to do this or I need to die. Those are my two choices.

THERAPIST: Well, why not die?

CLIENT: Well, if it comes down to it, I will.

THERAPIST: Um hmm, but why not now?

CLIENT: Because, this is my last hope. Because if I've got one last hope left, why not take it?

THERAPIST: So, in other words, all things being equal, you'd rather live than die, if you can pull this off.

CLIENT: If I can pull it off, yeah.

THERAPIST: OK, that's good; that's going to be your strength. We're going to play to that. You're going to have to remember that when it gets tough. But now I want to tell you about this program and how I feel about you harming yourself, and then we'll see if you still want to do this.

As illustrated by the foregoing segment, the therapist's relentless use of the devil's advocate strategy successfully "got a foot in the door" and achieved an initial client commitment. The therapist then "upped the ante" with a brief explanation of the program and its goals.

THERAPIST: Now the most important thing to understand is that we are not a suicide prevention program; that's not our job. But we are a life enhancement program. The way we look at it, living a miserable life is no achievement. If we decide to work together, I'm going to help you try to improve your life, so that it's so good that you don't want to die or hurt yourself. You should also know that I look at suicidal behavior, including drinking Clorox, as problem-solving behavior. I think of alcoholism the same way. The only difference is that cutting, burning, unfortunately—it works. If it didn't work, nobody would do it more than once. But it only works in the short term, not the long term. So to quit cutting, trying to hurt yourself, is going to be exactly like quitting alcohol. Do you think this is going to be hard?

CLIENT: Stopping drinking wasn't all that hard.

THERAPIST: Well, in my experience, giving up self-harm behavior is usually very hard. It will require both of us working, but you will have to work harder. And like I told you when we talked briefly, if you commit to this, it's for 1 year—individual therapy with me once a week, and group skills training once a week. So the question is, are you willing to commit for 1 year?

CLIENT: I said I'm sick of this stuff. That's why I'm here.

THERAPIST: So you've agreed to not drop out of therapy for a year, right?

CLIENT: Right.

THERAPIST: And do you realize that if you don't drop out for a year, that really does, if you think about it, rule out suicide for a year?

CLIENT: Logically, yeah.

THERAPIST: So we need to be absolutely clear about this because this therapy won't work if you knock yourself off. The most fundamental mood-related goal we have to work on is that, no matter what your mood is, you won't kill yourself or try to.

CLIENT: All right.

THERAPIST: So that's what I see as number one priority—not our only one but number one—that we will work on that. And getting you to agree—meaningfully, of course—and actually follow through on staying alive and not harming yourself and not attempting suicide, no matter what your mood is. Now the question is whether you agree to that.

CLIENT: Yes, I agree to that.

The therapist, having successfully obtained the client's commitment to work on suicidal behavior again employed the strategy of devil's advocate to reinforce the strength of the commitment.

THERAPIST: Why would you agree to that?

CLIENT: I don't know. (*Laughs.*)

THERAPIST: I mean, wouldn't you rather be in a therapy where, if you wanted to kill yourself, you could?

CLIENT: I don't know. I mean, I never really thought about it that way.

THERAPIST: Hmm.

CLIENT: I don't want to .. . I want to be able to get to the point where I could feel like I'm not being forced into living.

THERAPIST: So are you agreeing with me because you're feeling forced into agreeing?

CLIENT: You keep asking me all these questions.

THERAPIST: What do you think?

CLIENT: I don't know what I think right now, honestly.

A necessary and important skill for the DBT therapist is the ability to sense when a client has been pushed to his/her limits, as well as the concomitant skill of being willing and able to step back and at least temporarily refrain from further pressuring the client. In these instances, continued pressure from the therapist is likely to boomerang and have the opposite effect of what the therapist intends. Here the therapist noticed the client's confusion and sensed that further pushing was likely to result in the client's reducing the strength of her commitment. Consequently, the therapist stepped back and moved in with validation.

THERAPIST: So you're feeling pushed up against the wall a little bit, by me?

CLIENT: No, not really. (*Starts to cry.*)

THERAPIST: What just happened just now?

CLIENT: (*pause*) I don't know. I mean, I don't think I really want to kill myself. I think I just feel like I have to. I don't think it's really even a mood thing. I just think it's when I feel like there's no other choice. I just say, "Well, you know there's no other choice, so do it." You know. And so right now, I don't see any ray of hope. I'm going to therapy, which I guess is good. I mean, I know it's good, but I don't see anything any better than it was the day I tried to kill myself.

THERAPIST: Well, that's probably true. Maybe it isn't any better. I mean, trying to kill yourself doesn't usually solve problems. Although it actually did do one thing for you.

CLIENT: It got me in therapy.

THERAPIST: Yeah. So my asking you all these questions

makes you start to cry. You look like you must be feeling pretty bad.

CLIENT: Just overwhelmed, I guess the word is.

THERAPIST: That's part of the reason we're having this conversation, to try to structure our relationship so that it's very clear for both of us. And that way, at least, we'll cut down on how much you get overwhelmed by not knowing what's going on with me. OK?

CLIENT: Um hmm.

THERAPIST: And so I just want to be clear on what our number one goal is, and how hard this is because if you want to back out, now's the time. Because I'm going to take you seriously if you say, "Yes, I want to do it."

CLIENT: I don't want to back out.

THERAPIST: OK. Good. Now I just want to say that this seems like a good idea right now. You're in kind of an energized mood today, getting started on a new program. But in 5 hours, it might not seem like such a good idea. It's kind of like it's easy to commit to a diet after a big meal, but it's much harder when you're hungry. But we're going to work on how to make it keep sounding like a good idea. It'll be hell, but I have confidence. I think we can be successful working together.

Note how the therapist ended the session by preparing the client for the difficulties she was likely to experience in keeping her commitment and working in therapy. Cheerleading and relationship enhancement laid the foundation for a strong therapeutic alliance. The following session occurred approximately 4 months into therapy. The session target was suicidal behavior. The therapist used validation, problem solving (contingency clarification, didactic information, behavioral analysis, and solution analysis), stylistic (irreverent communication), dialectical (metaphor, making lemonade out of lemons), and skills training (distress tolerance) strategies.

The therapist reviewed the client's diary card and noted a recent, intentional self-injury, in which the client opened up a previously self-inflicted wound following her physician's refusal to provide pain medication. The therapist began by proceeding with a behavioral analysis.

THERAPIST: OK. Now you were in here last week telling me you were never going to hurt yourself again because this was so ridiculous, you couldn't stand it, you couldn't hurt yourself any more. So let's figure out how that broke down on Sunday, so we can learn something from it. OK. So when did you start having urges to hurt yourself?

CLIENT: My foot began to hurt on Wednesday. I started to have a lot of pain.

THERAPIST: It hadn't hurt before that?

CLIENT: No.

THERAPIST: So the nerves were dead before that or something, huh? So you started having a lot of pain. Now when did you start having the pain, and when did the urge to harm yourself come?

CLIENT: At the same time.

THERAPIST: They just come at the identical moment?

CLIENT: Just about.

The specification of an initial prompting environmental event is always the first step in conducting a behavioral chain analysis. Here the therapist began by directly inquiring when the urges toward suicide and NSSI began. Note also the therapist's use of irreverent communication early in the session.

THERAPIST: So how is it that feeling pain sets off an urge to self-harm? Do you know how that goes? How you get from one to the other?

CLIENT: I don't know. Maybe it wasn't until Thursday, but I asked my nurse. I go, "Look, I'm in a lot of pain, you know. I'm throwing up my food because the pain is so bad." And the nurse tried. She called the doctor and told him I was in a lot of pain, and asked if he'd give me some painkillers. But no! So I kept asking, and the answer kept being no, and I got madder and madder and madder. So I felt like I had to show somebody that it hurt because they didn't believe me.

THERAPIST: So let's figure this out. So is it that you're assuming that if someone believed it hurt as bad as you said it does, they would actually give you the painkillers?

CLIENT: Yes.

THERAPIST: OK. That's where the faulty thinking is. That's the problem. You see, it's entirely possible that people know how bad the pain is but still aren't giving you medication.

CLIENT: I believe firmly, and I even wrote it in my

journal, that if I'd gotten pain medication when I really needed it, I wouldn't have even thought of self-harming.

The therapist proceeded by obtaining a description of the events co-occurring with the onset of the problem. It was not completely clear what about not getting pain medication set off self-harm. In the following segment, the therapist used the dialectical strategy of metaphor to analyze what factors might have been important. Notice that the example is presented as an experiment in which different scenarios are given and responses elicited.

THERAPIST: Now let me ask you something—you've got to imagine this, OK? Let's imagine that you and I are on a raft together out in the middle of the ocean. Our boat has sunk and we're on the raft. And when the boat sank, your leg got cut really badly. And together we've wrapped it up as well as we can. But we don't have any pain medicine. And we're on this raft together and your leg really hurts, and you ask me for pain medicine, and I say no. Do you think you would then have an urge to hurt yourself and make it worse?

CLIENT: No, it would be a different situation.

THERAPIST: OK, but if I did have the pain medication and I said no because we had to save it, what do you think?

CLIENT: If that were logical to me, I'd go along with it and wouldn't want to hurt myself.

THERAPIST: What if I said no because I didn't want you to be a drug addict?

CLIENT: I'd want to hurt myself.

THERAPIST: OK. So we've got this clear. The pain is not what's setting off the desire to self-harm. It's someone not giving you something to help, when you feel they could if they wanted to.

CLIENT: Yes.

The therapist used contingency clarification to point out the effects of others' responses on the client's own behavior. In the following segment, the therapist again employed contingency clarification in a continued effort to highlight for the client the communication function of NSSI.

THERAPIST: So, in other words, hurting yourself is communication behavior, OK? So what we have to do is figure out a way for the communication behavior to quit working.

CLIENT: Why?

THERAPIST: Because you're not going to stop doing it until it quits working. It's like trying to talk to someone; if there's no one in the room, you eventually quit trying to talk to them. It's like when a phone goes dead, you quit talking.

CLIENT: I tried three nights in a row in a perfectly assertive way and just clearly stated I was in a lot of pain.

THERAPIST: You know, I think I'll switch chairs with you. You're not hearing what I'm saying.

CLIENT: And they kept saying, "No," and then some little light came on in my head.

THERAPIST: I'm considering switching chairs with you.

CLIENT: And it was like, "Here, now can you tell that it hurts a lot?"

THERAPIST: I'm thinking of switching chairs with you.

CLIENT: Why?

THERAPIST: Because if you were sitting over here, I think you would see that no matter how bad the pain is, hurting yourself to get pain medication is not a reasonable response. The hospital staff may not have been reasonable either. It may be that they should have given you pain medicine. But we don't have to say they were wrong in order to say that hurting yourself was not the appropriate response.

CLIENT: No, I don't think it was the appropriate response.

THERAPIST: Good. So what we've got to do is figure out a way to get it so that the response doesn't come in, even if you don't get pain medicine. So far, it has worked very effectively as communication. And the only way to stop it is to get it to not work anymore. Of course, it would be good to get other things to work. What you're arguing is "Well, OK, if I'm not going to get it this way, then I should get it another way."

CLIENT: I tried this time!

THERAPIST: Yes, I know you did, I know you did.

CLIENT: A lady down the hallway from me was getting treatment for her diabetes, and it got real bad, and they gave her pain medication.

THERAPIST: Now we're not on the same wavelength in this conversation.

CLIENT: Yes, we are. What wavelength are you on?

THERAPIST: I'm on the wavelength that it may have been reasonable for you to get pain medicine, and I certainly understand your wanting it. But I'm also saying that no matter what's going on, hurting yourself is something we don't want to happen. You're functioning like if I agreed with you that you should get pain medication, I would think this was OK.

CLIENT: Hmm?

THERAPIST: You're talking about whether they should have given you pain medication or not. I'm not talking about that. Even if they should have, we've got to figure out how you could have gotten through without hurting yourself.

As illustrated by the foregoing exchange, a client with BPD often wants to remain focused on the crisis at hand. This poses a formidable challenge for the therapist, who must necessarily engage in a back-and-forth dance between validating the client's pain and pushing for behavioral change. This segment also illustrates how validation does not necessarily imply agreement. Although the therapist validated the client's perception that the nurse's refusal to provide pain medication may have been unreasonable, she remained steadfast in maintaining the inappropriateness of the client's response.

CLIENT: I tried some of those distress tolerance things and they didn't work.

THERAPIST: OK. Don't worry, we'll figure out a way. I want to know everything you tried. But first I want to be sure I have the picture clear. Did the urges start building after Wednesday and get worse over time?

CLIENT: Yeah. They started growing with the pain.

THERAPIST: With the pain. OK. But also they started growing with their continued refusal to give you pain medicine. So you were thinking that if you hurt yourself, they would somehow give you pain medicine?

CLIENT: Yeah. 'Cause if they wouldn't listen to me, then I could show them.

THERAPIST: OK, so you were thinking, "If they won't listen to me, I'll show them." And when did that idea first hit? Was that on Wednesday?

CLIENT: Yeah.

THERAPIST: OK. Well, we've got to figure out a way for you to tolerate bad things without harming yourself. So let's figure out all the things you tried, and then we have to figure out some other things because those didn't work. So what was the first thing you tried?

At this juncture the behavioral analysis remained incomplete, and it would normally have been premature to move to the stage of solution analysis. However, in the therapist's judgment, it was more critical at this point to reinforce the client's attempts at distress tolerance by responding to the client's communication that she had attempted behavioral skills.

CLIENT: I thought that if I just continued to be assertive about it that the appropriate measures would be taken.

THERAPIST: OK, but that didn't work. So why didn't you harm yourself right then?

CLIENT: I didn't want to.

THERAPIST: Why didn't you want to?

CLIENT: I didn't want to make it worse.

THERAPIST: So you were thinking about pros and cons—that if I make it worse, I'll feel worse?

CLIENT: Yeah.

One aspect of DBT skills training stresses the usefulness of evaluating the pros and cons of tolerating distress as a crisis survival strategy. Here the therapist employed the dialectical strategy of turning lemons into lemonade by highlighting for the client how she did, in fact, use behavioral skills. Note in the following response how the therapist immediately reinforced the client's efforts with praise.

THERAPIST: That's good thinking. That's when you're thinking about the advantages and disadvantages of doing it. OK, so at that point the advantages of making it worse were outweighed by the disadvantages. OK. So you keep up the good fight here. Now what else did you try?

CLIENT: I tried talking about it with other clients.

THERAPIST: And what did they have to say?

CLIENT: They said I should get pain medication.

THERAPIST: Right. But did they say you should cut yourself or hurt yourself if you didn't get it?

CLIENT: No. And I tried to get my mind off my pain by playing music and using mindfulness. I tried to read and do crossword puzzles.

THERAPIST: Um hmm. Did you ever try radical acceptance?

CLIENT: What's that?

THERAPIST: It's where you sort of let go and accept the fact that you're not going to get the pain medication. And you just give yourself up to that situation. You just accept that it ain't going to happen, that you're going to have to cope in some other way.

CLIENT: Which I did yesterday. I needed a little Ativan to get me there, but I got there.

THERAPIST: Yesterday?

CLIENT: Yeah. I took a nap. When I woke up I basically said, "Hey, they're not going to change, so you've just got to deal with this the best that you can."

THERAPIST: And did that acceptance help some?

CLIENT: I'm still quite angry about what I believe is discrimination against borderline personalities. I'm still very angry about that.

THERAPIST: OK. That's fine. Did it help, though, to accept?

CLIENT: Um hmm.

THERAPIST: That's good. That's great. That's a great skill, a great thing to practice. When push comes to shove, when you're really at the limit, when it's the worst it can be, radical acceptance is the skill to practice.

CLIENT: That's AA.

During a solution analysis, it is often necessary that the therapist facilitate the process by helping the client "brainstorm," or by making direct suggestions for handling future crises. Here the therapist suggested a solution that is also taught in the DBT skills training module on distress tolerance. The notion of radical acceptance stresses the idea that acceptance of one's pain is a necessary prerequisite for ending emotional suffering.

THERAPIST: OK. Now let's go back to how you gave in to the urge. Because you really managed to battle all the way till then, right? OK. Usually, with you, we can assume that something else happened. So let's figure out Sunday and see if there wasn't an interpersonal situation that day that made you feel criticized, unloved, or unacceptable.

CLIENT: Well, on Saturday I was so pissed off and I went to an AA meeting. And it got on my brain how alcohol would steal away my pain. I went looking all around the neighborhood for an open store. I was going to go get drunk. That's how much my pain was influencing me. But I couldn't find a store that was open, so I went back to the hospital.

THERAPIST: So you got the idea of getting alcohol to cure it, and you couldn't find any, so you went back to the hospital. You were in a lot of pain, and then what happened?

CLIENT: I told the nurse, "I've been sober almost 10 years and this is the first urge I've had to drink; that's how bad my pain is." And that wasn't listened to.

THERAPIST: So you figured that should have done it?

CLIENT: Yeah.

THERAPIST: Yeah. 'Cause that's a high-level communication, that's like a suicide threat. Very good, though. I want you to know, that's better than a suicide threat because that means you had reduced the severity of your threats.

The response above was very irreverent, in that most clients would not expect their therapists to view making a threat as a sign of therapeutic progress. The therapeutic utility of irreverence often lies in its "shock" value, which may temporarily loosen a client's maladaptive beliefs and assumptions, and open the client up to the possibility of other response solutions.

CLIENT: And I just told her how I was feeling about it, and I thought that would do it. And the doctor still wouldn't budge.

THERAPIST: So what did she do? Did she say she would call?

CLIENT: She called.

THERAPIST: OK. And then what happened?

CLIENT: She came back. She was really sweet, and she just said, "I'm really sorry, but the doctor said no."

THERAPIST: Then did you feel anger?

CLIENT: I don't know if I was really angry, but I was hurt.

THERAPIST: Oh, really? Oh, that's pretty interesting. OK. So you were hurt .. .

CLIENT: Because I ended up hugging my teddy bear and just crying for a while.

THERAPIST: Before or after you decided to hurt yourself?

CLIENT: Before.

THERAPIST: OK. So you didn't decide right away to hurt yourself. You were thinking about it. But when did you decide to do it?

CLIENT: Later on Saturday.

THERAPIST: When?

CLIENT: After I got sick of crying.

THERAPIST: So you laid in bed and cried, feeling uncared about and hurt, abandoned probably, and unlovable, like you weren't worth helping?

CLIENT: Yes.

THERAPIST: That's a really adaptive response. That's what I'm going to try to teach you. Except that you've already done it without my teaching it to you. So how did you get from crying, feeling unloved and not cared about, and you cry and sob—how did you get from there to deciding to hurt yourself, instead of like going to sleep?

CLIENT: Because then I got angry. And I said, "Fuck this shit, I'll show him."

THERAPIST: Now did you quit crying before you got angry, or did getting angry make you stop crying?

CLIENT: I think getting angry made me stop crying.

THERAPIST: So you kind of got more energized. So you must have been ruminating while you were lying there, thinking. What were you thinking about?

CLIENT: For a long time I was just wanting somebody to come care about me.

THERAPIST: Um hmm. Perfectly reasonable feelings. Makes complete sense. Now maybe there you could have done something different. What would have happened if you had asked the nurse to come in and talk to you, hold your hand?

An overall goal of behavioral analysis is the construction of a general road map of how the client arrives at dysfunctional responses, with notation of possible alternative pathways. Here the therapist was searching for junctures in the map where possible alternative responses were available to the client.

CLIENT: They don't have time to do that.

THERAPIST: They don't? Do you think that would have helped?

CLIENT: I don't know. She couldn't help me.

THERAPIST: She could have made you feel cared about. That would have been a caring thing to do.

CLIENT: Yeah, but I don't think it would have helped.

THERAPIST: What would have helped?

CLIENT: Getting pain medication.

THERAPIST: I thought you'd say that. You have a one-track mind. Now listen, we've got to figure out something else to help you because it can't be that nothing else can help. That can't be the way the world works for you. There's got to be more than one way to get everywhere because we all run into boulders on the path. Life is like walking on a path, you know, and we all run into boulders. It's got to be that there are other paths to places. And for you, it really isn't the pain in your ankle that's the problem; it's the feeling of not being cared about. And probably a feeling that has something to do with anger, or a feeling that other people don't respect you—a feeling of being invalidated.

CLIENT: Yes.

THERAPIST: So I think it's not actually the pain in your ankle that's the problem. Because if you were out on that raft with me, you would have been able to handle the pain if I hadn't had any medicine, right? So it's really not the pain; it's the sense of being invalidated and the sense of not being cared about. That's my guess. Do you think that's correct?

CLIENT: Yes.

THERAPIST: See, the question is, is there any other way for you to feel validated and cared about, other than them giving it to you?

CLIENT: No.

THERAPIST: Now is this a definite, like "I'm not going to let there be any other way," or is it more open, like "I can't think of another way, but I'm open to the possibility?"

CLIENT: I don't think there's another way.

THERAPIST: Does that mean you're not even open to learning another way?

CLIENT: Like what?

THERAPIST: I don't know. We have to figure it out. See, what I think is happening is that when you're in a lot of pain and you feel either not cared about or not taken seriously, invalidated, that's what sets you up to hurt yourself, and also to want to die. The problem that we have to solve is how to be in a situation that you feel is unjust without having to harm yourself to solve it. Are you open to that?

CLIENT: Yeah.

As illustrated here, behavioral analysis is often an excruciating and laborious process for client and therapist alike. The therapist often feels demoralized and is tempted to abandon the effort, which may be likened to trying to find a pair of footprints hidden beneath layers of fallen leaves; the footprints are there, but it may take much raking and gathering of leaves before they are uncovered. With repeated analyses, however, the client learns that the therapist will not "back down." Such persistence on the part of the therapist eventually extinguishes a client's refusal to attempt new and adaptive problem-solving behaviors. As clients increasingly acquire new behavioral skills, more adaptive attempts at problem resolution eventually become discernible.

In the following session (approximately 10 months into therapy), the client arrived wearing mirrored sunglasses (again) and was angry because collection agencies were persistent in pressuring her for payment on delinquent accounts. In addition, her therapist had been out of town for a week. The session targets were emotion regulation and interpersonal effectiveness. Dialectical (metaphor), validation (cheerleading), problem solving (contingency clarification, contingency management), stylistic (reciprocal communication, irreverent communication), and integrated (relationship enhancement) strategies were used. In this first segment, the therapist used cheerleading, contingency clarification, and the contingency management strategy of shaping to get the client to remove her sunglasses and work on expressing her anger.

THERAPIST: It's not a catastrophe that the collector did this to you, and it's not a catastrophe to be mad at the collector. It's made your life a lot harder, but you can handle this. You can cope with this. This is not more than you can cope with. You're a really strong woman; you've got it inside you. But you've got to do it. You've got to use it. I'm willing to help you, but I can't do it alone. You have to work with me.

CLIENT: How?

THERAPIST: Well, by taking off your sunglasses, for starters.

The therapist began the exchange by attempting to normalize the issue ("It's not a catastrophe"), validat-

ing the client ("It's made your life a lot harder"), and cheerleading ("You can handle this. You can cope.. ..You're a really strong woman"). The therapist then moved to contingency clarification by pointing out that provision of the therapist's assistance was contingent on the client's willingness to work. She immediately followed this by requesting a response well within the client's behavioral repertoire.

CLIENT: I knew you'd say that.

THERAPIST: And I knew you knew I'd say that.

CLIENT: Sunglasses are your biggest bitch, I think.

THERAPIST: Well, how would you like to look at yourself talking to someone else? (*long pause*) They make it difficult for me. And I figure they make it harder for you. I think you do better when you're not wearing those sunglasses. It's like a step; you always do better when you go forward. And when you do, you feel better. I've noticed that. (*long pause*) So that's what you should do; you should take off your sunglasses, and then we should problem-solve on how to cope when you can't get angry. There's nothing freakish about that. Something has happened in your life that has made it so that you're afraid to be angry, and we just have to deal with that, you and me. It's just a problem to be solved. It's not a catastrophe; it's not the worst thing anyone ever did. It's just a problem that you have, and that's what you and I do. We solve problems; we're a problem-solving team. (*pause*)

CLIENT: (*Removes sunglasses.*) All right.

THERAPIST: Thank you. That's a big step, I know, for you.

The therapist's use of reciprocal communication informed the client of her feelings regarding the sunglasses. Note the matter-of-fact attitude taken by the therapist and her continued attempt to normalize the issue (i.e., "There's nothing freakish about that .. . it's not the worst thing anyone ever did"). Also note the framing of the issue as a problem to be solved, as well as the therapist's use of the relationship strategy to enhance the therapeutic alliance. The therapist also made a point of validating the client by letting her know that she realized this was difficult.

THERAPIST: Now, c'mon, I want you to find it inside yourself. I know you've got it; I know you can do it. You can't give up. You can't let your feet slip. Keep going. Just express directly to me how you feel. That you're angry at yourself, that you're angry at the collection agency, and that you're damn angry with me. (*long pause*)

CLIENT: (*barely audible*) I'm angry at you, at myself, and the collection agency.

The therapist continued to rely on cheerleading and praise as she continued the shaping process in an attempt to get the client to express her anger directly.

THERAPIST: Good, did that kill you? (*long pause*) That's great. Is that hard? (*long pause*) It was, wasn't it? Now say it with a little vigor. Can't you say it with a little energy?

CLIENT: (*Shakes her head no.*)

THERAPIST: Yes, you can. I know you've got it in you. I have a good feel for what your strengths are. I don't know how I've got this good feel, but I do. And I know you can do it and you need to do it, and you need to say it with some energy. Express how angry you are. You don't have to yell and scream or throw things. Just say it aloud—"I'm angry!" (*long pause*) You can scream, of course, if you want; you can say, "I'm angry!"

CLIENT: That's it. That's all I can do.

THERAPIST: Listen, you have to take the risk. You're not going to get past this or through this. You have to take the risk. You are like a person mountain climbing and we've come to this crevasse and it's very deep, but we can't go back because there's an avalanche, and the only way to go forward is for you to jump over this crevasse. You've got to do it. Tell me how mad you are, in a way that I can understand how you really feel.

CLIENT: (*long pause*) I can't do any of it.

THERAPIST: That is bullshit.

CLIENT: You want me to get angry at you, don't you?

THERAPIST: I don't care who you get angry at. I think you already are angry. I just want you to express it. I'm not going to ask you to do anything more today, by the way. I figure the only thing today you have to do is say "I'm angry," in a voice that sounds angry, and I figure you're capable of that. And I might be angry if you don't do it. I don't think I will, but I might. That's OK. I can be angry, you can be angry, we can be angry sometimes, and it isn't going to kill either one of us.

Cheerleading and metaphor were unsuccessful in moving the client to express her anger more forcefully. Consequently, the therapist switched to irreverent communication in an attempt to get the client to "jump track." Also note how the therapist communicated to the client the potential negative consequences of her continued refusal to express her anger (i.e., ".. . I might be angry .. ."). In this manner, the therapist used the relationship as a contingency in order to promote change in the client.

THERAPIST: OK, so how angry are you? On a scale of 1 to 100, how angry would you say you are? At 100, you're ready to kill. You're so enraged, you'd go to war if you could.

CLIENT: (*barely audible*) Maybe 100.

THERAPIST: Really?

CLIENT: They know my situation.

THERAPIST: Um hmm.

CLIENT: They're persistent.

THERAPIST: Um hmm. (*pause*) Who's the safest to be angry at? Yourself, me, or the collection agency?

CLIENT: Collection agency.

THERAPIST: OK, then, tell me how angry you are. You don't have to make it sound like 100. Try to make it sound like 50.

CLIENT: They really pissed me off! (*said in a loud, angry voice*)

THERAPIST: Well, damn right. They piss me off, too.

As illustrated by the foregoing exchange, a primary difficulty in working with clients who have BPD is their not uncommon tendency to refuse to engage in behavioral work. Thus, it is absolutely necessary that the therapist maintain persistence and not give up in the face of a client's "I can't" statements. In situations like these, the use of irreverent communication often succeeds in producing a breakthrough and gaining client compliance.

POSTVENTION BY LINEHAN

After completing the writing of Cindy's case history for publication in this *Handbook*, 14 months into therapy, Cindy died of a prescription drug overdose plus alcohol. I (M. M. L.) considered dropping the case history and replacing it with a more successful case. However, in Cindy's honor, and because I think much can be learned from both failed and successful therapy, I decided to leave the case in. The immediate precipitant for Cindy's overdose was a call to her estranged husband, during which she discovered that another woman was living with him. As Cindy told me during a phone call the next morning, her unverbalized hope that they might someday get back together, or at least be close friends, had been shattered. She phoned again that evening in tears, stating that she had just drunk half a fifth of liquor. Such drinking incidents had occurred several times before, and the phone call was spent "remoralizing" Cindy, offering hope, problem-solving how she could indeed live without her husband, and using crisis intervention techniques to get her through the evening, until her appointment the following day. Cindy's roommate was home and agreed to talk with her, watch a TV movie together, and go to bed (plans on which the roommate did follow through). Cindy stated that although she felt suicidal, she would stop drinking and would not do anything self-destructive before her appointment. She was instructed to call me back later that evening if she wanted to talk again. The next day, when Cindy did not arrive for her appointment, I called her home, just as her roommate discovered Cindy dead, still in bed from the night before. At this point, I was faced with a number of tasks. I called to inform other therapists who had been treating the client, and spoke with a legal consultant to review the limits of confidentiality when a client has died. Once the family (Cindy's parents and estranged husband) were alerted, I called each to offer my condolences. The next day, as the senior therapist and supervisor on the treatment team, I called a meeting of the treatment team to discuss and process the suicide. It was especially important to notify the individual therapists of the remaining members of Cindy's skills training group. Group members were notified of the suicide by their individual psychotherapists. Within minutes of the beginning of the next group session, however, two members became seriously suicidal, and one of them had to be briefly hospitalized. (By the third week following the suicide, however, both had regained their forward momentum.) A third group member took this occasion to quit DBT and switch to another therapy, saying that this proved the treatment did not work. In the days and weeks following the suicide, I attended the funeral and met with Cindy's roommate and with her parents.

What can we learn from this suicide? First, it is important to note that even when a treatment protocol is

followed almost to the letter, it may not save a client. Even an effective treatment can fail in the end. In this case, DBT failed. This does not mean that the progress made was unimportant or not real. Had this "slippery spot over the abyss" been negotiated safely, perhaps the client would have been able to develop, finally, a life of quality. Risk is not eliminated, however, just because an individual makes substantial progress. In this case, I did not believe during the last phone call that the client was at higher than ordinary risk for imminent suicide. In contrast to many previous phone calls and therapy sessions in which the client had cried that she might not be able to hold on, during the last call the client made plans for the evening, agreed to stop drinking and not to do anything suicidal or self-destructive, and seemed to me (and to the roommate) to be in better spirits following the phone call. Her roommate was home and available. Thus, I did not take extraordinary measures that evening to prevent suicide. Indeed, the problem behavior focused on during the call was the drinking. I brought up the topic of suicide while conducting a risk assessment.

Second, could I have known? Only (perhaps) if I had paid more attention to the precipitant and less to the affect expressed at the end of the phone call. In reviewing notes about the client, I saw that each previous nonlethal self-injury was a result of intense anger at her husband. Each previous near-lethal attempt was a result of the client's belief that the relationship with her husband had irrevocably ended. Although the client could tolerate losing her husband, she could not tolerate losing all hope for a reconciliation at some point, even many years hence. Had I linked these two ideas (complete loss of hope and suicide attempt), I might have been able to work out a better plan for a reemergence of the crisis later in the evening. I definitely would have handled the situation differently. "Oh that woman's obviously a floozy, we will figure out a way to get him back! I'm sure of it," I would have said. The value of both conducting thorough behavioral assessments and organizing them into a coherent pattern is highlighted in this case. In this sense, I provided DBT almost to the letter but not all the way.

Third, when all is said and done, an individual with BPD must ultimately be able and willing to tolerate the almost unimaginable pain of his/her life until the therapy has a chance to make a permanent difference. Ultimately, the therapist cannot save the client; only the client can do that. Even if mistakes are made, the client must nonetheless persevere. In this case, the DBT protocol of "no lethal drugs for lethal people" was violated, even though the client had a past history of near-lethal overdoses. Why was the protocol not enforced? There were two primary reasons. First, the client came into therapy with a strong belief that the medication regimen she was on was essential to her survival. Any attempt on my part to manage her medications would have been met by very strong resistance. Although the drugs were dispensed in small doses, the only safe alternative would have been to have the person living with her (her husband at first, then her roommate) manage her medications, which the client also resisted. In addition, some professionals disagree with the "no lethal drugs" protocol of DBT because they believe that psychotropic medications are a treatment of choice for suicidal clients. In the face of professional and client resistance I relented. The second reason was that behavioral analyses indicated that her preferred lethal behavior was cutting; thus, I allowed myself a false sense of safety in thinking that her use of drugs to commit suicide was not likely.

Fourth, a group member's suicide is extraordinarily stressful for clients with BPD who are in group therapy. Although it is easy to believe that alliances are not strong in a psychoeducational behavioral skills group, this has universally not been our experience. The suicide of one member is a catastrophic event and can lead to contagious suicide and NSSI behavior, and therapy dropouts. Thus, extreme care is needed in the conduct of group meetings for some time following a suicide. Similar care is needed with the treatment team, where the thread of hope that maintains therapists in the face of a daunting task is also strained. It is important that the personal reactions of therapists, as well as a period of mourning and grieving, be shared and accepted. Fears of legal responsibility, never far from the surface, must be confronted directly; legal counsel should be sought as necessary; and, in time, a careful review of the case and the therapy must be conducted, if only to improve treatment in the future.

ACKNOWLEDGMENTS

The writing of this chapter was supported by National Institute of Mental Health Grant No. MH34486 to Marsha M. Linehan. Parts of this chapter are drawn from Linehan (1993b), Linehan and Koerner (1992), Koerner and Linehan (1992), and Linehan (1997). The quotations from Linehan (1997) in the section on validation are reprinted with the permission of the American Psychological Association. Finally, this chapter is a revision of the same chapter in the previous edition of this book, with contributions made by previous authors Bryan M. Cochran, Constance A. Kehrer, and Liz Dexter Mazza.

REFERENCES

Adler, G. (1981). The borderline–narcissistic personality disorder continuum. *American Journal of Psychiatry, 138,* 46–50.

Adler, G. (1993). The psychotherapy of core borderline psychopathology. *American Journal of Psychotherapy, 47,* 194–206.

Adler, G., & Buie, D. H. (1979). Aloneness and borderline psychopathology: The possible relevance of child development issues. *International Journal of Psychoanalytic Psychotherapy, 60,* 83–96.

American Psychiatric Association. (1987). *Diagnostic and statistical manual of mental disorders* (3rd ed., text rev.).Washington, DC: Author.

American Psychiatric Association. (2000). *Diagnostic and statistical manual of mental disorders* (4th ed., text rev.). Washington, DC: Author.

American Psychiatric Association. (2013). *Diagnostic and statistical manual of mental disorders* (5th ed.). Arlington, VA: Author.

Aviram, R. B., Brodsky, B. S., & Stanley, B. (2006). Borderline personality disorder, stigma, and treatment implications. *Harvard Review of Psychiatry, 14,* 249–256.

Barlow, D. H. (1988). *Anxiety and its disorders: The nature and treatment of anxiety and panic.* New York: Guilford Press.

Barlow, D. H., Allen, L. B., & Choate, M. L. (2004). Toward a unified treatment for emotional disorders. *Behavior Therapy, 35,* 205–230.

Barnoski, R. (2002). *Preliminary findings for the Juvenile Rehabilitation Administration's Dialectic Behavior Therapy Program* (Document No. 02-07-1203). Olympia: Washington State Institute for Public Policy.

Bateman, A., & Fonagy, P. (1999). Effectiveness of partial hospitalization in the treatment of borderline personality disorder: A randomized controlled trial. *American Journal of Psychiatry, 156,* 1563–1569.

Bateman, A., & Fonagy, P. (2001). Treatment of borderline personality disorder with psychoanalytically oriented partial hospitalization: An 18-month follow-up. *American Journal of Psychiatry, 158,* 36–42.

Bateman, A. W., & Fonagy, P. (2004). Mentalization-based treatment of BPD. *Journal of Personality Disorders, 18,* 36–51.

Bateman, A., & Fonagy, P. (2008). Eight-year follow-up of patients treated for borderline personality disorder: Mentalization-based treatment versus treatment as usual. *American Journal of Psychiatry, 165(5),* 631–638.

Bateman, A., & Fonagy, P (2009). Randomized controlled trial of outpatient mentalization-based treatment versus structured clinical management for borderline personality disorder. *American Journal of Psychiatry, 166*(12), 1355–1364.

Beck, A. T., Brown, G., Berchick, R. J., Stewart, B. L., & Steer, R. A. (1990). Relationship between hopelessness and ultimate suicide: A replication with psychiatric outpatients. *American Journal of Psychiatry, 147*, 190–195.

Beck, A. T., & Freeman, A. (1990). *Cognitive therapy of personality disorders.* New York: Guilford Press.

Bedics, J. D., Atkins, D. C., Comtois, K. A., & Linehan, M. M. (2012). Treatment differences in the therapeutic relationship and introject during a 2-year randomized controlled trial of dialectical behavior therapy versus nonbehavioral psychotherapy experts for borderline personality disorder. *Journal of Consulting and Clinical Psychology, 80*(1), 66–77.

Benjamin, L. S. (1996). *Interpersonal diagnosis and treatment of personality disorders* (2nd ed.). New York: Guilford Press.

Blum, N., Pfohl, B., St. John, D., Monahan, P., & Black, D. W. (2002). STEPPS: A cognitive-behavioral systems-based group treatment for outpatients with borderline personality disorder—a preliminary report. *Comprehensive Psychiatry, 43*, 301–310.

Blum, N., John, D. S., Pfohl, B., Stuart, S., McCormick, B., Allen, J., et al. (2008). Systems Training for Emotional Predictability and Problem Solving (STEPPS) for outpatients with borderline personality disorder: A randomized controlled trial and 1-year follow-up. *American Journal of Psychiatry, 165*(4), 468–478.

Bohus, M., Haaf, B., Simms, T., Limberger, M. F., Schmahl, C., Unckel, C., et al. (2004). Effectiveness of inpatient dialectical behavioral therapy for borderline personality disorder: a controlled trial. *Behaviour Research and Therapy, 42*, 487–499.

Bohus, M., Limberger, M. F., Chapman, A. L., Kuhler, T., Stieglitz, R., & Frank, U. (2007). Psychometric properties of the Borderline Symptom List (BSL). *Psychopathology, 40*, 126–132.

Bohus, M., Limberger, M. F., Frank, U., Sender, I., Gratwohl, T., & Stieglitz, R. D. (2001). Development of the borderline symptom list. *Psychotherapies, Psychosomatik, Medizinische Psychologie, 51*, 201–211.

Bohus, M., Dyer, A. S., Priebe, K., Krüger, A., Kleindienst, N., Schmahl, C., et al. (2013). Dialectical behaviour therapy for post-traumatic stress disorder after childhood sexual abuse in patients with and without borderline personality disorder: a randomised controlled trial. *Psychotherapy and Psychosomatics, 82*(4), 221–233.

Bos, E. H., van Wel, E. B., Appelo, M. T., & Verbraak, M. J. (2010). A randomized controlled trial of a Dutch version of systems training for emotional predictability and problem solving for borderline personality disorder. *Journal of Nervous and Mental Disorders, 198*(4), 299–304.

Bos, E. H., van Wel, E. B., Appelo, M. T., & Verbraak, M. J. (2011). Effectiveness of Systems Training for Emotional Predictability and Problem Solving (STEPPS) for borderline personality problems in a "real-world" sample: Moderation by diagnosis or severity? *Psychotherapy and Psychosomatics, 80*, 173–181.

Bradley, R. G., & Follingstad, D. (2003).Group therapy for incarcerated women who experienced interpersonal violence: A pilot study. *Journal of Traumatic Stress, 16*(4), 337–340.

Bradley, R., Zittel, C. C., & Westen, D. (2005). The borderline personality diagnosis in adolescents: Gender differences and subtypes. *Journal of Child Psychology and Psychiatry, 46*, 1006–1019.

Brent, D. A., Johnson, B. A., Perper, J., Connolly, J., Bridge, J., Bartle, S., et al. (1994). Personality disorder, personality traits, impulsive violence, and completed suicide in adolescents. *Journal of the American Academy of Child and Adolescent Psychiatry, 33*, 1080–1086.

Brown, G. K., Newman, C. F., Charlesworth, S. E., Crits-Christoph, P., & Beck, A. T. (2004). An open clinical trial of cognitive therapy for borderline personality disorder. *Journal of Personality Disorders, 18*, 257–271.

Buie, D. H., & Adler, G. (1982). Definitive treatment of the borderline personality. *International Journal of Psychoanalytic Psychotherapy, 9*, 51–87.

Carter, G. L., Willcox, C. H., Lewin, T. J., Conrad, A. M., & Bendit, N. (2010). Hunter DBT project: A randomized controlled trial of dialectical behaviour therapy in women with borderline personality disorder. *Australian and New Zealand Journal of Psychiatry, 44*, 162–173.

Cavanaugh, M. M., Solomon, P. L., & Gelles, R. J. (2011). The dialectical psychoeducational workshop (DPEW) for males at risk for intimate partner violence: A pilot randomized controlled trial. *Journal of Experimental Criminology, 7*(3), 275–291.

Chesin, M. S., Jeglic, E. L., & Stanley, B. (2010). Pathways to high-lethality suicide attempts in individuals with borderline personality disorder. *Archives of Suicide Research, 14*, 342–362.

Cisler, J. M., Olatunji, B. O., Feldner, M. T., & Forsyth, J. P. (2010). Emotion regulation and the anxiety disorders: An integrative review. *Journal of Psychopathology and Behavioral Assessment, 32*, 68–82.

Clarkin, J. F., Levy, K. N., Lenzenweger, M. F., & Kernberg, O. F. (2007). Evaluating three treatments for borderline personality disorder: A multiwave study. *American Journal of Psychiatry, 164*, 922–928.

Conklin, C. Z., & Westen, D. (2005). Borderline personality disorder in clinical practice. *American Journal of Psychiatry, 162*(5), 867–875.

Cottraux, J., Note, I. D., Milliery, M., Genouihlac, V., Yao, S.

N., Note, B., et al. (2009). Cognitive therapy versus Rogerian supportive therapy in borderline personality disorder. *Psychotheray and Psychosomatics, 78*, 307–316.

Courbasson, C., Nishikawa, Y., & Dixon, L. (2012). Outcome of dialectical behaviour therapy for concurrent eating and substance use disorders. *Clinical Psychology and Psychotherapy, 19*(5), 434–449.

Crowell, S. E., Beauchaine, T. P., & Linehan, M. M. (2009). A biosocial developmental model of borderline personality: Elaborating and extending Linehan's theory. *Psychological Bulletin, 135*, 495–510.

Davison, G. C., & Neale, J. M. (1994). *Abnormal psychology* (6th ed.). New York: Wiley.

Dimeff, L. A., McDavid, J., & Linehan, M. M. (1999). Pharmacotherapy for borderline personality disorder: A review of the literature and recommendations for treatment. *Journal of Clinical Psychology in Medical Settings, 6*, 113–138.

Doering, S., Horz, .S, Fischer-Kern, M., Schuster, P., Benecke, C., Buchheim, A., et al. (2010). Transference-focused psychotherapy v. treatment by community psychotherapists for borderline personality disorder: Randomised controlled trial. *British Journal of Psychiatry, 196*, 389–395.

Ellis, A. (1973). *Humanistic psychotherapy: The rational–emotive approach.* New York: Julian Press.

Etkin, A., & Wager, T. D. (2007). Functional neuroimaging of anxiety: A meta-analysis of emotional processing in PTSD, social anxiety disorder, and specific phobia. *American Journal of Psychiatry, 164*, 1476–1488.

Evershed, S., Tennant, A., Boomer, D., Rees, A., Barkham, M., & Watson, A. (2003). Practice-based outcomes of dialectical behaviour therapy (DBT) targeting anger and violence, with male forensic patients: A pragmatic and non-contemporaneous comparison. *Criminal Behaviour and Mental Health, 13*(3), 198–213.

Farrell, J. M., Shaw, I. A., & Webber, M. A. (2009). A schema-focused approach to group psychotherapy for outpatients with borderline personality disorder: A randomized controlled trial. *Journal of Behavior Therapy and Experimental Psychiatry, 40*, 317–328.

Feigenbaum, J. D., Fonagy, P., Pilling, S., Jones, A., Wildgoose, A., & Bebbington, P. E. (2012). A real-world study of the effectiveness of DBT in the UK National Health Service. *British Journal of Clinical Psychology, 51*(2), 121–141.

Feldman, G., Harley, R., Kerrigan, M., Jacobo, M., & Fava, M. (2009). Change in emotional processing during a dialectical behavior therapy-based skills group for major depressive disorder. *Behaviour Research and Therapy, 47*(4), 316–321.

Foa, E. B., & Kozak, M. J. (1986). Emotional processing of fear: Exposure to corrective information. *Psychological Bulletin, 99*, 20–35.

Fossati, A., Madeddu, F., & Maffei, C. (1999). Borderline personality disorder and childhood sexual abuse: A meta-analytic study. *Journal of Personality Disorders, 13*, 268–280.

Giesen-Bloo, J., Van Dyck, R., Spinhoven, P., van Tilburg, W., Dirksen, C., van Asselt, T., et al. (2006). Outpatient psychotherapy for borderline personality disorder: Randomized trial of schema-focused therapy vs. transference-focused psychotherapy. *Archives of General Psychiatry, 63*, 649–658.

Goldberg, C. (1980). The utilization and limitations of paradoxical intervention in group psychotherapy. *International Journal of Group Psychotherapy, 30*, 287–297.

Gunderson, J. G. (1984). *Borderline personality disorder.* Washington, DC: American Psychiatric Press.

Harley, R., Sprich, S., Safren, S., Jacobo, M., & Fava, M. (2008). Adaptation of dialectical behavior therapy skills training group for treatment-resistant depression. *Journal of Nervous and Mental Disease, 196*(2), 136–143.

Harned, M. S., Chapman, A. L., Dexter-Mazza, E. T., Murray, A., Comtois, K. A., & Linehan, M. M. (2008). Treating co-occurring Axis I disorders in recurrently suicidal women with borderline personality disorder: A 2-year randomized trial of dialectical behavior therapy versus community treatment by experts. *Journal of Consulting and Clinical Psychology, 76*(6), 1068–1075.

Harned, M. S., Rizvi, S. L., & Linehan, M. M. (2010). Impact of co-occurring posttraumatic stress disorder on suicidal women with borderline personality disorder. *American Journal of Psychiatry, 167*(10), 1210–1217.

Harned, M. S., Korslund, K. E., Foa, E. B., & Linehan, M. M. (2012). Treating PTSD in suicidal and self-injuring women with borderline personality disorder: Development and preliminary evaluation of a dialectical behavior therapy prolonged exposure protocol. *Behaviour Research and Therapy, 50*, 381–386.

Herman, J. L. (1986). Histories of violence in an outpatient population: An exploratory study. *American Journal of Orthopsychiatry, 56*, 137–141.

Herman, J. L., Perry, J. C., & van der Kolk, B. A. (1989). Childhood trauma in borderline personality disorder. *American Journal of Psychiatry, 146*, 490–495.

Hill, D. M., Craighead, L. W., & Safer, D. L. (2011). Appetite-focused dialectical behavior therapy for the treatment of binge eating with purging: A preliminary trial. *International Journal of Eating Disorders, 44*(3), 249–261.

Hirvikoski, T., Waaler, E., Alfredsson, J., Pihlgren, C., Holmström, A., Johnson, A., et al. (2011). Reduced ADHD symptoms in adults with ADHD after structured skills training group: Results from a randomized controlled trial. *Behaviour Research and Therapy, 49*(3), 175–185.

Hollandsworth, J. G. (1990). *The physiology of psychological disorders.* New York: Plenum Press.

Isometsa, E. T., Henriksson, M. M., Aro, H. M., Heikkinen, M. E., Kuoppasalmi, K. I., & Lonnqvist, J. K. (1994). Suicide in major depression. *American Journal of Psychiatry, 151*, 530–536.

Katz, L. Y., Cox, B. J., Gunasekara, S., & Miller, A. L. (2004) Feasibility of dialectical behavior therapy for suicidal adolescent inpatients. *Journal of the American Academy of Child and Adolescent Psychiatry, 43*, 276–282.

Kegan, R. (1982). *The evolving self: Problem and process in human development.* Cambridge, MA: Harvard University Press.

Kellogg, S. H., & Young, J. E. (2006). Schema therapy for borderline personality disorder. *Journal of Clinical Psychology, 62*, 445–458.

Kernberg, O. F. (1984). *Severe personality disorders: Psychotherapeutic strategies.* New Haven, CT: Yale University Press.

Kernberg, O. F., Selzer, M. A., Koenigsberg, H. W., Carr, A. C., & Appelbaum, A. H. (1989). *Psychodynamic psychotherapy of borderline patients.* New York: Basic Books.

Keuthen, N. J., Rothbaum, B. O, Fama, J., Altenburger, E., Falkenstein, M. J., Sprich, S. E., et al. (2012). DBT-enhanced cognitive-behavioral treatment for trichotillomania: A randomized controlled trial. *Journal of Behavioral Addictions, 1*(3), 106–114.

Kleindienst, N., Krumm, B., & Bohus M. (2011). Is transference-focused psychotherapy really efficacious for borderline personality disorder? *British Journal of Psychiatry, 98*(2), 156–157.

Koerner, K., & Linehan, M. M. (1992). Integrative therapy for borderline personality disorder: Dialectical behavior therapy. In J. C. Norcross & M. R. Goldfried (Eds.), *Handbook of psychotherapy integration* (pp. 433–459). New York: Basic Books.

Kohlenberg, R. J., & Tsai, M. (1991). *Functioned analytic psychotherapy: Creating intense and curative therapeutic relationships.* New York: Plenum Press.

Koons, C. R., Chapman, A. L., Betts, B. B., O'Rourke, B., Morse, N., & Robins, C. J. (2006). Dialectical behavior therapy adapted for the vocational rehabilitation of significantly disabled mentally ill adults. *Cognitive and Behavioral Practice, 13*, 146–156.

Koons, C. R., Robins, C. J., Tweed, J. L., Lynch, T. R., Gonzalez, A. M., Morse, J. Q., et al. (2001). Efficacy of dialectical behavior therapy in women veterans with borderline personality disorder. *Behavior Therapy, 32*, 371–390.

Kring, A. M., & Bachorowski, J. A. (1999). Emotions and psychopathology. *Cognition and Emotion, 13*, 575–599.

Kring, A. M. & Sloan, D. M. (2010). *Emotion regulation and psychopathology: A transdiagnostic approach to etiology and treatment.* New York: Guilford Press.

Kring, A. M. & Werner, K. H. (2004). Emotion regulation and psychopathology. In P. Philippot & R. S. Feldman (Eds.), *The regulation of emotion* (pp. 359–408). Mahwah, NJ: Erlbaum.

Kyokai, B. D. (1966). *The teachings of Buddha.* Japan: Bukkyo Dendo Kyokai.

Lequesne, E. R., & Hersh, R. G. (2004). Disclosure of a diagnosis of borderline personality disorder. *Journal of Psychiatric Practice, 10*, 170–176.

Levy, K. N., & Scala, J. W. (2012). Transference, transference interpretations, and transference-focused psychotherapies. *Psychotherapy, 49*(3), 391–403.

Lieb, K., Völlm, B., Rücker, G., Timmer, A., & Stoffers, J. M. (2010). Pharmacotherapy for borderline personality disorder: Cochrane Systematic Review of randomised trials. *British Journal of Psychiatry, 196*, 4–12.

Lieb, K., Zanarini, M., Linehan, M. M., & Bohus, M. (2004). Seminar section: Borderline personality disorder. *Lancet, 364*, 453–461.

Linehan, M. M. (1987). Dialectical behavior therapy for borderline personality disorder: Theory and method. *Bulletin of the Menninger Clinic, 51*, 261–276.

Linehan, M. M. (1993a). *Cognitive-behavioral treatment of borderline personality disorder.* New York: Guilford Press.

Linehan, M. M. (1993b). *Skills training manual for treating borderline personality disorder.* New York: Guilford Press.

Linehan, M. M. (1997). Validation and psychotherapy. In A. Bohank & L. Greenberg (Eds.), *Empathy reconsidered: New directions in psychotherapy* (pp. 353–392). Washington, DC: American Psychological Association.

Linehan, M. M. (in press). *Skills training manual for treating borderline personality disorder* (2nd ed.). New York: Guilford Press.

Linehan, M. M., Armstrong, H. E., Suarez, A., Allmon, D., & Heard, H. L. (1991). Cognitive-behavioral treatment of chronically parasuicidal borderline patients. *Archives of General Psychiatry, 48*, 1060–1064.

Linehan, M. M., Bohus, M., & Lynch, T. R. (2007). Dialectical behavior therapy for pervasive emotion dysregulation: Theoretical and practical underpinnings. In J. J. Gross (Ed.), *Handbook of emotion regulation* (pp. 581–605). New York: Guilford Press.

Linehan, M. M., Comtois, K. A., Murray, A., Brown, M. Z., Gallop, R. J., Heard, H. L., et al. (2006). Two-year randomized trial + follow-up of dialectical behavior therapy vs. therapy by experts for suicidal behaviors and borderline personality disorder. *Archives of General Psychiatry, 63*, 757–766.

Linehan, M. M., Dimeff, L. A., Reynolds, S. K., Comtois, K., Shaw-Welch, S., Heagerty, P., et al. (2002). Dialectical behavior therapy versus comprehensive validation plus 12-step for the treatment of opioid dependent women meeting criteria for borderline personality disorder. *Drug and Alcohol Dependence, 67*, 13–26.

Linehan, M. M., & Heard, H. L. (1993). Impact of treatment accessibility on clinical course of parasuicidal patients: In reply to R. E. Hoffman [Letter to the editor]. *Archives of General Psychiatry, 50*, 157–158.

Linehan, M. M., Heard, H. L., & Armstrong, H. E. (1993).

Naturalistic follow-up of a behavioral treatment for chronically parasuicidal borderline patients. *Archives of General Psychiatry, 50,* 971–974.

Linehan, M. M., & Koerner, K. (1992). A behavioral theory of borderline personality disorder. In J. Paris (Ed.), *Borderline personality disorder: Etiology and treatment* (pp. 103–121). Washington, DC: American Psychiatric Association.

Linehan, M. M., McDavid, J. D., Brown, M. Z., Sayrs, J. H., & Gallop, R. J. (2008). Olanzapine plus dialectical behavior therapy for women with high irritability who meet criteria for borderline personality disorder: A double-blind, placebo-controlled pilot study. *Journal of Clinical Psychiatry, 69*(6), 999–1005.

Linehan, M. M., Rizvi, S. L., Shaw-Welch, S., & Page, B. (2000). Psychiatric aspects of suicidal behaviour: Personality disorders. In K. Hawton & K. van Heeringen (Eds.), *International handbook of suicide and attempted suicide* (147–178). Sussex, UK: Wiley.

Linehan, M. M., Schmidt, H., III, Dimeff, L. A., Craft, J. C., Kanter, J., & Comtois, K. A. (1999). Dialectical behavior therapy for patients with borderline personality disorder and drug-dependence. *American Journal of Addiction, 8,* 279–292.

Linehan, M. M., Tutek, D. A., Heard, H. L., & Armstrong, H. E. (1994). Interpersonal outcome of cognitive behavioral treatment for chronically suicidal borderline patients. *American Journal of Psychiatry, 151,* 1771–1776.

Livesley, J. W., Jang, K. L., & Vernon, P. A. (1998). Phenotypic and genetic structure of traits delineating personality disorder. *Archives of General Psychiatry, 55 ,* 941–948.

Loranger, A. W. (1995). *International Personality Disorder Examination (IPDE) manual.* White Plains, NY: Cornell Medical Center.

Lynch, T. R., Cheavens, J. S., Cukrowicz, K. C., Thorp, S. R., Bronner, L., & Beyer, J. (2007). Treatment of older adults with co-morbid personality disorder and depression: A dialectical behavior therapy approach. *International Journal of Geriatric Psychiatry, 22,* 131–143.

Lynch, T. R., Morse, J. Q., Mendelson, T., & Robins, C. J. (2003). Dialectical behavior therapy for depressed older adults: A randomized pilot study. *American Journal of Geriatric Psychiatry, 11,* 33–45.

Marlatt, G. A., & Gordon, J. R. (1985). *Relapse prevention: Maintenance strategies in the treatment of addictive behaviors.* New York: Guilford Press.

McDonell, M. G., Tarantino, J., Dubose, A. P., Matestic, P., Steinmetz, K., Galbreath, H., et al. (2010). A pilot evaluation of dialectical behavioural therapy in adolescent long-term inpatient care. *Child and Adolescent Mental Health, 15*(4),193–196.

McMain, S., Korman, L. M., & Dimeff, L. A. (2001). Dialectical behavior therapy and the treatment of emotion dysregulation. *Journal of Clinical Psychology, 57*(2), 183–196.

McMain, S. F., Links, P. S., Gnam, W. H., Guimond, T., Cardish, R. J., Korman, L., et al. (2009). A randomized clinical trial of dialectical behavior therapy versus general psychiatric management for borderline personality disorder. *American Journal of Psychiatry, 166,* 1365–1374.

Mennin, D. S. (2004). Emotion regulation therapy for generalized anxiety disorder. *Clinical Psychology and Psychotherapy, 11,* 17–29.

Mennin, D. S., Heimberg, R. G., Turk, C. L., & Fresco, D. M. (2005). Preliminary evidence for an emotion dysregulation model of generalized anxiety disorder. *Behaviour Research and Therapy, 43,* 1281–1310.

Merriam-Webster, Inc. (2006). Merriam-Webster online dictionary. Available online at *www.m-w.com.*

Merriam-Webster's New Universal Unabridged Dictionary. (1983). Cleveland, OH: Dorset & Baber.

Mintz, R. S. (1968). Psychotherapy of the suicidal patient. In H. L. P. Resnick (Ed.), *Suicidal behaviors: Diagnoses and management* (pp. 271–296). Boston: Little, Brown.

Nadort, M., Arntz, A., Giesen-Bloo, J., Eikelenboom, M., Spinhoven, P., van Asselt, T., et al. (2009). Implementation of outpatient schema therapy for borderline personality disorder with versus without crisis support by the therapist outside office hours: A randomized trial. *Behaviour Research and Therapy, 47,* 961–973.

Neacsiu, A. D., Eberle, J. E., Kramer, R., Weismann, T., & Linehan, M. M. (2013). *A treatment mechanism for emotion dysregulation across mood and anxiety disorders: A randomized controlled trial.* Manuscript under review.

Neacsiu, A. D., Rizvi, S. L., & Linehan, M. M. (2010). Dialectical behavior therapy skills use as a mediator and outcome of treatment for borderline personality disorder. *Behaviour Research and Therapy, 48*(9), 832–839.

Nisenbaum, R., Links, P. S., Eynan, R., & Heisel, M. J. (2010). Variability and predictors of negative mood intensity in patients with borderline personality disorder and recurrent suicidal behavior: Multilevel analyses applied to experience sampling methodology. *Journal of Abnormal Psychology, 119*(2), 433–439.

Nose, M., Cipriani, A., Biancosino, B., Grassi, L., & Barbui, C. (2006). Efficacy of pharmacotherapy against core traits of borderline personality disorder: Meta-analysis of randomized controlled trials. *International Clinical Psychopharmacology, 21,* 345–353.

Paris, J. (2005). Borderline personality disorder. *Canadian Medical Association Journal, 172,* 1579–1583.

Peng, K., & Nisbett, R. E. (1999). Culture, dialectics, and reasoning about contradiction. *American Psychologist, 54,* 741–754.

Pistorello, J., Fruzzetti, A. E., MacLane, C., Gallop, R., & Iverson, K. M. (2012). Dialectical behavior therapy (DBT) applied to college students: A randomized clinical trial. *Journal of Consulting and Clinical Psychology, 80*(6), 982–984.

Pretzer, J. (1990). Borderline personality disorder. In A. Freeman, L. Pretzer, B. Fleming, & K. M. Simon (Eds.), *Clinical applications of cognitive therapy* (pp. 181–202). New York: Plenum Press.

Rakfeldt, J. (2005). Dialectical behavior therapy with transitional youth: Preliminary findings. *Best Practices in Mental Health, 1*(2), 61–76.

Rathus, J. H., & Miller, A. L. (2002). Dialectical behavior therapy adapted for suicidal adolescents. *Suicide and Life-Threatening Behavior, 32*, 146–157.

Reiser, D. E., & Levenson, H. (1984). Abuses of the borderline diagnosis: A clinical problem with teaching opportunities. *American Journal of Psychiatry, 141*, 1528–1532.

Roepke, S., Schröder-Abé, M., Schütz, A., Jacob, G., Dams, A., Vater, A., et al. (2011). Dialectic behavioural therapy has an impact on self-concept clarity and facets of self-esteem in women with borderline personality disorder. *Clinical Psychology and Psychotherapy, 18*(2), 148–158.

Safer, D., Robinson, A., & Jo, B. (2010). Outcome from a randomized controlled trial of group therapy for binge eating disorder: Comparing dialectical behavior therapy adapted for binge eating to an active comparison group therapy. *Behavior Therapy, 41*, 106–120.

Safer, D. L., & Joyce, E. E. (2011). Does rapid response to two group psychotherapies for binge eating disorder predict abstinence? *Behaviour Research and Therapy, 49*(5), 339–345.

Safer, D. L., Telch, C. F., & Agras, W. S. (2001). Dialectical behavior therapy for bulimia nervosa. *American Journal of Psychiatry, 158*, 632–634.

Salbach-Andrae, H., Bohnekamp, I., Bierbaum, T., Schneider, N., Thurn, C., Stiglmayr, C., et al. (2009). Dialektisch behaviorale therapie (DBT) und kognitiv behaviorale therapie (CBT) für Jugendliche mit Anorexia und Bulimia nervosa im Vergleich [Dialectical behavior therapy and cognitive behavior therapy for anorexia and bulimia nervosa among adolescents: A randomized, controlled trial with a waiting control group]. *Kindheit und Entwicklung* [*Childhood and Development*], *18*(3), 180–190.

Shearin, E. N., & Linehan, M. M. (1992). Patient–therapist ratings and relationship to progress in dialectical behavior therapy for borderline personality disorder. *Behavior Therapy, 23*, 730–741.

Siever, L. J., & Davis, K. L. (1991). A psychobiological perspective on the personality disorders. *American Journal of Psychiatry, 148*, 1647–1658.

Silk, K. R., Lee, S., Hill, E. M., & Lohr, N. E. (1995). Borderline personality disorder symptoms and severity of sexual abuse. *American Journal of Psychiatry, 152*, 1059–1064.

Simpson, J. A., & Weiner, E. S. (1989). *Oxford English Dictionary* (2nd ed.) [Online]. Retrieved December 17, 2000, from *www.oed.com*.

Soler, J., Pascual, J. C., Campins, J., Barrachina, J., Puigdemont, D., Alvarez, E., et al. (2005). Double-blind, placebo-controlled study of dialectical behavior thera-

py plus olanzapine for borderline personality disorder. *American Journal of Psychiatry, 162*(6), 1221–1224. Erratum in *American Journal of Psychiatry, 165*(6), 777.

Soler, J., Pascual, J. C., Tiana, T., Cebria, A., Barrachina, J., Campins, M. J., et al. (2009). Dialectical behaviour therapy skills training compared to standard group therapy in borderline personality disorder: A 3-month randomised controlled clinical trial. *Behaviour Research and Therapy, 47*, 353–358.

Soloff, P. H., & Chiapetta, L. (2012). Subtyping borderline personality disorder by suicidal behavior. *Journal of Personality Disorders, 26*(3), 468–480.

Soloff, P. H., Lis, J. A., Kelly, T., Cornelius, J., & Ulrich, R. (1994). Risk factors for suicidal behavior in borderline personality disorder. *American Journal of Psychiatry, 151*, 1316–1323.

Stein, D. J., Simeon, D., Frenkel, M., Islam, M. N., & Hollander, E. (1995). An open trial of valproate in borderline personality disorder. *Journal of Clinical Psychiatry, 56*, 506–510.

Telch, C. F., Agras, W. S., & Linehan, M. M. (2001). Dialectical behavior therapy for binge eating disorder: A promising new treatment. *Journal of Consulting and Clinical Psychology, 69*, 1061–1065.

Thorberg, F. A., & Lyvers, M. (2006). Negative mood regulation (NMR) expectancies, mood, and affect intensity among clients in substance disorder treatment facilities. *Addictive Behaviors, 31*(5), 811–820.

Trupin, E. W., Stewart, D. G., Beach, B., & Boesky, L. (2002). Effectiveness of a dialectical behaviour therapy program for incarcerated female juvenile offenders. *Child and Adolescent Mental Health, 7*(3), 121–127.

Turner, R. M. (2000). Naturalistic evaluation of dialectical behavioral therapy-oriented treatment for borderline personality disorder. *Cognitive and Behavioral Practice, 7*, 413–419.

van Asselt, D. I., Dirksen, C. D., Giesen-Bloo, J. H., van Dyck, R., Spinhoven, P., van Tilburg, W., et al. (2008). Out-patient psychotherapy for borderline personality disorder: Cost-effectiveness of schema-focused therapy v. transference-focused psychotherapy. *British Journal of Psychiatry, 192*, 450–457.

Van den Bosch, L., Verheul, R., Schippers, G. M., & van den Brink, W. (2002). Dialectical behavior therapy of borderline patients with and without substance use problems: Implementation and long-term effects. *Addictive Behaviors, 2*, 911–923.

Van Dijk, S., Jeffrey, J., & Katz, M. R. (2013). A randomized, controlled, pilot study of dialectical behavior therapy skills in a psychoeducational group for individuals with bipolar disorder. *Journal of Affective Disorders, 145*(3), 386–393.

Verheul, R., van den Bosch, L. M. C., Koeter, M. W. J., de Ridder, M. A. J., Stijnen, T., & van den Brink, W. (2003).

Dialectical behaviour therapy for women with borderline personality disorder: 12-month, randomised clinical trial in The Netherlands. *British Journal of Psychiatry, 182,* 135–140.

Waltz, J., Dimeff, L. A., Koerner, K., Linehan, M. M., Taylor, L., & Miller, C. (2009). Feasibility of using video to teach a dialectical behavior therapy skill to clients with borderline personality disorder. *Cognitive and Behavioral Practice, 16*(2), 214–222.

Wasser, T., Tyler, R., McIlhaney, K., Taplin, R., & Henderson, L. (2008). Effectiveness of dialectical behavior therapy (DBT) versus standard therapeutic milieu (STM) in a cohort of adolescents receiving residential treatment. *Best Practices in Mental Health, 4*(2), 114–125.

Weinberg, I., Gunderson, J. G., Hennen, J., & Cutter, C. J., Jr. (2006). Manual assisted cognitive treatment for deliberate self-harm in borderline personality disorder patients. *Journal of Personality Disorders, 20,* 482–492.

Wells, H. (1972). Alienation and dialectical logic. *Kansas Journal of Sociology, 3,* 7–32.

Whitaker, C. A. (1975). Psychotherapy of the absurd: With a special emphasis on the psychotherapy of aggression. *Family Process, 14,* 1–16.

Wolf, M., Ebner-Priemer, U., Schramm, E., Domsalla, M.,

Hautzinger, M., & Bohus, M. (2011). Maximizing skills acquisition in dialectical behavioral therapy with a CD-ROM-based self-help program: Results from a pilot study. *Psychopathology, 44*(2), 133–135.

Young, J. E., Klosko, J. S., & Weishaar, M. E. (2003). *Schema therapy: A practitioner's guide.* New York: Guilford Press.

Zanarini, M. C. (2003). Zanarini Rating Scale for Borderline Personality Disorder (ZAN-BPD): A continuous measure of DSM-IV borderline psychopathology. *Journal of Personality Disorders, 17,* 233–242.

Zanarini, M. C., Frankenburg, F. R., & Parachini, E. A. (2004). A preliminary, randomized trial of fluoxetine, olanzapine, and the olanzapine–fluoxetine combination in women with borderline personality disorder. *Journal of Clinical Psychiatry, 65,* 903–907.

Zanarini, M. C., Frankenburg, F. R., Sickel, A. E., & Yong, L. (1996). *The Diagnostic Interview for DSM-IV Personality Disorders.* Belmont, MA: McLean Hospital, Laboratory for the Study of Adult Development.

Zanarini, M. C., Vujanovic, A., Parachini, E., Boulanger, J., Frankenburg, F., & Hennen, J. (2003). A screening measure for BPD: The McLean Screening Instrument for Borderline Personality Disorder. *Journal of Personality Disorders, 17,* 568–573.

CHAPTER 11

Bipolar Disorder

DAVID J. MIKLOWITZ

> Our goal in this book is to present creative and important psychological treatments with empirical support. This chapter on bipolar disorder by David J. Miklowitz presents his innovative approach called family-focused treatment (FFT), a treatment with substantial existing evidence for efficacy. Based on years of systematic research on psychological factors contributing to the onset and maintenance of bipolar disorder, this sophisticated family therapy approach targets the most important psychosocial factors linked to the disorder and associated with poor outcome (e.g., appropriate psychoeducation, communication enhancement training, and problem-solving skills training). This chapter, and especially the very useful case study, also illustrates an essential linkage between psychological and pharmacological approaches in the successful treatment of this very severe form of psychopathology.—D. H. B.

Bipolar disorder is one of the oldest and most reliably recognized psychiatric disorders. Our thinking about this disorder has evolved over the last 100 years, but the original descriptions (Kraepelin, 1921) of "manic–depressive insanity" greatly resemble our current conceptualizations. This chapter begins with a review of basic information about the disorder, its diagnosis, its longitudinal course, and drug treatment. This information about the illness is interesting in its own right, but it also provides the rationale for using psychosocial treatment as an adjunct to pharmacotherapy. The majority of the chapter describes a focused, time-limited, outpatient psychosocial treatment—family-focused treatment (FFT)—that comprises three interrelated modules: psychoeducation, communication enhancement training (CET), and problem-solving skills training (Miklowitz, 2008b; Miklowitz & Goldstein, 1997). It is designed for patients who have had a recent episode of mania or depression.

THE DIAGNOSIS OF BIPOLAR DISORDER

DSM-5 Criteria

The core characteristic of bipolar disorder is extreme affective dysregulation, or mood states that swing from extremely low (depression) to extremely high (mania). Patients in a manic episode have euphoric, elevated mood or irritable mood; behavioral activation (e.g., increased goal-directed activity, excessive involvement in high-risk activities, decreased need for sleep, increased talkativeness or pressure of speech); and altered cognitive functioning (grandiose delusions or inflated self-worth, flight of ideas or racing thoughts, distractibility)—typically for more than 1 week. For the diagnosis of a manic episode, there must be evidence that the person's psychosocial functioning (marital, occupational, or social) is disrupted, that hospitalization is required, or that psychotic features (e.g., grandiose delusions) are present (see the fifth edition of the *Diagnostic and Statistical Manual of Mental Disorders* [DSM-5; American Psychiatric Association, 2013]).

A patient in a hypomanic episode shows many of the same symptoms, but the duration is typically shorter (i.e., 4 days or more). Hypomanic symptoms also do not bring about severe impairment in social or occupational functioning and are not associated with the need for hospitalization or with psychosis. However, the symptoms must reflect a real change in a person's ordinary behavior—one that is observable by others. The distinction between mania and hypomania, which is really one of degree rather than type of illness, is difficult for clinicians to make reliably. Often the degree to which the behavioral activation affects a patient's functioning is underestimated by the patient, who can see nothing but good in his/her behavior. A theme of this chapter is the value of including significant others (i.e., parents, spouses/partners, and siblings) in patients' assessment and treatment.

In previous editions of the DSM, patients could be diagnosed with bipolar I disorder on the basis of a single "mixed" episode, in which the criteria for a major depressive episode and a manic episode are met nearly every day for 1 or more weeks. This definition has caused considerable confusion among clinicians, who may ignore the requirement that episodes of both poles be syndromal and use the mixed designation to describe patients with a variety of co-occurring subsyndromal depressive and hypomanic or manic symptoms (Frank, 2011). One large-scale population study found that "mixed hypomania" is particularly common among women with bipolar I or II disorder (Suppes et al., 2005). These considerations have relevance for prognosis as well as diagnosis. Patients with major depressive disorder (MDD) who have two or more co-occurring manic symptoms have more similarity to patients with bipolar depression than to patients with MDD without manic symptoms on features such as age at onset, family history of bipolar disorder, functional impairment, suicide attempts, and long-term conversion to bipolar I disorder (e.g., Sato, Bottlender, Schröter, & Möller, 2003; Fiedorowicz et al., 2011).

In DSM-5 the mixed episode criteria are a much broader course specifier in manic, depressive, or hypomanic episodes. The specifier *with mixed features* is applied when three or more subthreshold symptoms from the opposite pole occur during a mood episode. However, there are unanswered questions about the treatment implications of this definition, such as whether depression with subthreshold mixed symptoms should be treated with mood stabilizers in conjunction with antidepressants (First, 2010).

DSM-5 proceeds with the diagnosis of bipolar disorder somewhat differently than earlier DSM systems. First, the diagnostician determines whether the patient satisfies the cross-sectional criteria for a manic episode. If he/she does meet these criteria, the diagnosis of bipolar I disorder is applied. If the patient currently meets DSM-5 criteria for a major depressive episode, he/she is diagnosed as having bipolar disorder only if there is a past history of manic, mixed, or hypomanic episodes; otherwise, the diagnosis is likely to be MDD or another mood disorder, such as persistent depressive disorder. If the patient is in remission, there must be evidence of prior manic or mixed episodes. One implication of this rather complicated set of diagnostic rules is that a single manic (and in DSM-IV, a single mixed) episode, even in the absence of documentable depression, is enough to warrant the bipolar I diagnosis. The key word here is "documentable," because patients often underreport their depression histories and reveal them only upon careful questioning.

How Has the Diagnosis of Bipolar Disorder Changed?

Every version of the DSM has brought changes in the way we think about bipolar disorder, and modifications are likely to continue as new editions are published. One consistent area of controversy has been the proposal to use separate criteria for child- and adolescent-onset bipolar illness. Manic and hypomanic episodes among children appear to be shorter than those in adults, with more polarity switches and longer subthreshold mixed states (Birmaher et al., 2009). Previously, DSM-IV (American Psychiatric Association, 1994) used the same criteria to diagnose mania in adults and children, despite the clear developmental differences in presentation (Leibenluft, Charney, Towbin, Bhangoo, & Pine, 2003). However, DSM-5 includes a new category, disruptive mood dysregulation disorder, to characterize children with frequent and explosive temper outbursts and persistent irritability. The investigators who proposed this category believe it will reduce false-positive diagnoses of bipolar disorder in children (e.g., Leibenluft, 2011), although not all agreed with this new disorder (e.g., Axelson, Birmaher, Findling, et al., 2011).

DSM-5 distinguishes between bipolar I and bipolar II disorders. In the former, patients have fully syndromal manic episodes, but in bipolar II, patients must have had at least one major depressive episode and one hypomanic episode (in this chapter, the term "bipolar disorder" refers either to bipolar I or bipolar II disorder as defined in DSM-5, unless otherwise specified). DSM-5 also includes a course descriptor, "rapid cycling," which appears to characterize between 13 and 20% of patients (Calabrese, Fatemi, Kujawa, & Woyshville, 1996). Rapid cycling is applied when patients have had four or more discrete major depressive, manic, or hypomanic episodes in a single year. The confusion in applying this course descriptor lies in the fact that it is difficult to tell when one episode has ended and another begins: If a patient quickly switches from mania to depression in a 48-hour period (what some refer to as "ultrarapid cycling"), is this truly a new episode or just a different presentation of the same episode (perhaps with mixed features)? Rapid cycling appears to be a transient state of the disorder and not a lifelong phenomenon (Coryell, Endicott, & Keller, 1992).

Finally, DSM-5 deals with the thorny problem of patients with depression who develop manic or hypomanic episodes that are brought on by antidepressants or other activating drugs. Because of the effects of antidepressants on the serotonin, norepinephrine, and dopamine systems, there is the potential for these drugs to induce activation, particularly in a patient who is already biologically vulnerable to mood swings. If a patient has never had a manic episode but then develops one after taking an antidepressant, the likely diagnosis is a substance-induced mood disorder. The diagnosis of bipolar disorder is only then considered if the symptoms of mania preceded the antidepressant (a difficult historical distinction), or if the mania symptoms continue for at least a month after the antidepressant is withdrawn. Similar diagnostic considerations apply to patients who abuse drugs (e.g., cocaine, amphetamine) that are "psychotomimetics" and can induce manic-like states.

Epidemiology, Comorbidity, and Differential Diagnosis

Across studies, cultures, and age groups, bipolar I and bipolar II disorders affect at least 2% of the population. The National Comorbidity Survey Replication (NCS-R), an epidemiological study of 9,282 U.S. adults using a lay-administrator structured diagnostic interview, reported lifetime prevalence rates of 1.0% for bipolar I disorder, 1.1% for bipolar II disorder, and 2.4% for sub-

threshold bipolar illness (e.g., bipolar disorder not otherwise specified or cyclothymic disorder; Merikangas et al., 2007). In the international World Health Organization World Mental Health Survey Initiative, a study of 61,392 adults in 11 countries that used the same diagnostic instrument, lower lifetime prevalence rates were reported: 0.6% for bipolar I disorder, 0.4% for bipolar II disorder, and 1.4% for subthreshold bipolar disorder (Merikangas et al., 2011).

In a community sample of adolescents (ages 13–18), 2.5% met lifetime DSM-IV criteria for bipolar I or II disorder, with the prevalence increasing with age (Merikangas et al., 2012). Interestingly, 1.7% of adolescents met DSM-IV criteria for a manic episode without depression. Finally, in a meta-analysis of 12 studies across the world involving a total of 16,222 youth between ages 7 and 21, the rate of bipolar disorder was 1.8%, and did not differ across countries (Van Meter, Moreira, & Youngstrom, 2011).

Bipolar disorder virtually always co-occurs with other conditions, some of which become the focus of immediate treatment. The disorders with which bipolar disorder is comorbid have the common underpinning of affective dysregulation. When 1-year prevalence rates were considered in the NCS-R, the highest correlations were observed between mania/hypomania and anxiety disorders (62.9%), followed by behavior disorders (attention-deficit/hyperactivity disorder [ADHD] and oppositional defiant disorder; 44.8%) and substance use disorders (36.8%) (Merikangas et al., 2007).

Some studies have found that patients with pediatric onset have more comorbid disorders than patients with adult onset patients (Leverich et al., 2007). The comorbidity of bipolar disorder and ADHD in children is between 60 and 90%, even when overlapping symptoms are not considered (Kim & Miklowitz, 2002). Risk for substance use disorders is five times greater in adolescents with bipolar disorder than in healthy adolescents (Wilens et al., 2004). Comorbidity with anxiety disorders is approximately 44% (Masi et al., 2012; Sala et al., 2010). Interestingly, anxiety disorders are often first diagnosed in children of parents with bipolar disorder and may represent the first signs of major mood illness (Henin et al., 2005).

The distinction between bipolar disorder and personality disorders is especially difficult. Notably, the hallmark of borderline personality disorder is affective instability. Akiskal (1996) has argued that what is commonly seen by clinicians as personality pathology is actually undertreated subsyndromal mood disorder.

When studies of the overlap of bipolar disorder and personality disorders are done, the estimates of comorbidity are actually quite conservative. For example, George, Miklowitz, Richards, Simoneau, and Taylor (2003) found that only 29% of patients with bipolar disorder meet the diagnostic criteria for personality disorders during a period of remission. Furthermore, the comorbid personality disorder diagnosis was not always borderline personality disorder and was often a disorder from cluster C (e.g., avoidant or dependent personality disorder).

The boundaries between bipolar and unipolar illness are sometimes difficult to draw. Depressions in bipolar and unipolar disorders may look quite similar, but, on average, bipolar depression has a younger age of onset, more short-term mood variability, and is more treatment-resistant than MDD (Cuellar, Johnson, & Winters, 2005). In the National Epidemiologic Survey on Alcohol and Related Conditions ($N = 13,048$), patients with bipolar depression endorsed suicidal ideation and psychomotor disturbance more often than did patients with unipolar depression, and patients with unipolar depression were somewhat more likely to endorse fatigue (Weinstock, Strong, Uebelacker, & Miller, 2009). Thus, the differences between bipolar and unipolar depression are not large, and past history of mania or hypomania (or family history of mania in a patient who has not had a manic episode) may provide more information for the differential diagnosis.

Even more complicated is the distinction between agitated depression of the unipolar type and mixed mania of the bipolar type; both are characterized by sadness and a highly anxious, restless, activated state. Goldberg and Kocsis (1999) recommend that clinicians attempting to make these distinctions place emphasis on attributes such as goal-drivenness and undiminished energy (despite lack of sleep), both of which tip the scales toward bipolar disorder rather than unipolar depressive illness.

The distinction between bipolar disorder and schizophrenia can also be a surprisingly difficult clinical judgment. When a patient who has schizophrenia presents with a psychotic episode, he/she can appear acutely activated, grandiose in thinking and actions, and elated or depressed. In conditions once thought to be etiologically distinct, more and more studies are finding a significant degree of genetic overlap between bipolar disorder and schizophrenia or other psychotic conditions (Berrettini, 2003). For example, a recent genomewide association study found significant overlap in gene variants among patients with schizophrenia and patients with bipolar disorder who had mood-incongruent psychotic features (e.g., delusions or hallucinations that have no clear content related to sadness or elation) (Goes et al., 2012).

DSM-5 makes a distinction between schizoaffective disorder and major mood disorders with psychotic features. In schizoaffective disorder, delusions and hallucinations have been present for at least 2 weeks, in the absence of prominent affective symptoms. In major mood disorders, psychotic symptoms occur only during periods of significant mood disturbance. A 10-year follow-up of patients with schizophrenia, schizoaffective disorders, and major affective disorders (both bipolar and unipolar) found that "mood-incongruent" delusions and hallucinations (i.e., those whose content does not relate to feelings of grandiosity and elation or, alternatively, feelings of worthlessness) are a poor prognostic sign across diagnoses (Harrow, Grossman, Herbener, & Davies, 2000). Harrow and colleagues (2000) argue for a dimensional view of schizoaffective disorder, with some patients on the psychotic end and others on the mood end of the spectrum.

DSM-5 also describes a subsyndromal or subaffective condition: cyclothymic disorder. Patients with cyclothymic disorder alternate between periods of hypomanic symptoms and brief periods of depression that fall short of the criteria for major depressive illness. As soon as the person develops a full manic, mixed, or depressive episode, the diagnosis of bipolar I or II disorder is given. Again, these distinctions really concern the degree and duration of symptoms rather than their form. In my own experience, clinicians are prone to "push" patients with cyclothymia into the bipolar II category, especially if they feel that the patients are not reliable in their historical reporting. Sometimes it is better to observe the mood lability of a patient over time than attempt to distinguish cyclothymic disorder and bipolar disorder cross-sectionally.

DRUG TREATMENT AND THE COURSE OF BIPOLAR DISORDER

Standard Pharmacotherapy

The course of bipolar illness (its pattern of relapsing and remitting over time) is best considered with reference to the drug treatments that help stabilize patients and allow most to function in the community. In the prepharmacological era (i.e., prior to 1960), patients were hospitalized for years at a time (Cutler & Post, 1982). Nowadays, the availability of mood stabilizers such as lithium carbonate, the anticonvulsants (e.g., divalproex sodium [Depakote], lamotrigine [Lamictal], and other agents), and the atypical antipsychotics (e.g., olanzapine [Zyprexa], quetiapine [Seroquel], risperidone [Risperdal], ziprasidone [Geodon], or aripiprazole [Abilify]) has done much to ameliorate the course of bipolar illness (Goldberg, 2004; Malhi, Adams, & Berk, 2009). Some of these drugs not only control the acute episodes of the illness but also have "prophylactic value," which means that they help prevent future episodes or minimize the duration or severity of episodes that do occur.

Most psychiatrists describe three phases of drug treatment: an "acute phase," in which the goal is to control the most severe symptoms of the manic, mixed, or depressive disorder; a "stabilization phase," in which the goal is to help the patient recover fully from the acute phase, which often means treating residual symptoms (e.g., mild depression) or levels of social–occupational impairment; and a "maintenance phase," in which the goal is to prevent recurrences and continue to treat residual symptoms. The drugs recommended for bipolar disorder vary according to the phase of treatment. During the acute and stabilization phases, an antipsychotic medication may accompany a mood stabilizer. An antidepressant may be recommended after a manic episode has stabilized if a patient has ongoing, residual depression symptoms. These phases of treatment are also relevant to the psychosocial–psychotherapeutic treatment of bipolar disorder, which I discuss later.

Symptomatic Outcome

If drug treatment is so effective, then why do we need psychosocial treatment? The problem that consistently arises in the drug treatment of bipolar disorder is "breakthrough episodes." With lithium or anticonvulsant treatment, the rate of relapse over 1 year is about 37% (Gitlin, Swendsen, Heller, & Hammen, 1995). In 1,469 adults with bipolar I and II disorders, 49% had recurrences over 1 year; twice as many of these recurrences were of depressive (rather than manic or hypomanic) episodes. In a 12.8-year follow-up of 146 adult patients with bipolar I disorder, patients had syndromal or subsyndromal depressive symptoms for about 32% of the weeks of their lives, manic or hypomanic symptoms for 9%, and mixed or cycling symptoms states for 6%; patients were in remission only about half of the time (Judd et al., 2002).

Keck and colleagues (1998) examined the 12-month course of bipolar disorder among 134 patients who began in an acute manic or mixed episode. The majority of the patients (N = 104) were treated with mood stabilizers, with or without accompanying antipsychotics or antidepressants. The investigators made a distinction among "syndromic recovery," in which patients no longer met the DSM criteria for a manic, mixed, or depressive episode for at least 8 weeks; "symptomatic recovery," a tougher criterion by which patients had to have minimal or no mood disorder symptoms for 8 weeks; and "functional recovery," which required that patients regain their premorbid (preillness) level of employment, friendships, interests, and independent living status. Of the 106 patients who completed the study, 51 (48%) achieved syndromic recovery by 12-month follow-up. Only 28 (26%) achieved symptomatic recovery, and 25 (24%) reached functional recovery at follow-up. Predictors of poor outcome included low socioeconomic status, medication noncompliance, and longer duration of illness.

Social–Occupational Functioning

Patients with bipolar disorder experience significant impairment in work, social, and family functioning, and their chances of early illness recurrence increase dramatically when they have subsyndromal depressive symptoms (Altshuler et al., 2006; Gitlin, Mintz, Sokolski, Hammen, & Altshuler, 2011). Additionally, patients with persisting depressive symptoms often have cognitive impairment, which strongly affects social and occupational functioning (Altshuler, Bearden, Green, van Gorp, & Mintz, 2008). A study of 253 bipolar I and II patients revealed that only about 33% of the patients worked full time, and only 9% worked part time outside of the home; 57% of patients reported being unable to work or able to work only in protected settings (Suppes et al., 2001).

The relationship between mood symptoms and functioning appears to be bidirectional: Residual depressive symptoms are clearly associated with poorer social and occupational functioning (e.g., Gitlin et al., 2011), but other studies have shown that poor social functioning predicts a shorter time to mood disorder relapse (e.g., Weinstock & Miller, 2008).

Medication Nonadherence

Part of the reason why patients with bipolar disorder have so many "breakthrough episodes" is drug nonadherence. In one review, Colom, Vieta, Tacchi, Sanchez-Moreno, and Scott (2005) estimated that at least 60% of patients with bipolar disorder discontinue their medications at some point in their lives. Between 40 and 60% are partially or fully nonadherent in the year after their first hospitalization for a manic or mixed episode (Strakowski et al., 1998). One study of a large health maintenance organization found that patients took lithium for an average of only 76 days (Johnson & McFarland, 1996). Nonadherence has considerable implications for the course of the disorder: When patients stop their medications suddenly, they are at much higher risk for relapse or suicide (Baldessarini, Tondo, & Hennen, 2003).

The reasons that patients stop taking mood stabilizers are varied, and include side effects, lack of insight into the illness, younger age, lower socioeconomic status, lack of information about medications, negative feelings about having one's moods controlled by a medication, missing high periods, recent hospitalizations, and low family support (Colom, Vieta, Tacchi, et al., 2005). Some of these issues are amenable to modification through adjusting dosages or substituting one agent for another. Other problems related to nonadherence can be addressed in adjunctive psychotherapy.

Why Psychotherapy?

What is the role of psychosocial treatment in a disorder with such a heavy biological and genetic basis? There is little doubt that medication is the first-line treatment for bipolar disorder. The evidence that lithium, the anticonvulsants, and the atypical antipsychotics reduce relapse rates and improve functioning is substantial. But can we do better? An optimal and perhaps overly optimistic view of the outcome of patients with bipolar disorder would include symptom stability for extended periods, minimal disruptions in social functioning after episodes, and having consistent work and family lives. Indeed, these outcomes are highly valued by patients, who often devise their own self-management strategies to cope with the illness (Murray et al., 2011).

The roles of adjunctive psychotherapy can include teaching skills for symptom management, augmenting social and occupational role functioning, and keeping patients adherent to their drug regimens. Implicit in this objective is that the physiology and psychology of major psychiatric disorders are not fully separable. We know that changes in neural function (e.g., as revealed in functional magnetic resonance imaging scans) often occur among patients who respond to psychotherapy (e.g., Kumari et al., 2011). The time has come to think about psychotherapy and medication as working synergistically in the major mood disorders.

The strongest argument for including psychotherapy in an outpatient treatment program is to help patients to cope with stress triggers. As noted in the next section, certain forms of life events and family tensions are risk factors in the course of bipolar disorder. Psychotherapy can target these factors and teach patients adaptive coping mechanisms, which can then be brought to bear during periods of wellness to help stave off the likelihood of a future relapse.

A VULNERABILITY–STRESS MODEL OF RECURRENCES

Implicit in the notion that psychotherapy would be helpful to a patient with bipolar disorder is the notion that stress plays a role in eliciting symptoms of mood disorder. What is the evidence for this view? What are the targets for psychosocial intervention?

Life Events and Social Rhythms

Life events are consistently associated with relapses of bipolar depression, and in some studies, of mania as well (Johnson, 2005a). Two major pathways have been proposed for the association of life events and mood relapses. The first of these, the social rhythm stability hypothesis (Ehlers, Kupfer, Frank, & Monk, 1993), posits that major life events disrupt daily rhythms (i.e., when one wakes, eats, exercises, socializes, works, and sleeps) in mood disorders. Life events can act as *zeitstorers*, which disrupt established social and circadian rhythms (e.g., the production of neuroendocrines as a function of the time of day). For example, a previously unemployed patient who gets a job with constantly shifting work hours is forced to adopt a new pattern of daily routines, which may include changes in sleep–wake habits. Major events can also result in the loss of social *zeitgebers*—people or events that help maintain the stability of rhythms. For example, a spouse or partner helps to maintain a person on predictable sleep schedules. A relationship separation, in addition to being a significant emotional event, results in the loss of this human timekeeper.

Patients with bipolar disorder are exquisitely sensitive to even minor changes in sleep–wake habits. Studies by Malkoff-Schwartz and colleagues (1998, 2000) have revealed that manic episodes are often precipitated by life events that change sleep–wake habits (e.g., changing time zones due to air travel). However, depressive episodes were not differentially associated with rhythm-disruptive life events. One of the clinical implications of these findings is that if patients can be taught to regularize their social rhythms, especially in the face of life events that normally disrupt those rhythms, then the outcome of bipolar disorder should be improved. Thus, variability in the sleep–wake cycle is a target for treatment. This is a central tenet of interpersonal and social rhythm therapy (IPSRT; Frank, 2005), as discussed below.

Life Events, Goal Dysregulation, and Mania

Across more than 12 studies, people with a history of mania and students who are vulnerable to mania have described themselves as more likely to react with strong emotions to reward (Johnson, Edge, Holmes, & Carver, 2012). Self-reported reward sensitivity has been found to predict a more severe course of mania among those with bipolar I disorder (Meyer, Johnson, & Winters, 2001; Salavert et al., 2007), and of conversion from bipolar spectrum disorder to bipolar II or I disorder in high-risk college students (Alloy et al., 2012). A related construct, heightened ambition, is associated with a more severe course of mania among patients with bipolar I disorder (Johnson et al., 2012). Impulsive responding, in which people pursue rewards without awareness of potential negative consequences, becomes elevated during the escalation to mania (Swann, Dougherty, Pazzaglia, Pham, & Moeller, 2004).

Sheri Johnson and colleagues (2000) hypothesize that excess reward sensitivity may heighten reactivity to successes, such that manic symptoms would be more likely after life events involving goal attainment (e.g., getting a promotion). Goal attainment may increase confidence, which then fuels increased goal engagement and accelerates the development of manic symptoms (Johnson, 2005b). In two longitudinal studies of patients with bipolar I disorder, goal-attainment life events predicted increases in manic symptoms but not

depressive symptoms, even after excluding life events that could have been caused by manic symptoms (e.g., job loss; Johnson et al., 2000, 2008).

Family Stress

Family conflicts are also a breeding ground for increased cycling of bipolar disorder. One method of measuring family stress is to evaluate a family's level of "expressed emotion" (EE). In this procedure, a researcher administers the Camberwell Family Interview (Vaughn & Leff, 1976) to a family member (parent, spouse/partner, or sibling) for approximately 1 hour to assess the relative's reactions to the patient's psychiatric disorder, with particular emphasis on a recent illness episode. Later, a trained judge evaluates tapes of these interviews on three primary dimensions: critical comments (e.g., "When I talk to him, I get upset that he just shuts down. It's like there's no one there!"); hostility, or personal, generalized criticism of the patient (e.g., "I like nothing about him"); and emotional overinvolvement, or the tendency to be overconcerned, overprotective, or to use inordinately self-sacrificing behaviors in the patient's care (e.g., "I don't invite people to the house because Allen [son] doesn't like it"). Family members who score high on one or more of these dimensions are called "high-EE"; those who do not are called "low-EE."

EE is a well-established predictor of the course of schizophrenia. In Butzlaff and Hooley's (1998) meta-analysis of 28 longitudinal studies of EE in schizophrenia, 23 studies replicated the same core finding: Patients who return after an illness episode to high-EE families are two to three times more likely to relapse in 9-month to 1-year prospective follow-ups than those returning to low-EE families. Several studies have documented a link between high-EE families and relapse among patients with bipolar disorder followed either prospectively or retrospectively (Honig, Hofman, Rozendaal, & Dingemanns, 1997; Miklowitz, Goldstein, Nuechterlein, Snyder, & Mintz, 1988; O'Connell, Mayo, Flatow, Cuthbertson, & O'Brien, 1991; Priebe, Wildgrube, & Muller-Oerlinghausen, 1989; Yan, Hammen, Cohen, Daley, & Henry, 2004). A 2-year study of family EE among bipolar adolescents undergoing family treatment also replicated this longitudinal association (Miklowitz, Biuckians, & Richards, 2006).

On first examination, one might conclude that patients with bipolar disorder are sensitive to stress in the family milieu, and that levels of EE elicit an underlying biological vulnerability. But the relationship is far from simple. First, it appears that the high-EE relatives of patients with bipolar illness, unipolar illness, or schizophrenia are more likely than low-EE relatives to interpret the patients' negative problem behaviors as controllable by the patients (see, e.g., Hooley & Licht, 1997; Weisman, Lopez, Karno, & Jenkins, 1993; Wendel, Miklowitz, Richards, & George, 2000). Second, relatives and patients coping with bipolar disorder are often locked into verbally aggressive, negative cycles of face-to-face interaction. Simoneau, Miklowitz, and Saleem (1998) found that high-EE relatives of patients with bipolar disorder were more negative than low-EE relatives during face-to-face problem-solving interactions. The relatives and patients in high-EE families were also more likely to engage in counterproductive "attack–counterattack" cycles. Often the patients were provocateurs in these interchanges; they were not the "victims" of verbally aggressive or punitive relatives (Miklowitz, Wendel, & Simoneau, 1998; Simoneau et al., 1998).

Clearly, a psychosocial treatment program should consider aspects of the family's affective environment—such as high-EE attitudes in relatives or the negative interchanges that characterize relative–patient communication—to be targets for intervention. But does one attempt to change these attitudes and interaction patterns directly, or instead make an "end run" around them? Family members coping with a spouse/partner, offspring, or sibling who has bipolar disorder are understandably quite angry, and it makes little sense to tell them they should not be. Others feel that their overprotective behavior is more than warranted by the situation.

In developing FFT, my associates and I concluded that at least one component of dealing with these attitudes and transaction patterns is psychoeducation, which involves the provision of information to patients and family members about the disorder and its manifestations. As discussed earlier, relatives (parents, spouses, or siblings) need to realize that at least some proportion of the patient's aversive behaviors (e.g., irritability, aggression, inability to work, or low productivity) can be attributed to a biochemically driven illness state. This may seem obvious to us as clinicians, but to family members who deal with the patient on a day-to-day basis, it is easy to attribute aversive behaviors to personality factors or laziness, or to believe that "He/she is doing this to hurt me." In parallel, patients need to become more cognizant of the way they provoke anger and resentment in family members.

Negative face-to-face interactions cannot be eradicated, but they can be made more productive through the techniques of communication and problem-solving skills training. Thus, families or couples can be taught to stick with one problem topic rather than trying to solve many at a time, or to use listening skills to avoid counterproductive attack–counterattack cycles. Later in this chapter, I explain these methods with reference to a difficult treatment case.

TREATMENT OUTCOME STUDIES

Controlled psychotherapy outcome studies are new to the field of bipolar disorder and certainly have not kept pace with research on drug treatment. This section describes several randomized controlled trials (RCTs) of individual and family/marital interventions. More thorough reviews of the studies in this area are available (Geddes & Miklowitz, 2013; Miklowitz & Scott, 2009).

Individual Therapy

Two models of individual therapy deserve emphasis here. Cognitive-behavioral models focus on risk factors for relapse, including medication nonadherence, excessive risk taking (or reward overestimation) prior to mania, and behavioral inactivity during depression. Lam, Hayward, Watkins, Wright, and Sham (2005; Lam et al., 2003) examined a 6-month, 12- to 18-session cognitive-behavioral therapy (CBT) model with drug treatment versus drug treatment alone ($N = 103$). Patients had been in remission for at least 6 months but had had at least three episodes in the past 5 years. At a 1-year follow-up, 44% of patients in CBT had relapsed compared with 75% of the patients who received drug treatment alone. Twelve to 30 months after treatment, CBT did not prevent relapse relative to drug treatment alone, but it did continue to show a positive influence on mood and days spent in episodes. The effects on depression were more significant than the effects on mania.

A multicenter effectiveness trial of CBT in the United Kingdom ($N = 253$) indicated that not all subpopulations of patients with bipolar disorder are equally likely to benefit from CBT (Scott et al., 2006). The study compared 22 sessions of CBT plus pharmacotherapy to treatment as usual (TAU) plus pharmacotherapy. The patients had been in a variety of symptomatic states before study entry. No effects were found for CBT on time to recurrence. A post hoc analysis revealed that patients with less than 12 prior episodes had fewer recurrences in CBT than in TAU. However, patients with 12 or more episodes were more likely to have recurrences in CBT than in TAU. The authors concluded that CBT is most applicable to patients in the early stages of their disorder or in those whose course is less recurrent. However, a "metaregression" of six RCTs concluded that there was no evidence that relapses were moderated by number of prior episodes (Lam, Burbeck, Wright, & Pilling, 2009).

Cognitive rehabilitation, a form of behavioral treatment that emphasizes attention, concentration, and memory strategies, may be a useful adjunct to pharmacotherapy for patients with bipolar disorder who have cognitive impairment. In an 18-case open trial, Deckersbach and colleagues (2010) found that after 14 sessions of treatment, patients had improvements in depressive symptoms, occupational functioning, and executive functioning compared to their baselines. Randomized trials of cognitive rehabilitation in patients with neuropsychological impairments are warranted.

Ellen Frank and colleagues (2005) investigated the efficacy of IPSRT—a treatment that includes not only the core elements of Klerman, Weissman, Rounsaville, and Chevron's (1984) model of interpersonal psychotherapy for depression but also a component in which patients self-regulate their daily routines and sleep–wake cycles. Patients with a recent mood episode were randomly assigned to either 45-minute IPSRT sessions and mood-stabilizing medications or an active clinical management intervention, also with medications. The latter comprised 20-minute sessions with a psychotherapist who focused on drug side effects and symptom management. Randomization was done first during an acute phase of treatment, with sessions held weekly; and again at the beginning of a preventive, maintenance phase of treatment, with sessions held biweekly or monthly for up to 2 years. Patients who received IPSRT in the acute phase had longer intervals prior to recurrences in the maintenance phase than patients who received clinical management in the acute phase. IPSRT was most effective in delaying recurrences in the maintenance phase among patients who succeeded in stabilizing their daily routines and sleep–wake cycles during the acute phase (Frank et al., 2005). IPSRT also had a positive impact on vocational functioning (Frank et al., 2008). Thus, consistency of routines may protect against a worsening course of the disorder and enhance functioning.

Group Psychoeducation

The effects of group psychoeducation have been documented in several large-scale RCTs, including one at a Veterans Administration outpatient clinic (Bauer et al., 2006) and another at a health maintenance organization (Simon, Ludman, Bauer, Unutzer, & Operskalski, 2006). In both studies, psychoeducation groups were embedded in larger systems of care, including patient monitoring by a nurse care manager and monitoring of the physician's adherence to treatment guidelines. These systematic care models were shown to be highly effective in improving illness course and functioning compared to usual care for bipolar patients in these settings.

An RCT focused on the combination of pharmacotherapy and group psychoeducation was undertaken at the University of Barcelona (Colom et al., 2003). A total of 120 remitted patients with bipolar disorder who were receiving pharmacological treatment were allocated to (1) 21 sessions of structured group psychoeducation or (2) 21 sessions of an unstructured support group, both administered by psychologists. Psychoeducation sessions included lectures, role play, discussions of beliefs and attitudes, behavioral interventions and between-session homework assignments. Over 2 years, individuals who received group psychoeducation were significantly more likely than those allocated to the unstructured group to show lower relapse and hospitalization rates and higher, more stable plasma lithium levels (Colom et al., 2003; Colom, Vieta, Sanchez-Moreno, et al., 2005). Moreover, a 5.5-year follow-up of this sample revealed that the gains associated with group psychoeducation were sustained (Colom et al., 2009). Thus, group psychoeducation appears to be a cost-effective adjunct to pharmacotherapy for bipolar patients who begin in remission.

Family Therapy

There are now several studies of family interventions as adjuncts to medication for patients with bipolar disorder. Here, I focus on trials published after 2000; the reader is referred to more comprehensive reviews (Miklowitz, 2008a; Miklowitz & Scott, 2009) for coverage of earlier family and marital studies.

Five randomized trials have been completed on FFT. Two of these were conducted with adults recruited from hospital settings following an acute episode, one at the University of California, Los Angeles (UCLA;

Rea et al., 2003) and one at the University of Colorado (Miklowitz, George, Richards, Simoneau, & Suddath, 2003). One study was conducted in the context of the Systematic Treatment Enhancement Program for Bipolar Disorder (STEP-BD; Miklowitz et al., 2007b), which examined three intensive psychotherapies (FFT, IPSRT or CBT) in comparison with a control condition for patients with bipolar depression. Two RCTs have been conducted with pediatric-onset patients, one involving adolescents with bipolar disorder (Miklowitz et al., 2008) and the other with symptomatic children and adolescents (ages 9–17) who were genetically at risk for bipolar disorder (Miklowitz et al., 2013). These studies are examined in detail below.

The UCLA and Colorado Studies

These studies each examined a 9-month, 21-session FFT intervention that comprised psychoeducation, communication enhancement training, and problem-solving training. Participants were patients and their parents or spouses. Patients were recruited during an index episode of bipolar disorder and maintained on mood-stabilizing medications, with or without antipsychotic or antidepressive agents. However, the studies differed in an important respect: At Colorado, the comparison "crisis management" group received two sessions of family education and individual crisis sessions, as needed, over 9 months. In the UCLA study, patients in the comparison group received an individual case management and problem-solving intervention that was of similar intensity (21 sessions) to the FFT intervention.

Despite these design differences, the results that emerged from the Colorado and UCLA studies were quite similar. In the Colorado study (Miklowitz et al., 2003), FFT and medication led to lower frequencies of relapses and longer delays prior to relapses over a 2-year period than did crisis management and medication. FFT was also associated with more improvement in depression and mania symptoms—effects that did not appear until the 9- and 12-month follow-ups but continued for the full 24 months of follow-up. In the UCLA study (Rea et al., 2003), the effects of FFT were seen on hospitalization rates over a 2-year follow-up. The effects of FFT on time to relapse were not seen in the first year but did appear in the second year. Notably, rates of rehospitalization in the 1- to 2-year period following the 9-month treatment were 12% in the FFT group and 60% in the individual therapy group; for re-

lapse, the rates were 28% and 60%, respectively. Results of both studies suggest that there may be a delayed effect of FFT: Patients and family members may need to "absorb" the treatment and incorporate the education and skills training into their day-to-day lives before it has ameliorative effects on the illness.

This latter point was clarified further by Simoneau, Miklowitz, Richards, Saleem, and George (1999), who examined family interaction transcripts obtained in the Colorado study before and after FFT or crisis management treatment. Families (patients with their parents or spouses) participated in interactional assessments that comprised 10-minute problem-solving discussions that were transcribed and coded via the Category System for Coding Partner Interactions (Hahlweg et al., 1989). Forty-four families returned at 1 year for the same assessment, after the FFT or crisis management protocol had been completed. Interestingly, at the posttreatment (1 year) interactional assessments, patients in FFT and those in crisis management could not be distinguished on the basis of frequency of negative interactional behaviors (e.g., criticisms). But there were clear differences at posttreatment in positive interactional behaviors, particularly in the nonverbal sphere. After FFT, patients and relatives were more likely to smile at each other, nod when others were speaking, and lean toward each other when speaking. Moreover, the degree to which patients improved in their nonverbal interactional behavior over the course of psychosocial treatment was correlated with their degree of symptom improvement over the year of treatment.

FFT appeared to have ameliorated certain tensions within the family environments. Future studies using multiple, time-lagged assessments of family interaction and patients' symptoms would help to disentangle the directional relationship between improvements in family communication and patients' symptomatic outcomes.

The STEP-BD Study

STEP-BD examined the effectiveness of treatment with mood stabilizers in combination with psychosocial treatments in 15 participating sites in the United States (Miklowitz et al., 2007b). Patients with bipolar disorder in a depressive episode ($N = 293$) were randomly assigned to mood-stabilizing medications—with or without antidepressants—and 30 sessions of FFT, IPSRT, CBT, or collaborative care (CC), a three-session psychoeducational treatment. Patients assigned to any intensive psychotherapy had higher recovery rates over 1 year and recovered an average of 110 days faster than patients in CC. Patients in intensive therapy were also more likely to remain stable in mood over the yearlong study. In FFT, 77% of the patients recovered by 1 year; in interpersonal therapy, 65%; and in CBT, 60%. In the CC condition, 52% recovered. The differences between the intensive modalities did not reach statistical significance. It is worth noting that in STEP-BD, there was no evidence that patients randomly assigned to mood stabilizers with adjunctive antidepressants recovered any more rapidly from depression than patients assigned to mood stabilizers with adjunctive placebo (Sachs et al., 2007).

STEP-BD, one of the largest randomized treatment studies for bipolar disorder, suggests that psychotherapy is an essential component of the effort to stabilize patients with bipolar disorder in a depressive episode. When clinicians are treating bipolar, depressed patients with mood stabilizers or atypical antipsychotics, adding an intensive therapy may be associated with more rapid recovery than adding an antidepressant (Miklowitz et al., 2007a, 2007b). The common ingredients of intensive treatments—such as teaching strategies to manage mood, identifying and intervening early with prodromal symptoms, enhancing patients' compliance with medications, and working toward resolution of key interpersonal or family problems—may contribute to more rapid recoveries. FFT proved to be a particularly potent treatment in this study, although its limitations also became apparent: Only 54% of the patients assessed for the study had families who were accessible and willing to participate in treatment.

Family Psychoeducation in Early-Onset Bipolar Disorder

More recent applications of family psychoeducation have focused on patients with juvenile-onset bipolar disorder, who most frequently live with or are strongly connected with their families of origin. FFT for adolescents (FFT-A; Miklowitz et al., 2004) uses the same 21-session structure, adapted to the developmental needs of this age group (e.g., the occurrence of more frequent, briefer episodes, typically with a mixed presentation). A 2-year RCT of 58 adolescent patients with bipolar disorder revealed that, compared to patients who received three sessions of family psychoeducation (enhanced care, or EC), patients in FFT-A recovered more rapidly from their baseline depressive symptoms, spent less time

depressed at follow-up, and had greater improvements in depressive symptoms over a 2-year follow-up (Miklowitz et al., 2008). Furthermore, the effects of FFT-A were moderated by the level of EE in families during the pretreatment period. Adolescents from high-EE families showed greater improvement in both depressive and manic symptoms over 2 years in FFT-A than in EC; the effects of FFT-A in adolescents from low-EE families were not as robust (Miklowitz et al., 2009).

A version of FFT has been developed for children and adolescents who are at risk for developing bipolar disorder. These youth have (1) a first-degree relative (usually a parent) with bipolar I or II disorder and (2) significant mood dysregulation and impairment, in the form of major depression or bipolar disorder not otherwise specified (BD-NOS). Children with BD-NOS have brief (1–3 days) and recurrent periods of mania or hypomania that represent a change from baseline. A follow-up of children with BD-NOS and a positive family history of mania found that up to half "converted" to bipolar I or II disorder within 5 years (Axelson, Birmaher, Strober, et al., 2011).

In a 1-year RCT, 40 high-risk children (ages 9–17) with MDD or BD-NOS were randomly assigned to a high-risk version of FFT (FFT-HR) or to a one- to two-session education control (Miklowitz et al., 2013). The participants in FFT-HR had more rapid recovery from their initial mood symptoms, more weeks in remission from mood symptoms, and more improvement in hypomania symptoms over 1 year than participants in the education control. As was found in the adolescent sample, the magnitude of the treatment effect was greater among high-risk children in high-EE (vs. low-EE) families.

Other models of family intervention for pediatric bipolar disorder are showing promise. In a large (N = 165) wait-list trial, Fristad Verducci, Walters, and Young (2009) found that children with mood disorders who were assigned to multifamily groups showed greater mood improvement over 6 study months than children on a wait list. Moreover, children on the wait list who participated in the multifamily groups 1 year later showed the same amount of improvement between 12 and 18 months.

Finally, a family-focused CBT treatment developed for school-age children with bipolar disorder incorporates psychoeducation, cognitive restructuring, and affect regulation interventions (West & Weinstein, 2012). This 12-session treatment has shown positive effects in open trials. Results of an RCT are pending.

Summary

The addition of psychosocial treatment—family, group, or individual—to pharmacotherapy leads to more positive outcomes of bipolar disorder than can be achieved with pharmacotherapy alone. In drawing conclusions, we must keep in mind the different clinical conditions of patients at the outset of treatment. For example, the studies of CBT and group psychoeducation focused on patients in remission, whereas those of FFT and IPSRT focused on patients who were symptomatic and only partially recovered from an acute episode.

The remainder of this chapter is devoted to the specifics of delivering FFT. For whom is it intended? How does it proceed? How are families educated about bipolar disorder, and how do they learn new styles of communicating or solving problems? In reviewing these methods, the reader may wish to reflect on the various targets of family intervention (i.e., family attitudes or expectations, interpersonal conflict, medication nonadherence) and the various domains of outcome that are presumed to be influenced by family interventions via their impact on these targets.

CONTEXT OF THERAPY

Treatment Objectives and Structure

FFT has six objectives, all of which concern coping with an episode of bipolar disorder. These are summarized in Table 11.1. Some of these pertain to dealing with the current episode; others are more focused on anticipating episodes in the future, and the stress

TABLE 11.1. The Six Objectives of Family-Focused Treatment

Assist the patient and relatives in the following:

- Integrating the experiences associated with recent episodes of bipolar disorder
- Recognizing and accepting the patient's vulnerability to future episodes
- Accepting the need for mood-stabilizing medications for symptom control
- Distinguishing between the patient's personality and his/her bipolar symptoms
- Recognizing and learning to cope with stressful life events that trigger recurrences of mania or depression
- Reestablishing functional family relationships after a mood episode

triggers for these episodes. A strong case is made for the protective effects of medications and a stable, nonstressful family environment.

For patients with syndromal bipolar disorder, FFT is usually given in 21 outpatient sessions lasting 1 hour each. Sessions are given weekly for 3 months, biweekly for 3 months, and monthly for 3 months. Although the 21-session version is described here, shorter versions have been developed for high-risk populations: children at risk for bipolar disorder (12 sessions over 4 months) (Miklowitz et al., 2013) and adolescents/young adults at risk for psychosis (18 sessions over 6 months) (Schlosser et al., 2012).

This 9 month, 21-session structure was originally proposed by Falloon, Boyd, and McGill (1984) for the behavioral treatment of families of patients with schizophrenia. The session-by-session plan is more a guide for the clinician than a requirement because some families require less intensive contact at the beginning, others require more intensive contact later, and still others simply do not need this much treatment. The treatment is designed to parallel stages of recovery from a mood episode. During the stabilization phase, about seven sessions are devoted to psychoeducation, in which patients and their relatives become acquainted with the nature, course, and treatment of bipolar disorder. At this stage, patients are often still symptomatic and usually are functioning socially or occupationally at a level lower than their preepisode capabilities (Keck et al., 1998). Psychoeducation is an attempt to hasten clinical stabilization by reducing the family tensions that often accompany the stabilization phase. This is done through helping a patient and his/her family members make sense of the different events that have precipitated the acute episode, come to a common understanding of the causes and the treatment of the illness, develop plans for how the family will act if there are signs of a developing recurrence, and modulate expectations for the patient's and the family's functioning in the recovery period.

Once the family has begun the communication training module (seven to 10 sessions), the patient is usually fully stabilized from the acute episode, although he/she may still have residual mood symptoms. At this point, the patient is usually able to tolerate exercises oriented toward resolving family conflict and promoting behavior change. For example, he/she can practice listening while another family member speaks, and family members can do the same for him/her. These exercises can be difficult when a patient's emotions are still dysregulated, but the structure introduced by communication training can help the patient modulate how he/she expresses emotions.

During the final phase, problem-solving training (four to five sessions), the mood episode is largely remitted and the patient has moved into the maintenance phase of drug treatment. At this stage, and sometimes even earlier, the patient and family are motivated to identify and address quality-of-life issues that have been disrupted by the illness (e.g., how a married/cohabiting patient can find work; how parents can help a young adult offspring move out of the home and gradually become more independent). The last few sessions of FFT, held monthly, help to consolidate gains made during the 9-month treatment.

Setting

FFT has been done in a variety of outpatient settings, such as the Child and Adolescent Mood Disorders Program (CHAMP) at the UCLA School of Medicine; the Didi Hirsch Community Mental Health Services in Culver City, California; the Colorado Family Project in Boulder, Colorado; the Pediatric Bipolar Disorders program at Stanford University; and the Child and Adolescent Bipolar Services program at the University of Pittsburgh School of Medicine.

UCLA-CHAMP specializes in the treatment of adolescents and children who are on the bipolar spectrum (bipolar I, bipolar II, or BD-NOS). The staff comprises faculty members in psychology and psychiatry, psychiatry fellows and psychology interns, marriage and family therapists, and psychology graduate students. The clinic, opened in January 2010, evaluates 10–12 new patients and families per month.

Client Variables

FFT is conducted with patients with bipolar disorders (bipolar I, bipolar II, or BD-NOS) who live with (or in close proximity to) their parents, siblings, or, for adults, spouses/partners. Patients can be of any age. Family participants can also include combinations of parental and spousal relatives, or divorced parents of the person with bipolar disorder. In the latter case, we may conduct some of the sessions with the patient and one parent and other sessions with the patient and the other parent.

Patients with bipolar disorder can present as manic, mixed, hypomanic, depressed, or rapid cycling. The polarity of the most recent episode, however, is a moving target—it may change before the patient is seen next. Patients who are manic or hypomanic, particularly those who are elated and grandiose, are often in denial about whether they are really ill, and may believe that the disorder and its treatment are simply ways for others to control them. Depressed patients may be more motivated for psychosocial treatment but may have cognitive difficulty assimilating the educational content of sessions. Patients with a mixed episode or rapid-cycling bipolar disorder can be candidates for FFT. Any of these presentations may require emergency interventions such as changes in medications or hospitalization during treatment. Although there is no contraindication for offering FFT to patients who have been symptomatically recovered for lengthy periods, in our experience, they and their family members are less motivated for treatment than those who have recently coped with a mood episode.

Patients with comorbid alcohol or other substance use disorders pose special problems. These patients are usually resistant to psychosocial treatment and medication. They are also difficult to diagnose; the effects of drugs or alcohol can mimic the cycling of a mood disorder. Generally, patients with active substance use disorders are more successfully treated if they are "dry" before FFT commences. It is often necessary to supplement FFT with chemical dependency programs (e.g., dual-diagnosis Alcoholics Anonymous groups). Nonetheless, a protocol for treating adolescents with bipolar disorder and substance abuse has been developed (Goldstein, Goldstein, & Miklowitz, 2008; Miklowitz, 2012).

Concurrent Drug Treatment

We require that our patients be seen simultaneously by a psychiatrist, who monitors the patient's medications. Typically, a regimen includes a primary mood stabilizer, usually lithium carbonate, divalproex sodium (Depakote), or lamotrigine (Lamictal). The choice of these mood stabilizers is at least in part a function of whether the patient presents with clear-cut episodes of euphoric mania, in which case lithium is often recommended. Lamotrigine is increasingly used for bipolar depression. More and more, we are seeing patients treated with atypical antipsychotics (risperidone [Risperdal], quetiapine [Seroquel], aripiprazole [Abilify], ziprasidone [Geodon], or olanazapine [Zyprexa]) as either primary mood stabilizing agents or adjuncts to traditional mood stabilizers. There is strong evidence that these agents are highly effective in controlling mania (Scherk, Pajonk, & Leucht, 2007), and some (notably, quetiapine) have antidepressant properties as well (Malhi et al., 2009). These agents are particularly valuable if the patient is highly agitated or psychotic. Antidepressants (e.g., paroxetine [Paxil], venlafaxine [Effexor], bupropion [Wellbutrin]) are still recommended as adjuncts to mood stabilizers or atypical antipsychotics if the patient's depression does not remit, but they are given sparingly because of the risk of switching from depression into manic, mixed, or rapid-cycling states (Altshuler et al., 1995) and, in children, a concern about a slightly increased risk of suicidal ideation or behaviors (Vitiello & Swedo, 2004). However, there is little evidence that antidepressants cause mania among patients with bipolar depression who are simultaneously treated with mood stabilizers or atypical antipsychotic agents (Sachs et al., 2007).

A core principle of FFT is that the family therapist must have regular contact with the patient's psychiatrist. This contact is established early in treatment. A close affiliation between the psychosocial and pharmacological treatment team enhances the likelihood of the patient's remaining compliant with his/her medications; it also decreases the likelihood of "splitting," or the tendency for a patient (or even family members) to have a "good doctor" and a "bad doctor." For example, patients frequently complain about their physicians and say to their FFT clinicians, "I wish you could just monitor my medications." An FFT clinician who has a regular dialogue with a patient's physician can avoid the trap that is being set by encouraging the patient to bring up these problems with the physician directly.

Some patients who refuse all medications assume that coming to therapy will be a substitute for drug treatment. These patients often have had bad experiences with pharmacotherapy and psychiatrists, and may also believe that they are not ill, or that the illness they do have can be treated using "alternative medicine." We have generally taken a hard line with these patients and do not accept them into FFT unless they commit to standard pharmacotherapy (usually lithium, anticonvulsants, and/or atypical antipsychotics). Patients with bipolar disorder who are unmedicated are highly likely to have relapses, and it is not in their best interests for the clinician to imply that their illness can be managed with psychosocial treatment alone.

Therapist Variables

In our UCLA and Colorado studies, therapists' ages have ranged from 23 to 55 years, with from 1 to 30 years of clinical experience. The majority have been graduate students in clinical psychology or psychology interns, psychiatry fellows, or postdoctoral psychology fellows. Few have had extensive background in family therapy before learning FFT. The 15-site STEP-BD program involved both therapists with doctorates and social workers who varied considerably in treatment experience. In other words, there is no requirement that an FFT therapist has to have a certain amount of clinical training at the outset.

Although there have been no studies of therapist variables as predictors of the outcome of FFT, our clinical experience has been that two variables influence the uptake of this intervention. The first is the ability to think of a family or couple as a system in which members are interdependent and mutually influence other members' behaviors. Therapists who have trouble with FFT often have difficulty making the transition to this systemic way of thinking. They tend, for example, to conduct family sessions as if they were individual sessions, with one patient and several observers. Some of these same problems arise in learning other forms of family therapy.

The second positive predictor is the willingness to think *biopsychosocially*—that is, to see bipolar disorder as a biologically based illness that requires medications, even if its symptoms are partially evoked by concurrent stressors. Thus, a therapist often must argue for the patient's drug adherence even when psychosocial issues are more interesting and seem more pressing.

We have found that the following training protocol works well for learning FFT. First, therapists attend an FFT workshop conducted over 1–2 days. Then, they begin attending group supervision sessions in which trained FFT therapists discuss their cases, and in which they are able to observe sessions (or listen to tapes). They read the published treatment manual (Miklowitz, 2008b) and, when relevant, the adapted manuals for adolescents with BD or children at risk for BD. Then they serve as cotherapists to trained FFT therapists. After treating two cases with close supervision, they are usually ready to see families or couples independently, or even take on trainees themselves.

The cotherapy model has several advantages for training. It has a long history in the family therapy literature (see, e.g., Napier & Whitaker, 1988). Cotherapists have a way of keeping their fellow therapists on track. Also, if one person appears to be feeling "ganged up on" by one clinician and other family members, the other therapist can bridge the gap by allying him/herself with this family member. In-session dialogue between the clinicians can also provide effective modeling of communication skills for members of a family or couple.

PRETREATMENT ASSESSMENTS

Diagnostic Evaluation

Bipolar disorder is becoming an increasingly common diagnosis in inpatient and outpatient community settings. Although this is a positive development given its underidentification in the past, there is also an element of sloppiness in modern diagnostic evaluations. Nowhere is this more obvious than in the diagnosis of children and adolescents, who are now being called "bipolar" with little supporting evidence (Carlson et al., 2009). The inadequacy of community diagnostic evaluations derives in part from inadequate insurance reimbursement for the evaluation phases of patients' treatment. Some of the patients referred to us have been more aptly diagnosed as having cyclothymic disorder, borderline personality disorder, or even MDD. Many adolescents are referred with "rage attacks." Our colleagues in community practice have often noted the same problems when patients who presumably have bipolar disorder are referred to them.

Upon seeing a new patient, a clinician often finds it useful to determine the reliability of the diagnosis with a formal assessment, using all or part of a structured diagnostic interview. Within our research protocols, we have used the Structured Clinical Interview for DSM-IV—Patient Version (SCID; First, Spitzer, Gibbon, & Williams, 1995) as the diagnostic assessment device. The SCID is well described elsewhere (Spitzer, Williams, Gibbon, & First, 1992). When the patient is under age 18, we use the Schedule for Affective Disorders and Schizophrenia for School-Age Children—Present and Lifetime Version (K-SADS-PL), with the accompanying K-SADS Depression and Mania Rating Scales (Axelson et al., 2003; Chambers et al., 1985; Kaufman et al., 1997). The K-SADS-PL requires separate interviews with the child and at least one parent, followed by consensus ratings of each symptom item.

These instruments are being updated for DSM-5 to include changes such as the addition of disruptive mood dysregulation disorder or the broader definition of autism spectrum disorders.

Some of the factors that can affect the reliability of the data obtained from the SCID or K-SADS-PL include whether the patient is acutely ill or stable; acutely ill patients are less reliable in their symptom reports. Typically, patients in a manic state minimize their symptoms, whereas depressed patients may do the reverse. Patients with bipolar disorder also have trouble with retrospective reporting: "I've had over 1,000 episodes" and "I've been constantly manic–depressed since I was an infant" are common responses to diagnostic interviews.

Whether one uses the structured or an open-ended clinical interview, it is often difficult to determine whether a patient's mood dysregulations and associated changes in activity are at the subsyndromal or syndromal levels. Some patients report brief periods of hypomania or irritability that alternate with more severe depressions. These brief, activated periods do not always reach the DSM duration threshold for hypomania (4 days or more), especially among children and teens. In some cases, the patient is "one symptom short." Some of these patients are better characterized as having cyclothymic disorder or MDD. For children with manic symptoms who do not meet the duration or symptom count criteria, the diagnosis of BD-NOS is often given.

Hagop Akiskal (1996) has encouraged clinicians to consider a broader bipolar spectrum that includes core temperamental disturbances, including hyperthymia (exuberance, overoptimism, grandiosity, stimulus seeking, physical intrusiveness with others) or "sub-bipolar dysthymia." In FFT, the broadening of the bipolar spectrum to include these patients introduces a quandary: Does the clinician proceed with such patients in the same way as with patients with bipolar I or bipolar II disorder? How does the clinician educate the patient and family about the factors that bring about manic or depressive episodes if discrete episodes cannot be identified? If a patient has never had a full manic episode, should the therapist proceed under the assumption that the patient eventually will develop mania spontaneously? Do the same self-management techniques (e.g., using problem solving to minimize family conflict) apply?

Our general impression has been that patients who do not go through clear-cut cycles of mood episodes comprise a different population of patients than those with true bipolar disorder. Therefore, before we recommend a course of FFT, we require that there be evidence of an episodic course of illness, even if at the subthreshold level. Nonetheless, psychosocial interventions almost certainly have a role to play in the stabilization of patients with these broad spectrum presentations, an important direction for future research.

Mood Chart

Clarity on the diagnosis, as well as the patient's progress in treatment, is aided by asking the patient to keep a daily mood chart. One such instrument, the Social Rhythm Metric (Monk, Kupfer, Frank, & Ritenour, 1991), asks the patient to document daily mood on a –5 (*Depressed*) to +5 (*Euphoric/activated*) scale, along with social routines that may influence these moods (e.g., sleep–wake times, times when the patient socializes, the intensity of this social stimulation, the patient's exercise habits, and other factors).

Leverich and Post (1998) have developed a self-rated "life chart" that requires the patient to keep track of daily mood variations, medications, life stressors, and sleep. Data from mood/activity charts help the clinician and patient to evaluate collaboratively the type of cycling the patient experiences and the degree to which social stressors contribute to mood fluctuations. Figure

11.1 is an example of a mood chart; note the cycling of the disorder in relation to specific social stressors and sleep patterns reported by the patient. In this example, a stressor (a pet's illness) is associated with sleep disruption and the appearance of mixed mood symptoms at the subsyndromal level.

Family Assessments

FFT begins with a thorough assessment of family attitudes and behaviors to identify the targets of intervention. The research studies at UCLA have begun with the Camberwell Family Interview, the instrument for rating EE discussed earlier. This interview, usually done when the patient is acutely symptomatic, focuses on the prior 3-month period, which usually includes the prodromal phases of symptom buildup. The interview yields answers to the following questions: What is the current level of tension in the household and in the relative–patient relationship? Which of the patient's behaviors are eliciting stimuli for family arguments or hostility? Do family members understand that the patient has bipolar disorder, or are they likely to attribute the patient's negative behaviors to internal or controllable factors?

A problem with the EE/Camberwell Family Interview method is its lack of exportability to community

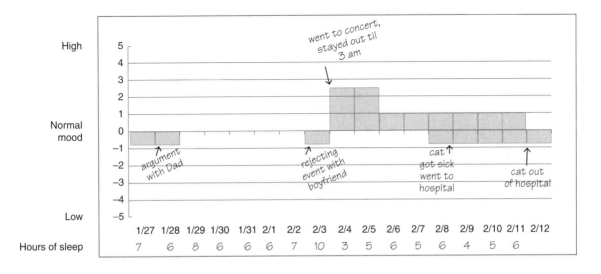

FIGURE 11.1. Example of a self-rated mood chart.

care settings. Interviews with two parents can total 3 hours, and the coding of interview tapes can add an additional 6 person-hours per family. If a clinician's purpose is treatment planning rather than research, he/she may be able to substitute a self-report measure such as the Perceived Criticism Scale (Hooley & Teasdale, 1989). This measure simply asks the patient to rate, on a 1- to 10-point scale, the degree to which close relatives express critical comments toward him/her, and the degree to which he/she expresses critical comments toward relatives. We evaluated the predictive validity of this scale in a sample of 360 bipolar adults followed over 1 year (Miklowitz, Wisniewski, Miyahara, Otto, & Sachs, 2005). The degree to which patients reported being upset or distressed by criticism from relatives was a strong predictor of their levels of depression over a 1-year prospective period. Interestingly, the *amount* of criticism they perceived from relatives was not prognostically significant.

In our research protocols, we typically bring the family in for an interactional assessment before treatment is initiated. First, each member of the family, including the patient, identifies one or several family problem topics. Then, the family discusses one or more of these topics while the clinician observes through a one-way mirror. Transcripts of these 10-minute problem-solving discussions can then be coded using manuals such as the Category System for Coding Partner Interactions (Hahlweg et al., 1989) or the Global Assessment of Relational Functioning (Dausch, Miklowitz, & Richards, 1996).

The clinician can also rely on simple observations of the family's communication and problem-solving behavior to inform the skills training modules of FFT. To quote Yogi Berra, "You can observe a lot by just watching." First, many family members or patients are unable to focus on a single problem, and instead "cross-complain" or accuse other family members to counteract the accusations directed at them. Some engage in attack–counterattack cycles. For any particular family, the clinician must first identify the form these interchanges take, which dyadic or triadic relationships they involve; the content areas that trigger the interchanges (e.g., medication-taking habits, independence, interpersonal boundaries); and whether members of the family are able to stop these cycles before they spiral out of control. Who criticizes whom, and how often? How does the target person respond? Does the original problem ever get solved? How clear (or disorganized) is the speech of patients or relatives?

PROCESS OF TREATMENT

Psychoeducation

Table 11.2 summarizes the topical domains that are covered in FFT. The initiation of the psychoeducation module of FFT requires three conditions. First, the patient must be seeing a psychiatrist and have begun a medication regimen. Second, a diagnostic assessment must have been completed. Third, the patient must be able to tolerate family sessions. There is no requirement that the patient be in remission or recovery.

TABLE 11.2. Family-Focused Treatment: Structure and Topical Outline

I. Psychoeducation

The symptoms and course of bipolar disorder
- The signs and symptoms of (hypo)mania and depression
- The development of the most recent mood episode
- The role of life events in most recent episode
- The course of the disorder over time

The etiology of bipolar disorder
- The vulnerability–stress model
  o The role of stress
  o Genetic and biological predispositions
- Risk and protective factors in the course of the disorder

Interventions and self-management
- Keeping a mood chart
- Types of medications
- Types of psychosocial treatments
- How the family can help
- Self-management of the disorder
- The relapse prevention drill

II. Communication enhancement training
- Expressing positive feelings
- Active listening
- Making positive requests for change
- Expressing negative feelings

III. Problem-solving skills training
- Define problems
- Generate solutions
- Evaluate advantages/disadvantages
- Choose one or a combination of solutions
- Develop an implementation plan
- Review the problem's status

In the seven or more weekly sessions that comprise the psychoeducation module, participants (patients and their close relatives) become acquainted with the symptoms of bipolar disorder; the way episodes develop; the roles of genetics, biology, and stress; pharmacological treatments; and the role of stress management strategies.

The Initial Sessions: Providing a Rationale

As in most other forms of therapy, the clinicians begin by explaining the rationale for FFT. Many participants ask why family or couple sessions should accompany medication for a patient adjusting to a recent episode of bipolar disorder. Particularly helpful in orienting participants is the "reentry model" (Miklowitz, 2008b, p. 104):

An episode of mood disorder can be quite traumatic to all members of the family. . . . In bipolar disorder, when the person returns home and begins to recover, there is a "getting reacquainted" period in which everyone has to get to know everyone else again, and when everyone tries to make sense of what happened. This is a tough time for any family, and part of our purpose here is to make this "reacquaintance period" less disturbing to all of you. We'd like during this year to get you, as a family, back to where you were before _____ became ill. We want to give you some tools to deal with this recovery period.

There are two purposes for this introduction. First, it communicates to the family members that their emotional reactions to the patient's illness—even if quite negative—are normal and expectable. Second, it implies that the therapy will include exploration and clarification of participants' emotional reactions to information about the disorder. This feature of the therapy can be made even more explicit:

If feelings come up for you when we're discussing this material, please bring them up. We're interested in knowing how this material applies to you and your own experiences. You may or may not agree with some of the material we present here. . . . The purpose of focusing on this material is to put your experiences into a context that will make sense. (p. 110)

Next, the treatment is previewed:

We're going to work with you on two different levels. One is on encouraging _____'s ongoing work with his psychiatrist so that he can get himself stabilized on medications. The second is on how you as a family can minimize stress. . . . We think there are several ways to do this, including acquainting you with the facts about bipolar disorder, and working with you on improving your communication and problem solving with each other. These strategies should increase _____'s chances of making a good recovery and help you as a family cope with the disorder. How does this sound to you? (p. 107)

The Symptoms of Bipolar Disorder

FFT proceeds with a series of handouts that are used as stimuli for generating family or couple discussions. These contain descriptions of the symptoms of manic, hypomanic, or depressive episodes, with illustrations. The purpose of these handouts is not for the participants to memorize the diagnostic criteria. Rather, they provide a starting point for destigmatizing the illness and breaking family taboos against talking about it. The patient is asked to look at the lists and describe to family members the way it feels when one is euphoric, irritable, unable to sleep, or activated by racing thoughts or grandiose plans. Likewise, family members describe the behaviors they observe when the patient cycles into mania or hypomania. A similar dialogue is undertaken for depression symptoms. Consider the following dialogue among a patient, mother, father, and therapist.

PATIENT: Well, the thing is, there's the manic and then there's the hypomanic. When I'm manic, I really should be hospitalized. I control the weather; I'm famous. When I'm hypomanic, well, I just can get into that from having too much stress, too much caffeine, and being all revved up. . .

MOTHER: I can tell when she's high because I start getting real mad at her. She provokes me.

FATHER: And she gets this look in her eyes. And she says we're not listening to her. . .

PATIENT: But you're not! That's when you're most likely to tune me out!

THERAPIST: Let's hold on that for now, about listening. It's very important, and certainly something we'll want to focus on as we go along, but what else do you notice when you get manic or hypomanic? [*Redirects the focus.*]

PATIENT: I get sort of, well, reactive. . . I experience

everything so intensely, but see, they know this as who I am.

Note the themes that arise in this discussion of symptoms, and how these relate to the six objectives of FFT outlined in Table 11.1. The patient's vulnerability to recurrences is made explicit by the family's identification of the prodromal signs of her episodes. The patient points to the role of disturbed family communication. She alludes to questions about whether some of her symptoms are really just personality traits (i.e., intensity and reactivity). There is a beginning discussion of stress factors that may play a role in triggering her episodes.

The Vulnerability–Stress Model and the Life Events Survey

Early in psychoeducation, the family clinicians make a strong argument for the conjoint influences of stress, biological imbalances of the brain, and genetic vulnerability in the course of bipolar illness. A handout illustrating these vulnerability–stress interactions is provided, and various risk and protective factors are reviewed. For example, the patient and family members are warned of the impact of "poor sleep hygiene" (i.e., keeping irregular hours, having unpredictable bedtimes); alcohol and drug use; stressful family interchanges; and provocative, overstimulating interpersonal interactions. They are encouraged to make use of available protective factors (e.g., social supports), and help the patient maintain adherence to his/her pharmacotherapy regimen. The purposes of the patient's various medications are given, and the role of blood level monitoring (where relevant) is reviewed. In outlining protective factors, a special emphasis is placed on keeping the family environment low in conflict and on maintaining reasonable performance expectations of the patient during the recovery period. In the following vignette, the clinician reminds the patient and his mother that depression is not the same as lack of effort, and that a period of recovery prior to regaining one's pre-illness occupational status is to be expected.

THERAPIST: (*to Gary, the patient*) I think you can't expect too much just yet. You're still recovering from your episode. It may take some time to get back on track.

MOTHER: How long? He's been like this now for a while.

THERAPIST: I'm sure that's frustrating, but you have to think of this as a convalescent period. When someone has a bad flu, he may need an extra day or two in bed to recover completely. For bipolar disorder, this period of time can average 3 to 6 months. But, Gary, with your medication treatments and our family sessions, and the fact that you've maintained your friendships, I have every expectation that you'll recover and be able to get back to work.

The clinician here offers hope but does not paint a rosy picture of the future. Often the family has been through these episodes before, and a clinician who offers an excessively optimistic view of the future will be dismissed as unrealistic.

Describing the biology and genetics of the disorder is critical to justifying the role of medications. However, it is not necessary for the clinician to go into detail about the neurophysiology of the disorder. Instead, the clinician begins by asking the participants to review their family pedigree and discuss any other persons in the family who have had episodes of depression or mania. In reviewing this history, the family is told that the vulnerability to bipolar disorder may take many forms, including major depression without mania, alcoholism, suicide, and dysthymia. Next, the clinician explains the notions behind neural dysregulation in bipolar disorder:

"We know that people with bipolar disorder have trouble regulating their emotional states, sleep, and arousal, all of which are regulated by the limbic system, an important circuit in your brain. In mania, we think that the limbic system becomes overactive, and the frontal cortex—the 'executive' in your brain—stops being able to do its job. It's almost like having your foot on the gas pedal when the brakes are not working. When a person gets depressed, the system shuts down, and the circuits become underactive. These changes in brain activity can't be controlled through your conscious efforts, but the medications you take can go a long way toward balancing the activity in your nervous system."

When family members begin to attribute the patient's aversive behaviors to willfulness (the "fundamental attributional error"), the clinician can remind them of the existence of neural dysregulation. But the family and patient should also be discouraged from overemphasizing the biological nature of the disorder, to the point of neglecting stress factors such as long-standing family conflicts. In other words, the patient is not entirely taken off of the hook: He/she is encouraged to self-monitor when getting into arguments with family members, and to determine whether his/her reactions to these conflicts reflect an unresolved symptom state or a reemergence of conflicts that would have been troublesome even before he/she became ill.

Clarifying the stress triggers for the most recent episode is aided by a handout describing life changes that may have occurred when the episode was developing. Some of these changes are quite severe and negative (e.g., death of a parent); others are mild but may have provoked changes in sleep–wake cycles (e.g., taking a vacation). The clinician engages the family or couple in a discussion about what stressors may have provoked the patient's current episode, with the caveat that the triggers for mania and depression may be quite different. It is not critical that the participants agree on a singular cause for the most recent episode, but they may benefit from the awareness that mood episodes are affected by environmental as well as neurobiological factors.

The Relapse Drill

Toward the end of psychoeducation, the family and patient are given their first exposure to problem solving. The task is to review the prodromal signs of a developing episode and go through the steps that are necessary to prevent a full relapse. Participants are asked to generate alternative courses of action should the patient relapse into mania or depression, which can include arranging emergency psychiatric services (e.g., calling the patient's psychiatrist), introducing behavioral activation exercises (e.g., assisting the depressed patient in scheduling more outdoor activity during the day). Each family member is asked to perform a function in the relapse prevention plan. For example, in some families it may make sense for a parent to undertake contact with the physician. In others, the patient may want the first opportunity to do so. The family or couple is encouraged to leave phone numbers of emergency contact people, including the family clinicians, in an easily accessible place.

Dealing with Resistance to the Illness Concept

Patients with bipolar disorder often have strong reactions to the psychoeducational materials, as do their family members. These materials require that the participants recognize bipolar disorder as an illness that will eventually recur. Younger patients are particularly likely to reject the notion of a recurrent illness, particularly if they are still hypomanic; they feel powerful and in control, and the idea of having an illness feels like shackles. Moreover, they are particularly attuned to the stigma associated with bipolar disorder or any other psychiatric diagnosis, and fear that their behavior will now be labeled as that of a crazy person. Resistance can also originate with family members. Relatives of depressed patients are apt to see the disorder as willfully caused and not the product of biochemical imbalances. Resistance from one member is often associated with intense family conflicts.

Accepting a psychiatric disorder is a painful process for patients and relatives. Often the psychoeducational materials raise questions, such as "Why me? Why now? What kind of life will I have? Will people treat me like I'm mentally ill from now on? Will I ever get back to normal?" Relatives ask themselves similar painful questions, such as "Will I always have to take care of him/her? Are my dreams and hopes for him/her gone?" Spouses/partners may ask, "Should I leave him/her?" When asking themselves these questions, some patients respond by "underidentifying," or denying the reality of the disorder, or by acknowledging the illness superficially but living their lives as if it were not real.

Others "overidentify" and unnecessarily limit themselves. For example, one woman avoided romantic relationships because "No one will ever be able to get close to me because of my mood swings." Likewise, family members can deny the realities of the disorder or, in contrast, overmonitor the patient's health status and try to limit his/her behavior unnecessarily. Family conflict reaches a maximum when there is a mismatch between coping styles, such as when patients underidentify and relatives overidentify, or the reverse.

FFT clinicians proceed with a sensitivity to the painful emotional issues underlying these reactions to the illness. One method for dealing with these reactions is to predict that denial will occur, and to reframe it as a sign of health. For example, consider a young man with hypomania who has accepted taking medications but denies being ill, and whose parents overcontrol and overmonitor his behavior. To this young man, the clinician might say:

"Although I appreciate that you're taking medication and going along with the treatment plan, I'm going to guess that you're not always going to want to do this. You probably have some questions about whether this diagnosis is right for you or whether you'll have more symptoms. I can understand why you'd have these questions. Coming to terms with having bipolar disorder—or really any illness—is a very painful process that can be hard to accept. This is a normal and a healthy struggle. So, as we're going through our material, you may find yourself reacting to it and feeling that it can't be relevant to you. But I'd like for you to agree that if you have these reactions, you'll bring them up so we can discuss them."

Note that this intervention has a paradoxical flavor, but that the clinician stops short of actually encouraging the patient to remain resistant or to increase his level of disagreement with the diagnosis. Instead, the clinician reframes this denial as healthy and expectable, and connects it with an underlying emotional struggle.

A second way to intervene is through "spreading the affliction." Being labeled as mentally ill can put a person in a one-down position vis-à-vis other family members, including siblings with whom he/she may already feel competitive. A possible side effect of psychoeducation is the exaggeration of these structural family problems. The clinician can avoid this trap by encouraging other members of the family to discuss their own experiences with depression, anxiety, or other problems. This process can help normalize mood problems and take the patient "off the hot seat."

The following vignette involves Josh, a 25-year-old with a recent manic episode. He reacted strongly because he thought everyone was telling him he was "whacked out." According to Josh, all he had done was "party too much." During one of the psychoeducation sessions, his father admitted to having had a depressive episode in college.

THERAPIST: Josh, you seem like you're reacting to something I just said about bipolar disorder. Were you offended?

JOSH: I dunno. It wasn't anything you said; just I get tired of being the only one in the family who has problems.

THERAPIST: Is that really true? Has anyone else in the family ever had any problems with depression? Or what I've called mania?

FATHER: (pause) I did, and I've told Josh about this. Remember what I told you about college?

JOSH: (sullen) I don't know. Why don't you clue us in?

FATHER: I had that long period when I couldn't sleep and eat, and I couldn't study. I dropped out for a semester.

The session then focused on the father and his own history of depression. He revealed a history of psychosis involving delusional thinking. Although the patient was sullen at first, he became more cooperative in the discussions that followed, and more willing to talk about how the illness label made him feel stigmatized.

A third method of dealing with resistance involves making analogies to medical disorders. The illness will feel less stigmatizing to patient and family if they can see it within the continuum of other kinds of chronic physical illness. Diabetes and hypertension are often good comparisons, particularly because the influence of stress can also be brought to bear:

"Bipolar disorder involves biological imbalances much like hypertension does, and it's affected by stress in much the same way. Most people have changes in blood pressure when something stressful happens. But people with hypertension have a vulnerability to extreme shifts in their blood pressure. In the same way, most people have mood changes when something important happens, but people with bipolar disorder operate at greater extremes."

In making these analogies, the clinician validates the patient's feelings about social stigma:

"Although there are some similarities with illnesses like hypertension, bipolar disorder can be tougher to live with because other people tend to be afraid of it and don't know what it means. They can think you're doing it on purpose. You have to take the time to educate other people—particularly those people who are most important to you—and explain it in a way that they won't be freaked out by it."

Communication Enhancement Training

The second module of FFT, CET, begins at approximately Session 8 and lasts for about seven or eight sessions (five weekly sessions, followed by two or three biweekly sessions). CET is guided by two assumptions. First, aversive family communication is a common sequel to an episode of a psychiatric illness and to a large extent reflects distress within the family or couple in members' attempts to deal with the disorder. Second, the frequency of aversive communication can be reduced through skills training.

CET uses a role-playing format to teach patients and their relatives four communication skills: expressing positive feelings, active listening, making positive requests for changes in others' behaviors, and giving negative feedback. These skills are central to the behavioral family management approach to schizophrenia of Falloon and colleagues (1984) and Liberman, Wallace, Falloon, and Vaughn (1981). The degree to which each of these skills dominates the role-play exercises varies according to the family assessments conducted earlier. Treatment of a family with much heated conflict and high-EE attitudes might focus on adaptive ways in which participants could ask for changes in each other's behaviors. Treatment of an emotionally disengaged couple might focus on positive feedback and listening skills to coax the partners into experimenting with a more interdependent relationship.

The module begins with an explication of the CET method for the family:

> A person can be at risk for another relapse of bipolar disorder if the home environment is tense. . . . Good communication and problem solving can be among those "protective factors" against stress that we talked about before. For a close relative, learning effective communication skills can be a way of decreasing tension and improving family relationships. . . . We want to help you communicate in the most clear and the least stressful way possible. . . . We'll be asking you to turn your chairs to each other and practice new ways of talking among yourselves. (Miklowitz, 2008b, pp. 208)

Note that CET is linked with two of the six objectives of the larger treatment program: helping participants to cope with stress triggers and restoring functional family relationships after an illness episode. The first two skills, positive feedback and active listening, generally foster a feeling of collaboration between members of the couple or family. In contrast, making positive requests for change and giving negative feedback are more conflict-oriented, and are only introduced once participants are used to the role-playing and behavioral rehearsal format.

For each skill, the clinician gives participants a handout that lists the skill's components (e.g., for active listening: make good eye contact, nod your head, ask clarifying questions, paraphrase/check out what you heard). Then the clinician models the skill for the family. For example, the clinician might compliment one member of the family for his/her cooperativeness with the treatment, or model effective listening while another family member talks about a problem. After the skill is introduced and modeled, participants are asked to practice the skill with each other, with coaching and shaping by the clinician. Typically the therapist coaches one participant at a time on appropriate ways to use a given skill. The feedback of other family members is actively solicited. The speaker or listener is then asked to try the skill again, until he/she has approximated its use. A homework assignment, in which participants keep a written log of their efforts in using the skills between sessions, facilitates generalization of the learning process to the home and work settings.

Many times, the skills are harder than they look. Consider Jessie, a 38-year-old woman with bipolar disorder who had had several episodes of psychotic mania and also a borderline level of mental retardation. She worked part-time as a gift wrapper in a department store. Jessie was trying to move into her own apartment and required help finding a moving van. She was instructed to learn to make positive requests of her father, with whom she and her sister lived.

THERAPIST: Maybe that's a good topic to ask your dad about. Can you look at this "Positive Requests" handout and use these steps to ask your dad to help you move?

FATHER: It won't help. There won't be anything to move because she still hasn't packed a single box! (*Laughs.*)

JESSIE: Well, get me the damn boxes and I'll do it.

THERAPIST: (*derailing this interchange*) Do you think you could ask your dad for something specific, like helping you find a moving company?

JESSIE: (*Looks at father, smirking.*) Dad, will you help me find a moving company? (*Giggles.*)

FATHER: (*more serious*) You're not. . . you're not looking at this. (*Indicates handout.*) You're supposed to say, "I'd appreciate it if you would. . ."

JESSIE: (*Shrugs.*) All right, I'd appreciate it if you would! Get me a phone number. Please.

THERAPIST: (*after a pause*) Well, you got part of it that time, Jessie. Dad, what did you like about what she just said to you?

FATHER: (*sarcastically*) Gee, all the sincerity.

JESSIE: (*Laughs nervously.*)

THERAPIST: Well, if you didn't care for it, can you say how she might say it to you?

FATHER: How about something like "I'd appreciate it if you'd get me those phone numbers. It'd make it a lot more comfortable for me to plan my move."

THERAPIST: Nice job, Dad. Jessie, what did your dad do that you liked or didn't like?

JESSIE: He followed the sheet. He did all the things you said.

THERAPIST: True, but you don't have to say it exactly the way he did. You can put your own spin on it. Do you feel you could try doing it one more time?

JESSIE: (*Gasps, giggles.*)

THERAPIST: I know it's hard being in the hot seat. But you're doing fine. Keep trying.

JESSIE: Dad, could you get me those phone numbers of the movers? I'd appreciate it. That way I could be. . . I wouldn't have to worry about the move, and, well, just thank you for your help.

THERAPIST: That was very good, Jessie. Dad, how did you like it that time?

FATHER: (*a little tentative*) That was better. It made a lot more sense.

These kinds of skills are most difficult to learn if the patient is highly symptomatic and/or cognitively impaired, or if the level of conflict in the family is so severe that productive conversations cannot ensue. This patient was moderately hypomanic and also had limited intellectual resources. Clearly, the skills training taxed her and made her nervous. However, with patience and practice, Jessie was able to adopt some of the communication skills, and her relationship with her father gradually improved. Her father, who was often quite critical, became more and more convinced that her limited functioning was a result of her bipolar disorder rather than lack of effort, as he had believed previously.

The FFT manual (Miklowitz, 2008b) describes "short-fuse" families. These families begin with apparently innocuous discussions, which quickly escalate into angry, back-and-forth volleys of criticism or hostility. Our research indicates that these are usually high-EE families or couples, but not invariably (Simoneau et al., 1998). We have been surprised that relatives who, on the surface, appear benign and supportive of the pa-

tient during the EE/Camberwell Family Interview become quite aggressive and confrontational when facing the patient in a one-to-one interaction. Not surprisingly, the likelihood that this will occur is greatly augmented if the patient is hypomanic and irritable. Short-fuse families typically have difficulty with communication training because the participants' emotions quickly get out of hand (see the case study presented later). But much can be accomplished by modifying the skills training to the family's natural styles. For example, the therapist can encourage the participants to use active listening skills during their arguments. After a negative, back-and-forth interchange involving a couple, a clinician said:

"I think this is an important discussion. You're a couple that really likes to get things out in the open. But I'm afraid that you're missing out on each other's viewpoints. So let's see if we can make it more productive. I want you each to paraphrase each other's statements before making your next argument, like we did in the active listening exercises. Also, why don't you turn your chairs to each other so that you can more easily keep eye contact?"

Note again the use of reframing. It is better to cast a couple's or family's ongoing dynamics (unless clearly abusive or threatening) as an adaptive way of coping that needs modification than to label these dynamics as "bad" or "dysfunctional."

A short-fuse family may also be able to make good use of positive requests for change or negative feedback exercises, in which the partners make constructive suggestions about specific aspects of each other's behavior (e.g., "I don't like it when you talk down to me about my health habits") and offer suggestions as to ways these behaviors could be improved (e.g., "Could you be more aware of your tone of voice?"). These exercises often set the stage for problem solving, the final module of FFT.

Problem-Solving Skills Training

Families of patients with bipolar disorder often have difficulty with problem solving, especially if the patient has recently been ill (e.g., Simoneau et al., 1998). Family problems in adjusting to the postepisode phases of bipolar disorder appear to fall into one of four categories: medication nonadherence, difficulty resuming prior work and social roles, repairing the financial and social damage done during manic episodes ("life trash-ing"), and relationship/living situation conflicts.

In FFT, the purposes of problem solving are three-fold: (1) to open a dialogue among family members about difficult conflict topics; (2) to allow them a con-text in which to share their emotional reactions to these problems; and (3) to help them develop a framework for defining, generating, evaluating, and implementing ef-fective solutions to problems. This module occupies the final four to five sessions of FFT, and usually begins by the fourth or fifth month, when sessions have been ta-pered to biweekly. Problem solving is positioned last in FFT because the patient is usually in remission by this point and is more able, both cognitively and emotion-ally, to experiment with new ways of behaving. Fur-thermore, if the psychoeducation and CET have gone well, family members are more ready to see their own role in generating or maintaining family conflicts and are more open to hearing each other's viewpoints.

In problem solving, families are taught to break broad problems down into smaller units that are more amenable to solution. Family members are given a problem-solving worksheet in which they are asked to take the following steps: define the problem (with each participant's input); "brainstorm" all possible solutions without evaluating them; consider each solution indi-vidually and weigh its advantages and disadvantages; choose a best solution or combination of solutions; and plan and implement the chosen solutions. Once they have had at least a moderately successful experience in solving a relatively minor problem, participants are given a homework task in which they record their at-tempts to solve a new, larger problem. Assignments are sometimes quite modest; some families are simply given the task of defining one or more problems to work on in the upcoming session.

The rationale for problem solving is presented as fol-lows:

> Up until now, we've been talking mainly about how you communicate with each other. Now we'd like to deal with some of the concrete problems of living you've all been alluding to. But rather than our just giving you suggestions about what to do about these—which prob-ably wouldn't work that well anyway—we'd like to teach you a way of solving problems cooperatively, as a family. (Miklowitz, 2008b, pp. 259)

This rationale is then followed by a review of the steps for solving problems and familiarizing the family or couple with a problem-solving worksheet. The clini-cian also reviews some of the problems the members raised during earlier phases of treatment.

Consider this case example of the problem-solving method. Karla, age 35, moved in with her new boy-friend, Taki, shortly after her divorce. She was in poor shape financially; she had a tendency to "spend to im-prove my self-esteem." In fact, most of her spending sprees occurred during hypomanic periods, and Karla had become hypomanic shortly after meeting Taki, who was quite well off. Perhaps due to eagerness to make the relationship work, he gave Karla access to his credit cards. During their first months together, his bills increased hugely. Karla's own employment was inconsistent. She had had trouble for years keeping to a budget and maintaining a checking account. They had begun to fight heavily about this problem. Karla argued that money was his way of controlling women, and Taki argued that she was taking advantage of him and being inconsiderate.

First, the clinician returned to the communication enhancement exercises. He encouraged the couple to expand on these broader issues before zeroing in on the more specific problem of spending. Karla voiced her opinion about what she felt was the "meat of the problem," while Taki listened. Then Taki described his take on the underlying issues, while Karla listened and paraphrased. The structure imposed by problem solv-ing eventually helped them define the issue more spe-cifically: Karla spent more on clothing and "comfort items" than either of them thought she should, but it was unrealistic for her to try to support herself given her unresolved symptomatic state. Various options were then considered: Taki doing most of the buying, Karla being assigned her own account with an upper limit negotiated each month, and the two of them sim-ply separating their finances. These and other options were evaluated as to their advantages and disadvantag-es. Finally, they agreed on a somewhat complicated but clever solution: Karla was to obtain three bank debit cards assigned to each of three accounts. Each card was labeled with an expense item (e.g., "doctor bills") and had a spending limit posted on it. They were to meet weekly to determine whether the solution was working, and to practice listening skills with each other when they began to disagree.

In this example, the problem was to some degree gen-erated by the patient's residual symptoms. There were also relationship dynamics: Karla tended to become overly dependent on men and then to devalue them, and

Taki tended to rescue women and then become angry about being in the rescuer role. The clinician decided to let them first "ventilate" about these larger relationship themes. Allowing a certain amount of emotional expression about loaded issues often reduces a family's or couple's resistance to dealing with more specific problems (in this case, disagreements about spending).

When taking families or couples through their first problem-solving exercises, FFT clinicians monitor participants' reactions to the method. Reactions can vary from "This is just what we need" to "Gee, how superficial." Patients with bipolar disorder and their family members seem to crave spontaneity and enjoy fast-paced, unpredictable interchanges. They get bored easily. The communication and problem-solving exercises impose structure and encourage goal-directedness but can also generate resistance. Resistance can take the form of changing the subject, "cross-complaining," or being unwilling to cooperate with the homework tasks.

When addressing resistances, a clinician reiterates the rationale for problem solving (e.g., "Sometimes you have to gain confidence from solving minor problems before you move on to bigger ones"). But often he/she must determine whether it is really the problem-solving method that family members object to or whether there are certain costs or painful consequences associated with attempting to solve a problem (e.g., a mother's fear that her son with bipolar disorder will be unable to handle agreed-upon tasks that require greater independence). Family members who fear the consequences of solving a problem often approach solutions, then quickly abandon the problem-solving process, arguing that "this is not really the issue." The therapist has a number of options available. One is to take responsibility for the unsolved problem. For example, he/she can say, "Perhaps it was wrong of me to encourage you to solve this problem. Maybe you have other things you want to deal with first. Would you like to table it for now?" Alternatively, the clinician may proceed more paradoxically, framing the family's difficulty as due to "healthy avoidance":

"Solving a problem as a family involves some costs–benefits thinking. There are certainly some benefits to solving this problem, but there may be some hidden costs as well. I think if the costs of solving this problem outweigh the benefits, it's certainly understandable that you'd want to avoid putting a solution in place. Is that what's happening here?"

Both of these interventions give the family members "permission" to leave the problem untouched. Later, when the pressure is off, they may be able to return to the problem and have more success the second time around.

Terminating FFT

FFT is terminated after 9 months. As termination approaches, a therapist reviews with the family members the six goals for treatment (discussed earlier) and the degree to which those goals were or were not realized. The status of the patient's bipolar disorder is evaluated relative to that at the beginning of treatment. In some cases, maintenance or "tune-up" FFT sessions are recommended.

Referrals for subsequent treatment for both the patient and other family members are discussed. For example, some patients follow up FFT with individual therapy or mutual support groups involving other persons with bipolar disorder. Family members may choose to attend support groups of the Depressive and Bipolar Support Alliance (*www.dbsalliance.org*) or the National Alliance on Mental Illness (*www.nami.org*). In our experience, it is unusual for families to request additional family or couple therapy after FFT, but referrals are made, if requested.

The clinicians reiterates the importance of continued medication adherence and incorporation of communication and problem-solving skills into the family's day-to-day life. Finally, a review of the relapse drill (see the earlier "Psychoeducation" section) is conducted: The patient's prodromal signs are reviewed, and the steps the patient and family can take to avert a relapse are reiterated.

CASE STUDY

Debra, a 36-year-old European American woman, lived with her husband Barry, age 46, and their 8-year-old daughter Jill. She had completed 2 years of college and worked part time as a sales clerk in a luggage shop. She had been married previously. Debra was referred for FFT by a university clinic, where she had been diagnosed with bipolar II disorder. The initial SCID confirmed this diagnosis. Her depression was marked by loss of interests and "being bummed" for several weeks at a time. She also complained of loss of appetite, waking several times each night, fatigue, guilt, and loss of concentration. She denied having suicidal thoughts. She recounted that her current depression was "a really big one" and had lasted on and off for a full year. Debra also said, "I've had tons of small ones." She dated the first onset of her depression to approximately 8 years earlier, following her divorce from her first husband.

Debra also admitted to having had a hypomanic episode in the previous month, including about 5 days of elevated and irritable mood. She explained, "My confidence level was up." She admitted to racing thoughts, increased activity and talkativeness, and becoming involved in many different projects. She had trouble dating the onset and offset of these periods, noting, "I've been this way all my life." She did admit that Barry had commented on these mood phases. Debra complained, "He now tells me I'm getting manic every time we get in an argument. . . . It's his newest weapon against me." She denied having delusions or hallucinations.

Debra had been treated previously with sertraline (Zoloft) and bupropion (Wellbutrin). Her psychiatrist had recently started her on divalproex sodium (Depakote) at 1,500 mg/day, a medication that she said had made a difference in stabilizing her mood.

Barry, an attorney, presented as a "no-nonsense" type of man. He responded to the clinicians in a very businesslike manner and insisted that he had no problems of his own to discuss "except those that relate to Debra's care." He denied any psychiatric history himself. He preferred to talk about FFT as an educational course and became defensive if his wife referred to it as "therapy." The FFT clinicians, a male–female cotherapy team, did not dissuade him from labeling the treatment this way, believing that they would need to work on building a rapport with him before addressing his defensive style.

Family Assessment

Based on the Camberwell Family Interview, Barry met the criteria for a high level of EE. He voiced nine criticisms during his 1-hour interview. He tended to complain at length about Debra's memory, work habits, and disorganization (e.g., "She never remembers about parent–teacher meetings," "She forgets to turn in her time sheet at work—it drives me crazy"). Barry admitted that he still loved Debra but found her very frustrating. He was convinced that she had ADHD as well as bipolar disorder.

Debra and Barry came in for the family interactional assessment well dressed and smiling. The clinicians interviewed them individually, and arrived at an important problem topic for them to discuss: Barry's claim that Debra lied to him. Her response was to apologize for her past misdeeds and to argue, "I'm not lying or withholding. . . . Those are usually things I've forgotten or just don't think are important." Upon discussing this issue, the couple's dynamics became apparent, with Barry speaking in an accusatory, scolding mode and Debra apologizing and justifying her behavior. As Barry became more accusatory, Debra looked more and more depressed.

BARRY: Lying is a way of life for you. You twist the truth and say you don't remember things.

DEBRA: But I really don't. I've been trying to tell you everything. Sometimes I just forget. (*Starts rocking her chair.*)

BARRY: (*holding Debra's chair still*) Why do you think it's OK to lie to me?

DEBRA: I don't. I'm being up front with you. Maybe you want to believe there's more, but there's not.

BARRY: I think you'll always do this. It's your bag. How would you like it if I lied to you? How would it make you feel? Would you want to stay married to me?

DEBRA: (*sullen*) No, probably not. But I'm trying to be open with my feelings, kinda with you as a practice case. (*Smiles awkwardly.*)

BARRY: You're doing that little smile again. The one you do when you're trying to get away with something.

DEBRA: (*defensive*) Oh, give me a break.

BARRY: Is it because we're talking so directly? I don't know if it's your personality or if it's the bipolar stuff acting up, but you have no tolerance for anything these days, especially people.

The therapists who viewed this assessment were struck by Barry's level of criticism, paired with Debra's tendency to take a one-down position. They also learned during the assessment that Barry doled out Debra's medications and made her doctor appointments for her, and also usually attended them with her. An initial appointment for FFT was set with two clinical psychologists, one of whom was a trainee.

Psychoeducation (Sessions 1–7)

During the initial session, the clinicians (Therapist 1 and Therapist 2 in the dialogues below) described the FFT program to Barry and Debra, with particular emphasis on the psychoeducational component. They previewed the communication enhancement and problem-solving modules. The couple listened politely but expressed skepticism.

BARRY: We've been in and out of therapy for years. I haven't been impressed.

THERAPIST 1: When you say "We," do you mean you as a couple?

BARRY: As a couple, and she's had her own therapy.

DEBRA: I thought Dr. Walker was good.

BARRY: Yeah, but you hadn't had the bipolar diagnosis yet. She was just treating you for depression. And she got into that whole "You were probably abused as a child and forgot about it" thing.

THERAPIST 1: What was your couple therapy like?

BARRY: A lot of digging into our childhoods and getting in touch with our feelings.

THERAPIST 1: Debra?

DEBRA: It wasn't that bad. I thought it was pretty useful.

THERAPIST 1: Well, it sounds like you've got different opinions on how helpful those sessions were. Let me tell you how this will be different. Our treatment is going to be focused mainly on the present, and we'll be working on how you as a couple are coping with bipolar disorder. Barry, you're going to be affected by the cycling of Debra's mood disorder, but Debra, you're also going to be affected by the way Barry responds to your symptoms. I'm not saying your past will be irrelevant, but it's just not our focus.

BARRY: I need help dealing with all of this. The more information I get, the better.

THERAPIST 1: I'm sure that's true. But we won't just throw a lot of information at you—we want to individualize it to your situation. I think you'll have a much easier time if you come to a common understanding of the disorder as a couple and learn to communicate about it.

In this dialogue, the therapist made a distinction between FFT and more generic forms of couple therapy. At this point, the clinicians already suspected that there would be resistance from Barry, especially around

tasks in which he was asked to look at his own behavior and its contribution to Debra's mood problems.

The psychoeducation itself began in the second session and continued through the seventh. The first task was to encourage the couple to come to a shared definition of "bipolar disorder." During the assessments, both had mentioned the term "cycling," but without apparent agreement on what it meant.

THERAPIST 1: I want to be sure we're all on the same page when we talk about the meaning of the term "bipolar." Debra, you did a great job just now of explaining what depression feels like. Let's talk about the other side now. (*Passes around a handout describing the symptoms of mania/hypomania.*) Barry, which of these have you observed when Debra gets hypomanic?

BARRY: (*surveying the handout*) Well, all of these except appetite disturbance. . . . I guess you could say she has grandioseness—she thinks one day she'll be wealthy. (*Laughs.*)

THERAPIST 2: When was the last time you think she was like that?

BARRY: Last time I was working on a case—she always gets like that when I'm working on a case.

DEBRA: I agree, but I think it's because I have a lot more to do when he's working all the time. . . . He thinks it's some "abandonment" thing, but I think he forgets the realities I face when he's gone. (*Looks at list.*) I get more energy, I feel uncomfortable in my own body, I jump outta my skin. . . probably a good day to go shopping! (*Giggles.*) I probably get crankier, don't have much tolerance for people in general.

BARRY: Especially me. (*Smiles.*)

This was the first time that Debra had defended herself, by commenting on how relationship problems fed into her mood swings. Interestingly, her assertive stance cut through some of her husband's negativity. The therapists soon realized that Barry and Debra lacked a consensus about what really constituted a bipolar episode. This is a critical point in FFT: The members of a couple or family need to come to a shared perception of when the patient is getting ill, so that they can institute procedures to keep the patient's episodes from spiraling (e.g., visits to the physician, reduction in the patient's workload, learning to deescalate negative verbal exchanges). But it was not yet clear that Debra had discrete episodes.

THERAPIST 2: Do you think you have what we're calling "episodes"? Like a couple of days of being wired?

DEBRA: There can be, like 2 or 3 days when I can do a lot of stuff, my memory gets better, and then 2 or 3 days when it's just not gonna work. I can. . .

BARRY: (*Interrupts.*) It's that household project thing. She starts redoing Jill's room over and over. She'll sponge-paint it purple and then wipe it out that same evening, put in new closets.

DEBRA: I can filter all my energy into housework instead of killing somebody. (*They both chuckle.*)

THERAPIST 1: Maybe I'm a little slow today, but I'm trying to figure out whether you both agree on when these high and low periods are. Debra, have you ever kept a mood chart?

The therapist then produced a written assignment in which Debra and Barry were asked to track independently, on a daily basis, the ups and downs of Debra's mood states, so that agreements and disagreements about what constituted the symptoms of the disorder (as opposed to personality traits) could be tracked.

The dynamics of this couple became more evident in Sessions 3–5. Debra was inconsistent about keeping her mood chart, and Barry felt that his conscientiousness in charting her mood was not being rewarded. "She won't take responsibility for her illness," he argued. Nonetheless, Debra had good recall of her mood swings, even though she had not written them down. The therapists offered the couple much praise for their somewhat half-hearted attempt to complete this assignment. Interestingly, Barry noted small changes in mood that he called her "manic-ness," which Debra argued were just her reactions to everyday annoyances.

BARRY: You were manic as hell on Saturday morning.

THERAPIST 2: What do you mean, Barry?

BARRY: I went to tell her that Jill needed to get to soccer, and she practically bit my head off!

DEBRA: Because you had told me eight times already. I wasn't manic, I was just getting annoyed. Even Jill said something about you overdoing it.

This became a theme throughout the treatment: Barry tended to overlabel Debra's mood swings, to the extent that he often called her "manic" when the real issue appeared to be her transient irritability. He also frequently called her "depressed" when Debra felt that she was just "relaxing. . . bored. . . trying to unwind and keep to myself for a while." The therapists were careful not to attribute blame or to take sides with either of them. Therapist 1 said:

"I think this is a very hard distinction to make. I wish I could give you a simple rule for determining when Debra is in and out of an episode. But as you've seen, it's not always so clear. I usually suggest that people go back to that symptom list and ask, 'Is there more than one of these symptoms? Does irritability go with more sleep disturbance? Racing thoughts?' Just being annoyed is not enough to be called 'manic,' unless it's ongoing, it cuts across different situations, or it goes along with some of these other symptoms and impairment in getting through your day."

The therapists outlined a vulnerability–stress model for understanding Debra's episodes. Debra recounted a family history of her mother's depression and her father's alcohol abuse: "My mom was probably bipolar, but we just didn't call it that back then." They also discussed eliciting stressors that may have contributed to Debra's prior depressions. Barry became very vocal when discussing her risk factors: He noted that crowded places (e.g., shopping malls) made her hypomanic, and that alcohol, even in small amounts, contributed to her sleep disturbance and in turn contributed to her hypomanias. The therapists offered a handout on risk factors (e.g., substance abuse, sleep irregularity, unpredictable daily routines, family conflict) and protective factors (e.g., regular medications, good family communication). Next, the clinicians helped Barry and Debra devise a relapse prevention plan:

THERAPIST 1: The clients we've worked with who've done best with this illness have been able to rely on their spouses and other close family members at times of crisis. It's a fine line you have to walk between being able to turn to your spouse and say, "I think I'm getting sick again," and to take some of their advice without giving up control altogether. Debra, when your moods are going up and down, you are going to want more control. Barry, maybe you sometimes feel like you're walking a fine line as well: You want to say "Yes, you are getting sick, and I'd like to help you," without rubbing it in, to be able to give suggestions without taking over.

BARRY: That's one thing we have in common. We're both control freaks. I guess likes attract.

THERAPIST 1: Well, maybe the fact that you both like to be in control of your own fate was part of what attracted the two of you in the first place [reframing]. But like many things that attract people initially, something like not wanting to give up control can become a problem in the relationship later.

The partners came to some agreements about what the prodromal signs of Debra's hypomania looked like (e.g., increased interest in household projects, getting up extraordinarily early, irritability that occurred in multiple situations) and some of her risk factors (e.g., alcohol). They conjointly developed a relapse prevention plan that involved keeping emergency phone numbers handy, avoiding alcohol, and avoiding high-stress interpersonal situations (e.g., conflicts between Debra and her mother). Barry and Debra also discussed how they could communicate if her symptoms started to escalate. Barry admitted that he "had to learn not to lash out" at such times, and not to "just blurt out everything I think." Interestingly, both showed resistance to the suggestion that Debra try to maintain a regular sleep–wake cycle, even on weekends, when she had her worst mood swings. Barry scoffed, "Maybe we should just join the Army," and both emphasized that they were not about to give up their love of late-night partying.

The psychoeducation module ended with a discussion of the effects of the illness label on Debra's self-esteem. She had been alluding throughout the first six sessions to her discomfort with the diagnosis of bipolar II disorder.

THERAPIST 1: Sometimes when we go through our symptom lists and talk about the causes of bipolar disorder, people can feel labeled or picked apart. Debra, have you ever felt that way in here?

DEBRA: When I first came in here, I felt picked on. I felt like it was "blame Debbie time," and now there was this real biological reason to pin all our problems on.

THERAPIST 1: I hope you don't think we're saying that all of your problems as a couple stem from your bipolar disorder.

DEBRA: No, I think you guys have been fair about that. It was hard for me to talk about, and sometimes I think Barry is just objecting to me, as a person.

THERAPIST 1: In other words, the line between your personality and your disorder gets blurred.

DEBRA: Yes, and to me they're very different.

THERAPIST 1: I'm glad you're bringing this up. I think that's very important, to be very clear on when we're just talking about you, your styles of relating to people. . . . Not everything you do has to be reduced to this illness.

BARRY: And I probably do bring it up [the illness] too much.

DEBRA: (*becoming activated*) Yes, and you bring it up in front of other people. . . . That can be a real problem for me. We used to have such great conversations! I get tired of talking with you about my disorder all the time. That's all you seem to wanna talk about.

BARRY: (*startled*) Why haven't you told me this?

DEBRA: I probably do need to tell you. . . . I just want more of a happy medium, between talking about it and not.

BARRY: So what do you want?

DEBRA: (*becoming tearful*) I'm not sure.

THERAPIST 1: I think it's understandable that you wouldn't know. . . . You're not always sure how much help you need from Barry. Maybe you're trying to find a good balance. That may take some time. I hope you don't feel that all *we're* interested in is your disorder, and not in you as a person [examines apparent resistance to the psychoeducational material].

DEBRA: I usually don't feel that way, except when I try to do that mood chart [acknowledges emotional pain underlying resistance to the therapeutic tasks]. I just want to have conversations with Barry like I have with my girlfriends. I'd like to talk about things other than my illness and my doctors.

Communication Enhancement Training (Sessions 8–14)

During Session 8, the therapists introduced CET to the couple. Barry and Debra both described a "demand–withdrawal" pattern in their communication. Barry would become intrusive in trying to understand Debra's mood state, and Debra would withdraw and become noncooperative. Debra admitted that she had a difficult time acknowledging being depressed and talking about it because "you just didn't do that in my family." She grew up in a Southern family, where "you didn't air your dirty laundry." In contrast, Barry was from Los Angeles, where "you might spill your guts to whoever was stuck in traffic next to you."

The therapists began by exploring the demand–withdrawal pattern:

THERAPIST 1: This is one of the dynamics we've seen in couples dealing with bipolar disorder. People with a mood disorder can get irritable with their spouses, and then their spouses react because they feel under attack, and when they react, the arguments can really spiral. The person with the disorder feels there's something he/she is legitimately angry about, and the spouse sees the anger as evidence of the bipolar illness.

BARRY: Well, my problem is that Debra's not aware of her symptoms.

DEBRA: I'm aware of them, but I wanna be left alone. You finish my sentences. . .

BARRY: And then you walk out of the room. You don't want to have anything to do with normal communication. It's just like it was with your parents. . .

DEBRA: When I'm in that state [depression], the last thing I want is a serious conversation or to have someone question what I want to do or why.

THERAPIST 2: Let's talk about what happens between the two of you [draws couple back to relationship focus]. When you try to talk about something, what happens? One of you just won't talk? You do talk, but it doesn't go well?

BARRY: She procrastinates, she won't deal with things; then I yell; then she won't be around me and she withdraws; and then I start thinking about how long I can live like this.

THERAPIST 2: Debra, how would you describe it?

DEBRA: Barry gets frustrated when I don't give him the answers he's looking for, and then I feel bad that I frustrated him, and he feels bad that he got upset at me, and then I feel bad that I made him feel bad about upsetting me.

THERAPIST 2: Is that something you'd like to work on—your communication as a couple?

BARRY: Yes. There's been no communication because of the bipolar disorder. I don't know if we'd have these problems if she weren't bipolar. She gets depressed, her thoughts don't get communicated, she never even tries. . . and that reminds me of what I was gonna ask you: Do you think she might have attention deficit disorder as well as being bipolar?

DEBRA: Oh, no, here we go. . .

THERAPIST 1: Barry, no one can tell for sure, but regardless of what the cause is, it sounds like you're ready for us to start focusing more on your relationship [redirects discussion but doesn't directly challenge Barry's definition of the problem]. At least part of what you're describing sounds like the habits you have communicating with each other as a couple. We'll be teaching you some fairly straightforward skills for talking to each other, like how to praise each other for things done well, how to listen, and how to ask for changes in each other's behavior. This will help you during these cycles, whether they be real mood cycles or just rocky periods in your relationship [provides rationale for upcoming communication module].

DEBRA: Yeah, I need to learn how to argue. He's a lawyer; he's a much better arguer than me.

BARRY: (*still angry*) But you see, no one ever said a damn thing in your family; no one was ever really there. So of course you're going to react to me because I'm passionate, and then when I get really pissed off, you finally take stock and listen. It's the only way I can get through to you.

THERAPIST 1: I think there's a lot for us to work with here. Debra, I'd like to take you off the "bipolar hook" for a while, and let's work on how you act and react with each other. We don't have to work on your communication just about bipolar disorder—maybe also how you talk about finances, friends. . .

BARRY: But that's all about doing it in here. . . . How are you gonna know how we communicate at home?

THERAPIST 1: We're gonna bug your house. (*Both chuckle*) We'll do some exercises in here that involve role playing new ways of talking, but you'll have to practice these new ways in between sessions at home. I personally think this will benefit you a great deal, if you have the time to do it [expresses optimism].

The therapists now had a better understanding of this couple's communication patterns. The demand–withdrawal pattern in part derived from their different family histories, but it was equally true that Barry was rewarded for being critical; it got results, even if these results were accompanied by Debra's resentment. They disagreed on the extent to which these communication patterns were driven by her bipolar disorder. Barry assumed that most or all of their problems could be attributed to the disorder, but Debra saw this assumption as just an attempt to blame her for everything. The therapists' take was that the marital dynamics existed independently of Debra's mood swings but became magnified by her hypomanic and depressive episodes. During hypomanic episodes she was more touchy and reactive, and when depressed she was more likely to withdraw.

In Session 9, the therapists began the skills training. FFT begins with positive communication skills to increase the likelihood that members of a couple or family will collaborate when dealing with more difficult issues. One therapist began by introducing a handout entitled Expressing Positive Feelings, in which each partner is directed simply to praise the other for some specific behavior the other has performed, and to tell the partner how this behavior makes him/her feel. The therapists first modeled the skill. One of them praised Barry, saying, "I appreciate you taking the long drive up here [to the clinic] and making an adjustment to your schedule to make this possible. . . . It makes me feel like you value what we do here." Barry expressed appreciation for the compliment. The therapist then asked Barry and Debra to turn their chairs toward each other and select a behavior to praise in each other. Interestingly, neither had trouble selecting a topic. The problem was in staying with positive emotions and not letting negative ones leak in.

BARRY: I appreciated your taking Jill to soccer on Wednesday. It made me feel like you. . . like you knew I was overwhelmed that day, and that, you know, I'm usually the one doing all the parenting while you. . .

THERAPIST 2: (*interrupting*) Barry, I'd like to stop you before we get into that. Debra, can you tell me what you liked so far about how Barry said that? Did he follow the instructions on this sheet?

DEBRA: Well, like you said, he was starting to get into it, but I liked the first part. I'm glad he feels that way.

BARRY: Do you feel I give you enough positive feedback?

DEBRA: (*pause*) You have your days.

THERAPIST 2: Barry, I thought you did that pretty well. Could you try it without the tail at the end?

BARRY: (*Chuckles.*) There you go, stealing my thunder. OK, um, Deb, thanks again for taking Jill to soccer. It made me feel like you. . . like my schedule is important to you, and that you're thinking of me.

THERAPIST 2: Good. Debra, what'd you think?

DEBRA: Much better.

BARRY: Sometimes I think I was put on this earth to learn tact.

Sessions 10 and 11 of CET focused on active listening skills. One member of the couple listened while the other spoke, first about issues outside of the marriage (i.e., work relationships), then about couple-related matters. Both Barry and Debra required restructuring of their listening skills. Specifically, Debra tended to "space out" when Barry spoke, and required prompting to stay with the issues. She acknowledged that she sometimes felt she was being tested by Barry when he talked to her, to determine whether she could come up with thoughtful, intuitive replies. Her "checking out" was a way of coping with the performance anxiety that she experienced when listening to him.

Not surprisingly, Barry's difficulty with listening centered on withholding his natural tendency to give advice. When Debra began to talk, he would listen reflectively for a minute or two, but then he would begin to ask questions, such as "Well, when are you gonna call that person?" or "Last time we talked you said you were going to finish that resumé. Why haven't you?" Repeated practice within sessions—supplemented by homework assignments to practice these skills—led Barry to become more aware of what he was doing. During a particularly poignant moment, he admitted, "I don't like the way I react to her. . . . I don't like the person I'm becoming."

As FFT passed the 3-month point and the frequency changed to biweekly, the clinicians introduced potentially more heated forms of communication, such as the partners making requests for changes in each other's behaviors and expressing negative feelings (Sessions 12–14). At this point, Debra was not as depressed as she had been during the assessment phase, although Barry continued to complain about her low functioning. He argued that she had become unable to tell him what she had and had not accomplished during the day, and that she often made it appear that she had done things that, in reality, she had not. He labeled this her "lack of follow-through" problem. In contrast, Debra became increasingly assertive about his "micromanagement" of her behavior.

THERAPIST 1: One of the things we'd like to work on with you is how you ask each other to change in some way. What's an appropriate way to ask someone to help you? (*Gives Barry and Debra the hand-out titled "Making a Positive Request."*) Try looking directly at each other; say what you would like the other person to do, and how it would make you feel. Debra, a minute ago you were talking about how Barry micromanages you. Can you turn this into a positive—ask him what you would like him to do? Phrase it in a way that he can help you? How can he ask you to follow through without nagging you?

DEBRA: Uh, Barry, it would really make me happy if you. . . in situations where there's a dilemma, if you'd give me a little more freedom.

BARRY: For example? Do you mean you want us to do things at your pace?

THERAPIST 1: Barry, let it come from her.

DEBRA: Um, like, if there's some shopping to do, it would help me out if I could just say, "Yes, this is on my list and I'll do it. . . if you could wait for me to get it done in my own time." That would help ease the tension.

THERAPIST 2: Barry, how did you feel about how Debra asked you? Did she follow this sheet?

BARRY: I think she asked me just fine, but my question is, will she then do the shopping?

DEBRA: I think it would really help me to have some plan—like agreeing that if I do this part of the shopping, you'll do that part. Maybe that would stop me from saying, "I'll show him. He's not gonna run my life; I'm not gonna do it his way."

THERAPIST 1: A person who feels one-down often reacts by refusing to go along with the plan, even though going along with it might be of help to them personally. Debra, do you get into that sometimes?

The therapists were encouraging assertiveness in Debra, and at the same time gently confronting what Barry had earlier called her "passive–aggressiveness." They then asked Barry to make a positive request of Debra.

THERAPIST 2: Barry, can you think of something you could ask Debra to do, to change her behavior?

BARRY: (*looking at clinicians*) OK, Deb, it's very important to me. . .

THERAPIST 2: Can you tell this to her?

BARRY: (*turns toward Debra*) OK, it's very important to me that you not just walk away when we have dis-

cussions. That you don't just withdraw. Especially when we talk about Jill and our differences about her. That really irritates me.

The therapists again observed Debra withdraw in reaction to Barry's "high-EE" behavior. They commented on her reactions.

THERAPIST 1: Debra, what's happening now? You seem like you're checking out.

DEBRA: (*Snaps back, smiles.*) Yeah, I guess I am. What were we talking about?

BARRY: You see, I think that's part of her attention deficit disorder. Do you think she needs Ritalin [medication for this condition]?

THERAPIST 1: Barry, in this case, I don't think so. I think that what happened, Debra, if I can speak for you for a moment, is that you withdrew because you felt you were under attack.

DEBRA: That's probably true. He got into his "You do this, you do that."

BARRY: (*frustrated*) Well, you just asked me to change something! Am I supposed to do all the work here?

THERAPIST 1: Barry, I'm going to encourage you to try again. Only this time, I'd like you to be more aware of how you phrase things. Notice you said what you didn't want her to do—withdraw when you were talking to her. That's quite important. But what would you like her to do instead?

BARRY: I want her to engage with me! To talk it out!

THERAPIST 1: Can you try again, only this time tell her what you want her to do?

BARRY: (*Sighs.*) Deb, when we talk, I'd really like. . . I'd really appreciate it if you'd hang in there and finish talking to me, especially about Jill. That would make me feel, I don't know, like we're partners.

THERAPIST 2: Barry, that was much better, and I'll bet it was easier to hear. Debra?

DEBRA: Yeah, I liked it. . . that's easier. We need to do more of this.

Much emphasis was placed throughout CET on between-session homework assignments. The couple was encouraged to hold weekly meetings and to record their efforts to use the skills. Both spouses reported a reduction in tension in the relationship by the time the problem-solving segment was initiated.

Problem Solving (Sessions 15–18)

FFT sessions were held less frequently (biweekly) in the fourth, fifth, and sixth months. At Session 15, problem solving was introduced. After explaining the rationale, the therapists asked the couple to identify several specific problems for discussion, then reviewed the problem-solving steps with them.

The first issue chosen by the couple seemed superficial at first. They had two cats, one of which belonged to Debra (and had come with her from a previous marriage) and the other of which Barry had bought. They disagreed on how much the cats should be fed: Debra "wanted mine to be fat" and fed it frequently, whereas Barry wanted his to be thin. As a result, Barry's cat was waking them up in the middle of the night, needing to be fed. The resulting changes in Debra's sleep–wake cycles had resulted in her becoming irritable, restless, and possibly hypomanic. Despite a conscientious literature search, the therapists were unable to find any research on the influence of cat diets on the cycling of bipolar disorder.

The couple considered various alternatives: feeding the cats equal amounts, keeping Barry's cat in the garage, giving away Barry's cat, and feeding both cats before the couple went to bed. They eventually settled on the last of these. The problem itself generated humor and playfulness between them, and they derived some satisfaction from being able to deal with it collaboratively.

A second and potentially more serious source of conflict concerned their night life. Both liked going to parties, but Barry liked to stay longer than Debra, who thought that parties contributed to her mood cycling. She tended to become overstimulated by the interactions with many people and would quickly become fatigued. They considered several alternatives: going to the parties in separate cars, Barry agreeing to leave earlier, Debra going to the car and sleeping when she felt tired, and Debra taking a cab home. They eventually decided to discuss and agree upon a departure time before going to a party.

The couple was able to apply the problem-solving method successfully to other issues, such as paying the bills and helping Jill get to her afterschool activities. They continued to have trouble breaking problems down into smaller chunks, and tended to "cross-complain" or bring up larger problems in the middle of trying to solve smaller ones. Barry often complained, "We aren't dealing with the source of these problems,

which is her bipolar disorder. We wouldn't have these problems if she weren't bipolar." Again, the therapists did not challenge his definition of the problem, but continued to offer the message that regardless of whether the source of the problems lay in Debra, the couple still needed to work collaboratively to generate acceptable compromises.

Termination (Sessions 19–21)

By 7 months, Debra, whose depression had largely remitted, had obtained a new job working in sales at a clothing store. The therapists began the termination phase of treatment, which focused on reviewing what the couple had taken away from the psychoeducation, CET, and problem-solving skills modules. Both reported that their relationship had improved, and that they "occasionally" used the communication skills at home. The therapists commented on how far they had come and encouraged them to pick a time each week to meet and rehearse one or more of the skills.

Barry was not entirely convinced of Debra's clinical improvement, however. In one of the final sessions, he returned to the issue of Debra's symptoms and her "unwillingness" to follow through on tasks such as cooking, depositing her paycheck, cleaning Jill's clothes, and doing other tasks they had agreed she would perform. The following interchange ensued:

BARRY: (*Laughs nervously.*) I had this dream the other night that I was getting married, and I knew that I was marrying Debra, but I couldn't see her face, and I wasn't sure it was really her. And I wasn't sure if I should be there.

THERAPIST 1: And you were standing in front of everyone wearing your pajamas as well.

BARRY: (*Laughs.*) Yeah, and I was about to take the exam that I hadn't studied for. But really, sometimes I feel like she's not the same person, especially when she doesn't want to follow through on things we've talked about.

THERAPIST 1: Let me give you some perspective on this. I think a dilemma many spouses face is "Should I stick it out with my husband or my wife, or should I leave and take care of me?" There are certainly people who do that, who leave, and then there are many others who hang out and wait for things to get better, which in fact they often do.

BARRY: And I think things have gotten better.

DEBRA: I think so. I don't know why you're being so negative.

BARRY: Well, if you. . .

THERAPIST 1: (*Interrupts.*) Let me finish this thought. Barry, I think it's critical for you to make a distinction in your own mind between what Debra can and can't control. That's sometimes vague between the two of you. When you say she doesn't want to follow through, that certainly sounds like an intentional behavior—something she's doing to hurt you or annoy you. Debra, do the problems with following through ever feel like they're about problems with your concentration? Your attention or your memory?

DEBRA: (*nodding emphatically*) Absolutely! If you could get him to realize that, we'd be a lot farther along.

BARRY: That memory stuff—is that her bipolar disorder or her attention deficit disorder?

THERAPIST 1: I'm not sure that's really the question. That's just a diagnostic distinction, and I'm not sure my answering one way or the other will help you. Maybe what you're really wondering is whether these problems are controllable by her or not. If I were in your position, the things that would really anger me would be those things I thought she was doing intentionally.

BARRY: Yeah, and I don't always think about that.

THERAPIST 1: If I thought what she was doing was due to a biological dysregulation, I might be more patient, more sympathetic—in the same way that if someone had a broken leg and had trouble walking up stairs, I might have more sympathy than if I thought she was deliberately trying to hold me up.

In this segment, the therapist was addressing directly what he felt was a major source of Barry's critical attitudes toward Debra: the belief that many of her negative behaviors were controllable and intentional (Hooley & Licht, 1997; Miklowitz et al., 1998). In some instances, Barry may have been right about Debra's motivations. But questioning the controllability of her symptoms forced him to consider a different set of causal explanations for her behavior. The distinction between controllable and uncontrollable behavior is a key point in the psychoeducational treatment of families of patients with bipolar disorder.

Barry and Debra's Progress

After completing FFT, Debra continued to have mild periods of depression despite her adherence to medication. Her depressions were unpleasant but not so severe that she was unable to keep her job or attend to her parenting duties. Her brief hypomanic periods sometimes caused arguments between Debra and Barry but were not debilitating. Barry and Debra were communicating better, and both agreed that Barry was more patient and less critical of her. But Debra frequently found herself reacting with the line from the now famous movie, "What if this is as good as it gets?" Although she was functional, she expressed chagrin that she could not have the life she had wanted—a successful career, a more intimate relationship with her husband, more friendships, an easier relationship with her daughter, and more financial success. The reality of her disorder and its psychosocial effects were difficult for her to accept. However, Debra felt that FFT had been helpful, as had her medication, which she showed no inclination to discontinue. The therapists offered her a referral for individual or group therapy, but Debra decided to forgo further psychosocial treatment for the time being. Barry was given the name of a local DBSA group for spouses of persons with mood disorders.

CONCLUSIONS

Family psychoeducational treatment appears to be a useful adjunct to pharmacotherapy. However, not all patients with bipolar disorder have families, and individual or group treatment approaches are important alternatives to consider. The finding that mood-stabilizing medications are more powerful in alleviating manic than depressive symptoms, whereas the reverse may be true for psychotherapy, is an argument for combining medical and psychosocial interventions in the outpatient maintenance of bipolar disorder.

There is limited research on which families are the best candidates for FFT. In several of our trials, patients in high-EE families have shown greater reductions in mood severity scores over 1–2 years than those in low-EE families. But reductions in relapses have been observed in patients from both high- and low-EE families treated with FFT. Our clinical observations also suggest that there are subgroups of patients who do not respond well to FFT. Specifically, patients who are unusually resistant to accepting the diagnosis of bipolar disorder often resent the educational focus of FFT. These patients usually see their troubles as having external origins (i.e., being mistreated by others) and resist interventions that require them to take more responsibility for their behavior. These patients may also reject pharmacotherapy. Sadly, we have seen many patients go through several hospitalizations before the reality of their disorder sets in.

A different kind of resistance originates from viewing the disorder as biologically based. Some patients prefer to limit their mental health contacts to a psychiatrist for medication, and regard psychotherapy as irrelevant. We see nothing wrong with this position; a subset of patients does function well on medication only. Future research needs to determine whether this self-selected group is different from patients who request psychotherapy, in terms of symptomatic, course-of-illness, or family/genetic variables. Equally importantly, some patients with bipolar II depression may recover just as quickly with psychotherapy as with medications (Swartz, Frank, & Cheng, 2012).

Family members are sometimes a major source of resistance. Their reasons can include a desire to distance themselves from the patient (whom they may have tried to help for years without reward), time or distance constraints, or the discomfort of talking about family or couple issues in front of a stranger. More subtle is the fear of being blamed for the disorder (Hatfield, Spaniol, & Zipple, 1987). The family therapy movement has come a long way, but it still has its roots in a culture that faulted parents for causing mental illness. The theoretical model underlying FFT does not in any way link poor parenting to the onset of bipolar disorder. Nonetheless, a clinician often needs to make clear early in treatment that he/she does not adhere to this antiquated position.

FUTURE DIRECTIONS

Important future research will include effectiveness studies, which examine the clinical impact of psychotherapy as delivered to patients in "real-world" (typically community mental health) settings, by the clinicians who work in these settings and the time constraints within which they work. As explained earlier, FFT was found to be effective in stabilizing depression

and maintaining wellness in the large-scale STEP-BD study of community effectiveness, which included therapists working in 15 outpatient sites (Miklowitz et al., 2007b). It remains to be seen whether FFT, along with other treatments whose evidence base includes STEP-BD (CBT, IPSRT), will be taken up by practicing clinicians.

A related problem is determining the proper structure of FFT. In many community settings, insurance companies only pay for six to eight sessions. FFT is rather time-intensive, and research is needed to determine which of its components predict the greatest proportion of variance in the clinical outcome of participants and the quality of life of family members. For example, it is possible that some families will benefit from just the psychoeducation module or just the communication module. Perhaps these modules could be streamlined without a great loss in treatment effect size. Ideally, decisions to modify treatments such as FFT will be based on clinical outcomes research rather than solely on the desire for cost containment.

A final direction is the applicability of FFT and other psychotherapy treatments to child and adolescent patients with bipolar disorder, or genetically vulnerable children who are showing early prodromal signs. The fact that bipolar disorder even exists in school-age or early adolescent youth is just now being recognized, and factors that predict the onset of the full disorder—such as the presence of a family history of mania—are being identified (Axelson, Birmaher, Strober, et al., 2011; Birmaher et al., 2009). Our current research is examining whether giving FFT in the earliest stages of the disorder reduces the risk of developing the full syndrome (Miklowitz et al., 2013). Possibly the negative symptomatic and psychosocial outcomes of adult bipolar disorder can be mitigated through early detection and carefully planned preventive interventions.

ACKNOWLEDGMENTS

Preparation of this chapter was supported in part by National Institute of Mental Health Grant Nos. MH43931, MH55101, MH42556, MH62555, MH073871, MH077856, MH093676, and MH097007; a Distinguished Investigator Award from the National Association for Research on Schizophrenia and Depression; and a Faculty Fellowship from the University of Colorado's Council on Research and Creative Work.

REFERENCES

Akiskal, H. S. (1996). The prevalent clinical spectrum of bipolar disorders: Beyond DSM-IV. *Journal of Clinical Psychopharmacology, 16*(Suppl. 1), 4–14.

Alloy, L. B., Urošević, S., Abramson, L. Y., Jager-Hyman, S., Nusslock, R., Whitehouse, W. G., et al. (2012). Progression along the bipolar spectrum: A longitudinal study of predictors of conversion from bipolar spectrum conditions to bipolar I and II disorders. *Journal of Abnormal Psychology, 121*(1), 16–27.

Altshuler, L. L., Bearden, C., Green, M., van Gorp, W., & Mintz, J. (2008). A relationship between neurocognitive impairment and functional impairment: A pilot study. *Psychiatry Research, 157,* 289–293.

Altshuler, L. L., Post, R. M., Black, D. O., Keck, P. E. J., Nolen, W. A., Frye, M. A., et al. (2006). Subsyndromal depressive symptoms are associated with functional impairment in patients with bipolar disorder: Results of a large, multisite study. *Journal of Clinical Psychiatry, 67*(10), 1551–1560.

Altshuler, L. L., Post, R. M., Leverich, G. S., Mikalauskas, K., Rosoff, A., & Ackerman, L. (1995). Antidepressant-induced mania and cycle acceleration: A controversy revisited. *American Journal of Psychiatry, 152,* 1130–1138.

American Psychiatric Association. (1994). *Diagnostic and statistical manual of mental disorders* (4th ed.). Washington, DC: Author.

American Psychiatric Association. (2013). *Diagnostic and statistical manual of mental disorders* (5th ed.). Arlington, VA: Author.

Axelson, D., Birmaher, B. J., Brent, D., Wassick, S., Hoover, C., Bridge, J., et al. (2003). A preliminary study of the Kiddie Schedule for Affective Disorders and Schizophrenia for School-Age Children mania rating scale for children and adolescents. *Journal of Child and Adolescent Psychopharmacology, 13,* 463–470.

Axelson, D. A., Birmaher, B., Findling, R. L., Fristad, M. A., Kowatch, R. A., Youngstrom, E. A., et al. (2011). Concerns regarding the inclusion of temper dysregulation disorder with dysphoria in the Diagnostic and Statistical Manual of Mental Disorders, Fifth Edition. *Journal of Clinical Psychiatry, 72*(9), 1257–1262.

Axelson, D. A., Birmaher, B., Strober, M. A., Goldstein, B. I., Ha, W., Gill, M. K., et al. (2011). Course of subthreshold bipolar disorder in youth: Diagnostic progression from bipolar disorder not otherwise specified. *Journal of the American Academy of Child and Adolescent Psychiatry, 50*(10), 1001–1016.

Baldessarini, R. J., Tondo, L., & Hennen, J. (2003). Lithium treatment and suicide risk in major affective disorders: Update and new findings. *Journal of Clinical Psychiatry, 64*(Suppl. 5), 44–52.

Bauer, M. S., McBride, L., Williford, W. O., Glick, H., Kinosian, B., Altshuler, L., et al. (2006). Collaborative care for bipolar disorder: Part II. Impact on clinical outcome, function, and costs *Psychiatric Services, 57,* 937–945.

Berrettini, W. (2003). Evidence for shared susceptibility in bipolar disorder and schizophrenia. *American Journal of Medical Genetics, Part C, 123,* 59–64.

Birmaher, B., Axelson, D., Goldstein, B., Strober, M., Gill, M. K., Hunt, J., et al. (2009). Four-year longitudinal course of children and adolescents with bipolar spectrum disorders: The Course and Outcome of Bipolar Youth (COBY) study. *American Journal of Psychiatry, 166*(7), 795–804.

Butzlaff, R. L., & Hooley, J. M. (1998). Expressed emotion and psychiatric relapse: A meta-analysis. *Archives of General Psychiatry, 55,* 547–552.

Calabrese, J. R., Fatemi, S. H., Kujawa, M., & Woyshville, M. J. (1996). Predictors of response to mood stabilizers. *Journal of Clinical Psychopharmacology, 16*(Suppl. 1), 24–31.

Carlson, G. A., Findling, R. L., Post, R. M., Birmaher, B., Blumberg, H. P., Correll, C., et al. (2009). AACAP 2006 Research Forum—Advancing research in early-onset bipolar disorder: Barriers and suggestions. *Journal of Child and Adolescent Psychopharmacology, 19*(1), 3–12.

Chambers, W. J., Puig-Antich, J., Hirsch, M., Paez, P., Ambrosini, P. J., Tabrizi, M. A., et al. (1985). The assessment of affective disorders in children and adolescents by semistructured interview: Test–retest reliability. *Archives of General Psychiatry, 42,* 696–702.

Colom, F., Vieta, E., Martinez-Aran, A., Reinares, M., Goikolea, J. M., Benabarre, A., et al. (2003). A randomized trial on the efficacy of group psychoeducation in the prophylaxis of recurrences in bipolar patients whose disease is in remission. *Archives of General Psychiatry, 60,* 402–407.

Colom, F., Vieta, E., Martinez-Aran, A., Reinares, M., Goikolea, A., Benabarre, A., et al. (2009). A randomized trial on the efficacy of group psychoeducation in the prophylaxis of bipolar disorder: A five year follow-up. *British Journal of Psychiatry, 194*(3), 260–265.

Colom, F., Vieta, E., Sanchez-Moreno, J., Martinez-Aran, A., Reinares, M., Goikolea, J. M., et al. (2005). Stabilizing the stabilizer: Group psychoeducation enhances the stability of serum lithium levels. *Bipolar Disorders, 7*(Suppl. 5), 32–36.

Colom, F., Vieta, E., Tacchi, M. J., Sanchez-Moreno, J., & Scott, J. (2005). Identifying and improving non-adherence in bipolar disorders. *Bipolar Disorders, 7*(5), 24–31.

Coryell, W., Endicott, J., & Keller, M. (1992). Rapidly cycling affective disorder: Demographics, diagnosis, family history, and course. *Archives of General Psychiatry, 49,* 126–131.

Cuellar, A. K., Johnson, S. L., & Winters, R. (2005). Distinctions between bipolar and unipolar depression. *Clinical Psychology Review, 25*(3), 307–339.

Cutler, N. R., & Post, R. M. (1982). Life course of illness in untreated manic–depressive patients. *Comprehensive Psychiatry, 23*, 101–115.

Dausch, B. M., Miklowitz, D. J., & Richards, J. A. (1996). A Scale for the Global Assessment of Relational Functioning, II: Reliability and validity in a sample of families of bipolar patients. *Family Process, 35*, 175–189.

Deckersbach, T., Nierenberg, A. A., Kessler, R., Lund, H. G., Ametrano, R. M., Sachs, G., et al. (2010). Cognitive rehabilitation for bipolar disorder: An open trial for employed patients with residual depressive symptoms. *CNS Neuroscience and Therapeutics, 16*(5), 298–307.

Ehlers, C. L., Kupfer, D. J., Frank, E., & Monk, T. H. (1993). Biological rhythms and depression: The role of *zeitgebers* and *zeitstorers. Depression, 1*, 285–293.

Falloon, I. R. H., Boyd, J. L., & McGill, C. W. (1984). *Family care of schizophrenia: A problem-solving approach to the treatment of mental illness.* New York: Guilford Press.

Fiedorowicz, J. G., Endicott, J., Leon, A. C., Solomon, D. A., Keller, M. B., & Coryell, W. H. (2011). Subthreshold hypomanic symptoms in progression from unipolar major depression to bipolar disorder. *American Journal of Psychiatry, 168*(1), 40-48.

First, M. B. (2010). DSM-5 proposals for mood disorders: A cost–benefit analysis. *Current Opinion in Psychiatry, 24*(1), 1–9.

First, M. B., Spitzer, R. L., Gibbon, M., & Williams, J. B. W. (1995). *Structured Clinical Interview for DSM-IV Axis I disorders.* New York: Biometrics Research Department, New York State Psychiatric Institute.

Frank, E. (2005). *Treating bipolar disorder: A clinician's guide to interpersonal and social rhythm therapy.* New York: Guilford Press.

Frank, E. (2011). Proposed revisions to the concept of mixed episodes in DSM-5: The path traveled (abstract). *Bipolar Disorders, 13*(1), 14.

Frank, E., Kupfer, D. J., Thase, M. E., Mallinger, A. G., Swartz, H. A., Fagiolini, A. M., et al. (2005). Two-year outcomes for interpersonal and social rhythm therapy in individuals with bipolar I disorder. *Archives of General Psychiatry, 62*(9), 996–1004.

Frank, E., Soreca, I., Swartz, H. A., Fagiolini, A. M., Mallinger, A. G., Thase, M. E., et al. (2008). The role of interpersonal and social rhythm therapy in improving occupational functioning in patients with bipolar I disorder. *American Journal of Psychiatry, 165*(12), 1559–1565.

Fristad, M. A., Verducci, J. S., Walters, K., & Young, M. E. (2009). Impact of multifamily psychoeducational psychotherapy in treating children aged 8 to 12 years with mood disorders. *Archives of General Psychiatry, 66*(9), 1013–1021.

Geddes, J. R. & Miklowitz, D. J. (2013). Treatment of bipolar disorder. *Lancet, 381*, 1672–1682.

George, E. L., Miklowitz, D. J., Richards, J. A., Simoneau, T. L., & Taylor, D. O. (2003). The comorbidity of bipolar disorder and Axis II personality disorders: Prevalence and clinical correlates. *Bipolar Disorders, 5*, 115–122.

Gitlin, M. J., Mintz, J., Sokolski, K., Hammen, C., & Altshuler, L. L. (2011). Subsyndromal depressive symptoms after symptomatic recovery from mania are associated with delayed functional recovery. *Journal of Clinical Psychiatry, 72*(5), 692–697.

Gitlin, M. J., Swendsen, J., Heller, T. L., & Hammen, C. (1995). Relapse and impairment in bipolar disorder. *American Journal of Psychiatry, 152*(11), 1635–1640.

Goes, F. S., Hamshere, M. L., Seifuddin, F., Pirooznia, M., Belmonte-Mahon, P., Breuer, R., et al. (2012). Genomewide association of mood-incongruent psychotic bipolar disorder. *Translational Psychiatry, 2*, e180.

Goldberg, J. F. (2004). The changing landscape of psychopharmacology. In S. L. Johnson & R. L. Leahy (Eds.), *Psychological treatment of bipolar disorder* (pp. 109–138). New York: Guilford Press.

Goldberg, J. F., & Kocsis, J. H. (1999). Depression in the course of bipolar disorder. In J. F. Goldberg & M. Harrow (Eds.), *Bipolar disorders: Clinical course and outcome* (pp. 129–147). Washington, DC: American Psychiatric Press.

Goldstein, B. I., Goldstein, T. R., & Miklowitz, D. J. (2008). *Integrating a substance use disorder (SUD) perspective into family-focused therapy of adolescents with bipolar disorder (FFT-A).* Pittsburgh, PA: Western Psychiatric Institute and Clinic.

Hahlweg, K., Goldstein, M. J., Nuechterlein, K. H., Magana, A. B., Mintz, J., Doane, J. A., et al. (1989). Expressed emotion and patient–relative interaction in families of recent-onset schizophrenics. *Journal of Consulting and Clinical Psychology, 57*, 11–18.

Harrow, M., Grossman, L. S., Herbener, E. S., & Davies, E. W. (2000). Ten-year outcome: Patients with schizoaffective disorders, schizophrenia, affective disorders and mood-incongruent psychotic symptoms. *British Journal of Psychiatry, 177*, 421–426.

Hatfield, A. B., Spaniol, L., & Zipple, A. M. (1987). Expressed emotion: A family perspective. *Schizophrenia Bulletin, 13*, 221–226.

Henin, A., Biederman, J., Mick, E., Sachs, G. S., Hirshfeld-Becker, D. R., Siegel, R. S., et al. (2005). Psychopathology in the offspring of parents with bipolar disorder: A controlled study. *Biological Psychiatry, 58*(7), 554–561.

Honig, A., Hofman, A., Rozendaal, N., & Dingemanns, P. (1997). Psychoeducation in bipolar disorder: Effect on expressed emotion. *Psychiatry Research, 72*, 17–22.

Hooley, J. M., & Licht, D. M. (1997). Expressed emotion and causal attributions in the spouses of depressed patients. *Journal of Abnormal Psychology, 106*, 298–306.

Hooley, J. M., & Teasdale, J. D. (1989). Predictors of relapse in unipolar depressives: Expressed emotion, marital distress, and perceived criticism. *Journal of Abnormal Psychology, 98*, 229–235.

Johnson, R. E., & McFarland, B. H. (1996). Lithium use and discontinuation in a health maintenance organization. *American Journal of Psychiatry, 153*, 993–1000.

Johnson, S. L. (2005a). Life events in bipolar disorder: Towards more specific models. *Clinical Psychology Review, 25*(8), 1008–1027.

Johnson, S. L. (2005b). Mania and dysregulation in goal pursuit. *Clinical Psychology Review, 25*, 241–262.

Johnson, S. L., Cuellar, A., Ruggero, C., Perlman, C., Goodnick, P., White, R., et al. (2008). Life events as predictors of mania and depression in bipolar I disorder. *Journal of Abnormal Psychology, 117*, 268–277.

Johnson, S. L., Edge, M. D., Holmes, M. K., & Carver, C. S. (2012). The behavioral activation system and mania. *Annual Review of Clinical Psychology, 8*, 143–167.

Johnson, S. L., Sandrow, D., Meyer, B., Winters, R., Miller, I., Solomon, D., et al. (2000). Increases in manic symptoms following life events involving goal-attainment. *Journal of Abnormal Psychology, 109*, 721–727.

Judd, L. L., Akiskal, H. S., Schettler, P. J., Endicott, J., Maser, J., Solomon, D. A., et al. (2002). The long-term natural history of the weekly symptomatic status of bipolar I disorder. *Archives of General Psychiatry, 59*, 530–537.

Kaufman, J., Birmaher, B., Brent, D., Rao, U., Flynn, C., Moreci, P., et al. (1997). Schedule for Affective Disorders and Schizophrenia for School-Age Children—Present and Lifetime version (K-SADS-PL): Initial reliability and validity data. *Journal of the American Academy of Child and Adolescent Psychiatry, 36*, 980–988.

Keck, P. E., McElroy, S. L., Strakowski, S. M., West, S. A., Sax, K. W., Hawkins, J. M., et al. (1998). 12-month outcome of patients with bipolar disorder following hospitalization for a manic or mixed episode. *American Journal of Psychiatry, 155*, 646–652.

Kim, E. Y., & Miklowitz, D. J. (2002). Childhood mania, attention deficit hyperactivity disorder, and conduct disorder: A critical review of diagnostic dilemmas. *Bipolar Disorders, 4*, 215–225.

Klerman, G. L., Weissman, M. M., Rounsaville, B. J., & Chevron, R. S. (1984). *Interpersonal psychotherapy of depression*. New York: Basic Books.

Kraepelin, É. (1921). *Manic–depressive insanity and paranoia*. Edinburgh, UK: Livingstone.

Kumari, V., Fannon, D., Peters, E. R., Ffytche, D. H., Sumich, A. L., Premkumar, P., et al. (2011). Neural changes following cognitive behaviour therapy for psychosis: A longitudinal study. *Brain, 134*(8), 2396–2407.

Lam, D. H., Burbeck, R., Wright, K., & Pilling, S. (2009). Psychological therapies in bipolar disorder: The effect of illness history on relapse prevention—a systematic review. *Bipolar Disorders, 11*(5), 474–482.

Lam, D. H., Hayward, P., Watkins, E. R., Wright, K., & Sham, P. (2005). Relapse prevention in patients with bipolar disorder: Cognitive therapy outcome after 2 years. *American Journal of Psychiatry, 162*, 324–329.

Lam, D. H., Watkins, E. R., Hayward, P., Bright, J., Wright, K., Kerr, N., et al. (2003). A randomized controlled study of cognitive therapy of relapse prevention for bipolar affective disorder: Outcome of the first year. *Archives of General Psychiatry, 60*, 145–152.

Leibenluft, E. (2011). Severe mood dysregulation, irritability, and the diagnostic boundaries of bipolar disorder in youths. *American Journal of Psychiatry, 168*(2), 129–142.

Leibenluft, E., Charney, D. S., Towbin, K. E., Bhangoo, R. K., & Pine, D. S. (2003). Defining clinical phenotypes of juvenile mania. *American Journal of Psychiatry, 160*, 430–437.

Leverich, G. S., & Post, R. M. (1998). Life charting of affective disorders. *CNS Spectrums, 3*, 21–37.

Leverich, G. S., Post, R. M., Keck, P. E. J., Altshuler, L. L., Frye, M. A., Kupka, R. W., et al. (2007). The poor prognosis of childhood-onset bipolar disorder. *Journal of Pediatrics, 150*(5), 485–490.

Liberman, R. P., Wallace, C. J., Falloon, I. R. H., & Vaughn, C. E. (1981). Interpersonal problem solving therapy for schizophrenics and their families. *Comprehensive Psychiatry, 22*, 627–629.

Malhi, G. S., Adams, D., & Berk, M. (2009). Medicating mood with maintenance in mind: Bipolar depression pharmacotherapy. *Bipolar Disorders, 11*(Suppl. 2), 55–76.

Malkoff-Schwartz, S., Frank, E., Anderson, B. P., Hlastala, S. A., Luther, J. F., Sherrill, J. T., et al. (2000). Social rhythm disruption and stressful life events in the onset of bipolar and unipolar episodes. *Psychological Medicine, 30*, 1005–1016.

Malkoff-Schwartz, S., Frank, E., Anderson, B., Sherrill, J. T., Siegel, L., Patterson, D., et al. (1998). Stressful life events and social rhythm disruption in the onset of manic and depressive bipolar episodes: A preliminary investigation. *Archives of General Psychiatry, 55*, 702–707.

Masi, G., Mucci, M., Pfanner, C., Berloffa, S., Magazù, A., & Perugi, G. (2012). Developmental pathways for different subtypes of early-onset bipolarity in youths. *Journal of Clinical Psychiatry, 73*(10), 1355–1341.

Merikangas, K. R., Akiskal, H. S., Angst, J., Greenberg, P. E., Hirschfeld, R. M. A., Petukhova, M., et al. (2007). Lifetime and 12-month prevalence of bipolar spectrum disorder in the National Comorbidity Survey Replication. *Archives of General Psychiatry, 64*(5), 543–552.

Merikangas, K. R., Cui, L., Kattan, G., Carlson, G. A., Youngstrom, E. A., & Angst, J. (2012). Mania with and without depression in a community sample of US adolescents. *Archives of General Psychiatry, 69*(9), 943–951.

Merikangas, K. R., Jin, R., He, J. P., Kessler, R. C., Lee, S., Sampson, N. A., et al. (2011). Prevalence and correlates of bipolar spectrum disorder in the World Mental Health

Survey Initiative. *Archives of General Psychiatry, 68*(3), 241–251.

Meyer, B., Johnson, S. L., & Winters, R. (2001). Responsiveness to threat and incentive in bipolar disorder: Relations of the BIS/BAS scales with symptoms. *Journal of Psychopathology and Behavioral Assessment, 23*, 133–143.

Miklowitz, D. J. (2008a). Adjunctive psychotherapy for bipolar disorder: State of the evidence. *American Journal of Psychiatry, 165*(11), 1408–1419.

Miklowitz, D. J. (2008b). *Bipolar disorder: A family-focused treatment approach* (2nd ed.). New York: Guilford Press.

Miklowitz, D. J. (2012). A family intervention approach to bipolar disorder and substance abuse in late adolescence. *Journal of Clinical Psychology: In Session, 68*(5), 502–513.

Miklowitz, D. J., Axelson, D. A., Birmaher, B., George, E. L., Taylor, D. O., Schneck, C. D., et al. (2008). Family-focused treatment for adolescents with bipolar disorder: Results of a 2-year randomized trial. *Archives of General Psychiatry, 65*(9), 1053–1061.

Miklowitz, D. J., Axelson, D. A., George, E. L., Taylor, D. O., Schneck, C. D., Sullivan, A. E., et al. (2009). Expressed emotion moderates the effects of family-focused treatment for bipolar adolescents. *Journal of the American Academy of Child and Adolescent Psychiatry, 48*, 643–651.

Miklowitz, D. J., Biuckians, A., & Richards, J. A. (2006). Early-onset bipolar disorder: A family treatment perspective. *Development and Psychopathology, 18*, 1247–1265.

Miklowitz, D. J., George, E. L., Axelson, D. A., Kim, E. Y., Birmaher, B., Schneck, C., et al. (2004). Family-focused treatment for adolescents with bipolar disorder. *Journal of Affective Disorders, 82*(Suppl. 1), 113–128.

Miklowitz, D. J., George, E. L., Richards, J. A., Simoneau, T. L., & Suddath, R. L. (2003). A randomized study of family-focused psychoeducation and pharmacotherapy in the outpatient management of bipolar disorder. *Archives of General Psychiatry, 60*, 904–912.

Miklowitz, D. J., & Goldstein, M. J. (1997). *Bipolar disorder: A family-focused treatment approach.* New York: Guilford Press.

Miklowitz, D. J., Goldstein, M. J., Nuechterlein, K. H., Snyder, K. S., & Mintz, J. (1988). Family factors and the course of bipolar affective disorder. *Archives of General Psychiatry, 45*, 225–231.

Miklowitz, D. J., Otto, M. W., Frank, E., Reilly-Harrington, N. A., Wisniewski, S. R., Kogan, J. N., et al. (2007a). Is psychosocial management effective?: In reply to Saddichha and Kumar. *Archives of General Psychiatry, 64*, 1452–1453.

Miklowitz, D. J., Otto, M. W., Frank, E., Reilly-Harrington, N. A., Wisniewski, S. R., Kogan, J. N., et al. (2007b). Psychosocial treatments for bipolar depression: A 1-year randomized trial from the Systematic Treatment Enhancement Program. *Archives of General Psychiatry, 64*, 419–427.

Miklowitz, D. J., Schneck, C. D., Singh, M. K., Taylor, D. O., George, E. L., Cosgrove, V. E., et al. (2013). Early intervention for symptomatic youth at risk for bipolar disorder: A randomized trial of family-focused therapy. *Journal of the American Academy of Child and Adolescent Psychiatry, 52*(2), 121–131.

Miklowitz, D. J., & Scott, J. (2009). Psychosocial treatments for bipolar disorder: Cost-effectiveness, mediating mechanisms, and future directions. *Bipolar Disorders, 11*, 110–122.

Miklowitz, D. J., Wendel, J. S., & Simoneau, T. L. (1998). Targeting dysfunctional family interactions and high expressed emotion in the psychosocial treatment of bipolar disorder. *In Session: Psychotherapy in Practice, 4*, 25–38.

Miklowitz, D. J., Wisniewski, S. R., Miyahara, S., Otto, M. W., & Sachs, G. S. (2005). Perceived criticism from family members as a predictor of the 1-year course of bipolar disorder. *Psychiatry Research, 136*(2–3), 101–111.

Monk, T. H., Kupfer, D. J., Frank, E., & Ritenour, A. M. (1991). The Social Rhythm Metric (SRM): Measuring daily social rhythms over 12 weeks. *Psychiatry Research, 36*, 195–207.

Murray, G., Suto, M., Hole, R., Hale, S., Amari, E., & Michalak, E. E. (2011). Self-management strategies used by "high functioning" individuals with bipolar disorder: From research to clinical practice. *Clinical Psychology and Psychotherapy, 18*(2), 95–109.

Napier, A. Y., & Whitaker, C. (1988). *The family crucible: The intense experience of family therapy.* New York: Harper & Row.

O'Connell, R. A., Mayo, J. A., Flatow, L., Cuthbertson, B., & O'Brien, B. E. (1991). Outcome of bipolar disorder on long-term treatment with lithium. *British Journal of Psychiatry, 159*, 132–129.

Priebe, S., Wildgrube, C., & Muller-Oerlinghausen, B. (1989). Lithium prophylaxis and expressed emotion. *British Journal of Psychiatry, 154*, 396–399.

Rea, M. M., Tompson, M., Miklowitz, D. J., Goldstein, M. J., Hwang, S., & Mintz, J. (2003). Family focused treatment vs. individual treatment for bipolar disorder: Results of a randomized clinical trial. *Journal of Consulting and Clinical Psychology, 71*, 482–492.

Sachs, G. S., Nierenberg, A. A., Calabrese, J. R., Marangell, L. B., Wisniewski, S. R., Gyulai, L., et al. (2007). Effectiveness of adjunctive antidepressant treatment for bipolar depression. *New England Journal of Medicine, 356*(17), 1711–1722.

Sato, T., Bottlender, R., Schröter, A., & Möller, H. J. (2003). Frequency of manic symptoms during a depressive episode and unipolar "depressive mixed state" as bipolar spectrum. *Acta Psychiatrica Scandinavica, 107*(4), 268–274.

Sala, R., Axelson, D. A., Castro-Fornieles, J., Goldstein, T. R., Ha, W., Liao, F., et al. (2010). Comorbid anxiety in children and adolescents with bipolar spectrum disorders:

prevalence and clinical correlates. *Journal of Clinical Psychiatry, 71*(10), 1344–1350.

Salavert, J., Caseras, X., Torrubia, R., Furest, S., Arranz, B., Duenas, R., et al. (2007). The functioning of the Behavioral Activation and Inhibition Systems in bipolar I euthymic patients and its influence in subsequent episodes over an eighteen-month period. *Personality and Individual Differences, 42*(7), 1323–1331.

Scherk, H., Pajonk, F. G., & Leucht, S. (2007). Second-generation antipsychotic agents in the treatment of acute mania: A systematic review and meta-analysis of randomized controlled trials. *Archives of General Psychiatry, 64*(4), 442–455.

Schlosser, D. A., Miklowitz, D. J., O'Brien, M. P., De Silva, S., Zinberg, J. L., & Cannon, T. D. (2012). A randomized trial of family-focused treatment for adolescents and young adults at risk for psychosis: Study rationale, design, and methods. *Early Intervention in Psychiatry, 6*(3), 283–291.

Scott, J., Paykel, E., Morriss, R., Bentall, R., Kinderman, P., Johnson, T., et al. (2006). Cognitive behaviour therapy for severe and recurrent bipolar disorders: A randomised controlled trial. *British Journal of Psychiatry, 188*, 313–320.

Simon, G. E., Ludman, E. J., Bauer, M. S., Unutzer, J., & Operskalski, B. (2006). Long-term effectiveness and cost of a systematic care program for bipolar disorder. *Archives of General Psychiatry, 63*(5), 500–508.

Simoneau, T. L., Miklowitz, D. J., Richards, J. A., Saleem, R., & George, E. L. (1999). Bipolar disorder and family communication: Effects of a psychoeducational treatment program. *Journal of Abnormal Psychology, 108*, 588–597.

Simoneau, T. L., Miklowitz, D. J., & Saleem, R. (1998). Expressed emotion and interactional patterns in the families of bipolar patients. *Journal of Abnormal Psychology, 107*, 497–507.

Spitzer, R. L., Williams, J. B., Gibbon, M., & First, M. B. (1992). The Structured Clinical Interview for DSM-III-R (SCID): I. History, rationale, and description. *Archives of General Psychiatry, 49*(8), 624–629.

Strakowski, S. M., Keck, P. E., McElroy, S. L., West, S. A., Sax, K. W., Hawkins, J. M., et al. (1998). Twelve-month outcome after a first hospitalization for affective psychosis. *Archives of General Psychiatry, 55*, 49–55.

Suppes, T., Leverich, G. S., Keck, P. E., Nolen, W. A., Denicoff, K. D., Altshuler, L. L., et al. (2001). The Stanley Foundation Bipolar Treatment Outcome Network: II. Demographics and illness characteristics of the first 261 patients. *Journal of Affective Disorders, 67*, 45–59.

Suppes, T., Mintz, J., McElroy, S. L., Altshuler, L. L., Kupka, R. W., Frye, M. A., et al. (2005). Mixed hypomania in 908 patients with bipolar disorder evaluated prospectively in the Stanley Foundation Bipolar Treatment Network: A sex-specific phenomenon. *Archives of General Psychiatry, 62*(10), 1089–1096.

Swann, A. C., Dougherty, D. M., Pazzaglia, P. J., Pham, M., & Moeller, F. G. (2004). Impulsivity: A link between bipolar disorder and substance abuse. *Bipolar Disorders, 6*, 204–212.

Swartz, H. A., Frank, E., & Cheng, Y. (2012). A randomized pilot study of psychotherapy and quetiapine for the acute treatment of bipolar II depression. *Bipolar Disorders, 14*(2), 211–216.

Van Meter, A. R., Moreira, A. L., & Youngstrom, E. A. (2011). Meta-analysis of epidemiologic studies of pediatric bipolar disorder. *Journal of Clinical Psychiatry, 72*(9), 1250–1256.

Vaughn, C. E., & Leff, J. P. (1976). The influence of family and social factors on the course of psychiatric illness: A comparison of schizophrenia and depressed neurotic patients. *British Journal of Psychiatry, 129*, 125–137.

Vitiello, B., & Swedo, S. (2004). Antidepressant medications in children. *New England Journal of Medicine, 350*, 1489–1491.

Weinstock, L. M., & Miller, I. W. (2008). Functional impairment as a predictor of short-term symptom course in bipolar I disorder. *Bipolar Disorders, 10*(3), 437–442.

Weinstock, L. M., Strong, D., Uebelacker, L. A., & Miller, I. W. (2009). Differential item functioning of DSM-IV depressive symptoms in individuals with a history of mania versus those without: An item response theory analysis. *Bipolar Disorders, 11*(3), 289–297.

Weisman, A., Lopez, S. R., Karno, M., & Jenkins, J. (1993). An attributional analysis of expressed emotion in Mexican-American families with schizophrenia. *Journal of Abnormal Psychology, 102*, 601–606.

Wendel, J. S., Miklowitz, D. J., Richards, J. A., & George, E. L. (2000). Expressed emotion and attributions in the relatives of bipolar patients: An analysis of problem-solving interactions. *Journal of Abnormal Psychology, 109*, 792–796.

West, A. E., & Weinstein, S. M. (2012). A family-based psychosocial treatment model. *Israeli Journal of Psychiatry and Related Sciences, 49*(2), 86–93.

Wilens, T. E., Biederman, J., Kwon, A., Ditterline, J., Forkner, P., Moore, H., et al. (2004). Risk of substance use disorders in adolescents with bipolar disorder. *Journal of the American Academy of Child and Adolescent Psychiatry, 43*(11), 1380–1386.

Yan, L. J., Hammen, C., Cohen, A. N., Daley, S. E., & Henry, R. M. (2004). Expressed emotion versus relationship quality variables in the prediction of recurrence in bipolar patients. *Journal of Affective Disorders, 83*, 199–206.

CHAPTER 12

Schizophrenia and Other Psychotic Disorders

NICHOLAS TARRIER
RUMINA TAYLOR

Among the most remarkable advances in the last decade is the direct treatment of "positive" symptoms of schizophrenia with psychological treatments. Many of these advances originally emanated from the United Kingdom, where a group of senior investigators working in the context of the National Health Service (NHS) developed and evaluated these approaches. Nick Tarrier was at the forefront of this group during this period. In the context of case management and antipsychotic medication, this very creative mix of treatment components has been proven effective for chronic patients who do not fully respond to medication, as well as for patients in an acute stage of the disorder. Evidence is now sufficient that government-sponsored treatment guidelines in both the United Kingdom and the United States have incorporated these approaches into comprehensive treatment recommendations. More recently, clear evidence has emerged supporting the use of these procedures for preventing the onset of the disorder for those at risk. The thrusts and parries of these techniques are illustrated in the case of "Jim," who had developed an intricate web of delusions reminiscent of Russell Crowe's character in *A Beautiful Mind*, concerning complex schemes by others, including friends and family, to take advantage of him and steal his money and his girlfriend. The therapist's skill in carrying out these new approaches is never better illustrated than in this chapter. These new, empirically supported psychological treatments represent the front line of our therapeutic work with these severely disturbed patients and are capable of further alleviating to some degree the tragedy that is schizophrenia.—D. H. B.

Schizophrenia is a serious mental illness that is characterized by positive symptoms of hallucinations, delusions, and disorders of thought. Typically, hallucinations are auditory, in the form of hearing voices that often talk about the person and in the third person, although hallucinations can occur in other senses. Delusions are frequently bizarre, are held with strong conviction, and often involve a misinterpretation of perception or experience. The content of delusions may include a variety of themes, including alien control; persecution; reference; and somatic, religious, or grandiose ideas. Disorders of thought are inferred from disruption and disorganization in language. Hallucinations and delusions, and sometimes thought disorders, are referred to as "positive symptoms" and reflect an excess or distortion of normal functioning. "Negative symptoms" are also frequently present and reflect a decrease in or loss of normal function, including restrictions in the range and intensity of emotions, in the fluency and productivity of thought and language, and in the initiation of behavior. The consequences of these symptoms can be dysfunction in personal, social, occupational, and vocational functioning. Comorbid disorders, especially depression and anxiety, are frequently present and further impair functioning. Suicide risk is high. Aspects of description, diagnosis, and classification of schizophrenia and psychotic disorders have stimulated much debate and controversy over the decades, and details can be found in most psychiatry textbooks. They do not concern us here except to say that there can be considerable variation in clinical presentation between patients and in the same patient over time. Furthermore, cognitive-behavioral therapy for psychosis (CBTp) in recent years has mainly focused on the reduction of positive symptoms and associated distress, and that is our major concern in most of this chapter. The standard treatments for schizophrenia remain antipsychotic medication and some type of case management, and CBTp described in this chapter is assumed to be in addition to this. Indeed, recent revisions to the National Institute for Health and Clinical Excellence (NICE; 2009) guidelines in the United Kingdom, and the Schizophrenia Patient Outcomes Research Team (Dixon et al., 2010) in the United States, have suggested that CBTp be offered alongside medication for all those with schizophrenia.

DEVELOPMENT OF COGNITIVE-BEHAVIORAL THERAPY FOR SCHIZOPHRENIA

Cognitive-behavioral therapy (CBT) for schizophrenia, although following a common theme and set of principles, has developed in a number of centers, mostly in the United Kingdom, and has been informed by a number of theoretical and conceptual perspectives. A dramatic expansion in the use of CBT in the 1980s and 1990s in the treatment of anxiety and affective disorders influenced clinical psychologists in the field of schizophrenia, who were trying to understand and treat schizophrenia from a psychological perspective. This was especially true in the United Kingdom, where clinical psychologists treated a range of disorders in adult mental health services and were able to transfer their treatment methods across diagnostic groups. The structure and function of a system of universal health care in the United Kingdom, the National Health Service (NHS), facilitated such skills transfer and multidisci-

plinary work. Furthermore, funding of the professional training of health professionals, especially clinical psychologists, has aided awareness and dissemination of CBT for patients in general and for psychotic patients in particular. However, dissemination of treatments into the health service and the universal availability of CBTp has been slow and not without its problems (Brooker & Brabban, 2006; Tarrier, Barrowclough, Haddock, & McGovern, 1999).

RESEARCH EVIDENCE

Clinical, ethical, and economic considerations have encouraged clinical practitioners to be guided by an evidence base produced from evaluations of treatments. The evidence develops from uncontrolled studies and small-scale projects to controlled studies, then to large randomized controlled trials (RCTs) of efficacy and effectiveness. In spite of criticisms of the appropriateness of RCTs in mental health (Richardson, Baker, Burns, Lilford, & Muijen, 2000; Slade & Priebe, 2001), they remain the "gold standard" by which all treatments are judged (Doll, 1998; Pocock, 1996; Salkovskis, 2002; Tarrier & Wykes, 2004). Once a database of controlled trials has been established, then meta-analysis can provide a measure of the average level of therapeutic effect for that treatment. For schizophrenia, a number of published meta-analyses indicate that CBTp is effective in treating positive psychotic symptoms in psychotic patients (e.g., Gould, Mueser, Bolton, Mays, & Goff, 2001; Pilling et al., 2002; Rector & Beck, 2001; Tarrier & Wykes, 2004; Zimmermann, Favrod, Trieu, & Pomini, 2005), although there have been conflicting findings (e.g., Lynch, Laws, & McKenna, 2010). Of the 20 controlled trials of CBT for schizophrenia identified by Tarrier and Wykes (2004), data were available from 19 studies on the effects of CBT on positive symptoms. These studies have a mean effect size of 0.37 ($SD = 0.39$, median = 0.32), with a range between −0.49 and 0.99. Using Cohen's (1988) convention for categorizing effect sizes, 14 (74%) studies achieved at least a small effect size, six (32%) at least a moderate effect size, and three (16%) achieved a large effect size. Overall these studies indicate a modest effect size in improving positive symptoms compared to standard psychiatric care (treatment as usual, or TAU), which is probably not surprising given the nature and severity of the disorder. An updated meta-analysis and review indicated that effect sizes were 0.476 for CBTp on positive symptoms from 30 trials, 0.474 for negative symptoms from 14 trials, 0.477 for social functioning from 11 studies, and 0.424 for depression from 11 studies (Wykes, Everitt, Steele, & Tarrier, 2008). A more recent meta-analysis has extended findings by examining the effectiveness of CBTp at follow-up (3 to 15 months after treatment), compared to TAU and other psychological treatments (psychoeducation and family intervention). Sarin, Wallin, and Widerlöv (2011) included 22 studies and 2,469 participants. When CBTp was compared to other psychological interventions at follow-up the outcome was statistically significant and in favor of CBTp having a small treatment effect on positive, negative, and general symptoms. When CBTp was compared to TAU at follow-up and to other psychological treatments immediately after ending, there was a trend in favor of CBTp but this was not statistically significant. Thus, there appeared to be a delay in the effects of CBTp.

Symptom Management in Chronic Schizophrenia

In spite of maintenance medication, a considerable percentage of patients with schizophrenia continue to have persistent hallucinations and delusions that do not respond further to medication. The majority of the CBTp studies have been carried out with patients who have chronic illnesses. These studies, for which data were available for 16, have a mean effect size of 0.4 (SD = 0.32, median = 0.33), with a range from –0.32 to 0.99 (Tarrier & Wykes, 2004). Another strategy has been to adopt a less generic approach and instead use CBTp to target a more defined participant group or specific symptoms. Fowler and colleagues (2009), for example, recruited young people with early psychosis and poor social functioning and unemployment, and offered a cognitive-behavioral intervention designed to improve social recovery. Compared to the TAU-alone group, those with nonaffective psychosis and social recovery problems who received CBT demonstrated significant increases in the number of weekly hours of constructive and structured activity. Moreover, this was achieved in association with clinically meaningful and significant reductions in symptoms and hopelessness. Similarly, Grant, Huh, Perivoliotis, Stolar, and Beck (2012) evaluated an 18-month recovery-focused cognitive therapy package to improve functioning and negative symptoms in people with schizophrenia who had neuro-

cognitive impairments. Those who received treatment showed significant improvements in global functioning and in positive and negative symptoms (motivation). In an earlier study, Trower and colleagues (2004) targeted harmful compliance in those with command hallucinations using cognitive therapy. Significant reductions in favor of the cognitive therapy group, which were found in perceived power and omniscience of voices, associated compliance behavior, and distress and depression, remained at 12-month follow-up. This study is currently being replicated in a large multicenter RCT with a longer follow-up to allow researchers to draw more definite conclusions regarding the effectiveness and durability of such an intervention (Birchwood et al., 2011). Recently, there have also been more successful approaches developed to treat delusional beliefs by addressing worry, insomnia, and reasoning biases, which are hypothesized to maintain the persistence of delusions and related distress (see Freeman, 2011, for a review of studies).

Symptom Recovery in Acute Schizophrenia

A handful of studies have investigated the use of CBTp in the treatment of acutely ill patients hospitalized for an acute psychotic episode. Because the participants are acutely ill and may well be suspicious, agitated, and unstable, the therapy is often implemented as a "therapy envelope," which comprises a range of durations of therapy that can be delivered in a flexible manner. Two studies have produced effect sizes of –0.49 and 0.93 (Drury, Birchwood, Cochrane, & Macmillan, 1996; Haddock, Tarrier, et al., 1999), indicating considerable variance in this small number of studies. The Study of Cognitive Reality Alignment Therapy in Early Schizophrenia (SoCRATES) (Lewis et al., 2002), which is by far the largest and methodologically most rigorous study, recruited 309 patients with early-onset schizophrenia and produced an effect size of 0.12. In an 18-month follow-up of this trial, both CBTp and supportive counseling continued to confer clinical benefit over TAU alone, although there was a trend toward significance for auditory hallucinations to respond better to CBTp (Tarrier, Lewis, et al., 2004). A more recent RCT included participants in the acute phase of their first episode of psychosis who either received CBTp or befriending. CBTp significantly improved functioning when compared to befriending at midtreatment and end of treatment with an effect size of 0.39, but it did not improve symptoms (Jackson et al., 2008). CBTp appeared to promote early recovery, similar to the SoCRATES study (Lewis et al., 2002). However, any differences between the CBTp and befriending groups were lost at 1-year follow-up. In addition, the lack of a TAU group meant any additional treatment participants were receiving as a result of their acute phase could not be considered (Jackson et al., 2008).

Relapse Prevention

A number of studies have investigated relapse prevention, or the ability of CBTp to prevent or delay future acute episodes. Relapse is an important outcome because of the disruption, distress, and economic costs that symptom exacerbation brings. Studies of CBTp interventions in which relapse prevention was just one of a series of components achieved little success, with four studies showing a mean reduction in relapse of only 1.4% compared to control treatments, whereas studies in which CBTp focused on and was dedicated to relapse prevention resulted in some success, with two studies showing a mean relapse reduction of 21% (Tarrier & Wykes, 2004). The latest meta-analysis by Sarin and colleagues (2011), which included a handful of studies examining relapse rates comparing CBTp to TAU and to other psychological interventions, did not show any strong evidence that CBTp had treatment effects in the prevention of relapse. Providing cognitive therapy in the acute phase was also found to be unsuccessful in reducing the number of admissions and the total number of days in hospital at 1-year follow-up (Jackson et al., 2008). A large, multicenter, methodologically robust RCT investigated the effectiveness of CBTp and family intervention specifically designed for relapse prevention and symptom reduction in patients with psychosis who had recently relapsed (Garety et al., 2008). Both interventions had no effects on remission or relapse at 12- or 24-month follow-up, although CBTp reduced depression and symptoms, and improved social functioning, and family work improved the distress associated with delusions. However, a later study by the same research group used novel statistical methodology to reexamine the data (Dunn et al., 2012). CBTp was found to be effective at increasing months in remission and reducing symptoms, but only when therapy was completed in full and included a range of cognitive and behavioral strategies targeting relapse prevention and symptoms.

Early Intervention

In addition to the effect on individuals with more established psychoses, there has been growing interest in diverting the course in schizophrenia at an early stage. Morrison and colleagues (2004) reported a study using CBT techniques in this early group to attempt to avert or postpone the first acute episode of the disorder by intervening during a prodromal period. Their technique focused not on frank positive symptoms, but on problem-solving difficulties. The results of this first RCT appeared promising. CBTp proved more beneficial than TAU in preventing progression into psychosis, preventing the prescription of antipsychotic medication, and reducing symptoms. However, in a more recent, much larger multisite RCT that compared cognitive therapy offered to young people at risk for serious mental illness and TAU, these findings were not replicated. There were no differences between the groups in terms of transition to psychosis over 12 to 24 months, although the authors discuss the possibility that their study lacked the power to detect a difference due to unexpectedly low conversion rates in the control group, and they questioned the at-risk mental state of their sample, as well as the impact of their active monitoring control condition (Morrison, French, et al., 2012). Therapy did confer clinically meaningful benefits in symptom frequency and intensity. This same research group has also evaluated the effectiveness of cognitive therapy for those within early interventions services who discontinued antipsychotic medication (Morrison, Hutton, et al., 2012). All participants received therapy, which was associated with improvements in positive and negative symptoms and functioning at the end of treatment and follow-up, and increases in self-rated recovery at follow-up. A recent meta-analysis of RCTs of early intervention services, CBT, and family interventions for those with early psychosis (3–5 years after illness onset) confirmed the positive effects of intervening in this crucial period. Early intervention services, which included CBTp, family work, and medication as part of the care package, allowed better access to and engagement with treatment, as well as reduced relapse rates, hospital admissions, and symptoms. CBTp alone improved symptom severity at 2-year follow-up, while family therapy improved relapse rates and hospital admissions at the end of treatment (Bird et al., 2010). Therefore, a holistic treatment plan provided by early intervention services appears advantageous during the initial stages of illness.

Summary of Evidence

The evidence for CBTp reducing positive symptoms in chronic, partially remitted patients with schizophrenia is good. Evidence that CBTp speeds recovery in acutely ill patients to the level of achieving a significant clinical benefit is more equivocal. Reductions in relapse rates are achieved when the intervention focuses on and is dedicated to relapse reduction, but they are disappointing for standard CBTp. There is positive evidence that CBTp and family intervention can benefit patients in early intervention services who are in the early stages of illness. Offering CBT in the prodromal phase appears to provide little additional benefit in terms of preventing full psychosis in vulnerable individuals, although symptoms can be improved.

THEORETICAL ADVANCES

There has been considerable debate about the theoretical understanding of schizophrenia, with biological explanations being dominant. However, psychological and social factors have consistently been shown to be influential, certainly in affecting the course of schizophrenia, and have been incorporated into stress–vulnerability models that have emphasized the importance of these psychosocial factors in precipitating and maintaining psychotic episodes (Nuechterlein, 1987). Cognitive models have been developed in tandem with advances in CBT (Garety, Kuipers, Fowler, Freeman, & Bebbington, 2001). It is expected that as these cognitive models develop and are subjected to empirical tests, further refinements of CBTp treatment will develop. For example, CBTp appears to have little significant effect in reducing suicide risk (Tarrier, Haddock, et al., 2006); however, with a greater conceptual understanding of the psychological mechanisms underlying such risk, more focused interventions to reduce risk will arise (Bolton, Gooding, Kapur, Barrowclough, & Tarrier, 2007; Johnson, Gooding, & Tarrier, 2008).

BASIC CLINICAL PRINCIPLES

A number of common clinical strategies underlie all variants of CBTp for schizophrenia: engagement and establishment of a therapeutic relationship; assessment based on an individualized case formulation that identifies psychotic experience (symptoms) and establishes associations between the patient's cognition,

behavior, and affect within the environmental context in response to this experience; and an intervention strategy based on this formulation that uses cognitive and behavioral methods to reduce psychotic symptoms and associated emotional distress. Patients are taught to be aware of their symptoms and to learn methods to manage them (e.g., learning to control auditory hallucinations by switching their attention away from them, or by thinking about alternative explanations for their experiences).

Patients can acquire coping strategies that are broken down into elements, learned individually, then aggregated into an overall strategy. To ensure that these coping strategies can be implemented outside of therapy, patients overlearn them during the therapy session. Learning such control techniques allows patients to challenge beliefs they may have had about voices, such as "The voices are uncontrollable," "The voices are all powerful," and "I must obey the voices." Thus, by learning to control basic psychological processes such as attention, through attention switching and distraction, patients also learn to challenge their beliefs about their experiences and symptoms. Behavioral experiments and reality tests may also be used to disprove delusional and inappropriate beliefs. Particular attention is paid to identifying avoidance and safety behaviors that reinforce inappropriate beliefs. Changing these behaviors is a powerful method of changing beliefs and delusions. Patients may be assisted in their attempts at behavior change by means of self-instruction and coping strategies that decrease arousal (e.g., breathing exercises; quick relaxation; guided imagery; and encouraging positive task-oriented internal dialogue). In some refractory cases, patients are convinced and unshakable in the belief that their delusions are true, and they are unwilling to examine the veracity of this subjective experience. In these cases, the clinician must negotiate treatment goals aimed at reducing distress rather than the symptoms themselves. A failure to do this will probably result in the patient disengaging and refusing treatment.

It is frequently the case that the patient's delusional beliefs persist in spite of evidence to contradict them, including evidence that occurs naturally and that is manufactured by the therapist through behavioral experiments and reality testing. To weaken these delusional explanations, the therapist should use all available opportunities, through guided discovery and Socratic questioning, to reappraise the evidence for the patient's explanation of events, thus weakening the delusions. Pointing out the contradictory evidence in a quizzical and puzzled manner, often known as the "Columbo technique," is advised, so the patient has to account for contradictions and review his/her explanation in light of this new and contradictory evidence. When delusions are strongly held, this can be a slow process, but the weakening of delusional beliefs can occur, or, as happens in some cases, the delusional interpretations remain or return, but their importance and distressing nature are greatly reduced. For example, an older adult female patient treated by one of the authors (N. T.) experienced auditory hallucinations that were of a blasphemous and obscene nature. She believed that her brain acted as a transmitter and broadcast her thoughts, so that other people in the vicinity could hear her blasphemous and obscene thoughts. Her main social contact was with her local church and associated social club. One Sunday, during the church service, she heard the voices and became convinced that her own thoughts about the voices were broadcast aloud to the congregation. She was mortified and so ashamed that she left the church and was unable to return or to have any contact with her friends. She was convinced that she had become ostracized by the church congregation. On being asked about the evidence for this, she replied that she had since met other members of the church congregation in town and they had totally ignored her, which had further reinforced her sense of exclusion, shame, and self-disgust. On further questioning, she revealed that she had been walking on the pavement and had seen her friends drive by some distance away. There was a high probability that they had not seen her. Thus, her evidence for being ostracized was challenged. We agreed upon a treatment goal that would test her interpretation of the situation. If the fear that the church congregation would shun her if she returned was real, then she should expect a negative reaction when she returned to church. If the fear was irrational, there would be no negative reaction; in fact, the others should be pleased to see her return. She experienced considerable anxiety at the thought of returning to church but managed the return using methods she had learned to cope with both the experience of auditory hallucinations and anxiety. To her surprise, far from being shunned or ostracized, she was greeted with warmth and concern. This experience considerably weakened her beliefs that others could hear her thoughts, and her delusions were rated as minimal. On being asked about the events some months later at follow-up, she said that she believed others could hear her thoughts, but because it did not

appear to bother them, she was no longer concerned about it either! In this case, her delusional explanation of past events had returned but no longer caused her any distress or disrupted her social functioning.

Emphasis has also been placed on improving the patient's self-esteem and feelings of self-worth. This more recent addition to the treatment has been found to be effective and well received by patients (Hall & Tarrier, 2003). In this chapter we have placed these methods after the treatment of symptoms, indicating a progression from symptom reduction to improved self-esteem. However, there is no reason why improvements in self-esteem cannot be initiated at the beginning of treatment, and in some cases this may be desirable.

The future may hold exciting new opportunities to use new technology such as smartphones to implement real-time assessment and interventions, and to individualize treatment protocols (Kelly et al., 2012).

BACKGROUND AND ASSOCIATED FACTORS

Phases of the Disorder and Relationship to Aims of Treatment

Schizophrenia, a complex disorder that may well be lifelong, passes through a number of phases. For example, the prodromal phase that occurs before a full-blown psychotic episode is characterized by nonspecific symptoms and symptoms of anxiety, depression, irritability, insomnia, and quasi-psychotic experience (e.g., magical thinking, feelings of paranoia). The prodromal phase develops into a psychotic episode, during which the most florid psychotic symptoms are present and seriously interfere with functioning. A psychotic episode usually requires acute management, frequently including hospitalization. Recovery from an acute episode of psychosis is followed by a period of remission or partial remission with maintenance doses of antipsychotic medication. It is not uncommon for residual symptoms to remain during the recovery and remission phase, and in some cases, there is little recovery at all. Treatment aims and strategies for CBTp vary depending on the phase of the disorder. For example, during the prodromal phase, the aim is to prevent transition into a full psychotic episode; during an acute episode, the aim is to speed recovery; during partial remission, the aim is to reduce residual symptoms and to prevent further relapse; and in full remission, the aim is to keep the patient well. The specifics of CBTp may vary depending on these aims and the phase of the disorder in which they are applied. For example, during an acute admission for a psychotic episode, the patient is often disturbed, distressed, and agitated. Thus, therapy sessions are often brief and frequent, whereas for chronically ill patients living within the community, therapy sessions follow the normal outpatient format. In all cases, therapy is tailored to the tolerance of the patient. In all but the most exceptional cases, CBTp is used in addition to appropriate antipsychotic medication. The various phases of the disorder and appropriate treatment strategies are outlined in Table 12.1.

Associated Features and Disability

It is important that the clinician attend to associated features and complicating factors, as well as the symptoms of the disorder. These vary from the effects of the disorder on basic psychological processes (e.g., attention) to clinical issues (e.g., suicide risk) to social issues (e.g., social deprivation and poor employment opportunities). These associated features are outlined in Table 12.2.

The crucial point is that the clinician be aware that these problems can arise. Some of them can be dealt with by keeping the message simple and brief, but with plenty of repetition (i.e., use of overlearning in teaching coping strategies). Writing down simple points for the patient as a memory aid can also be helpful, as can creating a small "workbook," so that the patient has a continuous record of these points. This is usually more effective than providing handouts, which are rarely

read and frequently are lost. It is important to balance the nature and duration of sessions against the patient's level of tolerance. Initially, it might be best to keep sessions brief or allow the patient to leave when he/she has had enough. The one-to-one nature of therapy is highly stressful, so initial sessions may serve merely to provide habituation to the social stress of being with the clinician. Teaching the patient simple strategies to deal with tension and anxiety (e.g., brief relaxation) may be helpful in habituating to the therapy situation and may also provide a concrete task on which to focus attention. Simple attention-focusing tasks, such as focusing on some item in the room for a short period, may be helpful in reducing the effect of irrelevant stimuli on the patient's conscious awareness. It is also important to recognize that the verbal and nonverbal cues the therapist might expect to indicate severe distress, depression, or suicidality may not be expressed by someone with schizophrenia. Affect may be flat or inappropriate, which may result in the therapist missing important signs of risk. This can be avoided, in part, by knowing the person and how he/she reacts, by never making assumptions about mental state, and by having the patient agree from the outset that he/she will inform the therapist of important changes in his/her life or mood.

Unfortunately, some issues, such as social conditions, are often beyond the therapist's power to change but may well have an impact on the treatment process. However, there is nothing wrong in assuming an advocacy role or in helping patients to empower themselves by aiding their attempts to improve their own circumstances. Finally, it is important that therapists adopt a

TABLE 12.1. Treatment Aims and Methods in Different Phases of the Schizophrenia Illness

Phase	Aim	Treatment method
Preillness prodrome	Prevention of translation into full psychosis	CBT for early signs and prevention of symptom escalation
Acute episode	Speed recovery	CBT and coping training
Partially remitted residual symptoms	Symptom reduction	CBT, coping training, self-esteem enhancement
Remission	Relapse prevention	CBT for staying well and family intervention
Relapse prodrome	Abort relapse	Early signs identification and relapse prevention

TABLE 12.2. Associated Features of Schizophrenia: Features That Need to Be Assessed and Considered as Potential Difficulties in the Psychological Treatment of Schizophrenia

Psychological

- Disrupted or slowed thought processes
- Difficulty discriminating signal from noise
- Restricted attention
- Hypersensitivity to social interactions
- Difficulty in processing social signals
- Flat and restricted affect
- Elevated arousal and dysfunctional arousal regulation
- Hypersensitivity to stress and life events
- High risk of depression and hopelessness
- Effects of trauma
- Stigmatization
- Low self-esteem and self-worth
- High risk of substance and alcohol abuse
- High risk of suicide and self-harm
- Interference of normal adolescent and early adult development due to onset of illness

Psychosocial

- Hypersensitivity to family and interpersonal environment (including that created by professional staff)
- Risk of perpetrating or being the victim of violence

Social

- Conditions of social deprivation
- Poor housing
- Downward social drift
- Unemployment and difficulty in competing in the job market
- Restricted social network
- Psychiatric career interfering with utilization of other social resources

noncritical approach and learn to accommodate their own frustrations if therapy is progressing more slowly than they had hoped. Aspects of schizophrenia can make some patients difficult to deal with, and the therapist needs to be aware of this and develop a tolerant approach. The lack of a positive relationship between case managers and patients has been shown to be associated with poorer prognosis (Tattan & Tarrier, 2000).

THE CONTEXT OF THERAPY

It is highly probable that by the time a referral is made for CBT the patient will be under the care of a multidisciplinary mental health team, and be receiving antipsychotic medication and some type of case management. People who develop a psychotic illness are usually diagnosed by a general practitioner or primary care team, or in an accident and emergency department, and referred on to mental health services. Mental health services are organized in different ways in different countries, depending on health care philosophies and structures, but what is delivered in terms of therapy content may be independent of how that service is organized. Thus, the therapeutic procedures described in this chapter can be utilized in different types of service structure and organization. We have provided CBTp to patients on closed and open wards, in hospital and health center outpatient facilities, in community facilities, and in the patients' own homes. It is probable that the more flexible the system, the more likely the patient will be engaged and attend. To this end we often deliver treatment in the patient's home, which is a common procedure in the United Kingdom.

Evidence from research trials indicates that cognitive-behavioral treatments are delivered over about 20 treatment sessions. These can be intensive, over 3 months, or less intensive, over 9 months or longer. Clinical impressions indicate that some patients benefit from continued, although less intensive treatment, whereas others benefit from booster sessions. The clinician should always be led by the clinical need of the patient and take a collaborative approach rather than adhering to a rigid "one size fits all" protocol. It should be remembered that CBT does not "cure" schizophrenia, but it does help the patient cope with a chronic illness.

The presence of possible associated factors, as outlined earlier, signifies that patients may present with a number of clinical difficulties, as well as psychotic symptoms. The clinician needs to be aware that this may be the case and be prepared to address or treat these presenting problems before moving on to treat the psychotic symptoms. It may be necessary to tackle clinical problems such as high levels of anxiety, depression, hopelessness, and suicidal behavior and risk because they are not only clinical priorities but also there may be important interactions between these other disorders and the psychosis.

The treatment described here is for individual CBTp. It is possible to deliver treatment in a group format. Groups are well received by some patients and are advantageous, in that patients can learn from each other. The results suggest clinical benefits in terms of enhanced self-esteem, but reductions in symptoms are modest compared to those in individual treatments (e.g., Barrowclough et al., 2006), and any improvements appear to get lost at follow-up (Lecomte, Leclerc, & Wykes, 2012).

Other psychosocial treatments may also be available, such as family interventions. There is a considerable literature on family interventions, which have been shown to reduce relapse rates in at-risk individuals, for those in the early stages, and in later psychosis (Bird et al., 2010; Onwumere, Bebbington, & Kuipers, 2011; Onwumere & Kuipers, 2011). Details of family intervention are beyond the scope of this chapter (for the clinical application of family interventions, see Barrowclough & Tarrier, 1992; Kuipers, Onwumere, & Bebbington, 2010; Mueser & Glynn, 1995; see also Miklowitz, Chapter 11, this volume). We have combined individual CBT and family intervention with some success and suggest that therapists consider whether this strategy would be clinically beneficial. Others have offered family therapy to those with co-occurring schizophrenia spectrum diagnoses and substance misuse, with some benefits in symptoms and functioning for both clients and their relatives (Mueser et al., 2013). Concomitant family intervention may reduce stressful home environments and help to sustain improvement. Many patients live alone or are estranged from their relatives, so family intervention may not be an option.

Patient Variables

Patients with schizophrenia represent a heterogeneous group of whom 20–45% may be resistant to medication treatment (Kane, 1999) and 5–10% show no benefit from antipsychotic medication (Pantelis & Barns, 1996). Although there is confusion among the terms "treatment-resistant," "incomplete recovery," and "treatment intolerance," it is clear that conventional treatment with antipsychotic medication is ineffective in a significant number of patients, in spite of well-publicized advances in antipsychotic medication. It is important, therefore, in tailoring and refining treatments to understand what factors predict a good response to psychological treatment and perhaps the converse, which patients do not derive benefit. Unfortunately, little is known in any great detail about which patients will or will not benefit from cognitive-behavioral treatments (Tarrier & Wykes, 2004). Factors that have been associated with poor outcome include negative symptoms of affective flattening and alogia (cognitive impoverishment) (Tarrier, 1996). Factors associated with better outcome include a shorter duration of illness, a younger age (Morrison, Turkington, et al., 2012), greater pretherapy coping ability (Premkumar et al., 2011) and better clinical and cognitive insight (Emmerson, Granholm, Link, McQuaid, & Jeste, 2009; Perivoliotis et al., 2010), less severe symptoms at pretreatment (Tarrier, Yusupoff, Kinney, et al., 1998), higher baseline functioning and educational achievement (Allott et al., 2011) and receptiveness to hypothetical contradiction (Brabban, Tai, & Turkington, 2009; Garety et al., 1997). These results suggest that those patients who are younger with less severe illness, fewer severe cognitive deficits, and better functioning may respond better, but no hard-and-fast rules are currently supported by evidence. Treatment dropout is a further issue of importance. There is some evidence that patients who drop out of treatment tend to be male, unemployed and unskilled, and single, with a low level of educational attainment and a low premorbid IQ. They have a long duration of illness but at the time of discontinuation are not necessarily severely ill and can function at a reasonable level. Fewer negative symptoms, cannabis or other drug use, and factors such as not having a family member involved with treatment have been found to predict disengagement (Stowkowy, Addington, Liu, Hollowell, & Addington, 2012). Dropouts suffer from both hallucinations and delusions, are paranoid, although not necessarily suspicious of the treating clinician, and depressed and moderately hopeless. The majority cannot see the point of psychological treatment or think that they will not personally benefit from treatment (Tarrier, Yusupoff, McCarthy, Kinney, & Wittkowski, 1998).

Therapist Variables

Therapist variables encompass a number of factors, including training, experience, competency, supervision, and personal style. There is a tendency for health care planners to expect, mainly on economic grounds, that these complex therapies will be delivered by minimally qualified clinicians. This may well be a mistake (Tarrier et al., 1999). Psychological treatment of someone with psychosis is complex, and besides having the skills and experience to treat the psychotic disorder itself, as outlined in this chapter, the clinician may well need to be able to treat a range of comorbid disorders, including anxiety, posttraumatic stress, depression, and addictive disorders. It seems reasonable that to treat successfully someone with a severe mental illness and very possibly a range of comorbid disorders, the clinician should be experienced and sufficiently well trained in CBT to be able to react to various clinical demands and levels of complexity. A recent study showed better outcomes from CBTp to be associated with therapists who spend the majority of their clinical time delivering this specific intervention, and who receive frequent supervision (Steel, Tarrier, Stahl, & Wykes, 2012). In our opinion the treatment of psychotic disorders does not lend itself well to merely following a highly prescriptive manual. As indicated in the previous section on associated features and disabilities, the clinician needs to be competent in recognizing and prioritizing a range of presenting clinical problems for treatment. Similarly, the clinician needs to have personal qualities that engage the patient, who may well be difficult to manage or disturbed, and to tailor the treatment to that individual. Previous research suggests that the absence of a positive relationship is associated with a poorer outcome (Tattan & Tarrier, 2000), so the clinician needs the experience and patience to develop that relationship and maintain engagement. A recent study used the Delphi method to examine what experts in the field viewed as important ingredients in CBTp. Elements such as a detailed assessment, use of a cognitive model and formulation, implementation of change strategies, and the attitudes that should be held by therapists (e.g., normalizing rationale) were agreed to be essential (Morrison & Barratt, 2010).

THE PROCEDURE OF CBT: THE MANCHESTER MODEL

A Clinical Model: The Coping–Recovery Model

The model developed and described by Tarrier bears many similarities to other models and has benefited from contact and discussion with other clinical researchers in the field. The basic tenet is the recovery model, in which patients are coping with a potentially persistent illness that may well change many aspects of their lives, affect their hopes and aspirations, and be associated with comorbid disorders such as depression and anxiety disorders. The therapist aids the patient in facilitating, as much as possible, the process of recovery. The coping model strongly resembles and uses many methods of other CBT approaches but emphasizes coping with symptoms rather than curing them, and intervenes to modify cognitive processes (e.g., attention), as well as cognitive content and behavior.

The clinical model that guides treatment is presented in Figure 12.1. It assumes that the experience of psychotic symptoms, hallucinations, and delusions is a dynamic interaction between internal and external factors. Internal factors may be either biological or psychological and can be inherited or acquired. For example, genetic factors may influence both the biochemical functioning of the brain and cognitive capacity. Alternatively, biological and psychological dysfunction may be acquired, for example, in deficits in cognitive flexibility and in the development of maladaptive attitudes. Such internal factors increase individuals' vulnerability to psychosis, and their risk is further increased through exposure to environmental stress, such as certain interpersonal or excessively demanding environments. The interaction between internal and external factors is important both in the origins of the disorder and in maintaining symptoms. A dysfunction in the processing of information, such as source monitoring

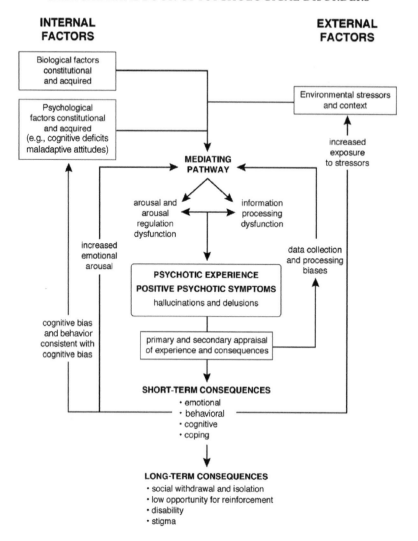

FIGURE 12.1. A clinical model of the origins and maintenance of psychotic symptoms.

in hallucinations (i.e., a belief about where the voice is coming from) and probabilistic reasoning in delusions, in combination with dysfunctions in the arousal system and its regulation, result in disturbances of perception and thought that are characteristic of psychosis. The individual is reactive to these experiences, and there is a process of primary and secondary appraisal in which the individual attempts to interpret these experiences and give them meaning, then react to their consequenc-

es. Often patients' appraisal of experience results in feelings of threat to their physical integrity or social standing and concomitant emotional reactions, and avoidant and safety behavior. The immediate reaction to the psychotic experience is multidimensional, including emotional, behavioral, and cognitive elements. Secondary effects, such as depressed mood, anxiety in social situations, and the effect of trauma may further compound the situation.

The important aspect of the model is that appraisal (including beliefs about experience) and reaction to the psychotic experience feedback through a number of possible routes and increase the probability of the maintenance or recurrence of the psychotic experience. For example, the emotional reaction to hearing threatening voices or experiencing strong feelings of paranoia may well be anxiety or anger. Both these emotions include elevated levels of autonomic arousal that act either directly, through sustained increased levels of arousal, or indirectly, through further disrupting information processing, to increase the likelihood of psychotic symptoms. Similarly, behavioral responses to psychotic symptoms may increase exposure to environmental stress or increase risk of trauma (e.g., becoming involved in violence or indulging in dangerous behavior) that maintains or aggravates psychotic symptoms. For example, paranoid thoughts may result in interpersonal conflict or, alternatively, social avoidance and withdrawal. Both situations are likely to increase the probability of symptoms occurring. Interpersonal conflict is likely to be interpreted as evidence for persecution, whereas withdrawal and isolation probably result in confirmatory rumination and resentment, with a lack of opportunity to disconfirm these paranoid beliefs. The appraisal of the content of voices or delusional thoughts as valid and true may result in behavior consistent with these beliefs and a confirmatory bias to collecting and evaluating evidence on which to base future judgments of reality.

Psychotic experiences can lead to dysfunctional beliefs that are then acted on in a way that leads to their confirmation or a failure to disconfirm. This can be termed the experience–belief–action–confirmation, or EBAC, cycle. It is suggested that such cycles maintain psychotic experience through reinforcement of maladaptive beliefs and behavior. The generic model indicated in Figure 12.1 provides an overarching picture of how the patient's problems arise and are maintained. Embedded within this model are the microelements of specific, time-linked events such as the EBAC cycle (see Figure 12.2).

Assessment

The clinician needs to be able to assess and develop a formulation of the determinants of the patient's psychotic symptoms. Clinicians may find the use of standardized assessment instruments helpful (there are many of

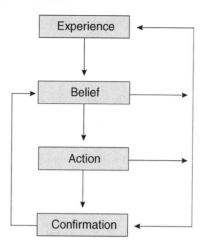

FIGURE 12.2. The experience–belief–action–confirmation (EBAC) cycle.

these, and they assess a range of functions; see Barnes & Nelson, 1994, for a detailed description and review of assessments). We recommend the Psychotic Symptom Rating Scales (PSYRATS; Haddock, McCarron, Tarrier, & Faragher, 1999) as an effective method of assessing the multidimensional nature of positive psychotic symptoms. The clinician needs to understand the individual variation in psychotic symptoms. This can be achieved by the use of a semistructured interview (the Antecedent and Coping Interview [ACI]; for more details, see Tarrier, 2002, 2006) that covers the nature and variation of positive psychotic symptoms experienced by the patient, including beliefs about psychotic symptoms, emotional reactions that accompany each symptom, antecedent stimuli and context in which each symptom occurs, consequences resulting from the symptoms and how the patient's behavior and beliefs are affected, and methods the patient uses to cope and manage his/her experiences. This allows the clinician to build up a comprehensive picture of how the patient experiences the psychosis on a daily basis and how his/her affect, behavior, and beliefs are changed. The clinician should be careful to identify avoidance and safety behaviors that occur because of psychotic symptoms, and examples in which the patient fails to disconfirm irrational or delusional beliefs. The clinician should use the clinical models shown in Figures 12.1 and 12.2 as a guide.

Intervention

Coping Strategies

When the clinician has constructed a comprehensive picture of the patient's psychotic experience, he/she can discuss this with the patient and present the rationale for CBTp. There may well be patients who are completely convinced of the truth of their delusional thoughts and will not accept any alternative view, in which case coping with distress should be advanced as a suitable goal.

The characteristics of CBTp and coping training are that

- They are based on an individualized assessment or formulation.
- They emphasize a normal and general process of dealing with adversity.
- They emphasize that this is part of the recovery process.
- They are carried out systematically through overlearning, simulation, and role play.
- They are additive in that different strategies can be added together in a sequence that progresses to *in vivo* implementation.
- They are based on providing a new response set that will be a method of coping with an ongoing problem rather than being curative.
- Cognitive coping skills are learned through a process of external verbalization that is slowly diminished until the required procedure is internalized as thought under internal control.
- They enhance executive function.
- The learning of cognitive and behavioral coping skills develops through a process of graded practice or rehearsal.
- They provide opportunities for reappraisal and reattributions.

These coping methods include the following changes in cognitive processes, cognitive content, and behavior.

ATTENTION SWITCHING

A process whereby patients actively change the focus of their attention from one subject or experience to another, "attention switching" involves inhibiting an ongoing response and initiating an alternative. Patients are trained within the session to switch attention on cue through rehearsal to external stimuli (e.g., an aspect of their environment, such as describing a picture or being aware of background traffic noise) or to internal stimuli, often to a set of positive images. For example, one patient who was asked to choose a positive scene to which to attend chose a restaurant in Blackpool, where he had had an enjoyable meal. He was trained to be able to elicit a visual image of the restaurant by describing the scene, furniture, decorations, and such in great detail. He was then asked to remember the experience of the meal in all his senses: the visual memory of the food; its smell and taste; the feel of holding the knife and fork in his hands; the experience of eating; and so on. He continually rehearsed the memory of the meal in the restaurant until he was able to elicit it at will. He then rehearsed switching his attention away from delusional thoughts to images of the meal. He was taught to use the onset of a delusion as a cue for attention switching (see "Awareness Training" below).

ATTENTION NARROWING

In "attention narrowing," a process whereby patients restrict the range and content of their attention, many patients talked about "blanking" their mind or focusing their attention as a method of coping. Evidence suggests that one problem faced by patients with schizophrenia is an inability to filter information input adequately, to distinguish signal from noise. Training patients to focus their attention and improve attentional control may assist them in overcoming this difficulty by narrowing and regulating their attention.

MODIFIED SELF-STATEMENTS AND INTERNAL DIALOGUE

That patients' use of self-statements can be incorporated successfully into intervention has been known for some years. The use of self-statements and internal dialogue may take on a number of functions in emotion control, such as teaching patients to overcome negative emotions associated with their voices and in cueing goal-directed behavior, and in cueing and directing reality testing. In each case the patient is taught statements that direct the appropriate response, such as "I don't need to be afraid," "I need to keep going and get on the bus," or "Why do I think that man is looking at me when I've never seen him before?" Within the session, the patient is first asked to repeat the set of statements or questions out loud when given the appropriate cue. The verbalized statements are then gradually reduced in loudness until they are internalized. The patient then practices these in simulated situations within the session. Learning such questioning statements is a useful stage in generating and evaluating alternative explanations for experience.

REATTRIBUTION

Patients are asked to generate an alternative explanation for an experience, then practice reattribution statements when that experience occurs. Initially, when we started coping training, we used reattributions that were illness related, such as "It's not a real voice, it's my illness." We have since abandoned this as unhelpful. We now try to use other, alternative explanations: "It may seem like a real voice, but it's just my own thoughts" and "It may seem as though people are looking at me, but they have to look somewhere." If patients do make changes that increase their control over their symptoms or circumstances, or challenge the omnipotence or infallibility of their voices, then these changes can be evidence for a reattribution concerning the nature of their symptoms or their ability to exert control—for example, "How can the voice be all powerful if it talks rubbish?" or "I don't have to believe it if it isn't true."

AWARENESS TRAINING

Patients are taught to be aware of and monitor their positive symptoms, especially their onset. Patients not only become aware of their experiences but they also try to accept these experiences but not react to them. Patients are aware of their voices but do not react to them or become captured by their content. One function of awareness training is to make patients aware of the form and characteristics of their thoughts and perceptions rather than the content—for example, to monitor the physical onset of a voice, then use attention switching to reduce the emotional impact of the content. The aim is twofold: to assist patients in becoming *mentally disengaged* from their symptoms, especially the content, and to use symptoms as a cue to alternative action.

DEAROUSING TECHNIQUES

Because high levels of arousal have been implicated in the psychopathology of schizophrenia and frequently occur as both antecedents and responses to psychotic experience, teaching patients to cope with these is im-portant. These coping strategies may be simple passive behaviors to avoid agitation, such as sitting quietly instead of pacing up and down, or they may be more active methods of arousal control, such as breathing exercises or quick relaxation. We have not favored lengthy relaxation training, such as traditional progressive relaxation exercises, because these are time-consuming and off the point. What is functional here is a quick, usable skill.

INCREASED ACTIVITY LEVELS

Many patients with schizophrenia are vulnerable to delusional thought or hallucinations during periods of inactivity, a problem to which they appear particularly prone. Many patients report that finding something to do is helpful. Thus, simple activity scheduling can be a powerful coping strategy, especially if implemented at the onset of the symptom, thus creating a dual task competing for attentional resources. Besides increasing purposeful activity this also reduces exposure to conditions under which symptoms are aggravated.

SOCIAL ENGAGEMENT AND DISENGAGEMENT

Although many patients tolerate social interactions poorly, surprisingly, many also find social engagement a useful method of coping. Possibly this may occur because social interaction serves as a dual task and source of distraction, and because it may help patients rationalize maladaptive thinking. It is beneficial to be able to titrate the amount of social stimulation involved in any interaction with the tolerance level of a particular patient, and to teach the patient that levels of social disengagement may be used to help develop tolerance of social stimulation. Social withdrawal and avoidance are common responses to experiencing overstimulation as a result of social interaction. However, patients can learn less drastic methods of disengagement, such as leaving the room for a short period and then returning, temporarily moving away from the social group, and practicing *functional disengagement* by not conversing for short periods or lowering their gaze. By using these methods, patients can control and tolerate social stimulation. Patients may also initiate social interaction more confidently as a method to reduce the impact of their symptoms, if they feel they have some control over the intensity of those interactions. Simple training in specific skills for interaction and role plays can facilitate this.

BELIEF MODIFICATION

Patients can learn to examine their beliefs and to challenge them if they are inappropriate by examining the evidence and generating alternative explanations. Many patients do this to some extent already, but the level of arousal experienced, or the level of isolation and avoidance, can make these attempts unsuccessful. These methods are very similar to those used in traditional cognitive therapy except that the patient may need more prompting, and the goal is to incorporate the skills of belief modification into a self-regulatory process. Patients can be encouraged to question their beliefs as they occur: "What would be the purpose of someone spying on me; how much effort and cost would it take; how would this be resourced and organized; and for what gain?" Similarly, patients can be encouraged to look for inconsistencies and use these to challenge their beliefs. For example, the patient who was involved in a fight 15 years earlier, and still avoids young men because he fears that the same group is out to get revenge, may be asked to reflect on the fact that because the members of the gang are now in their middle to late 30s, he has been vigilant for the wrong age group. This can be used to challenge his fear that he needs to be vigilant to stay safe. In effect, his safety behaviors have not protected him from the source of danger. Patients can also learn to examine evidence to challenge their beliefs about the voices they hear. When patients perceive their voices as omnipotent and truthful, clinicians can investigate to see whether they have been wrong or incorrect. For example, the patient whose voices told him he was going to be murdered because he was a spy, concluded that the voices must be true and that he must deserve this fate. However, the voices also told him that he was soon to be married, and because he could find no supporting evidence for this, he decided it was untrue. However, he had never thought to challenge the voices' veracity concerning the threat of murder. Realizing that he was unlikely to be married in the near future, as the voices had asserted, helped him to challenge the idea that he was to be murdered by doubting the truthfulness of the voices and to look for further supporting, objective evidence of the spy ring, which was not forthcoming.

REALITY TESTING AND BEHAVIORAL EXPERIMENTS

Probably the strongest way to test beliefs is to test them out in reality by some type of action; behavior change is probably the best way to produce cognitive change. Patients sometimes do this naturally, although a tendency toward biased interpretation and hypothesis protection may lead them to erroneous conclusions. Patients can learn to identify specific beliefs and to generate competing predictions that can be tested. The failure to do this in real life usually leads to patterns of avoidance, which can be reversed to challenge the beliefs that they underpin.

Enhancing Coping Strategies

Coping methods develop over time and vary in their complexity, from simple and direct attempts to control cognitive processes, such as attention, to more complex, self-directed methods that modify cognitive content and inference. Frequently, combinations of different coping strategies are built up, for example, the use of attention switching and dearousing techniques helps to dull the strength of a delusion, so that reality testing can be implemented. Without these initial coping methods the patient would not be able to undergo reality testing. Furthermore, the initial coping strategies can be used to challenge the strength of the delusion of the omnipotence of the voices and provide an increase in self-efficacy. The therapist may ask questions, such as "You've used these attention-switching methods to cope effectively with your voices. What does that tell you about them being in total control and you being helpless?" The patient may well make statements that indicate the voices have been demonstrated to be fallible and he/she has some control over the situation, which can then be used as self-statements or a modified internal dialogue to further enhance self-efficacy and coping.

Modification of Behavior or Cognition

Changes in behavior and cognition complement each other, and one is not necessarily better than the other. Changes in behavior should always be used to examine and potentially challenge maladaptive thoughts and beliefs or as learning experiences. Similarly, changes in cognition should be used as opportunities to change behavior and to establish new behaviors. The therapist should always look for opportunities to prompt patients to reappraise their beliefs. This can be carried out as part of formal behavioral experiments, naturally occurring changes, and frequent reflections on what has been achieved in treatment. In assessment and during formulation the therapist should always be alert to patients' avoidance or safety behaviors, or when patients do not behave in a way that could disconfirm their fears, delusions, or maladaptive cognitions. These can be used very early on in treatment as behavioral experiments to test out patients' beliefs or to provide opportunities for quick improvements to challenge despondent or hopelessness beliefs, such as "Nothing is worth it if I cannot change" or "I have no control over my life or circumstances." The belief of "no control" is often present and can be refuted by many small behavioral changes that may be repeated and referred to frequently. Finally, it is often helpful at the beginning of treatment to obtain some behavior changes, although often small, and increase activity that may have a number of associated benefits and provide the opportunity for reappraisal.

Modification of Cognitive Content or Cognitive Process

Therapists frequently face the choice of whether to try to modify the content of hallucinations or delusions, or the attentional processes that these phenomena have captured. Traditionally, in cognitive therapy the content of cognition is the main focus. In the coping model intervention, this is broadened to modification of cognitive processes because modifying cognitive processes provides greater clinical flexibility, and because deficits of the regulation of attention and executive function are often present in psychotic disorders. In practice, these tactics can work together. Initial modification of attentional processes through attention switching, for example, can decrease the emotional impact of the experience. A similar effect can be produced by attending to the physical characteristics of a hallucination rather than what the voice is actually saying. This can provide not only an opening to challenge the truth of the content of the voice or delusional thought but also a sense of control over these experiences. Take, for example, a young man who is experiencing voices that accuse him of having committed a murder and also say he is Russian. Initially, he can be taught to turn his attention away from the voices in a systematic way to reduce their emotional impact. This technique can be used to weaken the emotional strength of the experience, to elicit a sense of control, and to challenge the belief that the voices are all-powerful. With increased self-efficacy and a greater sense of power, the patient can later challenge the content of the voices that accuse him of murder by investigating the objective evidence that a murder has been committed. Furthermore, the untruthfulness of the voices in saying he is Russian can be used to challenge the veracity of the murder accusation; if the voices had been wrong about one issue, then they could be wrong about the other. Modification of cognitive process and content provides the therapist with two basic routes to intervention and the flexibility to move from one tactic to the other.

CASE STUDY

The following case example gives some indication of how CBTp works.

History

Jim, a 28-year-old man, developed a psychotic illness when he was 22. During his first episode, Jim became increasingly paranoid and accused people, including his friends, of stealing his money. He said that he could feel people taking money and his wallet from his pockets when he was socializing in his local pub and also when he was traveling by bus. The feeling that "something was wrong" had been with him for a few months, and Jim then began to hear voices warning him that people were against him and scheming to "do me down." These voices talked to Jim, warning him against "the schemes" and telling him who was involved and to be on his guard. These voices were especially insistent that those closest to Jim were the people most against him and the "worst schemers." The voices also told Jim that his girlfriend was unfaithful, and he experienced "visions," sent by the voices, of his girlfriend having sex with other men. He did not actually believe that his girlfriend was unfaithful, but he became very angry that the voices should make these accusations. On some occasions, Jim did lose control and confronted some male friends about having affairs with his girlfriend. Usually he accepted their denials.

Jim also heard voices talking about him. These different voices were usually "scheming" and making insulting and accusatory comments. Sometimes these voices would laugh at Jim because his girlfriend was cheating on him, and make remarks about his sexual inadequacy, to which they attributed her infidelity.

Jim's friends and family noticed that he began to withdraw and became increasingly disheveled. He was often found muttering to himself or making sarcastic comments to family members about how they were "growing rich on my hard work." The voices also told him to "look for signs that the scheming is coming to a head." Jim began to write down an account of everyday events, such as the time certain buses arrived near his house and the type of advertisements on their sides. His parents, who would find these writings left around the house with various passages heavily underlined, were increasingly worried about Jim and also concerned that he was drinking considerable amounts of alcohol. Jim's friends began to avoid him and he was increasingly isolated. He broke up with his girlfriend, who could no longer deal with his accusations of infidelity.

The situation deteriorated very rapidly during the summer months, and Jim was hospitalized one evening and detained under the Mental Health Act. He had gone out early to his local pub. A number of his friends were there, but he kept away from them, drinking alone in a corner. Suddenly Jim got out of his seat and began shouting at his friends, accusing them of stealing his money, undermining his confidence, and spreading rumors about him. He took some loose change from his pockets and threw it at his friends. They tried to ignore him, but Jim became increasingly agitated and aggressive, and finally physically attacked one of them. A number of people became involved, and the situation became more chaotic as a fight broke out. The police were called and Jim was arrested. He had suffered minor physical injuries, so he was taken to the accident and emergency department of the local hospital and from there was admitted to the psychiatric ward. Jim spent about 5 weeks in the hospital, during which time he was treated with antipsychotic medication. His health care plan included counseling, and his family received psychoeducation, in that they were given information about his diagnosis of schizophrenia and general advice on how to manage him at home. Jim's symptoms remitted during his hospital stay, and he was discharged, with frequent outpatient appointments with his psychiatrist and home treatment with the assertive outreach team.

Over the intervening years Jim had five more relapses, during which a similar pattern would follow. He would become paranoid, hear voices and become isolated, and have increasing difficulty in caring for himself. Each relapse was followed by a short period of hospitalization with increased medication. However, residual symptoms became common following an episode, and in spite of increased medication and changes to atypical antipsychotics, Jim continued to experience auditory hallucinations, paranoid delusions, and delusions of reference. He often avoided going out or contacting people because of his paranoia. He was able to initiate and maintain a relationship, although the voices continued to send him "visions" and to question his girlfriend's faithfulness.

Jim was referred for CBT to treat his persistent positive psychotic symptoms as part of a multidisciplinary approach to his care and to promote recovery.

Current Situation

Jim now lives in his own apartment. He has good relations with his parents, who live quite close by and whom he sees every few weeks. He is unemployed and receives disability benefits. Jim attends a day center for people with mental health problems 2 or 3 days a week. He had attended a local college to study computers but recently discontinued schooling because he found the social contact too stressful. Jim has a steady girlfriend, Sue, whom he sees regularly. He has lost contact with the friends he had before he became ill, and although he occasionally sees them, he avoids them and places he thinks they might go. He receives antipsychotic medication, attends monthly outpatient appointments with a psychiatrist, and is visited at home once a week by a community psychiatric nurse who provides counseling and support, and monitors his mental state.

Mental State at Referral

Jim experienced auditory hallucinations in the form of a variety of voices talking to and about him. He described these as "helpful" voices and "evil" voices. The "helpful" voices warned him of the "schemes" of others and told him about dangerous situations and times when he was under threat. They warned him to avoid "dodgy people" who might attack or assault him. Jim thought their warnings were very helpful and was convinced that acting upon these warnings kept him from harm. The "evil" voices generally spoke about him, saying that he was "stupid, useless, and no good," "not up to it sexually," and other personally defamatory statements.

There were voices that told Jim that his girlfriend Sue was unfaithful and cheating on him. He was unsure whether these voices were "helpful" or "evil." These voices also sent Jim pictures of Sue being unfaithful and simultaneously told him that he was stupid and useless to put up with it. He described these pictures as "visions" that he found extremely distressing. Although Jim said he did not believe that Sue was unfaithful, the voices became increasingly more intense and compelling, and he was unable to resist shouting back at them. Sue was able to reassure Jim that his fears were groundless.

Engagement

Initially Jim was resistant to contact with the clinician (in this case, Jim had been referred to a clinical psychologist for CBT). At the time of referral he was quite paranoid, and when he was visited at his home for the first appointment, having failed to attend his clinic appointment, Jim refused to open the door. (It is common practice for mental health professionals in the United Kingdom to do home visits.) A short conversation through the letter box ensued, ending with the clinician's statement that he would return at a more convenient time. Two further visits resulted in Jim refusing to open the door. The strategy here was just to make contact to reassure Jim that his views were perfectly valid and that another visit would be made at a later date to see how he felt about things then. In situations in which the initial engagement is problematic, the best strategy is to "roll with resistance" and try to defuse the situation and reduce any agitation, maintain contact, and return at another time.

On the next occasion Jim was more relaxed and allowed the clinician into his flat. Given Jim's paranoia, it was important for the clinician just to establish a positive interaction and relationship at this point, and not to introduce the topic of symptoms or psychological treatment until Jim was completely comfortable with him. So, in Jim's case, the first couple of sessions were kept brief and covered his general well-being and topics of interest for him. The clinician's primary focus was to keep Jim engaged and to develop the beginnings of a therapeutic relationship. It is not always the case that assessment and treatment cannot be embarked upon more quickly, but maintaining engagement is essential.

The fourth session was longer and the clinician introduced the possibility of psychological treatment. This necessitated a discussion of Jim's symptoms, along the following lines:

> "I understand you have been hearing voices when no one is there? What do you make of this? Have you any idea what these voices are? Are the voices a difficulty for you? Would you want to try and do something about these voices?"

These questions not only raise the topic of the psychotic experience and the suggestion of treatment but also attempt to obtain an idea of the patient's beliefs about the voices and whether they are perceived as real or not.

Similarly, the clinician can ask questions about the paranoid delusions:

> "It is true that you are having difficulties with people?"
>
> "Are you feeling that some people are against you? What do you make of these thoughts and feelings? Why do you think it is happening?"
>
> "Are they a difficulty for you?" "Would you want to try and do something about these thoughts and worries?"

Again, the clinician attempts to assess quickly how strongly Jim holds these delusions and whether he would consider treatment.

Jim was not enthusiastic about treatment. He thought that his fears, as well as the voices, were real, and that psychological treatment was not appropriate in his case. This reaction is often encountered in patients with residual and persistent psychotic symptoms. A number of important points should be considered:

- What needs to be done to maintain engagement?
- How can a clinically relevant problem be identified and mutually agreed upon?
- How can treatment be framed so that the patient sees it as achieving a positive and desired benefit?

First, it is important to validate the experience, but it is not necessary to agree on the cause. For example, in this case, it was important to agree that *Jim did hear voices* and *believe that some people were against him.* This can be done without agreeing that the voices come from a real entity or that people are actually against him. This helps to separate *Jim's belief* about what is happening to him from the experience; that is, that Jim has the belief is not the same as that belief being true. Similarly, that Jim hears voices is not the same as believing these voices exist as an independent and real entity. It may not necessarily be possible to agree on these points at this time, but the clinician can return to these issues. At the moment, engagement is more important.

Next, it is often helpful to investigate the consequences of the experience. Some of the voices cause distress, and Jim's paranoid ideas cause him to be fearful. Thus, distress and fear are more likely to be problems that Jim will be willing to address. This can be introduced as follows:

"You have told me that the voices sometimes make you feel very upset. Perhaps that upset is something I can help you with and that you would like to work on?"

"The thoughts that some people out there are against you and want to harm you make you very frightened. Perhaps that fear is something we can work on together, so you feel less afraid? Maybe if you were less afraid you could cope better with dealing with people. Would that be helpful to you?"

So in cases when patients are very deluded or lack insight into their symptoms, trying to persuade them to eliminate their symptoms and the experiences they believe to be real can be counterproductive and jeopardize engagement. However, trying to reduce distress may be a viable alternative for a collaborative goal. There is also an assumption from the model that reducing emotional reactions to symptoms may well weaken the symptoms themselves.

However, Jim remained unenthusiastic about this treatment goal as well. His view was that being fearful about people was a reasonable reaction given that there were people who would harm him, and this emotion kept him on his "edge," so that he was more vigilant for threat and danger. His belief was that such vigilance actually kept him safe from harm, so there was little motivation to change and put himself in harm's way.

To protect engagement, it is important not to dispute or argue with the patient, and most definitely not at this early stage, when the patient is not convinced that there is any benefit to be gained from treatment. The next strategy the clinician used to engage Jim was to ask about his goals in life.

CLINICIAN: Jim, what sort of goals do you have? Is there anything you would like to achieve personally? Is there anything you would like to do that you haven't been able to do, for whatever reason?

JIM: Yes, lots of things. I'd like to get a job that's well paid. I'd like to go back to college. That would help me get a good job.

CLINICIAN: Going to college would help you get a good job. That is a very good idea. Would you like to go back to college?

JIM: I would, but when I went before I had problems.

CLINICIAN: What sort of problems were they?

JIM: Well, I got scared of the people there. I thought some of them were scary, dodgy, money grubbers. The voices told me not to go. I have to do what the voices tell me.

CLINICIAN: So one of your important goals is to get to college so as to help you get a good job, but being scared of the people there and the voices is stopping you from going to college and achieving your goals. Is that about it?

JIM: Yes, I suppose you are right.

In this way Jim has realized that his important goals are being impeded by his psychosis, and he and the clinician are able to agree on a problem that needs to be addressed. Thus, Jim can see a benefit to receiving treatment.

As well as maintaining engagement, the clinician has learned quite a lot about Jim and his problems. The voices warn Jim about certain situations, and he listens to them and takes avoidant action; thus, he has developed a number of safety behaviors that protect him from perceived harm. Opportunities to test out or refute these threat cognitions by dropping safety behavior are not taken up. However, there are situations that lend themselves to reality testing. Jim experiences command hallucinations (voices that give him a direct order) to which he responds. The likelihood that Jim thinks the voices are powerful, and that he has little or no control over them, provides future opportunity to refute these attributions. Jim experiences some feelings of dissonance in that he is now aware that his valued goals are impeded.

Case Formulation

Treatment naturally follows from an accurate assessment of the patient's problems, and it is important to establish details of the antecedents and consequences of psychotic symptoms (see Tarrier & Calam, 2002, for a discussion of case formulation in general). In this case, Jim has many psychotic symptoms, and it is probably best to deal with them in stages.

Paranoid Delusions

Jim has paranoid delusions that occur in a number of situations. When alone in his flat, Jim worries that his old friends and family have stolen all his money and are scheming against him. This is reinforced by the voices telling Jim he needs to be on his guard. Jim also becomes very paranoid when he goes out. For example, in the street he scans the crowds for signs of his old friends, so that he can make good his escape if he sees them or "scary people" who might assault him. He is also paranoid at the day center, just as he was at college. The voices tell him the situation is dangerous, that there are dangerous people about, and that he must take care. Jim knows the voices will warn him of danger, so he listens out for them and is attentive to them when they occur. At the day center Jim becomes more agitated the longer he is there, and he usually goes home after a short time. In doing so he feels reassured that the voices have helped him and kept him from harm. Jim also wonders why the voices help him and concludes that it must be because he is special in some way. This puzzles him because the "evil" voices are unpleasant and nasty to him. Jim concludes that because he is special, he is being tested by the "evil" voices to see whether he is worthy of their help. Only special people would be helped and be tested. In thinking this way, Jim has resolved the dissonance posed by experiencing both "helpful" and "evil" voices.

The clinician and Jim decide jointly to focus on the difficult situation at the day center:

CLINICIAN: OK, Jim, I'd like you to talk me through what happens at the day center. The reason I ask this is because you remember that attending college was an important goal you wanted to achieve but couldn't because you felt suspicious of people there. Well, the situation at the day center is a lot like that at college, so we might learn how you can cope with returning to college if we examine the day center situation. Does that sound OK to you?

JIM: OK. Well one of the things that happens is that I know the voices know I'm vulnerable because they can tell when I'm like that, which is when they attack me, but they also want to help me, so they warn me about the scary people there.

CLINICIAN: How do the voices know you are vulnerable?

JIM: They can tell because they know how I feel.

CLINICIAN: How do you feel when you are vulnerable?

JIM: All shaky and on edge.

CLINICIAN: Is that like a feeling of being anxious or stressed?

JIM: Yes, a bit like that.

It appears that Jim becomes anxious in anticipation of going to the day center. There may be a range of reasons for this, such as anticipatory and situational anxiety, social anxiety, fear of being attacked, or general elevated levels of arousal. One hypothesis is that Jim picks up on this feeling of anxiety and misattributes it to being "vulnerable" to the voices. This is because his increased anxiety is associated with an increased probability of experiencing auditory hallucinations, but Jim attributes meaning to this association. Voices are imbued with attributes of power and intent.

CLINICIAN: OK, Jim, so you're feeling anxious and vulnerable. What happens next?

JIM: Well usually the voices will start. They can say a lot of things, but they will warn me about danger. I know that the voices will attack me, but I want to keep safe, and they will warn me so I listen out for them.

Here, Jim is indicating that not only do the voices occur in this situation but also his attention is focused on listening out for them, which may indicate that the threshold for detecting them is being lowered. This suggests that a redirection of attention may be a helpful method of coping with this situation. The clinician does not suggest this method at this stage but he may call upon it later.

CLINICIAN: When they warn you, how does it happen?

JIM: The voices will see someone that is dangerous and they will say, "See him? He's going to get you, he'll attack you. You better get out of here." When they say that, I can see this guy looks vicious and he's going to have a go at me, so I get out of there as fast as I can.

CLINICIAN: Then what happens?

JIM: I get out of there, and I feel real relieved that I've escaped. I feel real lucky that I've got the voices to keep me safe. Otherwise, I'd be in for it, I'd be in terrible trouble. The more I think about it, the more lucky and special I feel. They keep me safe.

It appears that Jim attributes both personal meaning to his voices and power to keep him safe. In fact he has developed a type of safety behavior that reduces his anxiety and helps him escape a feared consequence. His avoidant behavior also reinforces his feeling of being special.

This establishes a useful behavior cycle that the clinician may utilize to help Jim abandon his safety behaviors and to disprove his catastrophic predictions that he will be attacked. First, it is helpful to establish a little more detail.

CLINICIAN: You said that the voices warn you about danger at the day center most of the time. Does this always happen?

JIM: No, not every time. I always listen out very carefully for the voices, but sometimes they aren't there.

CLINICIAN: So when the voices aren't there, what happens?

JIM: Sometimes I still feel vulnerable, but I just get on with it.

CLINICIAN: Do you mean you don't leave, you stay there?

JIM: Yes, sometimes I get bored and go home, but usually I stay and have a chat and a cup of tea.

CLINICIAN: Tell me, Jim, is it pretty much the same people there whether you hear the voices or not?

JIM: Yes that's it, pretty much the same people all the time.

CLINICIAN: So sometimes the voices tell you someone is dangerous, and you get out pretty quick and feel relieved you weren't attacked, and at other times the voices aren't there, but you stay with the same people, those that you thought were dangerous before, and nothing happens. Doesn't that mean that at times they are dangerous and other times they're not dangerous? Isn't that strange?

JIM: Yes, I suppose it is. I'd not thought about that before.

Here, the clinician is looking for inconsistencies in situations that can be used to refute Jim's beliefs. The clinician highlights the inconsistency in the logical presence of threat and feeds it back to Jim, asking him what he makes of it. The clinician pursues the point about the inconsistency of the occurrence of the voices.

CLINICIAN: Sometimes the voices aren't there. Why is that?

JIM: I don't know that either. Maybe they have to look after someone else on that day. Yes, that must be it. There must be other special people that they have to look after and they are helping them. Just goes to show how important the voices are if they have lots of special people to look after. Means I'm really special, too, one of the real special people.

At this point Jim appears to be confabulating and absorbing this new information into his delusional thought network. New information is processed in a way that protects rather than challenges the delusional system. This is useful because an alternative explanation—that the voices occur when Jim attends to them and feels stressed and are less likely to occur if he is more relaxed and engaged—can be advanced and tested as an alternative belief.

The clinician now needs to motivate Jim to test out some of his beliefs. He compares the day center situation with college and the achievement of an important goal to motivate Jim to attempt to cope better at the day center. Furthermore, it is established that generally Jim enjoys going, although ambivalence is maintained by his fear of attack. Being taught how to manage his fear and be more relaxed in the situation is also a motivating factor.

Jim needs to have a plausible set of alternative explanations of what is going on, so that he may process any new information differently and not reinforce his delusions. In the past Jim has been told that he is paranoid because he has a mental illness involving an imbalance of biochemicals in his brain. This is not a particularly attractive explanation to Jim. It does not reflect his actual experience, and it is stigmatizing. Jim needs to be presented with an alternative model of his experiences that allows him to collaborate in his psychological treatment.

The clinician might suggest that paranoia is a result of misunderstanding or misinterpreting situations, and that if Jim feels stressed and anxious, as he does at the day center, then he may misattribute this physical state to a "vulnerability." He is more likely to experience the voices when he is anxious, but this does not mean that the voices know he is vulnerable. The clinician might also suggest that Jim ignore the voices when they tell him he is about to be attacked and just get on with what he is doing at the day center. Because the same people are there, and they do not attack him when the voices are absent, it is unlikely that he will be attacked when the voices are present. Thus, a behavior experiment can be established to test out whether the voices keep Jim safe. This may help challenge Jim's belief that the voices are both truthful and helpful, and that they are powerful and all knowing.

When Jim did enter these situations, he was acutely aware that his voices might occur, so that he developed an internal focus to monitor for feeling "vulnerable" and an external attention scan for hearing the voices. The former meant that he was more likely to amplify any internal sensations. The latter meant that he was more likely to verbalize what the voices usually said to him as a match and also, paradoxically, to focus his attention internally. This process of internal focus and attention scanning was more likely to trigger the voices. Intervention here involved persuading Jim to use other attentional strategies when he entered these situations. These strategies were rehearsed in the sessions and prompted with appropriate internal dialogue.

Jim also made a number of attributions about the voices. He believed that the voices warned him of threat because he "might be special"; he thought they might be able to do this through telepathy, and that he had little control over this process. Jim was troubled because the voices were often unpleasant, and he could not understand why they would be so if they were helping him to avoid danger. But Jim concluded that because he was special he needed to "be tested" by the voices, which in turn confirmed his belief that he was special. Of course, much of this explanation had been built up on the incorrect premise that the voices were actually warning him of a real danger, which could be challenged. An alternative explanation of his experience could be based on a normalization of this experience. Everyone has self-referent or bizarre thoughts at times, and in Jim's case these are perceived as external voices rather than being identified as part of the self and merely thoughts. Jim found this explanation plausible, although he was not entirely accepting of it. This is not unusual; however, it did seed doubt in his mind and could be referred to constantly, further weakening his delusional explanations.

Two difficulties arose with Jim. He did not have an alternative explanation for the voices other than they represented some, albeit vague and poorly defined, powerful entities or beings (delusional), or that they were the manifestation of a biochemical imbalance in his brain (disease). The clinician suggested to Jim that his voices might be his own thoughts or a leakage from memory into consciousness that was not identified as being part of his self. This was why the voices often reflected Jim's fears or concerns, or aspects of his past.

The voices warned Jim when he was in danger. He believed that the voices helped and protected him in these situations. For example, on one occasion when Jim was walking down a road, the voices told him that a man coming from the other direction was going to attack him. Jim crossed the road to avoid the man and believed that in doing so he had avoided being attacked. He also noticed that the man looked "suspicious," which further confirmed his belief that the voices had saved him from danger. Here is an example of an EBAC cycle to which we referred earlier in the chapter.

- Experience—Voices tell him of a suspicious person approaching.
- Belief—He is in imminent danger.
- Action—He crosses the road.
- Confirmation—He has avoided being attacked.

This can be used as another therapeutic example:

CLINICIAN: You've told me that when the man approached you in the street, he was looking at you and the voices told you you were in danger. What happened next?

JIM: Well, I knew he would go for me, so I crossed the street and got away.

CLINICIAN: When you crossed the street, did the man look at you or follow you, or say anything?

JIM: No, I don't think so.

CLINICIAN: Isn't that strange, if he was out to attack you?

JIM: Yes, I suppose so. I'd not thought about that before, I was so glad to get away.

CLINICIAN: Tell me, Jim, when you walk down the street, where do you look?

JIM: Well, where I'm going, of course. That's a daft question!

CLINICIAN: Well, it may seem so, but think where was the man going when you thought he was looking at you to attack you.

JIM: Well, he was walking toward me, and he was looking in that direction.

The clinician continues his questioning, so that Jim keeps returning to the conclusion that the man happened to be looking at him because Jim was in his line of vision, nothing more. There was no evidence of an intent to attack, and once Jim was out of his line of vision, the man paid no further attention to him. Experiments can be constructed to further emphasize this point. Sometimes Jim may be drawing attention to himself by his own actions, which make people look at him (the self-fulfilling prophecy). Again, this can be drawn out by a similar line of questioning and tested. A similar approach can be taken with other examples of Jim's paranoid behavior, and his behavior with friends and family. The clinician always comes back to these past examples of successful belief and behavior change, and asks Jim how he feels about them and whether he can identify any common factors between these past successes and current problems.

"Visions" Sent by the Voices

Jim was very upset with the "visions" he experienced of his girlfriend having sex with other people. He thought these visions were sent by the voices, also by a process of telepathy. Jim did not believe his girlfriend was unfaithful, but he became very upset and angry when the voices told him this. He tried to push the images out of his mind, but when this strategy failed, he became further convinced that the images were sent via telepathy. The more angry and upset Jim became, the more difficult he found it to resist the belief and to view the experience of the visions as collateral evidence. An alternative explanation was that the visions were mental images that had become very vivid and occurred in response to his catastrophic thoughts about his girlfriend's infidelity and persisted because Jim attempted to suppress them. The voices were his own thoughts, which again posed questions about his girlfriend's fidelity, because his constant ruminations on the topic had made Jim feel insecure about his relationship. This alternative explanation, in conjunction with a review of the objective evidence regarding the security of his relationship, significantly weakened Jim's delusional beliefs about infidelity, telepathy, and the reality of the voices. The clinician introduced thought suppression exercises to demonstrate the rebound effect of Jim pushing the images out of his mind. Exposure to the "visions" was also useful in this case (although it might not be in all cases), demonstrating that images held in attention fade with time, along with the distress they cause, which was further evidence of an internal phenomenon and not external telepathy. Jim was also taught to identify the onset of the voices and to switch his attention to alternative stimuli as a way to reduce their impact and to demonstrate that these experiences were more likely generated internally rather than coming from an external entity. The clinician compared these experiences with anxiety disorders in which catastrophic beliefs and images serve to fuel irrational and threatening beliefs, pointing out that vivid imagery of "what might happen" or an imagined "catastrophe" would produce a sudden cascade of intense emotions. These experiences could then be relabeled as unpleasant but highly improbable situations rather than reality.

Any slight reduction in the strength of a delusional belief was also used to challenge Jim's general beliefs about control, threat, and veracity.

LOW SELF-ESTEEM: A COMMON PROBLEM

Patients with schizophrenia frequently have a poor perception of themselves and low self-esteem. These global concepts can be hypothesized to be manifest in terms of a negative self-schema. This is postulated as being a consequence of severe mental illness and all that goes with this. This can involve suffering the stigma of a mental illness and even harassment and exclusion, the effects of social rejection and negative interpersonal environments, and the projected sense of being valueless and devalued. Patients with depression and suicidal ideation may feel increased feelings of low self-worth because of their depressed mood. Furthermore, an attribution process can make them think that if they feel they want to kill themselves, then they must be worthless and deserve to die.

The factors that potentially impact upon and maintain negative self-schemas are represented in Figure 12.3. As can be seen, the factors that influence and maintain negative self-schema are strong, multiple, and relentless. The consequence of having a severe mental

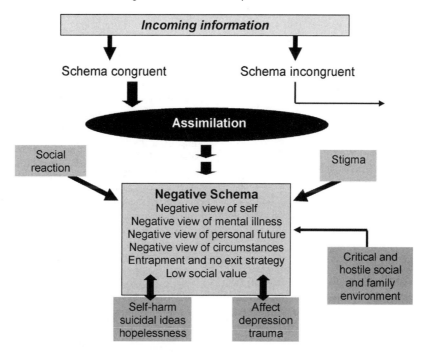

FIGURE 12.3. Maintenances of negative schemas.

illness is the formation of such negative self-schemas, which then serve to bias the way information is assimilated, so that these negative schemas are maintained and strengthened rather than being challenged and modified.

Feelings of low self-worth can both inhibit the effective use of coping strategies and increase the risk of depression and self-harm.

Improving the Patient's Self-Esteem

The aim of this set of techniques is to produce generalizations of positive attributes, challenge negative self-schemas, improve global self-esteem, and elicit positive emotional reactions. This method can be carried out in two stages. The first stage elicits positive cognitions about the self, and the second elicits a positive emotional response. Alternatively, the two stages can be combined, so that the processes of cognitive and emotional responding occur together. The procedure for the two-stage process is described for convenience as follows:

Stage 1: Cognitive Responding

• Ask the patient to produce up to 10 positive qualities about him/herself (the number can be varied dependent on the patient's capabilities; it is important that the patient not fail in generating the required number).

• Once the patient has produced a list of these qualities, ask him/her to rate each on how much he/she really believes it to be true on a 0- to 100-point scale (where 0 = *Not at all* and 100 = *Completely*).

• Ask the patient to produce specific examples of evidence of each quality; prompt specifically for actions that have occurred recently and can be time linked, such as "last week"; also use your knowledge of the patient to elicit examples. Prompt and list as many examples as possible.

• Ask the patient to rehearse the list of examples for each quality, which may be done through verbal description and mental imagery of the event, then to rerate his/her belief that he/she possesses this quality. (Usually the belief rating changes to show an increase;

it should be emphasized to the patient that his/her belief can change depending on the evidence on which he/she focuses attention.)

• The patient is given a homework exercise to monitor his/her behavior over the next week and to record specific evidence to support the contention that he/she has these qualities. The aim is to produce generalization and experiential learning of a number of positive attributes.

• At the next session, provide feedback on examples and prompt further examples. Again, ask the patient to rerate his/her belief that he or she actually has these qualities, and further point out any changes in these beliefs.

• Ask the patient to reflect on the effect that eliciting and focusing on specific behaviors and evidence has on beliefs and qualities about him/herself and how this could affect the general opinion of him/herself. Reinforce all positive attributes and the process whereby the patient comes to a more positive view of him/herself.

• Continue to repeat this procedure. Continually emphasize that the patient's beliefs about him/herself vary depending on what is the focus of attention, and that self-esteem can be greatly affected by belief and is thus amenable to change.

The case of "Dave" illustrates implementation of this procedure. Dave had very successfully learned to cope with his symptoms, which had been markedly reduced, and he had significantly improved his level of functioning. Dave produced a number of attributes that he thought he might have: "helpful," which he gave a belief rating of 60 out of 100; "friendly," which he rated 50; and "a good father," which he rated as 30. He was then asked to suggest concrete and specific evidence to support all of these. For "helpful," he cited having lent money to a friend some months before, opening a door to someone the previous week, and helping his father in the garden that week. He rerated this belief as 90.

For "friendly," Dave cited that he had had many friends of 10 to 20 years' standing; his friends contacted him regularly and enjoyed his company; he could talk comfortably to people in pubs or on buses. He got on well with the friends of his parents. Dave thought he got on well with the therapist and enjoyed speaking to him, and that he could talk to different types of

people from different backgrounds without difficulty or reserve. He rerated this belief as 100.

For being a "good father," Dave said that he enjoyed taking his son and daughter out every week (he was divorced from their mother, who had custody). He was upset when he did not see them. He liked to buy them presents. He was happy for them to decide on activities rather than doing things purely for convenience, and this in itself gave him pleasure. Dave rerated this belief as 60. However, at this point he introduced some negative evaluations. He felt that he could not be a good father because he did not live with his children. He did not get on with their mother. He said that it was always easier for absent fathers who saw their children for short periods of time and tended to spoil them. This was not responsible parenting in his view. At this point it was helpful for the clinician to go through the model of how negative views such as this are maintained (see Figure 12.3), to discuss these thoughts as being negative schema–congruent, and to indicate that the statements were "overgeneralizations," a process by which negatives are maximized and positives minimized. Furthermore, although these thoughts and beliefs had a depressing effect on his mood and maintained Dave's negative beliefs about himself, they did not accurately reflect circumstances. To challenge Dave's views of himself as a bad father, various exercises where undertaken: He was asked to define a "bad father" in explicit terms, then objectively compare his behavior to this definition. He was asked to compare his behavior with that of others in similar circumstances. Last, he was asked to give a realistic and objective appraisal of his performance and circumstances. While carrying out these exercises, the clinician emphasized the potential for negatively biased self-appraisals, along with strategies for coping with this in the future.

Stage 2: Affective Responding

Dave was also asked to explain why these qualities were important and the potential benefits of possessing them. The clinician used guided discovery and imagery during this process to ensure that the qualities selected were meaningful and important to Dave. He was then asked to generate practical examples of each quality. Particular emphasis was placed on describing specific behaviors associated with the quality and the context in which they were carried out. Attention was directed to Dave's emotional experiences when displaying that quality, thus generating the positive affect associated with that experience. Dave was asked to imagine the positive emotional reaction that another person would experience in interaction with him as he displayed a positive quality, and to vividly imagine the other person's experience and describe how he/she would feel and attempt to mimic this experience. Dave was then asked to describe how he himself felt when he had evoked the positive emotion in the other person.

For example, in displaying generosity by helping out a friend, Dave was asked to imagine through guided imagery how that friend felt when assisted by Dave. He was asked to intensify and sustain this positive emotion. Then, through a similar process, Dave was asked to imagine and describe how he himself felt when he realized how positive his friend had felt in being helped out. Again, Dave was asked to intensify and sustain this emotion. A similar process should be carried out for all positive characteristics and scenarios.

PREVENTION OF RELAPSE

Relapses rarely occur without any forewarning. They are usually preceded by a period of prodromal symptoms that can last for days, or more usually weeks, and in some cases, months; the average prodrome is, however, about 4 weeks (Birchwood, Macmillan, & Smith, 1994). Common prodromal signs and symptoms include nonpsychotic symptoms (e.g., mild depression or dysphoria, anxiety, insomnia, irritability, mood fluctuations and interpersonal sensitivity) and low-level psychotic symptoms (e.g., suspiciousness, magical thinking, ideas of reference, feelings that "something is strange or wrong" and that the individual does not "fit in" with others around him/her). During the prodromal phase, patients display behavior change, such as becoming more withdrawn, avoiding social contact, abandoning hobbies or interests, appearing more preoccupied, and being unable to continue with work or other routine or demanding activities. As the prodrome progresses, these signs and symptoms intensify and patients may exhibit strange and bizarre behavior, such as being unable to care for themselves, becoming socially or sexually inappropriate, making accusations against others, muttering to themselves, and disconnecting the television or telephone.

Patients may be asked to recall prodromal signs and symptoms that preceded previous episodes and relapses, which can be based on the onset of the episode or admission to the hospital, then identify when changes were first noticed, what changes occurred, and how they progressed and in what sequence. Each sign or symptom may be written on a card, and the patient may be asked to arrange them in temporal order of occurrence. In this way the patient's *relapse signature*, that is, the individual set of signs and symptoms that characterized the patient's prodrome and its time course leading to relapse, can be identified. Family members or professional mental health staff, if available, can help identify prodromal changes and their sequence. Clinicians may find the use of standardized assessments of prodromal symptoms helpful, such as the Early Signs Scale (Birchwood et al., 1989). Such instruments can also help the clinician cue or inquire about possible prodromal symptoms not spontaneously recalled by the patient. The patient needs to be able to discriminate between an actual relapse prodrome and normal mood fluctuations that do not signal a relapse. This is done through a process of discrimination training, whereby the patient monitors mood and experiences over a number of weeks, with a goal of learning to distinguish a real prodrome from the "false alarm" of a normal fluctuation in affect.

The next stage is to formulate a "game plan" to deal with a prodrome should one occur. Coping strategies can be formulated and rehearsed, the help of others can be elicited, and the assistance of psychiatric services can be requested, which may include an increase or change in medication. With an understanding of the time course of patients' prodromes, the clinician can identify different actions for different phases of the prodrome and the "window of opportunity" to intervene. An important part of the treatment approach is to plan for the future, especially for potentially stressful events that may occur and how to be aware of emerging symptoms and relapse. Patients can be monitored by returning to the clinician postcards that indicate they are well or that a prodrome may have started. Technology such as cell phones and e-mail may provide new, innovative platforms and methods for clinicians to monitor patients and maintain contact, to identify early signs of relapse, and to intervene at the optimal time. Such technological advances may also result in real-time assessment and intervention, and the development of intelligent systems to identify critical periods and deliver individualized interventions (Kelly et al., 2012).

CLINICAL PROBLEMS AND DIFFICULTIES

Thought Disorder

Thought disorder, typically characterized by disruption to language, makes it difficult to comprehend the meaning that the patient is imparting. However, with experience and patience, it is often possible to follow some internal logic in the patient's speech. This can be accomplished by asking the patient to explain the meaning, or by reflecting back one's own understanding, which is then rephrased in more coherent language. Progressing through these organized steps in a calm manner can help prevent the patient from feeling overloaded with the emotional content of the discussion, which can occur, especially when the material being discussed is emotionally salient.

Intractable Psychotic Symptoms

Regrettably, there are cases in which the therapist's best efforts and optimum medication produce little improvement in the patient's symptoms. A number of options are available in such intractable cases. First, it is necessary to ensure that appropriate support services are in place, so that the patient's quality of life is maximized. Second, there should be regular reviews of treatment, especially of medication and of environmental circumstances, so that excessive stresses are avoided. Last, it is always worth continuing with a few simple and direct cognitive-behavioral strategies because, over a long period of time, these may begin to have an effect.

Risk of Suicide and Self-Harm

The risk of suicide in patients with schizophrenia is significant. Risk factors include being young and male, having a chronic illness with numerous exacerbations, high levels of symptomatology and functional impairment, feelings of hopelessness in association with depression, fear of further mental deterioration, and excessive dependence on treatment or loss of faith in treatment. In one study, two paths to suicide risk, both of which were mediated by hopelessness, were also identified: (1) increased social isolation, to which longer illness duration, more positive symptoms, older age, and being unemployed contributed, and (2) greater negative views of the self, higher frequency of criticism from relatives, and more negative symptoms, to which being male, unmarried, and unemployed significantly contributed (Tarrier, Barrowclough, Andrews, & Gregg, 2004). A more recent cohort study and systematic review have confirmed and extended previous findings. Being young and male with a history of violent offending were identified as predictors of suicide, although this latter finding was restricted specifically to those with lower IQ (Webb, Långström, Runeson, Lichtenstein, & Fazel, 2011). A systematic review of 51 studies additionally identified important illness-related predictors such as depressive symptoms, hallucinations and delusions, and comorbid physical illness and substance misuse (Hor & Taylor, 2010).

It is important for therapists to be aware that suicide attempts are a very real possibility while treating someone with schizophrenia. Unfortunately, patients with schizophrenia often commit suicide impulsively and use lethal methods, such as jumping from heights, immolation, or firearms. The presence of suicidal ideation needs to be assessed, and the patient needs to be asked whether he/she has made any specific plans or taken any actions, and whether the normal barriers to self-harm and suicide have broken down. It is necessary to be aware of factors that can elevate risk, including erosion of self-esteem; increased sense of hopelessness and despair, especially related to the patient's perception of the illness and recovery; disruptive family or social relationships; and any changes in social circumstances or loss of supportive relationships (e.g., changes in mental health staff, staff holidays, or leave). Furthermore, the occurrence of major life events, loss, or shameful experiences can lead to despondency.

Some factors that can increase risk for suicide are quite unique to the psychotic disorders, such as the experience of command hallucinations telling patients to self-harm. Other examples are more idiosyncratic. One of the authors (N. T.) had a patient who experienced strange physical sensations that he interpreted as the Queen of England entering his body. As a loyal subject, he thought he should vacate his body to give her sole possession, and he attempted to kill himself by slashing his wrists. This was not the result of a will to die, but was more driven by some sense of social protocol toward royalty. Fortunately, the attempt was unsuccessful.

Many clinicians hypothesize that psychotic symptoms have a protective aspect in masking the harsh realities of the burden of serious mental illness. Improvement in insight and symptomatology can bring with it an increased exposure to this burden, thus increasing the probability of potential escape through suicide. The clinician needs to be aware of all these factors, to know his/her patients well, and to monitor changes in their circumstances or mood that may be problematic. It is important to be aware of predictable changes and plan for them, to establish good communication with other mental health workers, and to address depressed mood and hopelessness in an open manner. Assessing acute suicide risk is further complicated by patients' flat or incongruous affect, so that the cues a clinician would look for in a depressed patient may not be exhibited by a patient with schizophrenia. When risk is high, emergency psychiatric services should be called.

Dual Diagnosis: Comorbidity of Alcohol and Substance Use

Comorbid substance use disorders are an escalating problem in patients with schizophrenia. Dual-diagnosis patients tend to do worse than patients with schizophrenia alone on a range of outcomes. They tend to be more persistently symptomatic; to have more frequent and earlier relapse and readmission; to be more likely to present to the emergency services; and to have higher levels of aggression and violence, and greater risk of suicide and self-harm.

Motivational interviewing has been used effectively to enhance motivation to change substance use behavior in schizophrenia patients (Barrowclough et al., 2001; Haddock et al., 2003). Motivational interviewing has been termed a "style" rather than a specific intervention, and can be incorporated into a CBT approach to increase the patient's motivation to change substance or alcohol use behavior and concurrently address the psychosis. It is postulated that an important interaction between alcohol or substance use and psychotic symptoms requires this dual-treatment approach. Many patients do not consider their alcohol or substance use a problem and perceive the positive benefits, such as self-medication, peer identification, or enjoyment, as outweighing any negative consequences. The aim during the initial sessions is to elicit change or motivational statements from the patient. The therapist uses the motivational interviewing skills of reflective listening, acceptance, and selective reinforcement to elicit such statements. Once the patient identifies substance or alcohol use as a problem and expresses a desire to change, therapy can then progress to practical ways to achieve this goal. The largest RCT to date compared a combined condition of TAU, motivational interviewing, and CBT with TAU alone in those with psycho-

sis and co-occurring substance use. Results showed treatment to be beneficial in improving motivation to change substance use, and significantly reduced the amount of substance consumed per day, with this latter finding being maintained at 24-month follow-up. However, there were no effects on clinical outcomes such as relapse rates, symptoms, and functioning (Barrowclough et al., 2010).

CONCLUSION

CBTp does have significant benefits for patients with schizophrenia and psychosis. It should be carried out as part of a comprehensive care plan. It is unlikely to "cure" patients, but it may assist them in coping with and recovering from their illness. Intervention is based on a detailed assessment and formulation. It does require considerable skill, experience, and knowledge of CBT and psychosis, and it does not lend itself easily to a simple protocol format. Further research on theoretical aspects of understanding psychosis from a psychological perspective is important to inform and further develop CBT procedures. Research into dissemination and how new psychological treatments penetrate into mental health services and become accessible to patients are required.

REFERENCES

Allot, K., Alvarez-Jimenez, M., Killackey, E. J., Bendall, S., McGorry, P. D., & Jackson, H. J. (2011). Patient predictors of symptom and functional outcome following cognitive behaviour therapy or befriending in first-episode psychosis. *Schizophrenia Research, 132*, 125–130.

Barnes, T. R. E., & Nelson, H. E. (1994) *The assessment of psychoses: A practical handbook.* London: Chapman & Hall.

Barrowclough, C., Haddock, G., Lobban, F., Jones, S., Siddle, R., Roberts, C., et al. (2006). Group cognitive behaviour therapy for schizophrenia: Randomized controlled trial. *British Journal of Psychiatry, 189*, 527–532.

Barrowclough, C., Haddock, G., Tarrier, N., Lewis, S., Moring, J., O'Brian, R., et al. (2001). Randomised controlled trial of motivational interviewing and cognitive behavioural intervention for schizophrenia patients with associated drug or alcohol misuse. *American Journal of Psychiatry, 158*, 1706–1713.

Barrowclough, C., Haddock, G., Wykes, T., Beardmore, R., Conrod, P., Craig, T., et al. (2010). Integrated motivational interviewing and cognitive behavioural therapy for people with psychosis and comorbid substance misuse: Randomised controlled trial. *British Medical Journal, 341,* c6325.

Barrowclough, C., & Tarrier, N. (1992). *Families of schizophrenic patients: A cognitive-behavioural intervention.* London: Chapman & Hall.

Birchwood, M., Macmillan, F., & Smith, J. (1994). Early intervention. In M. Birchwood & N. Tarrier (Eds.), *Psychological management of schizophrenia* (pp. 77–108). Chichester, UK: Wiley.

Birchwood, M., Peters, E., Tarrier, N., Dunn, G., Lewis, S., Wykes, T., et al. (2011). A multi-centre randomised controlled trial of cognitive therapy to prevent harmful compliance with command hallucinations. *BioMed Central Psychiatry, 11,* 155–160.

Birchwood, M., Smith, J., MacMillan, F., Hogg, B., Prasad, R., Harvey, C., et al. (1989). Predicting relapse in schizophrenia: The development and implementation of an early signs monitoring system using patients and families as observers. *Psychological Medicine, 19,* 649–656.

Bird, V., Premkumar, P., Kendall, T., Whittington, C., Mitchell, J., & Kuipers, E. (2010). Early intervention services, cognitive-behavioural therapy and family intervention in early psychosis: Systematic review. *British Journal of Psychiatry, 197,* 350–356.

Bolton, C., Gooding, P., Kapur, N., Barrowclough, C., & Tarrier, N. (2007). Developing psychological perspectives of suicidal behaviour and risk in people with a diagnosis of schizophrenia: We know they kill themselves but do we understand why? *Clinical Psychology Review, 27,* 511–536.

Brabban, A., Tai, S., & Turkington, D. (2009). Predictors of outcome in brief cognitive behavior therapy for schizophrenia. *Schizophrenia Bulletin, 35,* 859–864.

Brooker, C., & Brabban, A. (2006). *Measured success: A scoping review of evaluated psychosocial interventions training for work with people with serious mental health problems.* London: National Health Service, National Institute for Mental Health in England.

Cohen, J. (1988). *Statistical power analysis for the behavioral sciences* (2nd ed.). Hillsdale, NJ: Erlbaum.

Dixon, L. B., Dickerson, F., Bellack, A. S., Bennett, M., Dickinson, D., Goldberg, R. W., et al. (2010). The 2009 schizophrenia PORT psychosocial treatment recommendations and summary statements. *Schizophrenia Bulletin, 36,* 48–70.

Doll, R. (1998). Controlled trials: The 1948 watershed. *British Medical Journal, 317,* 1217–1220.

Drury, V., Birchwood, M., Cochrane, R., & Macmillan, F. (1996). Cognitive therapy and recovery from acute psychosis: A controlled trial: I. Impact on psychotic symptoms. *British Journal of Psychiatry, 169,* 593–601.

Dunn, G., Fowler, D., Rollinson, R., Freeman, D., Kuipers, E., Smith, B., et al. (2012). Effective elements of cognitive behaviour therapy for psychosis: Results of a novel type of subgroup analysis based on principal stratification. *Psychological Medicine, 42,* 1057–1068.

Emmerson, L. C., Granholm, E., Link, P. C., McQuaid, J. R., & Jeste, D. V. (2009). Insight and treatment outcome with cognitive-behavioral social skills training for older people with schizophrenia. *Journal of Rehabilitation Research and Development, 46,* 1053–1058.

Fowler, D., Hodgkins, J., Painter, M., Reilly, T., Crane, C., Macmillan, I., et al. (2009). Cognitive behaviour therapy for improving social recovery in psychosis: A report from the ISREP MRC trial platform study (improving social recovery in early psychosis). *Psychological Medicine, 39,* 1627–1636.

Freeman, D. (2011). Improving cognitive treatments for delusions. *Schizophrenia Research, 132,* 135–139.

Garety, P. A., Fowler, D. G., Freeman, D., Bebbington, P., Dunn, G., & Kuipers, E. (2008). Cognitive-behavioural therapy and family intervention for relapse prevention and symptom reduction in psychosis: Randomised controlled trial. *British Journal of Psychiatry, 192,* 412–423.

Garety, P. A., Fowler, D., Kuipers, E., Freeman, D., Dunn, G., Bebbington, P., et al. (1997). London–East Anglia randomised controlled trial of cognitive-behavioural therapy for psychosis: II. Predictors of outcome. *British Journal of Psychiatry, 171,* 420–426.

Garety, P., Kuipers, E., Fowler, D., Freeman, D., & Bebbington, P. E. (2001). A cognitive model of the positive symptoms of psychosis. *Psychological Medicine, 31,* 189–195.

Gould, R. A., Mueser, K. T., Bolton, E., Mays, V., & Goff, D. (2001). Cognitive therapy for psychosis in schizophrenia: An effect size analysis. *Schizophrenia Research, 48,* 335–342.

Grant, P. M., Huh, G. A., Perivoliotis, D., Stolar, N. M., & Beck, A. T. (2012). Randomized trial to evaluate the efficacy of cognitive therapy for low-functioning patients with schizophrenia. *Archives of General Psychiatry, 69,* 121–127.

Haddock, G., Barrowclough, C., Tarrier, N., Moring, J., O'Brien, R., Schofield, N., et al. (2003). Randomised controlled trial of cognitive-behavior therapy and motivational intervention for schizophrenia and substance use: 18 month, carer and economic outcomes. *British Journal of Psychiatry, 183,* 418–426.

Haddock, G., McCarron, J., Tarrier, N., & Faragher, B. (1999). Scales to measure dimensions of hallucinations and delusions: The Psychotic Symptom Rating Scales (PSYRATS). *Psychological Medicine, 29,* 879–890.

Haddock, G., Tarrier, N., Morrison, A. P., Hopkins, R., Drake, R., & Lewis, S. (1999). A pilot study evaluating the effectiveness of individual inpatient cognitive behavioural therapy in early psychosis. *Social Psychiatry and Psychiatric Epidemiology, 34,* 254–258.

Hall, P. H., & Tarrier, N. (2003). The cognitive-behavioural treatment of low self-esteem in psychotic patients: A pilot study. *Behaviour Research and Therapy, 41,* 317–332.

Hor, K., & Taylor, M. (2010). Review: suicide and schizophrenia: A systematic review of rates and risk factors. *Journal of Psychopharmacology, 24*, 81–90.

Jackson, H. J., McGorry, P. D., Killackey, E., Bendall, S., Allott, K., Dudgeon, P., et al. (2008). Acute-phase and 1-year follow-up results of a randomized controlled trial of CBT versus befriending for first-episode psychosis: The ACE project. *Psychological Medicine, 38*, 725–735.

Johnson, J., Gooding, P., & Tarrier, N. (2008). Suicide risk in schizophrenia: Explanatory models and clinical implications, the schematic appraisal model of suicide (SAMS). *Psychology and Psychotherapy, 81*, 55–71.

Kane, J. M. (1999). Management strategies for the treatment of schizophrenia. *Journal of Clinical Psychiatry, 60*(Suppl. 12), 13–17.

Kelly, J. A., Gooding, P., Pratt, D., Ainsworth, J., Welford, M., & Tarrier, N. (2012). Intelligent real time therapy (iRTT): Harnessing the power of machine learning to optimise the delivery of momentary cognitive-behavioural interventions. *Journal of Mental Health, 21*(4), 404–414.

Kuipers, E., Onwumere, J., & Bebbington, P. (2010). Cognitive model of caregiving in psychosis. *British Journal of Psychiatry, 196*, 259–265.

Lecomte, T., Leclerc, C., & Wykes, T. (2012). Group CBT for early psychosis—Are there still benefits one year later? *International Journal of Group Psychotherapy, 62*, 309–321.

Lewis, S. W., Tarrier, N., Haddock, G., Bentall, R., Kinderman, P., Kingdon, D., et al. (2002). Randomised controlled trial of cognitive-behaviour therapy in early schizophrenia: Acute phase outcomes. *British Journal of Psychiatry, 181*(Suppl. 43), 91–97.

Lynch, D., Laws, K. R., & McKenna, P. J. (2010). Cognitive behavioural therapy for major psychiatric disorder: Does it really work?: A meta-analytical review of well-controlled trials. *Psychological Medicine, 40*, 9–24.

Morrison, A. P., & Barratt, S. (2010). What are the components of CBT for psychosis?: A Delphi study. *Schizophrenia Bulletin, 36*, 136–142.

Morrison, A. P., French, P., Stewart, S. L. K., Birchwood, M., Fowler, D., Gumley, A. I., et al. (2012). Early detection and intervention evaluation for people at risk of psychosis: Multisite randomised controlled trial. *British Medical Journal, 344*, e2233.

Morrison, A. P., French, P., Walford, L., Lewis, S., Kilcommons, A., Green, J., et al. (2004). A randomised controlled trial of cognitive therapy for the prevention of psychosis in people at ultra-high risk. *British Journal of Psychiatry, 185*, 291–297.

Morrison, A. P., Hutton, P., Wardle, M., Spencer, H., Barratt, S., Brabban, A., et al. (2012). Cognitive therapy for people with a schizophrenia spectrum diagnosis not taking antipsychotic medication: An exploratory trial. *Psychological Medicine, 42*, 1049–1056.

Morrison, A. P., Turkington, D., Wardle, M., Spencer, H.,

Barratt, S., Dudley, R., et al. (2012). A preliminary exploration of predictors of outcome and cognitive mechanisms of change in cognitive behaviour therapy for psychosis in people not taking antipsychotic medication. *Behaviour Research and Therapy, 50*, 163–167.

Mueser, K., & Glynn, S. M. (1995). *Behavioral family therapy for psychiatric disorders*. Needham Heights, MA: Allyn & Bacon.

Mueser, K. T., Glynn, S. M., Cather, C., Xie, H., Zarate, R., Fox Smith, L., et al. (2013). A randomized controlled trial of family intervention of co-occurring substance use and severe psychiatric disorders. *Schizophrenia Bulletin, 39*(3), 658–672.

National Institute for Health and Clinical Excellence (NICE). (2009). *Schizophrenia: core interventions in the treatment and management of schizophrenia in adults in primary and secondary care, updated guideline*. London: Author.

Nuechterlein, K. H. (1987). Vulnerability models for schizophrenia: State of the art. In H. Hafner, W. F. Gattaz, & W. Janzarik (Eds.), *Search for the cause of schizophrenia* (pp. 297–316). Heidelberg, Germany: Springer-Verlag.

Onwumere, J., Bebbington, P., & Kuipers, E. (2011). Family interventions in early psychosis: specificity and effectiveness. *Epidemiology and Psychiatric Sciences, 20*(13), 113–119.

Onwumere, J., & Kuipers, E. (2011). Cognitive-behavioral family intervention in psychosis. In M. Rimondini (Ed.), *Communication in cognitive behavioral therapy* (pp. 185–201). New York: Springer.

Pantelis, C., & Barns, T. R. E. (1996). Drug strategies in treatment resistant schizophrenia. *Australian and New Zealand Journal of Psychiatry, 30*, 20–37.

Perivoliotis, D., Grant, P. M., Peters, E. M., Ison, R., Kuipers, E., & Beck, A. T. (2010). Cognitive insight predicts favorable outcome in cognitive behavioral therapy for psychosis. *Psychosis, 2*, 23–33.

Pilling, S., Bebbington, P., Kuipers, E., Garety, P., Geddes, J., Orbach, G., et al. (2002). Psychological treatments in schizophrenia: I. Meta-analysis of family interventions and cognitive behaviour therapy. *Psychological Medicine, 32*, 763–782.

Pocock, S. J. (1996). *Clinical trials: A practical approach*. Chichester, UK: Wiley.

Premkumar, P., Peters, E. R., Fannon, D., Anilkumar, A. P., Kuipers, E., & Kumari, V. (2011). Coping styles predict responsiveness to cognitive behaviour therapy in psychosis. *Psychiatry Research, 187*, 354–362.

Rector, N. A., & Beck, A. T. (2001). Cognitive behavioral therapy for schizophrenia: An empirical review. *Journal of Nervous and Mental Disease, 189*, 278–287.

Richardson, A., Baker, M., Burns, T., Lilford, R. J., & Muijen, M. (2000). Reflections on methodological issues in mental health research. *Journal of Mental Health, 9*, 463–470.

Salkovskis, P. M. (2002). Empirically grounded clinical interventions: Cognitive behaviour therapy progresses through a multidimensional approach to clinical science. *Behavioural and Cognitive Psychotherapy, 30,* 3–10.

Sarin, F., Wallin, L., & Widerlöv, B. (2011). Cognitive behavior therapy for schizophrenia: A meta-analytical review of randomized controlled trials. *Nordic Journal of Psychiatry, 65,* 162–174.

Slade, M., & Priebe, S. (2001). Are randomised controlled trials the only gold that glitters? *British Journal of Psychiatry, 179,* 286–287.

Steel, C., Tarrier, N., Stahl, D., & Wykes, T. (2012). Cognitive behaviour therapy for psychosis: The impact of therapist training and supervision. *Psychotherapy and Psychosomatics, 81*(3), 194–195.

Stowkowy, J., Addington, D., Liu, L., Hollowell, B., & Addington, J. (2012). Predictors of disengagement from treatment in an early psychosis program. *Schizophrenia Research, 136,* 7–12.

Tarrier, N. (1996). A psychological approach to the management of schizophrenia. In M. Moscarelli & N. Sartorius (Eds.), *The economics of schizophrenia* (pp. 271–286). Chichester, UK: Wiley.

Tarrier, N. (2002). The use of coping strategies and self-regulation in the treatment of psychosis. In A. Morrison (Ed.), *A casebook of cognitive therapy for psychosis* (pp. 79–107). Cambridge, UK: Cambridge University Press.

Tarrier, N. (2006). A cognitive-behavioural case formulation approach to the treatment of schizophrenia. In N. Tarrier (Ed.), *Case formulation in cognitive behaviour therapy: The treatment of challenging and complex clinical cases* (pp. 167–187). London: Routledge.

Tarrier, N., Barrowclough, C., Andrews, B., & Gregg, L. (2004). Suicide risk in recent onset schizophrenia: The influence of clinical, social, self-esteem and demographic factors. *Social Psychiatry and Psychiatric Epidemiology, 39,* 927–937.

Tarrier, N., Barrowclough, C., Haddock, G., & McGovern, J. (1999). The dissemination of innovative cognitive-behavioural treatments for schizophrenia. *Journal of Mental Health, 8,* 569–582.

Tarrier, N., & Calam, R. (2002). New developments in cognitive-behavioural case formulation: Epidemiological, systemic and social context: An integrative approach. *Cognitive and Behavioural Psychotherapy, 30,* 311–328.

Tarrier, N., Haddock, G., Lewis, S., Drake, R., Gregg, L., & the Socrates Trial Group. (2006). Suicide behaviour over 18 months in recent onset schizophrenic patients: The effects of CBT. *Schizophrenia Research, 83,* 15–27.

Tarrier, N., Lewis, S., Haddock, G., Bentall, R., Drake, R., Kinderman, P., et al. (2004). Cognitive-behavioural therapy in first-episode and early schizophrenia 18-month follow-up of a randomised controlled trial. *British Journal of Psychiatry, 184,* 231–239.

Tarrier, N., & Wykes, T. (2004). Is there evidence that cognitive behaviour therapy is an effective treatment for schizophrenia: A cautious or cautionary tale? (Invited essay). *Behaviour Research and Therapy, 42,* 1377–1401.

Tarrier, N., Yusupoff, L., Kinney, C., McCarthy, E., Gledhill, A., Haddock, G., et al. (1998). A randomised controlled trial of intensive cognitive behaviour therapy for chronic schizophrenia. *British Medical Journal, 317,* 303–307.

Tarrier, N., Yusupoff, L., McCarthy, E., Kinney, C., & Wittkowski, A. (1998). Some reason why patients suffering from chronic schizophrenia fail to continue in psychological treatment. *Behavioural and Cognitive Psychotherapy, 26,* 177–181.

Tattan, T., & Tarrier, N. (2000). The expressed emotion of case managers of the seriously mentally ill: The influence of EE and the quality of the relationship on clinical outcomes. *Psychological Medicine, 30,* 195–204.

Trower, P., Birchwood, M., Meaden, A., Byrne, S., Nelson, A., & Ross, K. (2004). Cognitive therapy for command hallucinations: Randomised controlled trial. *British Journal of Psychiatry, 184,* 312–320.

Webb, R. T., Långström, N., Runeson, B., Lichtenstein, P., & Fazel, S. (2011). Violent offending and IQ level as predictors of suicide in schizophrenia: National cohort study. *Schizophrenia Research, 130,* 143–147.

Wykes, T., Everitt, B., Steele, C., & Tarrier, N. (2008). Cognitive behaviour therapy for schizophrenia: Effect sizes, clinical models and methodological rigor. *Schizophrenia Bulletin, 34,* 523–537.

Zimmermann, G., Favrod, J., Trieu, V. H., & Pomini, V. (2005). The effect of cognitive behavioural treatment on the positive symptoms of schizophrenia spectrum disorders: A meta-analysis. *Schizophrenia Research, 77,* 1–9.

CHAPTER 13

Alcohol Use Disorders

BARBARA S. MCCRADY

Clinicians working with individuals with alcohol use problems, as well as clinicians in training, have found this chapter to be an extraordinarily useful resource in guiding their treatment approaches. In this thoroughly updated and edited revision, the author begins by describing how recent societal trends and legislative initiatives have altered the nature of the clientele with drinking problems that comes for treatment. After briefly reviewing the available empirical evidence on treatment approaches that range from Alcoholics Anonymous to brief interventions to intensive inpatient treatment, the author describes the myriad factors that every clinician must consider in choosing and carrying out appropriate interventions for individuals with drinking problems. Using a variety of illuminating case vignettes, Barbara McCrady illustrates important therapeutic strategies, including methods for motivating these patients to begin treatment. In a manner that emphasizes the humanity of the couple and makes the partners come to life, the extended case study in this chapter illustrates the all-too-frequent tragic consequences of excessive drinking. In the context of this case description, the author describes in great detail what clinicians will not find in books that simply lay out various treatment procedures—that is, the thrusts and parries of a superb and experienced clinician in overcoming the roadblocks that inevitably emerge during treatment.—D. H. B.

Alcohol use disorders are a heterogeneous group of problems ranging in severity from the heavy-drinking college student who occasionally misses classes to the person with severe and chronic alcoholism who experiences serious medical and social consequences of drinking. Although the prevalence of alcohol use disorders is higher in males than in females and in younger than in older adults, these problems affect individuals from any sociodemographic, racial/ethnic, or occupational background. In mental health and medical settings, at least 25% of clients are likely to have an alcohol use disorder as part of their presenting problems (e.g., Zimmerman, Lubman, & Cox, 2012), so clinicians in health and mental health professions need to be competent to identify, assess, and plan an effec-

tive course of treatment for these clients. This chapter describes the social context of drinking and drinking problems, provides an integrative model for conceptualizing and treating alcohol use problems, and presents both a series of case vignettes and an extended case study to illustrate the clinical model.

The clinician functioning in the 21st century must provide treatment within a complex and contradictory treatment network; must have formal and systematic training in the treatment of alcohol and other drug use disorders; must have tools to work with involuntary and voluntary clients, those who adhere passionately to a traditional recovery perspective, and those who are offended by it; and must work either to promote major and enduring changes in alcohol use or to decrease the harm that individuals and groups may experience from their use. The need for clinicians who are competent in treating alcohol and other substance use disorders (AUDs and other SUDs) will increase because of two Federal laws passed in recent years. The Patient Protection and Affordable Care Act, passed in 2010 in the United States, mandates alcohol and drug screening and brief intervention in primary care settings as a covered benefit, and the Wellstone–Domenici Mental Health Parity and Addiction Equity Act of 2008 mandates comparable health care coverage for treatment for physical health, mental health, and addictions problems. If these laws are implemented successfully, more individuals with AUDs will be identified and referred to treatment.

Although the need for clinicians who are competent to treat AUDs is likely to increase, many clinicians may shy away from this population given the notorious reputation of persons with AUDs for being difficult and frustrating to treat. This chapter assumes that the clinician who has useful and effective tools for working with persons with drinking problems, and who has a bit of success with these tools, will find positive reasons to see these clients. Persons with drinking problems *are* treatable; they are both challenging and rewarding to treat; and when they change successfully, the clinician has the rare opportunity to participate in helping people make major and satisfying changes in their lives.

DEFINITIONS AND DIAGNOSIS OF ALCOHOL PROBLEMS

Diagnosis

The diagnosis of alcohol problems in the *Diagnostic and Statistical Manual of Mental Disorders*, fifth edition (American Psychiatric Association, 2013), treats AUDs as a single disorder, ranging along a spectrum of severity. Previous editions of the DSM discriminated between alcohol abuse and dependence; this distinction no longer applies. To be diagnosed with an AUD, an individual must meet at least two of 11 criteria, and the AUD is classified as mild (two to three symptoms), moderate (four to five symptoms) or severe (six to eleven symptoms). The 11 diagnostic criteria combine the DSM-IV criteria for alcohol abuse and alcohol dependence, eliminating "repeated alcohol-related legal consequences," and adding "craving." Thus, the diagnostic criteria include (1) failing to fulfill major social

role obligations, such as those related to work, home, or school; (2) drinking repeatedly in a ways that that have the potential to create physical harm (e.g., drinking and driving); (3) continuing to drink despite the fact that drinking is causing social or interpersonal problems; (4) having the desire to or attempting to cut down or stop without success; (5) drinking larger amounts or alcohol or drinking over longer periods of time than planned, (6) exhibiting signs of physical tolerance; (7) showing signs of physical withdrawal; (8) neglect of other activities; (9) spending considerable time obtaining alcohol, drinking, and recovering from its effects; (10) continuing to use despite knowing that alcohol is causing recurrent physical or psychological problems; and (11) experiencing persistent craving for alcohol. Alcohol dependence also may be classified as being in "partial remission" or in "full remission"; remission may be "early" (at least 3 months) or "sustained" (1 year or more).

Alternative Definitions

In contrast to the formal psychiatric diagnosis of an AUD, behavioral researchers and clinicians have suggested that alcohol problems represent one part of a continuum of alcohol use, ranging from abstinence through nonproblem use to different types and degrees of problem use. DSM-5 is more aligned with this perspective but still considers a cutoff indicative of a disorder. From the alcohol problems continuum perspective, problems may be exhibited in a variety of forms—some that are consistent with a formal diagnosis, and others that are milder or more intermittent. By using an alcohol problems perspective, the clinician can focus more clearly on the pattern of drinking, negative consequences that the client has accumulated, his/her behavioral excesses and deficits across various areas of life functioning, and his/her particular strengths. A de-emphasis on diagnosis forces the clinician to consider clients from a more individual perspective. Therefore, although formal diagnosis is useful for identifying and defining the severity of a client's problems and is necessary for formal record keeping, the approach to clinical assessment emphasized in this chapter attends less to diagnostic issues and more to problem identification.

This chapter views alcohol use problems as a multivariate set of problems, with alcohol consumption as a common defining characteristic. These problems vary in severity from severe alcohol dependence to mild and circumscribed problems. For some, alcohol consumption itself is a major presenting problem; for others, the consequences of alcohol use—such as disruption of a relationship, occupational problems, or health problems—are the major reason for seeking treatment. In viewing alcohol problems as multivariate, this chapter also assumes the existence of multiple etiologies for these problems, with genetic, psychological, and environmental determinants contributing in differing degrees for different clients.

Complicating Problems

Drinking problems are complicated by a variety of concomitant problems. Of significance is the comorbidity of AUDs with other psychiatric diagnoses. A high percentage of those diagnosed with an AUD also experience other psychological problems, which may be antecedent to, concurrent with, or consequent to their drinking (Rosenthal, 2013). The most common Axis I disorders are other SUDs, depression, and anxiety disorders, occurring in up to 60% of males in treatment. The most common Axis II disorder comorbid with an AUD in males is antisocial personality disorder, with rates ranging from 15 to 50%. Females more often present with depressive disorders; 25 to 33% of women with an AUD experience depression prior to the onset of their AUD.

Alcohol problems also are complicated by problems with cognition, physical health, interpersonal relationships, the criminal justice system, the employment setting, and the environment. Many people with alcoholism have subtle cognitive deficits, particularly in the areas of abstract reasoning, memory, cognitive flexibility, problem solving, and difficulties in emotional differentiation (for a review of this literature, see Oscar-Berman & Marinković, 2007). Because verbal functioning is usually unimpaired, these cognitive problems are not always immediately apparent. Heavy drinking also causes a variety of medical problems and can affect any organ system in the body. Heavy drinking may cause conditions such as cardiomyopathy, liver diseases, gastritis, ulcers, pancreatitis, and peripheral neuropathies. Even when obvious medical conditions are not present, the effects of heavy drinking can be insidious and debilitating. Many people eat poorly when drinking, which results in nutritional deficits, poor energy, or vague and diffuse physical discomfort. Mortality rates among persons of all ages are elevated with alcohol dependence, and are higher among women than among men.

Interpersonal relationships also may be disrupted. The rates of separation and divorce range up to seven times those of the general population (Paolino, McCrady, & Diamond, 1978); spousal violence is higher among both men and women with AUDs (Smith, Homish, Leonard, & Cornelius, 2012); and emotional and behavioral problems are more common among their spouses/partners and children (Moos & Billings, 1982; Moos, Finney, & Gamble, 1982). Health care utilization is elevated among the spouses and children of actively drinking individuals with AUDs (Spear & Mason, 1991).

Persons presenting for treatment of a drinking problem may be involved with the legal system because of charges related to driving while intoxicated (DWI), other alcohol-related offenses (e.g., assault), or involvement with the child welfare system. Drug-related charges also may bring a client to treatment. Clients vary in the degree to which they recognize that their drinking is creating problems, and in their degree of motivation to change their drinking patterns.

In conclusion, the client presenting for treatment may be drinking in a manner that creates concern, be formally diagnosed as having AUD, and also meet criteria for one or more Axis I or Axis II disorders. The person also may have other major problems, such as cognitive impairment, physical health problems, interpersonal or occupational problems, and/or legal problems. Problem recognition and motivation to change may be low. How does the clinician develop a rational approach to conceptualizing and treating this rather complicated clinical picture?

THEORETICAL MODEL

The model presented in this chapter assumes that treatment planning must be multidimensional, and that there is more than one effective treatment for alcohol problems. Unlike certain disorders for which one treatment approach has demonstrable superiority over others, in the alcohol field there are a number of legitimate and empirically supported approaches to treatment (for a review, see Hallgren, Greenfield, Ladd, Glynn, & McCrady, 2012). These treatments are based in different conceptualizations of the etiology, course, treatment goals, and length of treatment for alcohol problems. Among the treatments with the best support are brief and motivationally focused interventions, cognitive-behavioral treatment, 12-step facilitation treatment, behavioral couple therapy, cue exposure treatment, and the community reinforcement approach. A number of factors seem to be common to effective treatments. These are summarized in Table 13.1. A key therapist responsibility is to help a client find a treatment approach and treatment setting that is effective for him/her, rather than slavishly adhering to a particular treatment model or setting. A second and equally important therapist responsibility is to enhance the client's motivation to continue to try, even if the initial treatment setting is not effective. This treatment model takes into account seven major considerations: (1) problem severity, (2) concomitant life problems, (3) client expectations, (4) motivation and the therapeutic relationship, (5) variables maintaining the current drinking pattern, (6) social support systems, and (7) maintenance of change.

Problem Severity

Problem severity is relatively atheoretical, and is most important in decision making about the types of treatments to be offered, the intensity of the treatment, and the initial treatment setting. Severe alcohol dependence can best be conceptualized as a chronic, relapsing disorder (McLellan, Lewis, O'Brien, & Kleber, 2000), with relapses occurring even after extended periods of abstinence. As with other chronic disorders, such as diabetes, cardiovascular disease, or rheumatoid arthritis, the clinician necessarily takes a long-term perspective, and maximizing periods of positive functioning and minimizing periods of problem use should be the primary goals. In contrast, other individuals have alcohol-related problems that may be circumscribed and not progressive (Finney, Moos, & Timko, 2013). Epidemiological data suggest that for the majority of those with alcohol-related problems, the problems will resolve or remit without any need for formal treatment or intervention. The clinician encountering individuals at the mild end of the severity spectrum should plan a brief, motivationally enhancing intervention to complement the natural change process and inspire these individuals to make changes in their drinking.

Concomitant Life Problems

Clients with AUDs often have problems in multiple areas of life functioning—physical, psychological/psychiatric, familial, social/interpersonal, occupational, legal, child care, housing, and transportation. Assessment of multiple areas of life functioning is crucial for the planning and delivery of effective treatment. Research suggests that targeting client problem areas successfully can result in appreciable changes in these problems, even with clients who are severely alcohol dependent and homeless (Cox et al., 1998). Furthermore, providing treatment directed at multiple problem areas enhances positive alcohol and drug use outcomes as well (McLellan et al., 1997; Morgenstern et al., 2006; Rynes, McCrady, Morgan, Violette, & Pandina, 2012).

Client Expectations

Clinicians should provide clients with accurate expectations about the intensity of their treatment and the probable course of their problems. To date, limited research has examined ways to affect such client expectations, although the recent development of the Psychosocial Treatment Expectation Questionnaire suggests that clients have expectancies about the purpose and atmosphere of treatment, as well as the likelihood that treatment will impact their daily lives (Leite, Seminotti, Freitas, & Drachler, 2011). Because research is limited, the recommendations provided here derive only partly from empirical findings about the course and treatment of AUDs and remain to be tested.

The clinician can inform clients with circumscribed, less severe problems that treatment will be short in duration, that they are likely to be successful in reducing their drinking, and that the long-term prognosis is good. Such clients also can be told that now or at some point in the future they may decide to stop drinking completely (Miller, Leckman, Delaney, & Tinkcom, 1992), or that they may continue to drink in a moderated fashion.

Clients with more severe and chronic AUDs, however, should be given a different set of expectations about treatment and the likely course of their problems. It is fair to tell them that about 25% of clients maintain sustained abstinence for at least 1 year after treatment, that another 10% will use alcohol in moderation and without problems, that, on average, clients will reduce the amount they drink by about 87%, and that alcohol-related problems will decrease by about 60% (Miller, Walters, & Bennett, 2001). The challenge for such clients is to learn skills to manage their drinking in a way that makes it minimally disruptive to their lives. Chronic illness metaphors may be helpful. For example, like a patient with diabetes, a client with a severe AUD needs to make and maintain significant lifestyle

TABLE 13.1. Principles for Treatment of Substance Use Disorders

1. *Structure and organization of the treatment setting*
   - Clear and well organized
   - Actively involve the clients in the program
   - Provide a supportive and emotionally expressive environment
   - Emphasize self-direction, work, and social skills development
   - Expect clients to take responsibility for their treatment and follow through

2. *Type of provider and what the provider does*
   - Treatment by addictions specialists or mental health clinicians
   - Development of an effective therapeutic alliance is crucial
     - Accurate empathy
     - Respect for the experience of clients in therapy
     - Avoidance of confrontational struggles
   - Provide goal direction for the clients
   - Provide a moderate level of structure for the therapy
   - Handle ambivalence about changing or being in treatment:
     - Titrate level of confrontation to the level of clients' reactance
     - Avoid arguing with angry clients
     - Avoid pushing clients hard to accept their diagnosis or the need to change

3. *Level of care, continuity of care, and elements of treatment*
   - Pay attention to retaining clients in treatment
   - Determine the intensity and length of treatment partly by considering the severity of the substance use disorder.
     - For heavy drinkers with low alcohol dependence, less intense, briefer treatments are appropriate and intensive inpatient therapy yields poorer outcomes.
     - Clients with severe alcohol dependence have better outcomes with more intensive initial treatment, and respond most positively to treatment that focuses on 12-step counseling and involvement with 12-step groups.
   - Assess and arrange for attention to clients' other social service and medical care needs

4. *Contextual factors*
   - Involve a significant other
   - Help clients restructure their social environments to include persons that support change and abstinence.
   - With clients who have little commitment to remain in treatment or change their substance use, involve the family or other member of the social support system in the treatment to foster retention in treatment
   - In the treatment of adolescents with substance use disorders, use approaches that involve multiple systems, including the family, peers, and others

5. *Client characteristics*
   - Greater client readiness to change is associated with greater treatment success
   - Greater severity of the substance use disorder is associated with a poorer response to treatment

6. *Specific therapeutic elements*
   - Focus on client motivation
   - Help clients develop awareness of repetitive patterns of thinking and behavior that perpetuate their alcohol or drug use
   - Attend to the affective experiences of clients
   - Consider the role of conditioning in the development and maintenance of substance use disorders. Clinicians should carefully assess for indicators of specific conditioned responses to alcohol or drugs, and develop ways to change these conditioned responses
   - Enhance positive outcome expectancies

7. *Client–treatment matching*
   - Assess for comorbid disorders and use empirically supported treatments for additional presenting problems
   - Use female-specific treatment with women clients

Note. From Haaga, McCrady, and LeBow (2006). Copyright 2006 by Wiley Journals, Inc. Reprinted by permission.

changes to support healthy functioning. Like the patient with diabetes, the client with a severe AUD needs to know warning signs that he/she may be getting into trouble and know what to do. And neither individual can afford to forget or ignore his/her chronic problem.

Motivation and the Therapeutic Relationship

Clients vary in the degree to which they recognize their drinking is problematic and in their readiness to change. Motivational models suggest that individuals initiate change when the perceived costs of the behavior outweigh the perceived benefits, and when they can anticipate some benefits from behavior change (Cunningham, Sobell, Sobell, & Gaskin, 1994). Prochaska and DiClemente (2005) proposed a continuum of stages of readiness for change. The continuum includes the stages of "precontemplation," in which a person does not recognize a behavior as problematic; "contemplation," in which the person considers that a behavior pattern might be problematic; "determination" or "preparation," in which the individual resolves to change; and "action," in which a person initiates active behaviors to deal with the problem. Following "action" is "maintenance," if the behavior change is successful, or "relapse," if the person returns to the problem behavior. Miller and Rollnick (2002) suggested that several factors influence a person's readiness to change, including awareness of problem severity, awareness of positive consequences for changing the behavior, and the perception of choice in making changes. Clients' apparent stage of change and self-perception of their problems should guide a clinician's initial approach to treatment and treatment planning.

Contemporary models view motivation as a state that can be influenced by therapeutic behaviors and the client's life experiences. Therapeutic approaches to enhance motivation lead clients to talk more about changing their drinking than continuing to drink, and in turn this "change talk" predicts better outcomes (Moyers, Martin, Houck, Christopher, & Tonigan, 2009). Motivationally enhancing approaches appear to be particularly effective with clients who enter treatment very angry and hostile (Project MATCH Research Group, 1997b). Miller and Rollnick (1991) described six common elements to enhance motivation, summarized in the acronym FRAMES: personalized feedback (F) to the client about his/her status; an emphasis on the personal responsibility (R) of the client for change; provision of clear advice (A) about the need for change, given in a supportive manner; providing the client with a menu (M) of options for how to go about changing, rather than insisting upon one treatment or treatment goal; providing treatment in a warm, empathic (E), and supportive style; and enhancing the client's perceived self-efficacy (S) for change.

Factors Maintaining the Current Drinking Pattern

Case conceptualization for treatment planning focuses on factors maintaining the problematic drinking pattern. Different treatment models use different frameworks for conceptualizing current factors that maintain drinking. Presented here is a cognitive-behavioral approach to case conceptualization (see Epstein & McCrady, 2009). The cognitive-behavioral case formulation assumes that drinking can best be treated by examining current factors maintaining drinking rather than historical factors. Factors maintaining drinking may be individual, or related to environmental circumstances or interpersonal relationships. The model assumes external antecedents to drinking that have a lawful relationship to drinking through repeated pairings with positive or negative reinforcement, or through the anticipation of reinforcement. The model assumes that cognitions and affective states mediate the relationship between external antecedents and drinking behavior, and that expectancies about the reinforcing value of alcohol play an important role in determining subsequent drinking behavior. Finally, the model assumes that drinking is maintained by its consequences, and that the sources of these consequences may be physiological, psychological, or interpersonal.

To integrate these assumptions about drinking, my colleagues and I use a functional analytic framework, in which the drinking response (R) is elicited by environmental stimuli (S) that occur antecedent to drinking; that the relationship between the stimulus and response is mediated by cognitive, affective, and physiological, or organismic (O) factors; and that the response is maintained by positive or the avoidance of negative consequences (C) as a result of drinking. Various individual, familial, and other interpersonal factors are associated with drinking. At the individual level, environmental antecedents may be associated with specific drinking situations, times of the day, or the mere sight or smell of alcohol. Organismic variables may include craving for alcohol; withdrawal symptoms; negative affects such as anger, anxiety, or depression; negative self-evaluations or irrational beliefs; or positive expectancies about the effects of alcohol in particular situations. Individual reinforcers may include decreased craving or withdrawal symptoms, decreases in negative affect or increases in positive affect, decreased negative self-evaluations, or decreased focus on problems and concerns.

At the familial level, various antecedents to drinking occur. Alcohol may be a usual part of family celebrations or daily rituals. Family members may attempt to influence the problematic drinking behavior by nagging the person to stop or by attempting to control the drinking through control of the finances or liquor supply. These actions may become antecedents to further drinking. Families in which a member is drinking heavily may develop poor communication and problem-solving skills, as well as marital/couple, sexual, financial, and child-rearing problems that then cue further drinking. The person with the drinking problem may have a variety of reactions to these familial antecedents, experiencing negative affect, low self-efficacy for coping with problems, and/or retaliatory thoughts. Family behaviors may serve to reinforce the drinking. The family may shield the person from negative consequences of drinking by taking care of the drinker when intoxicated or assuming his/her responsibilities. A number of investigators have observed positive changes in marital/couple interactions associated with drinking, such as increases in intimate exchanges or increased assertiveness by the drinker, suggesting that these positive behaviors may reinforce the drinking (e.g., Frankenstein, Hay, & Nathan, 1985).

There also are other interpersonal antecedents to drinking. These may include social pressures to drink; work-related drinking situations; friendships in which alcohol consumption plays a major role; or interpersonal conflicts with work associates, friends, or acquaintances. The person may react to interpersonal antecedents to drinking with craving, positive expectancies for alcohol use, social discomfort, or negative self-evaluations for not drinking. Positive interpersonal consequences of drinking may include decreased craving or social anxiety, an enhanced sense of social connectedness or fun, or increased social comfort or assertiveness.

Social Support

The behaviors of family and other members of the client's social network are integral to the case conceptualization. The availability of general social support, as well as social support for abstinence or moderate drinking, is crucial to successful treatment. Support from the client's social network for abstinence is associated with better drinking outcomes; support for continued drinking is associated with poorer outcomes (Longabaugh, Wirtz, Zywiak, & O'Malley, 2010). Clients in a social network that is strongly supportive of drinking may need to take deliberate steps to detach from that social network and access new social networks that support abstinence or moderate drinking. Some data suggest that involvement with Alcoholics Anonymous (AA) can serve such a function (Longabaugh, Wirtz, Zweben, & Stout, 1998), and data on natural recovery from alcohol problems suggest that finding a new love relationship or involvement in religious activities also may be viable avenues for change (Vaillant & Milofsky, 1982).

Maintenance of Change

Implicit in much of the preceding discussion is a view that individuals with severe AUDs have a high probability of relapse, an ever-present consideration, both because long-term, ingrained habits are difficult to change, and because of the permanent physiological and metabolic changes stimulated by heavy drinking (Woodward, 2013). Several models have been proposed to conceptualize the maintenance or relapse process, with associated treatments. The most prominent maintenance models include the relapse prevention (RP) model (Marlatt & Gordon, 1985; Witkiewitz & Marlatt, 2004), and the disease model, best exemplified by the practices common to AA. The RP model, an extension of the functional-analytic model described earlier, focuses on the interplay among environment, coping skills, and cognitive and affective responses in maintaining successful change. In the RP model, relapse occurs in response to a high-risk situation for which the client either lacks or does not apply effective coping skills. Low self-efficacy for coping with the situation may contribute to the difficulties. If the client does not cope effectively, use of alcohol is likely. Marlatt and Gordon (1985) suggested that, following initial drinking, a cognitive factor, the "abstinence violation effect" (AVE), is activated. The AVE represents all-or-nothing thinking; after drinking, the client makes a cognitive shift to viewing him/herself as "drinking"; therefore, he/she continues to drink. RP treatment focuses on several points of intervention common to cognitive-behavioral treatment, such as identification of high-risk situations and acquisition of coping skills, as well as cognitive restructuring to help the client view a drinking episode as a "lapse" from which he/she can learn and return to abstinence rather than a "relapse" into previous drinking patterns. RP also focuses on lifestyle changes to decrease the presence of high-risk situations, and encourages development of a balance between pleasures and desires, and obligations and responsibilities (a "want–should" balance) in the client's life. In his more recent work, Marlatt (Marlatt & Donovan, 2005; Witkiewitz & Marlatt, 2004) described relapse as "multidimensional and dynamic" (Marlatt & Donovan, 2005, p. 21), and considered the influence of longer-term risk factors such as family history and social supports, and well as more proximal influences on relapse. He also suggested that there are reciprocal interactions among cognitions, coping skills, affect, and drinking.

Disease model perspectives view alcoholism as a chronic, progressive disease that can be arrested but not cured. Treatment based on the disease model focuses on helping the client recognize that he/she has this disease, that abstinence and a lifelong program of recovery are the only means to arrest the disease, and that involvement in AA or other 12-step groups is essential to successful maintenance of change (e.g., Slaymaker & Sheehan, 2013).

The model presented in this chapter is most closely allied with the RP model, but clinicians should be knowledgeable about the disease model underlying AA and recognize that some clients are drawn to it because they find the model and the program helpful and relevant to them.

CLINICAL APPLICATION OF THE THEORETICAL MODEL

Overview

The major elements of the treatment model have direct implications for facilitating problem recognition and entry into treatment, and for the planning and delivery of treatment. If an individual has not entered treatment, there are techniques to help that individual recognize his/her drinking as problematic and in need of change. For a client seeking alcohol treatment, the therapist must make decisions about the most appropriate setting in which to provide treatment and select the therapeu-

tic modalities most appropriate to him/her. Therapeutic techniques must be tailored to the client's needs related to drinking and other life problems. The therapist also must consider the social context in which drinking occurs, as well as the social context for change. He/she must be cognizant of the subtle and nonspecific aspects of providing treatment to clients with drinking problems and utilize a therapeutic stance that enhances the client's motivation to continue to engage in the change process. The therapist must attend to the client's own views about treatment and change, and provide the client with accurate long-term expectations about drinking outcomes. Core components of the treatment model are listed in Table 13.2.

Case Identification and Entry into Treatment

Before discussing applications of the model to active treatment, it is important to consider how to help clients enter the treatment system.

Case Identification and Screening

Many individuals who drink do not think they have problems related to drinking. They may be unaware of the high-risk nature of their drinking pattern, or unaware of the negative consequences that are occurring. Feeling ashamed or guilty, they may be reluctant to tell others about their problems, or they may perceive

TABLE 13.2. Steps in Treatment

1. Case identification and motivation to enter treatment
2. Assessment
3. Selection of treatment setting
4. Selection of treatment modalities
5. Enhancing and maintaining motivation to change
6. Selection of drinking goals
7. Initiation of abstinence
8. Developing a functional analysis
9. Early sobriety strategies
10. Coping strategies
11. Partner/family involvement
12. Long-term maintenance
13. Managing complicating conditions
14. Self-help groups

health care professionals as uninterested or unconcerned about drinking. Routine queries about drinking and its consequences in both medical and mental health care settings can obviate some of these difficulties. Given the high prevalence of drinking problems among individuals seeking health and mental health services, questions about drinking should be part of all clinicians' intake interviews. The Affordable Care Act will require screening for alcohol and drug problems of all patients who are seen in primary care settings. Given the increased integration of psychological services into primary care, mental health professionals may take the lead in introducing appropriate screening tools into these health care settings.

Many screening interviews and questionnaires have been developed to identify clients with alcohol problems. At a minimum, all clients should be asked whether they drink, and drinkers should be asked follow-up questions about the quantity and frequency of their drinking. Drinking should be considered as heavy or high-risk if a man drinks more than 28 standard drinks in a week, or a woman drinks more than 21 standard drinks in a week.[1] Concern should also be heightened if a client reports heavy drinking (five drinks for men, four for women) twice or more than per month. Follow-up questions may be used to inquire about subjective and objective consequences of drinking. The CAGE (cut down, annoyed, guilty, eye-opener; Mayfield, McLeod, & Hall, 1974; see Table 13.3) and the Alcohol Use Disorders Identification Test (AUDIT; Saunders, Aasland, Babor, de la Fuente, & Grant, 1993) are two useful screening measures. Two affirmative responses to the CAGE suggest a high probability of an AUD, but even one positive response warrants further clinical inquiry. The AUDIT includes both direct and subtle approaches to alcohol screening; therefore, it may be useful with clients who are reluctant to self-identify drinking problems. The CAGE and AUDIT questions are reproduced in Table 13.3.

Motivating a Drinker to Enter Treatment

The initial challenge for a clinician is to stimulate the client to initiate any change. Methods for motivating clients to enter treatment vary; a clinician may draw upon motivational interviewing techniques (Miller & Rollnick, 2002), may involve family and concerned others in collaborative, client-centered work (Miller, Meyers, & Tonigan, 1999; Smith & Meyers, 2004), or

may use confrontational approaches, such as an "intervention" (Liepman, 1993). Implementation of motivational principles and techniques in ongoing clinical practice, however, presents creative challenges to the clinician. Three examples illustrate the application of different approaches to motivating clients to enter treatment.

Bill was a retired chemist with a long history of heavy drinking, multiple phobias, and bipolar disorder. I was initially contacted by his wife Diana, who told me that her husband had a 20-year drinking history, that his drinking had increased since his retirement, and that she did not know what to do: The children were angry and threatening to break off contact with him; she and Bill were arguing frequently; and she was beginning to feel increasingly anxious and depressed herself. Diana had consulted with a certified addictions counselor, who told her that they should set up an "intervention"—a meeting in which Diana and the children would confront Bill about his drinking, insist that he get treatment, then take him directly to an inpatient treatment facility. When Diana was hesitant, the counselor told her she was codependent and enabling him. She left the counselor's office discouraged, certain that she did not want to initiate an intervention, but also certain that something should be done. I tried the most minimal intervention first. Over the telephone, I suggested that Diana speak with Bill one morning (before he had begun drinking) and say, "Bill, I am concerned about your drinking. I have spoken with a psychologist who specializes in alcohol treatment, and she said that she would be happy to see you for an evaluation. At the end of the evaluation, she'll give us feedback about what we could do." I told her not to elaborate on this statement, but simply to respond to Bill's questions. If he refused, she was to get back in touch with me.

I next heard from Diana a month later. Bill had refused her request, and she wondered what else she could do. I suggested an individual consultation with me to discuss how to change her own actions to motivate Bill toward change. Diana came in, and after some further assessment of both Bill's drinking history and her current functioning, I suggested three basic behavioral strategies, which I drew from Thomas's unilateral family therapy (Thomas, Yoshioka, & Ager, 1996) and the community reinforcement and family training (CRAFT) model (Smith & Meyers, 2004). First, I instructed Diana to leave Bill to his drinking as much as possible, to let negative consequences occur naturally.

TABLE 13.3. Questions to Screen for Alcohol Use and Problems

CAGE[a]

1. Have you ever felt you should cut (C) down on your drinking?
2. Have people annoyed (A) you by commenting on your drinking?

3. Have you ever felt bad or guilty (G) about your drinking?
4. Have you ever had a drink first thing in the morning (eye-opener [E])?

Alcohol Use Disorders Test (AUDIT)[b]

These 10 questions are about your use of alcohol *during the past 12 months.*

1. How often do you have a drink containing alcohol?
   0) Never [Skip to questions 9–10]
   1) Monthly or less
   2) 2 to 4 times a month
   3) 2 to 3 times a week
   4) 4 or more times a week

2. How many alcohol units do you have on a typical day when you are drinking?
   0) 1 or 2
   1) 3 or 4
   2) 5 or 6
   3) 7, 8, or 9
   4) 10 or more

3. How often do you have seven or more units on one occasion?
   0) Never
   1) Less than monthly
   2) Monthly
   3) Weekly
   4) Daily or almost daily

4. How often during the last year have you found that you were unable to stop drinking once you had started?
   0) Never
   1) Less than monthly
   2) Monthly
   3) Weekly
   4) Daily or almost daily

5. How often during the last year have you failed to do what was normally expected from you because of drinking?
   0) Never
   1) Less than monthly
   2) Monthly
   3) Weekly
   4) Daily or almost daily

6. How often during the last year have you needed a first drink in the morning to get yourself going after a heavy drinking session?
   0) Never
   1) Less than monthly
   2) Monthly
   3) Weekly
   4) Daily or almost daily

7. How often during the last year have you had a feeling of guilt or remorse after drinking?
   0) Never
   1) Less than monthly
   2) Monthly
   3) Weekly
   4) Daily or almost daily

8. How often during the last year have you been unable to remember what happened the night before because you had been drinking?
   0) Never
   1) Less than monthly
   2) Monthly
   3) Weekly
   4) Daily or almost daily

9. Have you or someone else been injured as the result of your drinking?
   0) No
   2) Yes, but not in the last year
   4) Yes, during the last year

10. Has a relative, friend, or a doctor or other health worker been concerned about your drinking or suggested you cut down?
   0) No
   2) Yes, but not in the last year
   4) Yes, during the last year

[a]From Mayfield, McLeod, and Hall (1974).
[b]From *http://whqlibdoc.who.int/hq/2001/who_msd_msb_01.6a.pdf.* Copyright by the World Health Association. Reprinted by permission. Complete scoring is available from this source.

Second, I encouraged her to give him factual feedback about negative behaviors related to his drinking, but only at times when he was sober. The structure of the feedback was as follows: "Bill, I am concerned that *X* happened last night when you were drinking." Third, I encouraged her to spend time with him in positive pursuits when he was not drinking. Given that they were going to Florida for the winter, I suggested that just before they returned, she should repeat her request that he come to see me for an evaluation.

I next heard from Diana in the spring, when she called me to make an appointment for the two of them to come in for an evaluation. They both attended. What follows is our initial discussion.[2] (In this and other dialogues in this chapter, I am the therapist.)

THERAPIST: I'm so glad to get to meet you. As you know, Diana first spoke with me a few months ago, so I feel as though I know you a bit. I understand that you were initially reluctant to come in, and I'm pleased that you decided to come. How did that come about?

BILL: Well, Diana asked me, and I know she's been concerned, so I agreed. But I only agreed to come today—I'm not making any kind of commitment here.

THERAPIST: I understand that and certainly won't try to push you to do anything you're not comfortable with. What I'd like to do today is to get a better understanding about your drinking and the kinds of problems it might be causing. At the end of our time together, I'll give you some feedback and we can discuss some options for you, if you decide you want to make any changes. If I ask you anything that you're not comfortable answering, just let me know. OK?

Bill was visibly uncomfortable, and pushed his chair as far back into the corner of my office as possible. He sat with his body turned away from Diana and often looked up at the ceiling or sighed when she was speaking. Despite his visible discomfort, he gave a clear account of his drinking. He had been drinking heavily for the past 25 years, and at one point had been drinking a pint of Jack Daniels whiskey each evening. He was diagnosed with colon cancer in his early 60s and treated surgically. Since the surgery, he had been concerned about his health and had attempted to reduce his drinking. His current pattern was almost daily drinking, in the evenings, ranging from two to four bottles of

Grolsch beer to an occasional (approximately twice per month) pint of Jack Daniels. He reported no withdrawal symptoms on days when he did not drink, and no apparent medical sequelae of his drinking. He said that he did not feel that he had control over his drinking, and expressed sadness that Diana was so upset. His love for her, apparent in his speech and demeanor, was clearly the primary reason he had come to see me.

Given Bill's discomfort, I did not try to complete any standardized assessment instruments or even to structure the initial interview as I might have with other clients. Instead, I followed his lead, made frequent comments reflecting the emotions he was expressing, and at times asked Diana not to interrupt, so that Bill could express himself. In the last 15 minutes of the 1-hour interview, we shifted to feedback and discussion:

THERAPIST: I'd like to stop asking you so many questions now, and see if we can talk about possible options. I am glad that you came in and appreciate that this was not easy for you. From what you and Diana have told me, it does seem that it makes sense to be concerned about your drinking. The amount you're drinking is above the recommended levels for safe and healthy drinking; you are concerned by your own feelings of lack of control; and your drinking has been upsetting to your family, which is painful to you. What do you think?

BILL: I guess talking about all of this at once makes it clearer that I'm drinking too much. I don't want to stop, though—I appreciate good beer, and look forward to having a bottle or two in the evening. I just don't want to overdo it to the point of hurting Diana.

THERAPIST: So you are concerned and think that some kind of change makes sense, but you're not sure exactly what those changes should be?

BILL: Exactly.

THERAPIST: I think you have a number of options. Making some kind of change makes sense given the problems we've discussed. Probably your safest choice is to stop drinking—you can't create future health problems from drinking if you don't drink, and in some ways it might be easiest given that you're in a pretty daily routine of drinking now. But if you don't want to stop, we could also work toward your reducing your drinking to a level that is safer and healthier, and one that Diana and your children are comfortable with. I'd be willing to work with you to try to reach that goal. I don't think that you need intensive treatment in a hospital program right now, but you would probably benefit from some help to make changes. What do you think?

BILL: I'm surprised that you think I could reduce my drinking. I have to think about this. I'll have Diana get back to you.

The discussion continued with input from Diana as well, and the session ended with a commitment only to think about our discussion. Several days later, Diana called to indicate that Bill wanted to begin treatment with me, and we scheduled an appointment.

Dorothy, a 78-year-old, widowed, retired schoolteacher, was hospitalized at a local medical center after a fall in her apartment. Her blood alcohol level (BAL) on admission was 185 mg%, and she had extensive evidence of old bruises, as well as a dislocated shoulder and broken wrist from the fall. She was immediately started on medication for alcohol withdrawal, and our addictions consultation team was called in to see her on the second day of her hospitalization. Dorothy's son John was in the room when I came to see her. With his assistance, I was able to obtain a lengthy history of alcohol consumption that dated back to her early 40s. Although Dorothy had wanted to stop drinking, she had never been successful for more than a few days at a time, and had never received any form of alcohol treatment. Since her husband's death 2 years earlier, she had been consuming a pint bottle of blackberry brandy each day. She had completely withdrawn from her previous social activities with friends, her hygiene had deteriorated, and she had had multiple accidents in her house. Dorothy provided this information tearfully, expressing a great sense of shame about her behavior. John described her home as "a mess" and said that he was angry and disgusted with her. Dorothy's family history revealed many family members with alcohol dependence, including her father, two brothers, and a maternal uncle. Despite the medication, she showed visible signs of alcohol withdrawal during the interview. Dorothy was tearful and stated repeatedly that she was a "sinful, bad" person. My interviewing style with her was empathic: I asked her about her concerns, inquired how she felt, and reflected back her obvious distress with her current situation. I then told her that there were treatments available to help people with problems like hers. Her immediate and strong reaction was to say that she was too bad, and that her drinking

was a sin. Although not usually a strong proponent of labeling alcohol dependence as a disease, I decided that this framework might in fact be acceptable and supportive to her. Given her long history of alcohol dependence with physiological dependence, and her heavy family history of alcohol dependence, such a framework seemed plausible and appropriate.

"Dorothy, it is clear to me that you are very, very upset by your drinking and by all the problems it has caused for you and your family. I understand that you blame yourself and seem to think your drinking shows that you are a bad person. There is another way of thinking about your drinking that I'd like to tell you about. You may or may not agree with me, but I hope you'll think about what I say. Some people say that alcoholism is a disease. In your case, I think that is true. You probably have genes that made you very vulnerable to alcohol—your father, your uncle, and your brothers all seem to have the same disease. We know that the vulnerability to alcoholism can be inherited, and I would guess that you inherited it. Over time, your body has become adapted to your drinking—it is more comfortable with alcohol than without it. If you try to stop, your body reacts badly. The shaking and nausea that you're experiencing now are signs that your body has become hooked on alcohol.

"What does all this mean? It means that your body reacts differently to alcohol than other people's, and probably has from the beginning of your drinking. It is no more your fault that you have a drinking problem than it is the fault of a diabetic that her body can't make insulin. People are not responsible for the diseases they develop. But they *are* responsible for making the decision to take care of their disease, for getting help, and for following the advice of the people who give them that help. Except for the problems your drinking has caused, you're healthy, and you obviously have people who care about you. If you can get help, you have a good chance of getting better."

Dorothy initially was skeptical of this reframing of her problems. Without my prompting, when her son left the hospital that day, he picked up some brochures about alcoholism as a disease and brought them back for his mother to read. When I came to see her the next day, she had many questions about this disease notion and about treatment, which I answered as factually as possible, still maintaining a motivational interviewing stance—not trying to push her into treatment, but reflecting her interest and concern. By my third visit, she agreed to enter a treatment program. She entered a short-term residential rehabilitation program, followed by longer-term outpatient group therapy. She began to volunteer at the hospital where I first saw her, and she remained sober and an active volunteer for several years, until advancing age required that she retire.

Dennis was a 41-year-old dentist with a history of abuse of alcohol, prescription opiates, and benzodiazepines. Dennis's case illustrates the need for a full armamentarium of clinical techniques to motivate individuals to enter treatment. At the time that I saw Dennis, our center had a contract with the state dental association to provide assessment, motivation, referral, and monitoring services for dentists with alcohol and drug problems. I was called about Dennis on a Friday afternoon by an emergency room physician. Dennis had taken an overdose of medications and had been rushed to the emergency room by his office staff. His condition had been stabilized, and he was now insisting that he leave the hospital. The physician wanted our program to "do something." In rapid succession, I received calls from the office staff, from Dennis's wife, and from another dentist, who had been serving as his AA sponsor. By telephone, they provided me with a horrific history of abuse of multiple substances, domestic violence, canceled afternoons of appointments with patients, extraction of the wrong tooth from a patient, and repeated failures in AA and outpatient treatment. Each caller described Dennis as intractable, and all were desperately concerned that he would kill himself. I asked them all to meet me at the hospital, and left my office to join them there. I informed the emergency room physician that I would be coming to the hospital, and asked him to hold Dennis there until I arrived.

When I arrived at the hospital, I first spoke with Dennis individually. He was alert, oriented, belligerent and angry, and utterly unwilling to speak with me at any length or to agree to any kind of plan of care. My best motivational interviewing skills failed completely with him. Given the crisis nature of the situation and his extremely severe SUD, I decided to utilize a more confrontational technique—the intervention (Liepman, 1993). Interventions are designed to confront the resistant client and create a forced plan of action. Research suggests that two-thirds of families will not follow through with an intervention (as was the case with Diana and Bill), but that if an intervention is implemented,

the probability of the client's entering treatment is very high (Miller et al., 1999). I gathered the office staff, Dennis's wife, and his AA sponsor together and asked them whether they would be willing to sit down to talk with Dennis about his problems. They were relieved and eager to do so. We spent about 30 minutes together, during which time I outlined the basic requirements for the intervention: (1) Each person's feedback should begin with an expression of caring or concern; (2) each should provide concrete, behavioral feedback related to Dennis's drinking and drug use (e.g., mentioning his canceling appointments rather than saying he was irresponsible); (3) at the end of his/her feedback, each person should repeat the expression of concern and request that Dennis get help. We then sat down with Dennis, and each person spoke. Dennis began to cry and after a lengthy period of time agreed that he needed help and would follow my recommendations for treatment.

Assessment

Once a client has entered treatment, the therapist should begin with an initial assessment of drinking, other drug use, and problems in other areas of life functioning. (Donovan, 2013, provides a comprehensive description of assessment for SUDs; Green, Worden, Menges, & McCrady, 2008, provide an evaluation of the psychometric properties of various assessment instruments for AUDs). Assessment of motivation, as well as resources that the client brings to the treatment, is important. If the therapist provides cognitive-behavioral treatment, assessment for a functional analysis of drinking is necessary. If the client's spouse/partner or other family members are involved in the treatment, their role in the drinking, as well as overall relationship functioning, should be assessed.

Drinking Assessment

The clinical interview is used to assess drinking history and client perceptions of his/her current drinking. Major topics to cover in the clinical interview are outlined in Table 13.4. Typically, we use a handheld breath alcohol tester at the beginning of each session to assess current BAL. In addition to the clinical interview, two structured interviews—the Timeline Follow-Back Interview (TLFB; Sobell & Sobell, 1995), designed to assess drinking and drug use behavior each day in a set window of time before treatment; and the alcohol and drug sections of the Structured Clinical Interview

TABLE 13.4. Topics to Cover in Initial Clinical Interview (If Both Partners Are Present)

1. Initial orientation
   a. Introductions
   b. Breathalyzer reading
   c. Brief questionnaires

2. Initial assessment
   a. Presenting problems
   b. Role of drinking/drug use in presenting problems
   c. Other concerns
   d. How the drinking has affected the partner
   e. How the drinking has affected the relationship

3. Drinking/drug use assessment
   a. Identified patient
      i. Quantity, frequency, pattern of drinking
      ii. Last drink/drug use
      iii. Length of drinking/drug problem
      iv. Negative consequences of drinking/drug use
      v. DSM-5 symptoms
      vi. Assessment of need for detoxification
   b. Partner
      i. Quantity, frequency, pattern of drinking
      ii. Last drink/drug use
      iii. Length of drinking/drug problem
      iv. Negative consequences of drinking/drug use
      v. DSM-5 symptoms
      vi. Assessment of need for detoxification

4. Assessment of other problems
   a. Psychotic symptoms
   b. Depression
   c. Anxiety
   d. Cognitive impairment
   e. Health status

5. Assessment of domestic violence
   a. This assessment is done privately with each partner alone
   b. Review of Conflict Tactics Scales
      i. Identification of episodes of physical aggression
      ii. Determination of level of harm/injury from aggression
      iii. Assessment of individual's sense of safety in couple therapy

for DSM-IV (SCID; Spitzer, Williams, Gibbon, & First, 1996)—provide standardized information about quantity, frequency, pattern of drinking, and other information needed to establish a formal diagnosis. Alternative structured interviews, such as the Form-90 (Tonigan, Miller, & Brown, 1997), may be used to obtain information about drinking history, patterns, and consequences of use. Self-report measures may be used to assess severity of alcohol dependence (the Alcohol Dependence Scale [ADS]; Skinner & Allen, 1982) and negative consequences of drinking (the Drinker Inventory of Consequences [DrInC] or the Short Inventory of Problems [SIP]; Miller, Tonigan, & Longabaugh, 1995).

Assessment of Other Problem Areas

The clinician can draw from a wide variety of measures to assess other life problems. Assessment may range from unstructured interviews to the use of simple problem checklists to formal interviewing techniques. The Addiction Severity Index (ASI; McLellan et al., 1992) is a widely used measure of client functioning across multiple domains; subscales include Medical, Psychological, Family/Social, Legal, Employment, Alcohol, and Drug. The ASI is in the public domain, and the instrument, instructions, and scoring programs can be downloaded from *http://triweb.tresearch.org/ index.php/tools/download-asi-instruments-manuals*. The ASI can be administered as an interview in about 45 minutes, and computer-assisted interview versions are available. The ASI, however, does not provide diagnostic information for any psychological disorders, and the cautious clinician should use formal diagnostic screening questions to assess for the possible presence of other psychological disorders.

Assessment of Motivation

Assessment of motivation should consider (1) reasons why the client is seeking treatment, with careful attention to external factors involved with help seeking; (2) the client's treatment goals; (3) the client's readiness to change; and (4) the degree to which the client sees negative consequences of his/her current drinking pattern and envisions positive consequences of change. Clinical interviewing provides information about reasons for seeking treatment, and drinking goals may be assessed either by asking the client directly or by using

We would like to know the **one GOAL** you have chosen for yourself about drinking at this time. Please read the goals listed below and choose the **ONE** goal that best represents your goal at this time by checking the box next to the goal and by filling in any blanks as indicated for that goal.

☐ I have decided not to change my pattern of drinking.

☐ I have decided to cut down on my drinking and drink in a more controlled manner—to be in control of how often I drink and how much I drink. I would like to limit myself to no more than _____ drinks (upper limit amount) per _____ (time period).

☐ I have decided to stop drinking completely for a period of time, after which I will make a new decision about whether I will drink again. For me, the period of time I want to stop drinking is for _____ (time).

☐ I have decided to stop drinking regularly, but would like to have an occasional drink when I really have the urge.

☐ I have decided to quit drinking once and for all, even though I realize I may slip up and drink once in a while.

☐ I have decided to quite drinking once and for all, to be totally abstinent, and to never drink alcohol ever again for the rest of my life.

☐ None of this applies exactly to me. My own goal is _____

FIGURE 13.1. Goal choice questionnaire.

a simple goal choice form (see Figure 13.1). The Readiness Ruler (Hesse, 2006) is a simple 10-point scale on which clients can indicate their readiness to change. It also can be used to assess the client's desire to change and confidence in being able to change. The University of Rhode Island Change Assessment Scale (McConnaughy, Prochaska, & Velicer, 1983), the Readiness to Change Questionnaire (Rollnick, Heather, Gold, & Hall, 1992), and the Stages of Change Readiness and Treatment Eagerness Scale (SOCRATES; Miller & Tonigan, 1996) all measure stage of change. Perception of negative consequences of drinking and positive consequences of change also may be assessed through the clinical interview, or by developing a Decisional Balance Sheet (Marlatt & Gordon, 1985) with the client (see Figure 13.2).

	Not Drinking	Drinking
Pros		
Cons		

FIGURE 13.2. Decisional Balance Sheet.

Urges			Drinks/Drugs				
Time	Strength (1–7)	Trigger?	Time	Type	Amount	% Alcohol	Trigger?

Relationship
satisfaction: 1 2 3 4 5 6 7
                       Worst   Greatest
                       ever   ever

FIGURE 13.3. Sample client self-recording card.

Functional Analysis

Two assessment techniques may be used to identify antecedents to drinking. A self-report questionnaire, the Drinking Patterns Questionnaire (DPQ; Menges, McCrady, Epstein, & Beem, 2008), lists potential environmental, cognitive, affective, interpersonal, and intrapersonal antecedents to drinking or drinking urges. The Inventory of Drinking Situations (Annis, Graham, & Davis, 1987), a shorter measure that assesses situations in which a client drinks heavily, also is available. Daily self-recording cards (Figure 13.3) are used throughout the treatment to record clients' drinks and drinking urges. Discussing events associated with drinking or drinking urges can help both client and clinician to develop a clearer picture of drinking antecedents and consequences. Self-recording cards also allow the clinician to track progress in terms of quantity and frequency of drinking, as well as frequency and intensity of urges to drink.

Partner Assessment

Questionnaires and self-recording cards can be used to assess how the client's partner has coped with the drinking. Each day, the partner who is involved with treatment records his/her perceptions of the drinker's drinking and drinking urges on a Likert scale (*None, Light, Moderate,* or *Heavy*; see Figure 13.4). In addition, the partner may complete the Coping Questionnaire (Orford, Templeton, Velleman, & Copello, 2005) to describe the variety of ways the partner has tried to cope with drinking. These include engaged, tolerant–inactive, and withdrawal coping. It also is important to assess other aspects of the couple's relationship, if both partners are to be involved in treatment. The Areas of Change Questionnaire (ACQ; Margolin, Talovic, & Weinstein, 1983) and the Dyadic Adjustment Scale (DAS; Spanier, 1976) are excellent self-report measures of relationship problems and satisfaction. The Revised Conflict Tactics Scales (Straus, Hamby, Boney-McCoy, & Sugarman, 1996) provides a succinct measure of relationship conflict, including physical violence.

Selection of Treatment Setting

Information from the assessment of drinking, concomitant problem areas, and motivation is used to determine the appropriate setting in which to initiate treatment. As with other areas of health and mental health care, the principle of least restrictive level of care should apply to alcohol and drug treatment. Residential rehabilitation of fixed length (usually 28–30 days) historically

Day	Date	Drinking	Drug use	Urge intensity	Relationship satisfaction
		No L M H	No L M H	0 1 2 3 4 5 6 7	0 1 2 3 4 5 6 7
		No L M H	No L M H	0 1 2 3 4 5 6 7	0 1 2 3 4 5 6 7
		No L M H	No L M H	0 1 2 3 4 5 6 7	0 1 2 3 4 5 6 7
		No L M H	No L M H	0 1 2 3 4 5 6 7	0 1 2 3 4 5 6 7
		No L M H	No L M H	0 1 2 3 4 5 6 7	0 1 2 3 4 5 6 7
		No L M H	No L M H	0 1 2 3 4 5 6 7	0 1 2 3 4 5 6 7

Note. Use the reverse side of the card to track behaviors you are learning to change.

FIGURE 13.4 Sample spouse self-recording card.

was seen as the treatment of choice. However, studies comparing the effectiveness of different levels of care (e.g., see Fink et al., 1985; Longabaugh et al., 1983; McCrady et al., 1986) have found that most clients can be treated effectively in an ambulatory treatment setting, and health care insurers typically require preauthorization of episodes of care. Outpatient treatment is the predominant form of treatment, with the ratio of clients seen in outpatient versus inpatient treatment at about 10:1 (Roman, 2013).

Both the Institute of Medicine (1990) and Sobell and Sobell (2000) have proposed stepped-care models for making decisions about level of care. The stepped-care model proposes brief interventions as the modal initial approach to treatment, with treatment "stepped up" to more intensive or extensive treatment based on the client's response to the initial treatment. Such models are economically conservative and maintain the principle of least restrictive level of care. However, some clients with more severe problems might not be served well by very brief treatment (e.g., Rychtarik et al., 2000), and studies using American Society of Addiction Medicine (ASAM) criteria suggest that patients have poorer outcomes if they receive less intensive treatment than suggested by these criteria (Magura et al., 2003).

Proposed decision-making models to determine level of care have been implemented in many states. The ASAM (2001) has proposed a multidimensional decision-making model for selecting initial level of care. ASAM criteria consider need for supervised withdrawal, medical conditions that might require monitoring, comorbid psychiatric conditions, motivation for change and degree of treatment acceptance or resistance, relapse potential, and nature of the individual's social environment in recommending an initial level of care. These criteria are mapped onto five major levels of care, including early intervention, outpatient, intensive outpatient/partial hospitalization, residential/inpatient, and medically managed intensive inpatient treatment. Table 13.5 summarizes how the major criteria are applied to level of care determinations. Studies of the ASAM criteria suggest a number of barriers to using the criteria in clinical practice. For example, among homeless individuals, treatment facilities may be inaccessible because of lack of insurance or money to pay. Also, such individuals often are placed on waiting lists because programs are full. Some programs also may lack adjunctive services needed by a homeless population, such as assistance with pragmatic issues (food stamps, housing, unemployment, medical care, mental health care, or family treatment) (O'Toole et al., 2004). Among other patients seeking alcohol treatment, some may receive treatment that is more intensive than that suggested by ASAM criteria because their insurance or Medicaid only covers inpatient treatment, there may have been pressure from the family for inpatient treatment, or a specific level of care was mandated by an external agency (e.g., Employee Assistance Program). Patients also may receive treatment that is less intensive than that suggested by ASAM criteria because of their work schedule or reluctance to commit to more (Kosanke, Magura, Staines, Foote, & DeLuca, 2002). Additional considerations in determining initial level of care are discussed below.

TABLE 13.5. American Society of Addiction Medicine General Guidelines for Selection of Treatment Settings

Level of care	Criteria
Level 0.5. Early intervention	• At risk for developing an SUD • Insufficient information to establish and SUD diagnosis
Level I. Outpatient treatment	• No serious risk for major withdrawal or withdrawal seizures • No acute or chronic medical or psychiatric problems that could interfere with treatment • Some openness to change • Some ability to maintain change • Reasonable environmental support for change
Level II. Intensive outpatient treatment	• No serious risk for major withdrawal or withdrawal seizures • No acute or chronic medical or psychiatric problems that could be managed with intensive supervision *and* • Some reluctance to change *or* • Limited ability to maintain change *or* • Limited environmental supports for change

Level III. Medically monitored intensive inpatient treatment	• At least two:
	  o Risk for withdrawal
	  o Some level of acute or chronic medical or psychiatric problems that could be managed with intensive supervision
	  o Reluctance to change
	  o Limited ability to maintain change
	  o Limited environmental supports for change

Level IV. Medically managed intensive inpatient treatment	• Serious risk for major withdrawal or withdrawal seizures *or* • Acute or chronic medical *or* psychiatric problems that could interfere with treatment

Need for Detoxification

If a client is physically dependent on alcohol, then he/she will experience alcohol withdrawal symptoms when drinking is decreased or stopped. A number of signs suggest that a client may be physically dependent on alcohol, including daily drinking, drinking regularly or intermittently throughout the day, and morning drinking. Awakening during the night with fears, trembling, or nausea, or experiencing such symptoms upon first awakening, also suggests dependence. Cessation or a substantial decrease in drinking will result in the appearance of minor withdrawal symptoms, such as tremulousness, nausea, vomiting, difficulty sleeping, irritability, anxiety, and elevations in pulse rate, blood pressure, and temperature. Such symptoms usually begin within 5–12 hours. More severe withdrawal symptoms (e.g., seizures, delirium, or hallucinations) may also occur, usually within 24–72 hours of the ces-

sation of drinking. If a client has not consumed alcohol for several days prior to initial clinical contact, concerns about alcohol withdrawal are not relevant. If the client has stopped drinking within the last 3 days, the clinician needs to inquire about and observe the client for signs of withdrawal. The Clinical Institute Withdrawal Assessment (CIWA, Sullivan, Sykora, Schneiderman, Naranjo, & Sellers, 1989) provides an objective measure of current withdrawal symptoms. If the client currently is drinking, the clinician must rely on drinking history, pattern, and the results of previous attempts to stop drinking to determine whether detoxification will be necessary.

If the client needs detoxification, five alternatives are available: inpatient or partial hospital medical detoxification, inpatient nonmedical detoxification, or outpatient medical or nonmedical detoxification. Inpatient, medically assisted detoxification is essential if the client has a history of disorientation, delirium, hallucinations, or seizures during alcohol withdrawal, or is showing current signs of disorientation, delirium, or hallucinations. If the client does not believe that he/she can stop drinking without being physically removed from alcohol, but does not show any major withdrawal signs, is in good health, and does not abuse other drugs, a social setting detoxification may be appropriate. If the client has some social supports, then detoxification can be initiated on a partial hospital or outpatient basis. The choice between these two latter settings is determined by how much support the person will need during withdrawal, and whether a structured program will be needed after detoxification. If the client needs a fairly structured program, then the partial hospital is the preferred setting for detoxification. If a client has a mild to moderate AUD, a program to reduce alcohol consumption gradually over several weeks also can be managed (Cohn et al., 2010).

Medical Problems

The clinician who is considering the best setting for detoxification should take into account the presence of other medical problems. A cautious approach dictates that every client should have both a thorough physical examination and blood and urine studies at the beginning of treatment. The clinician should routinely include questions about physical health in the first contact with a client, and if significant physical complaints are noted, the client should receive immediate medical attention. Some clients have medical problems that require hospitalization; if so, the hospitalization should initiate the treatment.

Treatment History

After physical health issues have been considered, the clinician should examine the client's previous treatment history. Questions to consider include the following:

1. Has the client attempted outpatient treatment in the past and been able to stop or decrease drinking successfully? If so, then another attempt at outpatient treatment may be indicated.
2. Has the client dropped out of outpatient treatment in the past? If so, and there is no indication that any variables have changed in the interim,

then a more intensive partial hospital or inpatient program should be considered.
3. Has the client dropped out of, or drunk repeatedly, while in a partial hospital program? If so, then inpatient treatment may be indicated.
4. Did the client relapse immediately after discharge from an inpatient program? If so, then a partial hospital or outpatient setting may be appropriate because relapse may have been associated with problems in generalization from the inpatient to the natural environment. Alternatively, a halfway house may be considered to provide a longer-term structured environment.

Previous Quit Attempts

Many clients have successfully decreased or stopped drinking on their own at some time. Outpatient treatment is more likely to be successful for a client with a history of stopping successfully on his/her own than for a client without any history of successful change.

Social Support Systems

Social support systems are a critical variable to consider in determining the appropriate setting for initial treatment. If a client has support from another person, and that person is perceived as an important source who is willing to provide support and reinforcement, then the client is a good candidate for ambulatory treatment. If the client is lacking in social support, or is in an environment that supports heavy drinking, then inpatient or partial hospital treatment may be advisable. Alternatively, a halfway house may provide a good treatment setting for persons who do not have current social supports and have not been successful at developing them in the past, even during periods of abstinence.

Personal Resources

The next area to consider encompasses the client's personal psychological resources. Has he/she been successful in other areas of life in setting goals, changing behavior, and completing tasks? If so, outpatient treatment is more feasible. Another aspect of personal resources is cognitive functioning. If the client shows significant cognitive deficits in memory, attention, abstraction, or problem solving, a higher level of care may be considered. Otherwise, the client may have difficulty with retaining information presented in treatment or generating successful ways to avoid drinking.

Other Psychological Problems

As noted earlier in the chapter, persons with drinking problems often have other, significant psychological problems. The clinician must not only assess these problems but also determine level of care based on the appropriate setting for treatment of these other problems. A client who presents with serious depression must be assessed for suicidality and appropriate precautions should be taken.

Attitudes about Treatment

Although difficult areas to assess, the client's commitment to treatment and desire to change are important factors in selecting level of care. The client who is ambivalent but willing to come to treatment may respond better to a more intensive program that provides higher density reinforcement for attending treatment and making changes. However, sometimes ambivalence makes it impossible to provide treatment in a more intensive setting because the client is unwilling to disrupt his/her life to the extent required for such a program.

Practical Concerns

There are a number of practical concerns that the clinician must consider. Although in certain therapeutic approaches these issues might be considered evidence of client "denial," I view practical matters as real barriers to treatment and work with the client to overcome these barriers. Some practical barriers revolve around employment—whether the client can get time off from work, whether the job is in jeopardy, whether the employer is willing to support treatment, or whether missing any more work would result in termination of employment.

A second concern is the client's financial condition. Can the client afford to take time off from work and experience a reduction in income while he/she collects temporary disability (if sick time is not available)? If not, outpatient treatment, or a partial hospital program that allows the person to work, is appropriate. Another financial concern is the client's ability to pay for treatment.

Other practical concerns revolve around transportation and child care. Can the client get to outpatient ap-

pointments? Does he/she have a driver's license, and if not, is other transportation available? Is child care available if the person has to be hospitalized? If not, a day treatment setting may be preferred. The clinician must consider a range of pragmatic barriers to treatment.

Personal Preferences

Finally, the client's own preferences about the treatment must be considered carefully. If the client feels strongly about wanting to be in a hospital or residential treatment program, the clinician should listen carefully to this request, even if the initial assessment suggests that outpatient treatment may be feasible. Similarly, if the client wants outpatient treatment, the clinician should perhaps attempt it, even if he/she believes that a more intensive treatment is preferable.

General Considerations

In general, the selection of the initial treatment setting must be seen as a tentative decision. Often an initial contract may be established that includes the client's preferred setting, but with specification of the circumstances that will dictate a different level of care. For example, if the clinician believes that the client will find it extremely difficult to discontinue drinking on an outpatient basis, but this is the client's desire, then an initial contract may involve a plan for reducing or stopping drinking, learning skills to support that plan, and a time limit. If the person is unsuccessful within the specified time frame, then the contract is reviewed and alternative settings are considered. Thus, although the initial setting decision is important, continuing to consider and discuss other treatment settings is an important early step in the treatment process.

Selection of Treatment Modalities

If a client is referred to inpatient, residential, or intensive outpatient treatment, a mixture of treatment modalities is included in the treatment. Six major treatment modalities are available for the provision of alcohol treatment: self-help groups, individual therapy, group therapy, couple therapy, family therapy, and intensive treatment programs. In the ambulatory setting, the clinician has more flexibility in selecting from among these treatment modalities.

Self-Help Groups

AA is the most commonly utilized self-help group. With groups in all 50 states, as well as more than 150 countries throughout the world, AA is widely available. It offers a specific approach to recovery, rooted in the view that alcoholism is a physical, emotional, and spiritual disease that can be arrested but not cured. Recovery is viewed as a lifelong process that involves working the 12 Steps of AA and abstaining from the use of alcohol (for a detailed description of AA, see McCrady, Horvath, & Delaney, 2003). The only requirement for membership in AA is a desire to stop drinking, and members do not have to pay dues or join the organization. Persons who become involved with AA usually attend different meetings; have a relationship with an AA sponsor who helps them with their recovery; and become involved with other AA-related activities, ranging from making the coffee before meetings to going on "commitments," in which members of one AA group speak at another group. More active involvement is correlated with more successful change (reviewed in McCrady & Tonigan, in press).

Research suggests that persons most likely to affiliate with AA have a history of using social supports as a way to cope with problems, experience loss of control over their drinking, drink more per occasion than persons who do not affiliate, experience more anxiety about their drinking, believe that alcohol enhances their mental functioning, and are more religious or spiritual (McCrady & Tonigan, in press). Outpatient treatment to facilitate involvement with AA (12-step facilitation) has been found to be as effective as other forms of outpatient therapy in controlled trials, and some evidence suggests that clients receiving 12-step facilitation are more likely to maintain total abstinence from alcohol than clients receiving more behaviorally oriented treatments (Project MATCH Research Group, 1997a). Twelve-step facilitation treatment appears to be particularly successful for individuals with social systems that support them in drinking heavily (Longabaugh et al., 1998).

Alternative self-help groups have developed in recent years. Self-Management and Recovery Training (SMART) is a self-help approach based largely on cognitive-behavioral principles. SMART offers several steps to recovery, emphasizing awareness of irrational beliefs, self-perceptions, and expectancies as core to successful change. SMART suggests abstinence as a preferred drinking goal but emphasizes personal choice. Secular Organizations for Sobriety/Save Ourselves (SOS) was developed largely in response to the spiritual aspects of AA and does not invoke a Higher Power as a part of the change process. Women for Sobriety, a self-help approach for women, emphasizes women's issues such as assertiveness, self-confidence, and autonomy as a part of the change process. Moderation Management (2006) draws on behavioral principles to accomplish moderate drinking outcomes. All of these alternative approaches are more compatible with behavioral approaches than is AA, but none are as widely available to clients.

Individual Treatment

Individual therapy is offered primarily on an outpatient basis. Few data are available to guide the choice of individual versus group therapy. The literature on women with alcoholism is replete with suggestions that women respond better to individual than to group therapy, but empirical support for that assertion is lacking. Similar assertions apply to the treatment of older persons who have alcoholism, with a similar lack of empirical support.

Group Therapy

There is a strong belief in the alcohol field that group therapy is preferable to individual therapy (but see the previous comments in regard to women and older adults). Group therapy is more economical to provide, and interaction among group members provides opportunities for modeling, feedback, and behavioral rehearsal that are less available in the individual setting. Behavioral models for providing group therapy (Monti, Kadden, Rohsenow, Cooney, & Abrams, 2002; Sobell & Sobell, 2011) are well documented. Clients who are able to function in a group setting and do not require intensive individual attention because of other psychological problems can be assigned to group therapy.

Couple Therapy

A number of studies have suggested that involving the spouse/partner in alcoholism treatment increases the probability of a positive treatment outcome (McCrady, Epstein, Cook, Jensen, & Hilderbrand, 2009; McCrady, Owens, & Brovko, 2013). Despite the empirical evidence, traditional alcoholism counselors prefer individual or group therapy over couple therapy, emphasizing the importance of a focus on personal change before relationship change. Models for treatments that integrate individual and relationship treatment are available (McCrady & Epstein, 2009). Couple therapy is most appropriate for clients who have a stable relationship in which the partner is willing to be involved in treatment and can function in a supportive manner in the early phases of treatment. Couples who have experienced severe domestic violence, or in which one partner's commitment to the relationship is highly ambivalent, are less appropriate for couple therapy.

Techniques also have been developed to provide treatment to partners of people with AUDs when the drinker will not seek help. Behavioral groups that emphasize personal decision making, communication, and limit-setting around drinking are effective in motivating individuals to seek treatment or to decrease drinking (Miller et al., 1999; Sisson & Azrin, 1986; Smith & Meyers, 2004; Thomas, Santa, Bronson, & Oyserman, 1987). Al-Anon offers a self-help approach to partners and other family members affected by alcoholism.

Family Therapy

Despite a strong interest in AUDs in the family therapy field, models for working with whole families in which an AUD is present are scarce. Within the self-help area, Alateen is available for teens affected by a family member's alcoholism, and Alatot is available for younger family members.

Intensive Treatment Programs

Although, technically, a treatment setting rather than a modality, intensive treatment programs have such a specific and defined role in alcohol treatment that they can be considered a treatment modality. The "Minnesota model" (Slaymaker & Sheehan, 2013) is an intensive treatment approach that includes group therapy, education, self-help group involvement, and some individual counseling. Programs based on the Minnesota model emphasize confrontation of denial, acceptance that one is an alcoholic who is powerless over alcohol, development of caring and interdependent relationships, and commitment to AA involvement. Over time, Minnesota model programs have incorporated many behavioral strategies and techniques, including social skills and relaxation training, as well as RP techniques. Minnesota model programs have been marketed as

the most effective approach to alcoholism treatment, but data to support these claims are lacking. Most research on these programs has involved the evaluation of a single treatment program, and all the evaluations have been of private treatment centers. The evaluations suggest substantial levels of abstinence among persons receiving treatment (see, e.g., Filstead, 1991; Stinchfield & Owen, 1998), but the subjects in these studies tend to be good-prognosis patients, and without appropriate controls, conclusions cannot be drawn about the relative efficacy of these treatments compared to other approaches. Slaymaker and Sheehan (2013) reviewed more recent experimental and quasi-experimental studies of intensive treatments based on the disease model that were similar to Minnesota model programs, concluding that these studies supported the efficacy of the treatment model. Their wide visibility has made them the choice of many individuals with alcoholism and their families.

Enhancing and Maintaining Motivation to Change

Once a decision has been made about the level of care and the client has entered treatment, the clinician needs to continue to focus on motivation to be in treatment and to change. Techniques to enhance motivation include feedback, use of motivational interviewing techniques, mutual goal setting and decision making, treatment contracting, and the instillation of hope. Three clinical examples illustrate some of these techniques.

Bill (described earlier in this chapter) began treatment quite tentatively. He was willing to complete a standardized assessment of his drinking, so we completed a 1-month TLFB (Sobell & Sobell, 1995), the DrInC (Miller et al., 1995), and a Decisional Balance Sheet (Marlatt & Gordon, 1985; see Figure 13.2). Based on this information, I provided him with a standardized feedback sheet (Figure 13.5) about his drinking. The sheet provided data about how his drinking compared to national norms (Epstein & McCrady, 2009), as well as information about his peak BAL, usual BAL, and negative consequences of his drinking. Bill found the feedback interesting and asked questions about alcohol metabolism, epidemiological surveys, and alcohol and health effects. Although his wife, Diana, was somewhat impatient with this conversation, I thought that Bill's interest in learning more about alcohol and its effects was a positive sign.

For the Drinker

1. Based on the information I obtained during the assessment, I calculated the number of "standard drinks" you consumed in a typical week, during the last month:

     Total number of standard drinks per week   _____

     Average number of standard drinks per day   _____

2. When we look at everyone who drinks in the United States, you have been drinking more than approximately ____ percent of the population of women/men in the country.

3. I also estimated your highest and average blood alcohol level (BAL) in the past month. Your BAL is based on how many standard drinks you consume, the length of time over which you drink that much, whether you are a man or a woman, and how much you weight. So,

     Your estimated peak BAL in an average week was   _____

     Your estimated average BAL in an average week was   _____

     This is a measure of how intoxicated you typically become. In New Jersey, the legal intoxication limit is 80 mg% or higher.

4. You have experienced many negative consequences from drinking. Here are some of the most important:

     _____   _____

     _____   _____

     _____   _____

For the Partner

1. You have been trying many ways to cope with your wife/husband's drinking. The things you have tried the most include:

     _____   _____

     _____   _____

     _____   _____

For the Couple

1. You have a number of areas of your relationship that you are concerned about. Some are concerns for both of you:

     _____   _____

     _____   _____

     _____   _____

2. Some concerns are mostly concerns for the husband:

     _____   _____

     _____   _____

3. Some concerns are mostly concerns for the wife:

     _____   _____

     _____   _____

FIGURE 13.5. Drinking feedback sheet for a couple.

We discussed drinking goals, and I suggested the Moderation Management (2006) drinking guideline for men of no more than 14 drinks in a week, no more than 4 days' drinking per week, and no more than four drinks per occasion. Bill indicated that he wanted to continue with daily drinking, but with a limit of three drinks per day. Diana was agreeable, saying that if he kept to this limit she would be "thrilled." Although his selected goal was higher than I would have liked, I agreed in order to engage him further in treatment. I then gave him his first "homework" assignment—to initiate self-recording of his drinking (see Figure 13.3). The assignment of homework serves as a useful behavioral probe for level of motivation, and I was pleased when Bill returned to the next session with completed self-recording cards.

Suzanne was a 39-year-old computer programmer whom I treated in outpatient therapy as part of a treatment research project. Suzanne drank daily, typically consuming three glasses of wine per day. She had made a number of unsuccessful attempts to stop drinking and felt that she had completely lost control over her drinking even though the amount she drank was not remarkably high. She was concerned about her ability to be alert and available to her children in the evenings when she was drinking, particularly since her husband traveled frequently for his business. Suzanne sought treatment voluntarily and wanted to abstain from drinking completely. Despite her self-referral to treatment and her self-defined need for abstinence, Suzanne reacted to the same structured feedback quite differently than Bill did. She had provided information for the TLFB and completed the Rutgers Consequences of Use Questionnaire (RCU), but when I gave her feedback that she had been drinking an average of 21.5 drinks per week, she told me that this figure was too high and that our measure was not very accurate. She also indicated that she was participating in a research study, not in therapy, which was why she thought it important that we have accurate data. I did not argue with her perspective, agreeing that she was in a research study, but that I hoped that the study would helpful to her. She continued with treatment, and several weeks later commented spontaneously, "You know, I know that I'm in treatment, and I really need it. I think I was just protecting my ego at the beginning by focusing on the research part so much."

Anne, a 32-year-old, married college graduate working as a cocktail waitress, was the mother of a 20-month-old daughter, Breanne. Her husband, Char-lie, was working full time and enrolled in a doctoral program in mechanical engineering. She entered treatment as part of our women's treatment research program. She was a daily drinker with a varying pattern of consumption. During the evenings, when her husband was at school, she drank one or two bottles of wine. When he was home, her typical consumption was one glass of wine with dinner. She also drank at the end of her shift at work, consuming four to six beers on those evenings. When I gave her the feedback about her alcohol consumption, indicating that her level of consumption placed her in the 99th percentile of women, her eyes filled with tears and she looked visibly distraught, saying repeatedly, "I knew it was bad, but I never knew it was this bad." As treatment progressed, Anne made few changes in her drinking. She canceled or changed appointments, and said on several occasions, "If I didn't like you, I'd probably just quit the whole thing." She continued:

ANNE: I really like to drink. When Charlie is at school, I make myself a nice dinner—a lamb chop, a salad—and have an excellent bottle of wine. No one bothers me, and I enjoy myself. But I know I should stop because of Breanne.

THERAPIST: [As part of the treatment protocol, we had completed a decisional matrix, and I suggest that we return to that form.] Anne, let's look at your decisional matrix again. We did this a few weeks ago. When you look at it now, what strikes you?

ANNE: Everything on it is still true. I'm not being a good mother with all this drinking. I'm out of it at night, and I have no energy during the day. I just plop her in front of the television, and she watches *Dora the Explorer*. I keep thinking about when she gets older, "Do I want her to have a drunken mother?"

THERAPIST: It seems as though those feelings are very strong right now, but it's hard for you to keep them in the front of your mind each day. I wonder if you could review this sheet every day at some point. Would that help?

ANNE: I think so. I can look at it while Breanne is eating her breakfast. My motivation would be sitting right in front of me then. I'll try that.

Anne began reviewing her decisional matrix every day. The task seemed helpful for about a month, and she began to decrease her drinking, joined a gym, and came to treatment regularly. However, these changes were short-lived, and she fairly quickly reverted to her pattern of erratic treatment attendance and heavy drinking.

Selection of Drinking Goals

The final major area to consider in treatment planning is the selection of drinking goals. Traditional approaches to alcoholism treatment view abstinence as the only appropriate drinking goal because these approaches view alcoholism as a progressive disease that can only be arrested with abstinence. Behavioral clinicians have examined alternatives to abstinence and have developed a number of strategies to teach clients how to drink moderately. Although better accepted as a goal for individuals who are hazardous drinkers or have a mild AUD, moderation training continues to be controversial, and the clinician who elects to provide such treatment may be vulnerable to criticism from the traditional, mainstream alcoholism treatment community. Earlier studies suggest that the long-term outcomes of alcoholism include reduced drinking (e.g., Helzer et al., 1985; Vaillant, 1983), but early data about the success of moderation training were more mixed. Two European studies found that giving clients the opportunity to select treatment goals increased compliance with treatment and might improve treatment outcome (Ojehegan & Berglund, 1989; Orford & Keddie, 1986). Two recent studies that have tested training in moderate drinking using a Web-based intervention (Hester, Delaney, Campbell, & Handmaker, 2009) or a women's therapy group (Walitzer & Connors, 2007) both found positive outcomes for moderation training with low dependence drinkers, with the results for the women's group sustained over 30 months of follow-up. In the past, I have argued in favor of abstinence as a preferred treatment goal (see, e.g., McCrady, 1992; Nathan & McCrady, 1987), and continue to view it as the preferred treatment goal for individuals with moderate to severe AUDs. Abstinence is clearly defined and is in accord with usual clinical practice in the United States. Also, agreeing readily to a goal of moderate drinking may reinforce a client's view that alcohol is important and necessary to his/her daily functioning.

Under certain circumstances the use of a reduced drinking goal is appropriate. Moderation may be used as a provisional goal to engage a client in treatment, or it may be used when the client will not agree to abstinence but does want assistance to change (as with Bill).

A moderate drinking goal also is more appropriate if a client shows few signs of alcohol dependence or withdrawal, has a history of being able to drink in moderation, does not have medical or psychological problems that would be exacerbated by continued drinking, is younger, and does not have a family history of alcoholism (Rosenberg, 1993). If clinician and client select a moderation goal, a period of initial abstinence usually makes it easier for the client to drink moderately. In selecting a moderation goal, the clinician should be careful to help the client recognize the current and potential negative consequences of excessive drinking, and make an informed and thoughtful choice in selecting a treatment goal. The clinician should view any initial drinking goal (abstinence or moderation) as tentative, to be reevaluated as therapy progresses.

Initiating Abstinence

For the client with a goal of abstinence, the clinician has a variety of alternatives to help him/her initiate abstinence. With a client whose goal is moderation, the most conservative approach is to initiate a period of abstinence, then gradually reintroduce alcohol. As noted earlier, several detoxification alternative strategies are available, including inpatient detoxification, ambulatory detoxification, "cold turkey" detoxification (in which the client simply stops drinking abruptly), or a graduated program of reduction of drinking over a period of weeks, until the client reaches abstinence. A case example illustrates a graduated program of reduction of drinking.

Steve, a 48-year-old, homeless, unemployed man with a long history of heroin, cocaine, and alcohol dependence, entered treatment after heroin detoxification but was still drinking an average of eight drinks per day (usually a half-pint of hard liquor plus one to two beers). He was healthy and had no history of alcohol withdrawal symptoms. No inpatient detoxification facility was available to him given his homeless and economically destitute state. Initial treatment focused on helping him achieve a stable housing situation and obtaining temporary General Assistance (welfare). Following these social interventions, the therapist (one of our practicum students) began to focus on his drinking. Steve expressed a strong preference for a program of graduated reduction in drinking. He was evaluated by a physician at the local free clinic and cleared medically. We had him record his drinking for 1 week to establish a clear baseline. We then set a program to reduce his drinking by 15% per week, or eight drinks per week. We discussed specific strategies to achieve this goal each week, and Steve continued to monitor his drinking. During the alcohol reduction period, Steve reestablished contact with a former long-term girlfriend who had terminated their relationship when he relapsed to alcohol and heroin use. She had heard that he was off heroin and expressed interest in being involved with him again. Her presence provided a strong incentive for him to follow the alcohol reduction program because she was unaware that he had been drinking. The program progressed smoothly, and he stopped drinking after 7 weeks.

Developing a Functional Analysis

As described earlier, completing a behavioral assessment of the factors associated with a client's drinking includes both a structured and a qualitative dimension, and incorporates clinical interviewing, questionnaires, and self-recording of drinking and drinking urges. Suzanne, described briefly earlier, provides an excellent illustration of the complexity and results of the behavioral assessment process.

Suzanne came from a large Jewish family, many members of whom made demands on her. She had three daughters, ages 10, 8, and 4 years old. Her drinking had increased 5 years prior to treatment after a car accident that took the life of her fraternal twin brother. They had gone out to a Bruce Springsteen concert together, and her brother had had several drinks at the concert. An autopsy after the accident revealed that he had also been using cocaine, but Suzanne had been unaware of his drug use. She blamed herself for allowing him to drive and for not insisting that he stop when he began to drive in a reckless manner. She began to drink immediately after the accident and quickly established a pattern of daily consumption of a half-bottle of wine per day.

Although the amount was not that great, she reported that the alcohol was very important because it helped her avoid her overwhelming sadness about her brother's death, especially at the end of the day. The results of the behavioral assessment revealed a more complex pattern of drinking antecedents. On the DPQ, Suzanne rated emotional antecedents as most important, endorsing feelings of sadness, hurt, and frustration. She also indicated that certain environments were triggers for drinking, such as specific restaurants, times of the day (evening), and activities (particularly watching televi-

sion). Other major triggers emerged from Suzanne's self-recording cards—her interactions with extended family members and with friends, and situations related to her children. Her parents were highly critical of how she was raising her children. Suzanne and her husband, Josh, were attending a conservative temple, kept kosher in their home, did not allow violent video games, and expected each daughter to participate in a fine arts activity (music, dance, or painting). Her parents believed that their grandchildren's upbringing and Suzanne and Josh's standards were too strict and conservative, and they were vocal in their criticisms. Other familial stressors included her interactions with a sister who was getting divorced and a cousin who was in economic straits. Each contacted Suzanne on a regular basis, demanding either her attention or her money. Suzanne's functional analysis is provided in Figure 13.6.

Early Sobriety Strategies

Early sobriety strategies help the client maintain abstinence from alcohol. Cognitive-behavioral techniques vary with the individual but may include stimulus control strategies to avoid or rearrange high-risk situations, development of skills to deal with urges to drink, learning to think differently about drinking and not drinking, identification of behaviors alternative to drinking in high-risk situations, developing alternative ways to obtain the reinforcers previously obtained from alcohol, and learning to refuse drinks.

Stimulus Control

Stimulus control strategies are designed to alter environmental cues for drinking by avoiding the cue, rearranging it, or implementing different responses in the same environment. Stimulus control strategies are compatible with the AA suggestion to be attuned to "people, places, and things." Work with Suzanne illustrates stimulus control strategies.

With Suzanne, stimulus control strategies served a major function early in treatment. She developed specific strategies to deal with a number of the environmental high-risk situations identified in her functional analysis. Her first approach was to avoid such situations whenever possible. She suggested to Josh that they eat only at restaurants without liquor licenses, and asked that they decline several social invitations to places where alcohol would be the main focus of the evening (e.g., cocktail parties). The one situation that she could

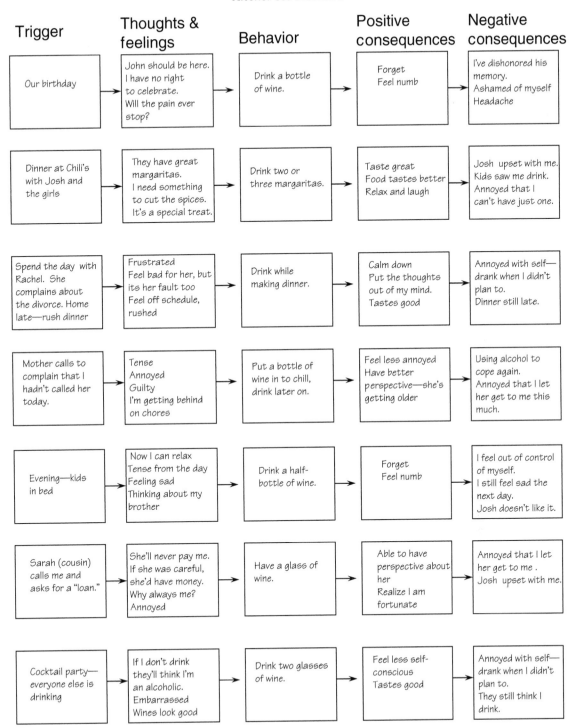

FIGURE 13.6. Suzanne's functional analysis.

not avoid was the end of the day, after the children had gone to bed. Her usual routine had been to complete the dinner dishes while Josh helped the girls get ready for bed, then to sit down in the den with her wine and the television after reading the children a story. She decided that she needed to disrupt this pattern and thought that if she got ready for bed herself, then curled up on the couch with a book and a cup of herbal tea, she would experience less urge to drink. It took her 3 weeks to get to a bookstore to buy some light novels, but once she had the books, Suzanne was able to implement this plan with success, except when she was upset.

Dealing with Urges

As individuals decrease their drinking or initiate abstinence, they may experience urges or cravings for alcohol. It is helpful to provide the client with a framework for understanding that urges are learned responses to drinking situations, and that urges abate if unfulfilled. Marlatt and Gordon (1985) suggested the use of imagery to help clients cope with urges, and described either acceptance-oriented imagery (e.g., surfing with the urge) or action-oriented imagery (e.g., attacking the urge with a samurai sword).

Suzanne struggled with urges to drink, particularly when anything reminded her of her twin brother's death. During therapy, we focused on a variety of aspects of her feelings about her brother's death and also addressed the urges more directly. Suzanne initially reacted to the imagery techniques negatively, saying that she was not a person who imagined things much. She clearly needed some way to cope with these rather strong urges, so I pushed her a bit to try:

THERAPIST: I appreciate that you don't think of yourself as imaginative, but maybe I can help you out. Just humor me for a minute, and let's see if we can come up with an image that grabs you. It doesn't matter what the image is—you could imagine climbing a mountain and coming down the other side, or spraying the urge with a fire extinguisher.

SUZANNE: (*smiling*) I know what I can imagine—I could picture you jumping out of the bottle and shaking your head at me.

THERAPIST: OK. Should I look mean?

SUZANNE: No, just having you there would help me deal with it.

THERAPIST: All right, I can live with that.

SUZANNE: In fact, I could picture a row of wine bottles—with you coming out of the first one, then showing me all the disgusting things in the other one.

THERAPIST: So what would be disgusting? Ticks?

SUZANNE: Ticks would be good, and maybe cockroaches, too.

THERAPIST: Let's try this out.

At that point, I had her practice using the imagery in an imagined urge situation. Remarkably, she used the imagery frequently and found it helpful.

A second technique for coping with urges is to enlist the assistance of a family member or friend. Persons involved with AA are told to call someone in the AA program when they feel the urge to drink, and they usually receive telephone numbers from several members. Clients not involved with AA can seek other sources of support. Suzanne, for example, asked her husband to help her when she had the urge to drink. She asked Josh to remind her of why she had stopped drinking and to say, "Of course, it has to be your decision."

Addressing Cognitive Distortions about Alcohol

People who drink heavily hold stronger positive expectancies about the effects of alcohol than do people who drink more lightly (Pabst, Baumeister, & Kraus, 2010). Clients may believe that drinking facilitates social interactions, enhances sexual responsiveness, allows them to forget painful events or feelings, or makes them more capable. These beliefs often are deeply held and difficult to challenge, particularly if a client continues to drink. Several cognitive strategies may help. First, effecting a period of abstinence allows the client to experience many situations without alcohol—an experience that often leads to reevaluation, with little input from the therapist. At some point, many clients are impressed with the vacuous nature of drunken conversation; the undesirable physical appearance, behaviors, and odors that accompany high BALs; and the shallow nature of drinking relationships. The wise therapist watches carefully for these observations and underscores their importance and self-relevance. If a client does not have such experiences spontaneously, the therapist facilitates new views of drunken comportment by developing a relatively safe way for the client to observe intoxicated behavior—through either movies or videotapes, or visits to a local bar (accompanied by someone who is aware of and supports the client's abstinence).

A second strategy reported in the self-change literature (Ludwig, 1985) is the ability to think past anticipated positive benefits of drinking to the clear, though often delayed, negative consequences of drinking. The therapist and client can generate a list of negative consequences of drinking and use imaginal rehearsal in the session to help the client pair positive thoughts with the list of negatives. Continued rehearsal in the natural environment is then important. Third, some clients develop a set of erroneous beliefs about their drinking that set them up for drinking. Common beliefs include "I've been doing so well, I can just drink tonight," or "I'll have just one." Although moderate drinking is possible for some clients, others have histories of drinking until they lose control, which is in direct opposition to a belief in control, and they need to learn to counter these beliefs.

Work with Steve provides a simple illustration of cognitive strategies to address positive expectations about drinking. Steve had a long history of loss-of-control drinking. After a period of abstinence, he began to think, "I could have just one beer, and that would be fine." His therapist questioned the accuracy of that belief. Steve readily acknowledged that he had never been able to control his drinking in the past, that if his girlfriend found out she'd be very upset and probably leave him, and that relapses to heavy drinking usually led him to use heroin. Steve and his therapist developed a simple cognitive formula to use when he thought about drinking: "1 = 32 = 10," meaning that for him, one drink would lead to a quart of liquor (32 ounces), which would lead to heroin use (10 bags a day).

Alternative/Distracting Behaviors

Drinking is a time-occupying activity, and clients may see few alternatives to help them through times when they previously would drink. Discussion of specific behavioral alternatives to drinking that are both time-occupying and mentally or physically absorbing is another helpful strategy early in treatment.

Steve's experiences provide a particularly powerful example of the alternatives that highly motivated clients may find. After Steve found a room in a rooming house and had begun the detoxification process, he was faced with the daunting prospect of filling his completely un-structured days. Some of his time was occupied with the time-consuming work of being poor—getting back and forth to the soup kitchen, waiting at the free clinic for medical services, getting an appropriate identification card so that he was eligible for other charitable programs, such as clothing distribution. But even with these necessary activities, Steve had hours and hours of free time. Steve began to address this challenge by creating his own activities. He obtained a library card and scheduled times for himself at the library. Instead of reading randomly or recreationally, he decided to read about the Crusades, which sparked an interest for him in medieval Christianity. A lapsed Catholic, he decided to attend Mass again, and began to attend daily. His daily attendance led to involvement in a Bible study group, and he became a thoughtful and passionate participant. A creative man, Steve then began to write short stories with religious themes.

Identifying Alternative Ways to Obtain Reinforcers

Among the more compelling aspects of alcohol and drug use are the psychoactive properties of the substances. In the short term, large quantities of alcohol effectively deaden negative affect, decrease obsessional thoughts, and decrease muscle tension, although these effects do not endure over the long term. Alcoholic beverages also have distinctive and desirable tastes that are difficult to replace with other beverages. An important aspect of the functional analysis is articulating the client's perception of positive consequences of drinking. The clinician can address the power of these perceived reinforcers in several ways: helping the client develop alternative means of obtaining the same types of positive experiences; challenging the client's belief that the desirable consequences will occur (e.g., questioning whether the client is in fact more socially adept and appealing after consuming a quart of vodka); helping the client reevaluate the importance of these reinforcers; and/or helping the client identify other classes of reinforcers that might be valued more highly in the long run (e.g., valuing spirituality more highly than hedonism).

Drink Refusal Skills

Some drinkers find the interpersonal aspects of abstinence difficult. For them, identification of interpersonal situations as high risk for drinking, development of effective responses, and rehearsal of these responses all form an important component of treatment. Early research (Chaney, O'Leary, & Marlatt, 1978) suggested that giving a quick response is strongly associated with successful change. More recent research has found that drink refusal training makes a unique positive contribution to treatment outcome (Witkiewitz, Donovan, & Hartzler, 2012). Suggested components of effective drinks refusal include indicating clearly that the one does not want an alcoholic beverage, requesting an alternative beverage, communicating confidence and comfort with the request, and being persistent in the face of social pressure (Foy, Miller, Eisler, & O'Toole, 1976). In addition, clients who face excessive social pressure may be advised to consider avoiding certain social situations or persons.

Although the guidelines for refusing drinks appear simple, client beliefs and expectations often make the drink refusal process difficult. Common cognitions include "Everyone will think I'm an alcoholic," "My host will be offended if I don't drink," or "People will think I'm too good for them if I don't drink." As with other distorted beliefs, the clinician can provide alternative frameworks for thinking about drink refusal situations, suggesting that most people really are uninterested in others' drinking, or that hosts are most concerned that guests are enjoying themselves. Many clients also experience ambivalence about not drinking and find that the most difficult part of the drink refusal process is internal rather than interpersonal. Another complicated aspect of drink refusal is how much personal information the client wishes to divulge. Most people share different levels of personal information, depending on the closeness of the relationship and their knowledge of the other person's behavior and attitudes. For persons to whom a client does not want to disclose his/her drinking problem, we encourage use of a simple "No, thank you," or, if pressed, a simple response that would discourage pushing without being revealing, such as "I'm watching my weight and can't afford the calories," "I'm on medication that doesn't allow me to drink," or "My stomach's been acting up—I better pass." None of these replies protects the client against future offers, but each is effective in the moment. For closer relationships, the client makes a decision about when, where, and how much to reveal. Two clinical examples illustrate these points.

Steve was living in a boarding house and had friendly, sociable neighbors who liked to drink on the front porch. These neighbors were from the Portuguese Azores and spoke virtually no English. After accepting a beer from them one day, he insisted to his therapist that he could not refuse because he did not speak Portuguese. The therapist suggested that perhaps the word "No," spoken with a smile and a hand gesture, might be understood even in Portuguese. Steve acknowledged that his difficulty with refusing the drink came from his desire to drink, and that a friendly "No" would certainly work.

Suzanne did not want anyone to know that she had a drinking problem, or that she was abstaining. This stance posed problems for an upcoming cocktail party. Strategizing, Suzanne decided ahead of time that she would drink seltzer water that evening, and that she would attempt to forestall offers of drinks by keeping a glass of seltzer in her hand at all times. If offered a drink, she decided to tell people that she had had some health problems that might be made worse by her drinking, so she was sticking to seltzer. Although she was concerned that one of her friends (a social worker) might surmise that she had an alcohol problem, the evening progressed uneventfully.

Coping Strategies

Clients face challenges beyond those directly related to their drinking. As do clients without drinking problems, clients with such problems face common life difficulties stemming from dysfunctional thoughts, negative affect, and interpersonal conflicts. As clients develop a greater ability to maintain abstinence or moderated drinking, the clinician may devote increasing attention to other problems clients are facing. Clinical techniques to deal with dysfunctional thoughts or social skills deficits can be used readily with clients with drinking problems.

Dealing with Negative Affect

There are multiple sources of negative affect in persons with alcohol abuse or dependence. As noted earlier in the chapter, comorbidity with other psychiatric disorders is high (e.g., mood and anxiety disorders are quite common). Rates of sexual and physical abuse are also elevated among those with AUDs (Cisler et al., 2011), and the sequelae of these problems often include a strongly negative affective component. In addition, persons who have used alcohol to cope with negative affect over an extended period of time may simply have limited experience, and limited skills, to cope with the pain that is a part of everyday life.

In focusing on negative affect, a careful assessment of the causes is essential. Intense negative affect associated with another disorder should be treated in accord with the appropriate approach for that disorder. Dealing with negative affect that is not necessarily disorder-based presents different challenges. Full behavioral mood management programs (e.g., Monti et al., 1990) have been developed, although a description of these is beyond the scope of the chapter. However, certain common principles are of value. When clients first reduce or stop drinking, they may experience all emotions as unfamiliar and intense. Cognitive reframing to help clients view these intense emotions as a natural part of the change process may be useful. For clients pursuing a moderation goal, avoidance of drinking at times of intense negative affect provides the opportunity to learn alternative coping strategies. Coping strategies may vary with the type of negative emotion, and may include relaxation, prayer or meditation; increasing the experience of pleasurable events to decrease depression; or use of anger management and assertiveness skills to cope with angry feelings.

Work with Suzanne illustrates several of these principles. Most difficult for Suzanne were any situations that reminded her of the death of her twin. Their birthday, the anniversary of his death, the celebration of Father's and Mother's Days, holiday celebrations, and special celebratory events for her children in which he would have been importantly involved with (e.g., a bat mitzvah) all elicited intense negative affect and a strong desire to drink. Given that Suzanne had begun drinking heavily right after her twin's death, she had spent little time experiencing grief or even discussing his death and her feelings about it. My initial approach in therapy was to give her opportunities to be exposed to these negative feelings by simply talking about him in the therapy session. The second approach was to discuss and identify ways to approach events that reminded her of him. I saw her over a 6-month period, during which a number of these situations arose naturally. For example, in the week prior to the anniversary of his death, we discussed ways that she could focus on his death and memories. Suzanne took one of her children to his gravesite, and they cleaned it up and planted flowers together. On the Saturday of the anniversary of his death, she went to temple with her family, and then cooked what had been her twin's favorite dinner. The day was sorrowful and Suzanne cried several times, but it was the first anniversary that she felt she had honored him rather than shaming his memory by getting drunk. We also addressed her repetitive, self-blaming thoughts about his death by using cognitive restructuring techniques. She found it difficult not to blame herself for his death, and few cognitive strategies had much impact on the self-blame. Suzanne finally was able to begin to think, "I cannot torture myself forever with this blame. If I don't let go of it, I won't be a good mother. He'd be disappointed with me if I let my children down."

Lifestyle Balance and Pleasurable Activities

Marlatt and Donovan (2005) suggest that long-term success is supported by lifestyle changes that enhance positive experiences and allow for a balance between responsibilities and pleasure. Although some studies of successful self-changers (e.g., Vaillant & Milofsky, 1982) have revealed that development of an "alternative dependency" (e.g., obsessive involvement with work or exercise) is associated with successful long-term abstinence, we typically work toward a more balanced approach. As they begin to change, some of our clients believe that they need to make up for their previous lack of responsibility with a very high level of responsibility to family, job, and home. Taking on major redecorating or remodeling projects, trying to spend every free moment with their children, or cleaning out 10 years' worth of messy drawers and cabinets is not uncommon. This zeal for responsibility can be a double-edged sword for both client and family. Unrelenting attention to responsibilities may be simultaneously satisfying and exhausting and unrewarding, and may lead the client to question the value of not drinking. Family members may be thrilled that the client is taking on responsibility but leery of the stability of the change and unwilling to give up responsibilities they have assumed for him/her. They also may experience the client's enthusiasm as an intrusion on their own independent lives and schedules. Clients should be prepared for such reactions, and the clinician can help reframe the family's response as understandable. With most clients, it is important for the clinician to suggest the importance of leisure time, pleasurable activities, and self-reinforcement for positive changes made.

Helping Suzanne identify a half-hour per day during which she could relax, read, or exercise was a challenge. She believed that she should devote herself to her daughters—a belief that resulted in her being with them virtually all the time when they were home. When they were at school, she focused on housecleaning, cooking, errands, paying bills, and other chores.

She was exhausted and tense at the end of the day, and commented that alcohol had been a good way to "come down." We finally agreed on a half-hour block before lunch, during which she would use her exercise bike, read a book of daily meditations, or take a walk. She was only partially successful in these efforts, often citing other responsibilities that took precedence.

Partner/Family Involvement and the Social Context of Treatment

The literature on the treatment of alcohol use disorders suggests that the involvement of some significant social system is associated with positive treatment results (reviewed in McCrady et al., 2013). Because of these findings, the clinician's first inclination should be to involve the client's spouse/partner or some significant other in the treatment. There are a number of ways to involve significant others: using them as sources of information, having them provide differential reinforcement for drinking and abstinence, helping them to provide emotional or practical support, involving them in relationship-focused treatment, providing treatment to them without the person who drinks, and/or helping them access new social systems.

Information

Folklore suggests that persons with alcoholism minimize or lie about their drinking and its consequences. The empirical literature suggests that such individuals provide relatively accurate data when sober, and when there are no strong negative consequences for telling the truth (e.g., Sobell & Sobell, 2003). Despite these results, a number of clinical considerations suggest that obtaining information from a family member may be useful in the assessment phase of treatment.

Clients who are referred to or coerced into treatment may be reluctant to provide full information about their drinking. Collecting data from the referring agent helps both client and clinician understand the reasons for the referral. Even with self-referred clients, significant others can provide information that may be unavailable to the clients because of problems with memory or recall. In addition, an intimate significant other usually has observed the drinker over a long period of time and in multiple environments, and may have valuable observations to contribute to the conceptualization of antecedents to drinking.

Responses to Drinking and Abstinence

A different type of social system involvement is the establishment of a network that provides differential reinforcement for abstinence and applies negative consequences for drinking. Such reinforcement may be relatively simple, such as positive comments and encouragement from friends and family, or it can involve the negotiation of detailed contracts that specify the consequences of drinking and abstinence. The "community reinforcement approach" (CRA; Meyers & Smith, 1995) helps clients access potential reinforcers (jobs, families, social clubs), teaches clients and partners behavioral coping skills, and may involve development of contingency contracts to make access to reinforcers contingent on sobriety. In addition, clients may be prescribed disulfiram or naltrexone, and compliance may be monitored by a significant other. Evaluations of the CRA approach suggest that clients are significantly more successful than controls in maintaining abstinence and employment, avoiding hospitalizations or jail, and maintaining a stable residence. In addition to formal treatments that focus on manipulation of environmental contingencies, the therapist also may teach spouses/partners and other family members how to allow the client to experience the naturally occurring negative consequences of drinking. Many spouses/partners protect the drinker from these consequences by covering for him/her at work, doing his/her chores, or lying to friends and family about the drinking (e.g., Orford et al., 2005). Experience of these negative consequences may increase the client's awareness of the extent and severity of his/her drinking problem, and provide further motivation for change.

Decreasing Cues for Drinking

Significant others also may engage in behaviors that cue further drinking. A wife who wants her husband to stop drinking may nag him repeatedly about the problems his drinking is causing, hoping that her concerns will motivate him to change. Or a husband may try to get his wife to stop drinking by limiting her access to alcohol or tightly controlling their money. Such behaviors may have an unintended and negative effect, eliciting anger or defensiveness from the person with the drinking problem, and leading to further drinking. Helping spouses/partners learn to identify such behaviors, recognize the results of these actions, and find alternative ways to discuss concerns about drinking may be helpful.

Support for Abstinence

Significant others can provide many kinds of support to clients. Support may involve helping a client to implement behavior change, discussing urges to drink, supporting a client's plan to avoid high-risk situations for drinking, or (upon the request of the client) assisting in the implementation of other coping skills that support sobriety.

Relationship Change

For many clients, interactions with their spouses/partners, children, parents, or close friends cue drinking. Thus, treatment that focuses on changing these interpersonal relationships is another way that significant others may become involved. These interventions may include couple or family therapy, or parent skills training. Data (McCrady et al., 2009; McCrady, Stout, Noel, Abrams, & Nelson, 1991) suggest that a focus on changing the couple relationship during conjoint alcoholism treatment results in greater stability of drinking outcomes, fewer separations, and greater couple satisfaction.

Accessing New Social Systems

Some clients have either no social support system or one that strongly supports heavy drinking. For such clients, it is important to access new systems that either reinforce abstinence or are incompatible with heavy drinking. Self-help groups are one potential source of such support. Because many religious groups are against the use of alcohol, serious involvement in such a group also may support abstinence. Many group activities are incompatible with drinking: Running, hiking, or cycling groups are examples. Unfortunately, alcohol can be involved in almost any activity, and therapist and client need to look carefully at activity groups to determine whether the group norm includes drinking.

In summary, decisions about the social context of alcoholism treatment are complicated. The initial assessment should involve at least one significant other. The results of the assessment should reveal persons who are most available for treatment, and who might be sources of support and reinforcement. For some clients with no readily accessible supports, new support systems need to be developed.

Long-Term Maintenance

Relapse Prevention

Marlatt and Gordon's (1985) RP model and Witkiewitz and Marlatt's (2004) revised RP model are comprehensive treatment models; Epstein and McCrady's (2009) cognitive-behavioral therapy (CBT) manual provides specific RP exercises in the last several treatment sessions. Many elements of the RP treatment model already have been described—identifying high-risk situations for drinking, developing alternative strategies to cope with high-risk situations, enhancing self-efficacy for coping, dealing with positive expectancies about the use of alcohol, and facilitating the development of a balanced lifestyle. An additional and important part of the RP model is addressing the possibility of relapse, and developing preventive and responsive strategies related to relapse.

Clients are told that use of alcohol after treatment is not uncommon, and treatment addresses this possibility. Two basic strategies are used. First, a client is helped to develop a list of signs of an impending relapse, including behavioral, cognitive, interpersonal, and affective signs. If a client's spouse/partner is part of the treatment, he/she contributes to the list. After this list is developed, a set of possible responses, should these signs arise, is developed. Most important is for the client to recognize that these warning signs should trigger action rather than inaction and fatalistic cognitions about the inevitability of relapse. A second set of strategies involves response to drinking or heavy drinking. The clinician attempts to address the possibility of the AVE by calling attention to the possibility that a client may have catastrophic thoughts if he/she drinks and helping him/her rehearse alternative thoughts. Marlatt and Gordon (1985) also suggested a series of behavioral steps: Introduce a behavioral delay (1–2 hours) between an initial drink and any subsequent drinks; get out of the immediate drinking situation; conduct a functional analysis of the drinking situation during that time; review possible negative consequences of drinking; and call someone who might be helpful. Some research evidence supports the use of such RP approaches. For example, we found in our own research (McCrady, Epstein, & Hirsch, 1999) that including RP procedures as part of conjoint alcoholism treatment was successful in reducing the length of relapse episodes compared to conjoint CBT without RP. O'Farrell, Choquette, and Cutter (1998), who incorporated RP techniques into their couple therapy treatment by providing additional therapy sessions over the 12 months after initial treatment, reported less frequent drinking among couples who received the additional therapy.

Maintaining Contact with Clients

Time-limited treatment is appropriate and effective for many clients, and there is good evidence of long-term, sustained improvement following a course of outpatient treatment (Project MATCH Research Group, 1998). However, periods of relapse are common. The clinical strategies I have described for RP are intended to minimize periods of problem use and to maximize positive outcomes. For some clients, however, alcohol dependence must be viewed as chronic, relapsing disorder (McLellan et al., 2000). As with other chronic health problems, such as diabetes or rheumatoid arthritis, acute care models that treat individuals and send them on their way may be inappropriate and ineffective. An alternative strategy provides longer-term, low-intensity contact over an extended time interval (McKay et al., 2011).

During the initial treatment of a client with a history of severe alcohol dependence, multiple treatment episodes, and difficulty maintaining successful change, the clinician may elect to set a different expectancy with that client—that some form of contact will be ongoing and long-term.

Lee, a 54-year-old married man, came to treatment with problems with alcohol dependence and agoraphobia. Treatment focused on both disorders, and he was successful in becoming abstinent from alcohol and in gradually increasing the distances that he could drive by himself. Lee's home was an hour's drive from my office, and treatment had gone on for almost 12 months before he could drive to my office without his wife accompanying him. By the end of the year, we were meeting every 2 to 3 weeks. Given that Lee had been abstinent for a year and was functioning well, we discussed the possibility of termination. His response was instructive:

LEE: Doctor, I've been drinking a long, long time. One year is just a drop in the bucket in comparison. I think that I need to keep seeing you.

THERAPIST: Lee, I understand your concerns, but you've been doing well for quite a long time now. Maybe we should just cut down more on how often you come in. How about an appointment in a month, and making it a bit shorter—a half-hour instead of an hour?

LEE: I think that's a good idea. Let's try it.

I gradually tapered the frequency and length of my sessions with Lee, and saw him twice per year, 15 minutes per session, for the last 3½ years of his 5-year course of treatment. He described the importance of the sessions: "I just know I'll have to see you and tell you what I've been doing. It keeps me honest."

Management of Complicating Conditions

As I described earlier in the chapter, clients with AUDs may present with myriad other complicating conditions. The clinician must assess and develop a treatment plan for the multiple needs of such clients. At a minimum, clinicians should consider possible problems related to housing, transportation, income, occupation/employment, the legal system, the family, child care, medical conditions, and comorbid psychological disorders. Knowledge of services and agencies in the local community and the development of working relationships with a range of agencies are essential to the treatment of complicated clients. Rose, Zweben, Ockert, and Baier (2013) provide a comprehensive framework for interfacing with other health and social systems.

The Role of Self-Help Groups

Types of self-help groups were described in an earlier section of this chapter. Various therapeutic strategies may facilitate involvement in a self-help group, when appropriate. The clinician should first assess whether a client may be a good candidate for self-help group involvement. Clients with very high social anxiety or social phobia, clients who believe that a person should take care of problems alone, and those with a history of negative experiences with self-help groups may be poorer candidates. Conversely, affiliative clients, those who are used to solving problems with assistance from others, those who are particularly anxious and concerned about their drinking, those whose social support systems strongly support continued heavy drinking, and those with more severe alcohol dependence are particularly good candidates for AA. Persons who are interested in the social support aspects of self-help but explicitly reject some of the constructs associated with AA (e.g., powerlessness or spirituality) may be best served by referral to an alternative self-help group.

As with all aspects of the therapy, the clinician should use a client-centered approach to the introduction of AA or other self-help groups. Such an approach suggests a dialogue between client and therapist, acknowledgment and discussion of the client's perceptions and concerns, and development of a mutually agreed-upon plan. Because many clients have misconceptions about AA and are unfamiliar with some of the alternative organizations, the clinician should be prepared to describe the organizations and answer questions. It also is helpful for the clinician to have some basic publications from each group available in the office. At times, I may encourage a reluctant client to try a few meetings to sample firsthand what actually occurs. We negotiate a very short-term agreement for a specified number of meetings in a specified length of time (e.g., six meetings in 3 weeks); we agree that if the client continues to be negative or reluctant after trying the groups, then we will abandon this idea; and we discuss the client's experiences and perceptions of the self-help group meeting in each therapy session. I use behavioral sampling with other aspects of therapy as well: Clients often cannot visualize how a strategy might work without trying it— be it a relaxation technique, an AA meeting, or an assertive response—and I encourage clients to be open to new strategies. In AA, newcomers may be told, "Your best thinking got you here," which suggests that their own coping strategies have been ineffective. Behavioral sampling is based on this same construct.

Therapist Variables

As with any form of therapy, the therapist's relationship and the therapeutic stance he/she assumes with the client are important. Empathy, active listening, instillation of hope, flexible application of therapeutic principles and techniques, and establishment of a sense that therapist and client are working toward mutually agreed-upon goals are essential. Research suggests that in contrast to a confrontational style, an empathic, motivational style is associated with better treatment outcomes, and that confrontational behaviors by the therapist tend to elicit defensive and counteraggressive behaviors by the client (Miller, Benefield, & Tonigan, 1993; Miller & Rollnick, 2002). Such responses are hardly conducive to a constructive therapeutic alliance.

Working with a client with an AUD often is difficult because of both the client's behavior during treatment and his/her history of drinking-related behaviors that the therapist may find repugnant or upsetting. The client may lie about or minimize drinking during treatment. If the spouse/partner is also involved in the treatment, the therapeutic relationship becomes even more complicated.

By treating a client with a drinking problem along with a spouse/partner who wants that client to stop or decrease drinking, the therapist is allied de facto with the spouse/partner. The partner may attempt to enhance his/her alliance with the therapist by echoing the therapist's comments, expressing anger at the client's behavior, being confrontational, or, alternatively, being submissive and allowing the client to be verbally aggressive or dominant.

Certain therapist attitudes and behaviors appear to be conducive to successful treatment. First is a sense of empathy with the client. The therapist must develop some understanding of the client's subjective experience of entering therapy and the difficulty of admitting behaviors that are personally embarrassing and often not socially sanctioned. In addition, the therapist needs to have some appreciation of the incredible difficulties involved with long-term change in drinking behavior. He/she may develop this appreciation by attempting to change his/her own deeply ingrained behavior pattern by attending meetings of some self-help group (e.g., AA, SMART Recovery) and listening carefully to clients.

A second important therapist skill is the ability to distinguish between the person and the drinking-related behavior. The client needs to be able to describe drinking-related actions without feeling either that the therapist is repulsed or that the therapist condones or accepts such behaviors. This is a delicate balance to achieve, especially when a client describes drinking episodes in a joking manner that may hide embarrassment or disgust with the behavior. The client's motivation to change may be enhanced by discussing negative, drinking-related behaviors and experiencing the negative affect associated with thinking about those actions. The therapist also should communicate a sense of hope to the client by anticipating positive changes that might be associated with changes in drinking, and by emphasizing that it is possible to change. Thus, the implied message to the client is as follows:

"You have done many things when drinking that are distressing to you and to the people around you. The fact that you are in treatment is a statement that you want to change. It is important to talk about things you have done when drinking because being aware of them will strengthen your desire to stop drinking and to stop doing these things. Making changes will take time and a lot of work on your part, but I believe that you will be successful if you stick with treatment."

In other words, the therapist's message is positive about change, but negative about drinking-related behavior.

A third important therapist quality is integrity. Both because of their discomfort and their reinforcement history, it is difficult for some clients to honestly report their drinking episodes, failed homework assignments, or their feelings and attitudes about being in treatment. The therapist can acknowledge how difficult it is to be honest given that lying was probably adaptive in the past, but he/she must make it clear that part of therapy involves learning how to be honest. The therapist also must provide a positive model of integrity. He/she should not ignore the smell of alcohol on a client's breath, and he/she should review the homework assigned each week. Attending to the client's behavior teaches the client the importance of following through on commitments and increases the chances that therapist and client will be able to identify problems and blocks to progress in treatment.

The therapist also must set clear expectations about both the client's and his/her own responsibilities to the therapy, and must be able to set appropriate limits. The therapist should set clear expectations for the client: coming to scheduled sessions on time, calling if unable to attend, paying the bill for therapy, coming in sober, and completing assigned homework. The therapist also should make his/her own commitment to therapy clear, by being at sessions on time, being reasonably available by telephone, providing coverage when away, and providing treatments with demonstrated empirical support for their effectiveness. Being clear about expectations for the client's behavior during therapy emphasizes the therapist's commitment to therapy as a serious process.

Client Variables

Only a few client characteristics are consistent predictors of treatment outcome (Haaga, McCrady, & Lebow, 2006). Clients who have positive expectancies about the outcomes of treatment tend to have better outcomes. Additionally, clients with greater readiness to change have more positive outcomes. Finally, clients with more severe problems have poorer outcomes. Both treatment expectancies and readiness to change can be influenced by the therapist.

The clinician must be aware of and sensitive to a number of issues that persons with drinking problems bring to treatment. The client's emotional experience, his/her beliefs, attitudes, and physical state (described in the section on treatment settings), and the social context of drinking (described in the section on the social context of drinking) are all important aspects of the therapeutic plan.

A person has a variety of reactions to the initial realization that his/her drinking is causing problems. Most commonly, as negative consequences accumulate, an individual begins to feel out of control and ashamed of the behavior. The person's actions may be unacceptable to his/her self-definition. Thus, financial or work irresponsibility, neglecting family members, engaging in physical violence, or verbal abuse all may be actions about which the individual feels intense guilt and self-blame. The prospect of admitting these actions to a stranger is frightening and embarrassing, making it difficult for a client to discuss drinking-associated problems. Because many clients ascribe their problems to weakness or lack of willpower, and believe that if they were only "stronger" these events would not occur, they blame themselves. Thus, clients are unusually sensitive to implied criticisms from the therapist. The therapist can attenuate this difficulty by making empathic comments while asking questions, letting clients know that their actions are common among people who drink heavily, and listening to clients' descriptions of drinking-related actions in an accepting manner. Clients also hold a number of beliefs and attitudes about alcohol and their ability to change that make change difficult. People with AUDs have positive expectancies about the effects of alcohol on feelings and behavior, and they hold these more strongly than do people without drinking problems. They may attribute their drinking to reasons external to themselves and believe that they are not personally responsible for either drinking or changing. They may have low self-efficacy beliefs about their ability to change their drinking or to handle alcohol-related situations without drinking, or they may have unrealistically high self-efficacy beliefs that are not grounded in actuality. Finally, if people stop drinking and then consume alcohol again, cognitive dissonance may occur; they may experience the AVE (Marlatt & Gordon, 1985), characterized by an excessively negative reaction to initial alcohol consumption, and a self-perception that they have "blown" their abstinence and will inevitably relapse to the previous drinking pattern.

CASE STUDY

In the preceding sections, I have presented case examples to illustrate the application of parts of our treatment model. In this section, I present a complete outpatient therapy case to illustrate a number of the issues described earlier in the context of ongoing treatment. The couple was part of a research project evaluating different approaches to the maintenance of change following conjoint behavioral alcoholism treatment (McCrady et al., 1999).

Couples in the study had to have been married or cohabitating for at least 6 months; neither partner could have a primary problem with the use of illicit drugs or show evidence of gross cognitive impairment or psychosis; and only the male partner could show evidence of alcohol abuse or dependence. All couples were seen by a therapist for 15–17 sessions of weekly outpatient treatment, and agreed to a baseline assessment and 18 months of posttreatment follow-up.

Carl and Maria were married, and both were 32 years old. They came to treatment because of Carl's drinking. Maria was of average height, had long, black, wavy hair and was heavy. Carl was also of average height, had blond hair, and was slim but showed the beginnings of a "beer belly." Both were neat and attractive. The couple had been married 5 years and had known each other for 12 years. They had two boys, ages 2 and 3. Both came from intact families, although Carl's father had died a number of years previously. Carl's family was primarily Polish; Maria's was Italian.

At the time of treatment, Carl and Maria had been separated for 5 months. He was living with his mother in her home; Maria was renting a one-bedroom apartment in a poor community, where she lived with the two boys. Maria was a trained cosmetologist; Carl was an electrician who worked out of the union hall. Carl was not working at the time because he did not want to establish a pattern of support for Maria or the children in case she filed for divorce. In addition, if he did not work for a certain period of time, Carl would be able to

withdraw his money from the union's pension plan, and he thought that would be an easy way to obtain money. Maria was not working because she had decided that Carl would have to babysit while she worked, and she did not think that he would be reliable about coming to her apartment to care for the children. She was supported by Aid to Families with Dependent Children (AFDC); Carl worked odd jobs "under the table." Both were high school graduates.

The couple came to treatment at Maria's urging. She was very concerned about Carl's drinking and cited it as the primary reason for their marital separation.

Behavioral Assessment and Case Conceptualization

Carl and Maria were assessed using several approaches. Their assessment was somewhat more extensive than is usual in clinical practice because of their involvement with the treatment research project. However, the main elements of the assessment are applicable to clinical practice as well.

Drinking Assessment

To assess his drinking, we used a clinical interview to ask Carl about his drinking history and perceptions of his current drinking. A handheld Breathalyzer was used at the beginning of each session to assess his current BAL. In addition, we used two structured interviews, the TLFB (Sobell & Sobell, 1995) and the Alcohol section of the Composite International Diagnostic Interview—Substance Abuse Module (CIDI-SAM; Robins et al., 1988), to obtain a more complete picture of his drinking. Maria was present for all interviews and contributed additional information.

The TLFB inquires about drinking behavior on each day in a set window of time before treatment. For this study, we asked about Carl's drinking in the prior 6 months, cueing his recall of drinking by noting other salient events in his and Maria's lives, such as social events, medical appointments, holidays, and other celebrations. The TLFB revealed that Carl had drunk alcohol virtually every day of the previous 6 months. His only abstinent day was when he and some friends were arrested for attempted breaking and entering. His preferred beverages were beer and vodka, and he reported that the most he drank on any single day was about 32 drinks. His usual consumption was in the range of 10–12 drinks daily. Carl met DSM-IV (the system in effect at the time of assessment) and DSM-5 criteria for a diagnosis of severe alcohol dependence with physiological dependence. He had been drinking since high school and reported having his first problems as a result of alcohol at the age of 25. Carl had experienced a variety of problem consequences of his use: three arrests for DWI, one arrest for breaking and entering, warnings from job supervisors for intoxication on the job, problems in his relationship with his wife, and the feeling that he had neglected his responsibilities to his wife and sons. He had experienced numerous blackouts and reported many signs of physical dependence, including morning drinking, a sense of "panic" when he thought he would not be able to obtain a drink when he wanted one, and drinking throughout the day. However, Carl said that he had never experienced any of the physical symptoms of alcohol withdrawal. He also reported no health or emotional problems associated with his drinking. When asked about his goals for treatment, Carl indicated that his own preference was to cut down and to drink moderately, but that his wife insisted on abstinence, and he was willing to work toward that goal.

We used two assessment techniques to identify antecedents to Carl's drinking, the DPQ (Menges et al., 2008) and self-recording cards. The DPQ was used to assess Carl's and Maria's perceptions of drinking antecedents. Carl completed the DPQ by checking off all antecedents that applied to his drinking in the previous 6 months, and Maria completed the measure as well, to indicate her views of his drinking. They also were asked to indicate what they thought were the most influential antecedents. Both perceived environmental influences as being most important to Carl's drinking, citing as the most salient settings bars and his home, afternoons when he was not working, any celebratory occasions, and being around others who were drinking.

The second most important set of drinking cues pertained to their relationship, with Carl citing arguments, anger, feeling nagged, or having a good time together as antecedents. The third area of concern that both Carl and Maria cited was physiological antecedents, primarily restlessness and fatigue.

Carl used daily self-recording cards throughout the treatment to record drinks and drinking urges. Reviewing the information he recorded and discussing events associated with drinking or drinking urges made it clear that being with heavy-drinking friends was an important component of Carl's drinking. The self-recording cards also clarified factors associated with

his feelings of "restlessness." When Carl and Maria were together and the children were being active, if he wanted to leave or go somewhere, then he would get restless and irritable, and want to drink to "take the edge off." Finally, it was apparent that Carl felt like drinking whenever Maria reminded him of a commitment that he had made (even something simple, such as bringing a book to her apartment), when she tried to get him to commit to any responsible course of action, or when he felt "trapped."

We used questionnaires and self-recording cards to assess how Maria coped with Carl's drinking. She recorded her perceptions of his drinking each day on a Likert scale (*None, Light, Moderate*, or *Heavy*) and recorded her daily marital satisfaction as well. Her responses antecedent to and consequent to drinking episodes were discussed in the therapy sessions. In addition, both partners completed a modified version of the Coping Questionnaire (Orford et al., 2005).

Data from these assessment sources made it apparent that Maria often questioned Carl about his actions, threatened him, or pleaded with him not to drink. She had reacted to his drinking in a number of negative ways—by separating from him, calling the police, and refusing to have sex with him. At the same time, she had made serious efforts to support him and encourage his abstinence by doing positive things with Carl when he did not drink, doing nice things for him, or talking about positive things they could do together if he did not drink.

Marital Relationship

We assessed the couple's relationship by administering the ACQ (Margolin et al., 1983) and the DAS (Spanier, 1976), and by viewing a videotape of the couple discussing a problem in their relationship. Maria had a number of major concerns about their relationship. In addition to Carl's drinking, she was concerned about his apparent lack of responsibility, citing his unwillingness to work, to care for the children, or to be independent of his mother. In general, Maria felt that Carl could not be relied upon for concrete or emotional support. A second concern that she expressed was their role definitions. She felt that Carl dictated her role to her, and that she allowed him to do so. She often felt angry and resentful as a result. Finally, she cited Carl's mother as a problem, describing her as an "enabler" who rescued Carl from his problems and made no demands upon him. She stated that when she and Carl first dated, they liked to drink, stay out late, ride motorcycles, and have a good time, but she felt that it was now time to "move forward" with their lives and "get somewhere."

Carl had fewer marital concerns. He disliked Maria's "nagging" him or discussing his drinking, stating at one point, "If I had a different wife, I wouldn't have a drinking problem." He also disliked her "persistence" in wanting to discuss topics at length and her "attitude change" when he drank.

A videotape of their interactions revealed several communication problems. Carl and Maria interrupted each other frequently and did not listen to each other's comments. Each made frequent sarcastic and biting comments about the other, usually stating these with a smile and a funny comment. Maria complained about her excessive responsibilities, and Carl criticized her for not fulfilling her responsibilities but refused to acknowledge any responsibilities of his own.

Despite these considerable marital problems, they enjoyed each other's company, shared many activities and pleasures (e.g., fishing, going to parks with the children), and had a very positive sexual relationship. Maria said of their relationship, "We get along great when I don't demand anything."

Behavioral Formulation

Carl's drinking appeared to have developed in a social context, with virtually all his drinking occurring within social groups with similar drinking patterns. The pattern was reinforced by these positive social interactions, both with friends and (early in their relationship) with Maria. He had developed significant tolerance for alcohol, so that he could consume increasingly large amounts, resulting in a pattern of daily drinking with some signs of physical dependence on alcohol. For Carl, alcohol provided a number of positive consequences: He enjoyed the tastes and sensations associated with drinking, the social context of drinking, and the feelings of relaxation that drinking engendered. Although he had accumulated a number of significant negative consequences of drinking, none had affected his internal perceptions of himself or of alcohol. From his perspective, negative consequences were imposed on him by others—the police, job supervisors, and his wife. In addition, Carl had been able to avoid responsibility for his actions in many areas of his life. When he did not work, he was able to live with his mother, who shielded him from the negative consequences of not working by providing shelter and food for him. When

Carl's wife made demands that he experienced as aversive, he avoided or ignored her. To some degree, his problems with alcohol were accentuated by their different developmental stages: Maria was ready to move to a more adult stage of life, with increased responsibilities and long-term goals; Carl, in contrast, wanted to maintain the lifestyle and behavior patterns of his early 20s.

Despite Carl's externalizing attributions for his problems and his tendency to avoid negative consequences and responsibility, his wife and children were important to him, and he did not want to lose them from his life. Therefore, he came to treatment to maintain these desired reinforcers, but not necessarily to make the behavior changes his wife saw as necessary for them to have a successful long-term marriage.

As treatment progressed (see below), Carl engaged in a variety of maneuvers to maintain the relationship but avoid behavior change, and his wife, and at times the therapist, reinforced these behaviors. Maria had a limited repertoire of effective ways to obtain positive reinforcers for herself. She appeared to expect most positive feelings to come from external sources, and nagging and criticizing were the only verbal behaviors she used to try to get what she wanted. She reinforced Carl's drinking by continuing to have contact with him but engaged in aversive negative verbal behavior at the same time. She placed responsibility for her happiness with Carl, stating that she could not work (something she enjoyed a great deal) until he stopped drinking and was more responsible, and that she could not lose weight until he stopped drinking and she was less upset.

As a couple, Carl and Maria lacked the verbal skills to discuss these very major problems. Aversive control, avoidance of responsibility, and lack of empathic communication characterized their interactions.

Preparing the Client for Change

Carl and Maria were seen together for all phases of the evaluation. In the initial evaluation, both spouses were asked to describe their perceptions of Carl's drinking, their relationship, and how each had attempted to cope with Carl's drinking. By seeing the couple together, I communicated my view that the drinking was intimately connected to their relationship, and that each spouse would need to examine his/her own behavior to effect positive changes. At the end of the evaluation, I provided them with feedback about the main difficulties that I perceived (as summarized earlier), and oriented them to the plan for treatment. In discussing the treatment plan, I covered the following:

"We have asked you to come to treatment as a couple. This is because drinking affects many areas of your life, including your marriage and your family. I know from what you have said, Maria, that you have tried many different ways to cope with Carl's drinking, and that you have been angry and frustrated at times. It is clear that you have tried to help, but it seems, Carl, that you mostly have resented it when Maria has said anything about your drinking. During treatment we will look at your drinking, how you have tried to cope with it, and how the two of you are getting along as a couple. Right now the two of you are separated, and you have a lot of concerns about your relationship. As we go along in the therapy, I will help you improve your communication, and I will ask you to try new ways to spend time together and discuss problems. The therapy will focus on three main topics—your drinking, Carl, how you, Maria, have coped with it, and how to cope in ways that work better for both of you, and for your relationship with each other."

In addition to this overall orientation, which both Carl and Maria felt captured their goals for the treatment, we discussed Carl's drinking goals in more detail and made plans for how to achieve those goals. As indicated earlier, Carl's preferred drinking goal was moderate drinking. However, Maria felt strongly that she wanted him to abstain, and he had agreed to that goal prior to coming to treatment. Since he had been drinking daily and showed evidence of tolerance to alcohol, I was concerned that he would not be able to stop drinking without assistance. I therefore discussed with him the possibility of being detoxified under medical supervision:

"I am concerned, Carl, that it will be difficult for you to stop drinking on your own. You drink every day and have been drinking a lot. On the questionnaires, you indicated that you 'panic' if you think that you will not be able to get any alcohol, and you typically drink throughout the day. All of these things suggest to me that you may be 'hooked' on alcohol, and that your body will have a strong reaction to going without any alcohol at all. The easiest way to get through the first few days without drinking is to check into

a hospital detoxification program, and I would like you to consider it."

Carl had a very negative reaction to the thought of being hospitalized. He was afraid of being "locked up," and said, "I know that I would go crazy. I can't stand being confined. After 24 hours I would just have to leave. It's not a good idea." I was most interested in engaging Carl in treatment, so I thought it inappropriate to try to force Carl to enter a detoxification center. I was certain that if I made brief hospitalization a prerequisite to further treatment, he would leave treatment completely. Therefore, we developed a plan to achieve abstinence. The plan had two major components: (1) Carl was to come to therapy sessions sober, and his BAL would be verified by breath alcohol test reading; and (2) Carl would set goals to reduce his drinking gradually, with a target date for abstinence 6 weeks hence. If he was not able to achieve either goal, then we would reevaluate the need for supervised detoxification. He was amenable to this agreement, as was Maria.

Process of Treatment

The course of treatment is described sequentially to provide the reader with the clearest picture of the progress and pitfalls of a fairly typical therapy case. The treatment covered several major areas: (1) helping Carl to reduce, then stop his drinking; (2) teaching Carl skills to maintain abstinence; (3) enhancing Carl's perception of his drinking as problematic; (4) teaching Maria more constructive coping strategies; (5) teaching the couple how to engage in positive interactions; and (6) teaching the couple mutual problem-solving techniques. In addition, as treatment progressed, we focused on some other areas of individual behavioral change for Maria.

Intake and Sessions 1–2

At the initial intake session, Carl had a BAL of greater than 400 mg%. Although he did not show gross signs of intoxication, he was belligerent, and the clinician doing the intake did not feel that he could conduct a reasonable intake interview. He suggested that Carl receive medical attention because his BAL was so high, but Carl refused, and the clinician rescheduled the intake. At the rescheduled appointment, Carl was sober and able to provide information, to give informed consent for the research aspects of the program, and to schedule the baseline data collection session.

At the first treatment session, however, Carl again had an elevated BAL (120 mg%). He acknowledged only having had "a couple of beers" and insisted that he was fine. We briefly discussed Carl's and Maria's concerns and goals, but I suggested that we would not be able to have a very productive session with Carl's BAL so high. (My general policy is to reschedule a treatment session if the client's BAL is greater than 50 mg%.) Carl agreed to come to the next session sober and to have no more than four drinks per day. I gave Carl and Maria self-recording cards, on which I asked them to record drinks, drinking urges, and marital satisfaction on a daily basis. Carl was given one card for each day and was asked to record each drink he actually consumed, to note urges to drink not followed by drinking, and to note on the back of the card the situations in which he drank or had urges to drink (see Figure 13.3).

Maria received one card to use for the entire week. I asked her to write on the card a daily estimate of Carl's drinking (*None, Light, Moderate,* or *Heavy*) and also to record her estimate of the strength of his urges to drink that day. She also made a daily rating of her marital satisfaction (see Figure 13.4).

When Carl and Maria came to the second session, his BAL was again elevated, at 60 mg%. He reported drinking about four beers during the day. We continued the discussion of detoxification, and Carl said that he felt he was addicted to alcohol. He said that he would consider detoxification, and we scheduled a phone conversation to discuss detoxification further. After we spoke twice by phone, Carl again decided that he did not want to be hospitalized. He did not use the self-recording cards during these first 2 weeks, although Maria completed his cards for him while they drove to the treatment session. I did not feel that I had a clear picture of Carl's drinking, but it was clear that he was continuing to drink daily.

Sessions 3–5

Carl came to the third session with a BAL of 0 mg%. He again reiterated his desire to stop drinking without hospitalization, and we worked out a plan for him to reduce his number of drinks gradually to zero over a 6-week time period. In addition to setting drinking goals, we began to discuss a behavioral-analytic view of drinking. To introduce the couple to a behavioral way of thinking about their drinking, I said:

> "Together we are going to observe carefully and analyze all the factors that seem to be part of your drinking. I think that we can look at your drinking and figure out what kinds of situations lead you to feel like drinking. If we can figure this out, then we can work together to come up with *alternatives* for these situations. We will be using these sheets, called 'triggers' sheets, to analyze your drinking. Let's go through one of these together."

I then asked Carl to identify a recent drinking situation. He indicated that he liked to drink when he went fishing. As we spoke, I completed the boxes on the "triggers" sheet, illustrated in Figure 13.7. Carl had a fairly nonpsychological view of his drinking. He described his thoughts as "I want to get some beer" and his feelings as "happy." He viewed drinking when fishing as having positive consequences—"I have a blast." He felt that the only negative consequences came from Maria, who would be angry when he came home.

Carl and Maria grasped the behavioral analysis quickly and found it a comfortable way to conceptualize his drinking. As homework, I then asked both of them to complete the DPQ and bring it to the next treatment session. I gave them additional self-recording cards to use for the week.

Carl also came to the fourth session sober but reported heavy drinking over the weekend. The graph of his weekly alcohol consumption during treatment is reproduced in Figure 13.8. Carl's and Maria's average weekly marital satisfaction ratings are reproduced in Figure 13.9. Carl expressed no concern about his continued heavy drinking, and showed no evidence that he was trying to cut down.

> "I am glad that you have come to the last two sessions sober—I know that's not easy for you, and it does show that you want treatment to succeed. However, I am concerned that you have not cut down at all between sessions. If anything, your drinking seems a bit heavier. It's not clear to me whether you don't really want to cut down, or whether you just don't know how."

Carl said that it was hard to cut down, but that he was committed to stop drinking because he wanted to have

FIGURE 13.7. "Triggers" sheet.

FIGURE 13.8. Carl's weekly alcohol consumption. Areas marked "a" represent missing self-recording data.

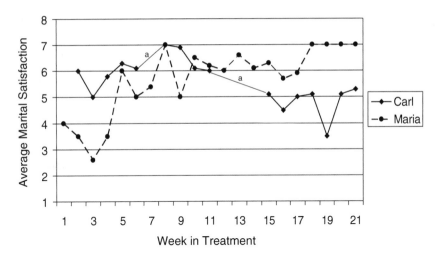

FIGURE 13.9. Carl and Maria's weekly marital satisfaction. Areas marked "a" represent missing self-recording data.

Maria and the boys back again. We then discussed a number of potential strategies to help him avoid drinking, such as sleeping (his suggestion) or having alternative beverages available in the house (my suggestion), or going back to work (Maria's suggestion). He was reluctant to commit to any plans, and Maria challenged whether he was really willing to stop drinking.

To respond to Carl's ambivalence, I suggested that we examine consequences of his drinking other than Maria's disapproval and the couple's arguments about his drinking. Carl was unable to think of any other adverse consequences. I asked him about his legal problems from the DWIs and the arrest for breaking and entering, but Carl said that he did not believe alcohol had anything to do with the latter charge, and that DWI laws were "ridiculous." He also indicated that he was still driving, even though he did not have a driver's license, and that he would continue to drive even if his license was revoked for 10 years (a real possibility, given that he had had three DWIs in less than 10 years, with two in the same month). Carl expressed a similar lack of concern about any other aspects of his drinking but again said that he was willing to stop because of his commitment to the marriage and his children. I made a list of the negative consequences that he or Maria had reported at various times and asked him to review the list at least twice daily, and to think about which of these consequences were of concern to him.

Carl reported looking at the list "once or twice" between sessions, but he was relatively indifferent to the content.

Despite my concern about Carl's relative lack of motivation to change, I decided to proceed with a behavioral analysis of his drinking. I thought that if we could identify a discrete set of antecedents to drinking, and if Carl could successfully avoid drinking in some of these situations some of the time, his motivation to change might increase as his self-efficacy increased. We discussed two other drinking situations in the session and, as homework, I had him complete two behavioral chains at home. A complete summary of the behavioral analysis of his drinking is provided in Figure 13.10.

Carl came to the next treatment session with a BAL of 118 mg% and reported drinking heavily for the last several days prior to the treatment session. After a lengthy discussion, he agreed to go for detoxification. Carl said he was afraid of the hospitalization and concerned that he would not be able to be abstinent after detoxification. I tried to emphasize that the detoxification was only the first step in treatment, and that we would be working together to help him learn ways of coping without drinking.

He also expressed his belief that life would not be fun if he did not drink. Maria oscillated between encouraging Carl to get detoxified and saying to me that he was only agreeing to the detoxification to get out

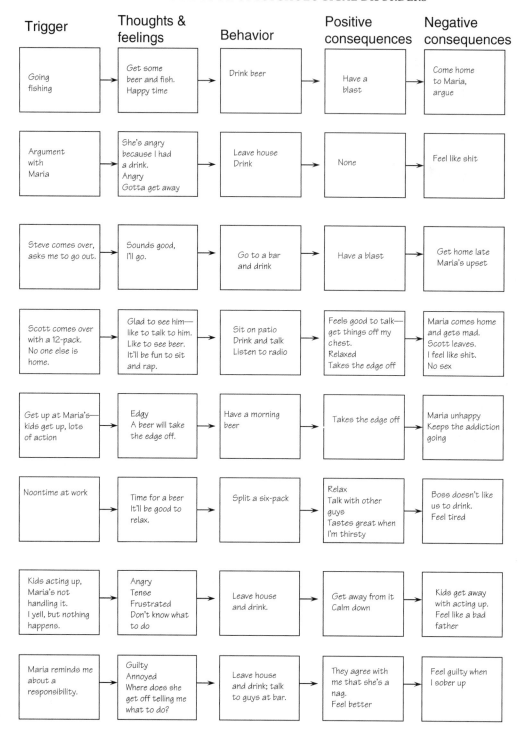

FIGURE 13.10. Sample behavioral analysis of Carl's drinking.

of my office. Because he was so concerned, I had him call the detoxification center from my office to ask any questions he had. He did so, and scheduled himself for admission the next day.

Sessions 6–8

Carl did not admit himself for detoxification and stated again that he could not face being "locked up." He was still drinking daily, making minimal efforts to decrease his drinking. I suggested outpatient detoxification and gave him the phone number of a physician colleague who supervised outpatient detoxification, but I had little expectation that he would follow through with that referral either. Carl continued to express willingness to be in treatment and to change his drinking, and I decided to continue despite my doubts about whether he had sufficient incentives to change. We completed the behavioral analysis of his drinking during the sixth session and identified several of Maria's actions that were antecedents to his drinking, including reminding him about responsibilities, her slow pace when they had an appointment and there was a lot to do to get themselves and their children ready to go out, and her comments about his drinking.

At one point during Session 6, Carl said, "You know, Maria has a real temper. You should ask her what she did to me at the beach." Maria responded immediately by saying, "Show Barbara your arms." Carl rolled up his sleeves, revealing a number of scratches and bruises covering his lower forearms. Maria then explained that she had been intensely frustrated with Carl because of his drinking, and often grabbed him, scratched him, or tried to hit him in the chest or abdomen when she was angry. The behavior had started in the last 4 months, and she found it very upsetting. She also indicated her concern that she might become abusive toward her children and admitted that she sometimes used physical punishment when she was angry at them. Although Maria's anger and frustration were not surprising and are common reactions of partners of people with alcoholism, the physical aggression, particularly in the absence of any physical abuse from Carl, was less usual. We discussed her behavior toward the children in great detail because I was concerned about whether there was any evidence of child abuse. She reported, and Carl confirmed, that she had never bruised, cut, or injured the children in any way, and that they had never had to take either of the children to a physician or emergency room because of her discipline. Both re-

ported the belief that physical punishment, in the form of "swats on the bum" or physically removing the child from a dangerous situation, was an appropriate form of discipline. However, Maria felt that she did not always discipline the children rationally, and that she would occasionally hit them on the arm, or pull too hard when removing them from a situation. From the couple's reports, I did not believe that Maria was abusing the children, but I thought it was important to address her concerns in the therapy. I instructed Maria to use the self-recording cards to write down any times in the next 2 weeks when she felt that she was reacting too strongly to the children or when she was physically aggressive toward Carl.

Over the next two sessions, Carl began to decrease his drinking substantially and was abstinent for each treatment session. Carl and Maria had begun to spend more time together, and they reported that their time together was more positive. They had a family barbecue and went fishing at the beach with the children.

Maria had been faithful in recording her reactions to her children, noting two times each week when she either slapped one of the children on the arm or felt that she grabbed him too hard. We discussed the antecedents to these incidents and identified several salient aspects: Maria was tired, the child was tired, and she attempted to tell him to do something when she could not enforce it (she was across the room or had her hands full). In each situation, she repeated her verbal instructions to the boy several times to no avail, then felt angry and stomped across the room and grabbed him. We discussed alternative strategies, and I emphasized the importance of being able to follow through on a verbal instruction immediately rather than allowing herself to get frustrated. She quickly picked up on my suggestions and also expressed relief at being able to discuss her concerns. After the 2-week period, Maria reported no further instances of excessive physical reaction to the boys, and reported feeling more in control of herself as a parent again. Carl's observations confirmed her reports.

At the same time that we discussed Maria's problems with disciplining the children, we began to implement some self-management planning techniques for Carl. I suggested to Carl that it would be easier not to drink if he had ideas about how to handle certain triggers without alcohol. He could avoid situations or rearrange them to minimize the importance of alcohol in the situation. We used a self-management planning sheet to assist in the process (see Figure 13.11).

Trigger	Plan	Pluses	Minuses	How Hard
1.				
2.				

FIGURE 13.11. Sample self-management planning sheet.

We selected fishing as a topic for self-management planning because it was a high frequency, high-drinking activity for him. Carl had a number of ideas about how to fish without alcohol. These included taking his older son, taking his wife, or inviting an older friend who was an excellent fisherman and did not drink at all. In addition, Carl thought that if he bought soft drinks the night before he went fishing and filled his cooler with the sodas before he left the house, he would be less tempted to stop by the liquor store at the end of his block. For homework, I asked Carl to implement this plan, and to develop another self-management plan for getting together with a friend without drinking.

Carl implemented the fishing plan successfully and also planned to ask his friend Scott to play tennis, then go to a fast-food restaurant to eat because alcohol would not be available there. Although Carl saw no obstacles to implementing this plan, he never used it, and could provide no reasons for not following it up. He did, however, tell Scott that he was trying not to drink, and his friend reacted positively and supportively.

The other major topic of these several sessions was reinforcement for changes in Carl's drinking. Because Carl was so ambivalent about changing his drinking, I thought it particularly important that he experience some positive consequences for decreased drinking and for abstinence. I also wanted to give Maria some positive rather than coercive ways to interact with Carl about his drinking. In introducing this topic, I suggested that they both should think about ways to make abstinence and reduced drinking more positive. I first suggested that Maria might give Carl positive feedback when he was not drinking, but he reacted quite nega-

tively to this suggestion, saying, "I would just think it was another one of her sneaky ways to try to pressure me to stop. I don't want her to say anything." In continuing with this discussion, I asked whether there was anything that Maria could *do* that would make abstinence worthwhile to him, and Carl suggested that she could refrain from talking about alcohol and spend time with him without being "picky." They decided on several mutually enjoyable activities to share when he was not drinking, such as sharing a shrimp dinner, and on having Maria tell Carl when she was enjoying their time together. They were able to implement these plans successfully, and although Carl drank while they were together, the amount was substantially less on these occasions.

Sessions 9–11

By this point in the treatment, Carl had reduced his drinking to approximately three to six drinks per day, but he had not abstained from drinking at all. His reports of urges to drink had also begun to decrease. Maria reported high marital satisfaction almost every day (a rating of 7 on a 1- to 7-point scale), and they were spending most of their free time either at her apartment or at the home of Carl's mother. However, in the therapy sessions they began to argue more frequently, with their conflict revolving around two major topics—Maria's desire to move to North Carolina and her feeling that Carl was not emotionally supportive of her. I began to implement some structured communication training with them, teaching them skills that included allowing the other to finish before speaking, reflective listening, and making specific positive requests. These sessions were supplemented with handouts about communication. After reading the first handout, which covered basic topics, such as the value of being polite and respectful of one's spouse, and some of the sources of bad communication, they came into the session absolutely surprised at the notion that calling each other names (e.g., "idiot," "asshole," or "shithead") could have any negative impact on their relationship. They had begun to use positive rather than negative communication at home and were pleased with the impact it had on their conversations.

Although we were making progress in the treatment, I was concerned that Carl was still drinking every day, and I relayed this concern to him. Carl stated that he believed he could now stop, and he agreed to be abstinent for 2 days in the following week. The first week that he agreed to this contract, Carl did not want to discuss strategies for abstinence, and he was unsuccessful. The second week we discussed very specific plans for how he would abstain. He planned to be with Maria and the children for part of each day, and he decided not to buy more beer to have in his mother's house those days. In addition, he would stock up on soft drinks and plan to go to bed early. I also suggested that he might use Maria as a support in his attempts to abstain. I often encourage a client to find someone with whom to discuss urges, and the partner can be a good source of support. He again was resistant to involving Maria, saying, "I wouldn't tell her that I wanted to drink—all I'd get is a lecture." I suggested that he usually disliked her comments because they were unsolicited, but in this situation, he would be in charge because he would be the person concerned about his drinking. He responded positively to this reframing. I then asked him whether there was anything Maria could say that would be helpful to him, and he suggested that she tell him it was his choice. Maria indicated that it would be difficult not to lecture, but she agreed to a role play. They imagined that they were driving to the beach, and Carl said, "I want to stop to pick up a six-pack on the way down." Maria answered, "It's your choice if you want to, but we could stop to get some sodas instead, if you want." Carl was amazed at how much he liked her response, and although Maria acknowledged that it was very difficult to be that neutral, she liked feeling that it was not her responsibility to prevent him from drinking. They agreed to try out such a discussion once during the coming week.

Carl was not successful in maintaining any abstinent days, although he did implement most of the rest of the plans and drank only one beer on each of the 2 target days. However, he did not tell Maria about any of his urges to drink. He again expressed little concern about not meeting his goals. During the session, Carl and Maria announced that they were going to North Carolina for a 2-week trip. Carl knew a contractor who had offered him work there, and Maria was intrigued with the possibility of moving to an area with a lower cost of living and more rural environment in which to raise the children. She stated that she would not move while Carl was still drinking, but they both decided that a trip to explore the possibilities was appealing.

Sessions 12–15

Carl and Maria returned from their 2-week trip very enthusiastic about North Carolina. They believed that work was available, the cost of living was clearly lower, and both of them liked the area they had visited. Maria said again that she would not move unless Carl had been abstinent for a considerable length of time because she did not want to leave her family if she could not depend on Carl. He again said that he would stop drinking. I had taken advantage of the break in the therapy to review all of my progress notes and to think about the couple with a bit more detachment. It was clear to me that although Carl had agreed to abstinence because of Maria's pressure, he wanted instead to reduce his drinking. However, he had dealt with this conflict by providing verbal reassurances that his behavior would change, without accompanying behavior changes. He had implemented only a few of the behavioral plans that we had developed, and I did not think that the lack of implementation reflected a skills deficit. I had decided to point out Carl's behavioral inconsistencies at this treatment session.

To initiate this discussion, I told Carl and Maria that I wanted to discuss their progress so far. I emphasized the positive changes that they had made so far: Carl had decreased his drinking substantially; he had developed some skills to assist him in drinking less; their communication had begun to improve; they were spending time together that was mutually enjoyable; and they had begun to consider possible long-term plans together. I noted, however, that Carl had made a series of promises about his drinking on which he had not followed through. I read them several passages from my progress notes, noting Carl's initial target date for abstinence, and his broken agreements about detoxification and abstinent days. I suggested two alternative explanations to them: Either Carl did not want to stop drinking completely but felt that he had to agree to abstinence to keep Maria happy or he really could not stop drinking and needed further assistance to do so. By framing my explanations this way, I tried to avoid labeling Carl as dishonest or unmotivated to change. I also suggested that Maria had helped Carl to keep drinking by reporting high marital satisfaction even though he was still drinking, and that perhaps reduced drinking really was acceptable to her as well. Both reacted quite strongly to my feedback. Carl said, "At first I didn't want to stop, but now it doesn't seem that bad. I'm not drinking enough now for it to mean anything, so I'll just quit. It's no big deal, and I don't want to disappoint you." Maria said, "I always feel like Carl is just saying whatever he has to say to get me or you off his back. But I have been so much happier since he cut down that I kind of lost sight of that fact that he's still drinking. I am afraid to move anywhere with him while he's still drinking at all. It was so bad before, I don't want to go back to that."

After this conversation, Carl denied that he preferred moderate drinking and announced that he was going to "quit for good." Over the next 2 weeks, Carl had one drinking day each week—one beer the first week and two beers the second week. Although we discussed a variety of behavioral coping strategies, such as developing behavioral alternatives for drinking situations, rehearsing strategies for refusing drinks, and using various strategies for coping with urges, Carl deemphasized their importance. Instead, he focused on cognitive coping strategies: When he had urges to drink, he would think about reasons not to drink ("It's not worth it—Maria and the kids are more important"). Or he would use delay tactics ("I won't have anything right now—if I still feel like drinking at 5:00 [or some other, later time during the day], then I'll have a beer"). Or he would deemphasize the positive aspects of alcohol ("One or two beers won't do anything for me, and I don't want to get blasted").

Carl and Maria also began to discuss their long-term goals. I asked them to write down how they would like their lives to be in 5 years. Carl wrote down the following[3]:

> Comfortable place to live for Maria and this kids. Good schools, backyard. Get finances in order; save money, consolidate bills, improve credit. Maintain stable income ie. steady construction work or other. Obtain a loving relationship with Maria. Self improvement: manage money better, listen to Maria more objectivly,

secure steadier employment. Maria: better self discipline, controll temper, improve self confidence, weight loss, less pestimistic in dialy matters. ie. scared of bugs, traffic, mishaps, etc.

Maria wrote down remarkably similar 5-year goals:

> Five years from now—37 years old; Jonathan 8 years, Marc 7 years. We are living in North Carolina in a rented house. I'm working, Carls working the boys are in school. We have two cars. Carl is 5 yrs sober. I'm 4 years thin. We are two yrs away from getting credit back from filing bankruptcy. Some nights we will be together as a family to relax or to go to a baseball or soccer game of Jonathan's or Marc's. Other nights I will be out to socialize or run errands. Other nights Carl will do the same. We will be somewhat financialy comfortable. Three things I want out of life:

Maria:	Carl:
calmness, thinness,	motivation, sobriety,
to feel secure, a car,	responsability,
money, independence,	contentedness
control over my life	

Because Carl and Maria's goals were so similar, I asked them if I could read them aloud. Both were amenable to this suggestion, and I did so. They reacted quite positively and felt encouraged; because their long-term goals were so similar, they could work together to achieve these goals. I began to teach them skills related to assertiveness and problem solving, discussing ways to implement these skills both in their relationship and in other interpersonal situations.

Sessions 16–18

Carl abstained from drinking from Session 15 to the end of the treatment. He reported a few urges to drink, but these soon decreased. However, he discussed very strong reactions to not drinking. He felt sad, saying that he missed drinking and felt that he had lost something important to him. He also said that it was frustrating because he always had been able to drink when he felt bad, but now he could not do so. I tried to reframe his feelings for him, noting that his ability to recognize that he missed alcohol was an important step toward being able to reorganize his life without it, and that his reaction suggested that he was serious about his intentions not to drink. Carl seemed to find the reframing helpful, but he continued to find abstinence uncomfortable.

As Carl remained abstinent, his marital satisfaction ratings decreased. Previously Carl had reported fairly high marital satisfaction, but as he stopped drinking he became increasingly unhappy. When I asked him about his ratings, he said that he felt they were "going nowhere" in terms of reconciling. We had begun assertion and problem-solving training, and I suggested that Carl could use these skills to express his feelings to Maria more directly. They had a positive discussion during the session about his feelings and about wanting to reconcile, and her concerns about how difficult that would be, with each using some of the positive skills on which we had worked. Both agreed that they now wanted to live together again, but it would be difficult to develop a plan to do so. We used structured problem-solving techniques over two treatment sessions to develop a plan. The major impediment to reconciliation was financial. Maria was receiving welfare, but if either she or Carl began to work, they would receive less public assistance. However, to be able to live together, they would have to save sufficient money for a security deposit and first month's rent. They finally decided that Maria would begin to work a few hours a week as a hairdresser, working "under the table," and that Carl would care for the children while she worked. If that worked well, then Carl would begin to look for work again; once both were working, they would move in with his mother for a limited period of time to save money for the deposits and rent, then either obtain an apartment together in New Jersey or find a trailer to rent in North Carolina and move. They also used problem-solving techniques to develop a plan to deal with their other debts.

Termination

Because Carl and Maria were part of a clinical research study, we had to terminate treatment after 18 sessions (including the sessions when he was intoxicated). They had made significant progress during treatment: Carl had been abstinent for more than a month; Maria had learned more effective ways to discipline the children and no longer reported concerns about being overly punitive to them; the couple's relationship was significantly improved; and they had a constructive plan for reconciliation. I was concerned that Carl was still uncomfortable with abstinence, and I thought that he had acquired only a few effective coping strategies to deal with triggers for drinking. We had not worked directly on Carl's style of avoiding responsibility except by fol-

lowing through on his commitment to abstinence and long-term goal setting. Whether Carl would implement his part of these agreements was relatively untested. The couple was fairly comfortable with termination but asked about possible follow-up treatment, inquiring specifically about AA or other support groups that focused on couples or on behavioral approaches to change. I referred them to SMART, and to a couples' AA group. The constraints of the clinical research protocol precluded any longer-term treatment with me, even though I thought continued treatment would be beneficial.

Comment

Carl and Maria were a fairly typical couple. Carl's ambivalence about change, his entry into treatment solely because of an external agent, and his resistance to many behavioral interventions are fairly representative. I believe that he began to engage in treatment when he stopped feeling that he was the sole focus of the treatment, after Maria began to discuss her aggressive behavior and feelings. The second critical point in treatment was addressing his continued drinking. I was willing to allow them to renegotiate for a goal of moderate drinking, but I did not think it therapeutic for Carl to feel that he could verbally agree to abstinence but then avoid the agreement. Addressing Carl's behavior directly forced him either to be assertive and renegotiate treatment goals or to follow through on his commitment.

The role of behavioral skills training in facilitating abstinence was less important with Carl than with some clients. He tried various skills introduced during the treatment but relied primarily on cognitive coping strategies. The role of reinforcement was probably more important in understanding his changed drinking behavior. Carl's marital relationship was important to him at the beginning of treatment, and focusing in the therapy on ways to improve that relationship increased its reinforcement value to him. Maria's consistency in saying that they could reconcile only if he were abstinent, in discussing long-term goals for the relationship, and in seeing the possible positive life they could live in North Carolina all contributed.

Finally, my relationship with the couple probably contributed to the positive changes they made. I found them a likable, appealing couple despite their difficulties. At times, I would tease or cajole Carl into compliance, and he commented at the end of the treatment,

"At first I didn't know if I liked you or not, but then I decided you were kind of cute, and then I realized that you weren't going to let up on me, so I decided that I'd give it a try." I tried to reinforce Maria's ability to take care of herself, and I suspect that she saw me as a female role model in some ways. She often asked me personal questions (whether I was married, how old my son was), and gave me a desk calendar as a thank-you gift at termination. Our research suggests that our more experienced therapists are more successful at keeping clients in treatment (Epstein, McCrady, Miller, & Steinberg, 1994; Raytek, McCrady, Epstein, & Hirsch, 1999), and I suspect that being able to deal with these complex relationships is one skill that our more experienced therapists have acquired more fully.

Typical Problems

The problems presented in this case are fairly typical—coming to treatment sessions intoxicated, continued drinking during treatment, ambivalence about change, noncompliance with assignments, and discovering new and major problems as the therapy progresses. Lying and failing to come to scheduled treatment sessions are other typical obstacles that clients with drinking problems sometimes present. By working with Carl and Maria together, I was able to minimize these particular difficulties because Maria was highly motivated for treatment and very responsible about keeping scheduled appointments. Also, by having them both record Carl's drinking and drinking urges, I had a clearer picture of his drinking and was able to maintain a clear idea of our progress (or lack thereof).

CLINICAL PREDICTORS OF SUCCESS OR FAILURE

A number of factors predict the success or failure of therapy. However, before I address these factors, it is important to discuss definitions of "success." In any treatment, a minority of clients maintain long-term, uninterrupted successful change (abstinence or nonproblem drinking). The proportion varies with the demographic characteristics of the population, and persons who are married, have stable employment, a stable residence, and no comorbid psychopathology have the best treatment outcomes. In addition, a person's posttreatment environment plays an important role (Moos, Finney, & Cronkite, 1990) in determining long-term outcomes.

Observations of the long-term instability of drinking outcomes have led many to consider alcoholism as a chronic, relapsing disorder, and to reconceptualize "success" as a process rather than a static outcome; that is, the client who learns not only effective skills to avoid drinking or heavy drinking but also ways to cope with relapses by minimizing their length and severity should be considered "successful" as well. In treatment outcome studies, investigators look at percentage of abstinent or moderate drinking days and length of periods of abstinence compared to periods of heavy drinking as ways to assess relative rather than absolute "success." From the individual clinician's perspective, certain client characteristics and behaviors bode well for the course of treatment. The client who has important incentives to change (either internal or external) and some recognition of a relationship between his/her drinking and life problems is easier to treat. Complying with early homework assignments, coming to sessions sober, and being honest about behavior outside of the treatment are also positive indicators. However, clinician behavior is another important predictor of success. Various studies have pointed to different aspects of clinician behavior —empathy, specific goal setting and treatment planning, developing drinking goals with the client rather than imposing goals, and providing the client with options for treatment—as all being associated with better compliance with treatment.

CONCLUSION

Providing treatment to persons with drinking problems is a complex and continuously fascinating process. The clinician is faced with decisions about matching each client to the appropriate level of care, the setting for treatment, and treatment modalities and techniques. Diagnostic skills to identify concomitant medical, psychological, psychiatric, and cognitive problems are challenged by these clients. Therapy requires knowledge of a range of treatment techniques, an ability to be able to form a positive therapeutic relationship with sometimes frustrating and difficult clients, and the ability to "think on your feet."

From the briefest, one-session treatments to motivate heavy drinkers to reduce their drinking to the complex and longer treatment provided to individuals with severe alcohol dependence, treatment is never dull or routine. The clinician has a large body of empirical literature to guide the selection of treatments and a significant clinical literature as well to illustrate clinical techniques and problems. And although many persons with drinking problems change successfully on their own or with minimal assistance, treatment also can provide an effective means for persons to change a major life problem.

So this chapter concludes as it began—as a "sales pitch" for clinicians to be knowledgeable about and receptive to providing thoughtful, informed treatment to persons with drinking problems.

NOTES

1. A standard drink is equal to one 12-ounce beer, one 5-ounce glass of wine, or a 1.5-ounce shot of 86-proof liquor.

2. All dialogue in this chapter is paraphrasing of actual therapist or client comments.

3. These verbatim transcripts include the clients' spelling of all words.

REFERENCES

American Psychiatric Association. (2013). *Diagnostic and statistical manual of mental disorders* (5th ed.). Arlington, VA: Author.

American Society of Addiction Medicine (ASAM). (2001). *ASAM patient placement criteria for the treatment of psychoactive substance use disorders* (2nd ed., rev.). Chevy Chase, MD: Author.

Annis, H. M., Graham, J. M., & Davis, C. S. (1987). *Inventory of Drinking Situations (IDS): User's guide.* Toronto: Centre for Addiction and Mental Health.

Chaney, E. F., O'Leary, M. R., & Marlatt, G. A. (1978). Skills training with alcoholics. *Journal of Consulting and Clinical Psychology, 46,* 1092–1104.

Cisler, J. M., Amstadter, A. B., Begle, A. M., Resnick, H. S., Danielson, C. K., Saunders, B. E., et al. (2011). PTSD symptoms, potentially traumatic event exposure, and binge drinking: A prospective study with a national sample of adolescents. *Journal of Anxiety Disorders, 25,* 978–987.

Cohn, A. M., Graff, F. S., Epstein, E. E., McCrady, B. S., Cook, S., Schneider, M., et al. (2010, June). *Alcohol use outcomes following "cold turkey" or graduated reduction among women with an alcohol use disorder enrolled in treatment.* Paper presented at the annual meeting of the Research Society on Alcoholism, San Antonio, TX.

Cox, G. B., Walker, R. D., Freng, S. A., Short, B. A., Meijer, L., & Gilchrist, L. (1998). Outcome of a controlled trial of the effectiveness of intensive case management for chronic public inebriates. *Journal of Studies on Alcohol, 59,* 523–532.

Cunningham, J. A., Sobell, L. C., Sobell, M. B., & Gaskin, J. (1994). Alcohol and drug abusers' reasons for seeking treatment. *Addictive Behaviors, 19,* 691–696.

Donovan, D. (2013). Evidence-based assessment: Strategies and measures in addictive behaviors. In B. S. McCrady & E. E. Epstein (Eds.), *Addictions: A comprehensive guidebook* (2nd ed., pp. 311–352). New York: Oxford University Press.

Epstein, E. E., & McCrady, B. S. (2009). *A cognitive-behavioral treatment program for overcoming alcohol use problems: Therapist guide.* New York: Oxford University Press.

Epstein, E. E., McCrady, B. S., Miller, K. J., & Steinberg, M. L. (1994). Attrition from conjoint alcoholism treatment: Do dropouts differ from completers? *Journal of Substance Abuse, 6,* 249–265.

Filstead, W. (1991). *Two-year treatment outcome: An evaluation of substance abuse services for adults and youths.* Park Ridge, IL: Parkside Medical Services.

Fink, E. B., Longabaugh, R., McCrady, B. S., Stout, R. L., Beattie, M., Ruggieri-Authelet, A., et al. (1985). Effectiveness of alcoholism treatment in partial versus inpatient settings: Twenty-four month outcomes. *Addictive Behaviors, 10,* 235–248.

Finney, J. W., Moos, R. H., & Timko, C. (2013). The course of treated and untreated substance use disorders: Remission and resolution, relapse and mortality. In B. S. McCrady & E. E. Epstein (Eds.), *Addictions: A comprehensive guidebook* (2nd ed., pp. 108–131). New York: Oxford University Press.

Foy, D. W., Miller, P. M., Eisler, R. M., & O'Toole, D. H. (1976). Social skills training to teach alcoholics to refuse drinks effectively. *Journal of Studies on Alcohol, 37,* 1340–1345.

Frankenstein, W., Hay, W. M., & Nathan, P. E. (1985). Effects of intoxication on alcoholics' marital communication and problem solving. *Journal of Studies on Alcohol, 46,* 1–6.

Green, K., Worden, B., Menges, D., & McCrady, B. S., (2008). Assessment of alcohol use disorders. In J. Hunsley & E. Mash (Eds.), *A guide to assessments that work* (pp. 339–369). New York: Oxford University Press.

Haaga, D. A. F., McCrady, B., & Lebow, J. (2006). Integrative principles for treating substance use disorders. *Journal of Clinical Psychology, 62,* 675–684.

Hallgren, K. A., Greenfield, B. L., Ladd, B., Glynn, L. H., & McCrady, B. S. (2012). Evidence-based practices for the treatment of adults with alcohol use disorders. In P. Sturmey & M. Hersen (Eds.), *Handbook of evidence-based practice in clinical psychology: Vol. II. Adult disorders* (pp. 133–166). Hoboken, NJ: Wiley.

Helzer, J. E., Robins, L. N., Taylor, J. R., Carey, K., Miller, R. H., Combs-Orme, T., et al. (1985). The extent of long-term moderate drinking among alcoholics discharged from medical and psychiatric treatment facilities. *New England Journal of Medicine, 312,* 1678–1682.

Hesse, M. (2006). The Readiness Ruler as a measure of readiness to change polydrug use in drug abusers. *Harm Reduction Journal, 3*. Published online at *www.harmreduction-journal.com/content/3/1/3.*

Hester, R. K., Delaney, H. D., Campbell, W., & Handmaker, N. (2009). A web application for moderation training: Initial results of a randomized clinical trial. *Journal of Substance Abuse Treatment, 37*, 266–276.

Institute of Medicine. (1990). *Broadening the base of treatment for alcohol problems.* Washington, DC: National Academy Press.

Kosanke, N., Magura, S., Staines, G., Foote, J., & DeLuca, A. (2002). Feasibility of matching alcohol patients to ASAM levels of care. *American Journal on Addictions, 11*, 124–134.

Leite, de C., Seminotti, J. C., Freitas, N. F., & Drachler, M. P. de L. (2011). The Psychosocial Treatment Expectations Questionnaire (PTEQ) for alcohol problems: Development and early validation. *European Journal of Psychological Assessment, 27*, 228–236.

Liepman, M. R. (1993). Using family influence to motivate alcoholics to enter treatment: The Johnson Institute Intervention approach. In T. J. O'Farrell (Ed.), *Treating alcohol problems: Marital and family interventions* (pp. 54–77). New York: Guilford Press.

Longabaugh, R., McCrady, B., Fink, E., Stout, R., McAuley, T., & McNeill, D. (1983). Cost-effectiveness of alcoholism treatment in inpatient versus partial hospital settings: Six- month outcomes. *Journal of Studies on Alcohol, 44*, 1049–1071.

Longabaugh, R., Wirtz, P. W., Zweben, A., & Stout, R. L. (1998). Network support for drinking, Alcoholics Anonymous and long-term matching effects. *Addiction, 93*, 1313–1333.

Longabaugh, R., Wirtz, P. W., Zywiak, W. H., & O'Malley, S. S. (2010). Network support as a prognostic indicator of drinking outcomes: The COMBINE study. *Journal of Studies on Alcohol and Drugs, 71*, 837–846.

Ludwig, A. M. (1985). Cognitive processes associated with "spontaneous" recovery from alcoholism. *Journal of Studies on Alcohol, 46*, 53–58.

Magura, S., Staines, G., Kosanke, N., Rosenblum, A., Foote, J., DeLuca, A., et al. (2003). Predictive validity of the ASAM Patient Placement Criteria for naturalistically matched vs. mismatched alcoholism patients. *American Journal on Addictions, 12*, 386–397.

Margolin, G., Talovic, S., & Weinstein, C. D. (1983). Areas of Change Questionnaire: A practical approach to marital assessment. *Journal of Consulting and Clinical Psychology, 51*, 921–931.

Marlatt, G. A., & Donovan, D. M. (Eds.). (2005). *Relapse prevention: Second edition: Maintenance strategies in the treatment of addictive behavior.* New York: Guilford Press.

Marlatt, G. A., & Gordon, J. R. (Eds.). (1985). *Relapse prevention: Maintenance strategies in the treatment of addictive behaviors.* New York: Guilford Press.

Mayfield, D., McLeod, G., & Hall, P. (1974). The CAGE questionnaire: Validation of a new alcoholism instrument. *American Journal of Psychiatry, 131*, 1121–1123.

McConnaughy, E. A., Prochaska, J. O., & Velicer, W. F. (1983). Stages of change in psychotherapy: Measurement and sample profiles. *Psychotherapy: Theory, Research, and Practice, 20*, 243–250.

McCrady, B. S. (1992). A reply to Peele: Is this how you treat your friends? *Addictive Behaviors, 17*, 67–72.

McCrady, B. S., & Epstein, E. E. (2009). *Overcoming alcohol problems: A couples-focused program.* New York: Oxford University Press.

McCrady, B. S., Epstein, E. E., Cook, S., Jensen, N. K., & Hildebrandt, T. (2009). A randomized trial of individual and couple behavioral alcohol treatment for women. *Journal of Consulting and Clinical Psychology, 77*, 243–256.

McCrady, B. S., Epstein, E. E., & Hirsch, L. (1999). Maintaining change after conjoint behavioral alcohol treatment for men: Outcomes at six months. *Addiction, 94*, 1381–1396.

McCrady, B. S., Horvath, A. T., & Delaney, S. I. (2003). Self-help groups. In R. K. Hester & W. R. Miller (Eds.), *Handbook of alcoholism treatment approaches: Effective alternatives* (3rd ed., pp. 165–187). Boston: Allyn & Bacon.

McCrady, B. S., Longabaugh, R. L., Fink, E., Stout, R., Beattie, M., Ruggieri-Authelet, A., et al. (1986). Cost effectiveness of alcoholism treatment in partial hospital versus inpatient settings after brief inpatient treatment: Twelve month outcomes. *Journal of Consulting and Clinical Psychology, 54*, 708–713.

McCrady, B. S., Owens, M., & Brovko, J. (2013). Couples and family treatment methods. In B. S. McCrady & E. E. Epstein (Eds.), *Addictions: A comprehensive guidebook* (2nd ed., pp. 454–481). New York: Oxford University Press.

McCrady, B. S., Stout, R., Noel, N., Abrams, D., & Nelson, H. F. (1991). Effectiveness of three types of spouse-involved behavioral alcoholism treatment. *British Journal of Addiction, 86*, 1415–1424.

McCrady, B. S., & Tonigan, J. S. (in press). Recent research into twelve step programs. In: R. Ries, D. Fiellin, S. Miller, & R. Saitz (Eds.), *Principles of addiction medicine* (5th ed.). Baltimore: Lippincott/Williams & Wilkins.

McKay, J. R., Van Horn, D., Oslin, D. W., Ivey, M., Drapkin, M. L., Coviello, D. M., et al. (2011). Extended telephone-based continuing care for alcohol dependence: 24-month outcomes and subgroup analyses. *Addiction, 106*, 1760–1769.

McLellan, A. T., Grissom, G. R., Zanis, D., Randall, M., Brill, P., & O'Brien, C. P. (1997). Problem–service "matching" in addiction treatment: A prospective study in four programs. *Archives of General Psychiatry, 54*, 730–735.

McLellan, A. T., Kushner, H., Metzger, D., Peters, R., Smith, I., Grissom, G., et al. (1992). The fifth edition of the Addiction Severity Index. *Journal of Substance Abuse Treatment, 9,* 199–213.

McLellan, A. T., Lewis, D. C., O'Brien, C. P., & Kleber, H. D. (2000). Drug dependence, a chronic medical illness: Implications for treatment, insurance, and outcomes evaluation. *Journal of the American Medical Association, 284,* 1689–1695.

Menges, D., McCrady, B. S., Epstein, E. E., & Beem, C. (2008). Psychometric evaluation of the Drinking Patterns Questionnaire: A measure of high-risk drinking situations. *Addictive Behaviors, 33,* 1061–1066.

Meyers, R. J., & Smith, J. E. (1995). *Clinical guide to alcohol treatment: The community reinforcement approach.* New York: Guilford Press.

Miller, W. R., Benefield, R., G., & Tonigan, J. S. (1993). Enhancing motivation for change in problem drinking: A controlled comparison of two therapist styles. *Journal of Consulting and Clinical Psychology, 61,* 455–461.

Miller, W. R., Leckman, A. L., Delaney, H. D., & Tinkcom, M. (1992). Long-term follow-up of behavioral self-control training. *Journal of Studies on Alcohol, 53,* 249–261.

Miller, W. R., Meyers, R. J., & Tonigan, J. S. (1999). Engaging the unmotivated in treatment for alcohol problems: A comparison of three strategies for intervention through family members. *Journal of Consulting and Clinical Psychology, 67,* 688–697.

Miller, W. R., & Rollnick, S. (1991). *Motivational interviewing: Preparing people to change addictive behavior.* New York: Guilford Press.

Miller, W. R., & Rollnick, S. (2002). *Motivational interviewing: Preparing people for change* (2nd ed.). New York: Guilford Press.

Miller, W. R., & Tonigan, J. S. (1996). Assessing drinkers' motivations for change: The Stages of Change Readiness and Treatment Eagerness Scale (SOCRATES). *Psychology of Addictive Behaviors, 10,* 81–89.

Miller, W. R., Tonigan, J. S., & Longabaugh, R. (1995). *The Drinker Inventory of Consequences (DrInC): An instrument for assessing adverse consequences of alcohol abuse.* Rockville, MD: National Institute on Alcohol Abuse and Alcoholism.

Miller, W. R., Walters, S. T., & Bennett, M. E. (2001). How effective is alcoholism treatment in the United States? *Journal of Studies on Alcohol, 62,* 211–220.

Moderation Management. (2006). The MM limits. Retrieved September 21, 2006, from *www.moderation.org/readings.shtml#mmlimits.*

Monti, P. M., Abrams, D. B., Binkoff, J. A., Zwick, W. R., Liepman, M. R., Nirenberg, T. D., et al. (1990). Communication skills training, communication skills training with family and cognitive behavioral mood management training for alcoholics. *Journal of Studies on Alcohol, 51,* 263–270.

Monti, P. M., Kadden, R. M., Rohsenow, D. J., Cooney, N. L., & Abrams, D. B. (2002). *Treating alcohol dependence: A coping skills training guide* (2nd ed.). New York: Guilford Press.

Moos, R. H., & Billings, A. (1982). Children of alcoholics during the recovery process: Alcoholic and matched control families. *Addictive Behaviors, 7,* 155–163.

Moos, R. H., Finney, J. W., & Cronkite, R. (1990). *Alcoholism treatment: Context, process, and outcome.* New York: Oxford University Press.

Moos, R. H., Finney, J. W., & Gamble, W. (1982). The process of recovery from alcoholism: II. Comparing spouses of alcoholic patients and matched community controls. *Journal of Studies on Alcohol, 43,* 888–909.

Morgenstern, J., Blanchard, K. A., McCrady, B. S., McVeigh, K. H., Morgan, T. J., & Pandina, R. J. (2006). A randomized field trial examining the effectiveness of intensive case management for substance dependent women receiving temporary assistance for needy families (TANF). *American Journal of Public Health, 96,* 2016–2023.

Moyers, T. B., Martin, T., Houck, J. M., Christopher, P. J., & Tonigan, J. S. (2009). From in-session behaviors to drinking outcomes: A causal chain for motivational interviewing. *Journal of Consulting and Clinical Psychology, 77,* 1113–1124.

Nathan, P. E., & McCrady, B. S. (1987). Bases for the use of abstinence as a goal in the behavioral treatment of alcohol abusers. *Drugs and Society, 1,* 109–132.

O'Farrell, T. J., Choquette, K. A., & Cutter, H. S. G. (1998). Couples relapse prevention sessions after behavioral marital therapy for male alcoholics: Outcomes during the three years after starting treatment. *Journal of Studies on Alcohol, 59,* 357–370.

Ojehegan, A., & Berglund, M. (1989). Changes in drinking goals in a two-year outpatient alcoholic treatment program. *Addictive Behaviors, 14,* 1–10.

Orford, J., & Keddie, A. (1986). Abstinence or controlled drinking in clinical practice: A test of the dependence and persuasion hypotheses. *British Journal of Addiction, 81,* 495–504.

Orford, J., Templeton, L., Velleman, R., & Copello, A. (2005). Family members of relatives with alcohol, drug and gambling problems: A set of standardized questionnaires for assessing stress, coping and strain. *Addiction, 100,* 1611–1624.

Oscar-Berman, M., & Marinković, K. (2007). Alcohol: Effects on neurobehavioral functions and the brain. *Neuropsychology Review, 17,* 239–257.

O'Toole, T. P., Freyder, P. J., Gibbon, J. L., Hanusa, B. J., Seltzer, D., & Fine, M. J. (2004). ASAM Patient Placement Criteria treatment levels: Do they correspond to care actually received by homeless substance abusing adults? *Journal of Addictive Diseases, 23,* 1–15.

Pabst, A., Baumeister, S. E., & Krause, L. (2010). Alcohol-expectancy dimensions and alcohol consumption at different ages in the general population. *Journal of Studies on Alcohol and Drugs, 71,* 46–53.

Paolino, T. J., Jr., McCrady, B. S., & Diamond, S. (1978). Some alcoholic marriage statistics: An overview. *International Journal of the Addictions, 13*, 1252–1257.

Prochaska, J. O., & DiClemente, C. C. (2005). The transtheoretical approach. In J. C. Norcross & M. R. Goldfried (Eds.), *Handbook of psychotherapy integration* (2nd ed., pp. 147–171). New York: Oxford University Press.

Project MATCH Research Group. (1997a). Matching alcoholism treatments to client heterogeneity: Project MATCH posttreatment drinking outcomes. *Journal of Studies on Alcohol, 58*, 7–29.

Project MATCH Research Group. (1997b). Project MATCH secondary a priori hypotheses. *Addiction, 92*, 1671–1698.

Project MATCH Research Group. (1998). Matching alcoholism treatments to client heterogeneity: Project MATCH three-year drinking outcomes. *Alcoholism: Clinical and Experimental Research, 22*, 1300–1311.

Raytek, H. S., McCrady, B. S., Epstein, E. E., & Hirsch, L. S. (1999). Therapeutic alliance and the retention of couples in conjoint alcoholism treatment. *Addictive Behaviors, 24*, 317–330.

Robins, L. N., Wing, J., Wittchen, H. U., Helzer, J. E., Babor, T. F., Burke, J., et al. (1988). The prevalence of psychiatric disorders in patients with alcohol and other drug problems. *Archives of General Psychiatry, 45*, 1023–1031.

Rollnick, S., Heather, N., Gold, R., & Hall, W. (1992). Development of a short "Readiness to Change" Questionnaire for use in brief opportunistic interventions. *British Journal of Addictions, 87*, 743–754.

Roman, P. (2013). Treatment for substance use disorders in the United States: An organizational technology perspective. In B. S. McCrady & E. E. Epstein (Eds.), *Addictions: A comprehensive guidebook* (2nd ed., pp. 597–621). New York: Oxford University Press.

Rose, S. J., Zweben, A., Ockert, D., & Baier, A. (2013). Interfaces of substance abuse treatment with other health and social systems. In B. S. McCrady & E. E. Epstein (Eds.), *Addictions: A comprehensive guidebook* (2nd ed., pp. 641–655). New York: Oxford University Press.

Rosenberg, H. (1993). Prediction of controlled drinking by alcoholics and problem drinkers. *Psychological Bulletin, 113*, 129–139.

Rosenthal, R. N. (2013). Treatment of persons with dual diagnoses of substance use disorder and other psychological problems. In B. S. McCrady & E. E. Epstein (Eds.), *Addictions: A comprehensive guidebook* (2nd ed., pp. 659–707). New York: Oxford University Press.

Rychtarik, R. G., Connors, G. J., Whitney, R. B., McGillicuddy, N. B., Fitterling, J. M., & Wirtz, P. W. (2000). Treatment settings for persons with alcoholism: Evidence for matching clients to inpatient versus outpatient care. *Journal of Consulting and Clinical Psychology, 68*, 277–289.

Rynes, K. N., McCrady, B. S., Morgan, T., Violette, N., &

Pandina, R. (2012). *Need-service matching predicts drug use outcomes in comprehensive treatment for mothers in the child welfare system.* Unpublished manuscript.

Saunders, J. B., Aasland, O. G., Babor, T. F., de la Fuente, J. R., & Grant, M. (1993). Development of the Alcohol Use Disorders Screening Test (AUDIT): WHO collaborative project on early detection of persons with harmful alcohol consumption—II. *Addiction, 88*, 791–804.

Sisson, R. W., & Azrin, N. (1986). Family-member involvement to initiate and promote treatment of problem drinkers. *Journal of Behavior Therapy and Experimental Psychiatry, 17*, 15–21.

Skinner, H., & Allen, B. A. (1982). Alcohol dependence syndrome: Measurement and validation. *Journal of Abnormal Psychology, 91*, 199–209.

Slaymaker, V., & Sheehan, T. (2013). The disease model. In B. S. McCrady & E. E. Epstein (Eds.), *Addictions: A comprehensive guidebook* (2nd ed., pp. 451–481). New York: Oxford University Press.

Smith, J. E., & Meyers, R. J. (2004). *Motivating substance abusers to enter treatment: Working with family members.* New York: Guilford Press.

Smith, P. H., Homish, G. G., Leonard, K. E., & Cornelius, J. R. (2012). Intimate partner violence and specific substance use disorders: Findings from the National Epidemiologic Survey on Alcohol and Related Conditions. *Psychology of Addictive Behaviors, 26*, 236–245.

Sobell, L. C., & Sobell, M. B. (2003). Alcohol consumption measures. In J. P. Allen & V. B. Wilson (Eds.), *Assessing alcohol problems: A guide for clinicians and researchers, second edition* (pp. 75–99), Bethesda, MD: National Institute on Alcohol Abuse and Alcoholism.

Sobell, L. C., & Sobell, M. B. (1995). *Alcohol Timeline Followback users' manual.* Toronto: Addiction Research Foundation.

Sobell, L. C., & Sobell, M. B. (2011). *Group therapy for substance use disorders: A motivational cognitive-behavioral approach.* New York: Guilford Press.

Sobell, M. B., & Sobell, L. C. (2000). Stepped care as a heuristic approach to the treatment of alcohol problems. *Journal of Consulting and Clinical Psychology, 68*, 573–579.

Spanier, G. (1976). Measuring dyadic adjustment: New scales for assessing the quality of marriage and similar dyads. *Journal of Marriage and the Family, 38*, 15–28.

Spear, S. F., & Mason, M. (1991). Impact of chemical dependency on family health status. *International Journal of the Addictions, 26*, 179–187.

Spitzer, R. L., Williams, J. B. W., Gibbon, M., & First, M. B. (1996). *Structured Clinical Interview for DSM-IV: Patient Edition (with Psychotic Screen—Version 1.0).* Washington, DC: American Psychiatric Press.

Stinchfield, R., & Owen, P. (1998). Hazelden's model of treatment and its outcome. *Addictive Behaviors, 23*, 669–683.

Straus, M., Hamby, S. L., Boney-McCoy, S., & Sugarman,

D. B. (1996). The Revised Conflict Tactics Scales (CTS2): Development and preliminary psychometric data. *Journal of Family Issues, 17*, 283–316.

Sullivan, J. T., Sykora, K., Schneiderman, J., Naranjo, C. A., & Sellers, E. M. (1989). Assessment of alcohol withdrawal: The revised Clinical Institute Withdrawal Assessment for Alcohol scale (CIWA-Ar). *British Journal of Addiction, 84*, 1353–1357.

Thomas, E. J., Santa, C., Bronson, D., & Oyserman, D. (1987}. Unilateral family therapy with the spouses of alcoholics. *Journal of Social Service Research, 10*, 145–162.

Thomas, E. J., Yoshioka, M., & Ager, R. D. (1996). Spouse enabling of alcohol abuse: Conception, assessment, and modification. *Journal of Substance Abuse, 8*, 61–80.

Tonigan, J. S., Miller, W. R., & Brown, J. M. (1997). The reliability of FORM 90: An instrument for assessing alcohol treatment outcome. *Journal of Studies on Alcohol, 58*, 358–364.

Vaillant, G. (1983). *The natural history of alcoholism*. Cambridge, MA: Harvard University Press.

Vaillant, G., & Milofsky, E. S. (1982). Natural history of male alcoholism: 4. Paths to recovery. *Archives of General Psychiatry, 39*, 127–133.

Walitzer, K. S., & Connors, G. J. (2007). Thirty-month follow-up of drinking moderation training for women: A randomized clinical trial. *Journal of Consulting and Clinical Psychology, 75*, 501–507.

Witkiewitz, K., Donovan, D. M., & Hartzler, B. (2012). Drink refusal training as part of a combined behavioral intervention: Effectiveness and mechanisms of change. *Journal of Consulting and Clinical Psychology, 80*, 440–449.

Witkiewitz, K., & Marlatt, G. A. (2004). Relapse prevention for alcohol and drug problems: That was zen, this is tao. *American Psychologist, 59*, 224–235.

Woodward, J. J. (2013). Alcohol. In B. S. McCrady & E. E. Epstein (Eds.), *Addictions: A comprehensive guidebook* (2nd ed., pp. 135–154). New York: Oxford University Press.

Zimmerman, A., Lubman, D. I., & Cox, M. (2012). Tobacco, caffeine, alcohol and illicit substance use among consumers of a national community managed mental health service. *Mental Health and Substance Use, 5*, 287–302.

CHAPTER 14

Drug Use Disorders

STEPHEN T. HIGGINS
STACEY C. SIGMON
SARAH H. HEIL

In this chapter we follow the case of "Bill," a 24-year-old individual with cocaine use disorder, who would ordinarily be considered to be among the most difficult types of patients for someone administering psychological interventions. As is typical with this population, Bill presented with not only cocaine but also alcohol use disorder; problems with anger management; heavy use of cigarettes and marijuana; suicidal ideation; and major interpersonal, social, and occupational problems (including a prohibition from visiting his 5-year-old daughter). The fact that Stephen T. Higgins and his team of close associates have been able to create a treatment protocol for individuals such as Bill—a protocol with strong empirical support—is in itself a remarkable achievement. But only those most familiar with this approach have a good idea of the multifaceted nature of this brief semistructured strategy, which includes attention to the full range of addictive behaviors, as well as mood disturbances, interpersonal relationships, and problems in living. Without this comprehensive approach, there seems to be no question that these treatment strategies would not enjoy the success that they do. Even clinicians or students not working directly with addictive behaviors will benefit from being familiar with this new generation of successful psychological approaches to drug use.—D. H. B.

Drug use disorders represent a highly prevalent and costly public health problem in the United States and virtually all other industrialized countries. To get a sense of the scope of the U.S. problem, an estimated 131.2 million persons 12 years and older (51.4%) report current alcohol use (past 30 days), 69.6 million (27.2%) report current tobacco use, and 22.7 million (8.9%) report current use of illicit drugs (United States Department of Health and Human Services [USDHHS], 2012). Of course, not all current users experience adverse effects, but a sizable proportion incur substantial problems. An estimated 22.2 million (8.7%) Americans 12 years and older meet formal *Diagnostic and Statistical Manual of Mental Disorders*, fourth edition, text revision (DSM-IV-TR; American Psychiatric Association, 2000) diagnostic criteria for drug abuse or dependence within the past year, and 1.5 million (0.6%) report being treated for a drug use problem within the past year (USDHHS, 2012). The annual costs to the U.S. economy associated with these problems are estimated to exceed $600 billion (Bouchery, Harwood, Sacks, Simon, & Brewer, 2011; Centers for Disease Control and Prevention, 2008; U.S. Department of Justice, 2011).

Clearly there is a tremendous need for effective treatments for drug use disorders. This chapter focuses on psychosocial treatments for illicit drug use disorders. Treatments for alcohol problems are covered by Mc-

Crady (Chapter 13, this volume) and there are several excellent reviews available on treatments for tobacco use disorders (e.g., Kenford & Fiore, 2004; Schnoll & Lerman, 2006). Because the focus is on empirically based interventions, we largely cover behavioral and cognitive-behavioral therapies. That said, effective contemporary treatments for drug use disorders often entail combining psychological treatments with medications, and this is reflected in this chapter as well. We use a multielement intervention to illustrate details of treatment implementation, namely, the community reinforcement approach (CRA) plus vouchers intervention that our group developed for outpatient treatment of cocaine dependence. Last, the National Institute on Drug Abuse (NIDA, 2009) has published 13 principles of effective treatment for illicit drug abuse based on more than 35 years of research and, when applicable, we underscore those principles throughout the chapter (Table 14.1).

DEFINING THE CLINICAL DISORDER

Before proceeding to discussions about treatment, we briefly discuss criteria for diagnosing drug use disorders. In the research discussed in this chapter we have used DSM-IV-TR (American Psychiatric Association, 2000), and we plan to use DSM-5 (American Psychiatric Association, 2013) in future efforts. DSM-5, published in May 2013, contains one major change from DSM-IV-TR that merits mention (O'Brien, 2011). The abuse and dependence diagnostic categories featured in DSM-IV-TR were replaced in DSM-5 by a single "substance use disorder" spectrum that comprises 11 symptoms. These symptoms, largely paralleling those found in DSM-IV-TR, are as follows: (1) use of substance in larger amounts or over a longer period than was intended; (2) a persistent desire or unsuccessful efforts to cut down or control substance use; (3) a great deal of time spent in activities necessary to obtain the substance; (4) craving; (5) a failure to fulfill major role obligations; (6) continued substance use despite having persistent or recurrent social or interpersonal problems; (7) cessation or reduction in important social, occupational, or recreational activities because of substance use; (8) substance use in situations in which it is physically hazardous, (9) continuation of substance use despite knowledge of having a persistent or recurrent physical or psychological problem that is likely to have been caused or exacerbated by the substance, (10)

TABLE 14.1. Principles of Effective Treatment

1. No single treatment is appropriate for all individuals.
2. Treatment needs to be readily available.
3. Effective treatment attends to multiple needs of the individual, not just his/her drug use.
4. An individual's treatment and services plan must be assessed continually and modified as necessary to ensure that the plan meets his/her changing needs.
5. Remaining in treatment for an adequate period of time is critical for treatment effectiveness (i.e., 3 months or longer).
6. Counseling (individual and/or group) and other behavioral therapies are critical components of effective treatment for addiction.
7. Medications are an important element of treatment for many patients, especially when combined with counseling and other behavioral therapies.
8. Addicted or drug-abusing individuals with coexisting mental disorders should have both disorders treated in an integrated way.
9. Medical detoxification is only the first stage of addiction treatment and by itself does little to change long-term drug use.
10. Treatment does not need to be voluntary to be effective.
11. Possible drug use during treatment must be monitored continuously.
12. Treatment programs should provide assessment for HIV/AIDS, hepatitis B and C, tuberculosis and other infectious diseases, and counseling to help patients modify or change behaviors that place themselves or others at risk of infection.
13. Recovery from drug addiction can be a long-term process and frequently requires multiple episodes of treatment.

tolerance; and (11) withdrawal. The milder end of the disorder spectrum (two to three symptoms) is comparable to the less severe abuse category in DSM-IV-TR, and the higher end of the spectrum (six or more symptoms) to the more severe dependence category. All of our research discussed below has involved individuals who fell along the more severe or "dependence" end of this spectrum.

Evidence does support a position that, on average, more severe drug use disorders are associated with poorer treatment outcome. Severity is influenced by frequency of use, amount of drug used and route of administration, and sociodemographics (e.g., educational attainment), among other factors. There seems to be little doubt that these factors will be positively correlated with the number of untoward signs and symptoms exhibited following a period of repeated drug use, and to that extent merit careful attention in a diagnostic assessment. For these and other reasons, we have found DSM-IV-TR helpful in assessing the severity of cocaine and other drug use disorders, and anticipate the spectrum approach of DSM-5 to be even more helpful in that regard.

ASSESSMENT

A comprehensive assessment is an essential first step in effective clinical management of drug use disorders. This section outlines the assessment practices we used in our specialty clinic for individuals who met DSM-IV-TR criteria for cocaine dependence and what in DSM-5 would represent the more severe end of the cocaine use disorder spectrum. The assessment framework is relatively generic and can be readily applied to other types of drug use disorders by substituting the cocaine-specific information with pertinent information on whatever other type of drug use disorder is the presenting problem.

All initial clinic contacts are handled by a receptionist, who establishes that the caller reports problems related to drug use, is age 18 years or more, and resides within the county in which the clinic is located. The CRA plus vouchers treatment that we use is intensive, requiring several clinic visits per week. Persons living outside the county are often unable to follow such a demanding schedule. A broader geographical range may be possible with other, less intensive interventions. The important matter is to have established the geographical range that is practical for the treatment being offered. Those who do not satisfy our basic inclusion criteria are referred to an appropriate alternative clinic. Those who meet the criteria receive an appointment for an intake assessment.

Every effort is made to schedule the intake assessment interview as soon as possible (Principle 2, Table 14.1). Scheduling the interview within 24 hours of clinic contact significantly reduces attrition between the initial clinic contact and assessment interview, which is a substantial problem among those with drug use disorders (Festinger, Lamb, Kirby, & Marlowe, 1996). Some patients cannot come in within 24 hours, so our secondary goal is to get them in within 72 hours.

Clients are informed that the intake interview will take about 3 hours. This initial session is one of the most important. Clinic staff should be aware of the client's potential uneasiness and try to make the person feel at ease. Being courteous, complimenting clients on taking this important first step toward change, respecting the fact that some clients might be physically ill or uncomfortable related to recent drug use and therefore being flexible with regard to tardiness, and so forth, can help. Accommodating the need for brief breaks, food or drink, or a brief phone call can help as well. Throughout all interactions we seek to be empathic and to convey a very upbeat, "You can do it" message.

During the intake assessment, we collect detailed information on drug use; evaluate treatment readiness; and assess psychiatric functioning, employment/vocational status, recreational interests, current social supports, family and social problems, and legal issues (see Principle 3, Table 14.1). The following instruments that we use to obtain such information are listed in the order in which they are typically administered. Modifications can be readily made to our list depending on the population being treated. We offer it only to provide an example of what we have found to be an effective assessment package, along with associated clinical rationales.

Self-Administered Questionnaires

We use several questionnaires that can be completed by the client upon arrival at the clinic for an initial intake assessment. The intake worker greets the client, introduces him/herself, brings the client into a private office, and briefly but carefully informs him/her about what to expect during the intake process. It is essential to ask about clients' reading ability prior to having them complete self-administered questionnaires. If there is doubt about reading capability, we discreetly ask clients to read several questions aloud to get an indication of whether they can complete the forms without staff assistance. With poor readers, the questionnaires can be read aloud by a staff member in a private setting. This must be done with care and positive regard for the discomfort that poor readers may feel under such circumstances. Competent readers are given approximately 45 minutes to complete the forms.

We have clients complete a routine, brief demographics questionnaire. Obtaining a client's current address and phone number is important, as is obtaining the number of someone who always knows the client's whereabouts. This information is important for purposes of outreach efforts during treatment should the client stop coming to scheduled therapy sessions or need to be contacted for other clinical purposes, and contacting clients for routine posttreatment follow-up evaluations.

The Stages of Change Readiness and Treatment Eagerness Scale (SOCRATES; Miller & Tonigan, 1996) provides information about clients' perceptions of the severity of their drug use problems and their readiness to engage in behavior to reduce their drug use. This questionnaire provides a quantitative index of motivation to change, which may be an important indicator of clients' willingness to comply with certain treatment goals. We use three versions of the SOCRATES that refer to specific substances (i.e., cocaine, alcohol, and other drug use) because clients' motivations to reduce substance use are often drug-specific. For example, almost all who seek treatment in our clinic are ready to act toward changing their cocaine use, but many are more ambivalent about changing their alcohol or marijuana use, which are the two other forms of drug use we deal with most frequently. Our approach is to reinforce action the patient is ready to take with regard to cocaine and to share empathically our empirical knowledge about the influence of other forms of drug use on the probability of successfully discontinuing cocaine use. Our recommendation is that at least short-term abstinence from all intoxicating substance use is the path with the greatest chance of success. Use of alcohol can directly increase the probability of cocaine use and predicts poor outcome. Use of marijuana, which does not predict poor outcome with regard to cocaine use per se, is associated with problems of its own.

We use an adaptation of the Cocaine Dependency Self-Test (Washton, Stone, & Hendrickson, 1988) as an efficient means to collect specific information regarding the type of adverse effects of cocaine that clients have experienced. Systematically collected information on the adverse effects of drug use is important. Such information is useful in helping clients to problem-solve regarding the pros and cons of cocaine use as part of efforts to promote and sustain motivation for change during the course of treatment.

A sizable proportion of clients with illicit drug use disorders are also problem drinkers, which makes assessment of that problem essential. As part of our alcohol assessment we use the Michigan Alcoholism Screening Test (MAST), a widely used, brief alcoholism screening instrument (Selzer, 1971). Considering that almost all clients entering treatment for cocaine abuse and dependence use alcohol and approximately 60% meet DSM-IV-TR diagnostic criteria for alcohol dependence, the MAST is useful for flagging clients with alcohol problems.

Depressed mood is another common problem among those presenting for treatment for drug use disorders. We use the Beck Depression Inventory–II (BDI-II; Beck, Steer, Ball, & Ranieri, 1996) to screen for depressive symptomatology and readminister it on a regular basis to monitor progress with those clients who score in the clinical range at intake. The average BDI-II scores of cocaine abusers entering treatment fall in the clinical range. For most clients, those scores decrease precipitously after 1 or 2 weeks in treatment. However, this is not true for all clients. Therefore, it is important to assess carefully and monitor depressive symptomatology, and to refer the client or intervene when symptoms do not remit. Assessing and monitoring for suicide risk are important as well. We do so using a protocol we developed in collaboration with our local mental health crisis service.

The Symptom Checklist 90—Revised (SCL-90-R; Derogatis, 1983) is also used to screen for psychiatric symptomatology more broadly and is helpful in determining whether a more in-depth psychiatric evaluation is warranted. The SCL-90-R also can be easily readministered to monitor progress or change in psychiatric status.

After clients complete these self-administered questionnaires, they are reviewed by clinic staff to be sure that all questions have been completed and that the information appears consistent. Any obvious inconsistencies are resolved with the client.

Program Description

We find it useful to break up the data-gathering aspects of the initial assessment between completion of the self-administered questionnaires and initiation of the structured interviews. We provide a brief description of the treatment program and its philosophy at this time. Clients are given the opportunity to ask questions or to express any concerns they may have. The goal here is to orient clients to what will happen in treatment, to create an atmosphere of optimism, and to help clients feel hopeful that they can succeed in treatment. This description and interaction is typically brief (10–15 minutes). A therapist provides more detailed rationales and descriptions during this same intake session, but after the structured interviews are completed. When asked questions about the treatment process, the intake worker provides brief answers and reassures the client that a therapist will soon be meeting with him/her to provide much more information about the program and how it works.

In providing the brief description, the intake worker explains that our program is confidential and specifically designed for persons who have problems with cocaine. For obvious reasons, users of illicit drugs are often quite concerned about confidentiality. Clients are informed about the overall duration of treatment, the recommended frequency and duration of clinic visits, and the general foci and orientation of our treatment approach (i.e., lifestyle changes). We explain that the primary goals of such changes are that clients discontinue cocaine use and make positive changes that result in greater life satisfaction. Examples of what might occur during treatment are provided:

"If you are interested in finding a job, the therapists will help you with the search, with a résumé, and with transportation and phone support, if necessary. If you would like to go back to school, we can help you obtain the applications, access funding and assistance, and even take you to an interview if you don't have transportation. If you are having relationship problems, relationship counseling is available. If you don't regularly participate in any fun activities, we have lots of suggestions and may even take you to some of these, like basketball, tennis, fishing, boating, arts and crafts classes, and so forth.

"Also, we provide coping skills training. So if you have problems controlling anger, we can help with anger management. If you have money problems, we can assist you with financial management. If you have difficulty with behavior problems with your children, we can assist you in get some help with that problem. If you have trouble relaxing, we can work on relaxation skills and stress management, and so forth."

In addition, the intake worker provides a very brief description of our clinic's incentive program:

"You also will participate in our incentive program. How this works is that if you provide urine samples that are cocaine-free, you earn points that can be used to support your goals. What that means is, if you stay clean, you accumulate points that can be used to pay for activities such as going to the mov-

ies, joining a gym, taking a class, buying a fishing rod, and so forth. Your therapist will tell you more about these things when you meet him/her after our interview."

Semistructured Interviews

A semistructured drug history interview (developed in our clinic) is used to facilitate collection of information on current and past drug use. Such detailed information is essential for proper treatment planning.

The goal in completing a drug use history is to obtain detailed information regarding the duration, severity, and pattern of the client's drug use. The accuracy of the client's report of drug use (amount and frequency) is facilitated by an effective technique for reviewing recent use (i.e., the Timeline Follow-Back Interview; Sobell & Sobell, 1992; for a review see Hjorthoj, Hjorthoj, & Nordendoft, 2012). Using a calendar as a prompt, clients are asked to recall on a day-by-day basis the number of days they used in the past week and the amount used per occasion. Grams are typically the best metric for determining amount of cocaine used. The same assessment is conducted for the past 3 weeks and as far back in time as needed for diagnostic reasons. This technique results in a good overview of the client's pattern of drug use during the past 30 days. The intake worker asks for as much clarification as possible to obtain an accurate assessment of drug use history. Diagnoses of abuse and dependence are made later by master's- or doctorate-level psychologists.

The Addiction Severity Index (ASI; McLellan, Cacciola, Alterman, Rikoon, & Carise, 2006) is designed to provide reliable, valid assessments of multiple problems commonly associated with drug use, and a quantitative, time-based assessment of problem severity in the following areas: alcohol and drug use; employment; and medical, legal, family, social, and psychological functioning. The information obtained in the ASI is quite useful for developing treatment plans that include lifestyle change goals. It is also a useful instrument for assessing progress at follow-up, in that it is time-based and yields quantitative composite scores for multiple problem areas. Training on ASI administration is necessary to ensure that the intake worker conducts a reliable ASI interview (for information on training in the use of the ASI, see *www.tresearch.org/training/ asi_train.htm*).

A Practical Needs Assessment Questionnaire (developed in our clinic) determines whether the client has any pressing needs or crises that may interfere with initial treatment engagement (e.g., housing, legal, transportation, or child care). The intake worker asks specific questions regarding current housing, child care, legal circumstances, medical issues, and other matters that might be of current and serious concern to the client. Detailed information is collected on any identified crisis. The rationale here is to identify matters that may need immediate clinical attention. The lives of many individuals entering treatment for drug dependence are in chaos. The probability of engaging and keeping such clients in treatment may be compromised if swift assistance relative to certain acute needs is not provided, typically in the form of referrals to community agencies for assistance.

After completing these interviews, the intake worker informs clients that they will be meeting with their therapist in a few minutes. During a brief break (5–10 minutes), the intake worker completes an intake summary sheet for the therapist taking on this new case, along with all of the supporting intake information. The intake worker meets briefly with the therapist to review the case. Patients are then introduced to their therapists. We try never to allow a patient to leave the intake interview without a brief meeting with a therapist, so that he/she can depart with the feeling that treatment has begun, and with concrete plans for abstaining from cocaine use until the next clinic visit.

In many ways this initial meeting is an orientation session to establish rapport with the client and provide further rationales for our treatment approach. Doing so permits clients to develop clear expectations about treatment. We continue with the "can do" approach, acknowledging how hard the client and clinic staff will have to work to succeed, but conveying a very confident message that success can be achieved by working together. The therapist and patient collaboratively begin formulating an initial treatment plan during this session. Clients are oriented to the rigorous urinalysis testing regimen that is a central component of this treatment. If it appears that a medication is indicated, initial steps are taken toward implementing the relevant medical protocols for making that happen. With the cocaine-dependent population, we routinely use a regimen of clinic-monitored disulfiram therapy to address problem drinking, which also reduces cocaine use (Carroll, Nich, Ball, McCance, & Rounsaville, 1998). Recently we have begun using a regimen of clinic-monitored naltrexone therapy because the prevalence of prescription opioid abuse has increased.

BEHAVIORAL AND COGNITIVE-BEHAVIORAL THERAPIES FOR ILLICIT DRUG USE DISORDERS

Conceptual Framework

Behavioral and cognitive-behavioral therapies are based largely on the concepts and principles of operant and respondent conditioning, and social learning theory. Within this conceptual framework, drug use is considered learned behavior that is maintained, at least in part, by the reinforcing effects of the pharmacological actions of drugs in conjunction with social and other nonpharmacological reinforcement derived from the drug-abusing lifestyle (Higgins, Heil, & Lussier, 2004). The reliable empirical observation that abused drugs function as reinforcers in humans and laboratory animals provides sound scientific support for that position (Griffiths, Bigelow, & Henningfield, 1980; Higgins et al., 2004). Cocaine, other psychomotor stimulants, ethanol, opioids, nicotine, and sedatives serve as reinforcers and are voluntarily self-administered by a variety of species. Moreover, through respondent and operant conditioning, environmental events that previously have been paired with drug use reliably lead to drug-seeking behavior. Physical dependence is not necessary for these drugs to support ongoing and stable patterns of voluntary drug seeking and use in otherwise healthy laboratory animals or humans. Commonalities do not end there. Effects of alterations in drug availability, drug dose, schedule of reinforcement, and other environmental manipulations of drug use are consistent and generalize across different species and types of drug abuse (Griffiths et al., 1980; Higgins et al., 2004). These commonalities support a theoretical position that reinforcement and other principles of learning are fundamental determinants of drug use, abuse, and dependence.

Within this conceptual model, then, drug use is considered a normal, learned behavior that falls along a frequency continuum ranging from patterns of little use and few problems to excessive use and many untoward effects, including death. The same processes and principles of learning are assumed to operate across the continuum. All physically intact humans are assumed to possess the necessary neurobiological systems to experience drug-produced reinforcement; hence, they develop patterns of drug use, abuse, and dependence. Said differently, individuals need not have any exceptional or pathological characteristics to develop drug abuse or dependence. Clearly, genetic or acquired characteristics (e.g., family history of substance dependence, other psychiatric disorders) can affect the probability of developing drug abuse or dependence (i.e., they are risk factors), but this model assumes that such special characteristics are not necessary for these disorders to emerge.

Treatment is designed to assist in reorganizing the physical and social environments of the user. The goal is to weaken systematically the influence of reinforcement derived from drug use and the related drug-using lifestyle, and to increase the frequency of reinforcement derived from healthier alternative activities, especially those that are incompatible with continued drug use. Below we describe the basic categories of empirically tested and efficacious behavioral and cognitive-behavioral therapies for achieving these overarching goals (Carroll & Onken, 2005).

Prototypical Behavioral and Cognitive-Behavioral Interventions and Empirical Support for Efficacy

At least four empirically based prototypical behavioral and cognitive-behavioral interventions are used in the treatment of illicit drug use disorders (Carroll & Onken, 2005). First is cognitive-behavioral/relapse prevention therapy, which has been shown to be effective with cocaine, methamphetamine, and other types of drug use disorders (e.g., Carroll et al., 1994; Rawson et al., 2004; Reback & Shoptaw, in press). Typically this approach entails functional analysis training through which clients learn to identify environmental antecedents and consequences that influence their drug use. Functional analysis is typically accompanied by skills training on how to rearrange one's environment to alter the probability of drug use by either avoiding high-risk settings or managing them effectively when contact cannot be avoided. Cognitive strategies are often used to identify and modify unrealistic expectations about drug use, to cope with craving for drug use, and to change thinking patterns that increase the likelihood of drug use. Social skills training is often incorporated when clients have used drugs to cope with social anxiety or when particular skills deficits limit clients' access to alternative, healthier sources of reinforcement (e.g., Monti, Rohsenow, Michalec, & Abrams, 1997). Systematic training is included to prevent relapse, with sufficient emphasis that the terms "cognitive-behavioral therapy" and "relapse prevention therapy" are often used inter-

changeably. There is good evidence that this approach is efficacious in treating illicit drug use disorders (for a meta-analysis, see Irvin, Bowers, Dunn, & Wong, 1999).

Second, contingency management is an efficacious behavioral treatment strategy commonly used to treat cocaine, opiate, and other types of illicit drug use disorders (Higgins, Silverman, & Heil, 2008), as well as other behavioral health problems (see Supplemental Issue of Preventive Medicine on "Incentives and Health"; Higgins, Silverman, Sigmon, & Naito, 2012). With contingency management, reinforcing and punishing consequences are systematically used to increase abstinence from drug use or to improve other therapeutic goals, such as treatment attendance or medication compliance (Higgins et al., 2008). A particular form of contingency management, wherein clients receive vouchers that are exchangeable for retail items contingent on objective evidence of recent abstinence from drug use, has become a common intervention for clients with illicit drug use disorders. We know of at least two meta-analyses supporting the efficacy of contingency management with methadone maintenance patients (Griffith, Rowan-Szal, Roark, & Simpson, 2000) and in the treatment of drug use disorders more generally (Lussier, Heil, Mongeon, Badger, & Higgins, 2006).

Third, motivational interviewing, an efficacious intervention with problem drinkers (Vasilaki, Hosier, & Cox, 2006), is being used more frequently to treat illicit drug use disorders as well. Motivational interviewing is a brief intervention designed to facilitate behavior change by helping clients to identify personal values and goals, to examine whether drug use may conflict with those values and goals, and to explore how to resolve any ambivalence or conflict between personal goals and values, and ongoing drug use (Miller & Rollnick, 2002). Results on the use of motivational interviewing with illicit drug use disorders are still mixed (e.g., Martino, Carroll, & Rounsaville, 2006; Smedslund et al., 2011).

Fourth, behavioral couple therapy has been effective in the treatment of illicit drug use disorders, although it has not been as extensively investigated as alcohol use disorders (Carroll & Onken, 2005; O'Farrell & Clements, 2012). Therapy typically emphasizes improved communication skills. Couples are taught how to negotiate for change in each other's behavior to make the relationship more reinforcing. A contract wherein the designated client agrees to abstain from drug use and/

or to comply with a recommended medication regimen is typically involved. There is also evidence that behavioral family counseling has efficacy with adolescents who have illicit drug use disorders (e.g., Azrin, Donohue, Besalel, Kogan, & Acierno, 1994) as do other family therapy interventions (e.g., Henggeler, Pickrel, Brondino, & Crouch, 1996; Liddle et al., 2001).

It is a common practice to provide multielement treatments for illicit drug use disorders that incorporate many of the specific interventions we have outlined (e.g., Bellack, Bennett, Gearson, Brown, & Yang, 2006). Indeed CRA plus vouchers, which we use to treat cocaine dependence, incorporates all of the interventions outlined earlier except for family therapies with adolescents. Below we describe the CRA plus vouchers intervention and its implementation in the treatment of cocaine dependence. With regard to efficacy, the meta-analysis supporting the efficacy of vouchers was noted earlier (Lussier et al., 2006). A meta-analysis supports the efficacy of CRA, with and without vouchers, in the treatment of drug use disorders (Roozen et al., 2004), and a randomized trial has demonstrated that the CRA component is an active element of the CRA plus vouchers treatment (Higgins et al., 2003).

CRA plus Vouchers

The recommended duration of CRA plus vouchers therapy is 24 weeks of treatment and 24 weeks of aftercare (Budney & Higgins, 1998). The influence of treatment duration has not yet been examined experimentally with this or other efficacious psychosocial treatments for drug use disorders, but a duration of 3 or more months of care is generally recommended (Principle 5, Table 14.1).

CRA therapy in this model is delivered in individual sessions, although CRA has been delivered effectively in a group therapy format with alcohol-dependent clients (Azrin, 1976). As we noted earlier, the treatment involves two main components: CRA and vouchers.

The Community Reinforcement Approach

Before we get into the specific elements of CRA, more general characteristics of the therapy style are worth mentioning. Therapists try to be flexible in appointment scheduling and goal setting, which we believe facilitates treatment retention and progress toward target goals. Particularly in the early stages of treatment, therapists try to work around client's schedules and generally make participation in treatment convenient. We try to tolerate tardiness to sessions and early departure from sessions, to be flexible in the time of day that sessions are scheduled, and we even meet with clients outside the office, if necessary. With especially difficult clients, improvements in these areas become part of the treatment plan.

Therapists must exhibit empathy and good listening skills. They need to convey a sincere understanding of the client's situation and its inherent difficulties. Throughout treatment, therapists avoid making value judgments, and instead exhibit genuine empathy and consideration for the difficult challenges that clients face.

Last, CRA requires both therapists and patients to develop an active, make-it-happen attitude throughout treatment. Active problem solving is a routine part of the therapeutic relationship. Within ethical boundaries, therapists are committed to doing what it takes to facilitate lifestyle changes on the part of clients. Therapists take clients to appointments or job interviews. They initiate recreational activities with clients and schedule sessions at different times of day to accomplish specific goals. They have clients make phone calls from their office, and they search newspapers for job possibilities or ideas for healthy recreational activities in which clients might be able to participate. In summary, the motto of CRA therapists is "We can make it happen," and they try their best to model that approach for patients.

CRA is delivered in twice-weekly 1- to 1.5-hour therapy sessions during the initial 12 weeks and once-weekly sessions of the same duration during the final 12 weeks of treatment. Sessions focus on the following seven general topics, depending on the needs of the individual client.

First, clients are instructed in how to recognize antecedents and consequences of their cocaine use, that is, how to functionally analyze their cocaine use. They are also instructed in how to use that information to reduce the probability of using cocaine. A twofold message is conveyed to the client: (1) His/her cocaine use is orderly behavior that is more likely to occur under certain circumstances than others, and (2) by learning to identify the circumstances that affect his/her cocaine use, the client can develop and implement plans to reduce the likelihood of future cocaine use. Our methods for teaching functional analysis are based on the work of Miller and Muñoz (e.g., 2005) and McCrady (Chapter 13, this volume), whose methods are used widely in substance abuse treatment.

Using the form shown in Figure 14.1, we help clients analyze instances of their own cocaine use. We explain the following:

"A functional analysis allows you to identify the immediate causes of your cocaine use. You have probably noticed that in certain situations you use cocaine, whereas in others you do not. The situations around us can powerfully control cocaine use, particularly if we are unaware of their influence.

"Some of the situations that can influence cocaine use are people you are with, places you go, time of day, the amount of money you have with you, how much alcohol you have consumed, and how you are feeling. The first step in understanding your cocaine use is to identify the situations in which you are likely to use. We call that identifying your 'triggers.' You will also want to identify consequences of your use; that is, identify the immediate, usually positive consequences (getting high, having fun), and the delayed, often negative consequences (blowing your money, unwanted sexual encounters, fights with your spouse). As you identify triggers and consequences, you will discover certain patterns to your cocaine use that are important targets for intervention."

Clients are assigned the task of analyzing at least three recent episodes of cocaine use. Learning to analyze one's cocaine use is emphasized during initial treatment sessions, but the exercise is used throughout the treatment process to help clients understand and modify any lapses to cocaine use, as well as to address problems with cocaine craving.

In conjunction with functional analysis, clients are taught self-management plans for using the information revealed in the functional analyses to decrease the chances of future cocaine use. Using the self-management planning sheet shown in Figure 14.2, clients are counseled to restructure their daily activities to minimize contact with known antecedents of cocaine use, to find alternatives to the positive consequences of cocaine use, and to make explicit the negative consequences of cocaine use.

A key part of self-management planning that is implemented with most clients is drug-refusal training. Most cocaine abusers who are trying to quit cocaine use continue to have contact, either planned or inadvertent, with individuals who are still using. Turning down cocaine or opportunities to go places where cocaine is available is more difficult than most clients anticipate. We approach this as a special case of assertiveness training (e.g., McCrady, Chapter 13, this volume; Meyers & Smith, 1995). The key components of effective refusal are shown in Table 14.2. Therapists should explain the rationale for drug-refusal skills training, engage the client in a detailed discussion of the key elements of effective refusal, assist the client in formulating his/her own refusal style (incorporating the key ele-

Trigger	Thoughts and feelings	Behavior	Consequences	
			Positive	Negative

FIGURE 14.1. Form for functional analysis of substance use.

Trigger	Plans	± Consequences	Difficulty (1–10)
1.	a		
	b		
	c		
	d		
	e.		

FIGURE 14.2. Self-management planning sheet. From Budney and Higgins (1998).

ments), and role-play some scenes in which the client is offered cocaine. The role-played situations should be very specific and realistic for the client in terms of people, times of day, location, and so forth. Client and therapist should alternate roles, so that the former has the opportunity to practice while receiving constructive feedback, and the latter has the opportunity to model effective refusal skills.

Second, all clients receive instruction in developing a new social network that supports a healthier lifestyle and getting involved with enjoyable recreational activities that do not involve cocaine or other drug use. Systematically developing and maintaining contacts

TABLE 14.2. Components of Effective Refusal

1. *No* should be the first thing you say.
2. Tell the person offering you drugs or asking you to go out *not to ask you now or in the future* if you want to do cocaine. Saying things like "maybe later," "I have to get home," or "I'm on medication," and so forth, just make it likely that he or she will ask again.
3. Body language is important:
   a. Making good eye contact is important; look directly at the person when you answer.
   b. Your expression and tone should clearly indicate that you are serious.
4. Offer an alternative, if you want to do something else with that person. Make sure that it is something that is incompatible with cocaine use (taking your children for a walk or to the park, going to work out, etc.).
5. Change the subject to a new topic of conversation.

with "safe" social networks and participation in "safe" recreational activities remain a high priority throughout treatment for the vast majority of clients. Specific treatment goals are set, and weekly progress on specific goals is monitored (Principle 4, Table 14.1).

Clearly, plans for developing healthy social networks and recreational activities must be individualized depending on the circumstances, skills, and interests of clients. For clients who are willing to participate, self-help groups (Alcoholics Anonymous or Narcotics Anonymous) can be an effective way to develop a new network of associates that supports a sober lifestyle. A clinic staff member often accompanies a client to his/her first self-help meeting or two. By no means do we focus exclusively on or mandate self-help involvement. We assist clients with getting involved in a wide variety of social groups that reinforce a healthy lifestyle (e.g., church groups). Clinic staff members accompany clients who are trying new, healthy activities. Some clients wish to reinitiate activities in which they engaged prior to becoming involved with cocaine use, or have clear ideas about activities they would like to pursue. We assist those clients in renewing or initiating participation in those activities. Many others either never engaged in recreation as adults without drug involvement or are simply unable to identify any activities they would currently like to pursue. We often have these clients complete a leisure interest inventory to prompt ideas about activities they might have liked previously or otherwise want to explore. We encourage clients to sample new activities even if they are unsure whether they will find them enjoyable. As we describe below, vouchers may be used to support costs of initiating recreational and other activities that support a healthy lifestyle.

Third, various other forms of individualized skills training are provided, usually to address some specific skills deficit that may influence directly or indirectly a client's risk for cocaine use (e.g., time management, problem solving, assertiveness training, social skills training, and mood management). For example, essential to success with the self-management skills and social/recreational goals discussed earlier is some level of time management skills. All clients are given daily planners to facilitate planning. Because clients may lose or forget their planners, providing photocopies to cover the next week of treatment is a good strategy. Therapists provide the following rationale:

"This part of your treatment involves learning to plan, schedule, and prioritize the events and activities in your life. Solving your cocaine problem requires making substantial lifestyle changes; it is important to develop efficient ways to do this. Some patients say they don't like to plan—they like to be spontaneous. But if they don't find a way to schedule and organize their lives, they often get overwhelmed and don't achieve their goals."

With most clients, time management in some form is worked on throughout treatment. The importance of writing down a schedule of activities that help to promote cocaine abstinence between therapy sessions is emphasized in each session. Planning for "high-risk" times is particularly important. Use of "to do" lists, daily planning, and prioritizing activities is addressed.

As other examples of skills training, we implement protocols on controlling depression (Lewinsohn, Muñoz, Youngren, & Zeiss, 1986; Muñoz & Miranda, 2000) with those clients whose depression continues after they discontinue cocaine use (see Principle 8, Table 14.1). We sometimes implement social skills and relaxation training with individuals who report social anxiety about meeting new people, dating, and so forth (Rodebaugh, Holaway, & Heimberg, 2004). Many clients report persistent problems with insomnia following discontinuation of drug use. With them we often implement a protocol based on those developed by Morin (2004). We often work with clients regarding money management. With many clients this might simply involve helping them arrange direct deposit for their paycheck, so that they are not tempted to use be-cause they have a large sum of cash on hand. For others, this might involve a plan to get out of debt, which can help to reduce stress. Because clients often have so many problems that could benefit from our assistance, we follow a rule of only treating those problems that we feel directly or indirectly affect the probability of initial and longer-term cocaine abstinence for individual clients. Here we rely heavily on functional analysis and other available information regarding the client's cocaine use. For problems that do not appear to be related to cocaine use but warrant professional attention, we generally make a referral. We work very hard to keep treatment focused on resolving the problem of cocaine use, and not being sidetracked by other pressing problems that may have no direct or indirect effect on the presenting problem of cocaine dependence.

Fourth, unemployed clients are offered Job Club, which is an efficacious method to help chronically unemployed individuals obtain employment (see the Job Club manual; Azrin & Besalel, 1980). The majority of people who seek treatment for cocaine dependence are unemployed, so we offer this service to many of our clients. We assist others in pursuing educational goals or new career paths. A meaningful vocation is fundamental to a healthy lifestyle, and we recommend goals directed toward vocational enhancement for all clients. Rules that we follow for several common types of vocational problems are outlined in Table 14.3.

Fifth, clients with romantic partners who are not drug abusers are offered behavioral couple therapy, an intervention designed to teach couples positive communication skills and how to negotiate reciprocal contracts for desired changes in each other's behavior. We attempt to deliver relationship counseling across eight sessions, with the first four sessions delivered across consecutive weeks and the next four delivered on alternating weeks. We introduce this aspect of therapy with the following rationale:

"As you well know, an important area of your life that is negatively affected by cocaine problems is your relationship with your partner. Those close to the person with the problem are typically most adversely affected by the problem. Many partners of cocaine-dependent individuals have tried many times to help their mate to stop using. Strategies for trying to help vary. Anger and frustration usually build up, and feelings of hopelessness and helplessness arise. Sometimes attempts to help are met with resentment and anger from the partner with the problem.

TABLE 14.3. Examples of Goals Set in Vocational Counseling

For the unemployed client:
- Eight job contacts per week.
- Develop a resume.
- Send out two resumes with a cover letter per day.
- Go to the job service twice per week.
- Enroll in a job training program.
- Enroll in a vocational exploration program.
- Take a job-skills-related class.
- Consider and collect information on educational possibilities.

For the client who works "too many" hours or has irregular schedule:
- Keep work hours between 35 and 50 hours per week.
- Establish a more regular schedule.
- Explore alternative work schedules.

For the person working in a "high risk" for drug use environment or the dissatisfied employee:
- Consider a job change.
- Submit applications for alternative employment while continuing to work.
- Modify the work environment to reduce risk of drug use or improve working conditions.
- Enroll in a career exploration class.
- Enroll in job-skills or alternative, career-related educational classes.

"In this part of treatment, we focus on how cocaine use has affected your relationship and how we can work to increase the positive aspects of your relationship. We also discuss ways that your partner can assist you in achieving and maintaining abstinence. We hope to be able to help you both deal more effectively with this cocaine problem.

"We have found that where there are drug abuse problems, there are usually communication problems. Usually, we see communication that is filled with anger, silence, apathy, or resentment, and many times partners try to get their needs met outside the relationship. By the time patients come to see us, there is little, if any, enjoyment left in the relationship."

The intervention involves a related series of exercises. Partners independently rate their current level of happiness across household responsibilities, child rearing, social activities, money, communication, sex and affection, academic progress, personal independence,

partner's independence, general happiness. These ratings are shared and discussed, then rerated weekly to monitor progress. Next, a system of "daily reminders to be nice" (i.e., express appreciation and affection toward one's spouse) is implemented. The obvious goal is to get the partners to take the time to be positive with each other. Each partner is expected to engage in a daily practice of "nice" gestures toward his/her spouse and to keep a daily compliance record of his/ her own behavior—not the spouse's compliance. That information is reviewed and shared during sessions. After some level of positive interaction is established, partners independently identify what a "perfect relationship" would entail in terms of the key elements of their relationship mentioned earlier—what that perfect relationship would look like. Finally, the partners begin to work on using positive communication skills to negotiate for reciprocal changes in each other's behavior to move toward that "perfect relationship." The terms "positive" and "reciprocal" are fundamentally important here. Requests are stated exclusively in positive terms, and both members have to be willing to make changes.

Sixth, HIV/AIDS education is provided to all clients in the early stages of treatment, along with counseling that addresses any specific needs or risk behavior of the individual patient (Herrmann et al., 2013). We address with all clients the potential for acquiring HIV/AIDS from sharing injection equipment and through sexual activity. This involves at least two sessions. First, clients complete an HIV/AIDS knowledge test. They next watch and discuss with their therapist a video on HIV/ AIDS. Points emphasized by therapists during the discussion are shown in Table 14.4. Clients are also provided HIV/AIDS prevention pamphlets and free condoms (if desired). The HIV/AIDS knowledge test is repeated, and any remaining errors are discussed and resolved. Finally, clients are given information about being tested for HIV antibodies and hepatitis B and C, and are encouraged to get tested (Principle 12, Table 14.1). Those interested in testing are assisted by clinic staff in scheduling an appointment.

Seventh, all who meet DSM-IV-TR diagnostic criteria for alcohol dependence or report that alcohol use is involved in their use of cocaine are offered disulfiram therapy (see Principle 7, Table 14.1), which is an integral part of the CRA treatment for alcoholism (Meyers & Smith, 1995), and decreases alcohol and cocaine use in clients who are dependent on both substances (Carroll et al., 1998). Clients generally ingest a 250-mg

TABLE 14.4. Points Emphasized in Discussions of HIV/AIDS

1. The fastest-growing risk group for HIV/AIDS is made up of people who use intravenous (IV) drugs and their sexual partners. At the start of the epidemic, this group made up just a small proportion of those getting infected, but these numbers are increasing rapidly at the present time. Not just gay men get infected!

2. Review the three ways that HIV is transmitted: (a) through sexual contact with an infected person, (b) through blood (as in needle sharing), and (c) from infected mothers to their babies during pregnancy or at the time of birth. Explain that the most efficient way for HIV to be transmitted is through blood (blood contains the highest concentration of the virus) and that sharing needles ("works") is an "easy" way for the virus to get from the system of one person to that of another.

3. Emphasize the point that people who are infected with HIV do not necessarily look sick and might not even know they are infected. You cannot tell by looking at someone whether that person has the virus.

4. If clients are currently using IV drugs, point out that the only safe thing to do if they tend to share needles is to use new needles or to clean them, if they are still using. Review the steps necessary for appropriate syringe cleaning.

5. Unprotected sexual intercourse with the exchange of body fluids (blood, vaginal fluids, semen, preejaculatory fluid) is also an efficient means of giving or receiving the virus. Sex can be made safer by using latex condoms for each and every sexual encounter (this includes oral, vaginal, and anal sex).

6. Point out that alcohol and other drug use contribute to risk because of (a) possible suppression of the immune system, and (b) impaired judgment, which can lead to increased risk taking (e.g., drug use, unsafe sex).

daily dose, observed by clinic staff on urinalysis test days, and, when possible, by a significant other on the other days. We encourage clients to sign a disulfiram contract, shown in Figure 14.3. Disulfiram therapy is only effective when implemented with procedures to monitor compliance with the recommended dosage of medication. We find that having staff monitor compliance on days that clients report to the clinic works very well. Having a significant other monitor compliance on the other days works well if the appropriate person is available to do so at the frequency needed. When that is not possible, we sometimes adopt a practice of having the client ingest a larger dose (500 mg) on days when he/she reports to the clinic and skip dosing on the intervening days.

Use of substances other than tobacco and caffeine is discouraged as well in CRA therapy. Anyone who meets DSM-IV-TR criteria for physical dependence on opiates is referred to an adjoining service located within our clinic for methadone or other opioid replacement therapy (see Bickel, Amass, Higgins, Badger, & Esch, 1997). We recommend marijuana abstinence because of the problems associated with its abuse, but we have found no evidence that marijuana use or dependence adversely affects treatment for cocaine dependence (Budney, Higgins, & Wong, 1996). Importantly, we never dismiss or refuse to treat a client due to other drug use. We recommend cessation of tobacco use but usually not during the course of treatment for cocaine dependence. That practice may change as new research begins to demonstrate that smoking cessation can be successfully integrated into simultaneous treatment for other substance abuse or dependence disorders.

Upon completion of the 24 weeks of treatment, clients are encouraged to participate in 6 months of aftercare in our clinic, which involves at least a once-monthly brief therapy session and a urine toxicology screen. More frequent clinic contact is recommended if therapist or client deem it necessary. These clinic visits might be considered booster sessions that monitor progress and address problems with cocaine use or other aspects of the lifestyle changes initiated during treatment. They also allow for a gradual rather than abrupt ending of the client's involvement with the clinic.

Voucher Program

As we noted earlier, the voucher program is a contingency management intervention designed to increase retention and abstinence. Many cocaine- and other drug-dependent individuals arrive in treatment with their lives in disarray. A reasonable assumption is that some time will be needed to assist these individuals in stabilizing and restructuring their lives, so that naturalistic sources of reinforcement for abstinence can exert some influence over their behavior. A protected environment is an option, but the voucher program is deemed a less expensive alternative. The goal is to have this incentive program play a major role during the initial 12 weeks of treatment, during which time CRA therapy is ongoing as well. CRA assists clients in restructuring their lifestyle, so that naturalistic rein-

I,_____, agree to take disulfiram at the regularly scheduled time outlined below. I agree to do this for _____ days. After this time, I agree to talk to my therapist and to discuss whether or not to continue taking disulfiram. I also agree to have the person designated below witness the administration of the disulfiram each time it is scheduled.

I,_____, agree to be present and witness each take-home administration of disulfiram.

Time: _____

Days: _____

Where: _____

In response to _____ taking disulfiram as scheduled, I agree to _____ as a means of reinforcing the taking of disulfiram.

_____   _____

Patient's Signature   Partner's Signature

_____   _____

Therapist's Signature   Date

FIGURE 14.3. Disulfiram contract.

forcers are in place to sustain cocaine abstinence once the vouchers are discontinued.

The voucher program is implemented in conjunction with a rigorous urinalysis monitoring program (see Principle 11, Table 14.1). We ask patients to sign an Abstinence Contract (Figure 14.4), which describes the voucher program and the urinalysis testing schedule. Urine specimens are collected from all participants according to a Monday, Wednesday, and Friday schedule during Weeks 1–12 and a Monday and Thursday schedule during Weeks 13–24 of treatment. Specimens are screened immediately via an onsite enzyme multiplied immunoassay technique (EMIT, Syva Company, San Jose, CA) to minimize delays in delivering reinforcement for cocaine-negative specimens. To decrease the likelihood of submitting bogus specimens, all specimen collection is observed by a same-sex staff member, and that staff member always reserves the right to request another specimen if he/she has any concerns regarding the integrity of a specimen. All specimens are screened for benzoylecgonine, a cocaine metabolite, and each

week one randomly selected specimen also is screened for the presence of other drugs of abuse. Breath alcohol levels (BALs) are assessed at the time urine specimens are collected. Failure to submit a scheduled specimen is treated as a cocaine-positive result. Participants are informed of their urinalysis and BAL results within several minutes after submitting specimens.

Urine specimens collected during Weeks 1–12 that test negative for benzoylecgonine earn points that are recorded on vouchers and given to participants. Points are worth the equivalent of $0.25 each. Money is never provided directly to clients. Instead, points are used to purchase retail items in the community. A staff member makes all purchases. The first negative specimen is worth 10 points at $0.25/point or $2.50. The value of vouchers for each subsequent, consecutive negative specimen increases by 5 points (second = 15 points, third = 20 points, etc.). To further increase the likelihood of continuous cocaine abstinence, the equivalent of a $10 bonus is earned for each three, consecutive negative specimens. A specimen that is cocaine-positive

This is an agreement between _____ (the client) and
_____ (the therapist) to help the client maintain abstinence from cocaine. By
this agreement I direct my therapist to establish a schedule for collecting urine specimens from me for 24 weeks. I will
provide urine samples three times per week on a Monday, Wednesday, and Friday schedule during the first 12 weeks of
treatment. During the second 12 weeks of treatment (Weeks 13–24), urine samples will be collected two times per week
on a Monday and Thursday schedule. A clinical staff member of my same sex will observe the urination. Half of each
urine sample will be submitted for immediate analysis and half will be saved at the clinic. Samples will be assayed for a
variety of drugs of abuse, among which are cocaine, amphetamines, opioids, marijuana, and sedatives.

Each specimen collection requires 3.0 ounces of urine. If the quantity is insufficient for analysis, that will be considered a
failure to provide a scheduled sample.

If I travel out of town due to an emergency, I will inform my therapist in advance of leaving. My therapist is authorized to
verify such absences with _____ . If I require hospitalization, my therapist
will arrange to collect urine in the hospital. If I am sick and do not require hospitalization, I will still arrange to produce
scheduled urine specimens. If I have difficulty with transportation, or inclement weather makes it difficult to travel, I will
work out (with the assistance of the clinical staff) a way to get to the clinic for urine collection. On certain major holidays
the clinic will be closed. My therapist and I will mutually agree to altered urine schedules on these occasions.

If for appropriate medical reasons a prescription for one of the drugs which sometimes is abused is written, I will supply
my therapist with copies of that prescription. The appearance of that drug in the urine will not be counted as a relapse
to drug use. I hereby direct my therapist to communicate by mail or telephone with the prescribing physician or dentist
when my therapist deems that action to be appropriate.

Cocaine-Free Urines: For each cocaine-negative urine sample collected during Weeks 1–12 of treatment, points will be
earned. Each point is worth the monetary equivalent of $0.25, although they may **not** be exchanged directly for cash. A
voucher stating the earned point value will be presented to me following the collection of a cocaine-negative sample. This
voucher will specify the number of points earned for that day, as well as the cumulative points earned to date and their
monetary equivalent.

During the first 12 weeks of treatment, the first cocaine-free urine sample will earn 10 points, with each consecutive
cocaine-free sample collected thereafter earning an increment of 5 points above the previously earned amount. For
example, if 10 points are received on Wednesday for a cocaine-free urine sample, Friday's cocaine-free sample will earn
15 points, Monday's will earn 20, and so on. As an added incentive to remain abstinent from cocaine, a $10 bonus will
be earned for each week of three consecutive cocaine-negative urine samples collected at our clinic. Assuming there are
no cocaine-positive urine samples collected, the monetary equivalent of $997.50 can be earned during the first 12 weeks
of treatment. Since a major emphasis in our program is on lifestyle changes, primarily increasing activities that effectively
compete with drug use, the money earned on this incentive system must be used toward social or recreational goods
and activities agreed upon by my therapist and myself. A list of acceptable uses of vouchers has been developed for this
purpose and will be shared with me. During the second 12 weeks of treatment, the incentive program will be changed.
Rather than earning vouchers for cocaine-negative samples, I will be earning lottery tickets for clean samples.

For the entire 24 weeks of treatment, immediately after the urinalysis test results indicate that the urine sample is
cocaine-negative, the following will happen. The vouchers (Weeks 1–12) or lottery tickets (Weeks 13–24) will be
delivered. Following the presentation of each voucher, I will be asked if I would like to "purchase" any goods or services.
Vouchers may be used at any time during the 24-week program. Earned vouchers cannot be taken away from me under
any circumstances. The procedure for dealing with cocaine-positive urine samples is discussed below.

Cocaine-Positive Urines: All urine samples will be screened for drug use. A record will be kept of all drugs screened
positive, although this contract will be in effect for cocaine only. For each cocaine-positive urine sample collected I will

(continued)

FIGURE 14.4. Sample abstinence contract.

not receive a voucher. In addition, the voucher earned for the next cocaine-free urine sample will be reset to 10. To reset the voucher value to where it was prior to the cocaine "slip," I must provide five *consecutive* cocaine-free samples. The fifth "clean" sample will then earn me the same monetary equivalent as that earned for the sample preceding the cocaine-positive one, and the system outlined earlier will continue to be in effect (i.e., each clean sample will earn 5 points more than the previous one).

Failure to Provide a Urine Sample: Failure to provide a urine sample on the designated date (without prior approval of my therapist) will be treated as a cocaine-positive sample and the procedures noted earlier will be in effect. Although clinic staff will make an attempt to obtain the sample by coming to my home (with my permission, of course), cocaine-negative urine samples collected in this manner will not earn voucher points, nor will they reset my voucher value to 10. In effect, cocaine-negative samples collected outside of our clinic (except in the case of hospitalization) are "neutral." On the other hand, if clinic staff obtain a sample from me outside of the clinic, and the sample is cocaine-positive, it will be treated in the manner outlined above for cocaine-positive urine samples.

My signature below acknowledges that I agree to the urinalysis monitoring system outlined above. This system has been carefully explained to me, and I understand the outcome of providing both cocaine-negative and cocaine-positive urine samples while I am a client at the clinic.

_____

Client

_____   _____

Date   Therapist

FIGURE 14.4. *(continued)*

or failure to submit a scheduled specimen resets the value of vouchers back to the initial $2.50, from which they can escalate again according to the same schedule. Submission of five consecutive cocaine-negative specimens following submission of a positive specimen returns the value of points to where they were prior to the reset. Points cannot be lost once they are earned.

Patients and therapists jointly select retail items to be purchased with points. The items commonly obtained are quite diverse, including YMCA passes, continuing education materials, fishing licenses, gift certificates to local restaurants, hobby materials, and so forth. Therapists retain veto power over all purchases. Purchases are only approved if therapists deem them to be in concert with individual treatment goals of increasing drug-free, healthy activities.

The voucher program is discontinued at the end of Week 12. During Weeks 13–24, participants receive a single $1.00 Vermont State Lottery ticket per cocaine-negative urinalysis test. Across the 24 weeks of treatment, patients can earn a maximum of $997.50 in vouchers during Weeks 1–12 and $24 in lottery tickets during Weeks 13–24. No material incentives are delivered during the recommended 6-month aftercare period. There is strong evidence that vouchers worth only several hundred dollars over the 12-week course of treatment are efficacious, although the magnitude of the treatment effect decreases significantly as the size of the incentive decreases (Lussier et al., 2006).

Getting Therapy Under Way

The therapist has many tasks to accomplish during the first two sessions (Week 1) of treatment, in addition to simply getting to know the client and developing rapport. These sessions are critical to enhancing motivation and setting the tone for treatment. Hence, we provide detailed descriptions of the specific tasks to accomplish during initial therapy sessions.

As discussed earlier, urinalysis and cocaine use test results are the first areas addressed. By starting the session with a direct assessment of cocaine use, the therapist provides a clear message that the focus of this treatment is the cocaine use disorder.

After a discussion of cocaine use and voucher earnings, the therapist should make sure that the client has completed all the intake materials. Here the therapist can also answer any new questions the client may have.

If practical needs, such as housing, transportation, or child care, are issues for treatment attendance, these needs should be a primary focus of the first session. Therapists should do everything possible to assist clients in finding solutions to these problems.

The therapist should discuss alternative activities or strategies for coping with high-risk situations for cocaine use, especially situations that are likely to arise during the upcoming week. As discussed earlier, having the client use appointment books or photocopies provided by the clinic is very helpful for scheduling alternative plans or activities. The next session should also be scheduled, and the client should record the day and time in the appointment book.

The therapist should begin to formulate a comprehensive treatment plan with specific goals and methods. He/she might introduce this task in the following way:

"A treatment plan will allow us to write down the things you and I think are important to accomplish and how we plan to go about trying to accomplish them. We will use the plan to keep us focused on the task at hand—that is, making lifestyle changes that will help you stop using cocaine and other drugs, and also increase your satisfaction with other important areas of your life. The treatment plan will be developed through a cooperative effort between you and me. It is important that you think the goals we set are important and will help you achieve what you want in life. My job in this process is to assist you in coming up with meaningful, effective goals, and to offer advice based on my knowledge and experience with treating persons with cocaine and other drug problems."

The therapist should then present ideas about which areas of the client's life need changes. For each suggested change, it is important that the therapist provide a rationale that draws from the information collected from the client, as well as from research findings and clinical experience. An open discussion and exchange of ideas should then follow.

If the client is reluctant to participate, the therapist should ask for his/her thoughts on each potential area for change. The therapist can facilitate client participation with questions such as "What do you think?"; "Do you have any thoughts on this?"; "Does this make sense to you?"; "Do you think this is important?"; and "Is this type of change possible?" It is important

for therapist and client to agree on which areas of life present problems and should be changed. If a client disagrees with the therapist's opinion, those areas should be dropped and discussed later in treatment if they continue to pose problems.

After the areas for change are agreed upon, therapist and client should discuss each one. Therapists should use active listening skills (reflection and empathy) and try to keep the focus on the specific areas. They should inform clients that they will focus on these problem areas in each session. Progress and problems are openly discussed, and additions or deletions to the plan are decided upon by therapist and client together.

Next, therapist and client together decide the order in which these problem areas should be addressed, always remembering that to increase cocaine abstinence is the primary goal. Mutual agreement is important, and a therapist may need to compromise to achieve such agreement.

Specific goals should then be set for each problem area. It is important that the therapist provide a rationale for setting specific goals:

"Setting specific goals is important. They will help us stay focused on the primary changes we agreed are important for stopping your drug use and achieving a more satisfying life without drugs. Specific goals also provide a way to measure progress. This can be very important because many times progress can be slow. You may feel you are getting nowhere. In reality, you may be progressing in making changes, but you don't feel much different. Information about specific goals will help us both see more clearly whether we are heading in the right direction, even if the progress is slow.

"This information can also show when you are not progressing as we planned and can lead us to either reconsider the goal or find other ways to meet the goal. Keeping track of progress on specific goals also provides us with a reminder to reward or praise you for the hard work you are doing. Lifestyle changes are often difficult to make. We would also like you to learn to pat yourself on the back and take credit if you are doing well."

These goals should be quantifiable, so that progress can be graphed. Targets for change should be set in the priority areas listed in the treatment plan and categorized as primary or secondary behavior change goals. Examples of typical goals are as follows:

- Five job contacts per week or making an appointment for vocational rehabilitation.
- Engaging in three recreational activities each week during high-risk times.
- Spending 4 hours each week engaging in fun activities with a family member or friend.
- Attending class one night each week.
- Doing 2 hours of homework toward obtaining a general equivalency diploma (GED).
- Planning and doing activities with a person who does not use drugs on nights when one typically used cocaine.

A therapist and client should mutually decide on these goals. Basic principles of effective goal setting should be followed:

- Set relatively low goals at first, so that the client can experience success early.
- Thoroughly analyze all possible barriers to achieving selected goals, so that unrealistic goals are avoided.
- Make sure that the client understands how a goal relates to the overall treatment plan.

It is essential to maximize the probability that the client will carry through and achieve the desired behavior change. The therapist's responsibility is to use the appropriate counseling style and behavioral procedures to increase the probability of compliance with a targeted behavior.

The treatment plan should be updated regularly because treatment planning is a process of constant re-evaluation, assessment, and change based on objective indices of progress (Principle 4, Table 14.1). The client and therapist together should review, discuss, and assess the treatment plan frequently as goals are achieved or as interventions fail, or as new information becomes available. These changes should also be reviewed at the regular clinical supervision meeting.

Implementing the treatment plan, monitoring progress, and modifying and updating the treatment plan according to client needs, progress, and problems are the "meat" of the remainder of treatment.

Clinical Supervision

Doctorate-level psychologists who have expertise in behavioral psychology and substance abuse treatment provide supervision in our clinic. Supervisors provide significant input into treatment plans and selection of targets for behavior change. The supervisor provides guidance about how to monitor progress.

Supervision is provided weekly in sessions that usually last 2–3 hours, during which all cases are reviewed. Therapists update the supervisor and other clinic therapists on each patient's progress based on specific treatment goals and whether progress has been made since the last supervision meeting. Progress is presented graphically for all goals.

A supervisor's style in this model should include a balance of support, feedback, problem solving, and instruction. Considering that CRA plus vouchers requires an active therapeutic approach that can be effortful, the supervisor must serve as a stable source of support, encouragement, and direction in implementing the treatment plan.

We follow a fixed protocol in reviewing cases. First, review begins with examination of a graph of the patient's cocaine urinalysis results from the start of treatment. Second, we review use of alcohol or any other drugs that are being targeted for change. Then we review attendance at therapy sessions, primary goals for lifestyle changes, and secondary goals for the same. Once those treatment targets have been reviewed and modified as necessary, any recent crises or relevant clinical issues, such as suicidal ideation or newly identified problem behaviors, are discussed.

At any point in treatment, treatment goals and targets may be changed. Changes in goals may be precipitated by achievement of prior goals, failure to make any progress toward a specific goal, and clear indication that the goal is not functionally related to cocaine use.

IMPLEMENTING THE CRA PLUS VOUCHERS TREATMENT: A CASE STUDY

In this section we review the case of a client treated in our clinic with the CRA plus vouchers treatment. We chose this case because it illustrates well a number of different aspects of using this treatment approach. Outcome was quite good but certainly not perfect, which is to be expected with this population. The case also illustrates the multifaceted problems with which cocaine-dependent clients present.

Bill, a 24-year-old, single (never married), European American male, was self-referred to the clinic for help with problems with cocaine use. He had been living with a friend, who also used cocaine, until several weeks prior to the intake interview, when Bill moved in with his parents. He had a 5-year-old daughter who lived with an estranged romantic partner. The client currently was without legal visitation rights with his daughter because of her mother's concerns over Bill's record of drug use.

Bill, a high school graduate, had been employed full-time in a retail business for the past 3 years. He reported that most of the individuals with whom he associated were drug abusers. Bill reported a history of healthy social and recreational activities, including golf and skiing, but he had not engaged in those activities with regularity for a number of years.

He had a history of involvement with the criminal justice system, with one conviction for a weapons offense. Bill was incarcerated for 3 months related to that charge but was not under criminal justice supervision at the time he sought treatment.

Presenting Complaint

Bill reported being on a 3-day binge prior to intake and wanted help with stopping cocaine use. He reported numerous prior attempts to stop on his own, but with minimal success. Bill reported being "fed up" with how he felt after bingeing episodes of cocaine use and was concerned about the financial problems his cocaine use caused. He also expressed serious concerns that his drug use and related lifestyle had resulted in the strained relationship with his child and ex-girlfriend that interfered with his getting visitation privileges.

Assessment

Cocaine Use

Bill met DSM-IV-TR criteria for cocaine dependence. He reported a 6-year history of intranasal cocaine use. In his most recent use, 7 days prior to intake, Bill used 10.5 grams of cocaine at home with friends, reporting that this was his typical pattern of use. At intake, Bill reported three episodes of cocaine use during the prior 30 days, with each episode lasting approximately 48 hours, usually during weekends. He typically used cocaine with friends at bars or at friends' houses.

His cocaine use was often preceded by spending time in bars or working excessive hours, or by certain moods that included feeling bored, depressed, anxious, or upset. Bill reported a number of serious consequences as a result of his cocaine use, including physical and financial problems; a relationship breakup; and psychiatric symptoms such as depression, anxiety, suicidal ideation, and violent impulses.

Other Drug Use

Bill's first use of alcohol was at age 16. He reported a pattern of weekly binge drinking, during which he would ingest 13–15 shots of hard liquor. He reported drinking 5 days out of the past 30 days. Bill's first use of cannabis was at age 14. He reported 10 years of daily use and having used cannabis on 30 of the prior 30 days. He reported limited prior use of amphetamines and hallucinogens but no regular or current use of those substances. A regular cigarette smoker, Bill smoked approximately 20 cigarettes per day. Bill reported no previous treatment episodes for substance abuse.

Bill also met DSM-IV-TR criteria for alcohol, cannabis, and nicotine dependence.

Other Psychiatric Problems

Bill reported a history of depression and suicidal ideation. He also noted problems with anger management, which he agreed had been a significant problem for him, and for which he had previously received counseling. His BDI score was 23 at intake (Beck, Ward, Mendelson, Mock, & Erbaugh, 1961), but he reported no suicidal ideation.

Motivation to Change

Bill's score on the SOCRATES at intake indicated a strong commitment to cocaine abstinence. He expressed a moderate commitment to alcohol abstinence but agreed to disulfiram therapy for the duration of treatment. He noted plans to return to social drinking after completion of treatment. He was uninterested in discontinuing marijuana use, which he did not consider a problem, and was not currently interested in discontinuing cigarette smoking.

Conceptualization of the Case

Bill worked long hours, sometimes holding several jobs simultaneously. That practice left little time for other types of activities and, as might be expected, he reported minimal involvement in any form of ongoing recreational activities. Aside from work, then, there were few alternative sources of reinforcement to compete with the reinforcing effects of Bill's cocaine and other drug use. These situations typically snowball, so that cocaine and related drug abuse monopolize more and more the person's activities. In this case, Bill's practices of working long hours, frequenting bars, and using drugs, and his difficulties with anger management, were sufficient to destroy his relationship with his romantic partner, thereby greatly restricting his time with his daughter. Losing those relationships further eliminated any competing sources of reinforcement and also freed up additional time and resources to allocate to the bar and cocaine use scenes. While we deemed Bill's long work hours to have likely increased his vulnerability to the drug-abusing lifestyle, his full-time employment also likely provided some protection against cocaine gaining even greater control over his behavior. Full-time employment is a positive prognostic variable with this and other treatments for cocaine dependence, as is the use of an intranasal route of cocaine administration, which was Bill's preferred route.

Treatment Plan

Cocaine abstinence was the first priority in Bill's treatment plan and is always the main focus in this treatment approach. Next, we recommended alcohol abstinence due to the close relationship between Bill's cocaine and alcohol use. As mentioned earlier, Bill was unwilling to change his use of marijuana despite the rationales we provided regarding both the benefits of doing so and potential adverse consequences of continuing to smoke. Our clinical approach was to look for opportunities during the course of treatment to reinforce any movement toward reducing or discontinuing marijuana use, but not to make Bill's reluctance to change this problem behavior a point of contention. Reestablishing a regular pattern of involvement in healthy recreational activities, especially activities that might substitute for cocaine and alcohol use on weekends, was a high-priority goal. The therapist provided the following rationale to Bill as to why we deemed participation in these activities to be a high priority:

THERAPIST: Many times, when cocaine or other drugs become a regular part of someone's life, they stop doing many of the nondrug activities they used to enjoy. That seems to be true in your case. You used to do lots of healthy recreational activities, but after getting into cocaine use you got away from those other activities.

BILL: No doubt. It's funny, too, because I'm not even sure how that happened. Just gradually got off into different things. Never really stopped liking the other stuff. Just seems like I sort of drifted away from them.

THERAPIST: That's a pretty common report. You have a lot going for you though, Bill. You have a history of doing these healthier activities and having liked them. That's a strength that you'll be able to build upon during treatment.

BILL: Good, haven't felt like I've had too many strengths lately. But how do we do this? What's the connection to my cocaine use?

THERAPIST: Healthy social and recreational activities are important in people's lives. They provide something positive to look forward to after work, a way to decrease boredom and to feel healthy, and a chance to be with people you like. Such activities can play an important part in becoming and staying cocaine free. When you give up using drugs, you have to do something else during the times you used to use. If the things you do are not satisfying or enjoyable, or you don't do anything but sit around and feel lonely or bored, you are more likely to use drugs. That is why we have a specific treatment component to assist you in developing a regular schedule of healthy social and recreational activities.

BILL: Yeah, that could be important for me. I don't find it easy to hang out around the house. I get bored, pretty antsy.

THERAPIST: OK, lets go right to work on these now. We gave you a daily planner. Lets plan some activities to do between today and your next clinic visit. We really have to think carefully about Friday night because that's a high-risk night for you. We'll be doing a lot of this throughout therapy.

Another high priority was to assist Bill in finding an alternative source of employment that would permit him to have a more reasonable work schedule, and that paid well enough that he would not feel compelled to hold several jobs simultaneously. To increase further Bill's involvement in activities that were incompatible with the cocaine-using lifestyle, we assisted Bill in petitioning for visitation privileges with his daughter. Regarding other psychiatric problems, we decided to monitor Bill's BDI scores weekly to see whether they followed the precipitous decline that typically occurs with cocaine-dependent patients within a couple of weeks of entering treatment. Because anger management had been a problem for Bill previously in dealing with his estranged partner, and because he would have to interact with her if he was to obtain visitation privileges, we deemed anger-management treatment appropriate.

Below we outline the progress made in implementing this treatment plan.

Cocaine Abstinence

Contingent vouchers, as the primary intervention for promoting initial abstinence, were made available to Bill according to our standard 12-week protocol. Functional analysis was also implemented with Bill during Sessions 1 and 2. Circumstances that increased the likelihood that Bill would use were being at a bar or at certain friends' houses, using alcohol, ending a particularly long work week, and experiencing depression or boredom. He identified going to the movies or to a

safe friend's house, hunting, fishing, and skiing as circumstances that decreased his likelihood of using. That information was updated and used throughout Bill's course of treatment in self-management planning and in planning for social and recreational activities.

Shown in Figure 14.5 is a cumulative record of Bill's cocaine use and urinalysis results during the 24-week treatment. His only instance of use occurred 7 weeks into treatment. Bill reported being surprised by the results and said that he had smoked marijuana with several friends, and that perhaps some cocaine had been in the pipe.

THERAPIST: Hi, Bill. How have things been going?

BILL: Pretty good.

THERAPIST: Look, the lab just called with your urinalysis results. You're positive for cocaine.

BILL: No way. That can't be right. Wow, I haven't used cocaine. Didn't do much of anything over the weekend.

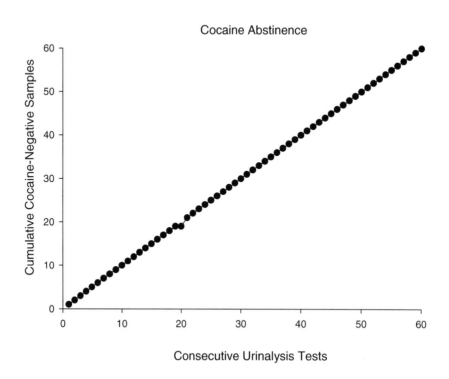

FIGURE 14.5. Shown is a cumulative record of Bill's urinalysis test results (*Y* axis) across 60 consecutive urinalysis tests (*X* axis) conducted during 24 weeks of treatment.

THERAPIST: That's how the machine read the sample. Let's talk more specifically about what you did over the weekend. Let's review what did you on each of the days, and perhaps that will give us some insights into what might be going on.

BILL: Just shut down the shop around midnight and went home and went to bed on Friday night. I worked Saturday morning. After I got off work, I hung out with some friends for a while.

THERAPIST: No gym like you planned?

BILL: Nah. Should have, but got sidetracked by running into some buddies I hadn't seen in a while.

THERAPIST: Any of those guys use cocaine?

BILL: Yeah, one does, but he knows I'm in treatment. I used to use cocaine with him. He doesn't do any cocaine around me now, though.

THERAPIST: What exactly did you guys do?

BILL: Just hung out at this one buddy's house, played video games, and watched some television. We smoked a couple of bowls of pot. You know, I'm still smoking. Could be that the bowl we used had been used to smoke cocaine in recently. Bet that was it.

THERAPIST: Could be. What is pretty clear is that by getting off track of what you had planned, you increased your vulnerability for problems.

BILL: Yeah, I agree. I'm not sure I understand why I did that. I've been doing really well with sticking with my plans even when I run into the guys. Was supposed to get a ride to the gym from my mom, but it was a nice day, so I told her I'd walk. Saw these dudes, started talking, and just sort of bagged my plans for the gym.

THERAPIST: I have no doubt about that. You've been doing a great job up to now with sticking with your plans. Bill, you've been doing terrific with abstaining from cocaine. That is not easy to do and you deserve a tremendous amount of credit for all of the work you've been doing.

BILL: Shoot, kind of blew it here.

THERAPIST: Important thing is to try to learn from what happened. As you know, my recommendation from the start of treatment has been to abstain from marijuana use. Marijuana has its own problems, plus it puts you into contact with other drug abusers, sometimes including cocaine users.

BILL: I agree with that to some extent, but I don't really think that marijuana was the problem here. I've been smoking regularly since starting treatment and have been able to stay away from cocaine. What is different here is that I hung out all day instead of sticking with my plan to go to the gym. That's where I screwed up. That's the big difference from what I had been doing on the other weekends.

THERAPIST: Good job with your analysis. Keep in mind though, if you weren't still smoking, you wouldn't have had any need to use a pipe—yours or theirs. Nevertheless, your point is well taken regarding what you did differently this weekend compared to the others since you've been in treatment. Sticking with the plans for alternative activities rather than just hanging out has really been working for you. I agree with you about that. The most important thing to do here is to learn from this situation and move on. What do you think you need to do to be sure you'll be cocaine-negative on Wednesday?

BILL: Well, I guess just keep doing what I've been doing—sticking to my plans: work, visit Mom, and I have a date tomorrow night. I'm scheduled to go to the gym tonight, and I'm definitely sticking with that. Being clean next time won't be a problem.

THERAPIST: How about minimizing your contact with any drug users, especially people you've used cocaine with in the past? We could even role-play how you might tell the guys how you have to be going, in case you run into them again.

BILL: I guess I could do that. I don't see most of those guys that often anyway. Yeah, sure.

THERAPIST: Good. As you know, we have to go by the urinalysis results. So you won't earn a voucher today and their value gets reset back to the original low value because of today's positive result. However, if you can get back on track with providing negative samples, five consecutive negatives mean that the value of the vouchers get reset back to where they were before today's positive.

BILL: That's fair enough.

Our experience is that there is little need to quibble over a client's denial of a single instance of cocaine use. If the client has resumed regular cocaine use, a pattern of positives will soon emerge. Instead, the therapist reviewed with Bill the risks of continuing to smoke marijuana while working on maintaining cocaine abstinence (continuing contact with drug-using friends, high-risk places, using marijuana rather than other possible activities or way to relax). They also reviewed the importance of sticking with planned activities and prepared to role-play some social skills that Bill could use to resist changing his plans should he run into drug-using friends again. Bill was very insightful about how he had deviated from what had been working for him up to this point—planning activities and sticking to the plans—and the therapist reinforced his analysis. The matter of denying cocaine use was not pursued further. Bill and the therapist carried on with implementing the treatment plan, with the few modifications mentioned. There were no further instances of cocaine use during Bill's 24 weeks of treatment. His record of documented cocaine abstinence was excellent.

Alcohol Abstinence

During the first session, the therapist discussed with Bill the rationale for disulfiram therapy:

THERAPIST: Bill, we want to go over a few reasons for you to give disulfiram therapy and alcohol abstinence a try. First, your history indicates that if you drink, you are more likely to use cocaine. You're not alone in that regard. The scientific evidence is very clear that for many individuals who seek treatment for cocaine dependence, alcohol and cocaine use are closely linked.

BILL: I don't want to get drunk any more. What about just a few drinks? Is that a problem, too?

THERAPIST: Use of even modest doses of alcohol, even just a few drinks, can significantly decrease your chances of successfully abstaining from cocaine use. Our experience, and the experience in other clinics around the country, is that you can make greater progress with cocaine abstinence by using disulfiram and abstaining from alcohol use than if you continue to drink.

BILL: How long are you suggesting I take the medicine? Are you saying I can never drink again?

THERAPIST: I'm not saying that you'll have to take this medicine forever or for years, or anything of that nature, or even that you can never go back to drinking. We can cross those bridges a ways down the road. But for now, if you want to give yourself the best chance to succeed with quitting cocaine, I recommend that you give disulfiram therapy a sincere try.

BILL: I'm not sure how much of a problem drinking is for me. I know it's caused some problems, but I'm just not so sure.

THERAPIST: Bill, the second thing I wanted to emphasize is that you also reported a history of depression and suicidal ideation. Substance use, particularly alcohol use, is a depressant and can worsen depressive symptoms and suicide risk. A period of abstinence may help a good deal with those problems. And still another point to consider is that agreeing to disulfiram therapy represents a concrete demonstration of your commitment to drug abstinence and substantial lifestyle changes. This would be helpful in general, but it could also be helpful in your pursuit of visitation privileges with your daughter.

BILL: Hey, I'm looking to make some progress here. When I've tried to quit cocaine on my own, it's not worked for beans. Maybe it's because I kept drinking, I'm not sure. I can't continue like this. How about I take the medicine during treatment? That's a pretty good commitment. What did you say, treatment is for 24 weeks? Lets say I'll go on the medicine for that amount of time.

Bill agreed to disulfiram therapy for the duration of treatment. A schedule was set up for Bill to ingest a 250-mg dose three times per week, under the observation of clinic staff, and to ingest the same dose under the observation of his father at home on alternating days.

In addition to disulfiram therapy, the therapist worked with Bill on a functional analysis of his alcohol use, similar to the preceding process for cocaine. They reviewed specific circumstances under which Bill was more likely or less likely to drink, and listed the negative consequences he had previously experienced from his alcohol use. The therapist and Bill then began to develop a plan for finding alternative ways to relax that did not involve the bar or drinking, as well as to rehearse how to refuse alcohol when it was offered, and how to identify times that Bill might be tempted to have a drink.

Bill was compliant with disulfiram therapy throughout treatment. He reported only one instance of alcohol use while on disulfiram therapy, when he did not take the medication on a Sunday morning and drank two beers at home that afternoon. On Monday, the therapist did a functional analysis with Bill to identify what set up the occasion for him to drink, and what had happened with his father serving as disulfiram assurance monitor. The therapist and Bill reviewed again his history of alcohol use and the negative consequences he had experienced in the past. Bill recommitted to alcohol abstinence and resumed disulfiram therapy.

When the end of the 24-week treatment approached (Week 23), Bill expressed a desire to "be able to have a drink if he wanted" and asked to discontinue disulfiram therapy, as planned. The therapist expressed his concerns about jeopardizing the substantial progress Bill had made.

THERAPIST: So you're due to end disulfiram therapy this week?

BILL: Yep, stuck to it like I promised, but now I'd like to be able to drink if I want to, like having a beer after work to relax. Nothing major.

THERAPIST: Bill, you've done really well so far with this current plan. Most folks are not as successful as you've been in stopping cocaine use.

BILL: Oh, I agree. I just feel like I've done really well in treatment and now that it's almost over, I'd like to be able to have that choice to drink if I want to.

THERAPIST: How risky do you think going off disulfiram is going to be for you in terms of continuing your success with abstaining from cocaine?

BILL: I really don't think it's going to be a problem. I'm feeling pretty confident about that.

THERAPIST: Bill, that's great. That sort of confidence is important to success. Let's talk about some specifics though. Remember, your alcohol history is still with you. In the past you've had periods of binge drinking combined with cocaine use. What's going to be different now from that past history?

BILL: Well, first of all, I don't plan on drinking like I used to. I'm not looking to get drunk. I'm not even sure I want to drink very often. Also, I'm not going to drink in bars. That's how I've gotten into trouble in the past. And I'm not going to drink with the same old crowd. I just want to know that if I go out to dinner on a date or something and want to have a drink, I can do that.

THERAPIST: You've given this careful consideration, which is good. Those kind of plans are important to continuing your success. Let's talk a bit more about how you can reduce your risk as much as possible

if you're going to resume drinking. By that, I mean how often you drink, how much you drink per occasion, where and with whom you drink—more or less, anything you can do to protect yourself from excessive drinking and, subsequently, cocaine use. Does this sound reasonable to you?

BILL: Yeah, sure, that sounds really good.

At this time, the therapist began the clinic's controlled drinking protocol (see Miller & Muñoz, 2005). Our primary clinical recommendation was abstinence, but Bill was not going to follow that recommendation. Hence, we felt that attempting systematically to provide him with some skills to decrease the likelihood of abusive or harmful drinking was indicated. The Miller and Muñoz approach aims to teach skills that enable the client to drink in a controlled manner. Some of these skills are the same as those involved with cocaine use, including functional analysis to identify the circumstances (location, people, times, feeling states) associated with heavy drinking. Others are specific to alcohol consumption (e.g., providing information about the alcohol content of common drinks, relationship between drinks consumed, body weight, and the blood alcohol curve). Bill and the therapist worked through some of the core elements of the controlled-drinking protocol during the final week of treatment, then covered the remaining parts during aftercare. Bill reported one instance of alcohol use during he final week of treatment. He had only two drinks and did not use cocaine. As we note below, Bill also has reported little drinking during posttreatment follow-up.

Other Drug Use

Bill continued the same pattern of marijuana use that he reported in the intake interview. He repeatedly asserted that marijuana use was not interfering with his other treatment goals. In turn, the therapist provided rationales for stopping or reducing marijuana use on numerous occasions but was not successful in initiating abstinence.

Recreational Activities

During the first several sessions, the therapist and Bill discussed the importance of developing new recreational activities. They decided on a goal of participating in four of these activities per week, as well as a plan to sample some new activities in the company of clinic staff. The therapist reminded Bill that the vouchers he would be earning during treatment for cocaine abstinence could be used to help pay for these activities.

During treatment, Bill consistently met his goal of four recreational activities per week. Those activities included movies, hunting, golf, and dinners at local restaurants. He used his vouchers to buy tickets to a performance at a local theater, greens fees to play golf, a gym membership, hunting and fishing licenses, and gift certificates to a local restaurant for dinner with a new girlfriend.

Family/Social Support

During the first few sessions, the therapist discussed with Bill the need to expand his social network to include family, friends, and other social contacts with non-drug-using people. Bill expressed a desire for increased contact with his daughter. Toward that end, Bill and his therapist completed a task analysis identifying the sequence of steps that would have to be taken to try to attain visitation privileges. These included requesting and completing legal forms from the court, the therapist helping Bill to discuss his wishes appropriately with his former partner, role plays in preparation for the court date, and accompanying Bill to court.

Bill succeeded in obtaining visitation privileges. His goal then became twice-weekly contact with his daughter, which he maintained consistently throughout the remainder of treatment.

Regarding other types of social support, Bill also increased contact with a couple of safe friends during the course of treatment. He also was able to meet several women through his new employment (discussed below), one of whom he began dating regularly.

Employment/Education

Bill came to treatment with a history of full-time employment, which is a good prognostic indicator in itself. However, his job upon entering treatment did not pay well and involved being around drinking. He expressed a desire to find a job that offered better pay, thereby allowing him to work fewer hours per week and to spend more time with his daughter, and to be at reduced risk for alcohol use. Therefore, Bill began participating in Job Club, coming to the clinic three times per week to go through local employment classifieds, complete a resume and cover letters with the help of staff, fill out job applications, and rehearse for job interviews. Bill successfully obtained a better paying job with fewer risks for alcohol use. Thereafter, his vocational goal was to focus on avoiding excessive hours.

Bill also expressed concern regarding the extensive debt he had accumulated during this prolonged cocaine use. The therapist began the clinic's money management protocol, including developing a budget for repayment of outstanding loans and skills for managing personal finances. Bill opened a savings account at a nearby bank and arranged for direct deposit of his paychecks. He used the phone in his therapist's office to arrange payback plans with several debtors. Bill consistently made payments on his debt throughout treatment, which the therapist graphed weekly and, by the end of treatment, had eliminated all back debt and was now paying current bills.

Bill had a long-term vocational goal of eventually opening his own retail business. He and his therapist completed a preliminary task analysis (see Sulzer-Azaroff & Meyer, 1991) related to that goal. They agreed that taking accounting and computer courses would be a good start. The therapist helped Bill collect information from the local community college on the classes being offered. Bill requested financial aid applications from the community college for assistance with tuition, which his therapist helped him complete.

Psychiatric Monitoring

Recall that Bill's BDI score at intake was 23. His BDI score had dropped precipitously by the second week of treatment, and reached a score of 2 by the end of treatment.

Bill and his therapist worked through an anger management protocol for substance abusers (Monti, Kadden, Rohsenow, Cooney, & Abrams, 2002) that helped Bill identify situations that would likely make him angry, develop coping skills to deal better with those triggers, and role-play those coping skills to gain proficiency. The therapist had Bill document when potential anger-provoking situations arose outside of the clinic and how he handled them. The therapist reviewed that information weekly, provided social reinforcement for those situations that were handled well, and problem-solved and role-played alternatives when Bill needed assistance.

Summary of Treatment Progress

Bill made substantial progress toward establishing a stable record of cocaine abstinence, eliminating problem drinking, increasing his involvement in social and recreational practices, improving his job situation, increasing his skill in managing anger, and improving his relationship with his daughter. The one area in which we were unable to make progress was Bill's use of marijuana and associated involvement with the illicit drug abuse community. This progress is reflected in the pre- to posttreatment changes in ASI composite scores shown in Table 14.5. Composite scores range from 0, representing *No problems* in the past 30 days to 1, representing *Severe problems*. Bill's scores at the end-of-treatment assessment generally reflected substantial improvements.

Follow-Up

Following completion of the 24-week treatment protocol, Bill participated in a 6-month aftercare program and completed periodic follow-up assessments for 4 years after treatment entry (see Table 14.5). Thus, we have a relatively good picture of his progress.

Bill largely sustained the excellent progress he made during treatment toward resolving his cocaine-use problems. All urine toxicology tests conducted during follow-up were negative for cocaine use. He reported two instances of cocaine use during the 3.5-year follow-up period, but they were separated in time, and neither resulted in a full-blown relapse. He reported moderate use of alcohol throughout follow-up, with only one instance of drinking to intoxication. He continued to smoke marijuana regularly, as he had done during treatment.

Regarding other areas of functioning, Bill sustained full-time employment throughout the follow-up period. There was an episode of criminal justice involvement at the 12-month assessment, which, according to Bill, was unrelated to substance abuse and was resolved before the later assessments. His depressive symptomatology remained well below intake levels throughout the follow-up period. Progress in other areas of functioning largely was sustained through follow-up, until the 48-month assessment, when a medical crisis arose. Bill developed a neuromuscular condition involving periodic episodes of full paralysis. He was also experiencing more routine but nevertheless painful dental problems. At the time of that assessment, Bill was still undergoing testing for the neuromuscular problem and did not have a diagnosis. This crisis had not precipitated a relapse back to cocaine or other drug abuse, which underscores the substantial progress Bill had made with those problems. The increases in ASI drug scale scores at that 48-month assessment were related to taking pain medication for the dental problems. Clearly, though, the medical conditions were having a destabilizing effect physically and psychologically. Although Bill recognized that the situation put him at increased risk for relapse, he did not deem the situation at that time to warrant reentry into treatment. Treatment staff commended Bill on his sustained progress in abstaining from cocaine and alcohol abuse, and reassured him that he could return to treatment if the need arose.

TABLE 14.5. ASI Subscale and BDI Scores at Intake, End of Treatment, and Posttreatment Follow-Up Assessments

Score	Intake	End of treatment	12 months	24 months	36 months	48 months
ASI subscales						
Medical	0.42	0.09	0.09	0.18	0.00	1.00
Employment	0.07	0.10	0.09	0.11	0.13	0.08
Alcohol	0.13	0.00	0.06	0.00	0.05	0.11
Drug (other than cocaine)	0.28	0.07	0.08	0.08	0.09	0.19
Cocaine	0.66	0.00	0.00	0.00	0.00	0.00
Legal	0.00	0.00	0.40	0.00	0.00	0.00
Family/Social	0.22	0.10	0.00	0.00	0.00	0.22
Psychological	0.36	0.00	0.09	0.09	0.18	0.53
BDI	23	1	3	5	10	6

CONCLUDING COMMENTS

In this chapter we have presented the most up-to-date scientific information available on effective clinical management of illicit drug use disorders. In the process, we have tried to illustrate what have come to be considered principles of effective treatment for illicit drug use disorders in general, using cocaine dependence as a specific exemplar. We have emphasized one efficacious, multielement treatment approach but have underscored how it contains elements of all of the empirically based behavioral and cognitive-behavioral therapies except behavioral family therapy. We realize that limitations in resources and other practical constraints will prevent many clinicians from utilizing the treatment practices just as we have outlined them in this chapter. Costs for the treatment provided to Bill were covered exclusively through a research grant. However, we hope that this information offers insights into the important elements of effective treatment for illicit drug use disorders. We also hope that this information makes the job of clinicians who are out there in the trenches treating the drug-dependent population a little easier and, we hope, their practices more effective.

ACKNOWLEDGMENT

Preparation of this chapter was supported in part by National Institute on Drug Abuse Grant Nos. DA09378, DA030534, and DA031928.

REFERENCES

American Psychiatric Association. (2000). *Diagnostic and statistical manual of mental disorders* (4th ed., text rev.). Washington, DC: Author.

American Psychiatric Association. (2013). *Diagnostic and statistical manual of mental disorders* (5th ed.). Arlington, VA: Author.

Azrin, N. H. (1976). Improvements in the community-reinforcement approach to alcoholism. *Behaviour Research and Therapy, 14,* 339–348.

Azrin, N. H., & Besalel, V. A. (1980). *Job Club counselor's manual.* Baltimore: University Park Press.

Azrin, N. H., Donohue, B., Besalel, V. A., Kogan, E. S., & Acierno, R. (1994). Youth drug abuse treatment: A controlled outcome study. *Journal of Child and Adolescent Substance Abuse, 3,* 1–16.

Beck, A. T., Steer, R. A., Ball, R., & Ranieri, W. (1996). Comparison of Beck Depression Inventories -IA and -II

in psychiatric outpatients. *Journal of Personality Assessment, 67,* 588–597.

Beck, A. T., Ward, C. H., Mendelson, M., Mock, J., & Erbaugh, J. (1961). An inventory for measuring depression. *Archives of General Psychiatry, 4,* 561–571.

Bellack, A. S., Bennett, M. E., Gearson, J. S., Brown, C. H., & Yang, Y. (2006). A randomized clinical trial of a new behavioral treatment for drug abuse in people with severe and persistent mental illness. *Archives of General Psychiatry, 63,* 426–432.

Bickel, W. K., Amass, L., Higgins, S. T., Badger, G. J., & Esch, R. A. (1997). Effects of adding behavioral treatment to opioid detoxification with buprenorphine. *Journal of Consulting and Clinical Psychology, 65,* 803–810.

Bouchery, E. E., Harwood, H. J., Sacks, J. J., Simon, C. J., & Brewer, R. D. (2011). Economic costs of excessive alcohol consumption in the U.S., 2006. *American Journal of Preventive Medicine, 41,* 516–524.

Budney, A. J., & Higgins, S. T. (1998). *The community reinforcement plus vouchers approach: Manual 2. National Institute on Drug Abuse therapy manuals for drug addiction* (NIH Publication No. 98-4308). Rockville, MD: National Institute on Drug Abuse.

Budney, A. J., Higgins, S. T., & Wong, C. J. (1996). Marijuana use and treatment outcome in cocaine-dependent patients. *Journal of Experimental and Clinical Psychopharmacology, 4,* 1–8.

Carroll, K. M., Nich, C., Ball, S. A., McCance, E., & Rounsaville, B. J. (1998). Treatment of cocaine and alcohol dependence with psychotherapy and disulfiram. *Addiction, 93,* 713–727.

Carroll, K. M., & Onken, L. S. (2005). Behavioral therapies for drug abuse. *American Journal of Psychiatry, 162,* 1452–1460.

Carroll, K. M., Rounsaville, B. J., Nich, C., Gordon, L. T., Wirtz, P. W., & Gawin, F. (1994). One-year follow-up of psychotherapy and pharmacotherapy for cocaine dependence: Delayed emergence of psychotherapy effects. *Archives of General Psychiatry, 51,* 989–997.

Centers for Disease Control and Prevention. (2008). Smoking attributable mortality, years of potential life lost, and productivity losses—U.S. 2000–2004. *Morbidity and Mortality Weekly Report, 57,* 1226–1228.

Derogatis, L. R. (1983). *SCL-90-R: Administration, scoring and procedures manual—II.* Towson, MD: Clinical Psychometric Research.

Festinger, D. S., Lamb, R. J., Kirby, K. C., & Marlowe, D. B. (1996). The accelerated intake: A method for increasing initial attendance to outpatient cocaine treatment. *Journal of Applied Behavior Analysis, 29,* 387–389.

Griffith, J. D., Rowan-Szal, G. A., Roark, R. R., & Simpson, D. D. (2000). Contingency management in outpatient methadone treatment: A meta-analysis. *Drug and Alcohol Dependence, 58,* 55–66.

Griffiths, R. R., Bigelow, G. E., & Henningfield, J. E. (1980).

Similarities in animal and human drug taking behavior. In N. K. Mello (Ed.), *Advances in substance abuse: behavioral and biological research* (pp. 1–90). Greenwich, CT: JAI Press.

Henggeler, S. W., Pickrel, S. G., Brondino, M. J., & Crouch, J. L. (1996). Eliminating (almost) treatment dropout of substance abusing or dependent delinquents through home-based multisystemic therapy. *American Journal of Psychiatry, 153*, 427–428.

Herrmann, E. S., Heil, S. H., Sigmon, S. C., Dunn, K. E., Washio, Y., & Higgins, S. T. (2013). Characterizing and improving HIV/AIDS knowledge among cocaine-dependent outpatients using modified materials. *Drug and Alcohol Dependence, 127*(1–3), 220–225.

Higgins, S. T., Heil, S. H., & Lussier, J. P. (2004). Clinical implications of reinforcement as a determinant of substance use disorders. *Annual Review of Psychology, 55*, 431–461.

Higgins, S. T., Sigmon, S. C., Wong, C. J., Heil, S. H., Badger, G. J., Donham, R., et al. (2003). Community reinforcement therapy for cocaine-dependent outpatients. *Archives of General Psychiatry, 60*, 1043–1052.

Higgins, S. T., Silverman, K., & Heil, S. H. (2008). *Contingency management in substance abuse use treatment.* New York: Guilford Press.

Higgins, S. T., Silverman, K., Sigmon, S. C., & Naito, N. A. (2012). Incentives and health: An introduction. *Preventive Medicine, 55*, S2–S6.

Hjorthoj, C. R., Hjorthoj, A. R., & Nordentoft, M. (2012). Validity of Timeline Follow-Back for self-reported use of cannabis and other illicit substances—systematic review and meta-analysis. *Addictive Behaviors, 37*, 225–233.

Irvin, J. E., Bowers, C. A., Dunn, M. E., & Wong, M. C. (1999). Efficacy of relapse prevention: A meta-analytic review. *Journal of Consulting and Clinical Psychology, 67*, 563–570.

Kenford, S. L., & Fiore, M. C. (2004). Promoting tobacco cessation and relapse prevention. *Medical Clinics of North America, 88*, 1553–1574.

Lewinsohn, P. M., Muñoz, R. F., Youngren, M. A., & Zeiss, A. M. (1986). *Control your depression.* New York: Simon & Schuster.

Liddle, H. A., Dakof, G., Parker, K., Diamond, G. S., Barrett, K., & Tejeda, M. (2001). Multidimensional family therapy for adolescent drug abuse: Results of a randomized clinical trial. *American Journal of Drug and Alcohol Abuse, 27*, 651–688.

Lussier, J. P., Heil, S. H., Mongeon, J. A., Badger, G. J., & Higgins, S. T. (2006). A meta-analysis of voucher-based reinforcement therapy for substance use disorders. *Addiction, 101*(2), 192–203.

Martino, S., Carroll, K. M., & Rounsaville, B. J. (2006). A randomized controlled pilot study of motivational interviewing for patients with psychotic and drug use disorders. *Addiction, 101*, 1479–1492.

McLellan, A. T., Cacciola, J. C., Alterman, A. I., Rikoon, S. H., & Carise, D. (2006). The Addiction Severity Index at 25: Origins, contributions, and transitions. *American Journal on Addictions, 15*, 113–124.

Meyers, R. J., & Smith, J. E. (1995). *Clinical guide to alcohol treatment: The community reinforcement approach.* New York: Guilford Press.

Miller, W. R., & Muñoz, R. F. (2005). *Controlling your drinking: Tools to make moderation work for you.* New York: Guilford Press.

Miller, W. R., & Rollnick, S. (2002). *Motivational interviewing: Preparing people for change* (2nd ed.). New York: Guilford Press.

Miller, W. R., & Tonigan, J. S. (1996). Assessing drinkers' motivation for change: The Stages of Change Readiness and Treatment Eagerness Scale (SOCRATES). *Psychology of Addictive Behaviors, 10*, 81–89.

Monti, P. M., Kadden, R. M., Rohsenow, D. J., Cooney, N. L., & Abrams, D. B. (2002). *Treating alcohol dependence: A coping skills training guide* (2nd ed.). New York: Guilford Press.

Monti, P. M., Rohsenow, D. J., Michalec, E., Martin, R. A., & Abrams, D. B. (1997). Brief coping skills treatment for cocaine abuse: Substance use outcomes at three months. *Addiction, 92*, 1717–1728.

Morin, C. M. (2004). Cognitive-behavioral approaches to the treatment of insomnia. *Journal of Clinical Psychiatry, 65*, 33–40.

Muñoz, R. F., & Miranda, J. (2000). *Individual therapy manual for cognitive behavioral treatment for depression.* Santa Monica, CA: RAND Corporation.

National Institute on Drug Abuse (NIDA). (2009). *Principles of addiction treatment: A research-based guide* (2nd ed.; NIH Publication No. 09-4180). Rockville, MD: Author.

O'Brien, C. (2011). Addiction and dependence in DSM-V. *Addiction, 106*, 866–867.

O'Farrell, T. J., & Clements, K. (2012). Review of outcome research on marital and family therapy in treatment for alcoholism. *Journal of Marital and Family Therapy, 38*, 122–144.

Rawson, R. A., Marinelli-Casey, P., Anglin, M. D., Dickow, A., Frazier, Y., Gallagher, C., et al. (2004). A multi-site comparison of psychosocial approaches for the treatment of methamphetamine dependence. *Addiction, 99*, 708–717.

Reback, C. J., & Shoptaw, S. (in press). Development of an evidence-based, gay-specific cognitive behavioral therapy intervention for methamphetamine abusing gay and bisexual men. *Addictive Behaviors.*

Rodebaugh, T. L., Holaway, R. M., & Heimberg, R. G. (2004). The treatment of social anxiety disorder. *Clinical Psychology Review, 24*, 883–908.

Roozen, H. G., Boulogne, J. J., van Tulder, M. W., van den Brink, W., De Jong, C. A., & Kerkhof, A. J. (2004). A systematic review of the effectiveness of the community reinforcement approach in alcohol, cocaine and opioid addiction. *Drug and Alcohol Dependence, 74*, 1–13.

Schnoll, R. A., & Lerman, C. (2006). Current and emerging pharmacotherapies for treating tobacco dependence. *Expert Opinion on Emerging Drugs, 11*, 429–444.

Selzer, M. L. (1971). The Michigan Alcoholism Screening Test. *American Journal of Psychiatry, 127*, 1653–1658.

Silverman, K., Robles, E., Mudric, T., & Stitzer, M. L. (2004). A randomized trial of long-term reinforcement of cocaine abstinence in methadone-maintained patients who inject drugs. *Journal of Consulting and Clinical Psychology, 72*, 839–854.

Smedslund, G., Berg, R. C., Hammerstrøm, K. T., Steiro, A., Leiknes, K. A., Dahl, H. M., et al. (2011). Motivational interviewing for substance abuse. *Cochrane Database of Systematic Reviews, 5*, CD008063.

Sobell, L. C., & Sobell, M. B. (1992). Timeline Follow-Back: A technique for assessing self-reported alcohol consumption. In R. Z. Litten & J. P. Allen (Eds.), *Measuring alcohol consumption: Psychosocial and biochemical methods* (pp. 41–72). Totowa, NJ: Humana Press.

Sulzer-Azaroff, B., & Meyer, G. R. (1991). *Behavior analysis for lasting change.* Fort Worth, TX: Holt, Rinehart & Winston.

U.S. Department of Health and Human Services (USDHHS). (2012). *National Survey on Drug Use and Health, 2010* (Substance Abuse and Mental Health Services Administration. Center for Behavioral Health Statistics and Quality). Ann Arbor, MI: Interuniversity Consortium for Political and Social Research [distributor].

U.S. Department of Justice. (2011). *The economic impact of illicit drug use on American society* [Product No. 2011-Q0317-002]. Washington, DC: United States Department of Justice, National Drug Intelligence Center.

Vasilaki, E. I., Hosier, S. G., & Cox, W. M. (2006). The efficacy of motivational interviewing as a brief intervention for excessive drinking: A meta-analytic review. *Alcohol and Alcoholism, 41*, 328–335.

Washton, A. M., Stone, N. S., & Hendrickson, E. C. (1988). Cocaine abuse. In D. M. Donovan & G. A. Marlatt (Eds.), *Assessment of addictive behaviors* (pp. 364–389). New York: Guilford Press.

CHAPTER 15

Evidence-Based Relationships and Responsiveness for Depression and Substance Abuse

JOHN C. NORCROSS
LARRY E. BEUTLER

Implicit in all chapters in this book is the necessity of tailoring the treatment in a flexible manner to the individual patient, as well as attending to patient, therapist, and relationship factors. Some chapters also purposefully integrate and "match" techniques from different approaches into the treatment protocols described to accomplish specific goals, such as motivational interviewing (see Payne, Ellard, Farchione, Fairholme, & Barlow, Chapter 6) or attention to the social and interpersonal context of the patient. But in this chapter the topics are made explicit by two senior and distinguished clinical investigators who have made it their life work to pursue these themes in a rigorous and empirical manner. The unique contribution of this chapter is that transdiagnostic patient and therapist factors, as well as matching the style of the treatment protocol (e.g., less directive or more directive depending on the level of resistance or "readiness" of the patient for therapy), are also evidence-based procedures and deserve description in this book. Thus, it is important not only to choose the most effective change procedure for a given disorder, such as panic disorder, but also to attend explicitly to relationship factors; to provide for consistent, bidirectional feedback between patient and the therapist; and to establish a transparent, collaborative therapeutic style. The authors demonstrate this integrative approach in the context of the fascinating case of "Amber," a young woman suffering from polysubstance abuse and depression. Awareness of this perspective will enrich the reader's appreciation of all of the chapters in this book.—D. H. B.

$\mathbf{P}$sychotherapy is a treatment method and a healing relationship fit to the individual patient and context. On this, virtually every practitioner (and patient) will agree. However, selection of the particular treatment method has received the lion's share of attention in the movement toward evidence-based practice (Norcross, Beutler, & Levant, 2006). Matching the treatment method to the patient is helpful indeed, but it is also clinically incomplete given that the therapy relation-ship frequently accounts for much of the success (and failure) of psychotherapy (Norcross, 2011). Moreover, psychological science directs us to which relationship behaviors and matches contribute to treatment outcomes across the spectrum of psychological disorders (Beutler, 2009).

As virtually every psychotherapist also knows, psychotherapy should be tailored to the individuality of the patient and the singularity of his/her context. As early as 1919, Freud introduced psychoanalytic psychotherapy as an alternative to classical analysis, based on the recognition that the more rarified approach lacked universal applicability (Wolitzky, 2011). The mandate for individualizing psychotherapy was embodied in Gordon Paul's (1967, p. 111, original emphasis) iconic question: "*What* treatment, by *whom*, is most effective for *this* individual with *that* specific problem, and under which set of circumstances?" Every psychotherapist recognizes that what works for one person may not work for another; we seek "different strokes for different folks."

Only in the past two decades has sufficient research been conducted to operationalize these noble intentions into specific matching guidelines. Particularly absent until recently has been research matching psychotherapy to the entire person of the patient, beyond his/her disorder. As Sir William Osler (1906), father of modern medicine, said: "It is sometimes much more important to know what sort of a patient has a disease than what sort of disease a patient has."

The process of creating this optimal fit in psychotherapy has been accorded multiple names: treatment adaptation, responsiveness, attunement, matchmaking, customizing, prescriptionism, treatment selection, specificity factor, differential therapeutics, tailoring, and individualizing. By whatever name, the goal is to enhance treatment effectiveness by tailoring it to the individual and his/her singular situation. In other words, psychotherapists endeavor to create a new therapy for each patient.

In this chapter, we apply our integrative psychotherapy to comorbid depression and substance abuse. We begin with an overview of the approach and its research evidence, particularly the evidence-based therapy relationship and responsiveness or fit to individual patients. The co-occurrence of mood disorders and substance abuse is outlined, and the step-by-step treatment selection is demonstrated. We conclude with a detailed case illustration of "Amber," a woman suffering from chronic depression, substance abuse, and a host of other psychological disorders.

OVERVIEW OF OUR APPROACH

Our approach to psychotherapy is broadly characterized as integrative and specifically labeled "systematic eclectic" or "systematic treatment selection." Psychotherapy integration is characterized by dissatisfaction with single-school approaches and a concomitant desire to look across school boundaries to see how patients can benefit from other ways of conducting psychotherapy (Norcross & Goldfried, 2005). We attempt to customize psychological treatments and therapeutic relationships to the specific and varied needs of individual patients as defined by a multitude of diagnostic and particularly nondiagnostic considerations. We do so by drawing on effective methods across theoretical schools (eclecticism), by matching those methods to particular clients on the basis of evidence-based principles (treatment selection), and by adhering to an explicit and orderly (systematic) model.

The clinical reality is that no single psychotherapy is effective for all patients and situations, no matter how good it is for some. Evidence-based practice has come to demand a flexible, if not integrative, perspective. Psychotherapy universally applied as one size fits all is proving impossible and, in some cases, even unethical. Of course, that would simplify treatment selection—give every patient the same brand of psychotherapy!—but it flies in the face of what we know about individual differences, patient preferences, and disparate cultures.

Imposing a parallel situation onto other health care professions drives the point home. To take a medical metaphor, would you entrust your health to a physician who prescribed the identical treatment (say, antibiotics or neurosurgery) for every patient and illness encountered? Or, to take an educational analogy, would you prize instructors who employed the same pedagogical method (say, a lecture) for every educational opportunity? Or would you entrust your child to a child care worker who delivers the identical response (say, a nondirective attitude or a slap on the bottom) to every child and every misbehavior? "No" is probably your resounding answer. Psychotherapy clients deserve no less consideration.

Concisely put, we believe that no theory is uniformly valid, and no mechanism of therapeutic action is equally applicable to all individuals. As a consequence, we select different methods and relationships according to the patient and the context. The result is a more efficient and efficacious therapy—and one that fits both the client and the clinician.

On the face of it, of course, virtually every clinician endorses matching the therapy to the individual client. After all, who can seriously dispute the notion that psychological treatment should be tailored to the needs of the individual patient? Indeed, treatment manuals increasingly focus on ways to be flexible—but they all still work within a confined set of theoretical parameters and technical procedures. In contrast, our integrative therapy goes beyond this simple acknowledgment of the need for flexibility in several ways:

- Our integrative therapy is derived directly from outcome research rather than from an idiosyncratic theory or seat-of-the-pants syncretism.
- Our therapy embraces the potential contributions of multiple systems of psychotherapy rather than working from within a single theoretical system.
- Our treatment selection is predicated on many diagnostic and nondiagnostic client characteristics, in contrast to relying on patient diagnosis alone.
- Our aim is to offer optimal treatment methods and healing relationships, whereas many therapists focus narrowly on selecting methods. Both interventions and relationships, both the instrumental and the interpersonal—intertwined as they are—are required in effective psychotherapy.
- Matching methods and relationships to the client occurs throughout the course of therapy, not only at pretreatment as a case formulation.
- As will be evident in the case illustration that follows, clients evolve and progress—and their initial complaints are not necessarily their primary disorders or goals at the conclusion of treatment. Our integrative therapy tracks their progress and evolves with them through termination.

RESEARCH EVIDENCE

The outcome research supporting our approach comes in several guises. First and most generally, the entire body of psychotherapy research has provided the foundation for the key principles on which integrative treatment rests. This is the basis from which we have systematized the process of treatment selection. A genuine advantage of being integrative is the vast amount of research attesting to the efficacy of psychotherapy and pointing to the differential effectiveness among different types of patients. Integration tries to incorporate state-of-the-art research findings into its open framework, in contrast to becoming yet another "system" of psychotherapy.

We embrace the robust common factors among the therapies and, at the same time, capitalize on their differences. Integration gathers, in the words of Abraham Lincoln, "strange, discordant, and even, hostile elements from the four winds." Diverse treatment methods are optimally employed with patients and in situations for which research has found evidence of effectiveness. We hasten to add that the incorporation of these treatments should occur within a systematic process and an integrative perspective, that is, be integrative, not syncretic.

A second and more specific source of research evidence is our ongoing programmatic research on treatment selection according to client characteristics (for details, see Castonguay & Beutler, 2006; Norcrosss, 2011). Below we summarize the research evidence underpinning evidence-based therapy relationships and responsive fit to transdiagnostic patient characteristics.

Relationships That Work

Decades of psychological science have identified many of the relational behaviors that contribute to and predict successful psychotherapy, and multiple meta-analyses have refined our understanding of which of these work to improve outcomes (Norcross, 2011). In fact, evidence-based therapy relationships have been highlighted on the National Registry of Evidence-Based Programs and Practices (NREPP; *www.nrepp.samhsa. gov/norcross.aspx*). Below we summarize the research evidence for those elements of the therapy relationship that are primarily provided by the psychotherapist.

The Alliance

The alliance is an emergent quality of partnership between therapist and client, built principally on a positive emotional bond between therapist and client, and their ability to agree on the goals of treatment and to reach a mutual consensus on the tasks. A meta-analysis of 201 studies, involving over 14,000 adult patients, found an effect size (d) of 0.60 (Horvath, Del Re, Flückiger, & Symonds, 2011), which describes the degree to which the alliance is related to and predicts psychotherapy outcome. (In all instances of reporting effect sizes in this chapter, we use d, where 0 indicates no effect; 0.20 represents a small effect; 0.50 represents a medium effect; and 0.80 and above, a large effect [Cohen, 1988].)

As in the adult research, the alliance in youth treatment is characterized as a collaborative bond between client and therapist, but the psychotherapist typically established two alliances: one with the youth and one with the parent or guardian. A meta-analysis of 29 studies with 2,202 youth clients and 892 parents estimated the association between alliance and outcome in youth therapy (Shirk & Karver, 2011). The effect size (d) was 0.39, between both the therapist and the youth, and the therapist and the parent/guardian.

Just as in individual therapy, the alliance in couple and family therapy (CFT) involves the creation of a strong emotional bond, as well as negotiation of goals and tasks with the therapist. However, family members often vary in the degree to which they like and agree with the therapist about treatment goals and tasks, thus creating multiple alliances that interact systemically. A meta-analysis of 24 studies (7 couples, 17 family studies; 1,461 clients) was conducted in which CFT alliances were used to predict treatment improvement midtreatment and final outcomes (Friedlander, Escudero, Heatherington, & Diamond, 2011). The effect size (d) was 0.53, indicating that the alliance accounted for a substantial proportion of variance in CFT retention and outcome. According to conventional benchmarks, this represents a medium effect size in the behavioral sciences; the success rate increases from 37 to 63% in low versus high alliance cases.

Cohesion in Group Therapy

Probably the closest parallel of the alliance in individual therapy is cohesion in group therapy. A meta-analysis of 40 studies, comprising 3,323 patients, was conducted on the association between cohesion and the success of group psychotherapy (Burlingame, McClendon, & Alonso, 2011). The effect size was a moderate d of 0.52. This indicates that, as cohesion levels increase in groups, client outcomes improve and psychological symptoms decrease. This correlation was found for therapy groups across different settings (inpatient and outpatient) and diagnostic classifications.

Empathy

Much of the research continues to follow Carl Rogers's (1957) definition of empathy as the therapist's sensitive ability to understand the client's thoughts, feelings, and struggles from the client's point of view and communicate that understanding to the client. A meta-analysis examined the association between therapist empathy and treatment outcome (Elliott, Bohart, Watson, & Greenberg, 2011). The analysis of 57 studies resulted in an overall d of 0.61, a medium effect, between therapist empathy and client success (suggesting a success rate of 57% compared to 43% for higher vs. lower empathy). Empathy predicted treatment outcome consistently

across different theoretical orientations (e.g., cognitive-behavioral, psychodynamic, humanistic).

Collecting Client Feedback

In this relational behavior, the therapist systematically monitors a client's mental health vital signs through the use of standardized scales and expected treatment response. Results of this monitoring are then fed back in real-time to the therapist and discussed in session with the client. A meta-analysis of nine studies on the impact of feedback methods on treatment outcomes showed effect sizes (d) between 0.49 and 0.70 (Lambert & Shimokawa, 2011). Rates of patient deterioration in psychotherapy were cut by two-thirds when client feedback was used with warning signals for at-risk patients. Accordingly, patients are better off when practitioners routinely monitor their ongoing mental health functioning. Such monitoring leads to increased opportunities to repair alliance ruptures, enhance motivation, and reduce premature termination. Systematic feedback is especially useful in helping clinicians identify the possible failure of ongoing treatment and collaborate with the client in restoring positive outcomes.

Goal Consensus

Agreement about the nature of the problem for which the client is seeking help, goals for treatment, and the way that the two parties work together to achieve these goals are the essence of goal consensus. A meta-analysis addressed how patient–therapist goal consensus relates to psychotherapy outcome (Tryon & Winograd, 2011). The goal consensus–outcome meta-analysis—based on 15 studies with a total sample of 1,302 patients—yielded an effect size (d) of 0.72. This substantial result reflects the meaningful positive outcomes that are associated with higher agreement between therapists and clients about the aims of treatment and how to accomplish such aims.

Collaboration

To help clients fulfill mutual treatment goals, professionals and patients should function as a team. The collaboration–outcome meta-analysis—based on 19 studies involving 2,260 patients—yielded an d of 0.70 (Tryon & Winograd, 2011). As with goal consensus, this result suggests that patient well-being is considerably enhanced with a better collaborative relationship.

Affirmation/Positive Regard

To investigate the association between therapists' positive regard and treatment outcome, Farber and Doolin (2011) performed a meta-analysis of 18 studies. The overall effect size among these studies was 0.57, indicating that positive regard has a moderate association with therapeutic outcomes. Thus, like many other relational factors, positive regard appears to be a significant but hardly an exhaustive part of the process–outcome equation.

Researchers cannot study all of these relationship behaviors simultaneously, and there is considerable overlap in these constructs and in the amount of variance they account for in psychotherapy. At the same time, it is demonstrably true that these relationship behaviors are important predictors and contributors to psychotherapy success that can be learned and, in most cases, taught.

Patient–Treatment Fits That Work

The question of fit or responsiveness becomes which patient transdiagnostic dimensions can reliably guide us in adapting psychotherapy to different clients or with the same client at different points in time. More than 200 client variables have been proposed as potential matchmaking markers, and at least 100 of these have been subjected to some research scrutiny (Clarkin & Levy, 2004). We commissioned a series of original meta-analyses on the research linking treatment outcome to patient characteristics, and the results of those analyses point to at least five potent matches: reactance level, stages of change, coping style, preferences, and culture (Norcross, 2011). Following are thumbnail descriptions of each, and we demonstrate their respective uses later in our case study.

Reactance Level

Research confirms what one would expect: High patient reactance or resistance is consistently associated with poorer therapy outcomes (in 82% of studies). But matching therapist directiveness to client reactance mightily improves therapy outcome. Specifically, clients presenting with high reactance benefited more from self-control methods, minimal therapist directiveness, and paradoxical interventions. By contrast, clients with low reactance benefited more from therapist directiveness and explicit guidance. This strong, consistent finding can be expressed as a large effect size (d) averaging 0.76 (Beutler, Harwood, Michelson, Song, & Holman, 2011).

Stages of Change

The amount of progress clients make in psychotherapy tends to be a direct function of their pretreatment stage of change—precontemplation, contemplation, preparation, action, and maintenance. A meta-analysis of 39 psychotherapy studies (Norcross, Krebs, & Prochaska, 2011) found a mean effect size (d) of 0.46, indicating that the stages reliably predict outcomes in psychotherapy. This effect has been found to be true for patients suffering from dozens of mental and medical disorders immediately following intervention, as well as 12 months afterward.

More importantly, research in behavioral medicine and psychotherapy converge in showing that different processes of change are differentially effective in certain stages of change. A meta-analysis (Rosen, 2000) of 47 studies examining relationships among the stages and the processes of change showed large effect sizes ($d = 0.70$ and 0.80). That is, adapting psychotherapy to the client's stage of change significantly improves outcome across disorders (Prochaska & Norcross, 2013).

These client markers provide prescriptive as well as proscriptive guidance to the psychotherapist. In reactance, the prescriptive implication is to match the therapist's amount of directiveness to the patient's reactance, and the proscriptive implication is to avoid meeting high client reactance with high therapist direction. In stages of change, action-oriented therapies are quite effective with individuals who are in the preparation or action stages. However, these same therapies tend to be less effective or even detrimental with individuals in the precontemplation and contemplation stages.

Coping Style

The research has been devoted primarily to the externalizing (impulsive, stimulation-seeking, extroverted) and internalizing (self-critical, inhibited, introverted) coping styles. Approximately 80% of the studies investigating this dimension have demonstrated differential effects of the type of treatment as a function of patient coping style. A meta-analysis of 12 of those studies, involving more than 1,000 patients, revealed a medium effect ($d = 0.55$) for matching therapist method to patient coping style (Beutler, Harwood, Michelson, et al., 2011). Specifically, interpersonal and insight-oriented therapies are more effective among internalizing patients, whereas symptom-focused and skill-building therapies are more effective among externalizing patients. This pattern is frequently known for child patients—say, a depressed internalizing girl versus a hyperactive externalizing boy—but less well known for the adult patients on whom the meta-analysis was conducted.

Preferences

Client preferences and goals are frequently direct indicators of the best therapeutic method and healing relationship for that person. Decades of empirical evidence attest to the benefit of seriously considering, and at least beginning with, the relational preferences and treatment goals of the client. A meta-analysis of 35 studies compared the treatment outcomes of clients matched to their preferred treatment to outcomes of clients not matched to their preference. The findings indicated a medium positive effect ($d = 0.31$) in favor of clients matched to preferences. Clients who were matched to their preference were one-third less likely to drop out of psychotherapy—a powerful effect indeed (Swift, Callahan, & Vollmer, 2011).

Culture

A meta-analysis of 65 studies, encompassing 8,620 clients, evaluated the effectiveness of culturally adapted therapies versus traditional, nonadapted therapies. The most frequent methods of adaptation in the studies involved incorporating cultural content and values, using the client's preferred language, and matching therapists of similar ethnicity. The results revealed a positive effect ($d = 0.46$) in favor of clients receiving culturally adapted treatments (Smith, Rodriguez, & Bernal, 2011). Cultural "fit" works, not only as an ethical commitment but also as an evidence-based practice.

DEPRESSION AND SUBSTANCE ABUSE

Depression is the most prevalent comorbid condition among the behavioral health disorders, co-occurring at very high rates in almost all behavioral and many medical disorders. It is especially likely to co-occur among those with substance abuse; posttraumatic stress disor-

der (PTSD) and other anxiety disorders; and heart disease, cancer, and many other physical diseases (Beutler, Clarkin, & Bongar, 2000; Kessler et al., 2005). As many as 80% of patients with chronic medical conditions suffer from comorbid (unipolar) depression. The prevalence rates of comorbid depression and substance abuse are so consistent that many have suggested that substance abuse may be a manifestation of depressive spectrum disorders). This may also be true for other disorders, such as PTSD, in which both depression and chemical abuse frequently seems to substitute for the PTSD symptoms following mass trauma (Housley & Beutler, 2007).

The lifetime prevalence rates for comorbid depression and substance abuse are high, reaching a figure of nearly 10%, closely approximating the lifetime prevalence rates of substance use disorders alone. What is more, co-occurring depression and substance abuse tend to follow similar patterns of response to treatment. Virtually all structured treatments produce similar effects among either depressed or substance-abusing patients (Beutler & Malik, 2002). Likewise, the course of recovery and relapse from depression is extremely variable and generally more similar to that of the extant comorbid conditions than to other instances of depression. Reviews of the literature conclude that there is little evidence of either a specific course of depression or a specific treatment that is uniquely effective (e.g., Cuijpers, van Straten, Andersson, & van Oppen, 2008; Cuijpers et al., 2010); rather, depression functions more as an indexing symptom of distress and impairment than as a separate disorder in its own right.

As we discuss throughout this chapter, it is also now relatively clear that the therapy relationship and matching strategies that positively impact the treatment of depression work in the same manner to ameliorate substance abuse. Beutler and colleagues (2003), for example, studied a group of patients with comorbid depression and substance dependence, comparing the relative and absolute influence of patient predisposing factors (e.g., reactance level, coping styles), treatment characteristics, the therapy relationship (as measured by the alliance), and the fit between the treatment characteristics and the patient factors. Cross-cutting categories of psychotherapy included therapist level of directiveness and the relative proportion of insight and symptom-focused interventions (Beutler et al., 2000).

Figures 15.1 and 15.2 show that all of these factors—patient factors, treatment methods, therapy relationship, and the degree of fit between the treatment and

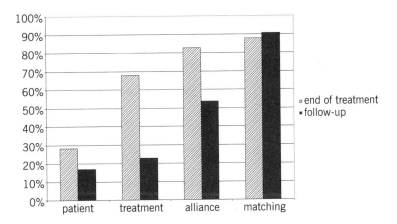

FIGURE 15.1. Relative contributions of patient, treatment, relationship, and treatment fit to changes in depression (Hamilton Rating Scale for Depression [HRSD]) among comorbid substance-abusing and depressed patients.

patient—contributed to the success of psychotherapy. Depression symptoms were somewhat easier to change at both the end of treatment and 6-month posttreatment follow-up, but the pattern and relative effects of each class of factors were similar and collectively added to the effectiveness of treatment. For both depression and substance abuse, maximal treatment gain was associated with a psychotherapy that fit both the treatment method and the healing relationship to the individual patient and context. That repeated research finding has become the leitmotif of applying our approach, to which we now turn.

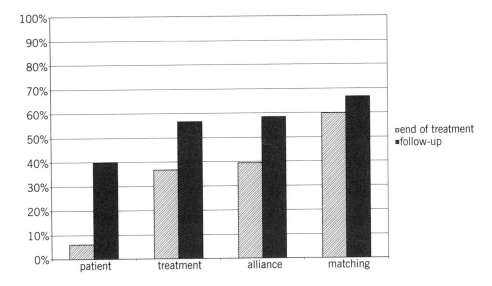

FIGURE 15.2. Relative contributions of patient, treatment, relationship, and treatment fit to changes in substance abuse (Addiction Severity Index [ASI]) among comorbid substance-abusing and depressed patients.

APPLICATION OF OUR APPROACH

Treatment selection invariably involves iterative, recursive decisions about setting, format, intensity, pharmacotherapy, therapy relationship, and treatment methods. Why? Because each client responds best to a different configuration or mix of components. We cannot and should not assume that the treatment will automatically be outpatient individual psychotherapy on a weekly basis. Below we consider each of these decisions, devoting more time to selection of treatment methods predicated on the patient's diagnostic and transdiagnostic features.

Treatment Settings

The setting is where the treatment occurs—a psychotherapist's office, a psychiatric unit, a halfway house, an outpatient clinic, a secondary school, or a medical ward. The choice of setting depends primarily on the relative need for restricting and/or supporting the patient given the severity of psychopathology and the amount of support in the patient's environment. As applied to depression and substance abuse, the urgent question is whether hospitalization or detoxification is required for either.

Each treatment decision is related to the other treatment decisions, as well as to certain patient characteristics. The optimal setting, for example, is partially determined by the level of functional impairment and partially reflects reactance level. Those clients who are most impaired and resistant have the greatest need for a restrictive environment. Outpatient treatment is always preferred over a restrictive setting; indeed, preference is nearly always for the least restrictive setting.

Therapy Formats

The format indicates who directly participates in the treatment, the interpersonal context within which the therapy is conducted. The typical treatment formats—individual, group, couples, and family—are characterized by a set of treatment parameters, all determined largely by the number and identities of participants.

Decades of research support the effectiveness and especially the cost-efficiency of group, couple, and family therapy. Therapy conducted in these formats is generally as effective as individual therapy, but patients and therapists usually prefer the individual format. Even so, a multiperson format is indicated when social support systems are low and if one or more of the major problems involves a specific other person.

Treatment Intensity

The intensity of psychotherapy is the product of the *duration* of the treatment episode, the *length* of a session, and the *frequency* of contact. It may also entail the use of multiple formats, such as both group and individual therapy or both pharmacotherapy and psychotherapy.

Intensity should be gauged as a function of problem complexity and level of impairment in the context of the patient's resources. For example, a patient with a multiplicity of treatment goals, severe functional impairment, few social supports, and a personality disorder is likely to require substantially longer, more intense, and more varied treatment than a patient with a simpler problem. Patients suffering from both mood disorders and substance abuse almost always require intense and long-term care.

Pharmacotherapy

Psychotropic medications are particularly indicated for more severe and chronic disorders, which is the case with the majority of depressed substance abusers. Unlike some systems of psychotherapy, integrative psychotherapies are well suited to the integration of pharmacotherapy and psychotherapy. This position, of course, is consistent with the pluralism underlying treatment selection. But like most health care professionals, integrative therapists are especially keen to avoid treating substance abuse with only another substance.

Thus, we offer a cautionary note here: Medication alone is not an integrative treatment. Tightening insurance reimbursements and restricting psychological services unduly favor pharmacotherapy at the expense of psychotherapy for virtually every disorder. This situation is clinically and empirically appalling to us because decades of research indicate that, in fact, there is frequently no stronger medicine than psychotherapy for both clinical depression and substance abuse (e.g., Antonuccio, 1995; Antonuccio, Danton, & DeNelsky, 1995; DeRubeis et al., 2005; Hollon, 1990). The preponderance of scientific evidence shows that psychotherapy is generally as effective as medications in treating nonpsychotic disorders, especially when patient-rated measures, side effect profiles, and long-term follow-up are considered. This is not to devalue the salutary impact of pharmacotherapy; rather, it is to underscore the reliable potency of psychotherapy.

Therapy Relationship

All psychotherapy occurs within the sensitive and curative context of the human connection. Although we emphasized this point and its research underpinnings earlier in this chapter, we hasten to dispute the unfortunate misperception of treatment selection as a disembodied, technique-oriented process. Our integrative approach attempts to fit not only therapy methods but also relationship stances to individual clients. One way to conceptualize the matter, paralleling the notion of "treatments of choice" in terms of techniques, is how clinicians determine "therapeutic relationships of choice" in terms of interpersonal stances (Norcross & Beutler, 1997). Conducting the best of evidence-based treatment all comes to naught unless the client feels safe, cared for, and connected.

Early on, then, we strive to develop a working alliance and to demonstrate empathy for the client's experiences and concerns. We proceed collaboratively in establishing treatment goals, in securing the patient's preferences, in allaying the initially expected distrust and fear, and in presenting ourselves as caring and supportive. Of course, the therapy relationship must also be matched or tailored to the individual patient and his/her cultures.

This imperative to fit or match psychotherapy to the patient can be misconstrued as an authority figure/therapist prescribing a particular form of psychotherapy for a passive client. The clinical reality is precisely the opposite. Our goal is for an empathic therapist to work toward an optimal relationship that enhances collaboration, is consistent with the client's preferences, and secures the patient's sense of safety and commitment. The nature of such an optimal relationship is determined by patient preferences, cultures, and personality. If a client frequently resists, for example, then the therapist considers whether he/she is pushing something that the client finds incompatible (preferences), or whether the client is not ready to make those changes (stage of change) or is uncomfortable with a directive style (reactance). We lead by following and respecting the client (Norcross, 2010).

Treatment Methods

When clinicians first meet clients, they are tempted to focus immediately and intensely on particular therapy methods and strategies. However, as we have noted, treatment selection always involves a cascading series of interrelated decisions. A truly integrated treatment requires that the therapist recursively consider these other decisions before jumping to therapy methods.

The selection of methods and strategies is the most controversial component of integrative therapy for depression and substance abuse. While there may be occasional professional disagreement about the ideal treatment setting and format, proponents of disparate theoretical orientations frequently endorse decidedly different positions on which methods should be used. Moreover, any given method can be used in different ways. Thus, rather than focusing on specific techniques per se, we prefer prescribing change principles. Principles are flexible, yet specific. Each principle can be implemented in a number of ways and with diverse techniques, depending on the predilections and skills of the therapist. By mixing and matching methods from different therapy systems, we tailor the treatment to the particular patient (Norcross, 2013).

Humans, including psychotherapists, cannot process more than a handful of matching dimensions at once (Halford, Baker, McCredden, & Bain, 2005). As discussed earlier, we principally consider five transdiagnostic patient characteristics (reactance level, stage of change, coping style, preferences, and culture) that have a proven empirical track record as prescriptive guidelines.

What about diagnosis in treatment selection? When it comes to the psychological treatment of unipolar depression and substance abuse, the diagnosis does not suggest a particular treatment, other than to favor those with the most research support. That is, diagnosis has the least evidence of differential treatment effects. In any case, we reiterate that reliance on diagnosis alone to select a treatment plan is empirically questionable and clinically suspect. Instead, as applied to depression and substance abuse, we select treatment methods on the basis of matching the outcome research to those transdiagnostic patient features of reactance, stage of change, preferences, coping style, and culture.

Clinical Assessment

Our approach strongly values clinical assessment that guides effective treatment (Harwood, Beutler, & Groth-Marnat, 2011). Such assessment is conducted early in psychotherapy to select treatment methods and therapy relationships that are most likely to be effective, throughout therapy to monitor the patient's response and to make midcourse adjustments as needed, and toward the end of psychotherapy to evaluate the outcome of the entire enterprise. Thus, assessment is continuous, collaborative, and invaluable.

Clinical assessment of the patient in integrative therapy is relatively traditional, with one major exception. The assessment interview(s) entail collecting information on presenting problems, relevant histories, and treatment expectations and goals, as well as building a working alliance. As psychologists, we also typically use formal psychological testing as a means of securing additional data and identifying disorders. We recommend both symptomatic rating forms (e.g., Beck Depression Inventory–II [BDI-II], Symptom Checklist 90—Revised) and broader measures of pathology and personality (e.g., Minnesota Multiphasic Personality Inventory–II, Millon Clinical Multiaxial Inventory–III).

The one way in which our assessment departs from the usual is that we collect, from the outset, information on multiple patient characteristics that will guide treatment selection.

The five patient characteristics identified in the research (as noted earlier) guide us in identifying a beneficial fit between patient and treatment. Of course, we are not confined to these five considerations, but they do illustrate our process of clinical assessment and treatment matching.

A free, online program has been developed (*www.innerlife.com*) to guide patients in selecting an optimal treatment and finding a clinician who can best implement that treatment. A companion program is available to clinicians (at the same website) for a modest cost to help them plan a research-informed treatment that is both broad and flexible in applying fundamental principles of change. Completing the assessment requires approximately 15 minutes and takes the person through a series of item-branching questions. At completion, the Innerlife STS renders a report to the patient that addresses treatment issues tailored to the person:

- Potential Areas of Concern
- Treatments to Consider
- Treatments to Avoid
- Compatible Therapist Styles
- Picking a Psychotherapist
- Self-Help Resources

A similar set of treatment issues are addressed in more detail in the parallel report directed to the clinician, and available through the same website. This more detailed report also includes programmatic considerations that should be addressed in structuring the environment and directing the staff of treatment centers in what is needed for effective change.

CASE STUDY: AMBER

Initial Encounters

Amber's father initially contacted our private practice office seeking psychotherapy for his 32-year-old, divorced European American daughter following her scheduled release from prison the next month. The father was informed of the 3-month waiting list, referred to an office mate psychiatrist to begin pharmacotherapy, and offered names of other psychologists. Amber and her parents decided to wait to see one of the authors (J. C. N.) but she began attending Alcoholics Anonymous (AA) meetings 5 days a week and started an antidepressant (fluoxetine, to 80 mg) and an anxiolytic (BuSpar, 20 mg three times a day) for 2 months before commencing individual psychotherapy. Although the delay was not clinically advisable, it did fortuitously provide a baseline and control comparison for the subsequent effects of psychotherapy. That is, at our initial evaluation, we were able to establish the extant effects of the medications and AA participation apart from and predating the psychotherapy. The two medications were continued over the course of psychotherapy and were monitored by a psychiatrist throughout.

At our first session, I began with standard open-ended questions:

THERAPIST: Ms. Smith, what brings you here today? What do you hope to accomplish?

CLIENT: Well, I am depressed and a recovering addict. I was released a couple of months ago from prison, where I was diagnosed with borderline personality disorder. I suppose I want to work on all of that.

We begin with Ms. Smith's story and with respect. I address the client as Ms. Smith until or if she grants me permission to call her Amber, which she does within 10 minutes. We also begin with the client's narrative story and concerns. The primary task in the first session is twofold: to cultivate an accepting, empathic relationship, one in which she will feel understood and prized, and to collect sufficient information to begin planning treatment together.

A tumultuous and complicated history pours out of Amber: For as long as she can remember, she has felt depressed, lonely, and incompetent despite having a loving and stable family. Three courses of psychotherapy, ranging from 3 months to a year each, and multiple antidepressants did little to relieve her misery. Approximately 5 years ago, she began embezzling funds from the legal firm where she worked as a paralegal and assisted with the bookkeeping. The stolen money was used to finance an escalating and expensive addiction to opiates, benzodiazepines, and alcohol. "They help me get numb." Her pathological gambling and shoplifting escalated as the drugs loosened her impulse control and impaired her judgment further. She descended into burglary to support her habit and into infidelity with men who supplied her with drugs. Her self-cutting, emotional lability, and fear of abandonment intensified. Amber's embezzlement was discovered by her law firm, the police caught her with stolen items, and her husband of 3 years learned of the serial affairs. Amber was fired, incarcerated, and divorced in a matter of weeks. She then spent 2 years in county and state prisons until she was released early for good behavior and sentenced to several years of parole.

An abbreviated mental status examination reveals that this well-oriented, well-nourished woman appears younger than her stated age. Amber is polite, deferential, and verbal throughout the interview. She is visibly distressed by her condition and acknowledges suicidal ideation, but no intentions or plans. Her mood is depressed and anxious but appropriate. There is no evidence or complaints of psychosis, mania, or aggression. Detailed assessment of her functioning will be undertaken between sessions and in subsequent visits.

Upon learning that Amber's three previous experiences with psychotherapy did not prove particularly successful, I began to explore what did and did not work in those treatments, thereby defining and aligning our collaborative relationship.

THERAPIST: From those experiences, Amber, you certainly learned how a psychotherapist could be most useful to you. What would he or she ideally do? And what should he or she not do?

AMBER: Well, I don't really know . . . (*sounding hesitant and incredulous*)

THERAPIST: I did not mean to put you on the spot [attributing her reluctance to voice preferences to my unexpected question rather than her core deference to authorities]. In our work together, I will be asking you to provide feedback on our progress and on what we do here. That's the honest partnership we hope to create. Perhaps you have had some thoughts about what worked and what did not in your previous treatment?

AMBER: Well, the one with Dr. *X* did not teach me anything, but he was very nice and supportive. I liked him but I did not make any progress. Dr. *Y* asked me to keep free associating and tell him my dreams. That was interesting, but did not leave me feeling any better.

THERAPIST: Do I have it right that we should not repeat those mistakes: only nice without teaching you new skills and leaving you too . . . unstructured?

AMBER: . . . and too passive. I need some skills, directions, ways to deal with all of this [her problems].

Amber nominates additional preferences for transparency in the process, between-session goals (also known as homework), and reading materials. Amber's preferences naturally segue into an exploration of our respective roles and her active collaboration in psychotherapy. She intellectually understands the importance of an active client but, emotionally, feels inadequate to undertake the task: "I've felt like this my entire life. I know what I want, but can't get there."

Thus, psychotherapy begins with both an explanation and an experience of the way we might proceed. To ensure that treatment proceeds with her informed consent and active collaboration, we jointly develop three between-session activities. First, Amber grants me permission to speak with the psychiatrist and to secure her psychological records from prison, and asks me to respond to her probation officer, should he contact me. Second, at my request, Amber agrees to complete a life history inventory and a series of comprehensive computer-administered psychological tests to cover the essential ground. We will review her test responses next session. And third, Amber will prioritize her treatment goals. Among the desirable changes, which would she like to focus on at the outset?

All of these activities are designed to jump-start the therapy process and to activate Amber's collaboration, despite her unsuccessful therapy experiences in the past. We both leave the first session feeling connected, more optimistic, but a bit overwhelmed by the magnitude of her conditions.

History and Background

Amber was the youngest of three children (girl, boy, girl), and experienced normal developmental milestones. According to her recollections and her mother's independent report, Amber had suffered pervasive anxiety "since birth" and throughout adolescence. Neither the patient nor her parents reported any history of trauma; instead, all agreed that family life was stable and relatively benign. Both parents were professionals, and both appeared to care deeply about Amber and her future.

The patient succeeded in academics but flailed at friendships. She completed high school with fine grades and went on to earn a college degree and another year of paralegal training. Starting early in school, Amber suffered from feelings of inadequacy, low self-esteem, avoidance, and school reluctance. It was the latter and a brief bout of being bullied that led her to the guidance counselor in elementary school for several sessions of counseling.

Her adolescence was punctuated by quiet academic achievement but a series of internalizing disorders: "secret" shoplifting, nonsuicidal self-mutilation, and alcohol use before high school classes ("to lift my mood and soothe my nerves"). In college, she became bulimic for a year. She related that "no one ever knew" about the eating disorder or the other dysfunctions, and that she was "keeping it all inside of me."

At that point Amber entered into individual therapy on three occasions over a span of about 5 years, while simultaneously working with two different psychiatrists. When those treatments did not materially reduce her distress, Amber reported that she "gave up" and began the downward spiral of addiction, impulse dyscontrol, and embezzlement that led to her being fired, incarcerated, and divorced in a matter of weeks.

Medical history was unremarkable: a bout of childhood asthma that she outgrew, a broken limb secondary to a sport accident, and seasonal allergies. With the exception of the psychotropic medications, Amber was not taking medications and was followed regularly by her primary care physician and gynecologist. She enjoyed robust physical health and was an avid exerciser. She had begun to smoke a few cigarettes daily since release from prison but had been abstinent from alcohol and drugs for 60 days when we first met.

By contrast, the family history was positive for multiple mental disorders. Her older sister was hospitalized for an eating disorder and suffers from anxiety disorders, for which she continues in psychotherapy. Her brother experiences clinical levels of anxiety and depression, which periodically leads him to psychotherapy and pharmacotherapy. Amber's mother, by multiple accounts, suffers from strong obsessive and agoraphobic tendencies, for which she has also sought professional care. Her father was characterized as "very anxious" but apparently did not receive treatment.

Assessment and Formulation

In addition to a mental status examination conducted during our second meeting and the life history inventory completed between meetings, Amber completed the Minnesota Multiphasic Personality Inventory–2 (MMPI-2), the BDI-II, and the Beck Anxiety Inventory (BAI). Scores on both the Beck instruments were in the severe range at intake (BDI-II = 37; BAI = 49), as shown in Figure 15.3. Amber's ratings of urge intensity in the last week on a 11-point visual analogue scale (0 = *None* to 10 = *The worst*) were 3 for alcohol, drugs 2, gambling 8, and shoplifting 9.

Amber's MMPI-2 profile was clinically elevated on multiple scales, including the D, Pt, and Sc scales, and suggested unusually severe psychological problems (Welsh code 87**21*<u>3460</u>"9+/5:F***+L-K/). Depression, anxiety, and social introversion were all spiking above the 99th percentile. So, too, were two scales measuring PTSD symptoms. The computer-generated interpretive report indicated that "a pattern of chronic psychological maladjustment characterizes individuals with this MMPI-2 clinical profile. The client is overwhelmed by anxiety, tension, and depression. She feels helpless and alone, inadequate and insecure, and she believes that life is hopeless and that nothing is working out right. She attempts to control her worries through intellectualization and unproductive self-analysis, but she has difficulty concentrating and making decisions." Her coping style was markedly introverted (at the 99th percentile) and avoidant (above the 95th percentile); her interpersonal relationships tended to be ambivalent, "never fully trusting or loving anyone. Many individuals with this profile never establish lasting, intimate relationships." The two negative treatment indicators were also quite elevated: Amber's low motivation and inability to disclose were both above the 95th percentile.

At the same time, several of Amber's strengths were evident despite the dismal symptom picture. Amber had survived years of incarceration, she was voluntari-

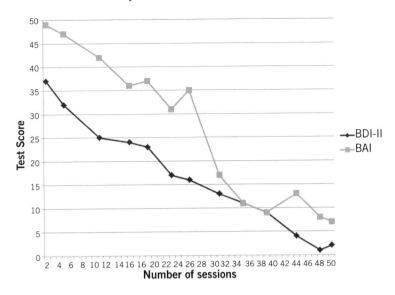

FIGURE 15.3. Amber's scores on the Beck Anxiety Inventory (BAI) and Beck Depression Inventory–II (BDI-II) across sessions.

ly seeking psychotherapy following three disappointing efforts, and she was pushing herself to relate to me in an honest, forthcoming manner. She was a resilient survivor with a keen intellect and a supportive family. And she knew in her heart, as she put it, "this time, it (psychotherapy) must work or I end up back in prison."

At the same time, our treatment approach is less concerned about formal diagnoses and more concerned with understanding Amber in her uniqueness and complexity. But this is not to say that diagnoses are inconsequential. At the second session, Amber and I reviewed her completed life history inventory and psychological test results. Although not flattering, the test results struck Amber as "exactly me." She appreciated the candid discussion of her multiple disorders, which she did not experience or recall occurring in her previous treatments. She was particularly struck by her high levels of anxiety, which she typically labeled depression, and multiple indications of PTSD stemming from her arrest and incarceration.

Her mental status examination, clinical history, and the psychological test results converged on a series of diagnosable DSM-5 disorders: major depressive disorder, polysubstance dependence, generalized anxiety disorder (chronic), PTSD, pathological gambling, klep-

tomania/shoplifting, borderline personality disorder, and prominent avoidant personality features. Her Global Assessment of Functioning (GAF) was 50.

But assessment falls short for treatment purposes if it stops with disorders and even strengths. What about Amber as a person, beyond a list of diagnoses? What are her treatment preferences, her reactance level, stage of change, coping style, and cultures? In terms of personality traits, Amber is low in reactance, almost pathologically unassertive and dependent, and her coping style is fundamentally internalizing. Although kleptomania and substance abuse typically indicate an externalizing style, she has kept most of her problems hidden from others. In terms of problem-specific stages of change, Amber is in the preparation stage for her anxiety, early action stage for depression, action stage for gambling and shoplifting, and in the early maintenance stage for her substance abuse. Two fear-charged exceptions arise from this pattern of "wanting to tackle problems:" Amber is in contemplation for the borderline personality disorder and PTSD. She acknowledges that she does not understand well the borderline diagnosis made in prison, and what she understands is scary and pessimistic. Nor is she willing yet to discuss treatment methods for her prison-related PTSD. We accede to her preferences and respect her early contemplation stage for those conditions. In terms of culture, Amber identifies herself as a female recovering addict of European American persuasion and heterosexual orientation.

Preparing the Patient

Amber presents for the second session looking more comfortable and less distressed. I share this observation, and Amber responds, "I did feel better this past week." I ask for her impressions of our first session, as a means of developing collaboration, collecting feedback, and communicating the need for goal and task consensus. We discuss Amber's experiences, including her perception of comfort with me and her feelings of shame and guilt in revealing her "awful mess of a life." I offer that I was impressed with her openness and honesty, particularly given her history of secrecy and the fact that it was our first meeting Within a few minutes, we agree that the therapist–patient fit is "good" and proceed to review the test results (as summarized earlier).

Consistent with her stages of change, Amber decides to focus in early sessions on treating her depression and maintaining her drug abstinence. I concur with these preferences because they coincide with the usual sequencing of treatment goals with multidisordered patients: Accord first priority to decreasing suicidal (and return-to-prison) behaviors, then to therapy-interfering behaviors, and then to decreasing behaviors that interfere with quality of life (Linehan, 1993a). We agree to begin with weekly individual psychotherapy with the caveat that we will increase the frequency if her distress and impairment do not decline soon.

Preparing the patient for psychotherapy occurs in two guises: one for the role demands of psychotherapy in general, and one for the specific treatment methods in particular. A good portion of the second session is occupied with laying the groundwork for psychotherapy—confidentiality, cancellations, contacting the therapist, handling crises, answering service, payment, and so on—and then Amber's role induction as an active, informed patient of the process. As an experienced therapy patient, Amber grasps this information rapidly, asks a few clarifying questions, and readily agrees to the frame of treatment. With a less experienced patient, more time would (and should) be devoted to these matters.

An additional element of preparation is introducing the view that psychotherapy is a single part of the more inclusive treatment plan. The research indicates that patients who are functionally impaired respond best to a comprehensive treatment. Specifically, more impaired or disabled patients profit from more treatment, lengthier treatment, psychoactive medication, multiple therapy formats (individual, couple, group), and explicit efforts to strengthen their social support networks (Beutler, Harwood, Alimohamed, & Malik, 2002). Patients suffering from both mood and substance disorders are cases in point; to put it simply, complex problems require complex treatments.

The second guise of preparation is explaining the particular treatment methods, in this instance, beginning with cognitive-behavioral therapy (CBT) for the depression and relapse prevention for the substance abuse, gambling, and shoplifting. These particular treatments immediately suggest themselves for Amber on several counts: They match her stage of change (action and maintenance, respectively), her low reactance level (calling for more directive and therapist guided treatments), and her preferences for change tools and homework assignments. And, of course, both CBT and relapse prevention enjoy solid research evidence of their effectiveness in treating Amber's disorders.

Psychotherapy is more effective when both the method and relationship are tailored to the client's stage of change and then evolve as the client moves along the stages during the course of treatment. With contemplators, the optimal role as therapist is akin to a Socratic teacher who encourages clients to achieve their own insights into their condition. Because Amber is into the action stage, the stance morphs into an experienced, supportive coach who has been through many crucial matches and can provide a fine game plan.

Although the research clearly indicates that Amber's action and maintenance stages and her low reactance favor the therapist's use of directive methods, the therapist must also sensitively broach the topic of transferring more responsibility and self-direction to the client over time. Amber, with a lifelong history of dependency and low reactance, will respond best to a directive stance on the part of the therapist. At the same time, we must be careful not to reenact, in conscious and unconscious ways, Amber's unassertive and subservient relationship with the powerful therapist. Thus, I broach this matter early in the third session and contract for an evolving relationship in terms of our respective roles.

THERAPIST: Last time, we agreed that I would be an active and directive therapist with action plans and homework in addressing your depression and drug use. (*Amber nods in agreement.*) The research evidence also supports that. My concern is that doing so may reinforce in here your tendency to behave dependently and defer to others. Does that make sense?

AMBER: Ummmm. Yes, I had not thought about that, but I see how that would probably happen. I would depend more on you.

THERAPIST: That will be fine in the short run, while we are reducing your depression and keeping you abstinent. In the long run, your depending too much on me compounds your unassertive personality style. Might I suggest this as a way out of the paradox? In our early sessions, I will be more directive, in the lead, so that you can become less depressed and certain in your sobriety. Once that happens, in the later sessions, then we will ask and teach you to become more assertive, more in the lead. It will sort of be like AA—right now you depend a lot on your sponsor, but one day you will be probably sponsoring others. How does that sound?

This distinction between mediating goals and ultimate goals is almost always enthusiastically received, as it was by Amber. The mediating goal is to reduce symptomatic distress; the ultimate is to restructure interpersonal behavior. Psychotherapy can be more directive in the short term to work toward more mature and assertive relationships in the long term.

Ongoing assessment will, of course, refine Amber's goals, and her early success will lead to further goals. Her immediate goals and, as she puts it, "where she is at" (in the stages of change) are to reduce depression and maintain her abstinence. Those goals reflect where her commitment and action lie, representing the best chances of reducing her suicidal ideation and her probability of returning to prison Her chronic anxiety, PTSD, and matrix of borderline personality symptoms are addressed more fully in later sessions.

Monitoring Progress

We routinely collect real-time client feedback over the course of psychotherapy regarding three crucial areas: patient functioning/symptoms; task and goal consensus; and satisfaction with the therapy relationship. In terms of symptom monitoring, Amber and I agree that she will complete the BDI-II and the BAI every four sessions (once a month) to monitor her progress. (Figure 15.3 presents these results). We have found that more frequent measurement in lengthier psychotherapy proves unnecessary and frequently annoys patients. In most sessions, Amber will rate her urges to drink, drug, gamble, and shoplift in the last week on a 11-point visual analogue scale, where 0 = *None* and 10 = *The worst.*

In terms of treatment and relationship satisfaction, we typically rely on asking direct questions of clients following the scoring and review of the measures of symptom outcome. These begin with broad, open-ended questions, such as "How is the psychotherapy going? How are we (the relationship) doing?" Then we follow up with more focused inquiries as the patient's responses and situations dictate. For Amber, these might be on the order of "What has been the most help so far? The least helpful? How are we doing on honoring your preferences? Do you experience me being directive enough and providing enough tools? How can we improve things?"

Several standardized measures are available for assessing two or more of these crucial areas: the COMPASS (Lueger et al., 2001), the Clinical Outcomes in Routine Evaluation (CORE) system (widely used in the United Kingdom; Barkham et al., 2001), the Partners for Change Outcome Management System (PCOMS; Miller, Duncan, Sorrell, & Brown, 2005), and the Outcome Questionnaire–45 (OQ-45; Lambert et al., 2004). Our favorite, the Innerlife STS system (*www.innerlife. com*), provides both clinician and client versions, and offers both pretreatment and across-treatment information. The important point here is not the particular outcome monitoring system but that the therapist regularly collects the information. For novice therapists unaccustomed to asking these questions, particularly those related to treatment and relationship satisfaction, we strongly encourage the use of the formal measurement systems.

Treatment Process

Having now created a sufficiently empathic alliance, collected sufficient diagnostic and transdiagnostic information to create a treatment plan, and prepared the patient, we proceed in the fourth session to conducting CBT for depression and relapse prevention.

The CBT follows a fairly standard protocol: The patient is oriented to the cognitive model of depression, guided in identifying depressogenic thoughts, asked to record those thoughts between sessions, and instructed in challenging and disputing those thoughts, replacing them with healthier attributions and coping statements. The patient also agrees to behavioral activation: getting out of her home for at least 3 hours a day initially (graduating to 6 hours later in therapy) and volunteering 4 hours a week (eventually progressing to 15 hours a week). Amber is presented with a list of psychologist-recommended and research-supported self-help books on depression (Norcross et al., 2013), and decides to read *Feeling Good: The New Mood Therapy* (Burns, 1999). She later decides to purchase the accompanying workbook and often brings it to session to review the worksheets.

We devote about half of the session time to the CBT for her depression and the other half to relapse prevention (RP) for her drinking, drugging, shoplifting, and gambling. Amber has become aware in her AA meetings that relapse is the most common long-term outcome in the treatment of addictions. More urgently, Amber feels the pressure of returning to prison if she is found taking drugs or shoplifting.

RP is self-management training designed to avoid recycling and to enhance the maintenance stage (Marlatt & Donovan, 2007). Through in-session discussions and between-session readings, Amber is taught how to understand relapse as a process, identify high-risk situations, learn to cope with cravings to engage in the addictive behavior, and achieve a balanced lifestyle. Her riskiest triggers pertain to inactivity, negative mood states, and a particular subset of friends. Fortunately, the first two of these are being fruitfully addressed by the CBT for her depression. A lot of time in session is spent on actualizing the "avoid people, places, and things" slogan of her AA meetings to minimize time spent with those friends. We also practice and rehearse urge-surfing for those times when, in spite of avoiding the triggers, Amber confronts the cravings.

As an eager computer user, Amber decides to search the Web for research reviews on RP and finds a meta-analysis (which she understandably does not fully comprehend) on its effectiveness in 26 studies representing a sample of 9,504 patients (Irvin, Bowers, Dunn, & Wang, 1999). The results reveal that RP is generally effective, certainly more so than no-treatment controls, and particularly effective for alcohol and polysubstance use disorders. "Just like me," Amber smilingly acknowledges in session.

In one session, the 13th or 14th, Amber appears uncharacteristically reticent to participate in the therapeutic work. I ask about her interest, and she unconvincingly responds, "Oh, I'm just tired today." The pattern persists into the next session:

THERAPIST: You do not seem into it [psychotherapy] today. It seems different to me, like last week. Not as much energy and zip like we usually have. What are you experiencing or feeling in session of late?

AMBER: Well .. . I don't know .. . feeling annoyed.

THERAPIST: Thanks for telling me. I realize that's a hard thing for you to do—voicing your annoyance, disappointment, with someone. Good for you.

AMBER: It's hard .. . (*about a 30-second pause*) Last time [session] I think that you did not understand how hard I have been working to do all of these things. You seemed critical of me like I'm not doing enough.

THERAPIST: You're feeling that I am not appreciating your hard work, in psychotherapy and at home, and that I'm critical of your efforts .. ..

AMBER: Yeah, that's right. But now I'm afraid that I'm disappointing you or making you angry .. .

THERAPIST: Certainly not, Amber. I'm feeling the opposite: I'm pleased and proud that you took the risk of being assertive and telling me how you feel today. That's a wonderful way for us to be, but not wonderful feelings inside you. Huh?

Amber concurs that these are troubling feelings for her: Assertion triggers her fear of rejection or abandonment. When I inquire when she has felt this way before, she immediately says—literally, immediately, speaking before I finish the question—"my father." That leads into an extended process of Amber speaking about how she perceives her father to be supportive in his remarks but critical and unaccepting of her in his behavior. Without prompting, she observes, "Ohh. That's what I am saying now about you.. .."

At the end of her psychotherapy, Amber and I both nominated this session as a memorable turning point for her. She found her voice to express her displeasure with me—a male authority figure—and discovered that she was transferring or projecting feelings originally associated with her father to me (and probably others).

It is quite possible that an empathic failure or a neutral look on my part sparked her feeling, but the underlying feelings certainly belonged to her father.

Beyond that self-awareness, this session also solidified our relationship in that it demonstrated *in vivo* a way for us to repair any ruptures in the alliance (Safran, Muran, & Eubanks-Carter, 2011). The therapist can respond nondefensively, attend emphatically and directly to the relationship, understand the mutual dynamics, adjust behavior (if necessary), and attend to the patient's conflictual relationship pattern. In several studies, rupture repair positively predicts treatment outcome (Safran et al., 2011). At the end of session, Amber said that she experienced "like a breakthrough," and I felt that is was one of the good moments in our work.

In approximately 20 to 22 sessions, Amber is less depressed. Her BDI-II score has been cut in half (Figure 15.3), and her suicidal ideation has disappeared. Her urges to use are down to 0–2, accompanied by no slips in drugging, drinking, gambling, or shoplifting.

Brimming with a new-found confidence and a genuine trust in the process, Amber is ready to address her anxiety and PTSD. However, she remains conflicted and fearful. "Depression" is her favored term, and understanding "anxiety" is novel and unsettling.

There are many therapeutic means to address ambivalence and resistance, of course, but I select motivational interviewing (MI) for Amber. MI fits our therapeutic relationship, matches Amber's contemplation stage, and comes with impressive research support for large effects in a small number of sessions (Hettema, Steele, & Miller, 2005). MI expands on person-centered therapy by providing specific methods to move the patient toward behavior change (Miller & Rollnick, 2002). Following the guiding spirit of MI, I try to:

- *Express empathy* by using reflective listening to convey understanding of Amber's ambivalence about tacking the anxiety problem and PTSD, and to communicate my respect for her need for self-preservation.
- *Develop discrepancy* between Amber's conviction that she suffers only from depression and substance abuse, and the clinical findings that she also experiences high anxiety.
- *Roll with resistance* by meeting it with reflection and curiosity rather than confrontation.
- *Support self-efficacy* by actively conveying the message that the client is capable of change.

MI leverages the inherent energy that resistance brings to the therapeutic interaction, seeking to redirect it in a manner that avoids a rupture in the therapeutic relationship and allows the emergence of client change talk. Just as a canoeist would probably not paddle upstream against a strong current, so, too, the motivational interviewer does not argue with clients. Instead, I roll with the resistance by using the energy in the client to steer the interaction (Moyers & Rollnick, 2002).

MI is used to enhance Amber's intrinsic motivation to change and to explore and resolve her ambivalence. After three sessions of primarily MI methods, Amber opts to confront her anxiety and PTSD. Just as Carl Rogers predicted, clients can go a long way in a short time when provided with facilitative conditions, an accepting therapist, and considerable autonomy. MI's flexibility of use permits it to be integrated into other psychotherapies to reduce client ambivalence and to minimize their resistance (Miller & Moyers, 2005).

The majority of session time now focuses on treating Amber's anxiety-fueled avoidance and her prison-related PTSD. The cognitive restructuring for depression has already prepared her for the cognitive work of exposure therapy in her daily life. Amber decides initially to target her fear of speaking in AA meetings and driving on highways. In order to promote her choice and autonomy, I ask Amber to read descriptions of two leading treatments for PTSD: prolonged exposure with response prevention and eye movement desensitization and reprocessing (EMDR). After doing so, Amber elects to try the EMDR, reasoning that whereas prolonged exposure requires extensive daily homework, EMDR does not.

Simultaneously, she begins to read *Getting Past Your Past* (Shapiro, 2012), a recent self-help book by EMDR's developer. When Amber mentions this to me, I congratulate her for taking the initiative, and then somewhat sheepishly admit that I should have thought of recommending it to her when she expressed interest in self-help materials. In an exchange that Amber nominated at the end of her therapy as a pivotal moment, she smiles and cautions me against thinking in terms of "shoulds." I laugh for a full minute, barely able to contain myself, congratulate her on mastering cognitive therapy, then observe that the "student is becoming the master." Amber responds deadpan, "Yes, grasshopper"—an allusion to an old television series (favored by her father!) in which the seasoned master calls the eager student "grasshopper."

We introduce breathing exercises and practice self-soothing skills before undertaking the EMDR proper. Amber then undergoes five elongated sessions (90 minutes) of EMDR to address a series of traumatic events during her incarceration. Amber tolerates the sessions well and successfully uses the breathing and self-soothing between sessions for a couple of nightmares and daytime flashbacks. Her anxiety noticeably drops, as do her subjective units of distress (SUDs) ascribed to the traumatic events. At the conclusion of the five EMDR sessions, the SUDS are 1 or 2 for each event, which she deems ecologically valid.

Meanwhile, the exposure to speaking in AA meetings and highway driving continues successfully. Amber participates verbally in a frequency of the "average person," which is her goal. Driving on the highway at or above the posted speed limit becomes "no big deal anymore." Quite apart from accomplishing these goals, Amber learns the larger lesson that avoidance reduces anxiety in the short run but brings far more misery in the long run.

The *in vivo* exposure work continues but occupies less of our attention in session as Amber now tackles the amorphous borderline personality disorder. Amber and I begin slowly and didactically with education about her unassertive, approval-seeking style through bibliotherapy. I offer a selection of assertion and borderline personality self-help resources rated highly by mental health professionals (Norcross et al., 2013), again asking Amber to choose actively instead of passively accepting a prescription. She selects not one but three: *Your Perfect Right* (Alberti & Emmons, 1995), *Sometimes I Act Crazy* (Kreisman & Straus, 2006) for her parents, and *Skills Training Manual for Treating Borderline Personality Disorder* (Linehan, 1993b) for herself.

We begin with assertion training in the behavioral and feminist traditions: exploring differences between assertion and aggression; cognitive restructuring for her guilt and fear of rejection when assertive; examining gender scripts in her family and in society about power; role-playing specific responses in session; tape-recording Amber during role plays to fine-tune her voice and words; and jointly developing homework assignments with family members. Assertion is a goal not only outside therapy but within it as well. I remind Amber of our compact several months earlier when we agreed that she would move forward and take more control over the work. She agrees, and I chuckle as I remind her, "I am the grasshopper now."

Amber's underlying identity or schema as inadequate is now more fully explored. It is difficult to summarize the constellation of intersecting therapy methods used for our final 20 sessions—emotional processing, cognitive restructuring, assertion training, transference interpretations, and active practice. The emotion-focused work follows in the experiential tradition, including a few two-chair dialogues between Amber's competent part and her inadequate part. The exercise provide, in Amber's words, "clarity—I can really see how they clash and result in strange behavior." Her symptoms continue to fade away.

Amber's emerging self is now confronted with endless choices in her life and in therapy. Should she secure employment? What about her love life? Would graduate school make sense? What would she like to tackle in therapy? I participate in these discussions, of course, but ultimately Amber will decide, knowing that I support Amber and her decisions.

By way of summary, here is how Amber courageously tackles these life challenges. She decides to continue her volunteer work (now at 20 hours per week) and to pursue part-time employment. Submitting job applications forces her to explain her legal and addiction travails, which prompts considerable anxiety, but she successfully avoids the avoidant pull and does so. She obtains part-time employment. Amber begins to date casually and decides that she is not ready yet for a romantic commitment; she is charmed that several men ask to date her and two of them seek something "deeper." She will make that decision "in time—when I am ready." She explores several career options with the assistance of a vocational interest inventory I administer and, like many clients engaged in psychotherapy and AA, decides to reorient her career trajectory to a human service field. Finally, the cumulative work on assertion deficits and borderline personality disorder prompts Amber to create different boundaries with her parents and to invite them in for a few conjoint sessions to renegotiate a competent adult to competent adult connection, in contradistinction to years of parent–crazy child relating.

Fifty or so sessions into the psychotherapy, Amber notes, "We have not rated my urges [to drink, drug, gamble, shoplift] lately." I reflect for a moment and respond, "There does not seem to be any need to do so, is there?" We mutually decide to recognize Amber's progress by changing from weekly sessions to sessions every 2 or 3 weeks.

As psychotherapy winds down, and as Amber consolidates and internalizes her progress, my mind turns to her future. I gently suggest that the best protection against slipping back into depression, substance abuse, avoidance, anxiety, and patterns of inadequacy is self-nurturance. Amber thinks on this for a few weeks, then at our next session presents a self-nurturance list. This includes reducing her cigarette smoking, continuing her AA attendance and physical exercise, and a host of assertive and social pursuits.

Maintenance or booster sessions are indicated when the problems are complex, when addictions are present, when the patient is highly impaired, and when a personality disorder is present. Those features certainly apply to Amber, at least the "old Amber," and constitute strong indicators of the tendency to relapse. For these reasons, Amber and I decide on a schedule of monthly maintenance sessions for several months.

Typical Problems

For patients undergoing integrative therapy, the typical problem entails the burden of a lot of work within and between sessions. As purposefully more inclusive and ambitious, integrative treatment probably asks more of the client. We routinely collaborate on homework—because the research strongly supports it (Kazantzis, Whittington, & Dattilio, 2010), and because Amber explicitly requested it. In collaboration with the client, the therapist must properly pace or "dose" the amount of work and ensure that the client's motivational distress remains motivating, not disabling. With Amber, the recurrent question was "Does this feel challenging but not overwhelming for you?"

For therapists conducting integrative therapy, a common problem involves retreat into their standard relationship style and default treatment method. When the research advises a more directive stance, for example, therapists may begin in a directive way but then gradually slip back into their customary less-directive stance. Or as another example, therapists more accustomed to working with patients in the action stage will start in a more exploratory stance compatible with the patient's contemplation stage, but subsequently provide action-oriented processes well before the patient is ready to plunge into the action stage. Periodic reevaluations, ongoing client feedback, and therapists' self-awareness to fit the patient (not only themselves) tends to correct these lapses.

For neophyte therapists, the core challenge in our approach is to avoid the extremes: overemphasizing either the treatment method or the healing relationship, adhering to either a rule-bound treatment manual or an intuitive seat-of-the-pants syncretism, relying exclusively on the empirical research or on participant preferences. We strive for balanced flexibility, the Aristotelian mean, that systematically incorporates all of these without succumbing to the human tendency of polarization. This can prove problematic for psychotherapists trained to think in either–or, binary ways about psychotherapy. It can also be daunting in a multidisorderd patient, like Amber, with multiple goals sequenced over time. "One treatment fits all" becomes an attractive, easier alternative to the hard work of tailoring psychotherapy to the unique individual and singular situation.

Outcome and Prognosis

Over the course of 50 weekly individual sessions and several maintenance sessions, Amber impressively reduced her depression and maintained her abstinence. Her depression consistently declined over time, as shown in Figure 15.3. The largest drop in her anxiety scores occurred between weeks 26 and 32, when the EMDR was conducted. Her cravings to drink, drug, and shoplift gravitated to 0 on the 0- to 10 scale after 3 months of psychotherapy, but her urge to gamble would periodically spike to the 3- or 4-point range. She did not behaviorally succumb to those temptations, however. Symptomatically, Amber's test scores were in the normal range, and she was better than ever.

Interpersonally, the patient achieved impressive gains as well. She was less impulsive, more emotionally self-regulating, more self-soothing, and increasingly assertive and expressive. She certainly no longer met the diagnostic criteria for borderline personality disorder, but she was susceptible to some behavioral avoidance and abandonment fears in her new dating relationships. She mourned the years lost to drugs and addressed her existential guilt and shame, as much as most humans can.

Her medications were gradually halved over the year of our psychological treatment, from 80 mg to 40 mg of fluoxetine and from 60 mg to 20 mg of BuSpar. She continues on those medications as maintenance with plans eventually to reduce them. And Amber continues to attend AA meetings twice a week and monthly maintenance psychotherapy sessions, where her most recent BDI-II and BAI scores were both 3, well within normal limits.

Despite all of these positive outcomes, as with most cases in psychotherapy, not all of Amber's goals were realized. She continues to smoke cigarettes (a maximum of 3 per day), and full-time employment has proven elusive because her felony record leaves her ineligible for many positions. She does work the equivalent of three-quarters time between two jobs and is applying to graduate school in a human service profession. And Amber is prone to occasional bouts of anxiety and avoidance when confronting new situations.

From all accounts, the prognosis is promising indeed. She is the "new" Amber as I phrased it, or, as she memorably put it, the Amber "2.0."

Case Commentary

We have chosen to illustrate our treatment approach for depression and substance abuse with a complex, multidisordered woman. As is typical, she suffered for many years and from more than two discrete disorders. The chronic course of comorbid disorders increases the need for integrative treatment, including, in Amber's case, individual psychotherapy, pharmacotherapy, support groups, self-help resources, and a few conjoint family sessions. The high rates of comorbidity of personality disorders and PTSD among substance abusers complicates psychotherapy and increases the need to sequence treatment methods and goals thoughtfully.

The psychotherapist can accept some credit for the salubrious outcomes in this case, but Amber deserves the lion's share. She worked hard to master new skills, prevent relapses, and intentionally expose herself to anxiety-provoking situations. She was a bright, motivated, and psychologically minded client who progressed from the contemplation stage to the action stage and ultimately to long-term maintenance. All these patient features predict more successful outcomes in all forms of psychotherapy.

Several circumstances also proved fortuitous. Amber participated regularly in AA meetings, was motivated by the "sobering" experiences of prison, and was supported by her parents, who contributed to payment for 50 sessions of psychotherapy. Fewer sessions with a therapist working in a public clinic would probably not have yielded the same benefits. Although Amber was not favorably impressed by her previous therapy experiences, it was clear the she had benefited from the so-cialization into psychotherapy and perhaps from moving from earlier stages of change to later stages before undertaking this course of treatment.

Where our integrative approach was probably most effective was in fitting or tailoring the therapy relationship and treatment methods specifically to Amber. The treatment proceeded stepwise in accordance with the research evidence, the patient's preferences, stage of change, and her other transdiagnostic characteristics. The therapist systematically addressed depression, substance abuse, and others disorders by combining therapy methods (those traditionally associated with person-centered, behavioral, cognitive, exposure, feminist, psychodynamic, and experiential traditions) and healing resources (psychotherapy, pharmacotherapy, self-help, and AA spirituality) in a seamless and responsive manner.

Predictors of Success and Failure

No therapy or therapist is immune to failure. It is at such times that experienced clinicians often wonder whether therapy methods from orientations other than their own might more usefully have been included in the treatment, or whether another orientation's strength in dealing with the particular problems might complement the therapist's own orientational weakness. Integrative therapies assume that each orientation has its particular domain of expertise and that these domains can be linked to maximize their effectiveness (Pinsof, 1995). In this way, rival therapy systems are increasingly viewed not as adversaries but as welcome partners (Landsman, 1974); not as contradictory but as complementary.

When integrative therapy fails, it may be a result of failure to follow the guiding integrative principles, a dearth of skill in implementing a particular treatment, a poor fit between the particular patient and the particular therapist, or inaccurate evaluation of the patient dimensions that indicate the optimal therapist style and objectives. Each of these alternatives should be considered when a patient is not accomplishing his/her goals at a rate expected among similar patients. Our approach embraces an initial evaluation of the transdiagnostic patient dimensions, as well as periodic review of treatment processes to ensure that the therapy methods are a good fit as defined by the research. Finally, formal feedback about progress is helpful and often initiates a discussion of things that slow or block progress and of procedures that may help move through such impasses.

In the past few years, we have begun sharing with the patient the results of serial testing (e.g., that presented in Figure 15.3) or the Innerlife STS progress graphs to illustrate points of impasse and success.

CONCLUSIONS

Psychotherapy is a treatment method and a healing relationship fit to the individual patient and context. In this chapter, we have endeavored to demonstrate how psychotherapists can do exactly that for patients suffering from depression and substance abuse, thereby increasing treatment effectiveness and efficiency. Such treatment selection must be systematic, flexible, and evidence-based. For these reasons, integrative psychotherapy seems particularly indicated for complex patients with comorbid disorders, such as Amber, and for patients whom pure form or monotherapies have failed or been only partially successful.

Our chapter presentation and case illustration may convey the impression that integrative psychotherapy can be thoroughly planned from the beginning, but clinical reality is not so accommodating. Although we try to formulate the case and plan treatment at the outset, we expect and welcome the invariable turn of events. Treatment selection is nonlinear and dynamic; a behavior or change at one point in time impacts all subsequent behavior. "You never know what to expect the next session" is one of the fascinations of psychotherapy. We are continuously moving with the patient and evolving with the unanticipated, but we do so informed by clinical experience and research evidence.

This chapter has outlined our integrative therapy and detailed its step-by-step process of systematic treatment selection in substance abuse and depression. This process applies research knowledge from multiple theoretical orientations on both diagnostic and transdiagnostic patient characteristics to the optimal choice of technical and relational methods. Such a therapy posits that many treatment methods and interpersonal stances have a valuable place in the repertoire of the contemporary psychotherapist. Their particular and differential place can be determined through outcome research, seasoned experience, and positioning the client at the center of the clinical enterprise. Integrative therapy offers the evidence-based relationships, treatments, and responsiveness to meet the multifarious needs of individual patients and their unique contexts well into the 21st century.

REFERENCES

Alberti, R., & Emmons, M. (1995). *Your perfect right: A guide to assertive living* (7th ed.). San Luis Obispo, CA: Impact.

American Psychiatric Association. (2013). *Diagnostic and statistical manual of mental disorders* (5th ed.). Arlington, VA: Author.

Antonuccio, D. O. (1995). Psychotherapy for depression: No stronger medicine. *American Psychologist, 50,* 450–452.

Antonuccio, D. O., Danton, W. G., & DeNelsky, G. Y. (1995). Psychotherapy versus medication for depression: Challenging the conventional wisdom with data. *Professional Psychology: Research and Practice, 26,* 574–585.

Barkham, M., Margison, F., Leach, C., Lucock, M., Mellor-Clark, J., Evans, C., et al. (2001). Service profiling and outcomes benchmarking using the CORE_OM: Toward practice-based evidence in the psychological therapies. *Journal of Consulting and Clinical Psychology, 69,* 184–196.

Beutler, L. E. (2009). Making science matter in clinical practice: Redefining psychotherapy. *Clinical Psychology: Science and Practice, 16,* 301–317.

Beutler, L. E., & Clarkin, J. (1990). *Systematic treatment selection: Toward targeted therapeutic interventions.* New York: Brunner/Mazel.

Beutler, L. E., Clarkin, J., & Bongar, B. (2000). *Guidelines for the systematic treatment of the depressed patient.* New York: Oxford University Press.

Beutler, L. E., & Harwood, T. M. (2000). *Prescriptive psychotherapy: A practical guide to systematic treatment selection.* New York: Oxford University Press.

Beutler, L. E., Harwood, T. M., Alimohamed, S., & Malik, M. (2002). Functional impairment and coping style. In J. C. Norcross (Ed.), *Psychotherapy relationships that work* (pp. 145–173). New York: Oxford University Press.

Beutler, L. E., Harwood, T. M., Kimpara, S., Verdirame, D., & Blau, K. (2011). Coping style. In J. C. Norcross (Ed.), *Psychotherapy relationships that work* (2nd ed., pp. 336–353). New York: Oxford University Press.

Beutler, L. E., Harwood, T. M., Michelson, A., Song, X., & Holman, J. (2011). Reactance/resistance. In J. C. Norcross (Ed.), *Psychotherapy relationships that work* (2nd ed., pp. 261–278). New York: Oxford University Press.

Beutler, L. E., & Malik, M. L. (2002). Diagnosis and treatment guidelines: The example of depression. In L. E. Beutler & M. L. Malik (Eds.), *Rethinking the DSM* (pp. 251–278). Washington, DC: American Psychological Association.

Beutler, L. E., Moleiro, C., Malik, M., Harwood, T. M., Romanelli, R., Gallagher-Thompson, D., et al. (2003). A comparison of the Dodo, EST, and ATI factors among comorbid stimulant-dependent, depressed patients. *Clinical Psychology and Psychotherapy, 10,* 69–85.

Burns, D. (1999). *Feeling good: The new mood therapy* (rev. ed.). New York: Avon.

Burlingame, G., McClendon, D. T., Alonso, J. (2011). Group cohesion. In J. C. Norcross (Ed.), *Psychotherapy relationships that work* (2nd ed., pp. 110–131). New York: Oxford University Press.

Castonguay, L. G., & Beutler, L. E. (Eds.). (2006). *Principles of therapeutic change that work*. New York: Oxford University Press.

Clarkin, J. F., & Levy, K. N. (2004). The influence of client variables on psychotherapy. In M. J. Lambert (Ed.), *Bergin and Garfield's handbook of psychotherapy and behavior change* (5th ed., pp. 194–226). New York: Wiley.

Cohen, J. (1988). *Statistical power analysis for the behavioral sciences* (2nd ed.). Hillsdale, NJ: Erlbaum.

Cuijpers, P., van Straten, A., Andersson, G., & van Oppen, P. (2008). Psychotherapy for depression in adults: A meta-analysis of comparative outcome studies. *Journal of Consulting and Clinical Psychology, 76*, 909–922.

Cuijpers, P., van Straten, A., Schuurmans, J., van Oppen, P., Hollon, S. D., & Andersson, G. (2010). Psychotherapy for chronic major depression and dysthymia: A meta-analysis. *Clinical Psychology Review, 30*, 51–62.

DeRubeis, R. J., Hollon, S. D., Amsterdam, J. D., Shelton, R. C., Young, P. R., Salomon, R. M., et al. (2005). Cognitive therapy vs medications in the treatment of moderate to severe depression. *Archives of General Psychiatry, 62*, 409–416.

Elliott, R., Bohart, A. C., Watson, J. C., & Greenberg, L. S. (2011). Empathy. In J. C. Norcross (Ed.), *Psychotherapy relationships that work* (2nd ed., pp. 132–152). New York: Oxford University Press.

Eysenck, H. J. (1970). A mish-mash of theories. *International Journal of Psychiatry, 9*, 140–146.

Farber, B. A., & Doolin, E. M. (2011). Positive regard. In J. C. Norcross (Ed.), *Psychotherapy relationships that works* (2nd ed., pp. 168–186). New York: Oxford University Press.

Friedlander, M. L., Escudero, V., Heatherington, L., & Diamond, G. M. (2011). Alliance in couple and family therapy. In J. C. Norcross (Ed.), *Psychotherapy relationships that work* (2nd ed., pp. 92–109). New York: Oxford University Press.

Halford, G. S., Baker, R., McCredden, J. E., & Bain, J. D. (2005). How many variables can humans process? *Psychological Science, 16*, 70–76.

Harwood, T. M., Beutler, L. E., & Groth-Marnat, G. (Eds.). (2011). *Integrated assessment of adult personality* (3rd ed.). New York: Guilford Press.

Hettema, J., Steele, J., & Miller, W. R. (2005). Motivational interviewing. *Annual Review of Clinical Psychology, 1*, 91–111.

Hollon, S. D. (1990). Cognitive therapy and pharmacotherapy for depression. *Psychiatric Annals, 20*, 249–258.

Horvath, A. O., Del Re, A., Flückiger, C., & Symonds, D. (2011). Alliance in individual psychotherapy. In J. C. Norcross (Ed.), *Psychotherapy relationships that work* (2nd ed., pp. 25–69). New York: Oxford University Press.

Housley, J., & Beutler, L. E. (2007). *Treating victims of mass disaster and terrorism*. Cambridge, MA: Hogrefe & Huber.

Irvin, J. E., Bowers, C. A., Dunn, M. E., & Wang, M. C. (1999). Efficacy of relapse prevention: A meta-analytic review. *Journal of Consulting and Clinical Psychology, 67*, 563–570.

Kazantzis, N., Whittington, C., & Dattilio, F. (2010). Meta-analysis of homework effects in cognitive and behavioral therapy: A replication and extension. *Clinical Psychology: Science and Practice, 17*, 144–156.

Kessler, R. C., Berglund, P., Demler, O., Jin, R., Merikangas, K. R., & Walters, E. E. (2005). Lifetime prevalence and age-of-onset distributions of DSM-IV disorders in the National Comorbidity Survey Replication. *Archives of General Psychiatry, 62*, 593–602.

Kreisman, J. J., & Straus, H. (2006). *Sometimes I act crazy: Living with a borderline personality disorder*. Hoboken, NJ: Wiley.

Lambert, M. J., Morton, J. J., Hatfield, D., Harmon, C., Hamilton, S., Reid, R. C., et al. (2004). *Administration and scoring manual for the Outcome Questionnaire–45*. Salt Lake City, UT: OQ Measures.

Lambert, M. J., & Shimokawa, K. (2011). Collecting client feedback. In J. C. Norcross (Ed.), *Psychotherapy relationships that work* (2nd ed., pp. 203–223). New York: Oxford University Press.

Landsman, J. T. (1974, August). *Not an adversity but a welcome diversity*. Paper presented at the annual meeting of the American Psychological Association, New Orleans, LA.

Linehan, M. M. (1993a). *Cognitive-behavioral treatment of borderline personality disorder*. New York: Guilford Press.

Linehan, M. M. (1993b). *Skills training manual for treating borderline personality disorder*. New York: Guilford Press.

Lueger, R. J., Howard, K. I., Martinovich Z., Lutz, W., Anderson, E. E., & Grissom, G. (2001). Assessing treatment progress of individual clients using expected treatment response models. *Journal of Consulting and Clinical Psychology, 69*, 150–158.

Marlatt, G. A., & Donovan, D. M. (Eds.). (2007). *Relapse prevention: Maintenance strategies in the treatment of addictive behaviors* (2nd ed., pp. 267–271). New York: Guilford Press.

Miller, S. D., Duncan, B. L., Sorrell, R., & Brown, G. S. (2005). The Partners for Change Outcome System. *Journal of Clinical Psychology: In Session, 61*, 199–208.

Miller, W. R., & Moyers, T. B. (2005). Motivational interviewing. In G. P. Koocher, J. C. Norcross, & S. S. Hill (Eds.), *Psychologists' desk reference* (2nd ed., pp. 267–271). New York: Oxford University Press.

Moyers, T. B., & Rollnick, S. (2002). A motivational interviewing perspective on resistance. *Journal of Clinical Psychology: In Session, 58*(2), 185–193.

Miller, W. R., & Rollnick, S. (2002). *Motivational interviewing: Preparing people for change* (2nd ed.). New York: Guilford Press.

Norcross, J. C. (2010). The therapeutic relationship. In B. L. Duncan, S. D. Miller, B. E. Wampold, & M. A. Hubble (Eds.), *Heart and soul of change* (2nd ed., pp. 113–142). Washington, DC: American Psychological Association.

Norcross, J. C. (Ed.). (2011). *Psychotherapy relationships that work* (2nd ed.). New York: Oxford University Press

Norcross, J. C. (2013). *Changeology: Five steps to realizing your goals and resolutions.* New York: Simon & Schuster.

Norcross, J. C., & Beutler, L. E. (1997). Determining the therapeutic relationship of choice in brief therapy. In J. N. Butcher (Ed.), *Personality assessment in managed care: A practitioner's guide.* New York: Oxford University Press.

Norcross, J. C., Beutler, L. E., & Levant, R. F. (Eds.). (2006). *Evidence-based practices in mental health: Debate and dialogue on the fundamental questions.* Washington, DC: American Psychological Association.

Norcross, J. C., Campbell, L. M., Grohol, J. M., Santrock, J. W., Selagea, F., & Sommer, R. (2013). *Self-help that works* (4th ed.). New York: Oxford University Press.

Norcross, J. C., & Goldfried, M. R. (Eds.). (2005). *Handbook of psychotherapy integration* (2nd ed.). New York: Oxford University Press.

Norcross, J. C., & Karpiak, C. P. (2012). Clinical psychologists in the 2010s: Fifty years of the APA Division of Clinical Psychology. *Clinical Psychology: Science and Practice, 19*, 1–12.

Norcross, J. C., Krebs, P. M., & Prochaska, J. O. (2011). Stages of change. In J. C. Norcross (Ed.), *Psychotherapy relationships that work* (2nd ed., pp. 279–300). New York: Oxford University Press.

Osler, W. (1906). *Aequanimatas.* New York: McGraw-Hill.

Paul, G. L. (1967). Strategy of outcome research in psychotherapy. *Journal of Consulting Psychology, 31*, 109–118.

Pinsof, W. M. (1995). *Integrative problem-centered therapy: A synthesis of biological, individual, and family therapies.* New York: Basic Books.

Prochaska, J. O., & Norcross, J. C. (2013). *Systems of psychotherapy: A transtheoretical analysis* (8th ed.). Pacific Grove, CA: Brooks/Cole.

Rogers, C. R. (1957). The necessary and sufficient conditions of therapeutic personality change. *Journal of Consulting Psychology, 21*, 95–103.

Rosen, C. S. (2000). Is the sequencing of change processes by stage consistent across health problems?: A meta-analysis. *Health Psychology, 19*, 593–604.

Safran, J. D., Muran, J. C., & Eubanks-Carter, C. (2011). Repairing alliance ruptures. In J. C. Norcross (Ed.), *Psychotherapy relationships that work* (2nd ed., pp. 224–238). New York: Oxford University Press.

Shapiro, F. (2012). *Getting past your past: Take control of your life with self-help techniques from EMDR therapy.* New York: Rodale.

Shirk, S. R., & Karver, M. (2011). Alliance in child and adolescent therapy. In J. C. Norcross (Ed.), *Psychotherapy relationships that work* (2nd ed., pp. 70–91). New York: Oxford University Press.

Smith, T. B., Rodriguez, M. D., & Bernal, G. (2011). Culture. In J. C. Norcross (Ed.), *Psychotherapy relationships that work* (2nd ed., pp. 316–335). New York: Oxford University Press.

Swift, J. K., Callahan, J. L., & Vollmer, B. M. (2011). Preferences. In J. C. Norcross (Ed.), *Psychotherapy relationships that work* (2nd ed., pp. 301–315). New York: Oxford University Press.

Tryon, G. S., & Winograd, G. (2011). Goal consensus and collaboration. In J. C. Norcross (Ed.), *Psychotherapy relationships that work* (2nd ed., pp. 153–167). New York: Oxford University Press.

Wolitzky, D. L. (2011). Psychoanalytic theories of psychotherapy. In J. C. Norcross, G. R. VandenBos, & D. K. Freedheim (Eds.), *History of psychotherapy* (2nd ed., pp. 65–100). Washington, DC: American Psychological Association.

CHAPTER 16

Treatment of Sleep Disturbance

KATHERINE A. KAPLAN
ALLISON G. HARVEY

Perhaps the best-kept secret among health and mental health practitioners everywhere is the marked superiority of brief psychological treatments for insomnia compared to popular and frequently advertised medications. With approximately 6% of members of the adult population suffering from insomnia to the degree that they meet diagnostic criteria, and as many as 12% reporting that insomnia interferes significantly with their daytime activities, the problem is significant and most often poorly treated. Insomnia very frequently accompanies other psychological disorders, and recent evidence indicates that insomnia predates and may contribute to or even cause these comorbid disorders, which is all the more reason why every health and mental health practitioner should be aware of the cutting-edge brief interventions presented in this chapter. Indeed, the American Academy of Sleep Medicine recommends these protocols as a first-line treatment for people with all forms of insomnia, including those currently using hypnotic drugs. Among the leaders in this burgeoning field, Kaplan and Harvey outline a state-of-the-art integrated behavioral and cognitive approach with strong evidence for both efficacy and durability that should be in the armamentarium of every health professional.—D. H. B.

Sleep disorders are common and associated with considerable morbidity and functional impairment. In this chapter we focus on insomnia, given its high prevalence and public health impact. We also briefly discuss hypersomnolence disorder given the rising possible role of psychological treatments for patients with this disorder. A wide range of other sleep disorders, which are beyond the scope of this chapter, are each prevalent and impairing. For example, obstructive sleep apnea/hypopnea involves transient closure of the upper airway during sleep that results in pauses in breathing, leading to daytime sleepiness and cardiovascular problems. Restless legs syndrome involves an involuntary urge to move one's legs during sleep that leads to partial or full awakenings, resulting in sleep fragmentation and daytime sleepiness. It is important for clinicians to have a working knowledge of these and other sleep disorders, as well as to know when to refer patients to a sleep center, neurologist, or other health professional (Kryger, Roth, & Dement, 2010).

Insomnia is a prevalent sleep disturbance that involves difficulty with falling asleep, staying asleep, or waking too early in the morning. It is associated with considerable functional impairment and health-related costs. Insomnia is often comorbid with, and predicts the development of, numerous psychological and medical conditions. As such, insomnia represents an important target for intervention. This chapter begins with a brief overview of human sleep, along with diagnostic and theoretical considerations, because this knowledge provides the basis for delivering cognitive-behavioral therapy for insomnia (CBT-I), which is the focus of this chapter.

SLEEP AND INSOMNIA

Sleep Stages

Human sleep can be divided into (1) non–rapid eye movement (or NREM) sleep that can be subdivided into three stages (N1, N2, and N3) through which sleep progressively deepens, and (2) rapid eye movement (or REM) sleep. In adults, each NREM–REM cycle spans 70 to 120 minutes (Kryger et al., 2010). NREM sleep is thought to be important for conservation of energy and restoration. This phase of sleep is associated with the most rapid cell division in some tissues, as well as increased protein synthesis (Kryger et al., 2010). The functions of REM sleep are understood to include a role in learning (Karni, Tanne, Rubenstien, Askenasy, & Sagi, 1994) and in the unlearning of irrelevant information (Crick & Mitchison, 1983), as well as memory consolidation (Walker & Stickgold, 2006), emotional processing, and mood/emotion regulation (Yoo, Gujar, Hu, Jolesz, & Walker, 2007). It is well established that sleep deprivation has detrimental effects in many domains of health (Zee & Turek, 2006), including the immune system, the neuroendocrine system, and the cardiovascular system (Banks & Dinges, 2010). Given these important functions, disorders of sleep have major public health implications.

Two-Process Model of Sleep

The two-process model of sleep regulation (Borbely, 1982) is important in that it underpins the treatment we describe later. In fact, many clinicians describe this model to clients as part of the rationale for delivering stimulus control and sleep restriction described below. The model proposes that sleep and wakefulness are dependent on two processes, a homeostatic process and a circadian process (Achermann & Borbely, 2010). The homeostatic process influences sleep likelihood. Sleep pressure increases with time spent awake, resulting in an increased tendency to sleep when a person has been sleep-deprived, and a decreased tendency to sleep after having had a substantial amount of sleep or a substantial nap. The circadian rhythm is an internal biological clock that operates on roughly a 24-hour basis. It is responsible for variations in melatonin, temperature, and other biological functions, including levels of alertness throughout the day (Lack & Bootzin, 2003). These two processes work together such that sleep is likely to occur when sleep pressure (the homeostatic process) is high and level of alertness (the circadian process) is relatively low. Thus, if a person naps in the afternoon, he/she may have difficulty falling asleep that evening because homeostatic sleep pressure is low; likewise, if a person goes to bed early following a poor night of sleep, even if sleep pressure is high, circadian arousal may prevent sleep onset from occurring.

Some, but not all, studies have found impaired sleep homeostasis in persons with insomnia (e.g., Besset, Villemin, Tafti, & Billiard, 1998; Stepanski, Zorick, Roehrs, & Roth, 2000). There is a similar lack of consensus in the research about whether circadian rhythm abnormalities play a role in insomnia. Environmentally induced phase shifts, such as those occurring as a result of shift work or jet lag, can cause acute insomnia. There is also evidence that hyperarousal, a central notion in theories of insomnia that we discuss below, may not be a 24-hour issue for some but rather may fluctuate according to circadian influences (Perlis, Smith, & Pigeon, 2005).

Sleep across the Lifespan

Sleep changes across the lifespan. This is very important because it impacts therapists' expectations of sleep outcomes when working with clients of different ages. With age, slow-wave sleep decreases, while lighter sleep and awakenings become more common across the night. Moreover, both circadian and homeostatic processes are influenced by age. For example, the circadian system grows increasingly less sensitive to *zeitgebers* such as melatonin and morning light with age (Van Someren, 2000). Throughout adolescence, there is a well-documented circadian shift in favor of later bedtimes and rise times, with a more slowly building homeostatic pressure to fall asleep (Jenni, Achermann, & Carskadon, 2005). This pattern can result in initial insomnia (difficulty falling asleep at night). In middle-to-older adulthood, circadian shifts can again favor of early bedtimes and rise times, resulting in terminal insomnia (early morning awakening with difficulty falling back asleep; Ancoli-Israel, 2009). Along with circadian rhythms, the homeostatic process also shows age-dependent changes across the lifespan. Individuals in their 60s and 70s showed reduced homeostatic pressure to sleep and achieve less total sleep time (TST) relative to members of a comparison group in their 20s (Klerman & Dijk, 2008).

THE INSOMNIA DIAGNOSIS

The following section describes diagnostic considerations, reviews prevalence and comorbidity, and presents several models of insomnia that have been influential in conceptualizing CBT-I treatment targets.

There are three main classification systems for sleep disorders: the second edition of the *International Classification of Sleep Disorders* (ICSD; American Academy of Sleep Medicine, 2005), the Research Diagnostic Criteria (RDC; Edinger et al., 2004), and the *Diagnostic and Statistical Manual of Mental Disorders* (DSM-5; American Psychiatric Association, 2013). Within DSM-5 criteria, a diagnosis of insomnia may be given when there is a subjective complaint of trouble falling or staying asleep. These difficulties must be associated with daytime impairment and must not be better accounted for by another medical or psychiatric condition.

The insomnia diagnostic criteria described earlier have been clarified with quantitative criteria. The quantitative criteria require that self-reported sleep-onset latency (SOL) and/or wake after sleep onset (WASO) must be greater than 30 minutes for at least 3 nights per week over a period of at least 6 months (Lichstein, Durrence, Taylor, Bush, & Riedel, 2003). Note that self-reports of insomnia complaints are sufficient for the diagnosis, without objective evidence for sleep disturbance (see "Assessment" below).

Insomnia Prevalence and Comorbidity

It is estimated that about 6% of the general adult population meets diagnostic criteria for a formal diagnosis of insomnia based on DSM-IV-TR criteria. Approximately 33% of the general population reports some significant symptoms of insomnia. Additionally, as many as 12% of individuals in the general adult population suffer from the daytime sequelae of sleep disturbance (Hohagen et al., 1993; Ohayon, 2002). More recent surveys suggest that health-related costs of insomnia are considerable, regardless of the diagnostic system used to define it (Roth et al., 2011).

Because insomnia can be associated with a wide range of medical illnesses and psychological disorders,

the previous DSM edition (i.e., DSM-IV-TR; American Psychiatric Association, 2000) made distinctions between "primary" and "secondary" or comorbid insomnia. The distinction between primary and secondary insomnia was blurred, however, by epidemiological research suggesting that insomnia may predate, and predict, psychological disorders (Breslau, Roth, Rosenthal, & Andreski, 1996; Ford & Kamerow, 1989). Indeed, a National Institutes of Health (NIH; 2005) state-of-the-science conference concluded that the term "secondary" should be replaced with "comorbid" on the basis of evidence that insomnia comorbid with another disorder likely contributes to the maintenance of the disorder (Harvey, 2001; Smith, Huang, & Manber, 2005). These conclusions were recognized in DSM-5, which does not distinguish between "primary" and "secondary" insomnia, but has only one "insomnia disorder."

For older adults, insomnia is often accompanied by medical illnesses, which may complicate issues of assessment and treatment, further compounding burden and cost (Morin et al., 2006). In a large epidemiological study, Ford and Kamerow (1989) found that there is approximately a 50% comorbidity rate between insomnia and other psychological disorders or medical illnesses; other studies have yielded a rate as high as 75% (Lichstein, 2000). In cases of comorbid insomnia, additional empirical and clinical attention may be especially important because there appears to be a cyclical influence of sleep disturbance and medical illness or psychological disorders, with worsening sleep problems leading to a decline in general health and increased psychiatric symptoms that, in turn, worsen sleep problems. Fortunately, evidence suggests that insomnia responds to CBT-I treatment even if the accompanying disorder is not under control (Rybarczyk, Lopez, Schelble, & Stepanski, 2005). Smith and colleagues (2005) concluded that treatment effects are generally moderate to large for CBT-I administered in the context of accompanying disorders or illnesses, and are comparable to treatment effects in primary insomnia.

Models of Insomnia

This section begins with a discussion of an influential overarching framework, the Spielman model. We then move on to describe several behavioral, cognitive, and combination models of insomnia that help to explain particular facets of the disorder that should be addressed and treated in CBT-I.

Spielman's Three-Factor Model

This is a diathesis–stress model often referred to as the three-factor or the three-P model. According to Spielman, Caruso, and Glovinsky (1987), acute or short-term insomnia occurs as a result of *predisposing* factors (e.g., traits) and *precipitating* factors (e.g., life stressors). This acute form can then develop into a chronic or longer-term disorder as a result of *perpetuating* factors (e.g., poor coping strategies). Predisposing factors (e.g., a tendency to worry) constitute a vulnerability for insomnia, and this vulnerability remains across the life of the disorder. Precipitating factors trigger acute insomnia, but their influence tends to wane over time. In contrast, perpetuating factors take hold of and maintain insomnia. CBT-I targets these perpetuating factors, seeking to reduce the additive effects of predisposing, precipitating, and perpetuating factors below the threshold for insomnia diagnosis.

Behavioral Models

One of the most important behavioral models for insomnia is the stimulus control model (Bootzin, 1972). It is based on the conditioning principle that insomnia occurs when the bed or bedroom ceases to be paired specifically with sleep, but has become paired with many possible responses (e.g., being awake and anxious about not sleeping). As will become evident later in this chapter, this theory has led to the development of "stimulus control," an intervention with strong efficacy (Morin et al., 2006).

Cognitive Models

Some of the earliest research on cognitive processes in insomnia noted that individuals with insomnia tended to overestimate wakefulness and underestimate TST (Bixler, Kales, Leo, & Slye, 1973; Carskadon et al., 1976), and researchers began to explore the role of cognitive arousal in insomnia (Borkovec, 1982; Lichstein & Rosenthal, 1980). Seminal work in the 1990s highlighted the importance of unhelpful beliefs about sleep (Morin, 1993) and delineated the content of presleep intrusive thoughts (Watts, Coyle, & East, 1994; Wicklow & Espie, 2000). The last decade has ushered in an increase in empirical attention to other cognitive mechanisms in insomnia, including attention to threat and the use of safety behaviors to allay perceived threats (Espie, 2002; Harvey, 2005; Harvey, Tang, & Browning, 2005).

One cognitive model of insomnia aims to specify the cognitive processes that serve to perpetuate insomnia (Harvey, 2002a) and represents an important component of CBT-I as outlined here. According to this conceptualization, contributors to the maintenance of insomnia include the following cascade of cognitive processes that operate at night and during the day: (1) worry and rumination, (2) selective attention and monitoring, (3) misperception of sleep and daytime deficits, (4) dysfunctional beliefs about sleep (based on Morin, 1993), and (5) counterproductive safety behaviors that serve to maintain beliefs. Many of the specific predictions generated by this model have been empirically tested, leading to refinement of the model (Harvey, 2005) and a new cognitive therapy treatment approach that has preliminary support in an open trial (Harvey, Sharpley, Ree, Stinson, & Clark, 2007).

Combination Models

Morin's (1993) cognitive-behavioral model of insomnia incorporates cognitive, temporal, and environmental variables as both precipitating and perpetuating factors, with hyperarousal as the key precipitating factor of insomnia. Conditioning can then exacerbate this arousal. For example, a person may associate temporal (e.g., bedtime routines) and environmental (e.g., bedroom) stimuli with fear of being unable to sleep. Worry and rumination may then result. Additional perpetuating factors may ensue, including, as in the cognitive model, daytime fatigue, worry, and emotional distress about sleep loss and maladaptive habits (e.g., excessive time in bed).

In summary, adequate treatment of insomnia targets both cognitive and behavioral processes to address their mutually maintaining effects. Each of the models reviewed earlier has been influential in conceptualizing the insomnia diagnosis and identifying treatment targets. In the next section, we review evidence for the effectiveness of CBT-I as a multicomponent treatment for insomnia.

EVIDENCE FOR CBT-I TREATMENT

CBT-I has been established as an effective treatment in multiple meta-analyses (e.g., Irwin, Cole, & Nicassio, 2006; Montgomery & Dennis, 2003; Morin, Culbert, & Schwartz, 1994; Murtagh & Greenwood, 1995) and in a review by the Standards of Practice Committee of the American Academy of Sleep Medicine (Chesson et al., 1999; Morin et al., 1999), which has been updated (Morin et al., 2006).

A number of randomized controlled trials (RCTs) have compared one or more components of CBT-I to each other and/or to placebo. A recent review found CBT-I to be highly effective and to have sustainable gains over long-term follow-up, up to 24 months in adult and older adult samples (Morin et al., 2006). This review used the American Psychological Association's Society of Clinical Psychology criteria for well-supported, empirically based treatments (Chambless & Hollon, 1998) and concluded that these criteria are met by stimulus control, paradoxical intention, relaxation, sleep restriction approaches, and the administration of multiple components in the form of CBT-I. The sleep hygiene intervention alone has not been found to be effective as a treatment for insomnia. Cognitive therapy for insomnia is a promising new approach, but randomized trials are still needed for it to meet criteria for an empirically supported treatment.

There are multiple classes of medications, both prescribed and over the counter, that can be used to treat insomnia (Kryger et al., 2010), including benzodiazepines, nonbenzodiazepine hypnotics (e.g., zolpidem, zaleplon, and eszopiclone), antidepressants (e.g., trazodone and doxepin), and over-the-counter antihistamines (e.g., diphenhydramine and doxylamine). However, there is evidence that nonpharmacological interventions for insomnia are more acceptable to clients (Morin, Gaulier, Barry, & Kowatch, 1992) and produce more durable effects (Morin et al., 2009; Sivertsen et al., 2006) than do hypnotic medications alone. In the case of comorbid insomnia, the optimal intervention would alleviate insomnia without causing adverse interactions with other prescribed medication; therefore, a nonpharmacological intervention may be the best choice for these cases of insomnia (Harvey, 2008).

In summary, CBT-I appears to be an efficacious and promising intervention to address sleep disturbance, particularly in treating comorbid insomnia. In the next section, we discuss treatment objectives, setting, and client–therapist variables that are considered when administering CBT-I.

THE CONTEXT OF THERAPY

Treatment Objectives and Structure

CBT-I aims to target and reverse the behavioral and cognitive processes that maintain insomnia. This is done in a time-limited format. Treatment usually comprises six to eight sessions, each 50 minutes in length. Because there are multiple targets to address in a limited period of time, it is essential that treatment be agenda-driven, goal-oriented, and center around an individualized case formulation derived for each client.

The overall treatment structure is illustrated in Figure 16.1. The first session of treatment focuses on explaining treatment rationale and objectives, deriving a case formulation, and providing psychoeducation on sleep and insomnia. This is generally followed by two to three sessions with a behavioral emphasis, and two to three sessions with a cognitive emphasis. However, the therapist will decide whether to pursue behavioral targets or cognitive targets, or some combination of both in tandem, based on the individualized case formulation. For example, a client who presents with excessive worry, rumination, unhelpful beliefs about sleep, and myriad safety behaviors is likely to benefit from treatment that begins with cognitive targets. A client whose sleep disturbance is characterized by schedule irregularity, daytime napping, and excessive time in bed is likely to benefit from treatment that begins with behavioral targets. The final session summarizes tools learned, and anticipates and plans for sleep setbacks.

Setting

The CBT-I overview presented here is an outpatient-based treatment, delivered in an individual rather than group setting. Sessions are typically held weekly. The therapist will find it helpful to have a table on which to spread out materials (diaries, handouts, thought records), along with a calculator to derive weekly sleep averages and sleep efficiency scores. The client is encouraged to keep all treatment-related materials in a binder or folder and reinforced for bringing this weekly to session.

Though treatment is conducted on an individual basis, the social and familial context of the sleep environment should not be ignored. Clients will have bedmates, children, or pets that may disrupt sleep, and often the therapist will have to improvise to adapt treatment guidelines to the lives of individual clients. Social contexts, when used strategically, can also facilitate treatment adherence and behavior change. Encouraging the use of friends, family, and technology to aid in adherence to sleep principles—for example, in regularizing sleep–wake times, sleep restriction, and stimulus control, each of which is described below—can be helpful. Many clients use cell phone alarms as reminders

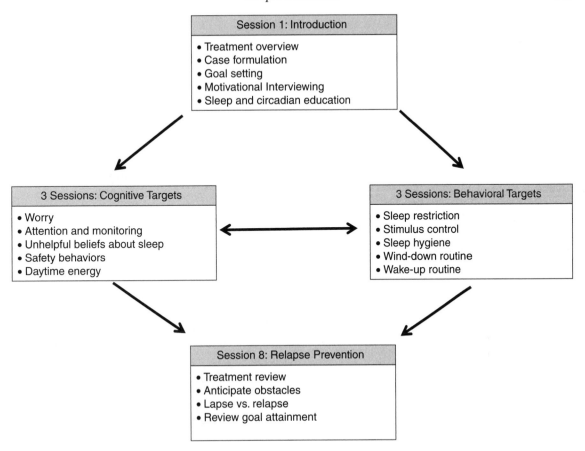

FIGURE 16.1. Treatment flow diagram. Note the practitioner's discretion in beginning with behavioral or cognitive targets as indicated by case conceptualization.

to begin a wind-down period or to wake up at the same time each morning. Likewise, recruiting the support of family and friends to call or visit in the morning so as to prevent oversleeping, or to respect a "no-calls" period in the hour before bed to promote a relaxing wind down, can be crucial to the success of the strategies.

Client Variables

The treatment described here is for individuals who experience "insomnia," defined as difficulty falling or staying asleep at least three nights per week. This treatment is equally suitable for men and women. Though we present a treatment here that is suitable for adults, adaptations can be readily made for teenagers (Clarke & Harvey, 2012; Harvey, 2009). This treatment is ef-

fective in clients who present with a variety of comorbid diagnoses, including anxiety, depression, and other psychological conditions, along with a variety of medical comorbidities. Special considerations are needed for clients with concurrent alcohol and substance use disorders given their myriad effects on sleep.

Many clients who present for treatment are taking concurrently a sleep medication, either prescribed or over the counter, and many of these medications are taken nightly. Clients may wish to reduce or cease their use of these medications. There is an evidence base for how to approach discontinuation of prescribed medication, and readers are referred to several protocols for more information (Belleville, Guay, Guay, & Morin, 2007; Lichstein et al., 1999). Any change to a prescribed medication regimen is made in collaboration with the prescribing provider. Over-the-counter sleeping agents do not appear to have substantial discontinuation effects (Morin, Koetter, Bastien, Ware, & Wooten, 2005) and may be stopped without physician collaboration.

Therapist Variables

It is essential to establish a collaborative working relationship between clinician and client. Along with genuine empathy and support, a strong therapist–client alliance is necessary because much of the treatment depends on the client's compliance with implementing different clinical recommendations. In this context, the therapist's role is one of facilitator and problem-solver. He/she provides specific guidelines, instructions, and corrective feedback. Therapy is directive, task-oriented, and teaches clients problem-solving skills to improve sleep and to cope with residual insomnia after completing treatment. In turn, the client is also actively engaged in the therapeutic process and is responsible for implementing clinical procedures.

The treatment is highly structured and requires time, effort, and diligent adherence with homework assignments. This cannot be overemphasized. Although some procedures may initially appear simplistic and straightforward, the client is cautioned that regular and consistent adherence to the entire program, including homework, is the key to successful outcome.

It is often necessary to contrast the CBT-I approach with medication treatment for insomnia. It is essential to point out that, with CBT-I, there is no "quick fix" for chronic insomnia. To avoid premature termination, the client is cautioned that no immediate results should be expected after one or two office visits. A time commitment of 6–8 weeks is required. This time-limited format is emphasized to maximize compliance. Considering that most clients will have suffered with insomnia for years, this represents a very short investment of time.

It is also important to convey a sense of hope and model a positive yet realistic attitude regarding outcome. An occasional poor night of sleep, particularly associated with a stressor, is normal and should be anticipated. Also, it is important to emphasize that a goal of treatment is to equip the client with tools and methods to continue making sleep gains once therapy is over.

Finally, therapists work with clients to encourage a system of regular rewards and positive reinforcement to facilitate behavior change. Clients can be motivated to comply with treatment recommendations with use of small daily rewards, such as a morning trip to the coffee shop or taking an enjoyable bath. Likewise, therapists are encouraged to highlight successes in sessions rather than failures. For example, if a client's weekly sleep diary reveals that naps were taken on 4 of 7 days, praise the client for the 3 days naps were *not* taken, and perhaps do a functional analysis of how naps were avoided. Point out positive nighttime sleep parameters (e.g., reduced time to fall asleep or nighttime wakefulness) on days that naps were not taken.

ASSESSMENT

Subjective Estimates

As is evident from the DSM-5 criteria, insomnia is defined subjectively. As such, three levels of self-reported sleep data are collected from clients during an assessment for insomnia (see Buysse, Ancoli-Israel, Edinger, Lichstein, & Morin, 2006, for further information on insomnia assessment). First, a clinical sleep history is taken to assess for diagnostic criteria and the presence of comorbid problems. Information gathered includes the duration, frequency, and severity of nighttime sleep disturbance, including estimates of the key sleep parameters: SOL, number of awakenings after sleep onset, total amount of time awake after sleep onset, TST, and an estimate of sleep quality (SQ). Information about the onset and duration of the insomnia and type of symptoms (i.e., sleep onset, sleep maintenance, early morning waking problem, or combinations of these) is collected. A description of the daytime correlates and consequences of insomnia is key. In addition, obtaining information about medications (prescription and over the counter) and screening for the presence of comorbid psychological disorders and medical problems (including other sleep disorders) are also important.

Second, one or more validated measures can be used to index the presence and severity of sleep disturbance (e.g., Pittsburgh Sleep Quality Index; Buysse, Reynolds, Monk, Berman, & Kupfer, 1989), insomnia (e.g., Insomnia Severity Index; Bastien, Vallieres, & Morin, 2001), and daytime sleepiness (e.g., Stanford Sleepiness Scale; Hoddes, Zarcone, Smythe, Phillips, & Dement, 1973). The Duke Structured Interview for Sleep Disorders (Edinger et al., 2009), a semistructured interview that assesses research diagnostic criteria for sleep disorders, may also be used to establish sleep disturbance diagnoses.

Third, asking the client to complete a sleep diary (Carney et al., 2012) each morning as soon as possible after waking for 2 weeks can provide prospective estimates of sleep. A sleep diary provides a wealth of information, including night-to-night variability in sleeping difficulty and sleep–wake patterns, and can be used to determine the presence of circadian rhythm problems, such as a delayed sleep phase or an advanced sleep phase. Also, sleep diaries reduce several problems associated with the methods just discussed that rely on retrospective report, such as answering on the basis of saliency (i.e., the worst night) or recency (i.e., last night) (Smith, Nowakowski, Soeffing, Orff, & Perlis, 2003). Interestingly, the "enhanced awareness" of sleep patterns facilitated by diary keeping can reduce anxiety over sleep loss and thus contribute to better sleep (Morin, 1993, p. 71). A sample sleep diary is illustrated in Figure 16.2.

Objective Estimates

Polysomnography (PSG) is used to classify sleep into various stages. It involves placing surface electrodes on the scalp and face to measure electrical brain activity, eye movement, and muscle tone. The data obtained are used to classify each epoch by sleep stage and in terms of sleep cycles (NREM and REM). Disadvantages associated with PSG include its expense, discomfort for participants, and labor-intensive nature. Although PSG is not needed for the routine assessment of insomnia (Reite, Buysse, Reynolds, & Mendelson, 1995), it is important if the client is suspected of having a comorbid sleep disorder, such as sleep apnea or periodic limb movement disorder.

Actigraphy is an alternative means of providing an objective estimate of sleep. An actigraph is a small, wrist-worn device that contains a sensor, a processor, and memory storage. The sensor samples physical motion and can be downloaded and analyzed to generate various estimates of sleep parameters, though it cannot differentiate stages of sleep. Correlation between actigraphy- and polysomnography-defined estimates of TST is quite strong, ranging from .88 to .97 in adult nonpatients (Jean-Louis et al., 1997). It is worth noting, however, that actigraphy validation for insomnia patients has been met with variable success. Actigraphy appears to be less accurate in populations with fragmented sleep (Paquet, Kawinska, & Carrier, 2007) and

in periods of quiet wakefulness, such as the sleep-onset period (Lichstein et al., 2006). Numerous studies have documented that actigraphy has a tendency to overestimate TST and underestimate wake time during sleep in insomnia (Lichstein et al., 2006; Vallieres & Morin, 2003). Thus, although actigraphy is not required for the assessment of insomnia and may be subject to overestimation of TST, it nonetheless provides an overview of the sleep–wake cycle in a way that is minimally intrusive (Morgenthaler et al., 2007).

INTRODUCING TREATMENT

Following an assessment of insomnia history, severity, and collection of 7–14 days of diary data, a first treatment session with the client should be scheduled. This first session has several critical treatment components: to provide a treatment overview and rationale, to derive an individualized case formulation, and to educate the client about basic sleep processes. After this initial session, behavioral and cognitive processes are selectively targeted. The treatment concludes with a review of tools and a focus on relapse prevention.

Treatment Overview

As a first introduction to treatment, the therapist presents an overview of the therapy in the first session. This can take the following format:

"The treatment that you will receive is called cognitive-behavioral therapy for sleep (CBT for short). CBT is a psychological intervention that is designed to help you change some behaviors (sleep habits, sleep schedules) and thoughts and beliefs (worries about sleeplessness and its consequences) that contribute to and perpetuate your sleep problem. These are selected as the target because research shows this is an effective strategy. The main characteristics of CBT for insomnia are that it is sleep-focused, relatively brief compared to other types of psychotherapy, and you take a very active role in your own treatment. Your treatment will involve six to eight weekly, 50-minute individual therapy sessions. The main agenda of each of these sessions will include reviewing your sleep diary from the previous week, providing practical recommendations and home projects to facilitate changes sleep habits, schedules, beliefs, thoughts, and so forth, and

In the morning, fill out the *night* information for the prior night . . . mo/day	Tuesday 3/25	/	/	/	/	/	/	/
1. Yesterday, I napped from ___ to ___ (Note the times of all naps.)	1:30 to 2:30 P.M.							
2. Yesterday, I took ___ mg of medication and/or ___ oz. of alcohol as sleep aid.	Ambien 5 mg							
3. Last night, I went to bed and turned the lights off at ___ o'clock (A.M. or P.M.).	10:45 P.M. 11:15 P.M.							
4. After turning the lights off, I fell asleep in ___ minutes.	40 min.							
5. My sleep was interrupted ___ times. (Specify number of nighttime awakenings.)	3							
6. My sleep was interrupted for ___ minutes. (Specify duration of each awakening.)	10 45							
7. Last night, I left my bed ___ times.	3							
8. This morning, I actually awoke at ___ o'clock. (Note time of last awakening.)	6:15 A.M.							
9. This morning I had planned to wake up at ___ o'clock A.M. or P.M. (or leave blank if you did not plan a specific time).								
10. This morning, I actually got out of bed at ___ o'clock (specify the time).	6:40 A.M.							
11. When I got up this morning I felt ___. (Answer on a 1- to 5-point scale: 1 = Exhausted, 5 = Refreshed.)	2							
12. Overall, my sleep last night was ___. (Answer on a 1- to 5-point scale: 1 = Restless, 5 = Very sound.)	3							

FIGURE 16.2. Sample sleep diary.

648

to help you solve problems that may interfere with your progress and homework assignments. The main objective is to help you improve your sleep and your daytime functioning. To achieve these goals, you will be provided with direct guidance, but you will be responsible for implementing the recommendations at home."

After presenting this overview, the therapist provides additional information about how this intervention was developed and about its clinical effectiveness. This information is useful to enhance treatment credibility and to induce a sense of hope in clients who have long-standing insomnia, and at the same time cautions others against expecting rapid changes in sleep.

"This treatment has been developed by psychologists as an alternative to medication therapies. It is based on clinical research and has been tested extensively throughout the world. This treatment has been shown effective with hundreds of individuals suffering from insomnia problems similar to yours. This treatment will help improve your sleep and, most importantly, develop self-management skills to regain control of sleep and cope more adaptively with occasional sleep difficulties you may encounter even after completing this program. Although it may take more time to improve your sleep with this approach than with medication, research has shown that CBT produces sleep improvements that are well maintained long after completing treatment."

Therapists are encouraged to emphasize the collaborative nature of the treatment and the importance of homework as core foundations in treatment. The cornerstone of this approach, which is common to most CBTs, is that the client assumes an active role in his/her treatment. As such, he/she is encouraged to develop new skills to achieve better control of his/her sleep.

Maintaining a daily sleep diary is an essential requirement of treatment, and this is made very clear during first therapy session. Therapists explain that a daily diary is important to (1) document the nature and severity of the initial sleep problem; (2) assess night-to-night variations in sleep patterns and identify factors that contribute to improved or worsened sleep; (3) monitor treatment progress; and (4) evaluate compliance with treatment procedures. The treatment can become difficult if a client fails to monitor his/her sleep or forgets to bring in his/her diary. As noncompliance with self-

monitoring is likely related to noncompliance with treatment procedures, therapists are encouraged to address this issue up front if it becomes a problem. There is no need for the client to monitor the clock in order to provide accurate times. Only one's "felt sense" of the timing of sleep is needed. If self-monitoring is overlooked on a particular day, clients should be discouraged from going back and estimating sleep parameters retrospectively. Compliance with the diary daily is often enhanced when completion time and place is identified. For example, the client and therapist can discuss a time (breakfast) and location (kitchen) for filling in the diary.

Functional Analysis and Case Formulation

To derive a case formulation, the therapist and client discuss frequency, intensity, and duration of insomnia and its antecedents. Sleep-related behaviors and consequences are assessed: before bed (e.g., bedtime routine), during the night (e.g., cell phone left on), on waking (e.g., sleepiness, lethargy) and during the day (e.g., caffeine use, napping). The relationship between sleep-specific thoughts, emotions, and behaviors is charted across the night and day. Figure 16.3 is an example of a case conceptualization form for the nighttime period.

The case formulation is designed to elicit the client's curiosity about his/her sleep and to start forming a picture of what is going on. The therapist can introduce the exercise as follows:

"It will be helpful in planning our sessions together to get a very detailed picture of what the experience of insomnia is like for you, almost like putting your sleep under a microscope. The way we do this is by identifying together a recent typical night and then after that a recent typical day. I'll ask you lots of questions about each, so that I can get a sense of the kind of things that are going on. It's like a fingerprint, everyone is a bit different so the treatment needs to be a bit different. Would that be all right?"

The first step is to help the client to choose a *very specific* recent example of an "insomnia episode" during the night. Make sure you work on deriving only one model (i.e., either the day or the night) at a time. A very specific episode is a situation that happened on one particular day and at a particular time. Be sure to check in regularly to ensure that the night was typical. Sometimes a selected night or day is not typical or it was not very distressing. The therapist should stop that

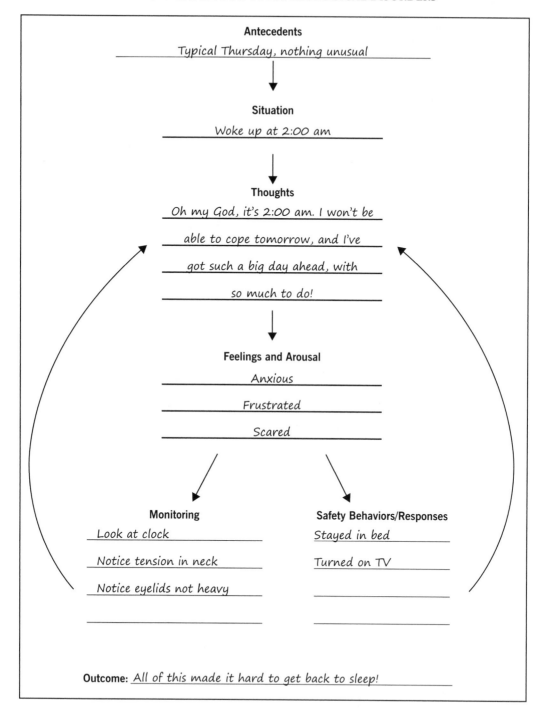

FIGURE 16.3. Case conceptualization form completed for the night.

model as soon as this becomes apparent and start again with a typical, distressing night. Examples of some very specific recent episodes may include "Last Tuesday night I worked until 1:00 A.M. and then I couldn't get to sleep" or "On Friday at work I had a terrible day, I felt sick, looked terrible and performed badly." Spend a few minutes asking information-gathering questions to explore the content of the nighttime or daytime model. The aim of this initial discussion is to obtain a very detailed description of *exactly* what happened, along with the consequences of it. The following is an example of a client who awoke at 2:00 A.M. (Figure 16.3):

THERAPIST: What woke you up?

CLIENT: Don't know.

THERAPIST: How did you know what time it was?

CLIENT: I looked at my clock and saw it was 2:00 A.M.

THERAPIST: When you looked at the clock and noticed it was 2:00 A.M. what ran through your mind?

CLIENT: I thought, "Oh my God."

THERAPIST: OK, so you looked at the clock and noticed it was 2:00 A.M. and you thought "Oh my God." Could you tell me more? What do you mean by "Oh my God?"

CLIENT: Oh my, I won't cope tomorrow, I've got such a big day ahead with so much to do.

THERAPIST: So when you thought, "Oh my, I've got such a big day ahead with so much to do," how did you feel?

CLIENT: Really anxious.

Drawing on classic treatment development work by David M. Clark's team (Clark et al., 1999, 2006), the following are useful questions to ask when deriving the model. The following illustrates questions for nighttime models, with analogous daytime questions in brackets [ ]:

For identifying negative thoughts:

- "What went through your mind/what were you thinking before getting into bed [on waking], as you got into bed [as you got ready for the day], and as you noticed you weren't getting to sleep [weren't performing well]?"
- "What did you think would happen as a result?"
- "What would that mean? What would be so bad about that?"

For identifying safety behaviors:

- "When you thought X might happen, did you do anything to try to prevent it from happening?"
- "Is there anything you do to ensure you get to sleep [perform well during the day]?"

For identifying feelings:

- "When you are afraid that X will happen, what do you notice happening in your body?"
- "What kind of emotions do you have as you think X?"
- "How about your energy level?"

For identifying monitoring:

- "How did you know that X would happen?"
- "How did you determine or measure how close to falling asleep you were or what the time was [that you were feeling so tired]?"
- "How do you monitor/measure when the insomnia is back?"
- "How do you know that you hadn't fallen asleep [were still tired]?"

It is important for the therapist to ask questions to illustrate the cyclical relationship among thoughts, feelings, and behaviors that is often evident in insomnia. These questions focus on the arrows. It is often important to connect "monitoring" and "safety behaviors" back to thoughts. Here are some questions that will help:

For connecting thoughts, feelings and behaviors:

- "When you are concentrating on (give examples of monitoring, like looking at the clock), what thoughts occur to you? Anything run through you mind?"
- "When you are concentrating on (give examples of safety behaviors, like remaining in bed for long periods of time), what is its impact on your getting back to sleep?"
- "When you monitor these things (when you cope by doing X), does that help you worry less or does it trigger more worries?"

Drawing out the consequences:

- "Does watching out for fatigue and tension have any consequences [for your day]?"
- "Were there any consequences of these thoughts,

emotions or behaviors for getting back to sleep [how the rest of your day went]?"

Once the model has been derived, the therapist shares the *personalized version* with the client, asking for feedback and reactions. The therapist might say the following:

"This has been very helpful. Let me show you what I have been scribbling here, and I'd like for you to give me feedback about which parts I understand and which parts I have got wrong. This is so similar to what we very often find. These kinds of thoughts [name some] seem to lead to these kinds of feelings [name them]. Both put together make it difficult to sleep. On top of that, the thoughts and feelings can put us into a state of vigilance. Then we start monitoring the environment and our bodies [name some examples of the kinds of monitoring in which client engages], which often triggers more thoughts, which triggers more feelings. Then, very understandably, we try to cope by doing things like [name some of the safety behaviors]. Now some of these really are likely to be helpful in getting us back to sleep, but sometimes during the treatment we will test out the extent to which they are helpful by doing an experiment, to double check. That's why we call them safety behaviors. Safety behaviors are things that people do in order to try and fix the problem they have but which, inadvertently, sometimes contribute to the problem. We may test out whether these behaviors are helpful or unhelpful. How does this model fit for you?"

Once the model has been completed, it is important to ask clients if they can think of ways to intervene. If an area is identified, draw a double line across the maintaining arrows to visually represent cutting into the cycle. Most often clients are not able to come up with ways to intervene, so the therapist can help them by saying something like the following:

"I suggest that one of our targets be these thoughts .. . if we can change them we will change your feelings. This alone will be very helpful for helping you get back to sleep. In addition, we'll also target the monitoring. When we change the monitoring people typically feel much more relaxed and sleep much better. Then, as I have already said, if you are interested, we'll test with experiments the things you are doing

to cope right now, just in case some are feeding into the cycle."

Summarize by pointing out that a change in one or more parts of the perpetuating cycle will shift the system.

Goal Setting

Once the case conceptualization/insomnia models are derived, specific goals are collaboratively identified and written down in session. Goals are clearly stated (e.g., "falling asleep within 30 minutes each night" instead of "falling asleep more quickly at night") and feasible (e.g., "sleeping through the night with only several brief awakenings" instead of "sleeping through the night without waking," as the latter is not biologically feasible). Practitioners and clients can establish goals for both the nighttime (falling asleep, staying asleep, advancing bedtime) and the daytime (increasing energy, reducing caffeine consumption). Goals are revisited briefly midway through treatment and at the conclusion of treatment.

Therapy goals are set in Session 1 but may need to be reevaluated and readjusted periodically as the intervention unfolds. It is important to set realistic, operational, and well-defined goals. Goal setting is useful to keep the therapy focused. By setting well-defined goals, the therapeutic alliance remains oriented to the client's needs and desires and minimizes diversion to irrelevant materials. It also provides useful information about the client's sleep expectations, which sometimes need to be adjusted during the goal setting process.

Motivational Interviewing

Motivational interviewing (MI) is a communication method that emphasizes accepting the client as an individual, avoiding argumentation/lectures, and focusing on the process of eliciting and shaping language in favor of change (i.e., change talk; Miller & Rollnick, 2002). MI also includes regular, straightforward reviews of perceived pros and cons of change because many sleep-incompatible/interfering behaviors are rewarding.

A straightforward review of perceived pros and cons of the change is conducted. For example, clients often struggle with waking up at around the same time on both weekdays and weekends. Allowing the client to generate advantages and disadvantages with therapist guidance facilitates behavior change. MI is revisited in future sessions as additional strategies are introduced.

Sleep and Circadian Education

Education on the circadian system and homeostatic sleep drive (see the earlier "Sleep and Insomnia" section) is presented to the client. This underscores the following two points: (1) Going to bed and waking up at the same time each day helps the circadian system adapt to the 24-hour sleep–wake cycle; and (2) daytime napping disrupts the natural buildup of homeostatic sleep pressure. Individuals across the age range may also benefit from education about specific changes in sleep across the lifespan. In adolescence and young adulthood, understanding the biological shift toward later bedtimes and rise times with puberty is helpful for later intervention. Likewise, explaining to adults that sleep grows lighter and more fragmented with age, and that sleep needs change with age, such that 7 hours of sleep per night may be sufficient, can go a long way to normalize and lay the foundation for intervention.

BEHAVIORAL COMPONENTS

Sleep Restriction

Sleep restriction, as developed by Spielman and colleagues (1987), rests on the general premise that time in bed should be limited to maximize the sleep drive, and so that the association between the bed and sleeping is strengthened. This behavioral treatment begins with a reduction of time spent in bed, so that time in bed is equivalent to the time the client estimates he/she spends sleeping. Thus, for instance, if an individual gets approximately 6 hours of sleep per night (an average across the week based on sleep diaries), but usually spends about an additional 2 hours trying to get to sleep, the sleep restriction therapy would begin by limiting his/her time spent in bed to 6 hours. This initial reduction in time spent in bed is intended to heighten a person's homeostatic sleep drive (Perlis & Lichstein, 2003) and reduce the association between the bed and wakefulness. Following this restriction, sleep gradually becomes more efficient, at which point time spent in bed is gradually increased.

Practitioners begin sleep restriction by calculating TST, time in bed, and *sleep efficiency* based on the prior week's sleep diary. "Sleep efficiency" is defined as TST divided by time in bed, multiplied by 100 to form a percentage. So, in the previous example, if a client sleeps an average of 6 hours per night over the week and spends an average of 8 hours in bed, sleep efficiency for the week will be $(6 \div 8) \times 100$, or 75%. The goal is to increase sleep efficiency to more than 85–90%. The therapist would set a "sleep window" equal to the prior week's TST (6 hours), choosing a bedtime and rise time with the client (e.g., 12:00 A.M. to 6:00 A.M.). Once sleep efficiency reaches 85%, client and therapist can gradually expand the window (e.g., by 30 minutes per week) toward an optimal sleep time.

Clients are often hesitant about implementing sleep restriction. Many individuals with insomnia believe that they need to spend a great deal of time in bed in order to "catch" a minimum amount of sleep. Still others worry about the short-term sleep deprivation that sleep restriction is likely to impart—after all, clients are presenting with the desire to get *more* sleep, and sleep restriction is a strategy that, in the short term, is likely to give them *less*. Explain to the client that his/her brain and body have developed habits that lead to time awake in bed and poor sleep efficiency. Sleep restriction is the most effective way to improve sleep efficiency by consolidating sleep time. Tell the client that, although initially he/she may not get more sleep, his/her sleep quality and sleep efficiency will likely improve. These are the first steps to remedying sleep problems. Reassure the client that, as his/her sleep efficiency improves, you will be expanding the "sleep window" to allow for more time in bed.

Stimulus Control

The rationale for stimulus control therapy lies in the notion that insomnia is a result of conditioning that occurs when the bed becomes associated with inability to sleep. The bed, bedtime, and bedroom have lost their properties previously associated with sleep, and the main therapeutic goal is to reestablish or strengthen the associations between sleep and the stimulus conditions under which it typically occurs. As described by Bootzin, Epstein, and Wood (1991), stimulus control requires clients to comply with a series of specific behavioral recommendations. These recommendations, along with suggestions for introducing them, are outlined below.

- *Only go to bed when sleepy.* To reestablish the association between the bed and sleep, clients are instructed to go to bed and to stay in bed only when sleepy and when sleep is imminent. Therapists explain that "sleepy" is different from "tired," and that although an individual may feel tired in the evening, he/she must wait until he/she feels sleepy before getting into bed. Note that, if a sleep window has been set as part of sleep restriction (described earlier), the client is instructed to *remain awake* until the start of the sleep window, even if he/she feels sleepy.

● *Get out of bed if unable to fall asleep.* Because time spent awake in bed can often be associated with worry, rumination, and arousal, clients are instructed to leave the bed if they do not fall asleep within 15–20 minutes, returning to bed only when they feel sleepy. This may be introduced in session as follows:

"If you are unable to fall asleep or return to sleep within 15–20 minutes, get out of bed, go into another room, and engage in a quiet activity that you find relaxing. You can read, listen to music, do a crossword puzzle, or find something else that is nonarousing. Return to bed only when sleepy, and repeat this step as often as necessary throughout the night—so that anytime you wake up and are awake for more than 20 minutes, you will be getting out of bed and going to another room. This regimen will help reassociate your bed/bedroom with falling asleep *quickly*."

● Therapists can brainstorm relaxing activities with clients and write them down in session, listening carefully for and discouraging potentially stimulating activities (Web browsing, watching certain TV programs, cleaning the house). Emphasize to clients that it will be difficult to comply with this recommendation. Encourage clients to put warm clothing by the bed to increase the desire to get out of bed. Brainstorm with clients who live in studios or single rooms to find an alternate place (a chair or pillow on the floor) to go to when getting out of bed.

● *Keep the bedroom for sleep and sex.* Eliminate all sleep-incompatible activities (upsetting conversations, studying, watching TV) from the bed and bedroom. Many individuals get into bed early and read or watch TV in order to facilitate sleep onset. Remind clients that this time in bed spent awake, however, dilutes the association between the bed and sleep.

● *Discourage napping.* Explain to clients that napping can offset homeostatic sleep pressure, making it more difficult to fall asleep or stay asleep at night. Often it can be helpful to point to specific examples in the sleep diaries where a daytime nap led to greater difficulty falling asleep, or more wakefulness throughout the night, to illustrate this point. If clients regularly nap at a certain time, brainstorm activities that can be scheduled as an alternative. Tell clients that although naps may feel helpful in the short term, they can disrupt sleep–wake rhythms and perpetuate insomnia in the long term.

Sleep Hygiene

Information about sleep and sleep incompatible behaviors, and the daytime consequences of sleep disturbance, is often given to inform clients of the basic steps that they can take to improve their sleep. Interventions targeting sleep hygiene are behavioral in nature and target sleep-incompatible routines. Sleep hygiene interventions typically include the following components (Morin & Espie, 2003). First, education on the sleep-disrupting effects of alcohol, tobacco, and caffeine use are introduced to the client, who is encouraged to avoid caffeine in the evening and alcohol/tobacco at bedtime. Clients are encouraged to have a small snack before bedtime but to avoid heavy meals. Likewise, exercise is known to enhance sleep continuity and quality, and is recommended to client; exercising within several hours of bedtime, however, can delay sleep onset. Finally, the client is encouraged to keep the bedroom environment quiet, dark, and cool. Although sleep hygiene education is typically included as one component of CBT-I, its use as the sole intervention in treating insomnia has not been empirically supported (Morin et al., 2006).

Wind Down, Wake Up, and Regularity

Wind-Down Routine

Clients need assistance to devise a "wind down" of 30–60 minutes in which relaxing, sleep-enhancing activities are introduced in dim lighting conditions. A regular wind-down routine is beneficial across multiple domains: It promotes relaxation, increases positive associations with the bed/bedtime, and, when done in dim lighting conditions, helps the circadian phase advance in clients who are evening-types, maintaining entrainment (Wyatt, Stepanski, & Kirkby, 2006). Activities that are encouraged in the wind-down routine include reading, grooming/hygiene, bathing, completing a light crossword, listening to soft music, and other relaxing activities of the client's choosing. A central issue is the use of interactive electronic media (Internet browsing, cell phone use, social networking). Though clients may acknowledge that these activities are stimulating, they may be reluctant to surrender them in the period before sleep. MI can often be helpful given that many clients are socially isolated and rely on prebedtime, Internet-based social interaction. A behavioral experiment stretching across the week (e.g., three nights of bedtime "as usual" followed by three nights with a "wind-down routine," with daily ratings of prebedtime relaxation and SOL) can be helpful to *illustrate* the sleep-promoting effects of a good wind-down routine (Harvey & Talbot, 2012a). Many clients voluntarily choose an electronics curfew and time at which the wind down will commence, opting to set an alarm on a cell phone as a reminder.

Wake-Up Routine

As mentioned earlier, clients benefit from education about sleep inertia upon waking, and about behaviors that can increase or decrease sleep inertia. Helpful behaviors to curb sleep inertia include not hitting "snooze," exposure to sunlight upon waking (e.g., opening the curtains to let sunlight in, eating breakfast outside), encouraging morning physical activity, showering, listening to upbeat music, and encouraging social contact. Behavioral recommendations may be introduced to combat the desire to sleep in, including placing an alarm away from the bed so that it is necessary to rise to turn it off, and making the bed, so the incentive to get back in bed is reduced. Encouragement from family and friends can also help a person to comply with morning rise times.

Regularizing and Shifting Sleep and Wake Times

Regularizing sleep and wake times across the week can be a helpful intervention, particularly if schedule variability appears to be a prominent feature of the sleep disturbance. Building motivation for the client to wake at the same time, including on weekends (Crowley & Carskadon, 2010) is a key focus. This promotes consistent sleepiness in the evening, particularly when naps are avoided.

Often it is helpful to frame schedule variability around the phenomenon of "jet lag" as follows:

THERAPIST: Have you ever experienced jet lag?

CLIENT: Yes, I have.

THERAPIST: When was the last time?

CLIENT: Oh, I guess the last time was flying out east to visit relatives.

THERAPIST: What did you notice?

CLIENT: Let's see . . . I felt kind of out of it, like I couldn't focus. It was difficult to fall asleep, even more than it usually is for me!

THERAPIST: And flying out east . . . that's a 3-hour time difference from here, correct?

CLIENT: Yes.

THERAPIST: Let's take a look at your sleep diary from last week. What do you notice from weekday to weekend?

CLIENT: Well . . . I went to bed at 2:00 A.M. on Friday and Saturday because I went out both nights. And I guess I slept in as a result.

THERAPIST: And what time did you go to bed on Sunday and Monday?

CLIENT: Looks like I tried to sleep at 11:00 P.M. because I have to get up for work.

THERAPIST: So you just went from 2:00 A.M. on the weekend to 11:00 P.M. on the weekday. You just flew across the country!

CLIENT: Huh. I guess I never thought of it that way.

THERAPIST: No wonder you had difficulty falling asleep on Sunday and Monday. Your body was jet lagged, and with the "time change" it was hard to fall asleep.

CLIENT: No wonder I have so much trouble on Sunday nights!

For clients who wish to advance their sleep schedules, we work to achieve behavioral adjustments to adapt to earlier bedtimes. We do this in small, systematic shifts (e.g., by advancing bedtime by 20–30 minutes each week) to ensure mastery. We encourage exposure to light upon waking, which will help the circadian system advance, and work with clients to minimize variability around wake times. We reassure clients that any sleep pressure (i.e., sleep loss) accumulated initially with bedtime advancement will actually help the sleep schedule align by increasing likelihood of earlier sleep onset on subsequent nights.

COGNITIVE COMPONENTS

Worry

It is well established that individuals with chronic insomnia worry while in bed about a range of topics, including the failure to fall asleep (Harvey, 2002b; Wicklow & Espie, 2000). Cognitive models implicating worry (e.g., Harvey, 2002a) posit that worry activates the sympathetic nervous system and corresponding physiological arousal, which hinders sleep onset (Espie, 2002). Therefore, an intervention targeting worry is an important clinical area in the treatment of insomnia.

Following well-established cognitive therapy approaches (Beck, 1995; Young, Rygh, Weinberger, & Beck, Chapter 7, this volume), the first step in addressing worry involves education on negative automatic thoughts (NATs) and mistakes in thinking. NATs can be introduced to clients as follows:

THERAPIST: Imagine there are two people outside of a movie theater, each waiting for a friend to arrive. The friend is late, and these two people have been waiting. Person 1 is thinking, "Gosh, I wonder why she is late. I hope everything is all right with her! Did she get into an accident on her way over?" Person 2 is thinking, "Gosh, I can't believe she is late. She always does this. She has no respect for my time. She is not a good friend." What kinds of emotions do you think Person 1 is feeling?

CLIENT: Probably some fear and concern.

THERAPIST: Right. And what about Person 2?

CLIENT: (*chuckling*) Anger, and maybe resentment.

THERAPIST: Exactly! So two people in the same situation can have *very* different emotional responses to an event based on what they were thinking. In other words, our thoughts can directly influence our emotions. Often we have dozens of thoughts, in rapid succession, and we don't even realize it. We accept them at face value without stopping to look at them. We're going to look for, and respond to, some sleep-related automatic thoughts over the next few weeks.

The therapist then provides further education on automatic thoughts: (1) They are often a train of thought that runs parallel with spoken thought; (2) we are often not fully aware of them; (3) automatic thoughts are extremely rapid, and sometimes only a few words rather than sentences; (4) they do not arise as a result of deliberation but just happen like a reflex; (5) they are often difficult to turn off; (6) we often accept their validity without stopping to question them; and (7) they often precede a powerful emotion. The therapist should underscore the point that we have hundreds and hundreds of NATs each day, and it is often helpful to look for NATs by paying attention to changes in emotion.

The therapist next works with a client to identify a recent powerful emotion from the previous 2 days, and use the emotion as the starting place to uncover related NATs. These are written down on a simple three-column form (Situation–Thoughts–Emotions). The client is asked to practice identifying additional NATs over the week by paying attention to changes in emotion and writing them down on the three-column form, emphasizing insomnia-related NATs ("I'm exhausted" or "I won't be able to cope today"). The therapist also provides psychoeducation on common cognitive distortions (black-and-white thinking, catastrophizing, personalizing, mistaking feelings for facts, etc.) and asks clients to categorize some of the NATs they spot over the week.

At the following session, the practitioner reviews the client's three-column NAT form and has a brief discussion/review of NATs and NAT themes. The practitioner then introduces an extended thought record that guides the client in evaluating the validity of the thought with a series of questions, including evidence for–against the thought; alternative ways of interpreting the thought; considering the worst that could happen and whether the client would be able to live through it; the helpfulness of the thought and the effect of thinking in this manner; how others might see the situation; how important the thought will be when the client is 80; and whether the thought falls into one of the "mistakes in thinking." Client and therapist pick a NAT together and work through the form together in session.

Once the client has fully grasped this procedure, the therapist assigns as homework completing one extended record daily or, at the very least, several examples each week. This is continued for several weeks. The therapist provides the following rationale for *continuing* to fill out the extended record on a daily basis: (1) By observing, reporting and evaluating NATs, it is easier to see them objectively and to get some distance from them; (2) observing, reporting, and evaluating NATs presents an opportunity to test their reality/logic and recognize that thoughts can be unreliable; and most importantly, (3) because it takes a long time to change thinking habits that have been around for many years, reversing the old habits will take practice. Completing one form daily over a period of weeks will make the new style of thinking habitual.

Helpful and Unhelpful Worry Strategies

A menu of other worry interventions is offered, so that the client gets to create a personalized list of helpful and unhelpful strategies to manage worry. Unhelpful strategies might include suppression (Harvey, 2003a), positive beliefs about worry (Harvey, 2003b), and "why" questions (Watkins & Baracaia, 2001). For suppression, introduce the adverse consequences of thought suppression whenever it becomes relevant, sometimes as early as Session 1. For example, as soon as the client mentions something along the lines of "I try to suppress my thoughts" or "I clear my mind," the therapist can do an in-session "white bear experiment" ("For the next minute, let's close our eyes and think about whatever we'd like, anything except a big white fluffy bear") to illustrate paradoxical effects of thought suppression. This helps the client become aware that suppression often leads to "thought rebound" or monitoring for the suppressed thought, which makes it more likely to occur. A helpful assessment for suppression and other thought control strategies is available (Ree, Harvey, Blake, Tang, & Shawe-Taylor, 2005). Therapists should also be on the lookout for clients who hold positive beliefs about the utility of presleep worry. Therapists can use Socratic questioning to discuss the pros and cons of presleep worry, or consider doing behavioral experiments to collect data on whether positive beliefs about worrying in bed are helpful or not. Finally, "why" questions are often implicated in the presentation of insomnia. Many clients ask questions such as "Why am I awake?" or "Why don't I sleep as well as my partner?" Give your client the rationale that experimental studies suggest that "why" questions block processing and promote rumination.

After reviewing what *not* to do to manage worry, consider alternative, more helpful thought management strategies with the client. First, suggest the idea of not controlling or suppressing thoughts. Do the opposite— let them come. Let them drift in and out. Letting the thoughts come and go may give the thoughts less strength and power, and may even move them into the category of being boring. Another helpful alternative involves catching the thoughts and evaluating them with the extended thought record described earlier. Introducing the importance of a wind-down or buffer zone to process and disengage from the day can be a helpful response to worry. Finally, practice "savoring" to focus on the positives in the client's life. Savoring involves attending to, appreciating, and enhancing positive experiences the client has had during the day. It can be a small/everyday event like looking out the window and noticing the lovely trees and flowers, reminiscing over a favorite vacation, or anticipating a family reunion or a date with one's spouse/partner. Encourage the client to focus on the positive experience, and when negative thoughts arise, return to the positive experience and savor it. The rationale is to associate bedtime with positive thoughts. Work with your client in the session to identify times in the present, past, and future that he/she can savor. Practice savoring together in the session and allow the client to reflect on the experience.

Set one or more of these alternative strategies as homework, introducing it as a behavioral experiment. Behavioral experiments, explained in Table 16.1, are powerful methods used across all of the cognitive components of CBT-I. (For further reading on behavioral experiments, see Perlis, Aloia, & Kuhn, 2012; Ree & Harvey, 2004a.) The goal is to give the client some experience and practice with each. Feel free to follow-up with additional experiments in subsequent sessions if needed.

Attention and Monitoring

As noted earlier, a number of studies have documented that individuals with insomnia underestimate their sleep time and overestimate time spent awake at night (e.g., Harvey & Tang, 2012). Individuals may become more anxious about their perceived sleep problem, and with increased vigilance towards the sleep state, may draw inaccurate conclusions about their prior sleep. Likewise, individuals may monitor for signs of daytime fatigue. A helpful measure of sleep-related monitoring is available (Neitzert Semler & Harvey, 2004). Behavioral experiments, both in and out of session, can be introduced to illustrate the effects of attentional bias and monitoring (Harvey & Talbot, 2012b; Ree & Harvey, 2004a).

To introduce the concept of monitoring, the therapist may wish to do the following:

THERAPIST: Close your eyes and focus on your knee joints and the sensations that are there. I'll do it, too. Let's both take 2 minutes to do this. (*after 2 minutes*) What did you notice?

TABLE 16.1. Steps Involved in Creating, Testing, and Processing Behavioral Experiments

Steps and description	Example
• *Step 1. Identify the thought, belief, behavior, or process the experiment will target.* The rationale for completing the experiment, along with the target or aim, should be clear. Targets can include challenging an unhelpful belief/behavior or testing a new belief/behavior. The target is written down in session.	Victor is unsure as to whether looking at the clock as he falls asleep is helpful. He believes that knowing the time, and calculating how much time he has left to sleep, may increase his anxiety at night; however, he also feels that *not* knowing the time could increase worry and anxiety throughout the night. Victor and his therapist set out to test the following: "Is looking at the clock at night helpful or harmful to my sleep?"
• *Step 2. Collaborate to brainstorm ideas for an experiment.* Encourage clients to be specific, defining a place and time for the experiment. Get creative and arouse clients' curiosity. Be open and flexible to ideas the clients have, as this may increase motivation to complete the experiment. Clients sometimes enjoy giving their experiments creative titles.	Victor and his therapist agree to set up an experiment to test the impact of clock watching on sleep. They agree to spend 3 nights watching the clock as usual, followed by 3 nights without looking at the clock. Victor states that he will be tempted to turn the clock around on the "no-clock" nights, so he and his therapist collaboratively brainstorm to move the clock across the room to reduce this temptation.
• *Step 3. Write down predictions about the outcome and devise a method to record the outcome as soon as possible after the experiment is completed.* This is very important: A delay in recording the outcome could lead to vague and inaccurate memory of the experiment itself.	Victor has the following prediction: "Not looking at the clock at night will increase my anxiety and keep me up longer because I'll be wondering what time it is all night." He and his therapist decide to record "last night's anxiety" on a scale of 1–10 *immediately upon waking* and use the sleep diary to look at time it takes to fall asleep.
• *Step 4. Anticipate problems and brainstorm solutions.* Ask your client what might prevent him/her from completing this experiment. Identify obstacles and collaborate on how to overcome them. If the experiment centers around a new skill, practice the skill together in session before making it a part of the experiment.	Victor and his therapist discuss obstacles to completing the experiment. Victor has a party to attend on one of the nights, which will delay his bedtime slightly; he and his therapist decide to skip the clock-watching experiment on this "nontypical" night and complete it the other six nights of the week.
• *Step 5. Conduct the experiment.*	Victor spends 3 nights looking at the clock and 3 nights not looking at the clock, recording anxiety and standard sleep variables on his sleep diary.
• *Step 6. Review the experiment.* Ask your client to summarize main points he/she has learned from the experiment. Assist him/her in filling in gaps, and write out conclusions together. Remind your client of the conclusions drawn from each experiment in future sessions. If the outcome is other than anticipated, ask follow-up questions to review any factors (mood, behavior, cognitions) that may have influenced the outcome in a manner other than expected. Typically, via careful questioning, learning can be derived from an experiment regardless of the outcome.	*Clock nights:* Anxiety ratings (on a scale of 1–10): 8, 6, 7 Time to fall asleep (in minutes): 120, 45, 60 *No-clock nights:* Anxiety ratings (on a scale of 1–10): 10, 6, 4 Time to fall asleep (in minutes): 140, 50, 15 At first glance, the numbers above do not appear to "solve" the experiment one way or the other. However, with careful questioning, a subsequent testable hypothesis is generated. Victor reports that his anxiety levels and length of time to fall asleep were consistent on the clock-watching nights. On the no-clock nights, Victor reports that his anxiety was initially very high as he wondered what time it was; by the third day, however, he acknowledged hardly thinking about the time. Victor and his therapist discuss the possibility that he was experiencing initial anxiety with the new behavioral change, and speculate that he may need more time in the no-clock condition to "get used to" the shift.
• *Step 7. Identify follow-up experiments if needed.* If the experiment was not completed in full, or if the outcome was ambiguous and/or raised another question, return to Step 1 and devise a further experiment.	Victor and therapist decide to extend the "no-clock" condition for another week, still rating anxiety and time to fall asleep immediately upon waking.

CLIENT: Hmm .. . some tingling, and pins and needles. Mild pain maybe.

THERAPIST: Imagine for a moment there was a lot of research to indicate that the things you mention are soft signs of a serious immune system disease. If you believed this were true, how would this impact your attention for the rest of the day?

CLIENT: I'd be paying attention to my knee all day!

THERAPIST: And how would you feel about those sensations?

CLIENT: Well, concerned, I guess. Wondering if they had gotten worse.

THERAPIST: What if your sleep is like that knee? And the more you look out for symptoms of tiredness or fatigue, the more they appear?

The therapist can use this dialogue to brainstorm with the client about the monitoring in which he/she may engage during the day and night. Then, the therapist can introduce one or more of the following behavioral experiments to assess monitoring.

Monitoring for Fatigue

Go for a brief walk together in session. Instruct the client to spend 5 minutes focusing internally to monitor how his/her body feels, paying particular attention to signs of tiredness and fatigue. Ask your client to rate how tired he/she feels. Then spend 5 minutes focusing externally on the trees, flowers, and sky. Ask your client to again rate how tired he/she feels. Go back to your office to debrief.

Monitoring for Sounds

To instruct the client about monitoring at night it is often helpful to use the metaphor of a "radar." One client who monitored for the garbage truck had her "radar" on all night for the sound of the garbage truck. She would wake up to many sounds during the night and think, "Oh no, it is the garbage truck, it must already be 5:00 A.M. I'm never going to get enough sleep." This thought led to anxiety that made it difficult for her to get back to sleep. We used multiple strategies to address this monitoring: (1) evaluating whether hearing the garbage truck was really an indication of wakefulness or whether the truck could have caused the client to wake from a light sleep; (2) discussing the pros and cons of having

a "radar" on during the night; and (3) asking the client to listen to sounds in the room, and further away, in the adjacent room, and still further away, to sounds on the road, and to sounds further away yet again, encouraging habituation to the full range of sounds.

Monitoring Physical Appearance

One client with whom we worked used to complain about her physical appearance on the days following poor nights of sleep. She would wake up and immediately look in the mirror, noticing bags under her eyes. When asked how bad the bags were on days when she had not slept poorly, the client admitted she never really looked for them. We devised a behavioral experiment whereby she was to look at the bags under her eyes upon waking every day of the week, regardless of how she had slept, and rate the appearance of baggy eyes. The client found that her bags did not really change from morning to morning, and that she had really just ignored them on days when her sleep was not poor.

Monitoring the Clock

Paying attention to the clock throughout the night can increase anxiety and vigilance, interfering with sleep. Client and therapist can create an experiment whereby the clock is displayed in full view 3 nights of the week, then hidden from view (i.e., turned to face the wall or placed under the bed) for 3 nights. Ask the client to rate overall anxiety about the prior night's sleep in the morning and record it on the sleep diary. The sleep diary can then be reviewed in the following session to compare anxiety and wakefulness on clock-watching nights versus clock-hidden nights.

Unhelpful Beliefs about Sleep

In seminal research on insomnia from the 1990s, Morin (e.g., 1993) highlighted the role of unhelpful beliefs about sleep. It has been suggested that these unhelpful beliefs may exacerbate intrusive and worrisome thoughts throughout the day and night, contributing to the development and maintenance of sleep disturbance (Harvey, 2002a). An unhelpful belief about insomnia might take the form of an individual believing that he/she needs to sleep through the night with no awakenings to feel refreshed. Such a belief is unhelpful in that awakenings are a natural part of nocturnal sleep (e.g., Akerstedt et al., 2002); worry related to this belief might take the form of an individual who, once awakened at night, believes that this fragmented sleep will result in impaired work performance the following day. One large-scale correlational study (Jansson & Linton, 2007) surveyed unhelpful beliefs about sleep, depression, anxiety, and arousal at two time points spaced 1 year apart. The researchers found that unhelpful beliefs about sleep—in particular, beliefs about the long-term negative consequences of insomnia—predicted a chronic pattern of poor sleep over and above arousal, depression, anxiety, and beliefs about short-term consequences. Such research suggests that targeting unhelpful beliefs about sleep is important for reversing chronic insomnia.

In addition to thought records, unhelpful beliefs about sleep can commonly be addressed in two ways: (1) gentle Socratic questioning to explore an unhelpful belief, and (2) creation of a survey to collect data related to the belief (Harvey & Eidelman, 2012). The following vignette illustrates how the therapist can use Socratic questioning to guide the client to explore and correct some unrealistic expectations about sleep needs and morning energy:

THERAPIST: Some of your responses suggest that you believe quite strongly about the need for 8 hours of sleep every night.

CLIENT: Well, I've always thought that we need 8 hours of sleep to stay healthy.

THERAPIST: Do all people you know have the same height?

CLIENT: Of course not!

THERAPIST: What is the normal height for an adult?

CLIENT: Well, there is no norm that applies to everyone. It varies.. ..

THERAPIST: It is similar for sleep. There are individual differences in the amount of sleep we need to feel rested and function well during the day. Although most people report about 7 or 8 hours of sleep, some can get by with less than that and still feel rested in the morning. It is possible that 6.5 hours of uninterrupted sleep be more satisfying and refreshing than 8 hours of broken sleep. So, it will be important to experiment with various sleep durations to determine what the optimal duration is for you. What do you think happens if you assume that you need 8 hours of sleep but you really only need 7?

CLIENT: I guess I'm awake an hour .. . and I spend that hour worrying about why I'm not sleeping!

THERAPIST: Exactly. Pursuing unrealistic goals is counterproductive and may actually make you anxious and, as a consequence, perpetuate the underlying sleep difficulties. I also noted that you are very concerned when you are not fully rested in the morning.

CLIENT: Well, this concerns me because I assume that if I am not well rested in the morning, it must mean that I have not slept well the night before.

THERAPIST: This may be a valid assumption. However, even the best sleepers do not always arise in the morning feeling well rested and full of energy.

CLIENT: So you're telling me that when I wake up in the morning feeling tired, it is not necessarily an indication of poor sleep.

THERAPIST: What I am suggesting is that you need to be careful with your expectations and interpretations. Even with good-quality sleep, you simply cannot expect to always feel refreshed and energetic during the day. There are day-to-day variations in how we feel and how energetic we are.

CLIENT: I guess I have noted that for myself.

THERAPIST: So, what alternative thoughts should you have the next time you catch yourself setting standards that may be unrealistic?

CLIENT: That 8 hours of sleep is not necessarily a "gold standard" that applies to everyone, and that even if on some days I am not fully rested, I may simply need to accept that and not jump to the conclusion that I slept poorly the night before and won't be able to function the next day.

THERAPIST: Very good! This should reduce your anxiety about sleep as well.

As the above vignette illustrates, many clients have unrealistic expectations about their sleep requirements and their daytime energy level. An important goal is to help these clients realize that diminished sleep and daytime energy are not always pathological, and that even good sleepers do not always get 8 hours of sleep or feel completely refreshed every morning. With gentle Socratic questioning, clients may benefit from reappraising their expectations regarding both sleep requirements and daytime energy.

Surveys can also be designed to evaluate unrealistic beliefs about sleep. Before the session, the therapist should have an idea of unrealistic beliefs to target (e.g., "Good sleepers get 8 hours of sleep," "Only people with insomnia feel tired in the daytime," or "I am not normal for waking up four times a night"). The Dysfunctional Beliefs and Attitude Scale (Morin & Espie, 2003) is a terrific measure to assess and document change in unhelpful beliefs about sleep. The therapist can introduce the survey by saying:

"One of the components of this treatment that we have found to be very effective is for us to collaborate together to create and administer a survey. There are a number of things we get from this: advice from good sleepers about why they sleep so well; a reminder as to how well good sleepers really sleep; and data on our beliefs about sleep. Most of us have developed our ideas about sleep from magazine articles, from a parent, or on the basis of our own experience. What or who has most influenced your ideas about sleep? [Allow the client to respond.] In order to start to become more data driven we are going to devise a survey together and administer it to people in your age group. This is always an interesting exercise and an opportunity to learn from others about how they manage their sleep. We focus on people around your age given that sleep changes so much across the lifespan. Here are some questions we have found to be helpful in the past."

At this point, the therapist asks questions that pertain specifically to the client's unhelpful beliefs about sleep. Survey questions may include the following:

- "Are you a good sleeper or someone with insomnia?" This question can be particularly useful to illustrate that individuals who regard themselves as "good sleepers" often feel tired in the morning, wake up at night, and feel sleepy in the afternoon.
- "How many hours of sleep per night do you get?"
- "How long does it take to fall asleep at night?"
- "How many times do you wake up at night?"
- "How alert do you feel upon waking, on a 1- to 10-point scale? What have you found helpful to increase alertness?"
- "How often do you nap? Does it affect your subsequent sleep?"

- "Do you have a bedtime routine? A morning routine?"
- "Do you feel tired in the daytime? When? What do you do to increase energy when you feel tired?" This question often generates many strategies suggested by others, and only a small proportion of the strategies involve resting or sleeping. Common alternatives include changing the environment, getting fresh air, going for a walk, drinking cold water, or having a snack. Clients often realize that energy can be increased by things other than rest and sleep, and that boredom is a big trigger for feeling tired.

Be sure to add questions of the client's choosing as well, so that the survey is truly collaborative and generates enthusiasm and interest. Clients are often curious about dreams, nightmares, or sleep patterns that can be added as questions to the survey. Also, questions about mood ("How often do you feel sad?" or "Have you noticed a relationship between your daytime mood and nighttime sleep?") can provide normalizing evidence that sleep and mood are interrelated, even in good sleepers.

Safety Behaviors

Closely related to unhelpful beliefs are so-called "safety behaviors," which are actions taken to avoid feared outcomes that are maladaptive in two ways: (1) They prevent disconfirmation of the unhelpful beliefs, and (2) they increase the likelihood that the feared outcomes will occur. Individuals with insomnia, in an attempt to cope with anxiety related to unhelpful beliefs about sleep, often employ safety behaviors (Salkovskis, 1991). In the previous section, we described an individual who endorsed the unhelpful belief that only solid, uninterrupted sleep would allow unimpaired work performance the next day. To prevent nocturnal awakenings, this individual might develop a routine of safety behaviors that include never going out in the evening, wearing earplugs, and using a sound machine as she sleeps. Engaging in these behaviors, while understandable in a general way, will clearly prevent her from learning that she can get adequate sleep even if the routine is broken. Paradoxically, these behaviors may make the feared outcome more likely to occur. Not going out in the evening increases the chance that she will become preoccupied with her sleep, and may contribute to rumination/worry and sad mood. Earplugs can be effective in certain circumstances, but they can also contribute to sleep problems if they are uncomfortable, or if they cause her to strain to try and hear things in the environment. A sound machine can facilitate awakenings in the night.

To work with safety behaviors, a helpful assessment tool is available (Ree & Harvey, 2004b). Behavioral experiments are designed in which the safety behavior is selectively adopted and then dropped, providing an often stunning demonstration of their adverse impact. For example, if a client avoids going out in the evenings because of feared impact on sleep, practitioner and client can set up a behavioral experiment in which two of the evenings in the week are spent at home (the "control" condition), and two evenings in the week are spent outside the home (socializing with others, going to a movie, etc.; the "experimental" condition). The practitioner instructs the client to rate not only standard sleep variables on the weekly diary (SOL, TST, etc.) but also to add a simple scale to measure evening satisfaction or mood each night. Often it is helpful to point out that mood and satisfaction increased on nights the client left the home, as well as to emphasize minimal (or inconsistent) changes in sleep as a result of leaving the home.

Daytime Energy

Individuals with disturbed sleep often monitor themselves for signs of fatigue upon waking or throughout the day. Normalizing feelings of grogginess upon waking (so-called "sleep inertia"), and introducing behavioral experiments and attention strategies for daytime monitoring can reduce anxiety and preoccupation with sleep. Often clients believe the only way they can feel less tired in the daytime is to sleep more. Hence, a behavioral experiment is devised to allow the client to experience the energy-generating effects of activity (Ree & Harvey, 2004a). This is also an opportunity to develop a list of energy-generating and energy-sapping activities that can be used to manage daytime tiredness and inevitable bouts of occasional sleep deprivation.

Many clients believe that energy progressively drains away throughout the day, and that the only way to generate energy is to sleep or rest. Accordingly, many clients work particularly hard at conserving energy after a poor night's sleep. As such, a behavioral experiment targets the following cognitions: "Energy is increased only by rest or sleep" and "I don't have much energy, so I need to take care to conserve it." We hope to use the experiment to illustrate that factors other than sleep influence energy levels.

To set up this behavioral experiment, client and therapist begin by using the sleep diary as a basis for discussing sleep and energy during the day. They note examples where nighttime sleep was good but energy levels in the day were poor, or where nighttime sleep was poor but energy levels during the day were good. The therapist may wish to say something like: "That is really interesting. So if sleep isn't the full account of how you feel during the day, then there must be other things that can account for it." Set up a 2-day experiment to test energy as follows: On the first day, spend one 3-hour block *conserving* energy, then a 3-hour block *using* energy. After each 3-hour block, the client rates his/her energy and mood. The following day, the client does this in the reverse order. Be careful to define what conserving energy means for your client. Examples include avoidance of socializing with colleagues, setting work tasks at a slow pace, attempting only mundane tasks, not going out for lunch with work friends, and not returning phone calls. Also, spend time in the session brainstorming strategies for using energy. These might include going for a 10-minute walk, returning all phone calls, arranging to have a coffee with a colleague, getting on top of the paperwork, going to the water cooler to get a drink, or walking to a local shop to buy a magazine or snack. Ask the client to rate his/her mood and fatigue on a form developed collaboratively in the session. The client typically finds that his/her mood and energy were *improved* by "using" energy, and using energy then becomes synonymous with generating energy. The therapist may comment that energy levels are like elastic that can be stretched quite easily.

TREATMENT SUMMARY AND RELAPSE PREVENTION

The final treatment session is oriented around consolidating skills and preparing for setbacks. Relapse prevention is designed to build skills to minimize or prevent the reoccurrence of sleep disturbance in the long term. At the end of treatment, the therapist guides the participant in identifying potential high-risk situations for insomnia in the future and discusses skills to prevent or cope with these high-risk situations. Client and therapist together discuss potential obstacles to maintaining gains, and they problem-solve around areas of future sleep disturbance. An individualized summary of learning and achievements guides relapse prevention work. Areas needing further intervention are addressed by setting specific goals and creating plans for achieving each goal.

In the final session, therapist and client distinguish between a lapse (an occasional night of insomnia), which is normal even for good sleepers, and relapse (return of frequent and chronic insomnia). Discuss with the client the inevitability of having an occasional poor night's sleep and caution against interpreting this as evidence that chronic insomnia has returned. Identifying situations that have been problematic in the past, and reviewing a "new" response to temporary setbacks, can be critical in maintaining gains.

The therapist can guide the client in imagining a typical scenario in which insomnia is present for two or three nights, then follow up by exploring strategies the client might use to handle this situation in the future. This is a good opportunity to check, once again, whether the client has integrated the necessary skills to cope with such insomnia nights. Discuss how he/she can avoid falling back in the old patterns of poor sleep.

Clients are strongly urged to review their materials from treatment and do their own assessment of the problem and identify the best course of action. Therapists also encourage clients to continue using tools after treatment has concluded. They work with clients to review tools, along with how the tools can be used to prevent insomnia reemergence. For example, the therapist can give the client multiple copies of the extended thought record or materials that the client found particularly helpful in session.

COMMON PROBLEMS IN TREATMENT

There are at least three common problems practitioners may encounter in delivering CBT-I for treatment of insomnia: difficulty regularizing the sleep–wake schedule, opposition to sleep restriction, and beliefs about the cause of insomnia that can hinder treatment compliance. We briefly discuss solutions to each problem below.

Clients are often reluctant to go to bed and wake up at the same time every day, including on weekends. This can be particularly problematic for teenagers or young adults who often socialize and/or schedule pleasurable activities in the weekend evening hours. As described earlier, MI that honestly reviews the pros and cons of regularizing a sleep schedule can be one way

to clarify ambivalence and prepare clients for change. Therapists may also find it helpful to guide clients in some general behavioral activity scheduling (e.g., encouraging clients to schedule a brunch, hike, or social visit on weekend mornings instead of weekend evenings, to enhance motivation). Finally, family members and friends can be instrumental to encouraging change. One client found it helpful to have a parent come in and turn on the overhead bedroom lights every morning, including weekends; another agreed to have a friend call at the same time every morning, and to keep her phone by the bed so that she knew to answer it.

In addition to regularizing sleep schedules, clients are often resistant to implementing sleep restriction. It is helpful to allow clients to voice their concerns with this component of treatment (e.g., fear of reduced sleep), then follow up with basic education and problem solving to address specific areas noted. Often it is helpful to characterize the mild sleep deprivation engendered by sleep restriction as a "tool" that will allows sleep pressure to build and the system to get back on track, or as a short-term side effect on the road to long-term, lasting gains. Encourage clients to experiment with their sleep.

Finally, clients may have a variety of beliefs about the cause of their insomnia that may shape treatment expectations and compliance. Some clients see their insomnia as purely biological; others recognize psychological components; and still others attribute emergence of their insomnia to environmental causes (e.g., the birth of a child, or experiencing a trauma). Each of these may influence motivation to implement components of CBT-I. The therapist can acknowledge the client's beliefs about his/her insomnia while explaining the Spielman model (see the earlier "Models of Insomnia" section), highlighting the fact that regardless of the predisposing/precipitating factors that initiated insomnia, perpetuating factors (excessive time in bed, worry, napping) are currently maintaining the insomnia. These perpetuating factors will be the focus of CBT-I treatment.

CONCLUSION AND FUTURE DIRECTIONS

CBT-I is emerging as an effective treatment option for insomnia. Administered as a brief, structured outpatient treatment, CBT-I targets behavioral, cognitive, and attentional processes that mutually maintain insomnia. Though it is structured, we wish to underscore the idea that CBT-I can be adapted *flexibly* according to the individualized conceptualizations of clients. Clinicians can use assessment data, sleep diaries, and clinical intuition to formulate a plan that emphasizes and addresses particular areas of concern (e.g., erratic sleep schedules, worry and rumination, or reliance on safety behaviors). Finally, CBT-I can be adapted for clients with comorbid conditions and even be used as a platform for addressing sleep problems such as hypersomnolence disorder. In this concluding section, we consider client–therapist variables that predict success or failure in treatment, issues specific to treating insomnia in mood disorders, and use of CBT-I principles to treat hypersomnolence.

Predictors of Clinical Outcome

There is limited research on factors that predict success or failure with CBT-I, though this represents an exciting area of future research. Evidence suggests that client factors predicting dropout from treatment include short sleep duration and elevated levels of baseline depressive symptomotolgy (Ong, Kuo, & Manber, 2008), though, in those who complete treatment, more severe insomnia and functional impairment at baseline actually predict clinical improvement (Van Houdenhove, Buyse, Gabriëls, & Van den Bergh, 2011). Clinical improvement is also predicted by changes in unhelpful beliefs about sleep (Edinger, Wohlgemuth, Radtke, Marsh, & Quillian, 2001; Morin, Blais, & Savard, 2002). Therapist qualities that appear to predict success in group CBT-I include client perceptions of therapist affiliation and warmth, while therapists perceived as confrontational have more client dropout (Constantino et al., 2007). In our own clinical experience, we have found that fostering a sense of curiosity and experimentation, and providing a clear rationale for homework completion, makes a big difference in client motivation and treatment outcome.

Treating Insomnia in Mood Disorders

Sleep disturbance is commonly comorbid with other mood disorders (Armitage, 2007), and CBT-I may be a particularly useful intervention to stabilize sleep and circadian rhythms. For example, individuals with bipolar disorder display night-to-night variability in TST (Gruber et al., 2009), along with reduced sleep efficiency and increased nighttime wakefulness (Eidelman, Talbot, Gruber, Hairston, & Harvey, 2010; Harvey, Schmidt, Scarna, Semler, & Goodwin, 2005) that may

respond particularly well to sleep restriction and stimulus control. Preliminary studies suggest that CBT-I improves unipolar depression when administered in combination with antidepressants (Manber et al., 2008) or as a stand-alone treatment (Taylor, Lichstein, Weinstock, Sanford, & Temple, 2007).

For practitioners who wish to address sleep problems in the context of depression or bipolar disorder, we offer the following recommendations. First, routinely monitor depression, anxiety, and/or mania symptoms, as applicable, at the start of each session. Negotiate a safety plan with the client prior to the start of therapy should his/her mood grow unstable during treatment. If symptoms of depression or mania emerge, evaluate changes in TST that may be contributing to decline and consider modifying or temporarily suspending sleep restriction or stimulus control if necessary. Finally, we encourage practitioners to monitor sleepiness regularly, using an instrument such as the Epworth Sleepiness Scale (Johns, 1991). When Epworth levels reach clinical significance (a score of 10), discourage clients from driving or engaging in other potentially unsafe behaviors during periods of drowsiness.

Adapting CBT-I to Treat Hypersomnolence

As with insomnia, several authors have raised the possibility that psychological mechanisms may contribute to the maintenance of hypersomnolence, or too *much* sleep (Billiard, Dolenc, Aldaz, Ondze, & Besset, 1994; Jacobson, Martell, & Dimidjian, 2001; Nofzinger et al., 1991). If these hypotheses are supported empirically, there may be utility in developing a psychological intervention for hypersomnolence. We have been developing a four- to eight-session multicomponent psychological intervention, briefly described below, though we emphasize that this approach awaits empirical evaluation. A number of the components used to treat hypersomnolence are adaptations or extensions of the interventions for insomnia reviewed earlier.

As in insomnia treatment, hypersomnolence treatment begins with a functional analysis and case formulation. Clinicians probe for the frequency, intensity, and duration of the hypersomnolence, as well as its antecedents, behaviors, and consequences. Clients complete a daily sleep diary, supplementing standard sleep diary questions with additional probes for energy, activity levels, and other contextual/psychological data of note. The first session also involves MI, including a straightforward review of pros and cons of working toward managing the hypersomnolence (Miller & Rollnick, 2002). The practitioner and client then set goals for treatment. The first and most obvious goal we set is for sleep (typically reducing sleep to approximately 8 hours per night), though we find it is equally critical to set goals for life. The latter is based on our clinical experience that "having nothing to get up for" is a key contributor to hypersomnolence in clients with mood disorders. Often the combination of the mood disorder and the sleep disorder has led to unemployment and disrupted social networks. Without work to get up for and family/friends to see, some individuals' motivation to reduce sleep seems to waver. After setting the "sleep" and "life" goals for the treatment, the client is asked to identify one small step toward these goals for the coming week. We engage in problem solving to limit the impact of these obstacles on reaching the goal, and a method is developed for monitoring the extent to which the goal is achieved (e.g., activity scheduling).

Clients with hypersomnolence also benefit from education about a range of issues relating to sleep. Two domains have been particularly important. The first involves education about the operation of the circadian system, the stimulating environmental influences acting on it (e.g., light), and the tendency, if left unchecked, to move toward a delayed phase. The second involves education about sleep inertia described earlier. Finally, we work with clients to establish a wind-down period, a "wake-up protocol" (e.g., not hitting "snooze" on the alarm; making the bed, so that the incentive to get back in is reduced; heading for the shower; taking a quick brisk walk; getting sunlight), and to minimize fluctuation in the sleep–wake schedule across the nights of the week.

Finally, many of the same behavioral experiments and surveys described in this chapter appear to effectively treat the decreased energy and fatigue that we see in hypersomnolence. For example, clients benefit from completing an "energy experiment" to experience how spending energy can be a useful way to generate energy. Other times, we structure an experiment in which clients are asked to rate their mood and energy before and after engaging in a social activity or leaving the house, to illustrate contextual variables that can improve mood and sleepiness. Creating a survey that emphasizes collecting data on what others do to generate energy, to get out of bed, or to fill their time when bored can offer helpful strategies. Finally, education and experiments on monitoring fatigue versus external stimuli can help to break attentional biases in hyper-

somnolence. As always, we conclude with a session on relapse prevention in which progress is reviewed, gains are consolidated, and possible setbacks are discussed. In this manner, many of the treatment principles useful for insomnia may also be used to treat hypersomnolence.

REFERENCES

Achermann, P., & Borbely, A. A. (2010). Sleep homeostasis and models of sleep regulation. In M. H. Kryger, T. Roth, & W. C. Dement (Eds.), *Principles and practice of sleep medicine* (5th ed., pp. 431–444). Philadelphia: Elsevier.

Akerstedt, T., Billiard, M., Bonnet, M., Ficca, G., Garma, L., Mariotti, M., et al. (2002). Awakening from sleep. *Sleep Medicine Reviews, 6*, 267–286.

American Academy of Sleep Medicine. (2005). *International classification of sleep disorders (ICSD): Diagnostic and coding manual* (2nd ed.). Westchester, IL: Author.

American Psychiatric Association. (2000). *Diagnostic and statistical manual of mental disorders* (4th ed., text rev.). Washington, DC: Author.

American Psychiatric Association. (2013). *Diagnostic and statistical manual of mental disorders* (5th ed.). Arlington, VA: Author.

Ancoli-Israel, S. (2009). Sleep and its disorders in aging populations. *Sleep Medicine, 10*(Suppl. 1), S7–S11.

Armitage, R. (2007). Sleep and circadian rhythms in mood disorders. *Acta Psychiatrica Scandinavica, 433*(Suppl.), 104–115.

Banks, S., & Dinges, D. F. (2010). Chronic sleep deprivation. In M. H. Kryger, T. Roth, & W. C. Dement (Eds.), *Principles and practice of sleep medicine* (5th ed., pp. 67–75). Philadelphia: Elsevier/Saunders.

Bastien, C. H., Vallieres, A., & Morin, C. M. (2001). Validation of the Insomnia Severity Index as an outcome measure for insomnia research. *Sleep Medicine, 2*, 297–307.

Beck, J. S. (1995). *Cognitive therapy: Basics and beyond.* New York: Guilford Press.

Belleville, G., Guay, C., Guay, B., & Morin, C. M. (2007). Hypnotic taper with or without self-help treatment of insomnia: a randomized clinical trial. *Journal of Consulting Clinical Psychology, 75*, 325–335.

Besset, A., Villemin, E., Tafti, M., & Billiard, M. (1998). Homeostatic process and sleep spindles in patients with sleep-maintenance insomnia: Effect of partial (21 h) sleep deprivation. *Electroencephalography and Clinical Neurophysiology, 107*(2), 122–132.

Billiard, M., Dolenc, L., Aldaz, C., Ondze, B., & Besset, A. (1994). Hypersomnia associated with mood disorders: A new perspective. *Journal of Psychosomatic Research, 38*(Suppl. 1), 41–47.

Bixler, E. O., Kales, A., Leo, L. A., & Slye, T. A. (1973).

A comparison of subjective estimates and objective sleep laboratory findings in insomnia patients. *Sleep Research, 2,* 143.

Bootzin, R. R. (1972). Stimulus control treatment for insomnia. *Proceedings of the American Psychological Association, 7,* 395–396.

Bootzin, R. R., Epstein, D., & Wood, J. M. (1991). Stimulus control instructions. In P. J. Hauri (Ed.), *Case studies in insomnia* (pp. 19–28). New York: Plenum Press.

Borbely, A. A. (1982). A two process model of sleep regulation. *Human Neurobiology, 1,* 195–204.

Borkovec, T. D. (1982). Insomnia. *Journal of Consulting and Clinical Psychology, 50,* 880–895.

Breslau, N., Roth, T., Rosenthal, L., & Andreski, P. (1996). Sleep disturbance and psychiatric disorders: A longitudinal epidemiological study of young adults. *Biological Psychiatry, 39*(6), 411–418.

Buysse, D., Ancoli-Israel, S., Edinger, J. D., Lichstein, K. L., & Morin, C. M. (2006). Recommendations for a standard research assessment of insomnia. *Sleep, 29,* 1155–1173.

Buysse, D. J., Reynolds, C. F., Monk, T. H., Berman, S. R., & Kupfer, D. J. (1989). The Pittsburgh Sleep Quality Index: A new instrument for psychiatric practice and research. *Psychiatry Research, 28,* 193–213.

Carney, C. E., Buysse, D. J., Ancoli-Israel, S., Edinger, J. D., Krystal, A. D., Lichstein, K. L., et al. (2012). The consensus sleep diary: Standardizing prospective sleep self-monitoring. *Sleep, 35*(2), 287–302.

Carskadon, M. A., Dement, W. C., Mitler, M. M., Guilleminault, C., Zarcone, V. P., & Spiegel, R. (1976). Self-reports versus sleep laboratory findings in 122 drug-free subjects with complaints of chronic insomnia. *American Journal of Psychiatry, 133*(12), 1382–1388.

Chambless, D. L., & Hollon, S. D. (1998). Defining empirically supported theories. *Journal of Consulting and Clinical Psychology, 1,* 7–18.

Chesson, A. L., Jr., Anderson, W. M., Littner, M., Davila, D., Hartse, K., Johnson, S., et al. (1999). Practice parameters for the nonpharmacologic treatment of chronic insomnia (An American Academy of Sleep Medicine report, Standards of Practice Committee of the American Academy of Sleep Medicine). *Sleep, 22,* 1128–1133.

Clark, D. M., Ehlers, A., Hackmann, A., McManus, F., Fennell, M., Grey, N., et al. (2006). Cognitive therapy versus exposure and applied relaxation in social phobia: A randomized controlled trial. *Journal of Consulting and Clinical Psychology, 74,* 568–578.

Clark, D. M., Salkovskis, P. M., Hackmann, A., Wells, A., Ludgate, J., & Gelder, M. (1999). Brief cognitive therapy for panic disorder: A randomized controlled trial. *Journal of Consulting and Clinical Psychology, 67,* 583–589.

Clarke, G., & Harvey, A. G. (2012). The complex role of sleep in adolescent depression. *Child and Adolescent Psychiatric Clinics of North America, 21*(2), 385–400.

Constantino, M. J., Manber, R., Ong, J., Kuo, T. F., Huang, J.,

& Arnow, B. A. (2007). Patient expectations and therapeutic alliance as predictors of outcome in group cognitive-behavioral therapy for insomnia. *Behavioral Sleep Medicine, 5*(3), 210–228.

Crick, F., & Mitchison, G. (1983). The function of dream sleep. *Nature, 304,* 111–114.

Crowley, S. J., & Carskadon, M. A. (2010). Modifications to weekend recovery sleep delay circadian phase in older adolescents. *Chronobiology International, 27,* 1469–1492.

Edinger, J. D., Bonnet, M. H., Bootzin, R. R., Doghramji, K., Dorsey, C. M., Espie, C. A., et al. (2004). Derivation of research diagnostic criteria for insomnia: Report of an American Academy of Sleep Medicine Work Group. *Sleep, 27,* 1567–1596.

Edinger, J. D., Wohlgemuth, W. K., Radtke, R. A., Marsh, G. R., & Quillian, R. E. (2001). Does cognitive-behavioral insomnia therapy alter dysfunctional beliefs about sleep? *Sleep, 24,* 591–599.

Edinger, J. D., Wyatt, J. K., Olsen, M. K., Stechuchak, K. M., Carney, C. E., Chiang, A., et al. (2009). Reliability and validity of the Duke Structured Interview for Sleep Disorders for insomnia screening. *Sleep, 32,* A265.

Eidelman, P., Talbot, L. S., Gruber, J., Hairston, I., & Harvey, A. G. (2010). Sleep architecture as correlate and predictor of symptoms and impairment in inter-episode bipolar disorder: Taking on the challenge of medication effects. *Journal of Sleep Research, 19*(4), 516–524.

Espie, C. A. (2002). Insomnia: Conceptual issues in the development, persistence, and treatment of sleep disorder in adults. *Annual Review of Psychology, 53,* 215–243.

Ford, D. E., & Kamerow, D. B. (1989). Epidemiologic study of sleep disturbances and psychiatric disorders. An opportunity for prevention? *Journal of the American Medical Association, 262,* 1479–1484.

Gruber, J., Harvey, A. G., Wang, P. W., Brooks, J. O., III, Thase, M. E., Sachs, G. S., et al. (2009). Sleep functioning in relation to mood, function, and quality of life at entry to the Systematic Treatment Enhancement Program for Bipolar Disorder (STEP-BD). *Journal of Affective Disorders, 114*(1–3), 41–49.

Harvey, A. G. (2001). Insomnia: Symptom or diagnosis? *Clinical Psychology Review, 21,* 1037–1059.

Harvey, A. G. (2002a). A cognitive model of insomnia. *Behaviour Research and Therapy, 40,* 869–894.

Harvey, A. G. (2002b). Trouble in bed: The role of pre-sleep worry and intrusions in the maintenance of insomnia [Special issue]. *Journal of Cognitive Psychotherapy, 16,* 161–177.

Harvey, A. G. (2003a). The attempted suppression of presleep cognitive activity in insomnia. *Cognitive Therapy and Research, 27,* 593–602.

Harvey, A. G. (2003b). Beliefs about the utility of presleep worry: An investigation of individuals with insomnia and good sleepers. *Cognitive Therapy and Research, 27,* 403–414.

Harvey, A. G. (2005). A cognitive theory of and therapy for chronic insomnia. *Journal of Cognitive Psychotherapy: An International Quarterly, 19*, 41–60.

Harvey, A. G. (2008). Sleep and circadian rhythms in bipolar disorder: Seeking synchrony, harmony, and regulation. *American Journal of Psychiatry, 165*, 820–829.

Harvey, A. G. (2009). The adverse consequences of sleep disturbance in pediatric bipolar disorder: Implications for intervention. *Child and Adolescent Psychiatry Clinics of North America, 18*(2), 321–338.

Harvey, A. G., & Eidelman, P. (2012). Intervention to reduce unhelpful beliefs about sleep. In M. Perlis, M. Aloia, & B. Kuhn (Eds.), *Behavioral sleep medicine treatment protocols* (pp. 79–90). New York: Academic Press.

Harvey, A. G., Schmidt, D. A., Scarna, A., Semler, C. N., & Goodwin, G. M. (2005). Sleep-related functioning in euthymic patients with bipolar disorder, patients with insomnia, and subjects without sleep problems. *American Journal of Psychiatry, 162*, 50–57.

Harvey, A. G., Sharpley, A. L., Ree, M. J., Stinson, K., & Clark, D. M. (2007). An open trial of cognitive therapy for chronic insomnia. *Behaviour Research and Therapy, 45*, 2491–2501.

Harvey, A. G., & Talbot, L. (2012a). Behavioral experiments. In M. Perlis, M. Aloia, & B. Kuhn (Eds.), *Behavioral sleep medicine treatment protocols* (pp. 71–78). New York: Academic Press.

Harvey, A. G., & Talbot, L. S. (2012b). Intervention to reduce misperception. In M. Perlis, M. Aloia, & B. Kuhn (Eds.), *Behavioral sleep medicine treatment protocols* (pp. 91–96). New York: Academic Press.

Harvey, A. G., & Tang, N. K. (2012). (Mis)perception of sleep in insomnia: A puzzle and a resolution. *Psychological Bulletin, 138*(1), 77–101.

Harvey, A. G., Tang, N. K. Y., & Browning, L. (2005). Cognitive approaches to insomnia. *Clinical Psychology Review, 25*, 593–611.

Hoddes, E., Zarcone, V., Smythe, H., Phillips, R., & Dement, W. C. (1973). Quantification of sleepiness: A new approach. *Psychophysiology, 10*, 431–436.

Hohagen, F., Rink, K., Kappler, C., Schramm, E., Riemann, D., Weyerer, S., et al. (1993). Prevalence and treatment of insomnia in general practice: A longitudinal study. *European Archives of Psychiatry and Clinical Neuroscience, 242*, 329–336.

Irwin, M. R., Cole, J. C., & Nicassio, P. M. (2006). Comparative meta-analysis of behavioral interventions for insomnia and their efficacy in middle-aged adults and in older adults 55+ years of age. *Health Psychology, 25*, 3–14.

Jacobson, N., Martell, C., & Dimidjian, S. (2001). Behavioral activation treatment for depression: Returning to contextual roots. *Clinical Psychology: Science and Practice, 8*, 255–270.

Jansson, M., & Linton, S. J. (2007). Psychological mechanisms in the maintenance of insomnia: Arousal, distress, and sleep-related beliefs. *Behaviour Research and Therapy, 45*(3), 511–521.

Jean-Louis, G., von Gizycki, H., Zizi, F., Spielman, A., Hauri, P., & Taub, H. (1997). The actigraph data analysis software: II. A novel approach to scoring and interpreting sleep-wake activity. *Perceptual and Motor Skills, 85*, 219–226.

Jenni, O. G., Achermann, P., & Carskadon, M. A. (2005). Homeostatic sleep regulation in adolescents. *Sleep, 28*, 1446–1454.

Johns, M. W. (1991). A new method for measuring daytime sleepiness: The Epworth sleepiness scale. *Sleep, 14*, 540–545.

Karni, A., Tanne, D., Rubenstien, B. S., Askenasy, J. J. M., & Sagi, D. (1994). Dependence on REM sleep of overnight improvement of a perceptual skill. *Science, 265*, 679–682.

Klerman, E. B., & Dijk, D. J. (2008). Age-related reduction in the maximal capacity for sleep—implications for insomnia. *Current Biology, 18*(15), 1118–1123.

Kryger, M. H., Roth, T., & Dement, W. C. (2010). *Principles and practice of sleep medicine* (5th ed.). Philadelphia: Saunders.

Lack, L. C., & Bootzin, R. R. (2003). Circadian rhythm factors in insomnia and their treatment. In M. Perlis & K. Lichstein (Eds.), *Treatment of sleep disorders: Principles and practice of behavioral sleep medicine* (pp. 305–343). New York: Wiley.

Lichstein, K. (2000). Secondary insomnia. In K. Lichstein & C. Morin (Eds.), *Treatment of late-life insomnia* (pp. 297–319). Thousand Oaks, CA: Sage.

Lichstein, K. L., Durrence, H. H., Taylor, D. J., Bush, A. J., & Riedel, B. W. (2003). Quantitative criteria for insomnia. *Behaviour Research and Therapy, 41*, 427–445.

Lichstein, K. L., Peterson, B. A., Riedel, B. W., Means, M. K., Epperson, M. T., & Aguillard, R. N. (1999). Relaxation to assist sleep medication withdrawal. *Behavior Modification, 23*(3), 379–402.

Lichstein, K. L., & Rosenthal, T. L. (1980). Insomniacs' perceptions of cognitive versus somatic determinants of sleep disturbance. *Journal of Abnormal Psychology, 89*, 105–107.

Lichstein, K. L., Stone, K. C., Donaldson, J., Nau, S. D., Soeffing, J. P., Murray, D., et al. (2006). Actigraphy validation with insomnia. *Sleep, 29*, 232–239.

Manber, R., Edinger, J. D., Gress, J. L., San Pedro-Salcedo, M. G., Kuo, T. F., & Kalista, T. (2008). Cognitive behavioral therapy for insomnia enhances depression outcome in patients with comorbid major depressive disorder and insomnia. *Sleep, 31*(4), 489–495.

Miller, W. R., & Rollnick, S. (2002). *Motivational interviewing: Preparing people for change* (2nd ed.). New York: Guilford Press.

Montgomery, P., & Dennis, J. (2003). Cognitive behavioural interventions for sleep problems in adults aged 60+. *Cochrane Database of Systematic Reviews, 1*, CD003161.

Morgenthaler, T., Alessi, C., Friedman, L., Owens, J., Kapur, V., Boehlecke, B., et al. (2007). Practice parameters for the use of actigraphy in the assessment of sleep and sleep disorders: An update for 2007. *Sleep, 30*(4), 519–529.

Morin, C. M. (1993). *Insomnia: Psychological assessment and management*. New York: Guilford Press.

Morin, C. M., Blais, F., & Savard, J. (2002). Are changes in beliefs and attitudes about sleep related to sleep improvements in the treatment of insomnia? *Behaviour Research and Therapy, 40*, 741–752.

Morin, C. M., Bootzin, R. R., Buysse, D. J., Edinger, J., D., Espie, C. A., & Lichstein, K. L. (2006). Psychological and behavioral treatment of insomnia: An update of recent evidence (1998–2004). *Sleep, 29*, 1396–1406.

Morin, C. M., Culbert, J. P., & Schwartz, S. M. (1994). Nonpharmacological interventions for insomnia: A meta-analysis of treatment efficacy. *American Journal of Psychiatry, 151*, 1172–1180.

Morin, C. M., & Espie, C. A. (2003). *Insomnia: A clinical guide to assessment and treatment*. New York: Kluwer Academic/Plenum Press.

Morin, C. M., Gaulier, B., Barry, T., & Kowatch, R. A. (1992). Patients' acceptance of psychological and pharmacological therapies for insomnia. *Sleep, 15*, 302–305.

Morin, C. M., Hauri, P. J., Espie, C. A., Spielman, A. J., Buysse, D. J., & Bootzin, R. R. (1999). Nonpharmacologic treatment of chronic insomnia: An American Academy of Sleep Medicine review. *Sleep, 22*, 1134–1156.

Morin, C. M., Koetter, U., Bastien, C., Ware, J. C., & Wooten, V. (2005). Valerian–hops combination and diphenhydramine for treating insomnia: A randomized placebo-controlled clinical trial. *Sleep, 28*(11), 1465–1471.

Morin, C. M., Vallieres, A., Guay, B., Ivers, H., Savard, J., Merette, C., et al. (2009). Cognitive behavioral therapy, singly and combined with medication, for persistent insomnia: A randomized controlled trial. *Journal of the American Medical Association, 301*(19), 2005–2015.

Murtagh, D. R., & Greenwood, K. M. (1995). Identifying effective psychological treatments for insomnia: A meta-analysis. *Journal of Consulting and Clinical Psychology, 63*, 79–89.

Neitzert Semler, C., & Harvey, A. G. (2004). Monitoring for sleep-related threat: A pilot study of the sleep associated monitoring index (SAMI). *Psychosomatic Medicine, 66*, 242–250.

National Institutes of Health. (2005). National Institutes of Health State of the Science Conference Statement: Manifestations and management of chronic insomnia in adults, *Sleep, 28*, 1049–1057.

Nofzinger, E. A., Thase, M. E., Reynolds, C. F., III, Himmelhoch, J. M., Mallinger, A., Houck, P., et al. (1991). Hypersomnia in bipolar depression: A comparison with narcolepsy using the multiple sleep latency test. *American Journal of Psychiatry, 148*(9), 1177–1181.

Ohayon, M. M. (2002). Epidemiology of insomnia: What we know and what we still need to learn. *Sleep Medicine Reviews, 6*, 97–111.

Ong, J. C., Kuo, T. F., & Manber, R. (2008). Who is at risk for dropout from group cognitive-behavioral theapy for insomnia? *Journal of Psychosomatic Research, 64*(4), 419–425.

Paquet, J., Kawinska, A., & Carrier, J. (2007). Wake detection capacity of actigraphy during sleep. *Sleep, 30*(10), 1362–1369.

Perlis, M., Aloia, M., & Kuhn, B. (Eds.). (2012). *Behavioral sleep medicine treatment protocols*. New York: Academic Press.

Perlis, M., & Lichstein, K. (Eds.). (2003). *Treating sleep disorders: Principles and practice of behavioral sleep medicine*. New York: Wiley.

Perlis, M. L., Smith, M. T., & Pigeon, W. R. (2005). Etiology and pathophysiology of insomnia. In M. H. Kryger, T. Roth, & W. C. Dement (Eds.), *Principles and practice of sleep medicine* (4th ed., pp. 714–725). Philadelphia: Elsevier/Saunders.

Ree, M., & Harvey, A. G. (2004a). Insomnia. In J. Bennett-Levy, G. Butler, M. Fennell, A. Hackman, M. Mueller, & D. Westbrook (Eds.), *Oxford guide to behavioural experiments in cognitive therapy* (pp. 287–305). Oxford, UK: Oxford University Press.

Ree, M., & Harvey, A. G. (2004b). Investigating safety behaviours in insomnia: The development of the Sleep-Related Behaviours Questionnaire (SRBQ). *Behaviour Change, 21*, 26–36.

Ree, M. J., Harvey, A. G., Blake, R., Tang, N. K., & Shawe-Taylor, M. (2005). Attempts to control unwanted thoughts in the night: Development of the thought control questionnaire-insomnia revised (TCQI-R). *Behaviour Research and Therapy, 43*, 985–998.

Reite, M., Buysse, D., Reynolds, C., & Mendelson, W. (1995). The use of polysomnography in the evaluation of insomnia. *Sleep, 18*, 58–70.

Roth, T., Coulouvrat, C., Hajak, G., Lakoma, M. D., Sampson, N. A., Shahly, V., et al. (2011). Prevalence and perceived health associated with insomnia based on DSM-IV-TR; International Statistical Classification of Diseases and related health problems, Tenth Revision; and Research Diagnostic Criteria/International Classification of Sleep Disorders, Second Edition criteria: Results from the America Insomnia Survey. *Biological Psychiatry, 69*, 592–600.

Rybarczyk, B., Lopez, M., Schelble, K., & Stepanski, E. (2005). Home-based video CBT for comorbid geriatric insomnia: A pilot study using secondary data analyses. *Behavioral Sleep Medicine, 3*, 158–175.

Salkovskis, P. M. (1991). The importance of behaviour in the maintenance of anxiety and panic: A cognitive account. *Behavioural Psychotherapy, 19*, 6–19.

Sivertsen, B., Omvik, S., Pallesen, S., Bjorvatn, B., Havik, O. E., Kvale, G., et al. (2006). Cognitive behavioral therapy vs zopiclone for treatment of chronic primary insomnia in older adults: A randomized controlled trial. *Journal of the American Medical Association, 295*, 2851–2858.

Smith, L. J., Nowakowski, S., Soeffing, J. P., Orff, H. J., & Perlis, M. L. (2003). The measurement of sleep. In M. L. Perlis & K. L. Lichstein (Eds.), *Treating sleep disorders: Principles and practice of behavioral sleep medicine* (pp. 29–73). New York: Wiley.

Smith, M. T., Huang, M. I., & Manber, R. (2005). Cognitive behavior therapy for chronic insomnia occurring within the context of medical and psychiatric disorders. *Clinical Psychology Review, 25*, 559–592.

Spielman, A. J., Caruso, L. S., & Glovinsky, P. B. (1987). A behavioral perspective on insomnia treatment. *Psychiatric Clinics of North America, 10*, 541–553.

Spielman, A. J., Saskin, P., & Thorpy, M. J. (1987). Treatment of chronic insomnia by restriction of time in bed. *Sleep, 10*, 45–56.

Stepanski, E. J., Zorick, F., Roehrs, T., & Roth, T. (2000). Effects of sleep deprivation on daytime sleepiness in primary insomnia. *Sleep, 23*, 215–219.

Taylor, D. J., Lichstein, K. L., Weinstock, J., Sanford, S., & Temple, J. R. (2007). A pilot study of cognitive-behavioral therapy of insomnia in people with mild depression. *Behavior Therapy, 38*(1), 49–57.

Vallieres, A., & Morin, C. M. (2003). Actigraphy in the assessment of insomnia. *Sleep, 26*, 902–906.

Van Houdenhove, L., Buyse, B., Gabriëls, L. & Van den Bergh, O. (2011). Treating primary insomnia: Clinical effectiveness and predictors of outcomes on sleep, daytime function and health-related quality of life. *Journal of Clinical Psychology in Medical Settings, 18*(3), 312–321.

Van Someren, E. J. (2000). Circadian rhythms and sleep in human aging. *Chronobiology International, 17*, 233–243.

Walker, M. P., & Stickgold, R. (2006). Sleep, memory, and plasticity. *Annual Review of Psychology, 57*, 139–166.

Watkins, E., & Baracaia, S. (2001). Why do people ruminate in dysphoric moods? *Personality and Individual Differences, 30*, 723–734.

Watts, F. N., Coyle, K., & East, M. P. (1994). The contribution of worry to insomnia. *British Journal of Clinical Psychology, 33*, 211–220.

Wicklow, A., & Espie, C. A. (2000). Intrusive thoughts and their relationship to actigraphic measurement of sleep: Towards a cognitive model of insomnia. *Behaviour Research and Therapy, 38*(7), 679–693.

Wyatt, J. K., Stepanski, E. J., & Kirkby, J. (2006). Circadian phase in delayed sleep phase syndrome: Predictors and temporal stability across multiple assessments. *Sleep, 29*, 1075–1080.

Yoo, S. S., Gujar, N., Hu, P., Jolesz, F. A., & Walker, M. P. (2007). The human emotional brain without sleep—a prefrontal amygdala disconnect. *Current Biology, 17*, R877–R878.

Zee, P. C., & Turek, F. W. (2006). Sleep and health: Everywhere and in both directions. *Archives of Internal Medicine, 166*, 1686–1688.

CHAPTER 17

Eating Disorders
A Transdiagnostic Protocol

Christopher G. Fairburn
Zafra Cooper

The fifth edition of the *Diagnostic and Statistical Manual of Mental Disorders* (DSM-5) clearly defines and separates anorexia nervosa and bulimia nervosa, and recognizes for the first time binge-eating disorder as a specific diagnosis. But many people with serious eating disorders do not quite fit these diagnostic criteria and would be lumped into an "other specified feeding or eating disorder" category. It is also the case that individuals with eating disorders change from one category to another over time. The authors of this chapter, involved over the years in the creation of the DSM eating disorder categories, are also among the originators of the most successful treatment yet devised for these disorders. Thus, it is significant that Fairburn and colleagues have moved ahead of the curve and created a "transdiagnostic" unified theory and treatment protocol applicable to all eating disorders, including those falling into the "other specified" category. (For a similar approach to emotional disorders, see Payne, Ellard, Farchione, Fairholme, & Barlow, Chapter 6, this volume.) In this chapter Fairburn and Cooper describe this state-of-the-art treatment. In what to some readers may be a surprising departure, the authors' note that the central problem requiring intervention is not necessarily dieting, bingeing, low weight, or purging, but rather the culturally reinforced abnormal attitudes and beliefs regarding shape and weight. The recommendation for applying various treatment components in a "modular" fashion speaks to the art of administering this treatment. The detailed explication of cognitive-behavioral therapy as applied to eating disorders should be extraordinarily useful to clinicians working with these difficult problems.—D. H. B.

Clinical eating disorders such as anorexia nervosa, bulimia nervosa, and binge-eating disorder are a cause of substantial physical and psychosocial morbidity among adolescent girls and young adult women. They are much less common among men. They typically begin in adolescence and may run a chronic course. Their effect is pervasive, since they interfere with psychological, physical, and social functioning. Once established, they are difficult to treat and impose a significant burden on health services. In this chapter we describe the psychopathology of the eating disorders and the mechanisms that cause them to persist. We then describe a transdiagnostic cognitive-behavioral treatment designed to disrupt these mechanisms.

CLASSIFICATION AND DIAGNOSIS

The DSM-5 Scheme

The DSM-5 scheme for classifying and diagnosing eating disorders recognizes three specific disorders: anorexia nervosa, bulimia nervosa, and binge-eating disorder. In addition, there are two residual categories termed "other specified feeding or eating disorder" and "unspecified feeding or eating disorder," respectively (American Psychiatric Association, 2013).

In essence, three features needed to be present to make a diagnosis of anorexia nervosa:

1. The overevaluation of shape and weight; that is, judging self-worth largely, or even exclusively, in terms of shape and weight.
2. This is often expressed as a strong desire to be thin, combined with an intense fear of gaining weight and becoming fat.
3. The active maintenance of an unduly low body weight (e.g., maintaining a body weight less than 85% of that expected or a body mass index $\leq$ 17.5[1]).

Amenorrhea (in postpubertal females), another requirement for the diagnosis of anorexia nervosa in the previous DSM edition, has been removed due to its questionable validity; that is, the majority of female patients who meet the other diagnostic criteria are also amenorrheic, and those who are not closely resemble those who are.

Three features also need to be present to make a diagnosis of bulimia nervosa:

1. The overevaluation of shape and weight, as in anorexia nervosa.
2. Recurrent binge eating. A "binge" is an episode of eating during which an objectively large amount of food is eaten, and there is a sense of loss of control at the time.
3. Extreme weight-control behavior, such as strict dietary restriction, recurrent self-induced vomiting, or marked laxative misuse.

In addition, to diagnose bulimia nervosa, there is an exclusionary criterion, namely, that the diagnostic criteria for anorexia nervosa not be met. This criterion ensures that it is not possible for patients receiving both diagnoses at one time.

Binge-eating disorder, which was a provisional diagnosis in DSM-IV, is now recognized as a full disorder in DSM-5. It is designed to denote an eating problem characterized by recurrent binge eating in the absence of the extreme weight control behavior seen in bulimia nervosa and anorexia nervosa.

No diagnostic criteria are specified for the two residual eating disorder diagnoses.

CLINICAL FEATURES

Anorexia nervosa and bulimia nervosa, and most cases of other specified eating disorders, share a distinctive "core psychopathology" that is essentially the same in females and males, adults and adolescents. This is the overevaluation of shape and weight. Whereas most people evaluate themselves on the basis of their perceived performance in a variety of life domains (e.g., the quality of their relationships; their work performance; their sporting prowess), people with eating disorders judge their self-worth largely, or even exclusively, in terms of their shape and weight, and their ability to control them. This psychopathology is peculiar to the eating disorders (and to body dysmorphic disorder) and is rarely seen in the general population. It should be distinguished from "body shape dissatisfaction," which refers to dislike of aspects of one's appearance. Some degree of body shape dissatisfaction is widespread and its presence is sometimes referred to as "normative discontent."

The overevaluation of shape and weight results in the pursuit of weight loss—note that it is usually weight loss that is sought, not a specific weight—and an intense fear of weight gain and fatness. Most other features of these disorders are secondary to this core psychopathology and its consequences (e.g., undereating; becoming severely underweight). Thus, in anorexia nervosa there is a sustained and successful pursuit of weight loss that results in patients becoming severely underweight. This pursuit is not seen as a problem: Rather, it is valued and, as a consequence, patients have little desire to change. For this reason it is often other people who are responsible for these patients' entry into treatment. In bulimia nervosa, equivalent attempts to restrict food intake are disrupted by repeated episodes of loss of control over eating (binges). Generally these binges are aversive and a source of distress, and they lead patients to seek help. Consequently those with bulimia nervosa are easier to engage in treatment, although because of the accompanying shame and secrecy, there is typically a delay of many years before they divulge their eating problem and enter treatment.

The core psychopathology of anorexia nervosa and bulimia nervosa has other expressions, too. Many patients mislabel adverse physical and emotional states as "feeling fat" and equate this with actually being fat. In addition, many repeatedly scrutinize their bodies, focusing on parts that they dislike. This may contribute to patients' overestimation of their size. Others actively avoid seeing their bodies, assuming that they look fat and disgusting. Equivalent behavior is seen with respect to weighing (weight checking), with many patients weighing themselves frequently. As a result these patients become preoccupied with trivial, day-to-day fluctuations, whereas others actively avoid knowing their weight but nevertheless remain highly concerned about it.

Anorexia Nervosa

In anorexia nervosa, the pursuit of weight loss leads patients to engage in a severe and selective restriction of food intake, avoiding foods viewed as fattening. Generally there is no true "anorexia" (loss of appetite) as such. The undereating may also be an expression of other motives, including asceticism, competitiveness, and a desire to attract the attention of others. In the early stages of the disorder, undereating may be a goal in its own right, with the patient valuing the sense of self-control that it confers. Some patients also engage in a driven type of exercising that contributes to their weight loss. This is characterized by a strong drive to exercise, a tendency to overexercise, and giving exercise precedence over other aspects of life. Self-induced vomiting and other extreme forms of weight control (e.g., the misuse of laxatives or diuretics) are practiced by a subgroup of these patients, and patients in an overlapping group have episodes of loss of control over eating, although the amount eaten may not be objectively large ("subjective binge eating"). Depressive and anxiety features, irritability, lability of mood, impaired concentration, loss of sexual appetite, and obsessional features are also frequently present. Typically these features get worse as weight is lost and improve with weight regain. Interest in the outside world also wanes as patients become underweight, with the result that most become socially withdrawn and isolated. This, too, tends to reverse with weight regain.

Bulimia Nervosa

The eating habits of those with bulimia nervosa resemble those seen in anorexia nervosa. The main distinguishing feature is that the attempts to restrict food intake are disrupted by repeated episodes of binge eating. The frequency of these episodes ranges from once a week (the DSM-5 diagnostic threshold) to several times a day, and the amount eaten per episode varies but is typically between 1,000 and 2,000 kilocalories (kcal). In most cases, each binge is followed by compensatory, self-induced vomiting or laxative misuse but there is a subgroup of patients who do not "purge." The weight of most patients with bulimia nervosa is in the healthy range (BMI between 18.5 and 25.0) due to the effects of undereating and overeating balancing each other. As a result, these patients do not experience the secondary psychosocial and physical effects of maintaining a very low weight. Depressive and anxiety features are prominent in bulimia nervosa—indeed, more than in anorexia nervosa—and there is a subgroup of patients who engage in substance misuse or self-injury, or both. This subgroup, which is also present in some anorexia nervosa patients who binge-eat, tends to attract the diagnosis of borderline personality disorder.

Binge-Eating Disorder

Patients with binge-eating disorder report recurrent binge eating, much as in bulimia nervosa, but their eating habits outside the binges are quite different. As noted earlier, in bulimia nervosa there is a high level of dietary restraint, with most patients attempting to adhere to a highly restricted diet when not binge eating. In contrast, in binge-eating disorder there is a tendency to overeat outside the binges. Indeed, the eating habits of patients with binge-eating disorder resemble those of people with obesity, albeit with binges superimposed. Thus, self-induced vomiting and laxative misuse are not present, nor is there any tendency to overexercise. Most people who seek treatment for binge-eating disorder are overweight or meet criteria for obesity (BMI ≥ 30.0).

Other Specified and Unspecified Eating Disorders

The psychopathology of the "other specified" and "unspecified" eating disorders in DSM-5, referred to as eating disorder NOS in DSM-IV, closely resembles that seen in anorexia nervosa, bulimia nervosa, and binge-eating disorder. It is also of comparable duration and severity (Fairburn et al., 2007). Conceptually, it is helpful to distinguish two subgroups within these categories, although there is no sharp boundary between them. The first comprises cases that closely resemble anorexia nervosa or bulimia nervosa but just fail to meet their diagnostic criteria; for example, body weight may be marginally above the threshold for anorexia nervosa or the frequency of binge eating may be just too low for a diagnosis of bulimia nervosa. These cases belong to the "other specified feeding or eating disorder" category. The second and larger subgroup comprises cases in which the clinical features of anorexia nervosa and bulimia nervosa are combined in a manner that is different than that seen in the two prototypical disorders. Such states may be described as "mixed" in character and they belong to the "unspecified feeding and eating disorder" category. Cases of this type are common (Fairburn & Cooper, 2011).

Readers may come across references to so-called "purging disorder," a term that refers to a state characterized by recurrent purging in the absence of binge eating. In DSM-5 these cases are placed in the "other specified feeding or eating disorder" category. In our experience, the great majority of people who meet these criteria experience subjective binges and are therefore best viewed as having a variant of bulimia nervosa.

Last, patients who describe overeating that is confined to the late evening or night are referred to as having "night eating syndrome," a relatively neglected state, and one that is outside the scope of this chapter. For information on night eating syndrome and its treatment readers are referred to the book by Lundgren, Allison, and Stunkard (2012).

DEVELOPMENT AND SUBSEQUENT COURSE

Anorexia nervosa typically starts in adolescence with the onset of dietary restriction that becomes progressively more extreme and inflexible. In its early stages the disorder may be self-limiting and treatment-responsive, but if it persists, it tends to become entrenched and requires more intensive treatment. In 10–20% of cases, it proves intractable and unremitting. Even in patients who recover, residual features are common, particularly some degree of overconcern about shape, weight,

and eating. A frequent occurrence is the development of binge eating and, in about half the cases, progression on to full bulimia nervosa. Most prominent among the favorable prognostic factors are early age of onset and short history, whereas unfavorable prognostic factors include a long history, severe weight loss, binge eating, and vomiting. Anorexia nervosa is the one eating disorder to be associated with a raised mortality rate, with the standardized mortality ratio over the first 10 years from presentation being about 10. The majority of deaths are either a direct result of medical complications or due to suicide.

Bulimia nervosa has a slightly later age of onset, typically in late adolescence or early adulthood. It usually starts in much the same way as anorexia nervosa—indeed, in about one-fourth of cases the diagnostic criteria for anorexia nervosa are met for a time. Eventually, however, episodes of binge eating interrupt the dietary restriction and, as a result, body weight rises to normal or near normal levels. The disorder is extremely self-perpetuating. Thus, patients often present with an unremitting history of 8 years or more of disturbed eating. No consistent predictors of outcome have been identified, although there is evidence that childhood obesity, low self-esteem, and signs of personality disturbance are associated with a worse prognosis.

Binge-eating disorder has a rather different age of presentation and course. Most of these patients are middle-aged and one-third or more are male. This is quite unlike patients with anorexia nervosa, bulimia nervosa, and the two groups of residual eating disorders, who are generally female (about 10% are male) and are adolescents or young adults. Clinical experience suggests that binge-eating disorder also differs in its course, in that it tends to be phasic rather than persistent, with most patients describing sustained periods lasting many months free from binge eating. Throughout, these patients have a general tendency to overeat and gain weight. Few report a history of either anorexia nervosa or bulimia nervosa.

Little is known about the development and course of the residual eating disorders. Most patients present in their adolescence or 20s, as in bulimia nervosa, and with a comparable length of history (Fairburn et al., 2007). Because between one-fourth and one-third of patients have had anorexia nervosa or bulimia nervosa in the past, their present state is simply the latest expression of an evolving eating disorder.

THE "TRANSDIAGNOSTIC" PERSPECTIVE

The DSM-5 scheme for classifying eating disorders encourages the view that anorexia nervosa, bulimia nervosa, and binge-eating disorder are distinct clinical states, each requiring its own form of treatment. It should be clear from consideration of their clinical features and course over time that the evidence does not support this (Fairburn & Harrison, 2003). With the possible exception of binge-eating disorder, the eating disorders have many features in common, most of which are not seen in other psychiatric disorders. Studies of their course indicate that patients migrate between these diagnoses over time: Indeed, temporal migration is the norm rather than the exception. This temporal movement, together with the fact that the disorders share the same distinctive psychopathology, suggests that common "transdiagnostic" mechanisms are involved in the persistence of eating disorder psychopathology (Fairburn, Cooper, & Shafran, 2003). If correct, this implies that treatments capable of successfully addressing these maintaining mechanisms should be effective with all forms of eating disorder rather than just one.

THE COGNITIVE-BEHAVIORAL THEORY

Bulimia Nervosa

In common with most evidence-based cognitive-behavioral treatments, the theory that underpins the cognitive-behavioral treatment for bulimia nervosa (CBT-BN) is primarily concerned with the *processes that maintain the disorder* rather than those responsible for its development. According to the theory, these patients' dysfunctional scheme for self-evaluation is central to the maintenance of the disorder. As noted earlier, whereas most people evaluate themselves on the basis of their perceived performance in a variety of life domains, people with eating disorders judge themselves largely, or even exclusively, in terms of their shape and weight, and their ability to control them. As a result, their lives become focused on shape, weight, and eating, with dietary control, thinness, and weight loss being actively pursued, while overeating, "fatness," and weight gain are assiduously avoided. Most of the other features of bulimia nervosa can be understood as stemming directly from this "core psychopathology," including the weight control behavior, the various forms of body checking and avoidance, and the preoccupation

with thoughts about shape, weight, and eating. Figure 17.1 provides a schematic representation (or "formulation") of the main processes involved.

The only feature of bulimia nervosa that is obviously not a direct expression of the core psychopathology is these patients' binge eating. The cognitive-behavioral theory proposes that the binge eating is largely a product of the particular way that these patients *attempt* to restrict their eating (i.e., their form of dietary restraint), irrespective of whether they actually undereat. Rather than adopting general guidelines about how they should eat, these patients try to adhere to multiple extreme, and highly specific, dietary rules. An accompanying tendency—one that involves reacting in an extreme and negative fashion to the frequent and almost inevitable breaking of these rules—leads to interpreting even minor dietary slips as evidence of lack of self-control. The result is that patients respond by temporarily abandoning their attempts to restrict their eating and instead give in to the urge to eat. This produces a highly distinctive pattern of eating in which attempts to restrict eating are repeatedly interrupted by episodes of binge eating. The binge eating maintains the core psychopathology by intensifying patients' concerns about their ability to control their eating, shape, and weight, and it encourages yet greater

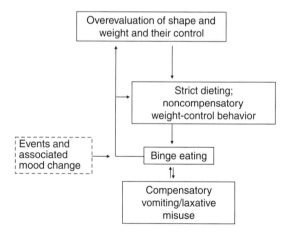

FIGURE 17.1. The cognitive-behavioral theory of the maintenance of bulimia nervosa. From Fairburn (2008, p. 19). Copyright 2008 by The Guilford Press. Reprinted by permission. This figure may be downloaded from *www.credo-oxford.com*.

dietary restraint, thereby increasing the risk of further episodes of binge eating.

It should be noted that these patients' dietary slips and binges do not come out of the blue; rather, they are particularly likely to occur in response to life difficulties and any associated mood change, in part because binge eating temporarily ameliorates negative mood states, and in part because it distracts patients from thinking about their difficulties.

A further process maintains binge eating in those patients who practice compensatory "purging" (i.e., those who induce vomiting or take laxatives in response to specific episodes of binge eating). Patients' mistaken belief in the effectiveness of purging in preventing calorie (i.e., energy) absorption undermines a major deterrent against binge eating. They do not realize that vomiting only retrieves part of what has been eaten, and laxatives have little or no effect on energy absorption (Fairburn, 2013).

This well-established cognitive-behavioral account of the maintenance of bulimia nervosa has clear implications for treatment. It suggests that if treatment is to have a lasting impact on binge eating and purging, then it also needs to address these patients' extreme attempts to restrict their eating, their overevaluation of shape and weight, and their tendency to eat in response to adverse events and negative moods.

Anorexia Nervosa and Other Specified Eating Disorders

The cognitive-behavioral account of the maintenance of bulimia nervosa can be extended to all eating disorders. As noted earlier, the "transdiagnostic" theory highlights the fact that anorexia nervosa and bulimia nervosa have much in common (Fairburn et al., 2003). They share essentially the same core psychopathology with both groups of patients who overevaluate shape and weight, and their control, and express this psychopathology in similar attitudes and behavior.[2] Thus, patients with anorexia nervosa restrict their food intake in the same rigid and extreme way as patients with bulimia nervosa, and they, too, may vomit, misuse laxatives or diuretics, and overexercise. Binge eating does not distinguish the two disorders because there is a subgroup of patients with anorexia nervosa who binge-eat (with or without compensatory purging). The major difference between the two disorders lies in the relative balance of the undereating and overeating, and its effect on body weight. In bulimia nervosa, body

weight is usually unremarkable, whereas in anorexia nervosa, undereating predominates, resulting in body weight that is extremely low and features of starvation contributing to the clinical picture and its maintenance. Particularly important in this regard is the pronounced social withdrawal seen in starvation, since this encourages self-absorption while isolating patients from external influences that might diminish their overconcern with eating, shape and weight. Figure 17.2 shows the cognitive-behavioral formulation of the classic "restricting" form of anorexia nervosa.

The processes that maintain bulimia nervosa and anorexia nervosa also appear to maintain the clinical presentations seen in other specified eating disorders. Figure 17.3 shows a composite transdiagnostic formulation. It is essentially a combination of the bulimia nervosa and restricting anorexia nervosa formulations. In our experience, this composite formulation represents the core processes that maintain any eating disorder, whatever its exact form. The specific processes operating in any individual patient depend on the nature of the eating disorder psychopathology present. In some cases, only a limited number of these processes are ac-

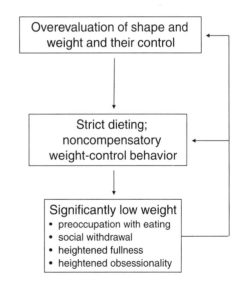

FIGURE 17.2. The cognitive-behavioral theory of the maintenance of anorexia nervosa. From Fairburn (2008, p. 21). Copyright 2008 by The Guilford Press. Reprinted by permission. This figure may be downloaded from *www. credo-oxford.com.*

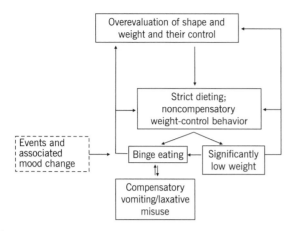

FIGURE 17.3. The "transdiagnostic" cognitive-behavioral theory of eating disorders. From Fairburn (2008, p. 21). Copyright 2008 by The Guilford Press. Reprinted by permission. This figure may be downloaded from *www.credo-oxford.com.*

tive (as in most cases of binge-eating disorder), whereas in others (e.g., cases of anorexia nervosa in which there is binge eating and purging) most of the processes are operating. In common with the cognitive-behavioral account of the maintenance of bulimia nervosa, this transdiagnostic account highlights the processes that need to be addressed in treatment, thereby helping the clinician design a bespoke treatment to fit the individual patient's psychopathology.

THE RESEARCH ON TREATMENT

Consistent with the current way of classifying eating disorders, the research on their treatment has focused on the particular disorders in isolation. This research has been reviewed by Hay and Claudino (2010), and an authoritative meta-analysis has been conducted by the U.K. National Institute for Clinical Excellence (NICE; 2004). The majority of the randomized controlled trials have focused on adults with bulimia nervosa, with the treatment of adolescents receiving far less attention. The findings indicate that there is a clear leading treatment, a specific form of cognitive behavior therapy for bulimia nervosa (CBT-BN). However, this treatment is far from being a panacea: At best, half the patients who start treatment make a full and lasting response.

Interpersonal psychotherapy (IPT) is a potential alternative to CBT-BN, but it takes 8 to 12 months longer to achieve a comparable effect. Antidepressant medication (especially fluoxetine at a dose of 60 mg in the morning) also has a beneficial effect, but this is not as great as that obtained with CBT-BN, and the limited evidence available suggests it is often not sustained. Combining CBT-BN with antidepressant medication conveys little, if any, advantage over CBT-BN alone.

There has been much less research on the treatment of anorexia nervosa, with no treatment supported by robust research evidence. In this case, most of the work has focused on adolescents, and much of it has been concerned with a highly specific form of family-based treatment (FBT; Lock, le Grange, Agras, & Dare, 2001). Despite widespread enthusiasm for FBT (often described as the "Maudsley method" because it was devised at the Maudsley Hospital in London), it is not without its limitations (Lock, 2011; Lock et al., 2010): The treatment is not acceptable to some families and patients; it renders some patients unable to eat without the encouragement of their parents; and fewer than half the patients make a full treatment response.

There is a growing body of research on the treatment of binge-eating disorder. Various psychological treatments seem reasonably effective and more so than when they are used to treat bulimia nervosa or anorexia nervosa (Wilson, Grilo, & Vitousek, 2007). Three treatments have the greatest support, an adaptation of CBT-BN, IPT, and a simplified version of CBT-BN termed "guided self-help." The effects of CBT-BN and IPT on binge-eating disorder are remarkably similar, both in their extent and time course, which is quite unlike the response seen in bulimia nervosa. Overall, it appears that binge-eating disorder is more treatment-responsive than the other eating disorders, and that shared "nonspecific" psychotherapeutic processes may have a potent influence. Perhaps most remarkable is the effect of guided self-help (Wilson & Zandberg, 2012). This brief intervention (typically 8–10, 20-minute sessions delivered by a nonspecialist "facilitator") has been shown to be as effective as 20, 50-minute sessions of IPT both at the end of treatment and at 2-year follow-up (Wilson, Wilfley, Agras, & Bryson, 2010). There is no drug treatment for binge-eating disorder. Finally, it should be noted that none of these treatments has a significant effect on comorbid obesity. This is not altogether surprising given that much of these patients' excess calorie intake comes from overeating outside their binges rather than the binges themselves.

There has been just one study of the treatment of the residual eating disorders, a remarkable omission given their prevalence. The findings of this study are discussed below.

The Research on Enhanced Cognitive Behavior Therapy

Relatively recently a transdiagnostic form of cognitive behavior therapy has been developed that is designed for the full range of clinical eating disorders seen in adults, including other specified eating disorders (Fairburn, 2008; Fairburn et al., 2003). It is based on the transdiagnostic theory outlined earlier and was derived from CBT-BN. The treatment—enhanced cognitive behavior therapy (CBT-E) —is described as "enhanced" because it uses a variety of new strategies and procedures intended to improve treatment adherence and outcome. In addition, it has modules designed to address certain obstacles to change that are "external" to the core eating disorder, namely, clinical perfectionism, low self-esteem, and interpersonal difficulties. Thus, there are two forms of CBT-E, a focused form that focuses exclusively on the eating disorder psychopathology, and a broad form that also addresses the three external obstacles to change.[3] The treatment also exists in two lengths, a 20-week version for patients who are not significantly underweight, defined as having a BMI of 18.5 or more, and a version that can be up to double this length for patients with a BMI below 18.5.

CBT-E, primarily an outpatient treatment, is designed to be delivered on an individual rather than a group basis, although day patient and inpatient versions have been developed (Dalle Grave, 2012). It has also been adapted for adolescents (Cooper & Stewart, 2008; Dalle Grave, Calugi, Doll, & Fairburn, 2013).

Research on CBT-E is still at a relatively early stage. In the first study of its kind, Fairburn and colleagues (2009) recruited from two community-based National Health Service centers in the United Kingdom a transdiagnostic sample of patients with eating disorders, all of whom had a BMI over 17.5 (i.e., in DSM-IV terms, they either had bulimia nervosa or eating disorder NOS). The patients were randomized to a waiting-list control condition, or to either the focused or the broad form of CBT-E, and they then entered a closed, 60-week period of follow-up. There were two main findings:

1. The two forms of CBT-E were equally effective overall. The size of treatment response suggested that CBT-E was more effective than its predecessor, CBT-BN, especially in light of the use of few trial exclusion criteria (Crow & Peterson, 2009).

2. There was no difference in treatment response between the patients with bulimia nervosa and those with eating disorder NOS.

A second (unpublished) study from Oxford has replicated these findings. In addition, an open transdiagnostic study from Australia obtained very similar results, at least among treatment completers (Byrne, Fursland, Allen, & Watson, 2011). Unfortunately, the therapists in this study were not trained or supervised by anyone expert in CBT-E, so it is difficult to have complete confidence in its findings.

The original U.K. study also included a planned moderator analysis (Fairburn et al., 2009). Its findings suggested that the broad version of the treatment was more effective with patients who had extreme external psychopathology of the type it was designed to target, whereas the focused version was more effective with the remaining patients.

One other study is worth mentioning. It involved a remarkable comparison of CBT-E (focused form, 20 sessions over 20 weeks) with a longer-term psychoanalytic treatment (about 100 sessions over 2 years) in the treatment of bulimia nervosa (Poulsen et al., in press). Two sets of therapists were used, and each was well trained and supervised. The findings were striking in that CBT-E was found to be far superior to the psychoanalytic treatment both after 20 weeks (the end of CBT-E) and at 2 years (the end of the psychoanalytic treatment). This was despite the marked discrepancy in the number of sessions received and the duration of treatment; moreover, it was contrary to any allegiance effect because the principal investigators were psychoanalysts. The finding is one of the clearest refutations of the so-called "dodo bird verdict," which concludes that all psychotherapies are equivalent in their effects (Luborsky, Singer, & Luborsky, 1975).

Until recently, the major outstanding question about CBT-E was whether it could be used to treat underweight patients (i.e., those with anorexia nervosa or underweight forms of other specified eating disorders). It is now clear that it can. Thus, it has been shown to be associated with a good outcome in three cohorts of patients with the disorder, two adult cohorts (total $N = 99$) (Fairburn, Cooper, Doll, Palmer, & Dalle Grave, 2013), and one adolescent cohort ($N = 49$) (Dalle Grave et al., 2013), all of whom were seriously underweight.

To conclude, there are three main points to note from the research on CBT-E:

1. CBT-E can be used to treat all forms of eating disorder in adults. Thus, CBT-E is truly transdiagnostic in its scope. This applies to no other evidence-based treatment for the eating disorders. Therefore, the availability of CBT-E renders redundant the need to learn different treatments for the different eating disorders (Fairburn & Wilson, 2013).

2. It needs emphasizing that there are good data on the use of CBT-E to treat adults with anorexia nervosa given that this is sometimes questioned. Indeed, there are more data on this application of CBT-E than on any other treatment.

3. CBT-E can also be used to treat adolescents with anorexia nervosa. This makes it a potential alternative to FBT. A comparison of the two approaches is definitely indicated (Dalle Grave et al., 2013).

The remainder of this chapter is devoted to a description of the main form of CBT-E, the focused version. This is the core version of the treatment, and it forms the basis of the variants of CBT-E. It is the version used to treat the great majority of adults with an eating disorder, so long as they can be managed on an outpatient basis. A full description of the focused treatment is provided in the complete treatment guide (Fairburn, 2008; Fairburn, Cooper, Shafran, et al., 2008b) together with details of the broad version (Fairburn, Cooper, Shafran, Bohn, & Hawker, 2008). A book by Dalle Grave (2012) describes how CBT-E may be modified to make it suitable for inpatient, day patient, and intensive outpatient settings, and there are two descriptions of the modifications needed for adolescents (Cooper & Stewart, 2008; Dalle Grave et al., 2013).

THE CONTEXT OF TREATMENT

The Patient

CBT-E is a treatment for patients with an eating disorder of clinical severity (i.e., the eating disorder psychopathology is persistent and significantly interferes with the patient's psychosocial functioning or physical health). It is designed for patients age 18 years or more, and it is equally suitable for men or women. Because it is an outpatient-based treatment, it is essential that it be safe for the patient to be managed this way, both in physical terms and from the psychiatric point of view. In practice this means that the patient's physical state must be stable and that he/she must not be at risk of suicide. The treatment is designed for patients with a BMI between 15 and 40. Although some patients with a BMI below 15 can be treated using outpatient CBT-E, this is probably best left to experienced therapists. The management of such patients is discussed by Dalle Grave (2012). The book edited by Mitchell and de Zwaan (2012) addresses the management of patients with a BMI over 40.

The Therapist

There are no specific professional qualifications needed to practice CBT-E, but certain background knowledge and experience are desirable. First, ideally, the therapist should be well informed about psychopathology in general and about eating disorder psychopathology in particular, and he/she should have experience working with patients with eating disorders. Second, therapists should also be aware of the medical complications of eating disorders and be able to manage them appropriately (Fairburn, Cooper, & Waller, 2008b). Third, therapists should be happy to implement a short-term, psychopathology-focused, treatment and, preferably, should have some experience working this way.

In contrast with many other applications of CBT, the gender of the therapist is of some relevance to the treatment of patients with eating disorders. Most of these patients are female; as a result, female therapists may have certain advantages. They may be viewed by patients as being more likely to understand their difficulties and, in addition, may serve as a role model in terms of the acceptance of shape and weight. These considerations are minor, however, in comparison with being competent at delivering the treatment. Our experience indicates that both women and men are capable of being excellent CBT-E therapists.

ASSESSING PATIENTS AND PREPARING THEM FOR TREATMENT

The Initial Evaluation Interview(s)

The initial assessment interview has three interrelated goals. The first is to put the patient at ease and begin to forge a positive therapeutic relationship. This is important for a number of reasons. First, many patients with an eating disorder are highly ambivalent about treatment because of the "ego-syntonic" nature of their psychopathology (especially true of underweight patients), because of shame (especially true of those who are binge eating), or because they have had adverse treatment experiences in the past. The assessing clinician needs to be sensitive to the patient's attitude to the assessment interview and ask directly about it. The goal is that it be a collaborative enterprise ending with the clinician being able to give the patient an expert opinion as to the nature of his/her problems and, if indicated, the treatment options.

The second goal is to establish the diagnosis. An apparent eating disorder may, for example, turn out to be an anxiety disorder (e.g., difficulty eating with others due to a social phobia), a presentation of a mood disorder (e.g., severe weight loss resulting from a clinical depression), or simple overeating (in cases of obesity). It is therefore critical to diagnose the problem or problems (if there is comorbidity) accurately and evaluate their severity in order to decide on the most appropriate next step.

The third goal is to ensure that the patient is safe to manage on an outpatient basis. This requires checking that there are no reasons to be concerned about the patient's physical health or the risk of suicide. Guidance for doing so is provided in the complete treatment guide (Fairburn, Cooper, Shafran, et al., 2008b; Fairburn, Cooper, & Waller, 2008b).

Patients are invited to bring others to the appointment if they wish. They may simply provide moral support (and stay in the waiting area) or also serve as informants. The informant's view is of interest, since it can provide a different perspective on the patient's difficulties. Problems may be described that were not disclosed by the patient (e.g., that the patient takes an inordinate time to eat meals or has extremely small portions). However, it is not appropriate to insist that informants attend given that some adult patients will have kept their eating problem hidden from others and would not attend if disclosure were required. The situation is different with younger patients when involvement of the parents is generally essential.

Toward the end of the first interview, we weigh patients and measure their height. This is an extremely sensitive matter for most patients, and some are resistant to it. As the patient must be weighed for the assessment to be complete, we explain this. We do not regard it as appropriate to rely on patients' self-reported weight or height, which can be inaccurate. In our experience, patients expect their weight to be measured, although many prefer that this not happen. At this stage we do not insist on patients knowing their weight if they do not wish to, but we like to tell them their BMI when discussing the outcome of the assessment.

We are not in favor of lengthy assessment appointments because they are exhausting for the patient. On the other hand, we routinely see patients twice as part of the assessment process, since we find that a second appointment, a week or two later, often adds new information of value. On the second occasion patients are more relaxed; they sometimes disclose material previously withheld; and there is an opportunity to pursue matters that require particularly careful exploration (e.g., the nature and extent of any comorbid depressive features). The second appointment is also a good time to discuss treatment options.

We routinely ask patients to complete certain questionnaires prior to the initial appointment. This is useful, since it gives us standardized information on the nature and severity of patients' eating problems. The two questionnaires we favor are the Eating Disorder Examination Questionnaire (EDE-Q; Fairburn & Beglin, 2008) and the Clinical Impairment Assessment (CIA; Bohn & Fairburn, 2008). The EDE-Q provides a measure of the severity of current eating disorder features, and the CIA assesses the impact of this psychopathology on psychosocial functioning. Both questionnaires are short and easy to fill in, and both focus on the previous 28 days and are sensitive to change. In addition, we include one of the well-established measures of general psychiatric features.

Outcome of the Evaluation

By the end of the second appointment it should be possible to decide on the best course of action. Generally there are five possible next steps:

1. Do "nothing." This is appropriate with minor eating problems that are likely to be self-limiting.
2. Observe. This is appropriate if the nature or severity of the problem is not clear; for example, if it seems to be remitting.
3. Recommend outpatient-based CBT-E. This is appropriate for the vast majority of patients. We recommend CBT-E for virtually all patients with

an eating disorder who have a BMI between 15.0 and 40.0.

4. Recommend more intensive treatment. We recommend more intensive treatment (mainly day patient or inpatient treatment) for patients whose BMI is below 15.0 and for those whose physical state is not stable. This can be followed by outpatient-based CBT-E. We may also recommend more intensive treatment when CBT-E fails to be of benefit.

5. Recommend referral elsewhere. This is appropriate when the problem is not an eating disorder (e.g., an anxiety or mood disorder).

If patients have not benefited from CBT in the past, it merits thought whether it is appropriate to offer them the same treatment a second time. On the other hand, it is possible that a patient's circumstances may now be more conducive to a good outcome than in the past, or the patient may be more motivated than before. It is important to note that while patients may report having had CBT before, it often emerges that it was quite different in character from CBT-E. It is always worth finding out exactly what the prior treatment involved.

Contraindications to Starting CBT-E Immediately

There are certain contraindications to embarking upon CBT-E straightaway. Most of these apply to any psychological treatment for an eating disorder. The main contraindications are as follows:

Comorbid Clinical Depression

Most patients with an eating disorder have secondary depressive features but a sizable subgroup has an independent, but interacting, clinical depression. The identification and management of clinical depression in patients with eating disorders is discussed in detail in the complete treatment guide (Fairburn, Cooper, & Waller, 2008a). The presence of a clinical depression interferes with psychological treatment in a number of ways. Depressive thinking results in patients being unduly negative about the possibility of change and the reduction in drive has a similar effect. Concentration impairment is also a problem, since it results in information not being retained. Once the depression has been treated, however, CBT-E can start and such patients are often particularly highly motivated.

It is important to add that other, co-occurring forms of psychopathology (e.g., anxiety disorders, personality disorders) are not contraindications to CBT-E. Thus, the research on CBT-BN has typically included patients with comorbid Axis I and Axis II disorders, neither of which has been shown to be consistent predictors of outcome.

Significant Substance Misuse

Intoxication in treatment sessions renders the sessions virtually worthless, and persistent intoxication outside sessions severely undermines the patient's ability to utilize CBT-E. Once the substance misuse has been addressed CBT-E can start.

Major Life Difficulties or Crises

These are distractions that interfere with treatment. It is often best to delay treatment until the crisis has passed.

Inability to Attend Regularly

A central feature of CBT-E is establishing and maintaining "therapeutic momentum." This requires that appointments be frequent (especially in the early stages) and regular. We ask patients to guarantee that there will be no breaks in their attendance in the first 6 weeks and no breaks of longer than two consecutive weeks throughout the rest of treatment. If this is impossible, say, because of a prebooked vacation, we prefer to defer starting treatment. Patients generally understand and respect the rationale behind this stance. They can see that we are taking their treatment seriously and do not want them to have a "false start."

Therapist Absence

The need to establish and maintain therapeutic momentum also places an obligation on the therapist. If the therapist is going to be away in the first 6 weeks of treatment, it is best to delay its start. Ways of minimizing the impact of therapist absence are discussed in the treatment guide (Fairburn, Cooper, Shafran, et al., 2008b).

Describing CBT-E to the Patient

If CBT-E is to be recommended, it is important that it be accurately portrayed. Once this has been done, possibly with the aid of an information sheet (obtainable from *www.credo-oxford.com*), and patients have had an opportunity to ask questions, it is our practice to ask them to think over what has been proposed and let us know within a week what they have decided. In our experience, virtually all of them say that they would like to proceed with the treatment.

OVERVIEW OF THE TREATMENT

Length of Treatment

CBT-E is a short-term, time-limited, highly individualized psychological treatment, which is why it is best delivered on a one-to-one basis. For patients who are not significantly underweight (which may be defined in this context as having a BMI above 18.5[4]) an initial assessment appointment followed by 20 fifty-minute treatment sessions over 20 weeks is generally sufficient. For patients below this weight, treatment needs to be longer, often involving about 40 sessions over 40 weeks. In this chapter, we describe the 20-week treatment first, then the adaptations needed for underweight patients.

The fact that CBT-E is usually time-limited might be thought to be inconsistent with the claim that it is individualized. To an extent this is true, but our experience is that the recommended number of treatment sessions is sufficient, but not excessive, for the great majority of patients. There are major advantages to working within a fixed time frame, and in our view these outweigh the potential disadvantage of standardizing the length of treatment. The main advantage is that a fixed time frame concentrates the minds of both patient and therapist. It encourages the establishment of the therapeutic momentum that is needed early on, and it helps to ensure that therapist and patient keep working hard to help the patient change. It also makes it much more likely that treatment will have a formal ending rather than fizzling out, as sometimes happens when treatment is open-ended. Having a definite endpoint is important, as it ensures that important future-oriented topics (e.g., how to minimize the risk of relapse) are covered in the final part of treatment.

There are circumstances under which it is appropriate to adjust the length of treatment. It rarely needs to be shortened, although this does apply in occasional cases in which change is so profound and rapid that there is little or no remaining psychopathology to address. Somewhat more often there is a case for extend-

ing treatment. The indications for doing this are described briefly towards the end of the chapter.

Structure of the Treatment

The 20-week version of the treatment has four stages:

- *Stage 1.* This is most important. The aims are to engage the patient in treatment and change, jointly create a formulation of the processes maintaining the eating disorder, provide education, address weight concerns, and introduce a pattern of regular eating. Following the initial preparatory session, the appointments are twice weekly for 4 weeks.
- *Stage 2.* The aims of this stage is to take stock, review progress, identify barriers to change, modify the formulation as needed, and plan Stage 3. This stage generally comprises two appointments, each a week apart.
- *Stage 3.* This is the main body of treatment. The aim is to address the key mechanisms that are maintaining the patient's eating disorder. There are eight weekly appointments.
- *Stage 4.* This is the final stage of treatment, and the focus is on the future. There are two aims: The first is to ensure that the changes made in treatment are maintained over the following months, and the second is to minimize the risk of relapse in the long term. Typically there are three appointments, each 2 weeks apart.

In addition, there is a single review appointment 20 weeks after treatment has finished.

The Implementation of CBT-E

CBT-E is designed to be a complete treatment in its own right. In our view it should not be combined with other forms of therapy, nor should it coexist with them. Both can detract from the treatment.

CBT-E should remain focused on the eating disorder, more or less, whatever happens. If the patient experiences a crisis during treatment that cannot be ignored—for example, the parents of one of our younger patients disappeared unexpectedly, leaving the patient at a loss as to what to do—we arrange one or more "crisis sessions" in addition to the CBT-E sessions to address the problem in question. This rarely happens, however. Very occasionally we suspend CBT-E for a few weeks if continuing seems inappropriate.

We have observed that some therapists are tempted to change therapeutic tack if progress is slow or difficult. We think that this is rarely appropriate. Although it might be tempting to switch over to another therapeutic modality, or add or try to "integrate" other techniques, we recommend that the therapist continues to work within the framework of CBT-E while trying to understand the basis of the relative lack of progress. Indeed, this is the strategy that led to the development of CBT-E and its broad form in particular (Cooper & Fairburn, 2011).

THE TREATMENT PROTOCOL

Stage 1: Starting Well

This is the initial intensive stage of treatment. There are a number of interrelated goals, all of which apply, regardless of the exact nature of the patient's eating problem.

The Initial Preparatory Session

The initial session is typically up to two hours long and has four major goals.

ENGAGING THE PATIENT IN TREATMENT
AND THE PROSPECT OF CHANGE

A particular challenge in working with patients with eating disorders is engaging them in treatment. Many come to treatment with misgivings and varying degrees of reluctance. It is essential that the therapist understand this and be sensitive at all times to the patient's likely ambivalence.

The initial session is especially important in this regard. The patient is evaluating the therapist just as much as the therapist is evaluating the patient. Some clinicians advocate an initial phase of "motivational enhancement." We agree that engagement in treatment, and more especially, in change, is crucial, but contend that competently administered CBT-E enhances motivation for change and overlaps significantly with the strategies of motivational interviewing (Wilson & Schlam, 2004). We do not view special non-CBT procedures as being required.

Integral to engaging patients is explaining what treatment will involve. With this in mind, it is important that patients be fully informed about the treatment on which they are embarking. Various topics need to be covered:

1. *The nature and style of the treatment.* Clearly, patients need to be told the name, nature, and style of the treatment.
2. *Treatment practicalities.* They should also be told the number, duration, and frequency of the treatment sessions.
3. *In-session weighing.* Patients need to be forewarned about the in-session weighing that is an element of treatment from Sessions 1 or 2 onward. The rationale needs to be explained (see "Establishing Collaborative Weighing"). We are often asked whether patients ever refuse to be weighed. The answer is that the occasional patient is very reluctant, but in the context of an "engaging" initial session and the rationale being well explained, we find that refusal is not a problem. Our experience is that if one accedes to the patient's fear of in-session weighing, it is difficult to introduce the procedure later.
4. *Instillation of "ownership," enthusiasm, and hope.* The notion that it is the patient's treatment, not the therapist's, also needs to be stated. Throughout treatment, patients should feel clear about what is happening and why. While many patients are keen to overcome their eating problem and eager for treatment to start, it is important to maximize enthusiasm and hope. Part of this involves conveying that one is knowledgeable about eating disorders in general and the patient's type of eating problem in particular.

Not infrequently we come across patients who have been told that they will never overcome their eating disorder. Rarely have we felt that such a statement was warranted. Saying something like this sets up a self-fulfilling prophecy because it undermines any hope of recovery that the patient might have had. Research has not generated reliable predictors of treatment outcome, and our experience over the years has taught us not to trust our clinical judgement in this regard. We are continually surprised (usually favorably) at our patients' response to treatment.

ASSESSING THE NATURE AND SEVERITY
OF THE PSYCHOPATHOLOGY PRESENT

Depending on the context within which one works, the person who conducts the initial evaluation interview(s) may or may not be the person who subsequently treats the patient. In our context, the therapist is often seeing the patient for the first time. This means that a second assessment of the eating disorder needs to take place, so that the therapist is fully in the picture. Inevitably, this assessment overlaps to an extent with the initial one. This cannot be avoided.

This particular assessment is treatment-oriented rather than diagnostic, so it differs somewhat from the one conducted when the patient was first seen. While a broad range of topics is covered, the main focus should be on the patient's present state. Mainly, an information-gathering style of interviewing is used, but the therapist remaining aware of the patient's likely sensitivity to certain topics (e.g., binge eating, self-induced vomiting).

JOINTLY CREATING THE FORMULATION

The next step is the creation of the "formulation," that is, a personalized visual representation (i.e., a diagram) of the processes that appear to be maintaining the patient's eating problem. This is done in the initial session unless the patient is significantly underweight (see below) or the eating disorder is unusual and difficult to understand, in which case it is best delayed until the next session, so that the therapist has ample time to think over its likely form.

The creation of the formulation has a number of purposes: It helps to engage the patient in treatment; it involves "decentering," which is central to helping patients change; it conveys the notion that eating problems are understandable and maintained by a variety of interacting self-perpetuating mechanisms; and by highlighting the maintaining mechanisms, it provides a guide to what needs to be targeted in treatment.

A composite transdiagnostic formulation was shown in Figure 17.3. This should be used by the therapist as a template from which the personalized formulation can be derived, one that matches the particular clinical features present. The more familiar the therapist becomes with the template formulation, the easier it is to create an individualized one. We have not encountered any patients whose eating problems cannot be formulated in this way.

The formulation should focus on the main mechanisms that appear likely to be maintaining the patient's eating problem. It does not need to be comprehensive (as this risks the formulation being over-detailed and confusing), and it is not concerned with the origins of the problem.

The formulation, usually referred to as the "diagram" or "picture," should be drawn out, step by step,

in an unhurried manner, with the therapist taking the lead but with the patient's active involvement. It is best to start with something that the patient wants to change (e.g., binge eating) or something that is clearly a problem (e.g., very low weight). Whenever possible and appropriate, the patient's own terms should be used. Since the formulation is based on information only just obtained, the therapist should make clear that it is provisional and will be modified as needed during treatment. It is important that patients accept the formulation as a credible explanation of their eating problem. Most resonate with it.

Once the formulation has been created, the therapist should discuss its implications for treatment. The points to be made are that to overcome the eating disorder, the patient will need to address not only the things that he/she would like to change (e.g., loss of control over eating) but also the mechanisms responsible for maintaining them (the "vicious circles"). Thus, for example, with patients who binge-eat, treatment commonly needs to focus on more than simply stopping binge eating; instead, it may also need to address the patient's various forms of dieting, his/her ability to deal with adverse events and moods without binge eating, and his/her concerns about shape and weight. Not addressing the range of maintaining processes markedly increases the likelihood of relapse.

ESTABLISHING REAL-TIME SELF-MONITORING

The final task in the initial session is to establish real-time self-monitoring. This is the ongoing, "in-the-moment" recording of relevant behavior, thoughts, feelings, and events. It needs to be initiated from the outset of treatment and fine-tuned in Session 1. It continues throughout treatment and is central to it. It has two main purposes: First, it helps the patient identify precisely what is happening on a day-to-day basis; second, by gaining such awareness of their thoughts, feelings, and behavior at the time it happens, patients learn that they have choices, and that many things they thought were automatic and beyond their control can be changed.

The monitoring record that we employ is simple for patients to complete and to use. Exactly what is recorded evolves during treatment. At the beginning, the emphasis is largely on the patient's eating habits. When describing how to monitor eating habits, it is our practice to go over an example (created for this purpose) that roughly matches in form the eating habits of the patient in question. Table 17.1 shows our instructions for monitoring, and Figure 17.4 shows a completed monitoring record.

We do not recommend using smartphone apps for recording. In our experience they provide a far less rich source of information and as a result they impede therapy.

Fundamental to establishing accurate real-time recording is going over the patient's records in detail, especially in Session 1, when the patient brings them back for the first time. Reviewing the records should be a joint process, with the patient taking the therapist through each day's record in turn. There are two aspects to the review in Session 1: assessing the quality of monitoring and assessing the information gained about the patient's eating habits. In subsequent sessions, the focus is largely on what has been recorded, although the therapist should intermittently ask the patient about the

TABLE 17.1. Instructions for Self-Monitoring

During treatment, it is important that you record *everything* that you eat or drink, and what is going on at the time. We call this "self-monitoring." Its purpose is twofold: First, it provides a detailed picture of how you eat, thereby bringing to your attention and that of your therapist the exact nature of your eating problem; and second, by making you more aware of what you are doing at the very time that you are doing it, self-monitoring helps you change behavior that may previously have seemed automatic and beyond your control. Accurate "real-time" monitoring is central to treatment. It will help you change.

At first, writing down everything that you eat may be irritating and inconvenient, but soon it will become second nature and of obvious value. We have yet to encounter anyone whose lifestyle made it truly impossible to monitor. Regard it as a challenge.

Look at the sample monitoring record to see how to monitor. A new record (or records) should be started each day.

- The first column is for noting the time when you eat or drink anything, and the second is for recording the nature of the food and drink consumed. Calories should not be recorded: Instead, you should write down a simple (nontechnical) description of what you ate or drank. Each item should be written down as soon as possible after it is consumed. Recalling what you ate or drank some hours afterwards will not work, since it will not help you change your behavior at the time. Obviously, if you are to record in this way, you need to carry your monitoring sheets with you. It does not matter if your records become messy or if the writing or spelling is not good. The important thing is that you record *everything* you eat or drink, as soon as possible afterwards.
- Episodes of eating that you view as meals should be identified with brackets. Snacks and other episodes of eating should not be bracketed.
- The third column should specify where the food or drink was consumed. If this was in your home, the room should be specified.
- Asterisks should be placed in the fourth column, adjacent to any episodes of eating or drinking that you felt (at the time) were excessive. This is your judgment, regardless of what anyone else might think. It is essential to record all the food that you eat during "binges."
- The fifth column is for recording when you vomit (write "V") or take laxatives (write "L" and the number taken) or diuretics (water tablets; write "D" and the number taken).
- The last column is used in various ways during treatment. For the moment it should be used as a diary to record events and feelings that have influenced your eating: For example, if an argument precipitated a binge or led you not to eat, you should write that down. Try to write a brief comment every time you eat, recording your thoughts and feelings about what you ate. You may want to record other important events or circumstances in this column, even if they had no effect on your eating. The last column should also be used to record your weight (and your thoughts about it) each time you weigh yourself.

Every treatment session will include a detailed review of your latest monitoring sheets. You must therefore remember to bring them with you!

Day ......Thursday...........   Date .....March 21..........

Time	Food and drink consumed	Place	*	p	Context and comments
7.30	Glass water	Kitchen			[118 pounds—really gross] Thirsty after yesterday
8:10	Whole cinnamon raisin bagel Light cream cheese Black coffee	Cafe	*		Should have only had half the bagel. Must not binge today.
10:35	Half banana Black coffee	Work—at desk			Better—on track
11:45	Smoked turkey on wheat bread Light mayo Diet coke	Cafe			Usual lunch
6:40 to 7:30	Piece of apple pie 1/2 gallon ice cream 4 slices of toast with peanut butter Diet coke Raisin bagel 2 slices of toast with peanut butter Diet coke Peanut butter from jar Raisin bagel Snickers bar Diet coke—large	Kitchen	* * * * * * * *	V V	Help—I can't stop eating. I'm completely out of control. I hate myself.
					I am disgusting. Why do I do this? I started as soon as I got in. I've ruined another day.
9:30	Rice cake with fat-free cheese Diet coke	Kitchen			Really lonely. Feel fat and unattractive. Feel like giving up.

FIGURE 17.4. A completed self-monitoring record. V, vomiting. A blank monitoring record may be downloaded from *www.credo-oxford.com*.

process of recording and the accuracy of the records. In these subsequent sessions the review of the records generally takes no longer than 10 minutes. Therapists need to remember not to address identified problems while doing this, but to acknowledge the problems and put them on the session agenda.

The Main Body of Stage 1

Following the initial preparatory session, there are eight twice-weekly appointments. We find that twice-weekly appointments are needed in order to build up therapeutic momentum and to begin making inroads into the patient's disturbed way of eating. Once-weekly sessions are simply not sufficient for most patients. Stage 1 has four distinct elements.

ESTABLISHING COLLABORATIVE WEIGHING

The collaborative weighing intervention has a number of purposes. First, as the patients' eating habits will be changing in treatment they are likely to be anxious about any resulting change in their weight. In-session weighing provides good, week-by-week data on their weight. Second, regular in-session weighing provides an opportunity for the therapist to help patients interpret the number on the scale, which they otherwise are prone to misinterpret. Third, collaborative weighing addresses one form of body checking, namely, weight checking. Many patients with eating disorders weigh themselves at frequent intervals, sometimes many times a day. As a result they become concerned with day-to-day weight fluctuations that would otherwise pass unnoticed. Others actively avoid knowing their weight but remain highly concerned about it. Generally these patients weighed themselves frequently in the past but switched to avoidance when they found frequent weight checking too aversive. Avoidance of weighing is as problematic as frequent weighing, since it results in patients having no data to confirm or disconfirm their fears about weight gain.

Patients need to learn how to assess and interpret their weight. They should be informed that body weight fluctuates throughout the day and from day-to-day according to their state of hydration, the state of their bowels and bladder, their point in the menstrual cycle, and other factors, too. (All this information may be found in the second edition of *Overcoming Binge Eating* [Fairburn, 2013]; see the next section.) Frequent weighing results in preoccupation with inconsequential weight fluctuations that tend to be misinterpreted. This leads many patients to restrict their eating, whatever the reading on the scales. This important maintaining process is disrupted by the collaborative weighing intervention.

Collaborative weighing involves the therapist and patient together checking the patient's weight at the outset of the session. This is done once a week (for underweight patients, see below). Therapist and patient then plot the latest data point on an individualized weight graph and jointly interpret the emerging pattern, placing particular emphasis on trends over the past 4 weeks rather than focusing on the latest reading. A crucial element of the intervention is that patients do not weigh themselves outside these times.

Patients are also educated about the BMI. They are told their BMI and its significance from a health point of view. They are advised against having an exact desired weight, since this does not allow for natural, day-to-day fluctuations. Instead they are advised to accept a weight range of approximately 6 lb (or 3 kg) in magnitude.

Almost all patients are anxious about the effects of treatment on their weight. Patients with bulimia nervosa or other specified eating disorders (who are not underweight) generally do not change much in weight. Patients should be told that the aim of treatment is to give them control over their eating, and thus they will

have as much control over their weight as possible. It is best that patients postpone deciding upon a specific goal weight range until near the end of treatment, when their eating habits should have stabilized and they should be less sensitive about their weight and shape. Later in treatment patients are advised against having a goal weight (range) that necessitates anything more than slight dietary restraint, since dietary restraint will maintain preoccupation with food and eating and increase their risk of binge eating.

EDUCATING THE PATIENT ABOUT EATING PROBLEMS

Myths abound about eating and weight control, and some serve to maintain many patients' eating problem. To ensure that they have a reliable source of information, we recommend that they read one of the authoritative books on eating disorders. We use *Overcoming Binge Eating* because it provides all the information needed and it is popular with patients.[5] In addition, it has a CBT-E orientation and so is highly compatible with the treatment—indeed, some therapists use it as a workbook for patients as they progress through CBT-E. It should be noted that *Overcoming Binge Eating* is relevant to all patients with eating disorders, whether or not they binge-eat because it discusses and addresses all eating disorder psychopathology and not just binge eating.

It is our practice to provide the patient with a copy of the book; this way we can ensure that they have it at exactly the right point in treatment (generally Week 2). We ask patients to annotate the book in the margins, putting ticks by sections that particularly apply to them, crosses by sections that do not, and question marks by sections that they do not understand or would like to discuss. We term this procedure "guided reading." It allows patients to be educated in an efficient, thorough, and personalized way.

ESTABLISHING "REGULAR EATING"

Regular eating is fundamental to successful treatment, whatever the form of the eating disorder. For patients who binge-eat, it reliably results in a rapid decrease in frequency. For patients who have a high level of dietary restraint, it addresses an important type of dieting, socalled "delayed eating," that is, putting off eating during the day. And for patients who are underweight, it introduces regular meals and snacks that can be subsequently increased in size (see below).

Regular eating is introduced around Session 3. It is the first time that patients are asked to change the way that they eat. There are two aspects to the intervention: First, the patient should eat at regular intervals through the day (usually three planned meals each day, plus two planned snacks); second, patients' eating should be largely confined to these meals and snacks. A number of points about the intervention need to be stressed:

1. Patients should be allowed to choose what they eat in their planned meals and snacks. The only condition is that the meals and snacks must not be followed by vomiting, laxative misuse, or any other compensatory behavior.
2. Patients should not be put under pressure to change what, or how much, they eat at this point in treatment, since doing so tends to result in being unable to adopt the pattern of regular eating.
3. If patients seek advice on what to eat, they should be told that the priority is their pattern of eating and not what they eat. Nevertheless, if patients want guidance, they should be told that it would be ideal if they adopted a varied diet with the minimum number of avoided foods.
4. While the new eating pattern should be adhered to whatever the patients' circumstances or appetite, it should be adjusted to suit patients' day-to-day commitments.
5. Patients should plan ahead. They should always know when they are going to have their next meal or snack, and there should rarely be more than a 4-hour interval between the meals and snacks. If the day is going to be unpredictable, they should plan ahead as far as possible and identify a time when they can take stock and if necessary replan the rest of the day.
6. Patients whose eating habits are either chaotic or highly restrictive may need to introduce this pattern in stages. Patients should be told that their sensations of appetite, hunger, and fullness are all likely to be disturbed at present and for the time being should not be used to determine what they eat. Instead, they should adhere to the agreed pattern of eating.

Two rather different strategies may help patients resist eating between the planned meals and snacks. The first is to help them identify activities that are incompatible with eating or make it less likely. They should try to predict when difficulties are likely to arise and

intervene early by arranging activities that are likely to help them adhere to the regular eating pattern. Advice on how to do this is contained in *Overcoming Binge Eating*. The other strategy is very different. It involves asking patients to focus on the urge to eat, recognize that it is a temporary phenomenon, and that one does not have to give in to it. In this way patients can learn to decenter from the urge and simply observe it rather than try to eliminate it. As with feelings of fullness, they will find that the urge dissipates over time. This latter strategy is a difficult one for most patients, especially in the early stages of treatment. If it is to be used at all, it is best left until later on in treatment, when urges to eat between meals and snacks are intermittent and less overwhelming.

INVOLVING SIGNIFICANT OTHERS

CBT-E was developed as an individual treatment for adults; hence, it does not actively involve others. Despite this, it is our practice to see "significant others" if this is likely to facilitate treatment and the patient is willing for this to happen. We do this with the aim of creating the optimum environment for the patient to change. There are two specific indications for involving others:

1. If others can be of help to the patient in making changes.
2. If others are making it difficult for the patient to change, for example, by commenting adversely on his/her appearance or eating.

Typically the sessions with others last about 45 minutes and take place immediately after a routine session. We hold up to three such sessions with about three-fourths of our patients (with underweight patients there may be more such sessions, as we discuss below). Topics other than the eating disorder are not usually addressed. With adolescent patients there is far greater involvement of others (Cooper & Stewart, 2008; Dalle Grave et al., 2013).

Stage 2: Taking Stock

Stage 2 is a transitional stage in treatment. It has three aims:

1. To conduct a joint review of progress.
2. To revise the formulation, if need be.
3. To design Stage 3.

At the same time the therapist continues to implement the procedures introduced in Stage 1. The sessions are now held once weekly.

The reason for conducting this formal review of progress is that there is strong evidence across a variety of psychiatric disorders (Wilson, 1999), including bulimia nervosa (Fairburn, Agras, Walsh, Wilson, & Stice, 2004) and binge-eating disorder (Masheb & Grilo, 2007), that the degree of change during the first few weeks of treatment is a potent predictor of outcome. Thus, if progress is limited, this needs to be recognized early on, and its explanation sought, so that treatment can be adjusted as needed.

Conducting a Joint Review of Progress

The review of progress is best done systematically, with the patient completing once again the EDE-Q, the CIA, and the measure of general psychiatric features. In this way patient and therapist can both review the extent of change. Reviewing the patient's monitoring records can also be helpful. In addition, patient and therapist should consider the degree to which the patient has been complying with the various elements of treatment.

Generally patients' views on their progress are unduly negative. An important task for the therapist is therefore to help the patient arrive at a balanced appraisal of what has changed and what has not. Typically there will have been a decrease in the frequency of any binge eating and compensatory purging, and an improvement in the pattern of eating, whereas concerns about shape will not have changed (to a large extent because they have not been addressed).

One important, and sometimes overlooked, reason for progress not being as great as might be expected is the presence of a clinical depression. Ideally, such depressions should be detected and treated before treatment but inevitably some are missed and others develop afresh. If there appears to be a clinical depression, it is our practice to treat it with antidepressant medication (Fairburn, Cooper, & Waller, 2008a) and consider suspending CBT until the patient has responded.

Revising the Formulation

It is important to review the formulation in light of what has been learned during Stage 1. Often no change is indicated, but sometimes problems and processes are detected that were not obvious when the formulation was originally created. For example, it may have emerged that overexercising is a far greater problem than had been thought. If so, the formulation may need to be revised. Also, if the patient is receiving the "broad" form of CBT-E, it is at this point that the contribution of clinical perfectionism, core low self-esteem, and interpersonal difficulties is considered (see Fairburn, Cooper, Shafran, Bohn, & Hawker, 2008a).

Designing Stage 3

Last, Stage 2 is the time when Stage 3 should be designed. It is at this stage the treatment becomes highly individualized. The therapist has to decide which elements of Stage 3 will be of most relevance to the patient and in what order they should be implemented (see below).

Stage 3: Addressing the Key Maintaining Mechanisms

This is the main part of treatment. The focus is on addressing the key mechanisms that are maintaining the patient's eating problem. These may be categorized under six headings:

1. Overevaluation of shape and weight
2. Overevaluation of control over eating
3. Dietary restraint
4. Event- and mood-related changes in eating
5. Dietary restriction
6. Being underweight

The relative contributions of these mechanisms vary from individual to individual. Only a few of the mechanisms operate in those with binge-eating disorder, whereas most operate in cases of anorexia nervosa in which there is binge eating and purging. The first four are considered here. Dietary restriction and being underweight are addressed separately, when we discuss the adaptations required for those who are underweight. The order in which these mechanisms are addressed depends on their relative importance in maintaining the patient's psychopathology and the length of time it takes to address them. Generally it is best to start by addressing the concerns about shape and weight because this is the most complex mechanism, and it takes the longest.

At the same time the therapist needs to continue implementing the procedures introduced in Stage 1. If the patient is receiving the broad form of CBT-E, one or more of the additional treatment modules will also be employed (Fairburn, Cooper, Shafran, et al., 2008a).

Addressing the Overevaluation of Shape and Weight

At the heart of most eating disorders is the distinctive "core psychopathology," the overevaluation of shape and weight, that is, the judging of self-worth largely, or even exclusively, in terms of shape and weight, and the ability to control them. As described earlier, most of the other features of these disorders are secondary to this psychopathology and its consequences. This psychopathology occupies a central place in most patients' formulation and is a major target of treatment. Clinical experience and research evidence suggest that unless this psychopathology is successfully addressed, patients are at substantial risk of relapse. There are five aspects to this process:

1. Identifying the overevaluation and its consequences
2. Developing marginalized self-evaluative domains
3. Addressing body checking
4. Addressing body avoidance
5. Addressing "feeling fat"

Other than the initial aspect, they are not necessarily introduced in this order. In addition, towards the end of Stage 3 it is important to develop patients' skills at dealing with setbacks.

IDENTIFYING THE OVEREVALUATION AND ITS CONSEQUENCES

The starting point is educating the patient about the notion of self-evaluation. The therapist then helps the patient identify his/her scheme for self-evaluation. Finally, the implications of this scheme are discussed and a plan for addressing the expressions of the overevaluation is devised. Because therapists are often unsure how to broach the subject of self-evaluation, the complete treatment guide provides a detailed dialogue demonstrating how to explain this to patients.

Briefly the therapist starts by explaining that most people tend to judge themselves on the basis of meeting personal standards in the areas of life they value. The patient is then helped to generate a list of areas in his/her life that make an important contribution to his/her self-evaluation. Almost invariably this will include appearance and perhaps also controlling eating. The therapist then goes on to explore the relative importance of these domains of self-evaluation; the clue to their relative importance is the magnitude (in terms of intensity and duration) of the patient's response to things going badly in the area. In this way the various areas of life that have been listed can be ranked and represented by means of a pie chart, which the therapist and patient draw together. The pie chart of someone without an eating disorder is shown in Figure 17.5 and this may be contrasted with one typical of someone with an eating problem (Figure 17.6), in which there is a large "slice" representing the overevaluation of shape and weight.

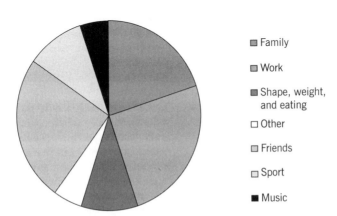

■ Family

▨ Work

■ Shape, weight, and eating

☐ Other

▥ Friends

☐ Sport

■ Music

FIGURE 17.5. The pie chart of a young woman without an eating problem. From Fairburn (2008, p. 99). Copyright 2008 by The Guilford Press. Reprinted by permission.

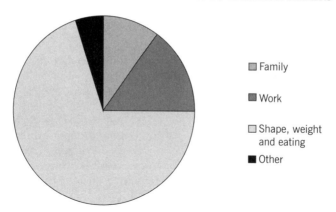

FIGURE 17.6. The pie chart of a young woman with an eating problem. From Fairburn (2008, p. 98). Copyright 2008 by The Guilford Press. Reprinted by permission.

It is useful for the patient to review his/her pie chart on several occasions before the next session, so that it can be discussed further and adjusted as needed. Generally, any revision takes the form of expanding the size of the slice representing the importance of shape and weight.

The next step is to ask the patient to consider the implications of his/her scheme for self-evaluation (as represented by the pie chart) and reflect on whether there might be any problems inherent to it. This discussion generally leads to the identification of three main problems:

1. Having a pie chart with a dominant slice is "risky." A dominant slice makes people particularly vulnerable should anything threaten their ability to meet their personal standards in the area concerned.
2. Judging oneself largely on the basis of appearance is particularly problematic because this aspect of life is only controllable to a limited extent. It therefore results in the person feeling like a failure at times.
3. Placing great importance on shape and weight drives people to diet, and in the patient's case, this maintains his/her eating problem.

This discussion naturally leads to the final step in the examination of self-evaluation, namely, the creation of a formulation that includes the consequences of the overevaluation (the "extended formulation"). The ther-

apist starts by asking the patient what he/she does, or experiences, as a result of the importance placed on shape and appearance. The goal is to derive a figure resembling that in Figure 17.7, with the therapist adding the upward feedback arrows and explaining that these consequences of the overevaluation also serve to maintain the overevaluation.

Having done this, the therapist needs to devise with the patient a plan to address the concerns about shape and weight, with two overarching strategies:

1. To develop new domains for self-evaluation.
2. To reduce the importance attached to shape and weight.

Both are important and they complement one another.

DEVELOPING MARGINALIZED DOMAINS FOR SELF-EVALUATION

Tackling expressions of the overevaluation of shape and weight gradually reduces the extent of the overevaluation: The shape and weight-related "slice" of the pie chart begins to shrivel. But, at the same time, it is most important to increase the number and importance of other domains for self-evaluation to diminish the relative importance of shape and weight. To achieve this, patients need help to begin to get actively involved with other aspects of life. There are six steps to this process, which needs to be a running theme throughout the rest of the treatment:

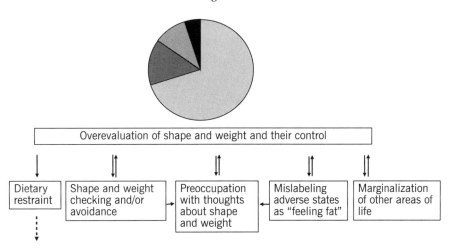

Overevaluation of shape and weight and their control

| Dietary restraint | Shape and weight checking and/or avoidance | Preoccupation with thoughts about shape and weight | Mislabeling adverse states as "feeling fat" | Marginalization of other areas of life |

FIGURE 17.7. The overevaluation of shape and weight: an "extended" formulation. From Fairburn (2008, p. 101). Copyright 2008 by The Guilford Press. Reprinted by permission. This figure may be downloaded from *www.credo-oxford.com.*

1. Explaining the rationale for developing new domains for self-evaluation.
2. Helping the patient identify new activities that might be engaging.
3. Agreeing on one, or possibly two, activities that the patient can try.
4. Ensuring that the patient actually does try the activity identified, often using a problem-solving approach (described later in the chapter).
5. Reviewing progress each week, with the therapist being encouraging and facilitative.
6. Simultaneously, directly targeting the patient's overevaluation of shape and weight, usually starting with body checking, which is often of central importance in maintaining the patient's concerns.

ADDRESSING BODY CHECKING

The importance of body checking and avoidance has only recently been appreciated. The reason is quite simple: Few clinicians know about it. This is because patients do not disclose the behavior unless asked, and many are not even aware of it.

The first step in addressing body checking is to provide information about body checking, body avoidance, and their consequences, stressing the following two points:

1. Everyone checks his/her body to some extent but many people with eating problems repeatedly check their bodies and often in a way that is unusual. Such checking can become "second nature," so that patients may not be aware they are doing it. In people with eating problems this checking can maintain dissatisfaction with appearance.
2. Some people with eating problems avoid seeing their bodies and dislike other people seeing them too. Usually these people engaged in body checking in the past but switched over to avoidance because the repeated checking became intolerable. Body avoidance is problematic because it allows concerns and fears about shape and appearance to persist in the absence of any accurate information. Therefore it too needs to be tackled.

Next, the therapist needs to find out what checking and avoidance the patient engages in. A specific monitoring record may be used for this purpose (see *www.credo-oxford.com*). Since recording body checking is highly distressing for some patients, it is best to ask patients to do it for only two 24-hour periods, one on a working day and the other on a day off work. It may be useful to forewarn patients that although it might be distressing, it will yield information that is helpful in overcoming their eating disorder. It is common for patients to be taken aback by how often they check their shape.

Having identified patients' various forms of body checking, they are then best divided into two groups, according to whether they are "normative."

Unusual Forms of Body Checking. Unusual forms of body checking are best stopped altogether. Examples include measuring the dimensions of certain body parts and photographing oneself. Patients can usually do this if the rationale is well explained and they are provided with support. There are two points to emphasize:

1. Body checking usually involves focusing on aspects of one's appearance that one dislikes, and it generally has adverse effects.
2. Stopping unusual forms of checking is generally experienced (after a week or so) as a relief.

Addressing More Normative Forms of Body Checking. A different strategy needs to be adopted with more normative forms of body checking. Here the problem is the frequency of checking, the way that it is done, and patients' interpretations of what they find. The therapist needs to help patients consider the following questions each time that they are about to check themselves:

- What are they trying to find out?
- Can checking in this way produce the information they are seeking?
- Might there be adverse effects from such checking?
- Is there a better alternative?

Mirror use deserves particular attention because mirrors have the potential to provide misleading, but highly credible, information and as a result they are likely to play an important role in the maintenance of many patients' body dissatisfaction. Education about mirrors and mirror use is therefore of importance. One point to stress is that apparent flaws that would normally go unnoticed become the focus of attention when people study in detail aspects of their appearance that they dislike. Another is that scrutiny is prone to magnify apparent defects. Patients therefore need to question their use of mirrors as they are the main way that we determine how we look. Mirrors are useful for applying makeup, brushing/styling hair, shaving, and so forth. Full-length mirrors are helpful to see whether clothes go well together. But the therapist should ask patients whether there is ever a case for looking at themselves

naked in a full-length mirror. If they are already dissatisfied with their appearance, doing so is likely to risk increasing their dislike of their shape through the magnification process mentioned earlier. This is not to say that total avoidance of mirrors is recommended; rather, the advice is (for the time being) to restrict the use of mirrors to the purposes listed earlier.

Another form of body checking that actively maintains dissatisfaction with shape involves comparing oneself with other people. The nature of these comparisons generally results in the patient concluding that his/her body is unattractive relative to those of others. As noted earlier, the patient's appraisal of his/her shape often involves scrutiny and selective attention to body parts that are disliked. The scrutiny is liable to result in the magnification of perceived defects, and the selective attention increases overall dissatisfaction with shape. In contrast patients' assessment of others is very different. They tend to make superficial and often uncritical judgements about other people. Furthermore, when making these comparisons, they tend to choose a biased reference group, generally people who are thin and attractive.

The steps involved in addressing comparison-making are as follows:

1. The therapist helps patients identify when and how the patient makes comparisons.
2. Once this information has been collected, the therapist helps the patient consider whether the comparison was inherently biased in terms of the person chosen and how their shape was evaluated. Two points are worth highlighting:
   - Body checking provides patients with a perspective on their bodies that is difficult, if not impossible, to get on someone else's body. For example what they see when looking at themselves in the mirror is quite unlike what they see when looking at someone else.
   - Comparing themselves with people portrayed in the media (models, film stars, and other celebrities) is problematic since they are an unrepresentative subgroup and images of them may well have been manipulated.
3. Certain homework tasks usefully complement these discussions; for example, patients may be asked to be more scientific when choosing someone to compare themselves with. Instead of selecting thin people, the therapist may ask them to select every third person (of their age and gender) they walk past in a busy street. They can

also experiment with scrutinizing other people's bodies. One way of doing this is for the patient to go to a changing room (e.g., of a swimming pool or gym), select someone nearby of about the same age and gender who seems at first glance attractive, then unobtrusively scrutinize their body, focusing exclusively on the parts that the patient is personally most sensitive about. What patients discover is that even attractive people have apparent flaws when scrutinized.

4. Assuming the patient's comparison-making is biased (as it almost invariably is), the therapist should explore the implications of this bias in terms of the validity of the patient's views relative to his/her appearance. The goal is that patients become aware that their checking and making comparisons has yielded misleading information about other peoples' bodies and their own.

ADDRESSING BODY AVOIDANCE

"Exposure" in its technical and literal sense is the strategy here. Therapists need to help patients get used to the sight and feel of their bodies and to learn to make even-handed comparisons of their own bodies with those of others. They need to get used to seeing their own bodies and letting others see them, too. Dressing and undressing in the dark needs to be phased out, and patients should gradually abandon wearing baggy, shape-disguising clothes. Participation in activities that involve a degree of body exposure can be helpful (e.g., swimming). Depending on the extent of the problem, tackling body avoidance may take many successive sessions. As there is a risk of a patient returning to repeated body checking, the therapist needs to help the patient adopt normative and risk-free forms of checking.

ADDRESSING "FEELING FAT"

"Feeling fat" is an experience reported by many women, but the intensity and frequency of this feeling appears to be far greater among people with eating disorders. It is an important target for treatment, since it tends to be equated with being fat, whatever the patient's actual weight or shape. Hence, feeling fat is not only an expression of overconcern with shape and weight but it also maintains it.

There has been almost no research on feeling fat, and little has been written about it. What is striking is that it tends to fluctuate markedly from day-to-day

and even within a single day. This is quite unlike many other aspects of these patients' core psychopathology, which is relatively stable. It is our impression that in people with eating disorders, feeling fat is a result of the mislabeling of certain emotions and bodily experiences. It is important to stress that "feeling fat" and "being fat" are quite different, but they can co-occur. Many people with obesity are not troubled by feeling fat, despite being dissatisfied with their shape, but some are dissatisfied, and in the same way as people with an eating disorder. Since feeling fat contributes to the maintenance of their body dissatisfaction, it is essential that this be addressed in these patients, too.

In general it is best to focus on feeling fat once one has begun to make inroads into body checking and avoidance, but this is not invariably the case. In patients in whom feeling fat is a particularly prominent feature, it is advisable to address it before tackling body checking and avoidance.

There are five steps in addressing "feeling fat":

1. The therapist should first explain that "feeling fat" should not be equated with "being fat," and that feeling fat may mask other feelings or sensations occurring at the same time.
2. Patients should be asked to record times when they have particularly intense feelings of fatness. This can be done as part of the normal recording process, using the right-hand column of the recording sheet for this purpose. This requires accurate real-time recording. When patients record feeling fat, they should also think (and record) what else they are feeling at the time.
3. Once patients have mastered this, they should ask themselves two questions each time they feel fat:
   - What has happened in the last hour that might have triggered this feeling?
   - What else am I feeling just now?
4. It usually emerges that the patient's experiences of feeling fat are triggered either by the occurrence of certain negative mood states or physical sensations that heighten body awareness. Examples of these two types of stimulus include the following:
   - Feeling bored, depressed, lonely, or tired.
   - Feeling full, bloated, or sweaty; feeling one's body wobble or one's thighs rubbing together; clothing that feels tight.
5. Over subsequent weeks patients should continue to do this whenever they have strong feelings

of fatness. In addition, they should address any masked problem (e.g., feeling bored) using the problem-solving approach (described later in this chapter). In some patients, problem solving will already have been taught in the context of addressing event-triggered changes in eating. In others, the approach needs to be introduced at this point. With regard to tackling patients' response to heightened body awareness, therapists should help them appreciate that the problem is their negative interpretation of these sensations rather than the sensations themselves.

Addressing feeling fat typically takes many weeks and will be a recurring item on the session agenda. What generally happens is that the frequency and intensity of feeling fat progressively decline, and patients' "relationship" to the experience changes, such that it is no longer equated with being fat. This metacognitive change is important, since once it happens, feeling fat ceases to maintain body dissatisfaction.

Addressing Dietary Restraint and Food Avoidance

Dieting is one of the most prominent features of patients with eating disorders. A major goal of treatment is to reduce, if not eliminate altogether, the strong tendency of these patients to diet. As noted earlier, attempts to restrict eating ("dietary restraint") may or may not be successful. Thus, it is far from inevitable that they result in true undereating in physiological terms ("dietary restriction") and weight loss. In this section we focus on addressing dietary restraint and dietary rules. The tackling of dietary restriction is addressed in a later section on treatment of those who are underweight.

The dietary restraint of patients with eating disorders is both extreme in intensity and rigid in form. These patients set themselves multiple demanding dietary rules. These may concern when they eat (e.g., not before 6:00 P.M.), how much they should eat (e.g., less than 600 kcal per day) and, most especially, what they should eat, with most patients having a large number of foods that they are attempting to avoid ("food avoidance"). Many have all three types of dietary rule. As a result of these rules, patients' eating is inflexible and restricted in nature. Despite this, dietary restraint is valued, and patients tend to be oblivious to its adverse effects.

When addressing dietary restraint, an important first step is for the therapist to help patients to see that their dieting is indeed a problem. This can be done with reference to their formulation, which in most cases shows that dieting plays a central role in the maintenance of their eating problem. If this is the case, it will need to be addressed to overcome the problem. Second their dieting may well have many adverse effects on their day-to-day life. These may be uncovered using the CIA (Bohn & Fairburn, 2008); for example, it may preclude eating out; it may result in tension about mealtimes; and it may cause preoccupation with thoughts about food and eating.

Once it has been agreed that dietary restraint is a problem, therapist and patient need to identify the various dietary rules present. Many will be evident by this stage in treatment. The principles that underlie addressing these rules are as follows:

1. Identifying a specific rule and what is motivating it.
2. Exploring with the patient the likely consequences of breaking the rule. The patient may believe that breaking the rule will lead to weight gain or invariably result in binge eating.
3. Devising a plan with the patient for breaking the rule in question in order to explore the consequences of doing so, and helping the patient implement this plan.
4. Analyzing the implications of the planned rule-breaking.
5. Planning further occasions of breaking the same rule, until the rule ceases to have significance.

With patients who binge-eat it is important to pay particular attention to food avoidance. The first step is to identify any foods being avoided. A good way of doing this is to ask patients to visit a local supermarket and write down all foods they would be reluctant to eat because of their possible effect on their shape or weight, or because they fear that eating them might trigger a binge. The patient and therapist should rank these foods (often comprising 40 or more items) according to the difficulty the patient would experience eating them. Patients should be helped to introduce these foods progressively into their diet, starting with the easiest and gradually moving on to the most difficult. The amount eaten is not important, although the eventual goal is that the patient should be capable of eating normal quantities with impunity. The systematic introduction of avoided foods should continue until patients are no longer anxious about eating them. Often this will take the remainder of treatment and sometime beyond it.

Other dietary rules should be tackled in a similar fashion, with a focus on both the belief that is maintaining the rule and breaking the rule itself. It is especially important to address rules that interfere with social eating.

Addressing Event- and Mood-Related Changes in Eating

In patients with eating disorders, eating habits may change in response to outside events and moods. This is particularly true of binge eating. The variety of different mechanisms involved include the following:

- Binge eating or vomiting, or both, to cope with negative events or adverse moods. Binge eating has two relevant properties: It is distracting and may take the patient's mind off aversive thoughts, and it has a direct mood-modulatory effect, in that it dampens strong mood states. The latter property is also true of vomiting and intense exercising.
- Eating less or stopping eating to gain a sense of personal control when external events feel outside the patient's control. This is seen most often in underweight patients.
- Eating less to influence others; for example, it may be a way of exhibiting feelings of distress or anger, or it may be an act of defiance.

If in Stage 3 events and moods appear to contribute to the maintenance of the eating disorder, this contribution needs to be assessed and in all likelihood addressed, with the goal of helping patients deal with events and moods directly and effectively, without influencing patients' eating. With most patients, the first step is to identify such changes in eating through real-time recording, and in the following session go over in detail one or more examples in an attempt to identify the triggers involved. Then, the patient should be trained in a variant of standard cognitive-behavioral technique of problem solving, termed "proactive problem solving." The distinctive feature of this approach is its emphasis on spotting problems early. It is described in detail in the complete treatment guide and it is also covered from the patient's perspective in *Overcoming Binge Eating*. The approach, if well taught, is remarkably effective in most cases. The exception is those patients who have difficulty tolerating mood states that

involve arousal. These patients (who tend to attract the diagnosis of borderline personality disorder) have what we term "mood intolerance." They benefit from proactive problem solving, but they also need more direct help coping with their moods. To this end we use an approach that overlaps with elements of dialectical behavior therapy (Linehan, 1993) and is described in the treatment guide.

Setbacks and Mindsets

The core psychopathology of eating disorders may be viewed as a "mindset" or frame of mind. While normally one's "mind-in-place" varies with changing circumstances, in people with eating disorders it tends to get locked in, and patients' thinking becomes persistently dominated by eating disorder thoughts. It leads patients to filter both internal and external stimuli in a distinctive way; it leads to the forms of behavior characteristic of eating disorders; and it results in the mislabeling of various physical and emotional experiences as "feeling fat."

The cognitive-behavioral strategies used in CBT-E are designed to address both the key features of the eating disorders and, most importantly, the processes that are maintaining them. In patients who are making good progress these mechanisms gradually erode during Stage 3, with the result that healthier and situationally more appropriate mindsets start to move into place, albeit temporarily at first. Such shifts in mindset usually become evident during the last third of treatment. They are reported by patients with surprise, using statements such as "On Sunday evening I forgot I had an eating disorder!" At first, the eating disorder mindset is prone to come back into place with even minor provocations (e.g., a friend discussing a diet she has just started) and with it returns the patient's eating disorder behavior, thoughts, and feelings. These "setbacks" can readily escalate into full-blown relapse unless they are promptly nipped in the bud. It is therefore import to raise the topic of mindsets at this stage in treatment so that patients can learn to spot their eating disorder mindset coming into place by detecting the characteristic early changes in their behavior. Once patients can do this, they can then go on to learn how to "eject" the mindset, thereby preventing the setback from becoming established. Practice spotting the mindset coming back into place and dealing with it effectively is of great value, as this skill—intervening very early at the beginnings of a setback—may account for the low relapse rate following CBT-E. It is therefore helpful if patients experience occasional setbacks later in treatment because this gives them the opportunity to utilize these strategies and procedures while still in treatment. Full details of how to help patients manipulate their mindset and address setbacks are provided in the treatment guide.

Stage 4: Ending Well

This is the final stage in treatment. With patients who are receiving 20 sessions of treatment, it comprises three sessions over 5 weeks (i.e., the sessions are 2 weeks apart). It has two broad aims:

1. To ensure that the changes made in treatment are maintained and built upon
2. To minimize the risk of relapse in the future

At the same time, patients discontinue self-monitoring and transfer from in-session weighing to weighing themselves at home.

Ensuring that the Changes Made in Treatment Are Maintained

The first step in doing this is to review in detail the patient's progress and what problems remain. This can be done in much the same way as in Stage 2, using the EDE-Q and CIA as a guide. Then, depending on what problems remain, therapist and patient jointly devise a specific short-term plan for the patient to follow until the posttreatment review appointment in 5 months' time. Typically, this includes further work on body checking and food avoidance, as well as encouraging the patient to maintain efforts to develop new interests and activities.

Minimizing the Risk of Relapse in the Future

Relapses are not all-or-nothing phenomena. They occur in degrees and may start as a "slip" or setback that then becomes established. Commonly, the slip comprises the resumption of dietary restraint, often triggered by an adverse, shape-related event (e.g., a critical comment, clothes feeling tighter than usual). In patients who were previously prone to binge-eat, this return of dietary restraint may lead to an episode of binge eating through the mechanisms described earlier, which in turn will encourage yet greater dietary restraint, thereby increasing the risk of further episodes of binge eating. Within

days, most aspects of the eating disorder may have returned. The patient's reaction to this sequence of events is crucial in determining what happens. If it is detected early on, as discussed earlier, it is relatively easy to intervene, but if it is not, it becomes progressively more difficult to deal with the setback.

To minimize the risk of relapse in the long term, the therapist needs to do the following:

1. *Educate the patient about the risk of relapse, highlighting common triggers and the likely sequence of events in the patient's case.* There is in some patients a tendency to hope that they will never have an eating problem again. This is especially common in those who have ceased to binge-eat, but it is seen in other patients, too. Without casting a negative light on patients' hopes for the future, therapists need to ensure that patients' expectations are realistic; otherwise there is a risk that patients will not take seriously the need to devise a "maintenance plan." Also, they will be vulnerable to react negatively to any emerging setback. Patients should learn to view their eating disorder as their Achilles' heel: that is, their responses to stress in general and to certain triggers.

2. *Stress the importance of detecting problems early, before they become entrenched.* With this in mind, therapist and patient should identify likely early warning signs of an impending relapse. For patients who are prone to binge or purge, these forms of behavior occur early on in the course of any setback and are readily noticeable. Patients whose eating disorder is primarily characterized by dietary restriction may need help to spot ominous signs.

3. *Construct with the patient a plan of action (a written personalized "long-term maintenance plan") for use in the future should problems arise.* There are two important elements: focusing on the emerging eating problem and correcting it, and addressing the trigger of the setback. In general the former is achieved by doing what was learned in treatment (doing the right thing), possibly following the guidance in *Overcoming Binge Eating*, while the latter is achieved using problem solving.

4. *Discuss when the patient should seek further help.* It is important that patients seek further help if it is needed. The strategy described earlier should get patients back on track within a few weeks. If, after some weeks of trying to correct matters, the problem has

not substantially resolved, we suggest that the patient should seek outside help.

Ending or Extending Treatment

It is unusual not to end CBT-E as planned. So long as patients have got to the point where the central maintaining mechanisms have been disrupted, treatment can and should finish. Otherwise, patients (and therapists) are at risk of ascribing continued improvement to the ongoing therapy rather than natural resolution of the eating disorder. In practice, this means that it is acceptable to end treatment with patients who are still dieting to an extent, perhaps binge eating and vomiting on occasions, and having residual concerns about shape and weight.

At times there are grounds for extending treatment. In our view, the main indication for doing this is the presence of eating disorder features that continue to interfere significantly with the patient's functioning and are unlikely to resolve of their own accord. Another reason to extend treatment is to compensate for the deleterious impact of disruptions to treatment, generally due to the emergence of a clinical depression or the occurrence of a life crisis.

The occasional patient benefits little from CBT-E. It is our practice to refer such patients for day patient or inpatient treatment.

The Posttreatment Review Appointment

We routinely hold a posttreatment review appointment about 20 weeks after the completion of treatment. During the intervening period, patients do not receive any further therapeutic input. The review session has several purposes:

1. To reassess the patient's state and need for further treatment. If residual eating disorder features are significantly interfering with the patient's functioning, then further treatment should be considered. If there has been a setback, a few brief sessions may be needed to get the patient back on track.
2. To review the patient's implementation of the short-term maintenance plan. The therapist should review the plan with the aim of identifying residual eating disorder features that the patient needs to continue to address.
3. To discuss how any setbacks have been handled.

The patient's ability to detect and address setbacks should be reviewed in detail.
4. To review the long-term maintenance plan.

CBT-E FOR UNDERWEIGHT PATIENTS

The great majority of patients with an eating disorder undereat at some stage and many may become underweight for a time. Generally this does not last, and they regain the lost weight, but a minority maintain strict control over their eating and stay underweight. A proportion of these patients meet current diagnostic criteria for anorexia nervosa, whereas others are eligible for one or other of the two residual eating disorder diagnoses.

CBT-E for underweight patients does not require major modifications because the core psychopathology and behavior of these patients is very similar to that of the majority of patients with an eating disorder. However, it does need to be adjusted to accommodate three problems seen in this group, but not necessarily confined to it:

1. Limited motivation to change
2. Being underweight
3. Undereating ("dietary restriction").

To do this, CBT-E needs to be extended in length because it takes time to engender motivation to change and even more time to regain weight. Hence, as mentioned earlier, for those with a BMI between 15.0 and 18.5, treatment generally takes up to 40 weeks, with sessions generally held twice weekly until the patient is consistently gaining weight. Once this is happening, sessions are weekly; then, toward the end of treatment, they are every 2–3 weeks.

Patients' health and safety are always of paramount importance, and this is especially true of patients who are underweight because their physical health is invariably compromised. Therapists need to be aware of potential physical complications, and those who are not medically qualified should have good access to a physician who can advise on the management of medical problems.

Overview

The four stages of the 20-week version of CBT-E do not neatly map onto the version for underweight patients.

Treatment for these patients may be thought of as having three phases:

- *Phase I.* This lasts up to 8 weeks and the focus is on engaging patients and helping them arrive at the decision that they need to regain weight.
- *Phase II.* This is the weight-gain phase. The goal is that patients gain weight at the rate of about 0.5 kg per week. Therefore, the length of this phase is determined by the amount of weight to be regained. During this phase the patient's eating disorder psychopathology is addressed.
- *Phase III.* This is the weight-maintenance phase, in which patients practice maintaining their new healthy weight. It lasts about 8 weeks.

As a result of the particular emphases of these phases, patients' weight graphs generally have a distinct three-phase pattern to them, as shown in Figure 17.8.

Phase I

The first two treatment sessions are similar to those of the 20-week treatment, although there are certain modifications to accommodate education about the ef-

fects of being underweight and to incorporate this information in the formulation. In practice this involves the following:

- Inquiring carefully in the initial assessment about the features that are likely to being underweight. This inquiry should be embedded within the usual assessment.
- Providing personalized education about the effects of being underweight before jointly creating the formulation. This involves delaying the formulation to the second treatment session rather than creating it in the initial session as in the 20-week version.
- Jointly creating a formulation that highlights the likely contribution of being underweight to the maintenance of the patient's eating problem (e.g., preoccupation with food and eating, increased need for routines and predictability, indecisiveness, heightened feelings of fullness, low mood, social withdrawal). A patient-oriented description of these features is provided in the second edition of *Overcoming Binge Eating* (Fairburn, 2013).
- Discussing the implications of the formulation for treatment. The major point is that almost all of the

FIGURE 17.8. The weight graph of a patient with anorexia nervosa. From Fairburn (2008, p. 180). Copyright 2008 by The Guilford Press. Adapted by permission.

effects identified will resolve if the patient regains weight, and at the same time patients will discover their true personality, which has been masked by being underweight. Simultaneously it is emphasized that treatment will involve much more than mere weight regain.

The emphasis then moves on to helping patients decide to change. The goal is that patients make this decision themselves rather than having the decision imposed on them. The aim is to interest the patient in the benefits of change and the possibility of a "fresh start." There are five steps in this process:

1. Creating a "Current Pros and Cons of Change" table.
2. Creating a "Future Pros and Cons of Change" table.
3. Creating a "Conclusions" table. An example is shown in Table 17.2.
4. Helping the patient identify and accept the implications of these conclusions.
5. Helping the patient decide to act and "take the plunge."

At the same time, collaborative weighing and regular eating are also introduced, much as in the 20-week treatment. One difference is that weighing takes place every session because patients' low weight is a significant health problem and a major target of treatment. Another is that the pattern of regular eating should include three meals and three snacks; that is, patients should have six episodes of eating rather than five, as in the 20-week treatment.

If the patient decides to regain weight, then Phase II begins. If, however, the patient never reaches this decision despite extensive nondirective exploration of the topic (over at least 8 weeks), then CBT-E has failed and other treatment options should be considered. This applies in about one in five cases.

Phase II

In Phase Two the focus is on weight regain while at the same time addressing the patient's eating disorder psychopathology in much the same way as described earlier. Thus, there will be emphasis on modifying the overevaluation of shape and weight, dietary restraint, and event- and mood-related changes in eating.

TABLE 17.2. Pros and Cons of Change: A Patient's "Conclusions"

I want to get better and regain weight because . . .

- *I will be able to have a full-life not one that is just about eating and weight.*
- *I will be healthier: my bones and heart will be stronger; I won't be cold and faint and will be able to sleep properly. I won't be ill!*
- *I will be able to have good relationships with other people and hopefully a partner and children who I can be a good role model to.*
- *I will be able to enjoy my job and be successful at it.*
- *At the moment the eating problem stops me from being able to do things well. When I am better I won't need an excuse.*
- *Regaining weight will mean that I will become slim and healthy. It does not mean that I will become fat.*
- *Getting better won't be giving in. Not getting better would be giving in. Getting better is about choosing to give myself a life.*
- *I want to show how strong I can be by eating as right now not eating is the easy thing.*
- *Eating enough food to be a healthy weight isn't greedy. It is being normal.*
- *Being a healthy weight and eating enough will help to give me true control over my eating. I will be able to make choices about what I eat. At the moment the eating problem has control over me. Becoming well will protect me from out-of-control eating and uncontrolled weight gain.*
- *Being well will enable me to develop my talents as a person and to discover my true self.*
- *Getting better will give me choices in life. The eating problem has been holding me back. Change can only be good.*

Note. From Fairburn (2008, p. 167). Copyright 2008 by The Guilford Press. Reprinted by permission.

Weight regain is very difficult for these patients. It is a long and laborious process. It requires that patients maintain an energy surplus each day of about 500 kcal if they are to regain weight at a rate of about 0.5 kg per week.

It is our practice to have as a goal a BMI over 19.0. This figure ensures that the great majority of patients are free from the psychobiological effects of being underweight, while still being slim. It is important not to compromise on this figure. Many female patients want to stop regaining weight when their BMI is in the 17.0–18.0 range, possibly because this is when their shape begins to become more feminine. This is a serious mistake because they are still experiencing the adverse effects of being underweight and have experienced few of the advantages of the weight regain. Patients with a BMI at this level also tend to go on to lose weight.

Full details of how to help patients regain weight are provided in the complete treatment guide.

Phase III

The goal of this phase is to help patients maintain a weight, such that their BMI fluctuates between 19.0 and 20.0. Patients and therapists have opposite concerns at this point. While patients are afraid that their weight will continue to rise, therapists fear that it will fall. The therapists' fears are usually the more realistic ones. The risks and dangers of weight loss should be discussed openly with patients.

This phase of treatment usually runs smoothly, and certainly so in comparison with Phase II. Therapists should encourage patients to live life fully now that they are free from the debilitating effects of being underweight. Patients should be helped to flourish, take risks, and enjoy themselves, while not forgetting the importance of maintaining their new healthy weight.

The final few sessions need to cover the same topics as those covered in the 20-week version. Thus, they address (along the same lines):

1. Mindsets and setbacks.
2. Ensuring that achieved changes achieved are maintained.
3. Procedures for minimizing the risk of relapse in the future.

CONCLUDING REMARKS

Myths and misconceptions concerning CBT abound. Two are particularly prevalent. The first is that treatment is diagnosis-driven; that is, the form of the treatment is almost exclusively determined by the patient's DSM diagnosis. The second is that the treatment is rigidly structured. We hope that it is clear that neither criticism applies to CBT-E. In CBT-E, the form of the patient's treatment is dictated by a highly personalized formulation that is diagnosis-independent. It is based on patients' eating disorder psychopathology, not their

DSM diagnosis. Moreover, this formulation is modified and further personalized as treatment progresses and the patient's psychopathology evolves. What happens in Session 10 with Patient A may bear little relation to what happens in Session 10 with Patient B. What is specified in CBT-E are the strategies and substrategies used, and the procedures employed to bring about change, but how and when they are applied varies markedly from case to case. As a result, CBT-E is more of a challenge to learn than more prescriptive treatments, but the compensation is that it is more rewarding to implement, not least because of its effectiveness.[6]

ACKNOWLEDGMENTS

We are grateful to the Wellcome Trust for its support: Christopher G. Fairburn is supported by a Principal Research Fellowship (046386), and Zafra Cooper is supported by a strategic award (094585). Our research on eating disorders is supported by a programme grant from the Wellcome Trust (046386). Sarah Collins provided valuable feedback on the manuscript.

NOTES

1. Body mass index (BMI) is a widely used way of representing weight adjusted for height. It is weight in kilograms divided by height in meters squared [i.e., $wt/(ht)^2$]. The BMI applies to adults of both sexes between the ages of 18 and 60. The healthy range is 18.5–25.0.

2. If there is a difference in their core psychopathology, it is that some patients with anorexia nervosa are primarily concerned with controlling their eating per se, rather than their shape and weight. This is especially true of younger cases of short duration.

3. Originally, the broad version of the treatment addressed a fourth obstacle to change, termed "mood intolerance." This has subsequently been incorporated into the focused form of CBT-E.

4. Our research on the 20-week version of CBT-E has included patients with a BMI over 17.5, but our clinical experience suggests that patients who are somewhat underweight do better with a longer treatment. We are therefore recommending a lower BMI threshold of 18.5.

5. C. G. F. acknowledges the obvious conflict of interest.

6. The website *www.credo-oxford.com* provides up-to-date information on the empirical status of CBT-E and opportunities to obtain training. All the materials needed to implement CBT-E may be downloaded free of charge from this website.

REFERENCES

American Psychiatric Association. (1994). *Diagnostic and statistical manual of mental disorders* (4th ed.). Washington, DC: Author.

American Psychiatric Association. (2013). *Diagnostic and statistical manual of mental disorders* (5th ed.). Arlington, VA: Author.

Bohn, K., & Fairburn, C. G. (2008). The Clinical Impairment Assessment Questionnaire (CIA 3.0). In C. G. Fairburn, *Cognitive behavior therapy and eating disorders* (pp. 315–317). New York: Guilford Press.

Byrne, S. M., Fursland, A., Allen, K. L., & Watson, H. (2011). The effectiveness of enhanced cognitive behavioural therapy for eating disorders: An open trial. *Behaviour Research and Therapy, 49*, 219–226.

Cooper, Z., & Fairburn, C. G. (2011). The evolution of "enhanced" cognitive behavior therapy for eating disorders: Learning from treatment non-response. *Cognitive and Behavioral Practice, 18*, 394–402.

Cooper, Z., & Stewart, A. (2008). CBT-E and the younger patient. In C. G. Fairburn, *Cognitive behavior therapy and eating disorders* (pp. 221–230). New York: Guilford Press.

Crow, S., & Peterson, C. B. (2009). Refining treatments for eating disorders. *American Journal of Psychiatry, 166*, 266–267.

Dalle Grave, R. (2012). *Intensive cognitive behavior therapy for eating disorders*. New York: Nova Science.

Dalle Grave, R., Calugi, S., Doll, H. A., & Fairburn, C. G. (2013). Enhanced cognitive behaviour therapy for adolescents with anorexia nervosa: An alternative to family therapy? *Behaviour Research and Therapy, 51*, R9–R12.

Fairburn, C. G. (2005). Evidence-based treatment of anorexia nervosa. *International Journal of Eating Disorders, 37*, S26–S30.

Fairburn, C. G. (2008). *Cognitive behavior therapy and eating disorders*. New York: Guilford Press.

Fairburn, C. G. (2013). *Overcoming binge eating* (2nd ed.). New York: Guilford Press.

Fairburn, C. G., Agras, W. S., Walsh, B. T., Wilson, G. T., & Stice, E. (2004). Early change in treatment predicts outcome in bulimia nervosa. *American Journal of Psychiatry, 161*, 2322–2324.

Fairburn, C. G., & Beglin, S. J. (2008). Eating Disorder Examination Questionnaire (EDE-Q 6.0). In C. G. Fairburn, *Cognitive behavior therapy and eating disorders* (pp. 309–313). New York: Guilford Press.

Fairburn, C. G., & Bohn, K. (2005). Eating disorder NOS (EDNOS): An example of the troublesome "not otherwise specified" (NOS) category in DSM-IV. *Behaviour Research and Therapy, 43*, 691–701.

Fairburn, C. G., & Cooper, Z. (2011). Eating disorders, DSM-5 and clinical reality. *British Journal of Psychiatry, 198*, 8–10.

Fairburn, C. G., Cooper, Z., Bohn, K., O'Connor, M. E., Doll, H. A., & Palmer, R. L. (2007). The severity and status of eating disorder NOS: Implications for DSM-V. *Behaviour Research and Therapy, 45*, 1705–1715.

Fairburn, C. G., Cooper, Z., Doll, H. A., O'Connor, M. E., Bohn, K., Hawker, D. M., et al. (2009). Transdiagnostic cognitive-behavioral therapy for patients with eating disorders: A two-site trial with 60-week follow-up. *American Journal of Psychiatry, 166*, 311–319.

Fairburn, C. G., Cooper, Z., Doll, H. A., Palmer, R. L., & Dalle Grave, R. (2013). Enhanced cognitive behaviour therapy for adults with anorexia nervosa: A UK–Italy study. *Behaviour Research and Therapy, 51*, R2–R8.

Fairburn, C. G., Cooper, Z., & Shafran, R. (2003). Cognitive behaviour therapy for eating disorders: A "transdiagnostic" theory and treatment. *Behaviour Research and Therapy, 41*, 509–528.

Fairburn, C. G., Cooper, Z., & Shafran, R. (2008). Enhanced cognitive behavior therapy for eating disorders ("CBT-E"): An overview. In C. G. Fairburn, *Cognitive behavior therapy and eating disorders* (pp. 23–34). New York: Guilford Press.

Fairburn, C. G., Cooper, Z., Shafran, R., Bohn, K., & Hawker, D. M. (2008a). Clinical perfectionism, core low self-esteem and interpersonal problems. In C. G. Fairburn, *Cognitive behavior therapy and eating disorders* (pp. 197–220). New York: Guilford Press.

Fairburn, C. G., Cooper, Z., Shafran, R., Bohn, K., Hawker, D. M., Murphy, R., et al. (2008b). Enhanced cognitive behavior therapy for eating disorders: The core protocol. In C. G. Fairburn, *Cognitive behavior therapy and eating disorders* (pp. 47–193). New York: Guilford Press.

Fairburn, C. G., Cooper, Z., & Waller, D. (2008a). "Complex cases" and comorbidity. In C. G. Fairburn, *Cognitive behavior therapy and eating disorders* (pp. 245–258). New York: Guilford Press.

Fairburn, C. G., Cooper, Z., & Waller, D. (2008b). The patients: Their assessment, preparation for treatment and medical management. In C. G. Fairburn, *Cognitive behavior therapy and eating disorders* (pp. 35–44). New York: Guilford Press.

Fairburn, C. G., & Harrison, P. J. (2003). Eating disorders. *Lancet, 361*, 407–416.

Fairburn, C. G., & Wilson, G. T. (2013). The dissemination and implementation of psychological treatments: Problems and solutions. *International Journal of Eating Disorders, 46*, 516–521.

Hay, P. J., & Claudino, A. M. (2010). Evidence-based treatment for the eating disorders. In W. S. Agras (Ed.), *The Oxford handbook of eating disorders* (pp. 452–479). Oxford, UK: Oxford University Press.

Linehan, M. M. (1993). *Cognitive behavioral treatment of borderline personality disorder*. New York: Guilford Press.

Lock, J. (2011). Evaluation of family treatment models for

eating disorders. *Current Opinion in Psychiatry, 24,* 274–279.

Lock, J., le Grange, D., Agras, W. S., & Dare, C. (2001). *Treatment manual for anorexia nervosa: A family-based approach.* New York: Guilford Press.

Lock, J., le Grange, D., Agras, S., Moye, A., Bryson, S. W., & Jo, B. (2010). Randomized clinical trial comparing family-based treatment with adolescent-focused individual therapy for adolescents with anorexia nervosa. *Archives of General Psychiatry, 67,* 1025–1032.

Luborsky, L., Singer, B., & Luborsky, L. (1975). Comparative studies of psychotherapies. *Archives of General Psychiatry, 32,* 995–1008.

Lundgren, J. D., Allison, K. C., & Stunkard, A. J. (Eds.). (2012). *Night eating syndrome: Research, assessment, and treatment.* New York: Guilford Press.

Masheb, R. M., & Grilo, C. M. (2007). Rapid response predicts treatment outcomes in binge eating disorder: Implications for stepped care. *Journal of Consulting and Clinical Psychology, 75,* 639–644.

Mitchell, J. E., & de Zwaan, M. (2012). *Psychosocial evaluation and treatment in bariatric surgery.* New York: Routledge.

National Institute for Clinical Excellence. (2004). *Eating disorders: Core interventions in the treatment and management of anorexia nervosa, bulimia nervosa and related eating disorders.* London: Author.

Poulsen, S., Lunn, S., Daniel, S. I. F., Folke, S., Mathiesen, B. B., Katznelson, H., et al. (in press). A randomized controlled trial of psychoanalytic psychotherapy versus cognitive behavior therapy for bulimia nervosa. *American Journal of Psychiatry.*

Wilson, G. T. (1999). Rapid response to cognitive behavior therapy. *Clinical Psychology: Science and Practice, 6,* 289–292.

Wilson, G. T., Grilo, C. M., & Vitousek, K. M. (2007). Psychological treatment of eating disorders. *American Psychologist, 62,* 199–216.

Wilson, G. T., & Schlam, T. R. (2004). The transtheoretical model and motivational interviewing in the treatment of eating and weight disorders. *Clinical Psychology Review, 24,* 361–378.

Wilson, G. T., Wilfley, D. E., Agras, W. S., & Bryson, S. W. (2010). Psychological treatments of binge eating disorder. *Archives of General Psychiatry, 67,* 94–101.

Wilson, G. T., & Zandberg, L. (2012). Cognitive-behavioral guided self-help for eating disorders: Effectiveness and scalability. *Clinical Psychology Review, 32,* 343–357.

CHAPTER 18

Couple Distress

ANDREW CHRISTENSEN
JENNIFER G. WHEELER
BRIAN D. DOSS
NEIL S. JACOBSON

The second edition of this book presented, for the first time, a substantially different approach to couple therapy—different both in conceptualization and in treatment strategies. It was noted that these changes in technique and conceptualization were profound enough to warrant a new name for the approach: "integrative behavioral couple therapy" (IBCT). As described in this fifth edition, IBCT has matured into a sophisticated and intuitively appealing set of strategies. These strategies are very nicely illustrated in this chapter in the context of the comprehensive treatment of one couple in substantial distress. Because these strategies require considerable clinical skill and talent, beginning therapists in particular should learn much from the case descriptions presented in this very readable and engaging chapter.—D. H. B.

Unlike other chapters in this *Handbook*, the term "couple distress" does not refer to a specific clinical or personality disorder. In DSM-5, couple distress is handled as it was in DSM-IV-TR: not considered a "mental disorder" but relegated to the category of "other conditions that may be a focus of clinical attention" and assigned a lesser "V code" of "relationship distress with spouse or intimate partner." Yet it is certainly arguable that couple distress creates as much psychological and physical pain as many, if not most, of the DSM disorders (e.g., Beach et al., 2006). Furthermore, couple distress can initiate, exacerbate, and complicate DSM disorders such as depression, or trigger their relapse (Whisman, 2007; Whisman & Bruce, 1999). Additionally, couple distress can have a major impact on children, and can trigger or exacerbate externalizing and internalizing disorders (Buehler et al., 1997). Indeed, there was a push to give relationship processes such as couple distress greater attention in DSM-5, and perhaps include some relationship problems as disorders; however, such efforts seem to have faltered (American Psychiatric Association, 2013; Beach et al., 2006). Whatever the merits and outcome of these efforts, there is no doubt that couple distress has serious psychological consequences and is deserving of therapeutic attention.

In this chapter we describe one promising approach to the treatment of couple distress called integrative behavioral couple therapy (IBCT; Christensen & Jacobson, 2000; Christensen, Jacobson, & Babcock, 1995; Jacobson & Christensen, 1998). We briefly review the development of this approach from its origins in traditional behavioral couple therapy, followed by a description of IBCT theories and techniques. Then we describe the application of IBCT, including the stages of therapy and the use of specific interventions. Finally, we discuss the empirical evidence in support of IBCT and provide a case example to demonstrate the application of IBCT to the treatment of couple distress.

TRADITIONAL BEHAVIORAL COUPLE THERAPY

The term "couple therapy" (as opposed to "individual" or "group" therapy) refers to clinical approaches for improving the functioning of two individuals within the context of their romantic relationship to one another.[1] Although couple therapy is unique in its emphasis on a specific dyad, by its very definition, it is a contextual approach to the treatment of two *individuals*. Accordingly, successful treatments for couple distress have emphasized the assessment and modification of each individual's contribution and response to specific interactions in their relationship (e.g., Baucom & Hoffman, 1986; Gurman, Knickerson, & Pinsof, 1986; Holtzworth-Munroe & Jacobson, 1991; Jacobson, 1978a, 1984; Jacobson & Holtzworth-Munroe, 1986; Jacobson & Margolin, 1979; Stuart, 1980; Weiss, Hops, & Patterson, 1973).

For over three decades, the "gold standard" for the treatment of couple distress has been behavioral couple therapy (for reviews of couple therapies, see Baucom, Shoham, Kim, Daiuto, & Stickle, 1998; Christensen & Heavey, 1999; Jacobson & Addis, 1993; Snyder, Castellani, & Whisman, 2006). First applied to couple distress by Stuart (1969) and Weiss and colleagues (1973), traditional behavioral couple therapy (TBCT) uses basic behavioral principles of reinforcement, modeling, and behavioral rehearsal to facilitate collaboration and compromise between partners. With an eye toward facilitating changes in the partners' behavior, TBCT teaches them how to increase or decrease target behaviors (behavior exchange), to communicate more effectively (communication training), and to assess and solve problems (problem solving) to improve overall relationship satisfaction. The monograph by Jacobson and Margolin (1979) is a commonly used treatment manual for TBCT.

In early studies, TBCT demonstrated significant empirical success (Jacobson 1977, 1978b) and soon became the focus of numerous treatment manuals, programs, and publications supporting the application of behavioral techniques to the treatment of couple distress (e.g., Floyd & Markman, 1983; Gottman, Notarius, Gonso, & Markman, 1976; Jacobson & Margolin, 1979; Knox, 1971; Liberman, 1970; Liberman, Wheeler, deVisser, Kuehnel, & Kuehnel, 1981; Stuart, 1980). Subsequent outcome research has consistently supported the efficacy of behavioral approaches for the treatment of couple distress (Baucom & Hoffman, 1986; Gurman

et al., 1986; Jacobson, 1984; Jacobson, Schmaling, & Holtzworth-Munroe, 1987). Research has even shown the positive impact of TBCT for couples in which one partner has an individual disorder, such as depression (Gupta, Coyne, & Beach, 2003), alcoholism (O'Farrell & Fals-Stewart, 2000), and/or anxiety (Baucom et al., 1998).

Despite the apparent success of TBCT, however, outcome research also revealed some limitations in its efficacy and generalizability. For example, approximately one-third of couples failed to show measurable improvement in relationship quality following treatment with TBCT (Jacobson et al., 1987). Furthermore, many couples who initially responded to treatment relapsed within 1 or 2 years after therapy (Jacobson et al., 1984, 1987). Four years after therapy, Snyder, Wills, and Grady-Fletcher (1991) found a divorce rate of 37% in couples treated with TBCT.

Findings about the limited effectiveness of TBCT encouraged the development of additional therapeutic approaches. Various modifications and enhancements have been made to TBCT in an effort to improve its effectiveness (e.g., Baucom & Epstein, 1990; Baucom, Epstein, & Rankin, 1995; Epstein & Baucom, 2002; Floyd, Markman, Kelly, Blumberg, & Stanley, 1995; Halford, 2001), yet the existing comparative treatment studies have failed to demonstrate any incremental efficacy in various enhancements to TBCT. For example, the addition of cognitive strategies created a treatment that was as good as but not better than TBCT (e.g., Baucom et al., 1998).

In addition to examining treatment outcome, couple therapy research aimed at understanding how "treatment successes" differ from "treatment failures." Early research on treatment response identified several factors that appear to affect the success of TBCT. Compared to couples who responded positively to TBCT, couples who were regarded as "treatment failures" or "difficult to treat" were generally older, more emotionally disengaged, more polarized on basic issues, and more severely distressed (Baucom & Hoffman, 1986; Hahlweg, Schindler, Revenstorf, & Brengelmann, 1984; Jacobson, Follette, & Pagel, 1986; see Jacobson & Christensen, 1998, for a review). Despite the fact that these couples arguably had the greatest need for effective treatment, each of these factors has an obvious deleterious effect on their ability to collaborate, compromise, and facilitate behavioral change. Older couples, for example, have had more time than younger couples to become "stuck" in their destructive behavioral patterns; couples who are more polarized on fundamental issues (e.g., how traditional they are with respect to their gender roles) may never be able to reach a mutually satisfying compromise; and extremely disengaged couples may be unable to collaborate. Each of these factors is likely to be associated with long-standing, deeply entrenched, and seemingly "unchangeable" behavioral patterns. Thus, it should come as no surprise that the change-oriented techniques of TBCT are ineffective for these couples.

AN "INTEGRATIVE" THERAPY

These findings served as the impetus for the development of IBCT. Evidence on the limited success of TBCT, particularly during follow-up, spurred an effort to find a treatment with more enduring effects. Evidence on TBCT's failures spurred efforts to find treatments that would be applicable even to these difficult cases. Three developments in IBCT are directed toward making treatment more enduring and more broadly applicable: (1) a focus on the couple's relational "themes" rather than on specific target behaviors; (2) an emphasis on "contingency-shaped" versus "rule-governed" behavior; and (3) a focus on emotional acceptance.

The first aspect that is intended to make IBCT's effectiveness more broadly applicable and more enduring is its focus on a couple's relational "themes," that is, their long-standing patterns of disparate yet functionally similar behaviors. Although this focus is similar to TBCT in that it requires a comprehensive assessment of the couple's behavioral patterns, it differs from TBCT in that multiple and complex behavioral interactions—and not just specific behavioral targets—are considered for therapeutic intervention.

A highlight of all behavioral approaches, and certainly of TBCT, is an assessment process that transforms broad, global complaints into specific, observable behaviors. For example, a wife may come into therapy complaining that her husband does not love her, while her husband complains that his wife does not believe in him. The TBCT therapist would assist the wife in defining her general complaint into specific behavioral targets for her husband, such as kissing and hugging her more often. The therapist would also assist the husband in defining his general complaint into specific behavioral targets for his wife, such as complimenting his achievements more often. However, IBCT suggests that valuable information may be lost in the transfor-

mation of a global complaint into a specific behavioral target. By quickly narrowing down global complaints into specific behavioral targets, TBCT inadvertently limits the means by which partners may satisfy each other. For example, if "feeling loved" is defined solely in terms of physical affection and the husband has difficulty in increasing and/or sustaining a higher level of physical affection, then his wife's desires to feel loved will not be satisfied. Indeed, the husband could perform a variety of other behaviors in addition to physical affection that function to make his wife feel loved, such as calling her during work to see how she is doing, listening to her troubles with her family, or noticing that the air in her car tires is dangerously low. She may not be able to articulate many behaviors that might function in ways to make her feel loved, either because she is not aware of the desired behaviors or perhaps she feels too vulnerable to express this need. Without more elaborate exploration of and functional analysis of the wife's and husband's thoughts, feelings, and behaviors, such important opportunities for facilitating therapeutic change may be lost. Furthermore, these very specific behavioral definitions may have iatrogenic effects. In the previous example, the wife may begin to define her husband's love more and more in terms of his limited ability to be affectionate because this is how "love" was operationalized in the context of the TBCT intervention. If the husband is unable to make her feel "loved" via physical affection alone, then her anger and sense of loss could be heightened rather than ameliorated by the treatment.

In contrast to TBCT's emphasis on specific behavioral targets, IBCT focuses on broader "themes" in the couple's history, that is, developing a shared understanding of the many circumstances in which the wife has felt loved and unloved, and in which the husband has felt that his wife believed or did not believe in him. Certainly this shared understanding includes some specific behavioral examples illustrating what makes the wife feel unloved and what would make her feel loved, and what makes the husband feel that his wife does not believe in him and what would make him feel that she does. However, IBCT tries to keep open all possibilities of behaviors that function to provide each spouse with his/her desired emotional state. Thus, if one partner has difficulty performing a particular behavior (e.g., physical affection), he/she may still be able to perform other, perhaps less obvious behaviors that serve the same function (e.g., calling one's wife from work). By focusing on the broader emotional "theme" (her history of feeling unloved, his history of feeling not believed in), rather than attempting to operationalize that theme completely into one or more specific behaviors, IBCT maintains its functional roots, while increasing the chances that each partner is able to meet the other's needs.

A second development that is designed to make IBCT applicable to more couples and to create more enduring change is based on the distinction between "rule-governed" versus "contingency-shaped" behavior (Skinner, 1966). In the former, an individual is provided with a rule to guide his/her behavior and is then reinforced when he/she follows the rule. Using the previous example, a therapist could develop a list of possible affectionate behaviors for the husband, such as giving his wife a kiss when he leaves for work and when he returns, then encourage the husband to implement these behaviors. Upon implementing them, the husband would be reinforced by both his wife and the therapist. TBCT is largely based on employing "rule-governed" strategies to create positive change. Not only is behavioral exchange a "rule-governed" strategy, but even more importantly, the TBCT strategies of communication training and problem-solving training are also dominated by "rule-governed" strategies. In both, the TBCT therapist teaches the partners certain rules of good communication or good problem solving to use during their discussions of problems. The guidelines to use "I statements" and to "define the problem clearly before proposing solutions" are examples.

With "contingency-shaped" behavior, naturally occurring events in the situation serve to elicit and reinforce the desired behavior. For example, the husband would be affectionate with his wife when something in their interaction triggered a desire for him to hug or kiss her; the experience of closeness or physical contact in the affectionate gesture itself, or his wife's response to his gesture, would serve to reinforce his affectionate behavior. In contrast to TBCT, IBCT engages in "contingency-shaped" behavior change. IBCT therapists try to discover the events that function to trigger desired experiences in each partner, then attempt to orchestrate these events. For example, IBCT therapists might hypothesize that a wife's criticisms push her husband away, but that her expressions of loneliness could bring him toward her. The IBCT therapist listens to her criticisms (e.g., that her husband ignores her), suggests that she may be lonely (as a result of feeling "ignored"), and, if she acknowledges such a feeling, encourages her to talk about it. The therapeutic goal is that this "shift"

in her conversation (from criticism to self-disclosure) might also "shift" her husband's typically defensive posture in listening to (or ignoring) his wife. Although such a strategy of emphasizing "contingency-shaped" behavior makes intervention more complicated and less straightforward than a purely "rule-governed" approach, IBCT suggests that a "contingency-shaped" approach leads to more profound and enduring changes in the couple's relational patterns.

A third development in IBCT that is designed to make it applicable to more couples and to create more enduring change is its focus on emotional acceptance. In TBCT, the approach to solving couple problems is to create positive change. If the husband in the couple we discussed could be more physically affectionate, and the wife more verbally complimentary, then the couple's problems would presumably be solved. However, if the husband is unable or unwilling to be more physically affectionate, and if the wife is unable or unwilling to be more complimentary, then the case will be a treatment failure. If the husband and wife are able to make these changes initially but are unable to maintain them over the long run, then the case becomes a temporary success followed by relapse.

In contrast to TBCT, the focus of IBCT is on emotional acceptance, as well as change. Unlike the change-oriented goal of TBCT, the primary goal of IBCT is to promote each partner's *acceptance* of the other and their differences. Rather than trying to *eliminate* a couple's long-standing conflicts, a goal of IBCT is to help couples develop a new understanding of their apparently irreconcilable differences, and to use these differences to promote intimacy, empathy, and compassion for one another. With its focus on *acceptance* rather than *change*, IBCT creates an environment for couples to understand each other's behavior before deciding whether and how they might modify it. In the earlier example, IBCT would explore the husband's difficulties in expressing affection and the wife's difficulties in giving him compliments—difficulties that may have little to do with how much love they feel for one another. Through this exploration of the individuals, the partners may come to a greater understanding of one another and experience more emotional closeness, thus achieving the feelings of love they previously pursued by requesting changes in each other's behavior (i.e., increased physical affection and verbal compliments).

While there *is* an expectation of "change" in IBCT, this expectation differs significantly from that of TBCT in regard to *which* partner and *what* behavior is expected to change. In TBCT, the "change" involves Partner A changing the frequency or intensity of a specified behavior in response to a complaint from Partner B. But in IBCT, the therapeutic "change" also involves Partner B modifying his/her *emotional reaction* to Partner A's "problem" behavior. When a difference between partners is identified to be "irreconcilable," the therapeutic strategy of IBCT is to change the "complaining" partner's response to the "offending" partner's behavior rather than directing all therapeutic efforts at attempting to change what has historically been an essentially "unchangeable" behavior. Ideally, through exploration of the thoughts and feelings underlying Partner A's behaviors, Partner B develops a new understanding of his/her partner's behavior, and the "complaint" is transformed into a less destructive response. In turn, this change in Partner B's reaction often then has a salutary impact on the frequency or intensity of Partner A's behavior. Using this approach, as opposed to an exclusively change-focused approach, even the most polarized, disengaged, and "unchangeable" couples have an opportunity to increase their overall marital satisfaction.

It is important to note that in this context acceptance is not confused with resignation. Whereas "resignation" involves one partner grudgingly giving in and giving up on the hope for a better relationship, "acceptance" involves one partner "letting go" of the *struggle to change* the other. Ideally, partners "let go" of the struggle not grudgingly but as a result of a new appreciation for their partner's experience. By understanding their couple distress in terms of their individual differences, and by learning to accept each other's differences, it is hoped that the distress that has historically been generated by their struggle to change one another will be reduced. Thus, for IBCT to be effective in treating couple distress, it is important for partners to understand the factors that have contributed to the development and maintenance of their distress.

THE ETIOLOGY OF COUPLE DISTRESS

According to IBCT, relationship distress develops as a result of two basic influences—decreases in reinforcing exchanges, such as through reinforcement erosion, and the development of punishing exchanges, such as through conflict development. "Reinforcement erosion" refers to the phenomenon whereby behaviors that were once reinforcing become less reinforcing with repeated

exposure. For example, demonstrations of physical affection may generate powerful feelings of warmth and pleasure for each partner during the early stages of their relationship. But after partners have spent many years together, the reinforcing properties of these affectionate behaviors may disappear. For some couples, once-reinforcing behaviors may become "taken for granted," whereas for others, once-reinforcing behaviors may actually become aversive. In some cases, behaviors that were once considered attractive, endearing, or pleasing become the very same behaviors that generate or exacerbate the couple's distress.

As with the erosion of reinforcing behaviors, conflicts may emerge as couples spend more and more time together. In the early stages of a relationship, differences in partners' backgrounds, goals, and interests may initially be downplayed or ignored. For example, if Partner A prefers to save money and Partner B prefers to spend money, this difference may not be apparent during courtship, when spending money is a tacit expectation of both partners. If this difference *is* detected early on, perhaps it is be regarded as a "positive" difference, in that each partner is encouraged to be a little more like the other in his/her spending habits. Or perhaps each partner expects the other to eventually compromise or change to his/her way of doing things. But over time, these incompatibilities and their relevance to the relationship are inevitably exposed. Differences that were once regarded as novel, interesting, or challenging may ultimately be perceived as impediments to one's own goals and interests. Furthermore, in addition to any extant incompatibilities, other unanticipated incompatibilities may emerge with new life experiences (e.g., having children, changing careers). Thus, even those couples who had initially made a realistic appraisal of their differences may discover unexpected incompatibilities over time.

These incompatibilities, while challenging in their own right, can be further exacerbated by each partner's emotional sensitivities or vulnerabilities. Returning to our earlier example, if our "saver" comes from a background of economic deprivation and has developed a justifiable fear of being destitute, then the issues related to saving may be motivated by powerful emotions, which may impair his/her ability to understand the partner's desire to spend and enjoy what they have. Incompatibilities can also be exacerbated by external stressors. For example, if one member of our "saver–spender" couple loses his/her job, that might put their differences into even sharper relief. Efforts by the partners to deal with their struggle over money might paradoxically make the problem worse. If the saver, for example, engages in behaviors such as investigating and interrogating the spender while the spender avoids and hides his/her purchases from the other, their problem might increase in intensity. One goal of IBCT is to help the partners identify and reframe their incompatibilities in a way that minimizes the destructive nature of these incompatibilities, by encouraging a more effective way of communicating about them, while maximizing their level of intimacy and relationship satisfaction.

APPLICATION OF IBCT

The Formulation

The most important organizing principle of IBCT is the "formulation," a term used to describe how the therapist conceptualizes and describes the couple's problems. The formulation is based on a functional analysis of the couple's problems and comprises three basic components: a *theme*, a *DEEP analysis*, and a *mutual trap*. The therapist refers back to the formulation and its components throughout the treatment process, whenever couples have conflicts during or between therapy sessions.

One of the most basic goals of IBCT is for the partners to adopt the formulation as part of their relationship history. From that point forward, they can use the formulation as a context for understanding their relationship and their conflicts. The formulation also gives couples a language to discuss their problems, and allows partners to distance themselves from their problems. It is important to remember, however, that the formulation is a dynamic concept that may require alteration and modification (or "reformulation") throughout treatment.

The Theme

The "theme," the description of the couple's primary conflict, is usually described by a word or phrase that captures the issues with which the couple struggles. For example, a common theme of many distressed couples is that of "closeness–independence," in which one partner seeks greater closeness, whereas the other seeks greater independence. Other common themes center around trust, sexuality, money, and parenting. A couple may struggle about any particular topic and cer-

tainly with many issues, but often their struggles center around one or two broad themes.

The DEEP Analysis

In IBCT, therapists conduct a DEEP analysis of the couple's theme or issue, an acronym that outlines the four major factors contributing to a couple's problems: Differences, Emotional sensitivities, External circumstances, and Patterns of interaction. IBCT suggests that partners have their primary conflict, or theme, because of Differences between them and because of each partner's Emotional sensitivities or vulnerabilities linked to those differences, both of which can be exacerbated by External circumstances. For example, in the theme of closeness–independence, Partner A may want more closeness and connection, and Partner B may want more independence simply because they are different people with different genes and different social learning histories. Perhaps this difference was not readily apparent early on because both partners were enchanted by their developing relationship. Or perhaps there really was little difference in their desires for closeness and independence until they had children, or until one partner's career took off. Whatever the basis for the difference, it creates problems for the couple as Differences are perceived as deficiencies. For example, the closeness seeker may see the other as being "afraid of intimacy"; the independence seeker may see the other as being "neurotically dependent." Partners find that they cannot both get their needs fully satisfied. Compromise may be relatively easy unless Emotional sensitivities or vulnerabilities are also present, which provide emotional fuel for the differences. If Partner A wants greater closeness than Partner B and is emotionally vulnerable to easily feeling abandoned, then negotiations about closeness may be threatening to Partner A. Similarly, if Partner B wants greater independence and is emotionally vulnerable to easily feeling controlled and restrained, then negotiations about closeness may be threatening for Partner B as well. External circumstances may conspire to make the problem even greater. If the couple lives in an area where Partner A, who wants more closeness, is far away from other sources of social support, and where Partner B, who wants more independence, is close to leisure activities in which he/she wants to engage independently, the struggle between them will be even greater. The combination of their differences (D), their emotional sensitivities (E), and the external circumstances (E) may lead the two to engage in a destructive pattern (P) of interaction that can polarize them even further.

The "pattern of interaction" refers to the often frustrating and destructive communication that ensues when a distressed couple enters into a theme-related conflict. A natural response for partners confronted with their differences is for each partner to try to change the other. In many cases these efforts at changing each other may be successful. However, many times the result may be that their differences are exacerbated and the two partners become polarized in their conflicting positions. When partners have become polarized on an issue, further attempts to change each other only increase the conflict and perpetuate their polarized stance. For example, in a couple whose theme is closeness–independence, the polarization process is likely to occur when the independence seeker "retreats" from attempts by the closeness seeker to gain more intimacy, which then creates more "intrusive" efforts by the closeness seeker. The more the one partner "advances," the more the other partner "retreats"; the more that partner "retreats," the more the other partner "advances." Furthermore, being deprived of a desired goal can make that goal seem even more important: Partners can become desperate, escalating their futile efforts, and their differences become magnified. It can begin to look like the closeness seeker has no needs for independence and the independence seeker has no needs for closeness. Through their interaction, they have become more different than they were originally.

The Mutual Trap

The mutual trap, which describes the outcome of the polarization process, is called a "trap" because it typically leaves the partners feeling "stuck" or "trapped" in their conflict. Partners in a mutual trap feel that they have done everything they can to change the other, and nothing seems to work. But they are reluctant to give up their efforts to change each other because this would mean resigning themselves to a dissatisfying relationship. As a result, they become more entrenched in their respective positions.

The experience of partners who are so polarized is one of helplessness and futility, and this experience is rarely discussed openly between them. As a result, each partner may be unaware that the other also feels trapped. Making each partner aware of the other's sense of entrapment is an important part of acceptance work, and encouraging each partner to experience the other's sense of "stuckness" can sometimes be the first step toward promoting empathy and intimacy between partners.

Stages of Therapy

In IBCT there is a clear distinction between the assessment phase and the treatment itself. The *assessment* phase comprises at least one conjoint session with the couple, followed by individual sessions with each partner. It is followed by a feedback session, during which the therapist describes his/her *formulation* of the partners and their problems as well as the therapist's plan for their treatment. The feedback session is followed by the *treatment* sessions, the exact number of which should be determined on a case-by-case basis depending on each couple's treatment needs. However, the protocol used in a recent clinical trial of IBCT for seriously and chronically distressed couples (discussed below) was a maximum of 26 sessions, including both the assessment and treatment phases.

The Use of Objective Measures

Objective assessment instruments (see Table 18.1) may be useful for both initial assessment and for monitoring a couple's progress at various points throughout treatment. Although such objective measures are not necessary to conduct IBCT, they may provide additional information about areas of disagreement that have not been covered in the session, or they may provide objective data about a couple's levels of distress and satisfaction. Additionally, research has shown that sharing and actively discussing a couple's progress (or lack thereof) in therapy can improve therapy outcomes (e.g., Halford et al., 2012). For example, a couple's relationship satisfaction can be assessed using the Couples Satisfaction Index (Funk & Rogge, 2007); partners' commitment to the relationship and steps taken toward separation or divorce can be assessed using the Marital Status Inventory (Crane & Mead, 1980; Weiss & Cerreto, 1980); partner's areas of conflict and troubling behaviors can be assessed with the Problem Areas Questionnaire (Heavey, Christensen, & Malamuth, 1995) and the Frequency and Acceptability of Partner Behavior Inventory (Christensen & Jacobson, 1997; Doss & Christensen, 2006), and the couple's level of physical violence, with the Revised Conflict Tactics Scales (CTS2; Straus, Hamby, Boney-McCoy, & Sugarman, 1996).

TABLE 18.1. Useful Assessment and Screening Instruments

- Couples Satisfaction Index (Funk & Rogge, 2007): Measures relationship distress. (To obtain this freely available measure, go to *www.courses.rochester.edu/surveys/funk.*)

- Couple Questionnaire (Christensen, 2009): Brief screening assessment for couple satisfaction, intimate partner violence, and commitment, as well as open-ended descriptions of typical positive and negative interactions. (To obtain this freely available measure, go to *http://ibct.psych.ucla.edu.*)

- Frequency and Acceptability of Partner Behavior Inventory (Christensen & Jacobson, 1997; Doss & Christensen, 2006): Assesses frequency and acceptability of behavior for 24 categories of spouse behavior. (To obtain this freely available measure, go to *http://ibct.psych.ucla.edu.*)

- Marital Status Inventory (Crane & Mead, 1980; Weiss & Cerreto, 1980): Assesses commitment to the relationship and steps taken toward separation or divorce. (To obtain this measure, contact Robert L. Weiss, PhD, Oregon Marital Studies Program, Department of Psychology, University of Oregon, Eugene, OR 97403-1227; *darkwing.uoregon.edu/~rlweiss/msi.htm.*)

- Problem Areas Questionnaire (Heavey, Christensen, & Malamuth, 1995): Assesses common problem areas or areas of disagreement in couples. (To obtain this freely available measure, go to *http://ibct.psych.ucla.edu.*)

- Revised Conflict Tactics Scales (Straus, Hamby, Boney-McCoy, & Sugarman, 1996): Assesses domestic violence. (To obtain this measure, contact Multi-Health Systems, P.O. Box 950, North Tonawanda, NY 14120; *www.mhs.com.*)

- Weekly Questionnaire (Christensen, 2010): Assesses significant positive and negative events since the last session and includes a brief form of the Couples Satisfaction Index. (To obtain this freely available measure, go to *http://ibct.psych.ucla.edu.*)

We recommend that, at a minimum, clinicians administer measures that assess relationship satisfaction, intimate partner violence, commitment, and problem areas. The measure of relationship satisfaction serves as a measure of outcome and should be repeated periodically. Measures of violence, commitment, and problem areas are needed because partners may indicate concerns on a questionnaire that they do not bring up spontaneously. For example, couples often do not mention topics such as violence or sexual problems during therapy, even when these are present. Christensen

(2010) has developed a brief Couple Questionnaire (Christensen, 2010) that clinicians can use to assess baseline satisfaction, violence, and commitment. Typically, partners are given questionnaires at their first session to complete then return at their individual sessions. In addition to being part of the assessment phase, the questionnaires can be administered later in treatment, at the end of treatment, and at follow-up to assess changes from partners' presenting baseline levels of distress and satisfaction.

Assessment of Domestic Violence

Objective measures are particularly useful in assessing a couple's history of physical violence. Assessing for domestic violence is a critical part of every couple's intake—not only to determine whether the personal safety of either partner is in imminent danger but also because couple therapy may actually be *contraindicated* for some violent couples (Jacobson & Gottman, 1998; Simpson, Doss, Wheeler, & Christensen, 2007). Couple therapy requires that both partners take some degree of responsibility for their problems, but such a perspective is inappropriate when a couple's problems include domestic violence because perpetrators of violence must assume sole responsibility for their behavior. Furthermore, because therapy sessions can elicit strong emotions, the couple therapy itself may trigger postsession violence in some couples. In such cases, treatment that focuses on the violent behavior of the perpetrator—and not the interactive distress of the couple—is indicated. The CTS2 (Straus et al., 1996) and the Couple Questionnaire (Christensen, 2010) are useful screening tools for evaluating the frequency and severity of a couple's physical aggression, and to determine whether couple therapy is contraindicated. Finally, a couple's history of violence should be directly addressed during the assessment phase, primarily during the individual sessions, when each partner can talk freely without fearing consequences from the other.

Assessment

The *assessment* phase typically comprises one joint session with the partners (Session 1), followed by individual sessions with each partner (Sessions 2 and 3). The primary goal of the assessment phase is for the therapist to evaluate whether the couple is appropriate for therapy and, if so, to develop the *formulation*. However, the therapist should also use the assessment period to orient the couple to the therapy process. In addition, although the IBCT therapist is not actively intervening during the assessment phase, it is possible for the therapist to have a therapeutic impact in these first few sessions.

Orientation (Session 1)

After greetings and introductions, the couple is oriented to the upcoming therapy process. This orientation likely includes reviewing and signing an informed consent form, which explains billing procedures, defines confidentiality and its exclusions, and outlines the possible risks and benefits of participating in IBCT.

In addition to the general information provided during informed consent, the couple is also oriented to the specific process of IBCT. Therapists should explain the difference between the assessment and treatment phases of therapy, and ask the couple whether this is different from the couple's expectations in coming to therapy. Therapists should be prepared for couples' disappointment when they learn that therapy is not going to begin immediately. Therapists may need to explain to couples why an assessment period is needed before therapists can provide any useful help to them.

Also during the first session, couples are introduced to their manual, *Reconcilable Differences* (Christensen, Doss, & Jacobson, 2014; Christensen & Jacobson, 2000). Couples are asked to complete Part I of this book prior to the feedback session. Ideally, this reading helps couples begin to conceptualize their problems in a way that is similar to how their therapist will frame them during the feedback session.

Therapists should be aware that at least one partner, if not both, may likely be ambivalent about participating in therapy. Such ambivalence should be normalized and validated, and the therapist should explain to partners that the assessment period is also *their* opportunity to get to know the therapist and to determine whether this treatment is going to be a "good match" for them.

Problem Areas (Sessions 1, 2, and 3)

After the couple has been oriented to the therapy process, the therapist begins the evaluation by reviewing the couple's presenting problem(s). Much of this information can be gathered from objective measures and also during each partner's individual session, so this discussion during Session 1 should not consume the entire session. However, it is important during the first session that the partners feel heard and validated, and that their problems and distress are clearly understood by the therapist.

From the information gathered from objective measures and during the evaluation sessions, therapists should be able to describe the partners' problem areas and develop their formulation. The following six questions provide a guideline for this assessment, and each should be answered by the end of the assessment period.

1. How distressed is the couple?
2. How committed is this couple to the relationship?
3. What issues divide this couple?
4. Why are these issues a problem for them (the DEEP analysis)?
5. What strengths keep this couple together?
6. What can treatment do to help them?

The first three questions can be addressed with objective questionnaires. However, even questions that can be addressed with questionnaires should usually be explored in further detail in interviews. For example, the individual sessions may be particularly useful for assessing whether distress is so great that separation is imminent, for assessing each partner's level of commitment to the relationship and the possible presence of affairs, and for assessing the couple's history of physical violence.

The assessment of problem areas should also include a determination of the couple's "collaborative set" (Jacobson & Margolin, 1979). This term refers to the couple's joint perspective that they *share* responsibility for the problems in their relationship, and that *both* will have to change if the relationship is to change. The strength of this set determines whether change- or acceptance-oriented interventions are indicated. The stronger the couple's collaborative set, the more successful initial change-oriented interventions are likely to be. But partners who lack this collaborative set—who enter therapy believing they are the innocent victim of the other's behavior—first need to focus on acceptance work.

The fourth question—why the partners' issues are a problem for them—requires a functional analysis along the lines of the DEEP analysis described earlier. It is usually possible to obtain initial information about all four aspects of the DEEP analysis in the joint interview, but more nuanced understandings about these factors, particularly Emotional sensitivities and Patterns of interaction, are typically best left to the individual interviews. Because adults are often unaware of the contingencies controlling their behavior, or may be embarrassed to admit those contingencies even if they know them, a functional analysis of emotions and patterns involves much more than a simple, straightforward inquiry. The therapist must be particularly sensitive to the emotional reactions of partners, which may indicate important reinforcers and punishers. For example, let us assume that our partners with the closeness–independence theme argue frequently about the amount of time they spend together. However, that specific issue may not be where the most powerful contingencies are found. Perhaps the wife's history includes having been abandoned by her family members at a time when she was in particular need of their support and comfort. Her fear in her marital relationship is that her husband may do likewise. For her, the time they spend together is simply a poor proxy for her concerns that he may not always be there when she needs him. If she felt confident of that, then she could tolerate much less time together. For her husband's part, let us assume that his social learning history has led him to be especially sensitive to being controlled or restricted by another person. Therefore, he battles his wife over their time together not so much because he does not want the time together, but because he feels controlled by her and naturally resists. In such a situation, the IBCT therapist needs to move the discussion away from the repetitive arguments about time spent together, toward the more important contingencies that affect each spouse's behaviors, for example, the emotional sensitivities that each partner brings to the relationship and the pattern of interaction that triggers their emotional responses.

Answers to the fifth question, about the couple's strengths, also come from the joint and individual interviews. It is helpful for couples to keep their strengths in mind even as they focus on their difficulties. Sometimes there is an interesting relation between a couple's strengths and its problems, in that the latter may involve some variation of the former. For example, let us assume that two partners were initially attracted to each other in part because of their different approaches to life. He is much more spontaneous; she is more deliberate and planful. Those differences may be attractive and helpful at times, but they can also be a source of irritation and conflict.

In answering the final question, what treatment can do to help, the therapist must first be sure the couple is appropriate for couple therapy. If the couple has serious violence or a substance dependence problem, for example, then couple therapy as usual will not be the recommendation. Treatment directed at those particular problems will be necessary. If the couple is appropriate for couple therapy, the therapist will need to outline the focus of the therapy and what it comprises.

The Couple's History (Session 1)

After the partners have been oriented to therapy and their problem areas have been assessed, the therapist then takes the history of the couple's relationship. The therapist's obvious objective for taking this history is to gain a good understanding of the partners' attachment to one another. Often the distress has escalated to the degree that it has overshadowed the reasons the two became a couple in the first place. In addition, this history can provide some immediate therapeutic benefit to the couple. Generally, when partners discuss the earlier (and usually happier) stages of their relationship, their affect is likely to become more positive. They have been focused for so long on the negative aspects of their relationship that they probably have not thought about their early romance, courtship, and attraction to each other for a very long time. In this way, having couples describe the evolution of their relationship can be therapeutic in and of itself. Although some couples may be in too much pain to discuss their history without blaming and accusatory remarks (in which case the therapist should abandon the following guidelines and instead use the session to validate their pain), most couples enjoy reminiscing about their happier times.

The following series of questions provides the therapist with useful information about the couple's history and allow the partners an opportunity to reflect on the reasons they fell in love in the first place:

- "How did you get together?"
- "What was your courtship like?"
- "What attracted each of you to the other?"
- "What was your relationship like before your problems began?"
- "How is your relationship different *now* on days when you are getting along?"
- "How would the relationship be different if your current problems no longer existed?

These and other, related questions may also reveal useful information about each partner, such as his/her hopes and dreams for the future. Information about the couple's history is useful for the therapist in developing the couple's formulation, which is presented to the partners during their feedback session.

Individual History (Sessions 2 and 3)

Each partner's individual history can often provide useful information for the formulation, in that it provides a context for each partner's behavior and illuminates possible emotional vulnerabilities in each. For example, perhaps the husband experienced his mother as very demanding of him and learned to cope with this through withdrawal, so the withdrawal continues in response to his wife's demands. Or perhaps the wife had two previous boyfriends who cheated on her, so she is sensitive to any indication of betrayal by her husband.

The following questions may be useful in guiding a discussion of each partner's individual history:

- "What was your parents' marriage like?"
- "What was your relationship with your father like?"
- "What was your relationship with your mother like?"
- "What were your relationships with your siblings like?"
- "What were your relationships with previous important romantic partners like?"

Each of these questions could potentially take an inordinate amount of time. The IBCT therapist tries to elicit features of these early relationships that are similar to or may inform the current relationship. For example, if the therapist were aware of a difference between husband and wife in terms of how comfortable they were with conflict, he/she would guide the husband away from details about where his family lived and focus on the expression of conflict that occurred in his family.

Feedback

From the information gathered during the assessment sessions and from the questionnaires, the therapist develops the couple's formulation, which is discussed with the couple in the feedback session (usually Session 4). The feedback session can follow the outline of the six questions above used to assess the couple's problem areas. It is important that the feedback session be a dialogue and not a lecture from the therapist—with the therapist continually getting feedback from the couple about the formulation being presented. The partners are the experts on their relationship and should be treated as such.

The feedback session is also used to describe the proposed treatment plan for the couples, based on the therapist's formulation. The therapist describes for the couple the goals for treatment and the procedures for accomplishing these goals. The goals for therapy are to create an in-session environment in which the couple's problems can be resolved through some combination of acceptance and change techniques. In relation to the DEEP analysis, IBCT promotes emotional acceptance for the partners' Differences and Emotional Sensitivities, in that these factors are likely to change only slowly, if at all. External stressors can sometimes be changed but often they too require acceptance. It is the Pattern of interaction that can be changed and is the focus of change efforts in IBCT. The procedures for meeting these goals of acceptance and change are usually (1) in-session discussions of incidents and issues related to the formulation, and (2) homework to be conducted outside the session to further the in-session work. During the feedback session, the therapist introduces the couple to the Weekly Questionnaire (Christensen, 2010), goes over it, and asks that each partner to complete it prior to each session. It provides information on the couple's experiences since the last session and serves as the basis for treatment sessions. This questionnaire includes the four-item version of the Couples Satisfaction Index (Funk & Rogge, 2007), so therapists can monitor the couple's relationship satisfaction on a weekly basis. The questionnaire asks whether there have been any major changes in the couple's life, and whether any incidents of violence, or any problematic incidents of substance/drug use have occurred. Then the questionnaire asks each partner to describe the most positive or meaningful interaction they had in the last week, the most difficult or negative interaction in the last week, and whether they anticipate any upcoming, challenging events. Finally, the partners rank what they think would be most important to discuss: the positive, negative, or upcoming event, or some issue not tied to a particular incident (e.g., saving money). Finally there is a place for the couple's homework assignment, if there is any. These positive, negative, and challenging upcoming events, as well as the general issues the partners indicate on their questionnaires, provide the usual content for the therapy sessions.

The purpose of the feedback session is to orient partners to the goals of change and acceptance through open communication and finding new ways of looking at their problems. In addition, the feedback session gives partners some idea of what they can expect from therapy, and it elicits their willingness to participate. Finally, the feedback session may be used to implement some interventions. The first intervention is the therapist's description of the couple's strengths. From this discussion, partners may be able to see some solutions to their problems. The therapist can begin assigning relevant chapters from Part II of *Reconcilable Differences* (Christensen & Jacobson, 2000; Christensen et al., 2014), which specifically addresses the topic of acceptance. After the formulation and treatment plan have been described and the partners have agreed to proceed with therapy, the remaining sessions are devoted to building acceptance between partners and promoting change in each partner.

Treatment

IBCT Techniques for Building Emotional Acceptance

Typically, treatment begins with a focus on promoting acceptance. The exception is when partners are able to collaborate with one another ("the collaborative set") and both want to make specific changes in their relationship. In that case, the therapist begins with change strategies.

In the context of acceptance work, the actual content of each session is determined by the partners and what they "bring in" every week. The therapist looks for emotionally salient material that is relevant to the formulation. Recent negative or positive events listed on the Weekly Questionnaire and related to the formulation are often the topics of discussion. For example, a couple with a closeness–independence theme might discuss a difficult incident in which the independence seeker wanted to spend the night out with friends and the closeness seeker protested. Discussions also may be centered around upcoming events listed on the Weekly Questionnaire, such as a weekend trip for the couple, in which the independence seeker fears that there will not be space for him/her to be alone. Broad issues related to the formulation and listed on the questionnaire are also appropriate for discussion, such as whether separate weekend trips apart with friends are acceptable for the couple.

Sometimes salient events relevant to the formulation occur between partners during the session, and the therapist should generally make these the top priority because the emotions involving events during sessions tend to be more accessible than events that occur between sessions. For example, when the independence seeker turns away as the closeness seeker gets emotionally agitated during a discussion, the IBCT therapist focuses on this "in the moment" example of their closeness–independence theme and explores and frames it using the DEEP analysis. The therapist might also structure interactions during the session that mimic their difficulties or create possibilities for a different kind of interaction. For example, the therapist may have the couple replay a recent, difficult interaction to learn from it, or encourage the couple to attempt a different and more positive interaction around the topic. All of these topics are useful means for implementing the three acceptance-building strategies of *empathic joining, unified detachment from the problem,* and *tolerance building.* Because they can create greater closeness, as well as greater acceptance, the first two strategies are more commonly employed than the last one.

EMPATHIC JOINING

"Empathic joining" refers to the process by which partners cease to blame one another for their emotional suffering and instead develop empathy for each other's experience. To foster empathic joining, the IBCT therapist reformulates the couple's problem as a result of common differences rather than deficiencies in either partner, and highlights the emotional sensitivities that make these differences especially difficult to handle. Partners' behaviors are described in terms of their differences from one another, and their responses to these differences are validated as normal and understandable, especially given the emotional sensitivities that each may possess.

In making this reformulation of each partner's behavior, it is important that the IBCT therapist emphasize the pain that each partner is experiencing rather than the pain each has delivered. One strategy for building empathy between partners is through the use of "soft disclosures." Often partners express their emotional pain by using "hard" disclosures of feelings such as anger or disgust. Although hard disclosures are easier to make because they do not reveal vulnerability, they are more difficult for the other partner to hear because they imply blame. It is the combination of "pain and blame" that results in discord. But if the therapist can encourage partners to express their pain *without* expressing blame, the result may be increased acceptance from the other partner. IBCT therapists often encourage soft disclosures by suggesting "soft" feelings, such as the fear, hurt, and shame that may underlie each partner's behavior. Although soft disclosures are more difficult to make because they reveal vulnerability, they are easier for the other partner to hear and arouse more empathy. Thus, empathic joining is promoted by (1) *reformulation* of a couple's discord as a result of partners' common *differences* and their understandable emotional reactions to those differences, and (2) the use of *soft disclosures* to express painful emotions. These disclosures can come through interaction between the therapist and each partner or the therapist can prompt the partners to make these disclosures directly to each other, increasing the emotional intensity of the disclosure and allowing the partners to have the conversation they did not have but could have had (Wile, 2008).

UNIFIED DETACHMENT FROM THE PROBLEM

This IBCT technique allows partners to "step back" from their problems and describe them without placing blame—or responsibility for change—on either partner. In this way, partners engage in "unified detachment" from their problems. This strategy can be used to engage a couple in a DEEP discussion about their Differences (how these differences resulted from their backgrounds), their Emotional sensitivities (what past experiences may have understandably led to these sensitivities), their External stressors (how these stressors came to be), and their Patterns of interaction (how each interacts in ways that make sense from his/her perspective). However, most often it is used to help the couple understand, accept, and eventually alter their Patterns of interaction. For example, the therapist may engage partners in a dialogue in which they use nonjudgmental terms to describe the sequence of a particular conflict, including what factors typically trigger their reactions, how specific events are connected to one another, and how they can defuse or override the conflict in the future. The approach is an intellectual analysis of the problem that is described in an emotionally detached manner as a third-party "it" rather than in terms of "you" or "me." When possible, the therapist should give the couple's theme, pattern of interaction, or mutual trap a name, and use this to define the problem further as an "it." By detaching themselves from the problem, partners have an opportunity to discuss their conflict without becoming emotionally "charged" by it. In this way, they can try to understand the conflict from a more neutral, objective stance. They engage in a kind of joint mindfulness about their problem. The therapist can also use metaphor and humor to distance the couple emotionally from the problem, as long as the humor does not in any way belittle either partner.

TOLERANCE BUILDING

Building acceptance may be most challenging when one partner experiences intense emotional pain as a result of the other partner's behavior. In these circumstances, the IBCT therapist must help one partner build tolerance for the other partner's "offending" behavior. By building tolerance, the partner ideally experiences a reduction in the pain caused by the behavior. To build tolerance, however, the partner must cease efforts to prevent, avoid, or escape the "offending" partner's behavior. Instead, by exposing him/herself to the behavior without the associated struggle, the partner reduces his/her sensitivity to the behavior and, ideally, experiences the "offending" behavior as less painful.

One strategy for building tolerance is through "positive reemphasis," or focusing on the *positive aspects of a partner's negative behavior*. This strategy may be relatively easy when a negative behavior is in some way related to a quality the partner once found attractive about the other. For example, what she sees as her partner's "uptightness" might be the "stability" that first attracted her. Alternatively, what he sees as her "flakiness" or "irresponsibility" might be the "free-spiritedness" or "rebelliousness" that so attracted him in the beginning of their relationship. The positive reemphasis does not deny the negative qualities of the behavior in question, but it helps partners gain the perspective that any quality often has both good and bad features.

Another strategy for building tolerance for differences is to focus on the *ways these differences complement each other*, and to present these differences as part of what makes the relationship "work." One partner's stability might balance the other's free-spiritedness. The therapist might describe for the partners the ways they would be "worse off" if those differences did not exist. The differences can become a positive aspect of the relationship, something in which the partners take pride rather than something they see as a destructive threat.

A third technique for building tolerance to a partner's behavior is to *prepare couples for inevitable slip-ups and lapses* in behavior. This is especially important when the partners first begin to detect changes in their behavior and begin to feel positive about the progress they are making in therapy. It is during this time that the therapist should congratulate them for their hard work and progress, then warn them that "backsliding" is still a likely occurrence. The partners should be asked to imagine some of the circumstances in which a slipup is likely to occur, and to consider possible responses to the slipup in advance. Working out how they will face such lapses helps partners build their tolerance for them.

A related strategy for building tolerance is to instruct couples *to fake negative behavior* while they are in session or at home. Each partner is instructed to engage in a designated "bad behavior"—with the stipulation that he/she is to engage in this behavior only when he/she does not feel like doing so. The instructions are given to the couple, so that each partner knows that a bad behavior he/she is about to witness in session or may see in the future might actually be faked. Ideally this introduces an ambiguity about future negative behaviors that may mitigate the partner's emotional response to them. More importantly, however, is that faking behavior gives both partners an opportunity to observe the effects of their negative behavior on the other. Specifically, because they are performing the "bad behavior" during a time when they do not feel like it, they make these observations when they are in a calm emotional state that allows them to be more sympathetic. When done in session, the therapist can help debrief the reactions to the "bad" behavior. When done at home, the faker is instructed to let the other partner know about the faked behavior soon after is it performed, so the situation does not escalate and the partners have an opportunity to "debrief" following their "experiment."

One unavoidable source of pain for many partners is the feeling that the other fails to meet their needs in some important way. However, rarely is a partner able to fulfill all of the needs of the other. An important aspect of acceptance building is for partners to increase their own self-reliance, or *self-care*, in getting their needs met. They should be encouraged to find alternative ways to care for themselves when their partners are not able to do so. Partners may need to learn to seek support from friends and family in times of stress, or to find new ways to define and solve a problem on their own. As their self-reliance increases, reliance on partners to meet all of their emotional needs decreases. Ideally, this results in decreased sensitivity to their partners' failure to meet their needs, thereby reducing conflict.

Traditional Strategies for Promoting Change

For some couples, change interventions may be indicated. Whether an IBCT therapist begins by implementing "acceptance" rather than "change" techniques depends primarily on the couple's collaborative set and the partners' specific treatment needs. In general, however, change techniques are most effective if implemented later in therapy, after acceptance work has been done. Often acceptance work is sufficient for bringing about change by itself: Once the collaborative set is restored through acceptance, the couple is able to bring about change by applying skills and strategies they already possess. In these situations, no deliberate change strategies need to be employed.

BEHAVIOR EXCHANGE

The primary goal of behavior exchange (BE) is to increase the proportion of a couple's daily positive behaviors and interactions. These techniques are instigative, in that they are intended to increase each partner's performance of positive behaviors. Because BE requires a great deal of collaboration between partners, it is best implemented later in therapy, after acceptance work has been done. In addition to using BE to increase a couple's positive interactions, the IBCT therapist should also consider BE a diagnostic tool for assessing possible areas in need of more acceptance work.

The three basic steps in BE are (1) to identify behaviors that each partner can do for the other that would increase relationship satisfaction, (2) to increase the frequency of those behaviors in the couple's daily behavioral repertoire, and (3) to debrief the experience of providing and receiving positive behaviors. Partners are often given a homework assignment to generate a list of actions to do for the other to increase his/her satisfaction. Partners are instructed not to discuss these lists with each other to reduce the threat of criticism from the other and to keep each partner focused on his/her own assignment. In the next session, partners' lists are reviewed and discussed. Their next assignment might be to perform one or more of the actions on the list during the next week, but they are not to tell the partner which action they are performing. In the subsequent therapy session, partners review the success of their assignment and whether it had the desired effect on the other. The list can be modified to eliminate items that do not seem to have an effect, and in later sessions each partner can elicit feedback from the other to optimize the benefit of the actions on the list.

COMMUNICATION TRAINING

Although many couples are effective communicators without having had any formal "training," poor communication may exacerbate or even cause many problems for distressed couples. In their attempts to get the other to change, partners may resort to maladaptive communication tactics such as coercion (crying, threatening, withholding affection). Although coercion may be effective in the short term, in that the other may eventually comply with the demand, the use of coercion is likely to escalate such that increasingly coercive tactics are required to achieve the desired effect. Also, coercion tends to beget coercion, so that coercion by one partner leads to coercion by the other. The inevitable result of such interactions is that partners become extremely polarized. The goal of communication and problem-solving training is to teach couples how to discuss their problems and to negotiate change without resorting to such destructive tactics. Ideally, these skills will be useful to couples even after therapy has ended.

As part of communication training, couples are taught both "speaker" and "listener" skills. To become more effective "speakers," couples are instructed to (1) focus on the self by expressing "I statements"; (2) focus on expressing emotional reactions, such as "I feel disappointed . . . " or "I feel angry . . . "; and (3) focus on the partner's specific behaviors that lead to emotional reactions, such as "I feel disappointed when you don't call me when you are away." To become more effective listeners, partners are instructed to paraphrase and reflect what the other has just said. Paraphrasing ensures that neither partner is being misread during the conversation, and it decreases the tendency to jump to conclusions about what is being said, in addition to generally slowing down the interaction.

Once partners have been given some instruction in these communication skills, they are directed to use these skills in practice conversations in the therapy session. Communicating with these guidelines may feel awkward during practice conversations, so therapists should try to adapt the guidelines to the couple's style of conversation and explain that following the guidelines will feel more natural with increased use. The therapist should be prepared to interrupt and make corrections if the partners deviate from the guidelines and engage in destructive communication. The therapist should provide the couple with feedback after each practice session, and the exercise should be adequately debriefed. When the therapist is confident that the partners have improved their in-session communication skills, he/she then encourages them to practice these skills as homework.

These basic communication skills often enable partners to share their feelings with one another and to discuss difficult issues that arise, such as when one partner gets upset with the other's action. However, sometimes partners need to do more than share feelings or debrief an event. They need to solve an upcoming or recurrent problem, which is the purpose of problem-solving communication skills.

PROBLEM-SOLVING TRAINING

Often what is more damaging in partners' struggles around daily problems than the problems themselves is their destructive attempts to solve them. These attempts may begin with an accusation by one partner, which is met by defensiveness and anger from the other. Soon the argument may escalate to counterblaming and character assassination—and the problem itself gets lost in the conflict around it. In problem-solving training, couples are taught to have constructive problem-solving discussions while employing three sets of skills: problem definition skills, problem solution skills, and structuring skills.

First, partners are taught to *define* the problem as specifically as possible by specifying the behavior of concern and the circumstances surrounding it. Partners are encouraged to describe some of the emotions they experience as a result of the problem, in an effort to increase emotional acceptance. Finally, both partners are asked to define their respective roles in perpetuating the problem.

Once the problem has been defined, the couple can begin working toward problem *solution*. The first step in problem solution is brainstorming, in which the couple tries to come up with as many solutions to the problem as possible. The couple is told that any and all solutions may be considered, even impossible or silly ones. Immediate evaluative comments about the brainstormed solutions are discouraged, and discussions of which options are actually viable are held off for later. Suggestions are written down so that they can be reviewed later. This exercise can be lighthearted and playful, often generating positive affect during the session. After the list has been generated, the couple goes through the list, eliminating those suggestions that are obviously impossible, silly, or unlikely to be effective. After the list is pruned, each item is considered for its potential to solve the problem. For each item, the couple considers the pros and cons, and the list is further modified, until a final list of options has been generated. The remaining items are used to formulate a possible solution to the problem. The agreement that is made about this solution is written down and sometimes signed by each partner. Finally, the couple is asked to consider any obstacles to executing the agreement, and to work out strategies for combating these. The partners are told to post the agreement in a place where they both can see it often, and a date is set to review their progress in solving the problem. During the next few sessions, the therapist checks in with them on their progress, and the agreement may be renegotiated, if necessary.

Finally, the partners learn *structuring skills* for their problem-solving discussions. They structure these discussions by setting aside a specific time and place to have them. They are also instructed not to discuss the problem at the "scene of the crime," that is, to hold off discussing a problem until the designated time. Finally, the couple is instructed to focus on only one problem at a time. Throughout their problem-solving discussions, partners are asked to follow the basic guidelines of paraphrasing each other's statements, and to avoid both negative inferences about each other's intent, and negative verbal and nonverbal communication.

The couple's first attempts at using these problem-solving skills should occur in session, under the supervision of the therapist. But after the partners have practiced and received feedback about their problem-solving skills, they are encouraged to apply these techniques at home to help them discuss and negotiate their problems.

In implementing these behavior change skills, the IBCT therapist tries to adapt them to the particular needs of the couple. For example, if a couple finds it helpful to go back and forth between definition and solution while discussing a problem, the therapist would eliminate the guideline specifying that the problem be carefully defined before solutions are considered. Or if a couple finds it distracting to generate silly or impossible solutions, the therapist would not encourage that.

The therapist also tries to adapt these strategies to the formulation for the couple. For example, if the closeness seeker tends to dominate discussions and make proposals for solving a problem about time together, while the independence seeker tends to withdraw from the discussion, the therapist might shift the focus on problem solving to the independence seeker.

Therapist and Client Variables Relevant to IBCT

As in any therapy, it is important that IBCT therapists maintain a nonjudgmental stance toward their clients. But in the context of IBCT, it is particularly important that the therapist practice acceptance with both partners in the same way that partners are asked to practice acceptance with one another. The IBCT therapist must validate the experiences and responses of both partners, and find ways to develop empathy and compassion for them no matter how challenging this may be.

In addition to practicing acceptance, it is important that IBCT therapists listen carefully to couples' in-session interactions and look for the functions of their various problematic behaviors. IBCT therapists must be particularly attentive to subtle verbal and nonverbal cues that may be relevant to the formulation of couples' problems. IBCT therapists must also be prepared to abandon any prescribed agenda to address the immediate needs of the couple at any given time. When destructive interactions occur in session, the IBCT therapist must not only be able to maintain a nonconfrontational demeanor but also stop the interaction effectively. Other important IBCT skills include using couples' language and jargon when making interventions. Finally, it is not a goal of IBCT therapists to "cheerlead" for the success of the relationship; rather, they create an environment in which couples can experience the hope of finding a different way of being, and safely discuss and evaluate their own relationships.

The Efficacy of IBCT

Three studies attest to the efficacy of IBCT—two small pilot investigations and one major outcome study. Wimberly (1998) randomly assigned eight couples to a group format of IBCT and nine couples to a waiting-list control group, and found superior results for the IBCT couples. Jacobson, Christensen, Prince, Cordova, and Eldridge (2000) randomly assigned 21 couples to either IBCT or TBCT. At the end of treatment, 80% of couples who had received IBCT showed clinically significant improvements in relationship satisfaction compared to 64% of couples who received TBCT.

To date, the largest study of couple therapy in general and of IBCT in particular was reported by Christensen and colleagues (2004). In a two-site clinical trial conducted at UCLA and the University of Washington, Christensen and colleagues randomly assigned 134 seriously and chronically distressed couples to either IBCT or TBCT. Couples received a maximum of 26 sessions of couple therapy delivered by professional PhD-level therapists, who provided both IBCT and TBCT treatments and were carefully supervised in both. Adherence and competence data provided evidence that treatments were delivered as expected. At termination, 70% of IBCT couples and 61% of TBCT couples had clinically significant improvements in relationship satisfaction. Pre- to posttreatment effect sizes on marital satisfaction were $d = 0.90$ for IBCT and $d = 0.71$ for TBCT (see Christensen, Atkins, Baucom, & Yi, 2010) Although the termination results were not significantly different, the trajectory of change was different for both IBCT and TBCT couples. IBCT couples improved steadily in satisfaction throughout treatment, but TBCT couples improved more rapidly early on in treatment, with their gains flattening out more than those of IBCT couples later in treatment.

Atkins and colleagues (2005) examined the predictors of response to treatment in the previous study. A variety of interpersonal variables, such as quality of communication, predicted the initial status of couples, but precious few variables predicted change from intake to termination. Couples who were married longer showed greater improvements in satisfaction, and exploratory analyses indicated that sexually dissatisfied couples showed slower initial gains but overall more consistent gains in IBCT than in TBCT.

Doss, Thum, Sevier, Atkins, and Christensen (2005) analyzed the mechanisms of change in this study of couple therapy. Early in therapy, changes in the frequency of targeted behaviors were associated with increases in satisfaction for both treatment conditions. However, later in therapy, changes in the acceptance of targeted behaviors were associated with increases in satisfaction for both treatment conditions. TBCT generated significantly greater increases than IBCT in targeted behaviors early in treatment. However, IBCT generated significantly greater increases in the acceptance of targeted behaviors throughout treatment. Thus, the study validated some of the putative mechanisms of change

and differences between the treatments in their impact on these mechanisms.

Subsequently, studies have examined these couples over follow-up: Christensen, Atkins, Yi, Baucom, and George (2006) looked at relationship satisfaction data in couples every 6 months over a 2-year follow-up; Baucom, Sevier, Eldridge, Doss, and Christensen (2011) looked at observational data at 2-year follow-up; and Christensen and colleagues (2010) examined relationship satisfaction and relationship status approximately every 6 months over a 5-year follow-up. Couples generally maintained their treatment gains in satisfaction over 2 years, and IBCT couples had significantly superior relationship satisfaction compared to TBCT couples at each time point during the first 2 years of follow-up. Although TBCT couples, having been trained explicitly in communication, showed greater improvements in observed communication at termination than IBCT couples (Sevier, Eldridge, Jones, Doss, & Christensen, 2008), IBCT couples showed greater maintenance of gains over 2 years (Baucom et al., 2011). Over the subsequent 3 years, couples lost some of their gains, and results from IBCT and TBCT converged. At 5-year follow-up, results for marital satisfaction relative to pretreatment revealed effect sizes of $d = 1.03$ for IBCT and $d = 0.92$ for TBCT; 50.0% of IBCT couples and 45.9% of TBCT couples showed clinically significant improvement. Relationship status, obtained on all 134 couples, revealed that 25.7% of IBCT couples and 27.9% of TBCT couples were separated or divorced. None of these findings at 5-year follow-up were statistically significant. These follow-up data compared favorably to other, long-term results of couple therapy.

Baucom, Atkins, Simpson, and Christensen (2009) examined predictors of 2-year follow-up. As in the earlier prediction study, there were few predictors of outcome. Perhaps because of greater commitment, length of marriage predicted better outcomes at 2-year follow-up. Two objective predictor variables not used in the earlier prediction study were used here: a measure of arousal obtained from voice recordings during the observational data, and measures of influence tactics obtained through linguistic analysis of transcribed observational data. Using these measures, moderately distressed couples in which the wife had lower levels of arousal during problem-solving discussions and in which hard influence tactics (that give the partner little room to respond) were used less frequently tended to perform better in treatment than moderately distressed couples with higher levels of arousal or those who used more hard influence tactics. Couples in IBCT tended to do better than their counterparts in TBCT when the wife had higher levels of arousal and when couples used soft influence tactics. Clearly these findings need to be replicated, However, it may be that the strategies of IBCT, which emphasize emotional expression, work better than TBCT strategies when there is high emotional arousal and when partners are more open to influence.

It is important to note that this sample, although designed to include seriously and chronically distressed couples, excluded couples in which one or both partners were experiencing bipolar disorder, schizophrenia, or serious suicidality; met criteria for current drug or alcohol abuse or dependence; met criteria for borderline, antisocial, or schizotypal personality disorders; or had a history of severe physical violence. The rationale for these exclusionary criteria is that for such individuals, a primary treatment other than couple therapy is likely to be indicated. However, the sample did *not* exclude couples in which one or both partners suffered from other psychological disorders, such as anxiety or depression. The rationale for including these couples is that their relationship can still be treated despite partners having such individual problems. Furthermore, some of the couples' relationship problems may even be *contributing* to these individual problems. Thus, preliminary data suggest that IBCT can be successfully applied to many couples, including those in which a partner has certain other psychological disorders. For example, the preceding predictor studies found that indices of mental illness, including Structured Clinical Interview for DSM-IV diagnoses, were *not* related to improvements during couple therapy. Furthermore, Atkins, Dimidjian, Bedics, and Christensen (2009) found that depression in this sample improved as relationship satisfaction improved.

Ongoing research with this sample will examine in greater detail the process of couple therapy, potential mechanisms of change as they relate to 5-year outcome, and predictors of 5-year outcome. Apart from research on this particular sample, additional research is being done to expand the reach of IBCT. Brian Doss and Andrew Christensen have adapted IBCT for an online treatment and with support from the National Institute of Child Health and Development are testing the efficacy of this treatment. Also, IBCT has been chosen as one of the evidence-based treatments that the U.S. Veteran's Administration (VA) is implementing nation-

wide. VA therapists throughout the country are being given intensive training that involves several days of workshop followed by 6 months of weekly supervision as therapists see two or more couples using IBCT. A trained IBCT consultant listens to therapists' recorded sessions; therapists must reach proficiency on a rating scale of IBCT criteria in order to complete the training program successfully. Program evaluation data are being collected as part of that work, and initial results suggest positive outcomes for IBCT with this VA population of couples. For additional information on IBCT, including access to online research articles and a national database of therapists trained in the approach, see *ibct.psych.ucla.edu.*

CASE STUDY

We use the case example of Anne and Mark[2] to demonstrate the application of IBCT. We have included excerpts from the assessment and feedback sessions, in addition to treatment sessions selected for their effective use of IBCT acceptance-building interventions.[3]

Anne and Mark were a middle-aged couple married for 10 years at treatment onset. Anne had three children from her previous marriage.

Assessment

Session 1

After greetings and introductions, Anne and Mark's therapist (Dr. S) began Session 1 by orienting them to the assessment process as follows:

"We'll be working together for the next 25 sessions. You have already done the first step of the assessment process by completing all of those questionnaires. Your next three visits, including today, will be the second step of the assessment phase. Today I'm meeting with the two of you to get to know you, to hear about your relationship . . . as you share some of the history about meeting and dating, and bring us up until today. Then over the next two visits, I'd like to meet with the two of you individually. After that, at the fourth visit, I'll give you feedback. That's where I'll put together all of the information from the questionnaires and our time together today, as well as our time individually, to paint a picture to present some understanding of what could be going on."

Particularly if the couple expresses hesitation or ambivalence about being in therapy, the therapist should include the following:

"This assessment period is also your opportunity to get to know me and the kind of therapy we'll be doing, so that you can get a feeling for whether this is going to be a good match for your needs right now."

After checking in with Anne and Mark to see whether they understood this explanation, Dr. S elicited from them a brief description of their presenting problems:

"Before we get into your history, maybe you could give me a sense of some of the problems that have been going on that led you to decide, "Let's get some help.""

After Mark and Anne took turns describing their sides of the problems in the relationship, Dr. S gathered the couple's developmental history, using probing phrases such as the following:

"Let's start at the beginning. Why don't you tell me where and how the two of you met?"

"Mark, what was it about Anne that attracted you initially? What about you, Anne?"

"Anne, how could you tell that Mark was interested in you? . . . What kinds of things did he say? . . . How did you flirt with him? Which one of you made the first move?"

"When you decided to go from living together to getting married, how did that happen?"

In the course of their description, Anne and Mark had many opportunities to say complimentary things about each other. Mark described Anne as sensual, a quality that he found very attractive, and Anne described Mark as very nice and easygoing. Dr. S was very thorough and specific when eliciting details of Mark and Anne's behavior during courtship, such as the fact that both partners agreed that their first kiss was very good.

Even during this part of the assessment phase, opportunities for building acceptance may present themselves. At one point during Session 1, Anne made a soft disclosure when she discussed a time when she had initially rejected Mark (who had asked her to dance). Anne said that when Mark did not get angry with her after she rejected him, she felt safe with him because she could be herself and he would not get mad at her. She reported that this quality about Mark attracted her to him. Mark, who had initially reported feeling humiliated by Anne's rejection, responded to Anne's soft disclosure by saying, "I'm kind of surprised by that. I know that is an important feeling for her, but I didn't realize she was feeling that back then." Anne said that she had not realized she felt that way either, until describing the incident in the therapy session.

By the end of Session 1, Dr. S had a good understanding of Anne and Mark's history together, the qualities that first attracted each to the other, and some idea of their problem areas. The next two individual sessions helped Dr. S "fill-in" any missing information that he needed for their formulation.

Sessions 2 and 3

Dr. S introduced these individual sessions with a brief orientation, followed by an introduction to the ongoing assessment of the couple's problem areas:

"There are a lot of different topics that we'll be covering today as we go along. I'd like to spend some time clarifying some of the problems both you and [Anne/Mark] have had. In our first meeting, you described some problems that you've perceived about [problem area]. Can you tell me what you meant by that?"

In addition to the problems that Anne and Mark raised in their conjoint session, Dr. S used the individual sessions to address problem areas that Anne and Mark had indicated on the Frequency and Acceptability of Partner Behavior Questionnaire:

"When I looked over your list of problem areas, the item of most concern to you was [problem area]. Can you describe that to me?"

Dr. S was very specific in his efforts to get Anne and Mark to describe their disagreements and arguments. To encourage Mark and Anne to be behaviorally specific in these descriptions, Dr. S used probing questions:

"Do the two of you have fights about [problem area]? What do those fights look like?"

"When you are both angry, what do *you* tend to do?"

"Describe for me your most recent argument. Describe for me the worst argument you've ever had. If I had a video camera there with you, what would I have seen?"

In addition to understanding their conflict patterns, Dr. S also asked how problems were addressed in their families growing up ("How did your own parents deal with conflict?"). This information may be useful in understanding the developmental history and emotional vulnerabilities that each partner brings into a conflict, and the patterns that each may risk repeating or is trying to avoid (e.g., physical violence).

When eliciting descriptions of Anne and Mark's arguments, Dr. S also assessed whether the couple had ever engaged in physical violence. This assessment is a critical part of every couple therapy evaluation, and it is a major rationale for conducting these individual interviews. A simple direct question is useful here:

"Have your arguments ever led to pushing, shoving, or any type of physical violence?"

If either partner endorses this question, or has indicated violence on a questionnaire such as the CTS2, a more thorough assessment of violence should be conducted, and appropriate referrals should be made as indicated (Jacobson & Gottman, 1998). In this case example, violence was not an issue for Anne and Mark.[4]

Finally, the individual sessions provide a good opportunity for the therapist to assess each partner's level of commitment to the relationship. This assessment also includes inquiry as to whether one or both partners are engaging in extramarital affairs. Affairs require special treatment in IBCT (Jacobson & Christensen, 1998), which is beyond the scope of this chapter. Fortunately, Anne and Mark's relationship was not troubled by affairs. With Anne and Mark individually, Dr. S asked:

"On a scale of 1 to 10, how would you rate your level of commitment to [Mark/Anne]?"

By the end of Anne's and Mark's respective assessment sessions, Dr. S had sufficient information about their problem areas, patterns of conflict (including their

lack of a history of violence), relevant family history, and level of commitment to come up with their formulation and proceed with their feedback session.

Feedback and Formulation

Session 4

Dr. S began the feedback session by orienting Anne and Mark about what to expect, and also eliciting their participation in giving him feedback about his formulation and description of their problem areas:

"During this session, I'd like to share with you some feedback, as I mentioned in our first session together. I've spent some time looking over your questionnaires, and we've spent some time talking, which has been very helpful in helping me get a better sense of the two of you. As I go along, I'd really like your input, your reactions, because that's an important part of our work together—with you both responding, as opposed to me directing, interjecting any thoughts you have, as well as adding any information that fits or telling me when information doesn't fit."

Dr. S began giving Anne and Mark feedback by explaining the information gathered from questionnaires they completed:

"The measures we gave you were designed to give us a sense of where you are as a couple, in terms of the range of couples, from the very happily married to those with "everyday," normal distress, to the other end of the spectrum—couples who are very similar to ones who have divorced. Both of you are in the area of couples who are experiencing distress, couples who would like things to be better. You are both distressed, although Anne reported higher levels of distress."

Dr. S moved on to summarize Anne's and Mark's levels of commitment, which he characterizes as a strength for their work on therapy:

"With regard to commitment, both of you are committed to the relationship, which is very important to both of you. And that is very important in couple work—that in spite of everything that has gone on, there is still the commitment. That is very telling—you've both shown and expressed that."

Dr. S then moved on to summarize the content of Anne and Mark's problem areas. Dr. S had distilled their questionnaire data and their in-session descriptions to the following three basic problem areas:

"So let's talk about the areas of your relationship that are troubling. One area is finances; that tends to be an area of dispute. For you, Anne, feeling resentful sometimes, feeling the burden of the responsibility, and for you, Mark, feeling guilty about how things are financially. This area really brings out lots of different feelings—feelings of resentment, feelings of guilt, feelings of burden—and rather than feelings of closeness and togetherness, feelings of control. Does that sound accurate? Are there any other aspects of finances that the two of you can think of?

"The other area I saw was with regard to Anne's children. You both feel very differently about the subject of Anne's children: Anne, you feel like Mark is not involved with your children, and Mark, you feel as though you have not been invited. For you, Mark, the experience of being rejected [by the children] is Anne's fault. This is an area that brings out very strong feelings for both of you, whether it gets expressed directly or not. You may not talk about it, but I definitely got the sense that this is a real pressure cooker for both of you. This is an area that I imagine will come up in different ways, especially with the holidays coming up.

"The third area I saw concerns responsiveness. 'How responsive are you to me?' Whether you are being physical ('You're not responsive enough' or 'You're too responsive'), listening ('Are you listening to me?'), touching, or asking a question, your actions can carry a message of what you want to express, or a feeling that you are having. So part of what we will work on is expressing those feelings you are having. Those may be a surprise for each of you."

Throughout each of his descriptions, Dr. S checked in with Anne and Mark for their feedback about each problem area, and the ways that they might add to his description.

Even during this part of the feedback session, an opportunity for acceptance work presented itself. When Mark discussed his relationship with Anne's children, he was initially making only "hard" disclosures, by describing her children as rude, and only able to talk about themselves. Because Mark made such critical statements about Anne's children, Dr. S elicited from

Mark some softer disclosures about his emotions with regard to Anne's children:

DR. S: Besides them being rude, what is the feeling you are left with when [Anne's children] don't talk to you?

MARK: The feeling I'm left with is being ignored.

DR. S: Besides being ignored, how did it feel?

MARK: Like I don't matter, like I am only there to serve them.

DR. S: Like you are not a part of the family.

MARK: Yeah. I think I've just resigned myself to hoping that they'll show their love for their mother.

DR. S: So it upsets you that they don't take an interest in their mother? So it isn't just about *you*, you have some feelings about how Anne's sons interact with *her*?

MARK: Yeah, yeah, I do.

DR. S: And that upsets you?

MARK: Yeah, it does. I feel protective. I'd like them to show more appreciation to her. But then, I'd like myself to show more appreciation to her. I don't think I show enough appreciation to her. Maybe they're related . . . it's a reminder of the things *I'm* not doing well.

By moving Mark from criticizing Anne's children to making softer statements about his feelings, Dr. S gave Mark an unexpected opportunity to make important realizations about his own behavior—his emotional sensitivity.

After reviewing their problem areas, Dr. S proceeded to describe the two themes he had observed from his assessment of Anne and Mark:

"It seems to me from what you've both described in your individual sessions, your questionnaires, and even today, there are two themes that come up for you. When I say 'theme,' it's like in our sessions; whatever the topic is for the day, there's usually a theme. The theme is something I'll bring up from time to time. Again, it's clearly something that we'll work on together. It may take a different form, so I want to share it with you to make sure that it's on the mark, OK?

"I think the first theme is that you both have feelings of being unloved and unappreciated. You have an idea of what it means to be loved. You have an idea of what it means to be appreciated. But your definitions are different. And because of those different definitions, because of your different experiences, if something does happen, it leaves you feeling unappreciated and unloved. Within the arguments about finances or children, there is something about that—about feeling unappreciated. How does that sound to you?

"The second theme is that you both have your insecurities. You both have feelings of insecurity, for whatever reason. Some of the arguments, the differences, the conflicts, the big fights, come from that also. That feeling comes up and can create the whole battle. A concrete example is that you, Anne, described feeling insecure about yourself in relation to some of your family members. That affects how you feel about yourself in comparison to other women. Mark, you described feeling insecure about the fact that Anne has not annulled her previous marriage. That may affect how confident you feel in comparison to other men. Again, these feelings of insecurity, feeling not loved, unappreciated—these are the themes."

After Dr. S described each theme—some of the related differences, emotional sensitivities, and external stressors—and received feedback from Anne and Mark about these themes, he moved on to discuss their pattern of communication or polarization and the resultant mutual trap:

"Now, what is this thing we call the 'trap' that you both get into? You each have different ways of responding to feeling unloved and insecure. The sense that I get is that, Mark, when you start to feel those things, you use distance. The sense I get from you, Anne, is that you become critical. Put the two of you together, and you have a cycle: The feelings come up, Mark gets distant, and Anne gets critical. Mark feels criticism, he gets distant. Anne experiences the distance, she gets critical. Distance, criticism, criticism, distance. That's what we call the trap. It may be that you take turns being critical and distant, and that each response makes the other person feel even more insecure."

After reviewing the polarization process and mutual trap, Dr. S proceeded to explain to Anne and Mark what to expect from the upcoming therapy sessions:

"So this is what we're going to do in the upcoming weeks, the kinds of things we've talked about today. We'll talk about whatever is going on for the two of you on a given day. It isn't going to be structured in terms of things we *have* to do each day—it's up to you, whatever you bring in.

"What I hope to do is create in here a place of comfort, enough that you can both take risks in opening up, in sharing—sharing some of your reactions, your questions, your experiences. There is a desire for closeness here that is going to take some sharing and some risk taking. Now, there's no guarantee about how the other person is going to react. It may not always be pleasant. But on the other hand, that's the price we have to pay to get there, to open up. You can do some more thinking about this and from week to week we can reformulate, and we'll keep getting a clearer, better picture."

Having set the stage with the formulation, including the themes, the DEEP analysis, and mutual trap, Dr. S is prepared to begin work on building acceptance.

Treatment: Building Acceptance

Most of Anne and Mark's subsequent sessions were focused on building acceptance. Below are excerpts from a few sessions in which Dr. S helped Anne and Mark to increase acceptance by using techniques such as empathic joining, unified detachment, and tolerance building.

Session 12

The content of this session is about Anne and Mark's search for a condominium, and some of the difficulties they were experiencing. The discussion includes Mark's admission that he feels inadequate and insecure because he does not make enough money for them to afford Anne's dream condo. This led to an opportunity to explore Anne and Mark's theme of insecurity:

MARK: If we settle for a condominium that we don't really want, it will forever be a monument to my inability to get the condo she wants.

DR. S: I'm wondering if there's another part that wonders, "Will I ever really be able to give her what she wants?"

MARK: Yeah. If she married somebody who had a lot of money, she could get whatever condo she wanted.

ANNE: But if you married someone who was gorgeous, who was 20 years younger, you could have a trophy wife, but that's not what happened. (*Both laugh.*)

DR. S: So that may be part of your insecurity. If you looked the way that you experience as "the way he wants things," then maybe he'd be happier.

MARK: (*to Dr. S*) I think that's how she feels about herself at her worst moments. Like maybe all men are attracted to younger women and that you have to harness yourself not to lose what's important to you . . . (*to Anne*) maybe that's how you look at your desire to have your dream condo. How do you keep from saying, "There's that rich lawyer who looks at me all of the time"? . . . (*to Dr. S*) I think that would be a pretty natural thing for her to think about.

This dialogue also reveals the unified detachment Anne and Mark are developing, when they both laugh at Anne's comment about a "trophy wife." What has previously been a very painful subject for Anne is becoming something about which they can joke. The discussion then moved to exploring Anne's insecurities about Mark's relationships with other women:

DR. S: So what in your eyes is Mark's ideal "bill"? You made reference to a "bill" that is his ideal.

ANNE: Well, probably someone younger, who is able to have children, someone who plays tennis, who goes running and also cooks and cleans, makes a good living, is very good in bed . . .

DR. S: (*to Mark*) Because this is comparable to the richer man that you view with Anne. (*to Anne*) For you, it's the woman who . . .

ANNE: But that woman's out there. A lot of women are like that.

DR. S: And the way that you see and experience Mark talking to women. And at times you kind of wonder to what extent he enjoys it, and you think it's just a matter of time if you're not willing to live up to it . . .

ANNE: Right, that some other women is going to be able to step right in there without a problem.

DR. S: When the insecurities come up for both of you. For you, Mark, it's the rich man who could come along and provide what Anne longs for, and for you, Anne, it's that you don't compete physically—with

the workout—so it's just a matter of time until a woman comes along and decides, "I'm going after him." Anne, can you tell me some of the things Mark does that make you feel threatened?

ANNE: When he makes comments about how attractive a woman is, like I'm one of the guys. When he tells me I'm fat, or makes comments like I have a double chin . . .

DR. S: Which then tells you that you're not cutting it.

ANNE: Yeah.

Dr. S then brought back the subject of condominium buying, and used this as a metaphor for Anne and Mark's concerns about "settling" for less than what they want in making a major commitment:

DR. S: When you make a commitment, whether it's committing to a condo, committing to a relationship—it's settling, you're settling—you're saying, "This is it."

ANNE: That's a good way of looking at it. I hadn't thought of that. That's what we're having trouble with . . . the reality that we're not going to get everything that we want. The insecurity, the scariness of making the purchase, is knowing that we're never going to get what we want.

MARK: Part of it is our concern that the next condominium we see is going to be the one we want.

ANNE: Right, it's the condo over the next hill.

MARK: So you have to think, "Is 60% of what we want what we should settle for?" I'm thinking, 60? I was thinking it's more like 90. So I don't know when you're supposed to cut your losses and say we have to go for this—this is what reality dictates.

DR. S: And if we can take it a step further, it might be that when you both decided to get married, you both made a settlement. You both start to wonder whether the other settled for 60 or 90%. You wonder, "What did I settle for? Did I settle for 60 or 90%?"

MARK: Yeah.

ANNE: Right.

DR. S: Now let's put yourselves in a situation where you're insecure. What's gonna happen? When you're in an insecure place, that 90% might feel like . . .

ANNE: 50%.

DR. S: Exactly. When you're feeling good, you think, "She got 90% of what she wanted in me," or "I got

90%." But when you're in an insecure place, you think, "I settled for 50%." Then when you look at your own insecurity, you think, "My God, she settled for 35 or 40%." You both made a settlement when you married each other. You decided, "This is it, we're gonna get married," and you settled.

MARK: But "settled" has such negative connotations.

DR. S: I think there's some feelings associated with that. And a parallel to the word "settlement" is "acceptance."

MARK: Oh, I see.

DR. S: When you go through the settlement, you think, "This is who this person is." Whether it's 90, 80, 60, or 35%, you've settled—you've basically said, "I accept this."

By using condominium buying as a metaphor, Dr. S has underscored how Anne and Mark's theme of insecurity feeds itself, and how it leads them both to question whether each has "settled" for less than he/she wanted in the relationship. Adding the additional component of "insecurity about settlement" to their theme helped Anne and Mark understand the things each of them do that "threaten" the other (e.g., when Mark talks about his attraction to younger women), and also build a bridge toward working on acceptance.

Session 17

In this session, Dr. S continues to process the theme of insecurity with Anne and Mark. In this particular part of the dialogue, when Anne and Mark are discussing a familiar polarization process, Mark suggests to Anne that she work out more. Anne interprets Mark's suggestion as a criticism about her appearance, which makes her feel insecure and threatened. Anne then "fights back" against Mark's suggestions by becoming depressed and "doing nothing," which in turn makes Mark more critical of her.

Here Dr. S uses two IBCT acceptance-building techniques. The first technique is empathic joining. As Dr. S tries to "get to the bottom of" Mark's suggestions/criticisms of Anne's appearance, Mark makes the following soft disclosure about his own insecurities:

DR. S: This is a real, central question. There are some basic limits that you have, where you say, "Up to here, I accept you, but beyond that, you'd better change." On the other hand, this is who you are. *This is who*

you are. But the irony of it is, that once we accept, change can come about. But there's that push to determine within ourselves not only the other person's limits but also our own. I get the sense that you're both exploring yourselves and your own limits.

ANNE: Perhaps, yes.

DR. S: You're both looking at your own limits. With you, Anne, it's about your looks, your appearance. And for you, Mark, it's about you as a financial provider. And the temptation is, when that gets uncomfortable, that's where your partner comes in kind of, to redirect your focus from that versus being able to talk about how you're feeling.

ANNE: Yeah.

MARK: Yeah, I think I've noticed, since we've started therapy, that's what I do. When I get insecure about myself, I start looking outwards, saying, "You should do this," and that makes me feel better.

DR. S: Right, it's active. It can be advice giving—it can be a real male thing, "Do this, do that."

MARK: Right, I do that with her kids, too. I know I do.

Instead of focusing on the critical nature of Mark's suggestions, Dr. S has placed an emphasis on *why* Mark becomes critical. Mark is encouraged to consider the *reasons* for his behavior, and as a result he discloses that he becomes critical when he himself is feeling insecure. Mark recognizes that this happens not only with regard to his attempts to direct Anne's behavior but also in his interactions with Anne's children.

The second acceptance-building technique Dr. S uses in this portion of the session is a tolerance intervention: emphasizing the positive aspects of a partner's negative behavior. Dr. S continues:

DR. S: In some situations it might work really well [to give advice]. People might like that—like in your work as a counselor, Mark. You feel really productive.

MARK: Yeah, I change people's lives. I know I do.

DR. S: On the other hand, there might be some circumstances where it's experienced as being critical, and I think of this in terms of the two of you. It feeds into Anne's feeling criticized.

ANNE: Yes.

DR. S: And then it feels threatening, like "If you don't do something about it, then . . ."

Here Dr. S has positively reemphasized Mark's suggestions to Anne as his attempts to give her guidance or advice. Mark, an employment counselor, is used to giving such suggestions to others as a way of being constructive or helpful. Dr. S underscores this aspect of Mark's behavior—that this same "counselor" quality makes Mark very good at what he does in his career. However, Dr. S does not try to reframe Mark's behavior as *completely* positive. Dr. S also underscores how Mark's "advice" is experienced by Anne as critical and threatening.

At the end of the session, Dr. S recharacterizes Anne and Mark's polarization process in terms of the information that has emerged from these two interventions:

DR. S: I think you put it really well, Mark. When you start to feel uncomfortable, this is your process, this is what you do. You start to look outside yourself. From your end, it might be like you're being a counselor when you start with Anne. You want to advise. But from her end, it might be like you're being authoritarian, the drill sergeant, rather than the counselor. And you, Anne, start to feel you're being berated. You start to feel worse about yourself.

ANNE: Yeah.

DR. S: So you feel like you've gotta either take it, or you've gotta fight back.

MARK: I think I can . . . the fighting back is . . . well, I can understand that. I really can.

Session 25

In their final session, Anne described a recent insight she had had about feeling "undeserving" of happiness, and her belief that happiness comes at a cost of some kind. She said that happiness made her feel guilty because she felt that someone else must be suffering for her happiness, or that somehow she would suffer negative repercussions for being happy. Anne connected some of these feelings to her bout with an eating disorder as a teenager, and to the depressive episodes she sometimes experienced as an adult.

In the dialogue below, Dr. S uses several IBCT techniques to discuss Anne's insights and the way that her feelings contribute to the couple's polarization process. First, Dr. S uses empathic joining to help Mark understand the experience Anne is having when she gets depressed (a time when Mark regularly makes suggestions about how Anne "should" think, feel, or be-

have). Then Dr. S detaches Anne and Mark from their problem—that Anne feels criticized whenever Mark makes these suggestions. Rather than engaging Anne and Mark in their emotional responses to each other's behavior, Dr. S framed this problem as a consequence of basic communication problems. By describing their problem in terms of their methods of communication, Dr. S detaches Anne and Mark from the problem itself, and provides each with a new way of reacting to an old problem (without doing any formal communication training):

DR. S: I think the idea around the conflict over happiness—having the happiness—is like savoring a good meal, and that it will cost you: "OK, so it has some high fat, but I'm going to enjoy it because I deserve this, I deserve this moment—the same way that I deserve this moment of happiness, even if so-and-so doesn't have it together. I deserve this happiness." And that's going to be the struggle, to be able to react to Mark in a way that expresses, "God, I'm really feeling guilty."

ANNE: When I'm on the couch, and I'm totally immobile in my depression, that's a lot of what's going on. I'm beating myself up.

DR. S: And so Mark needs to listen, to just *listen* and say, "Gee, that must be really hard." Now there may be a pull, Mark, to problem-solve, to say, "Well, you shouldn't feel that way," or "So-and-so is that way because . . . ," but that will only bring out Anne's self-criticism and it could become argumentative. When you sense the pain, Mark, and what it's costing Anne, the reaction that you have is "Let me show you what to do." But that is only going to bring out in Anne the feeling of "You see, you idiot, you're not doing it right," which will then feed into the self-criticism. So it's going to help to just listen, and simply to paraphrase, and she will hear that it's not reasonable. If, rather than criticizing, you just say, "Gee, you really don't feel worthy of these things," if you just paraphrase those themes of her insecurity, her self-criticalness, that is kind of maintaining a connection.

Finally, Dr. S uses tolerance interventions to allow Anne and Mark to see their problem as a difference in their communication styles. As he continues to describe their problem in terms of communication difficulties, Dr. S describes Anne as responding to situations based on how she *feels*, while Mark is more likely to use logic or *reason* to determine his responses to situations. Dr. S also points out how Anne and Mark's problem is often a result of this difference, and that these differences actually complement one another:

DR. S: (*to Mark*) And that's what I want to encourage, maybe a new way of responding rather than using *reason* when you start to feel like Anne's feelings don't make sense. Rather than saying, "This doesn't make sense," say instead, "What I'm hearing you say is that you don't deserve this"—whatever it is. And what I'm expecting, Anne, is that to hear Mark express that he understands you would make you feel close to him.

ANNE: Yeah, and it would definitely not be the wedge of "you should." (*Mark laughs.*)

DR. S: Anne, you talk about things from the emotional experience, and Mark, you talk about things from the rational experience—and both are needed, both are important.

This section of the dialogue also reveals how Anne and Mark have developed unified detachment from their problem. Anne uses the phrase "the wedge of 'you should' " to describe what had previously been the "hot topic" of feeling criticized by Mark, and Mark is able to laugh about his own behavior.

CONCLUSION

Although a single case study is useful for illustrative purposes, it obviously does not establish generalizable conclusions about treatment outcome. However, the studies we have described give some promising results for the efficacy of IBCT.

IBCT is part of what Hayes (2004) has called the "third wave" of behavior therapy. The "first wave" encompassed traditional classical and operant conditioning approaches. The "second wave" incorporated cognitive strategies. The third wave emphasizes "contextual and experiential change strategies in addition to more direct and didactic ones" (p. 6). Acceptance and mindfulness are key aspects of these third-wave therapies. Although these therapies have generated considerable enthusiasm and confirming data, only additional outcome research will establish whether these therapies in general or IBCT in particular will work to alleviate human suffering, including the substantial suffering that occurs in couple relationships, in more powerful ways than the first two waves of behavior therapy.

NOTES

1. We use the more inclusive term "couple therapy" rather than the more limited "marital therapy," because "couple therapy" can refer to unmarried couples, gay and lesbian couples, as well as married couples.

2. Identifying information has been changed to protect confidentiality, but clinical dynamics are accurately portrayed and quotations are taken directly from tapes of the therapy sessions but altered slightly to increase readability.

3. Not included here are case examples of the application of TBCT interventions, which can be found elsewhere (e.g., Cordova & Jacobson, 1993; Jacobson & Margolin, 1979).

4. In our project we assessed for violence using the CTS2 and excluded any couple in which the wife reported moderate to severe violence from the husband. We excluded the partners prior to their seeing one of our project therapists, and we referred them to appropriate individual treatment for violence. Dr. S could proceed with the knowledge that the wife had not endorsed this kind of violence from her husband on the CTS2 (although she could still do so in the individual session). In a clinical setting, we recommend that practitioners give the Couple Questionnaire or the CTS2 to all clients and follow up with individual sessions, in which they focus specifically on violent items on the questionnaire that the individual has endorsed as committing or receiving. Based on these interviews, the practitioner should refer clients when appropriate (Jacobson & Gottman, 1998).

REFERENCES

American Psychiatric Association. (2013). *Diagnostic and statistical manual of mental disorders* (5th ed.). Arlington, VA: Author.

Atkins, D. C., Berns, S. B., George, W., Doss, B., Gattis, K., & Christensen, A. (2005). Prediction of response to treatment in a randomized clinical trial of marital therapy. *Journal of Consulting and Clinical Psychology, 73,* 893–903.

Atkins, D. C., Dimidjian, S., Bedics, J. D., & Christensen, A. (2009). Couple discord and depression in couples during couple therapy and in depressed individuals during depression treatment. *Journal of Consulting and Clinical Psychology, 77,* 1089–1099.

Baucom, B. R., Atkins, D. C., Simpson, L. E., & Christensen, A. (2009). Prediction of response to treatment in a randomized clinical trial of couple therapy: A 2-year follow-up. *Journal of Consulting and Clinical Psychology, 77,* 160–173.

Baucom, D. H., & Epstein, N. (1990). *Cognitive behavioral marital therapy.* New York: Brunner/Mazel.

Baucom, D. H., Epstein, N., & Rankin, L. A. (1995). Cognitive aspects of cognitive behavioral marital therapy. In N. S. Jacobson & A. S. Gurman (Eds.), *Clinical handbook of couple therapy* (pp. 65–90). New York: Guilford Press.

Baucom, D. H., & Hoffman, J. A. (1986). The effectiveness of marital therapy: Current status and application to the clinical setting. In N. S. Jacobson & A. S. Gurman (Eds.), *Clinical handbook of marital therapy* (pp. 597–620). New York: Guilford Press.

Baucom, D. H., Shoham, V. M., Kim, T., Daiuto, A. D., & Stickle, T. R. (1998). Empirically supported couple and family interventions for marital distress and adult mental health problems. *Journal of Consulting and Clinical Psychology, 66*(1), 53–88.

Baucom, K. J. W., Sevier, M., Eldridge, K. A., Doss, B. D., & Christensen, A. (2011). Observed communication in couples two years after integrative and traditional behavioral couple therapy: Outcome and link with five-year follow-up. *Journal of Consulting and Clinical Psychology, 79,* 565–576.

Beach, S. R. H., Wamboldt, M. Z., Kaslow, N. J., Heyman, R. E., First, M. B., Underwood, L. G., et al. (2006). *Relational processes and DSM-V: Neuroscience, assessment, prevention, and treatment.* Washington, DC: American Psychiatric Publishing.

Buehler, C., Anthony, C., Krishnakumar, A., Stone, G., Gerard, J., & Pemberton, S. (1997). Interparental conflict and youth problems behaviors: A meta-analysis. *Journal of Child and Family Studies, 6,* 233–247.

Christensen, A. (2009). Couple Questionnaire. Unpublished questionnaire. (To obtain this freely available measure, contact Andrew Christensen, PhD, UCLA Department of Psychology, Los Angeles, CA 90095; *christensen@psych. ucla.edu.*)

Christensen, A. (2010). Weekly Questionnaire. Unpublished questionnaire. (To obtain this freely available measure, contact Andrew Christensen, PhD, UCLA Department of Psychology, Los Angeles, CA 90095; *christensen@psych. ucla.edu.*)

Christensen, A., Atkins, D. C., Baucom, B., & Yi, J. (2010). Marital status and satisfaction five years following a randomized clinical trial comparing traditional versus integrative behavioral couple therapy. *Journal of Consulting and Clinical Psychology, 78,* 225–235.

Christensen, A., Atkins, D. C., Berns, S., Wheeler, J., Baucom, D. H., & Simpson, L. E. (2004). Traditional versus integrative behavioral couple therapy for significantly and chronically distressed married couples. *Journal of Consulting and Clinical Psychology, 72,* 176–191.

Christensen, A., Atkins, D. C., Yi, J., Baucom, D. H., &

George, W. H. (2006). Couple and individual adjustment for two years following a randomized clinical trial comparing traditional versus integrative behavioral couple therapy. *Journal of Consulting and Clinical Psychology, 74,* 1180–1191.

Christensen, A., & Heavey, C. L. (1999). Interventions for couples. *Annual Review of Psychology, 50,* 65–102.

Christensen, A., & Jacobson, N. S. (1997). *Frequency and Acceptability of Partner Behavior Inventory: Unpublished measures.* Los Angeles: University of California, Los Angeles.

Christensen, A., & Jacobson, N. S. (2000). *Reconcilable differences.* New York: Guilford Press.

Christensen, A., Doss, B. D., & Jacobson, N. S. (2014). *Reconcilable differences* (2nd ed.). New York: Guilford Press.

Christensen, A., Jacobson, N. S., & Babcock, J. C. (1995). Integrative behavioral couple therapy. In N. S. Jacobson & A. S. Gurman (Eds.), *Clinical handbook of couple therapy* (pp. 31–64). New York: Guilford Press.

Cordova, J., & Jacobson, N. S. (1993). Couple distress. In D. H. Barlow (Ed.), *Clinical handbook of psychological disorders* (2nd ed., pp. 481–512). New York: Guilford Press.

Crane, D. R., & Mead, D. E. (1980). The Marital Status Inventory: Some preliminary data on an instrument to measure marital dissolution potential. *American Journal of Family Therapy, 8*(3), 31–35.

Doss, B. D., & Christensen, A. (2006). Acceptance in romantic relationships: The Frequency and Acceptability of Partner Behavior Inventory. *Psychological Assessment, 18,* 289–302.

Doss, B. D., Thum, Y. M., Sevier, M., Atkins, D. C., & Christensen, A. (2005). Improving relationships: Mechanisms of change in couple therapy. *Journal of Consulting and Clinical Psychology, 73,* 624–633.

Epstein, N., & Baucom, D. H. (2002). *Enhanced cognitive-behavioral therapy for couples: A contextual approach.* Washington, DC: American Psychological Association.

Floyd, F. J., & Markman, H. J. (1983). Observational biases in spouse observation: Toward a cognitive/behavioral model of marriage. *Journal of Consulting and Clinical Psychology, 51,* 450–457.

Floyd, F. J., Markman, H. J., Kelly, S., Blumberg, S. L., & Stanley, S. M. (1995). Preventive intervention and relationship enhancement. In N. S. Jacobson & A. S. Gurman (Eds.), *Clinical handbook of couple therapy* (pp. 212–230). New York: Guilford Press.

Funk, J. L., & Rogge, R. D. (2007). Testing the ruler with item response theory: Increasing precision of measurement for relationship satisfaction with the Couples Satisfaction Index. *Journal of Family Psychology, 21,* 572–583.

Gottman, J., Notarius, C., Gonso, J., & Markman, H. (1976). *A couple's guide to communication.* Champaign, IL: Research Press.

Gupta, M., Coyne, J. C., & Beach, S. R. H. (2003). Couples treatment for major depression: Critique of the literature and suggestions for some different directions. *Journal of Family Therapy, 25,* 317–346.

Gurman, A. S., Knickerson, D. P., & Pinsof, W. M. (1986). Research on the process and outcome of marital and family therapy. In S. L. Garfield & A. E. Bergin (Eds.), *Handbook of psychotherapy and behavior change* (3rd ed., pp. 565–624). New York: Wiley.

Hahlweg, K., Schindler, L., Revenstorf, D., & Brengelmann, J. C. (1984). The Munich Marital Therapy Study. In K. Hahlweg & N. S. Jacobson (Eds.), *Marital interaction: Analysis and modification* (pp. 3–26). New York: Guilford Press.

Halford, W. K. (2001). *Brief therapy for couples: Helping partners help themselves.* New York: Guilford Press.

Halford, W. K., Hayes, S., Christensen, A., Lambert, M., Baucom, D. H.,& Atkins, D. C. (2012). Toward making progress feedback an effective common factor in couple therapy. *Behavior Therapy, 43,* 49–60.

Hayes, S. C. (2004). Acceptance and commitment therapy and the new behavior therapies. In S. C. Hayes, V. M. Follette, & M. M. Linehan (Eds.), *Mindfulness and acceptance: Expanding the cognitive-behavioral tradition* (pp. 1–29). New York: Guilford Press.

Heavey, C. L., Christensen, A., Malamuth, N. M. (1995). The longitudinal impact of demand and withdrawal during marital conflict. *Journal of Consulting and Clinical Psychology, 63,* 797–801.

Holtzworth-Munroe, A., & Jacobson, N. S. (1991). Behavioral marital therapy. In A. S. Gurman & D. P. Knickerson (Eds.), *Handbook of family therapy* (2nd ed., pp. 96–133). New York: Brunner/Mazel.

Jacobson, N. S. (1977). Problem solving and contingency contracting in the treatment of marital discord. *Journal of Consulting and Clinical Psychology, 45,* 92–100.

Jacobson, N. S. (1978a). A review of the research on the effectiveness of marital therapy. In T. J. Paolino & B. S. McGrady (Eds.), *Marriage and marital therapy: Psychoanalytic, behavioral, and systems theory perspectives* (pp. 395–444). New York: Brunner/Mazel.

Jacobson, N. S. (1978b). Specific and nonspecific factors in the effectiveness of a behavioral approach to the treatment of marital discord. *Journal of Consulting and Clinical Psychology, 46,* 442–452.

Jacobson, N. S. (1984). A component analysis of behavioral marital therapy: The relative effectiveness of behavior exchange and problem solving training. *Journal of Consulting and Clinical Psychology, 52,* 295–305.

Jacobson, N. S., & Addis, M. E. (1993). Research on couple therapy: What do we know? Where are we going? *Journal of Consulting and Clinical Psychology, 61,* 85–93.

Jacobson, N. S., & Christensen, A. (1998). *Acceptance and change in couple therapy: A therapist's guide to transforming relationships.* New York: Norton.

Jacobson, N. S., Christensen, A., Prince, S. E., Cordova, J., & Eldridge, K. (2000). Integrative behavioral couple therapy: An acceptance-based, promising new treatment for couple discord. *Journal of Consulting and Clinical Psychology, 68*(2), 351–355.

Jacobson, N. S., Follette, W. C., & Pagel, M. (1986). Predicting who will benefit from behavioral marital therapy. *Journal of Consulting and Clinical Psychology, 54,* 518–522.

Jacobson, N. S., Follette, W. S., Revenstorf, D., Baucom, D. H., Hahlweg, K., & Margolin, G. (1984). Variability in outcome and clinical significance of behavior marital therapy: A reanalysis of outcome data. *Journal of Consulting and Clinical Psychology, 52,* 497–564.

Jacobson, N. S., & Gottman, J. (1998). *When men batter women: New insights into ending abusive relationships.* New York: Simon & Schuster.

Jacobson, N. S., & Holtzworth-Munroe, A. (1986). Marital therapy: A social learning/cognitive perspective. In N. S. Jacobson & A. S. Gurman (Eds.), *Clinical handbook of marital therapy* (pp. 29–70). New York: Guilford Press.

Jacobson, N. S., & Margolin, G. (1979). *Marital therapy: Strategies based on social learning and behavior exchange principles.* New York: Brunner/Mazel.

Jacobson, N. S., Schmaling, K. B., & Holtzworth-Munroe, A. (1987). Component analysis of behavioral marital therapy: Two-year follow-up and prediction of relapse. *Journal of Marital and Family Therapy, 13,* 187–195.

Knox, D. (1971). *Marital happiness: A behavioral approach to counseling.* Champaign, IL: Research Press.

Liberman, R. P. (1970). Behavioral approaches to family and couple therapy. *American Journal of Orthopsychiatry, 40,* 106–118.

Liberman, R. P., Wheeler, E. G., deVisser, L. A., Kuehnel, J., & Kuehnel, T. (1981). *Handbook of marital therapy: A positive approach to helping troubled relationships.* New York: Plenum Press.

O'Farrell, T. J., & Fals-Stewart, W. (2000). Behavioral couples therapy for alcoholism and drug abuse. *Journal of Substance Abuse and Treatment, 18,* 51–54.

Sevier, M., Eldridge, K., Jones, J., Doss, B., & Christensen, A. (2008). Observed communication and associations with satisfaction during traditional and integrative behavioral couple therapy. *Behavior Therapy, 39,* 137–150.

Simpson, L. E., Doss, B. D., Wheeler, J., & Christensen, A. (2007). Relationship violence among couples seeking therapy: Common couple violence or battering? *Journal of Marital and Family Therapy, 33,* 270–283.

Skinner, B. F. (1966). *The behavior of organisms: An experimental analysis.* Englewood Cliffs, NJ: Prentice Hall.

Snyder, D. K., Castellani, A. M., & Whisman, M. A. (2006). Current status and future directions for couple therapy. *Annual Review of Psychology, 57,* 317–344.

Snyder, D. K., Wills, R. M., & Grady-Fletcher, A. (1991). Long-term effectiveness of behavioral versus insight-oriented marital therapy: A 4-year follow-up study. *Journal of Consulting and Clinical Psychology, 59,* 138–141.

Straus, M. A., Hamby, S. L., Boney-McCoy, S., & Sugarman, D. B. (1996). The Revised Conflict Tactics Scales (CTS2): Development and preliminary psychometric data. *Journal of Family Issues, 17*(3), 283–316.

Stuart, R. B. (1969). Operant interpersonal treatment for marital discord. *Journal of Consulting and Clinical Psychology, 33*, 675–682.

Stuart, R. B. (1980). *Helping couples change: A social learning approach to marital therapy.* New York: Guilford Press.

Weiss, R. L., & Cerreto, M. C. (1980). The Marital Status Inventory: Development of a measure of dissolution potential. *American Journal of Family Therapy, 8*(2), 80–85.

Weiss, R. L., Hops, H., & Patterson, G. R. (1973). A framework for conceptualizing marital conflict, technology for altering it, some data for evaluating it. In L. A. Hamerlynck, L. C. Handy, & E. J. Mash (Eds.), *Behavior change:* *Methodology, concepts, and practice* (pp. 309–342). Champaign, IL: Research Press.

Whisman, M. A. (2007). Marital distress and DSM-IV psychiatric disorders in a population-based national survey. *Journal of Abnormal Psychology, 116*, 638–643.

Whisman, M. S., & Bruce, M. L. (1999). Marital dissatisfaction and incidence of major depressive episode in a community sample. *Journal of Abnormal Psychology, 108*, 674–678.

Wile, D. B. (2008). *After the honeymoon: How conflict can improve your relationship* (Rev. ed.). Oakland, CA: Collaborative Couple Therapy Books.

Wimberly, J. D. (1998). An outcome study of integrative couples therapy delivered in a group format (Doctoral dissertation, University of Montana, 1997). *Dissertation Abstracts International B: Sciences and Engineering, 58*(12), 6832.

Author Index

I

J

Subject Index

Page numbers followed by *f* indicate figure, *t* indicate table.

751